Diagnostic Medical Sonography

A GUIDE TO CLINICAL PRACTICE

VOLUME III

Abdomen

VOLUME I Obstetrics and Gynecology

Edited by
MIMI C. BERMAN, PH.D., R.D.M.S.
Associate Professor, Diagnostic Medical Imaging Program
College of Health Related Professions
State University of New York
Health Science Center at Brooklyn
Brooklyn, New York

VOLUME II Echocardiography

Edited by
MARVEEN CRAIG, R.D.M.S.
Founder
International Ultrasound Institute
Dallas, Texas

VOLUME III Abdomen

Edited by
DIANE M. KAWAMURA, M.ED., R.T.(R), R.D.M.S.
Professor, Radiological Sciences
Weber State University
Ogden, Utah

Diagnostic Medical Sonography

A Guide to Clinical Practice

VOLUME III **Abdomen**

Edited by
DIANE M. KAWAMURA, PH.D., R.T.(R), R.D.M.S.

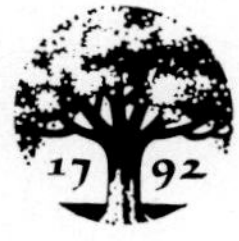

J. B. Lippincott Company

PHILADELPHIA NEW YORK
LONDON HAGERSTOWN

Acquisitions Editor: Charles McCormick, Jr.
Developmental Editor: Kimberley Cox
Production Manager: Janet Greenwood
Production: Editorial Services of New England, Inc.
Compositor: University Graphics, Inc.
Printer/Binder: Halliday Lithograph

3 5 6 4

Library of Congress Cataloging-in-Publication Data

Abdomen / edited by Diane M. Kawamura.
p. cm.—(Diagnostic medical sonography : v. 3)
Includes bibliographical references and index.
ISBN 0-397-50951-0
1. Abdomen—Ultrasonic imaging. I. Kawamura, Diane M.
[DNLM: 1. Abdomen—ultrasonography. WB 289 D5355 v. 3]
RC78.7.U4D48 vol. 3
[RC944]
616.07'543 s—dc20
[617.5'507543]
DNLM/DLC
for Library of Congress 91-23658
CIP

ISBN 0-397-50951-0
ISBN 0-397-50954-5 (set)

The authors and publisher have exerted every effort to ensure that drug selection and dosage set forth in this text are in accord with current recommendations and practice at the time of publication. However, in view of ongoing research, changes in government regulations, and the constant flow of information relating to drug therapy and drug reactions, the reader is urged to check the package insert for each drug for any change in indications and dosage and for added warnings and precautions. This is particularly important when the recommended agent is a new or infrequently employed drug.

To Bryan, Stephanie, Nathan, and to my family, colleagues, students, and friends who helped produce this book by giving of themselves.

And to those who will use this book:

"Any piece of knowledge I acquire today has a value at this moment exactly proportioned to my skill to deal with it. Tomorrow, when I know more, I recall that piece of knowledge and use it better."
Mark Van Doren—Liberal Education (1960)

Contributors

Jim Baun, R.T., R.D.M.S.
Faculty Instructor,
Foothill College Diagnostic Medical Sonography Program,
Los Altos Hills, California;
Co-Founder and Administrative Director,
Diagnostic Color Imaging Center,
San Mateo, California

Sue Ellen Beavers, R.T.(R), R.D.M.S.
Vice President/Clinical Director,
Institute of Ultrasound Diagnostics, Inc.,
Mobile, Alabama

Mimi C. Berman, Ph.D., R.D.M.S.
Associate Professor,
Diagnostic Medical Imaging Program,
College of Health Related Professions,
State University of New York,
Health Science Center at Brooklyn,
Brooklyn, New York

Rosemarie P. Cann, R.D.M.S.
Sonographer,
Huntington Hospital,
Huntington, New York

Catherine Carr-Hoefer, R.T., R.D.M.S., R.D.C.S.
Chief Sonographer,
Corvallis Radiology, P.C.,
Corvallis, Oregon

Marveen Craig, R.D.M.S.
Founder,
International Ultrasound Institute,
Dallas, Texas

Marie DeLange, B.S., R.D.M.S.
Program Director,
School of Allied Health Radiation Sciences,
Diagnostic Medical Sonography Program;
Chief Sonographer,
Loma Linda University Medical Center,
Loma Linda, California

Loriann D. Forbush, R.D.M.S., R.D.C.S., B.S.R.T.
Sonographer,
Primary Children's Medical Center,
Good Samaritan Medical Center,
Salt Lake City, Utah

Kathy A. Gill, R.T., R.D.M.S.
Program Director,
Institute of Ultrasound Diagnostics, Inc.,
Mobile, Alabama

John A. Guida, R.D.M.S., R.V.T.
Ultrasound Supervisor,
Meridian Park Hospital,
Tigard, Oregon

Diane M. Kawamura, Ph.D., R.T.(R), R.D.M.S.
Professor, Radiological Sciences,
Weber State University,
Ogden, Utah

Wayne C. Leonhardt, R.T.(R), R.D.M.S.
Staff Sonographer,
Merritt-Peralta Medical Center,
Oakland, California;
Clinical Ultrasound Instructor,
Foothill College,
Los Altos, California

Sherman S. Lipschitz, M.D.
Director, Ultrasound,
State University of New York,
Health Science Center at Brooklyn,
Brooklyn, New York

Joyce E. Lukken, R.T.(R), R.D.M.S., R.D.C.S.
Sonographer,
Primary Children's Medical Center,
Salt Lake City, Utah

Laura D. Newren, R.T., R.D.M.S., R.D.C.S.
Clinical Advisor,
Weber State College,
Ogden, Utah;
Ultrasound Supervisor,
Primary Children's Medical Center,
Salt Lake City, Utah,

Jerry R. Pearson, R.D.M.S.
Program Director,
Diagnostic Medical Sonography Programs,
Medical College of Georgia;
Instructor,
Department of Radiologic Technologies,
Medical College of Georgia,
Augusta, Georgia

Barbara S. Reid, M.D.
Associate Clinical Professor,
Univeristy of Utah,
Pediatric Radiologist,
Primary Children's Medical Center,
Salt Lake City, Utah

Sharon Roberts, R.T., R.D.M.S.
Independent Sonographer,
Loma Linda, California

Glenn A. Rouse, M.D.
Assistant Professor of Diagnostic Radiology,
School of Medicine,
Loma Linda University,
Loma Linda University Medical Center,
Loma Linda, California

Barbara Wajsbrot-Kandel, M.D.
Assistant Professor,
Department of Radiology,
State University of New York,
Health Science Center at Stony Brook,
Stony Brook, New York

Preface

Technical advances in diagnostic ultrasound equipment have produced so many rapid changes in the field of sonography that we felt a current textbook on adult and pediatric abdominal scanning and superficial structures was needed. This textbook addresses these advances and, recognizing that sonographers and sonography students have diverse backgrounds and experiences, also includes material on anatomy, physiology, and pathophysiology. A better understanding of these disciplines can only enhance the sonographer's role as a valuable member of the health care team.

The first chapter introduces terminology on anatomy, scanning planes, and patient positions. Adopting universal terminology permits every sonographer to communicate consistent information on how they positioned and scanned the patient and how anatomy and pathology are represented sonographically.

The next three sections are divided into specific content areas. This organization allowed the contributors to focus attention on a specific organ or system. It also simulates application in that while scanning, the sonographer systematically investigates each organ or system, and completes the examination by synthesizing all of the information to obtain the total picture.

We made every attempt to produce an up-to-date and factual textbook while capturing the reader's attention with an interesting and enjoyable format. To do this, we provide detailed descriptions of anatomy, physiology, pathology, and the normal and abnormal sonographic representation of these anatomical and pathologic entities, including illustrations, summary tables, and images, many of which incorporate valuable case study information.

Our goal is to present as complete a text as possible, while recognizing that by tomorrow, this book must be supplemented by current journal readings. With every technological advance made in equipment, the sonographer's imagination must stretch to create new applications. With the comprehensive foundation available in this text, the sonographer can meet that challenge.

DIANE M. KAWAMURA, M.ED., R.T.(R), R.D.M.S.
MIMI C. BERMAN, PH.D., R.D.M.S.
MARVEEN CRAIG, R.D.M.S.

Acknowledgments

Throughout the process of collaborating on the three volumes of *Diagnostic Medical Sonography,* I have appreciated the support and enthusiasm of Mimi Berman and Marveen Craig. Their continued input of ideas, coupled with the contributions by all the authors, made it possible to provide this three-volume textbook to the profession. My thanks go to all of them.

Thanks also go to Cristi Krames and Debra Stout for producing many of the medical illustrations, to Clark Taylor for photographing what may have materialized into endless stacks of sonograms, and to Doug Amussen for contributing so many cases.

Thanks to J. B. Lippincott Company for their major role in the project, especially to Jay Lippincott, who approved the project; to Lisa Biello and Delois Patterson who understood the need for the project; to Charles McCormick and Kimberley Cox for their support, encouragement, patience, and follow-through; and to all other individuals who helped edit, produce, promote, and deliver all three volumes.

To my friends, colleagues, and students who provided continued sources of encouragement, enthusiasm, and inspiration, thank you. Final recognition must go to my husband Bryan and to our two children, Stephanie and Nathan, for their continued love, support, patience, and understanding and for their belief that, someday, this project would be completed.

D.M.K.

Contents

Diagnostic Medical Sonography

A Guide to Clinical Practice

Volume III

Abdomen

CHAPTER 1

Introduction

DIANE M. KAWAMURA

This is a reference chapter for abdominal and superficial structure ultrasonographic examinations. It was written to assist sonographers and physicians in acquiring, using, and understanding the sonographic imaging terminology used in the remainder of this textbook. Accurate and precise terminology allows communication among professionals.

Anatomic Definitions

DIRECTIONAL TERMS

Sonographers have adopted standard nomenclature from the anatomists' terminology to communicate anatomic direction. Table 1-1 and Figure 1-1 illustrate how these simple terms help avoid confusion and convey specific information.

ANATOMIC POSITION

A body in the conventional anatomic position is standing erect, feet together, with the arms by the sides and the palms and face directed forward, facing the observer (see Fig. 1-1).[2,4,5] Whenever sonographers use directional terms or describe regions or anatomic planes, it is assumed that the body is in the anatomic position.

ANATOMIC PLANES

Anatomic planes are imaginary flat surfaces passing through a body in the anatomic position. Sonographers commonly use three: transverse, sagittal, and coronal (Fig. 1-2). The transverse plane divides the body into superior and inferior portions and runs parallel to the surface of the ground.[4,5,7] The word *sagittal* literally means "flight of an arrow" and refers to the plane that runs vertically through the body and separates it into right and left portions.[4,5] The plane that divides the body into equal right and left halves is referred to as the median sagittal or midsagittal plane.[3,5,7] Any vertical plane on either side of the midsagittal plane is referred to as a parasagittal plane (*para* means "alongside of").[3,4] The coronal plane runs vertically and divides the body into anterior and posterior portions.[3,5,7]

Scanning Definitions

TRANSDUCER ORIENTATION

When articulated-arm, static imaging systems are used, most abdominal and superficial structures are scanned utilizing the midsagittal, parasagittal, and transverse flat body surface planes. The results are a number of images that provide a global depiction of the area of interest; specific organs or structure location and position are evaluated after all images are obtained.

Most abdominal and superficial structure examinations are now scanned with real-time systems, which have a more limited field of view. Since many of these organs and structures lie oblique to the imaginary body surface planes, sonographers

TABLE 1-1. Directional terms[2–5]

Superior (cranial)	Toward the head, closer to the head, the upper portion of the body, the upper part of a structure, or a structure higher than another structure. Example: The left lobe of the lung is superior to the left lobe of the liver.
Inferior (caudal)	Toward the feet, away from the head, the lower portion of the body, toward the lower part of a structure, or a structure lower than another structure. Example: The lower pole of each kidney is inferior to the upper pole.
Anterior (ventral)	Toward the front or at the front of the body or a structure in front of another structure. Example: The main portal vein is anterior to the inferior vena cava.
Posterior (dorsal)	Toward the back or the back of the body or a structure behind another structure. Example: The main portal vein is posterior to the common hepatic artery.
Medial	Toward the middle or midline of the body or the middle of a structure. Example: The middle hepatic vein is medial to the right hepatic vein.
Lateral	Away from the middle or the midline of the body or pertaining to the side. Example: The right kidney is lateral to the inferior vena cava.
Ipsilateral	Located on the same side of the body or affecting the same side of the body. Example: The gallbladder and right kidney are ipsilateral.
Contralateral	Located on the opposite side of the body or affecting the opposite side of the body. Example: The pancreatic tail and pancreatic head are contralateral.
Proximal	Nearer the attachment of an extremity to the trunk or the origin of a body part. Example: The thoracic aorta is proximal to the abdominal aorta.
Distal	Farther from the attachment of an extremity to the trunk or the origin of a body part. Example: The iliac arteries are distal to the abdominal aorta.
Superficial	Toward or on the body surface or external. Example: The testicles are considered superficial structures.
Deep	Away from the body surface or internal. Example: The prostate is a deep structure.

must identify anatomy accurately to utilize specific organ and structure orientation for scanning surfaces. These scanning planes are described by the transducer's orientation to the anatomic plane or to the specific organ and structure (Fig. 1-3).

PATIENT POSITION

Positional terms refer to the patient's position relative to the surrounding space. Patient position terminology for ultrasonography was adopted from radiography (Table 1-2).[1,2] The eight positions are illustrated in Figure 1-4. In clinical practice, patients are scanned in a recumbent, semierect (head elevated), or sitting position. On occasion, the patient may be placed in other positions, such as Trendelenburg (head lowered) or standing, to obtain unobscured images of the area of interest.

Sonographers frequently convey information on patient position and transducer placement simultaneously. This terminology was adopted from radiography, where it describes the path of the x-ray beam through the patient's body. In sonography, this terminology describes the path of the sound beam. Table 1-3 illustrates how these terms are used and should clarify some terminology for readers who have no radiography background. There is no evidence in the literature that this terminology has been adopted as a professional standard.

IMAGE PRESENTATION AND LABELING

When describing sonographic images, body, organ, or structure plane terminology, coupled with transducer placement conveys a very descriptive view of sectional anatomy. Real-time imaging utilizes the same presentation and labelling protocol that was established with the static, articulated-arm instruments.

The anterior, posterior, right, or left body sur-

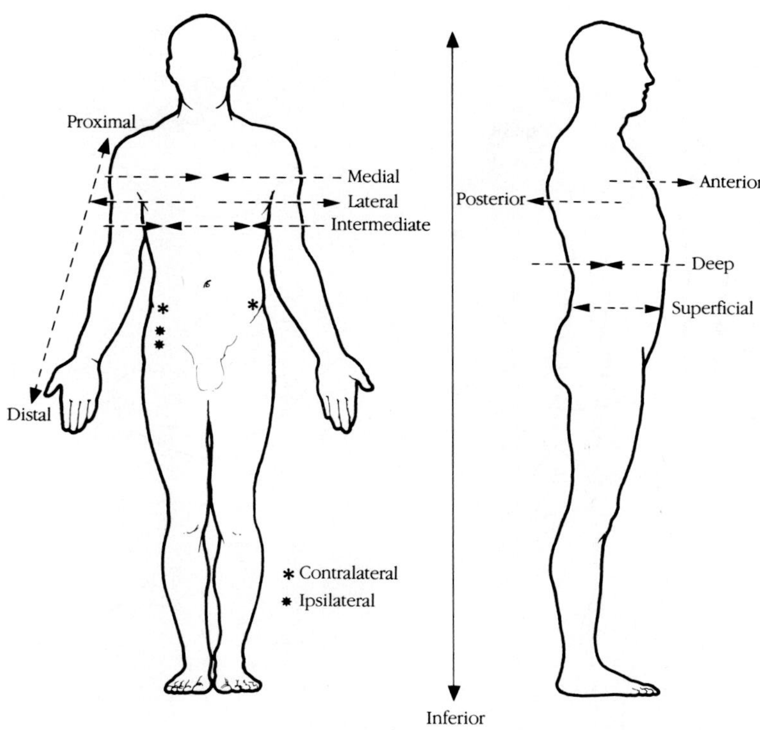

FIGURE 1-1. A schematic drawing of a body in the anatomic position (standing erect, arms by the side, face and palms directed forward) with the directional terms.

face is usually scanned in the transverse, sagittal, and coronal planes. The scanning surface is presented on the top of the image for abdominal and superficial structures.[1] Transverse images are viewed from caudad to cephalad, or from the feet looking toward the head. This places the patient's right side to the viewer's left and the patient's left side to the viewer's right. The superior scanning surface is presented at the top of the image and is used for neurosonography where the transducer is placed on the head. The orientation for viewing endovaginal and endorectal images based on transducer placement has not yet been resolved. Labeling these images will help orient the viewer.

These six scanning surfaces coupled with three anatomic planes produce a combination of twelve different image presentations.[1] Figure 1-5 illustrates how to view and label them.

Image Quality Definitions

Evaluating sonographic image quality is learned and communicated using specific definitions. Normal tissue and organ structures have a characteristic echographic appearance relative to surrounding structures. An understanding of the normal appearance provides the baseline against which to recognize variations and abnormalities. These definitions describe and characterize the sonographic image.

An echo is the recorded acoustic signal. It is the reflection of the pulse of sound emitted by the transducer. Prefixes or suffixes modify the quality of the echo, describing characteristics and patterns on the image.

Echogenic describes an organ or tissue that is capable of producing echoes, of reflecting the acoustic beam. This term does not describe the quality

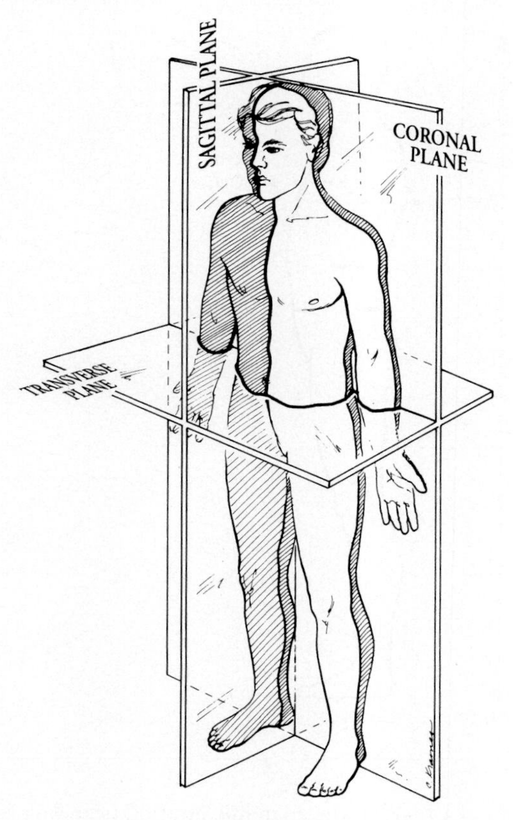

FIGURE 1-2. The anatomic position depicting the three imaginary anatomic flat surface planes: transverse, sagittal, and coronal.

of the image; it is often used to describe relative tissue texture (e.g., more or less echogenic than another tissue; Fig. 1-6). An aberration from normal echogenicity patterns may signify a pathologic condition or poor examination technique such as incorrect gain settings.

Anechoic describes the portion of an image that appears echo free. A urine-filled bladder, bile-filled gallbladder, and a clear cyst all appear anechoic (Fig. 1-7). The terms *echolucent* and *sonolucent* are misnomers that are often substituted for anechoic.

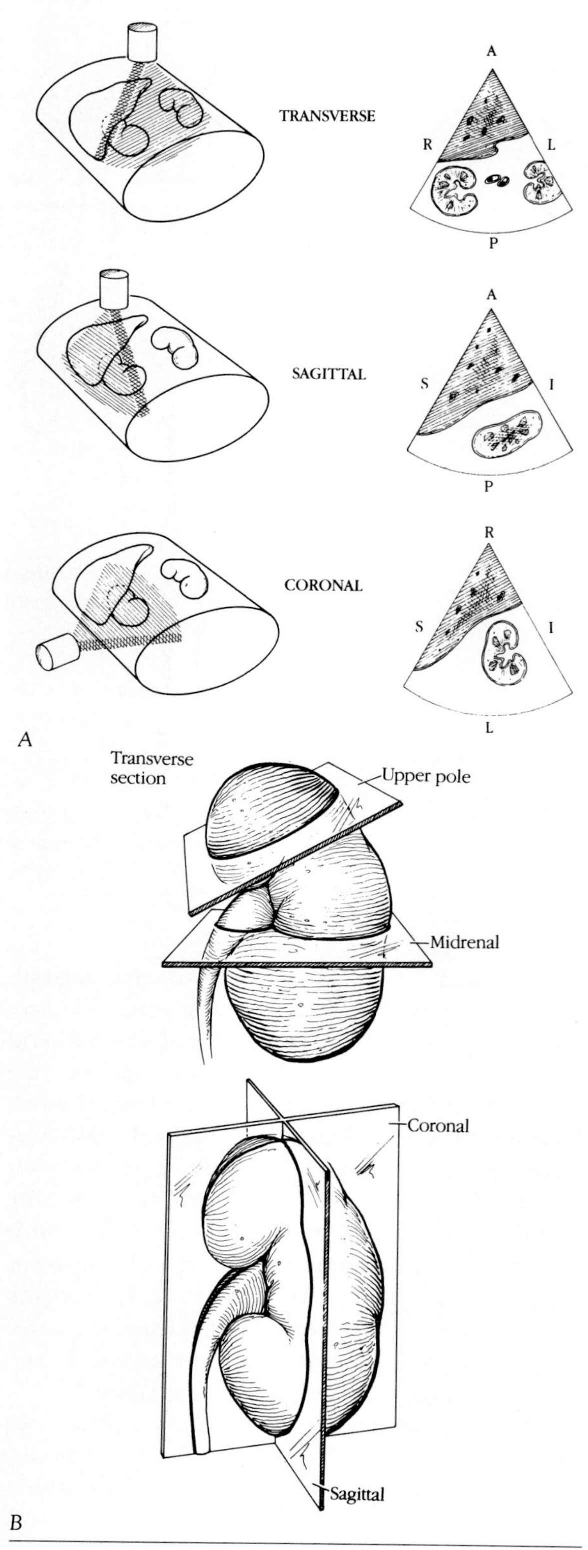

FIGURE 1-3. (*A*) The transverse, sagittal, and coronal scan planes and their display through the upper abdomen. (*B*) The transverse, sagittal, and coronal scan planes through the left kidney.

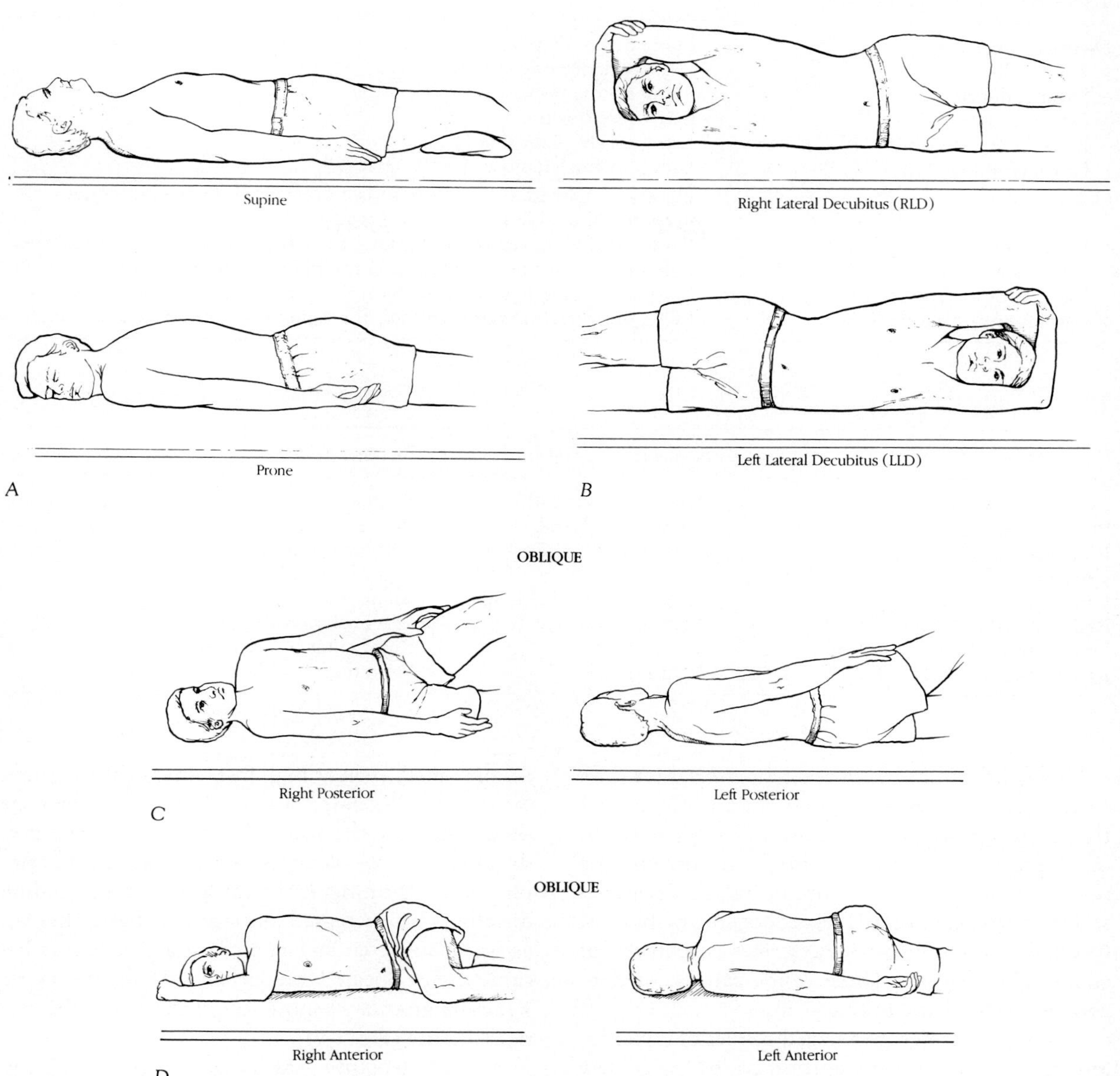

Figure 1-4. (*A*) The supine and prone recumbent patient positions. (*B*) The right lateral decubitus and left lateral decubitus patient positions. (*C*) The right posterior oblique and left posterior oblique patient positions. (*D*) The right anterior oblique and left anterior oblique patient positions.

TABLE 1-2. Patient positions[1,2]

Decubitus, recumbent	Lying down. (The adjective before the word describes the most dependent body surface.)
Supine, dorsal	Lying on the back.
Prone, ventral	Lying face down.
Right lateral decubitus (RLD)	Lying on the right side.
Left lateral decubitus (LLD)	Lying on the left side.
Oblique	Slanting, inclined. (Oblique positions are named for the body side nearest the table.)
Right posterior oblique (RPO)	Lying on the right posterior surface, the left posterior surface is elevated.
Left posterior oblique (LPO)	Lying on the left posterior surface, the right posterior surface is elevated.
Right anterior oblique (RAO)	Lying on the right anterior surface, the left anterior surface is elevated.
Left anterior oblique (LAO)	Lying on the left anterior surface, the right anterior surface is elevated.

TABLE 1-3. Path of insonating sound

DESCRIPTOR	SCANNING SURFACE	PATIENT POSITION
Anteroposterior (AP)	Anterior or ventral	Supine, semierect, Trendelenburg, standing
Posteroanterior (PA)	Posterior or dorsal	Prone, semierect, Trendelenburg, standing
Right lateral (RL)	Right side	Left lateral decubitus
Left lateral (LL)	Left side	Right lateral decubitus
Left anterior oblique (LAO)	Left anterior	Right posterior oblique
Right anterior oblique (RAO)	Right anterior	Left posterior oblique
Left posterior oblique (LPO)	Left posterior	Right anterior oblique
Right posterior oblique (RPO)	Right posterior	Left anterior oblique

Hyperechoic describes image echoes brighter than surrounding tissues or brighter than is normal for that tissue or organ. *Hypoechoic* describes portions of an image that are not as bright as surrounding tissues or are less bright than normal. *Echopenic* describes a structure that is less echogenic or has few internal echoes. *Isoechoic* describes structures of equal echo density. These terms can be used to compare echo textures (Fig. 1-8).

Homogeneous refers to imaged echoes of equal intensity. A homogeneous portion of the image may be anechoic, hypoechoic, hyperechoic, or echopenic. Heterogeneous describes tissue or organ structures that have several different echo characteristics. A normal liver, spleen, or testicle has a homogeneous echo texture, whereas, a normal kidney is heterogeneous, with multiple different textures.

Interpretation of Sonographic Characteristics

Three other definitions are frequently used to describe internal echo patterns: cystic, solid, and complex. A cystic structure or mass retains an anechoic center even at high instrument gain settings. Smooth, well-defined walls and side wall or edge shadowing may be seen. The echoes of structures distal to the cyst demonstrate increased echo amplitudes, beginning at the far wall and proceeding distally. This increased amplitude is better known as the acoustic enhancement artifact. It occurs because tissue located on either side of the cystic structure attenuates more sound than does the cystic structure (Fig. 1-9).

A solid structure may have a hyperechoic, hypoechoic, echopenic, or anechoic homogeneous echo texture; or it may be heterogeneous because it contains many different types of interfaces. Usually, solid structures exhibit the following characteristics: (1) internal echoes that increase with an increase in instrument gain settings; (2) irregular, often poorly defined walls and margins; and (3) low-amplitude echoes or shadowing posterior to the mass due to increased acoustic attenuation by soft tissue or calculi (Fig. 1-10).

A complex structure usually exhibits both anechoic and echogenic areas on the image, originat-

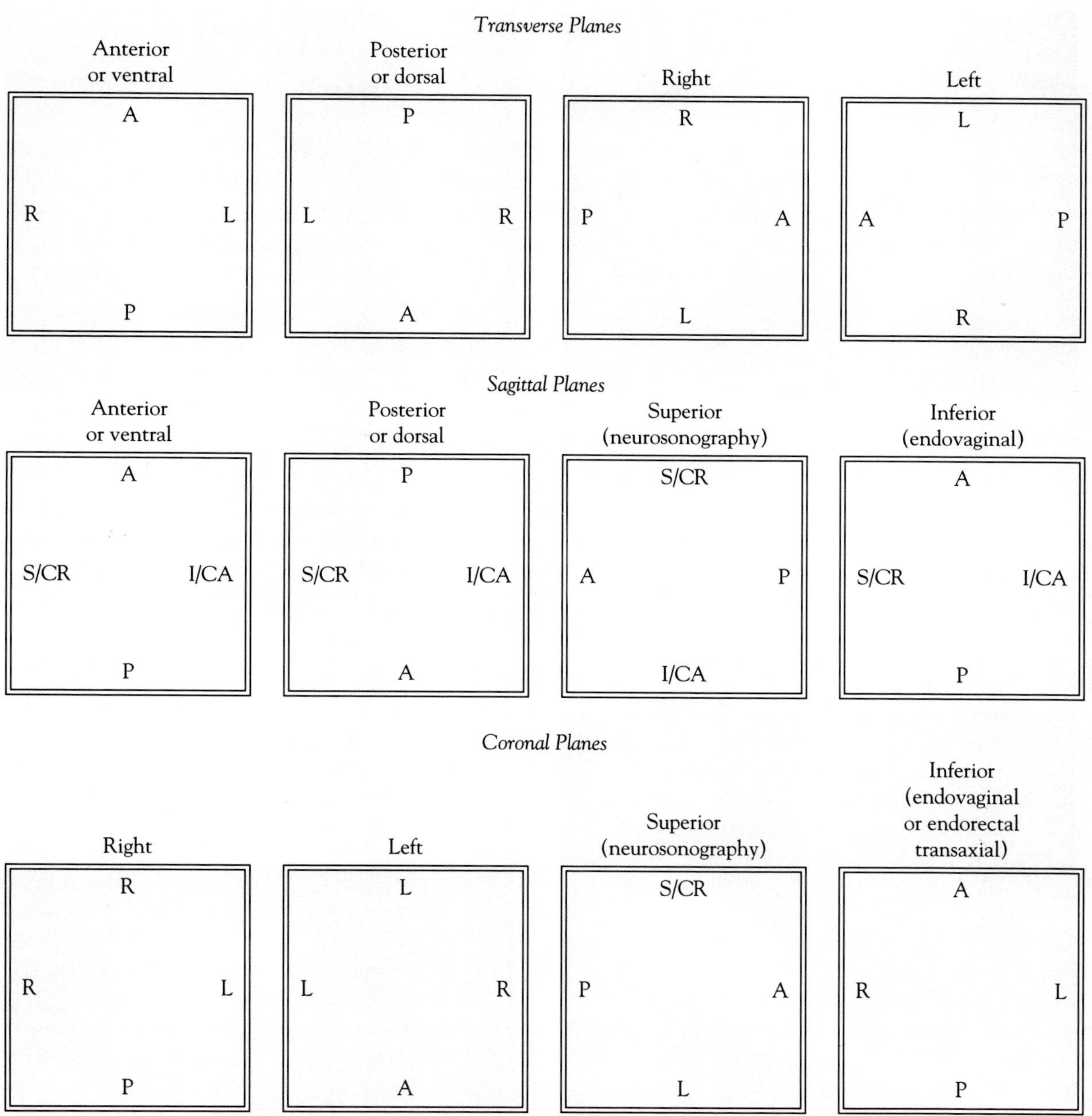

FIGURE 1-5. Image presentation: The scanning surface is presented on top, except for endovaginal. (A, anterior or ventral; P, posterior or dorsal; L, left; R, right; S, superior; CR, cranial; I, inferior; CA, caudal.)

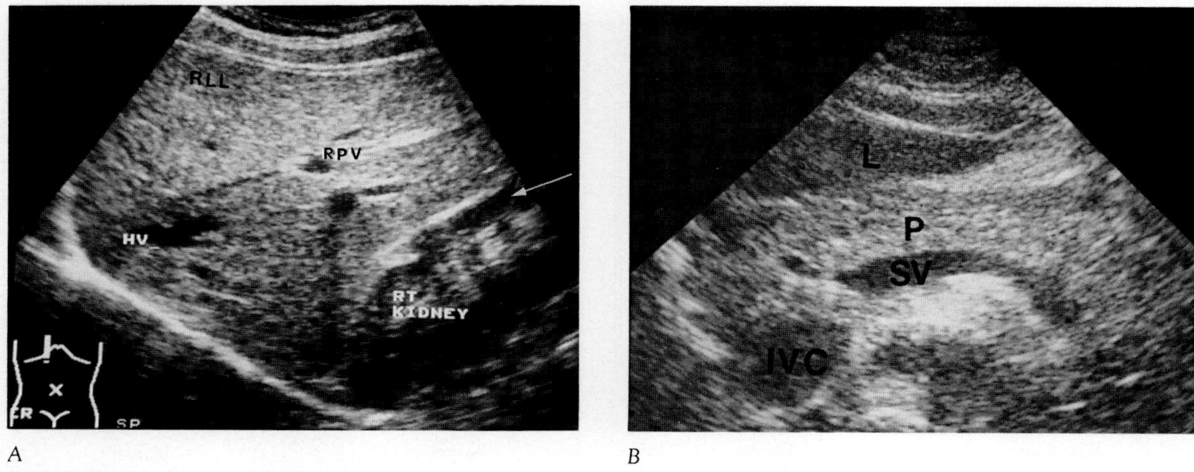

A B

FIGURE 1-6. (*A*) On this sagittal section made in a supine patient position, the normal texture of the right liver lobe (RLL) is described as more echogenic than the renal parenchyma *(arrow)*. (RPV, right portal vein; HV, hepatic vein.) (Courtesy Doug Amussen, Logan, UT.) (*B*) On this transverse section made in a supine patient position the normal texture of the liver (L) is described as less echogenic than the pancreas (P). (SV, splenic vein; IVC, inferior vena cava.)

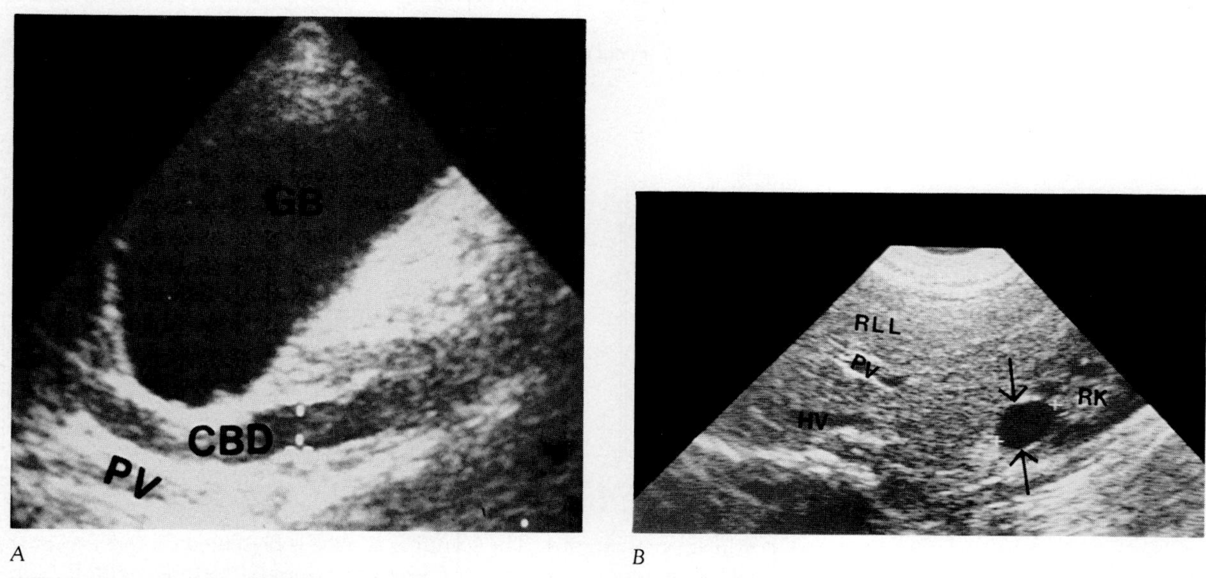

A B

FIGURE 1-7. (*A*) On this sagittal section made in a supine patient position the gallbladder (GB) is anechoic. This patient has a dilated common bile duct (CBD) measuring 9.3 mm seen anterior to the portal vein (PV). (*B*) A 2.5 cm cyst *(arrows)* in the upper pole of the right kidney (RK) and both the portal vein (PV) and hepatic vein (HV) in the right liver lobe (RLL) are described as anechoic since they produce no echoes.

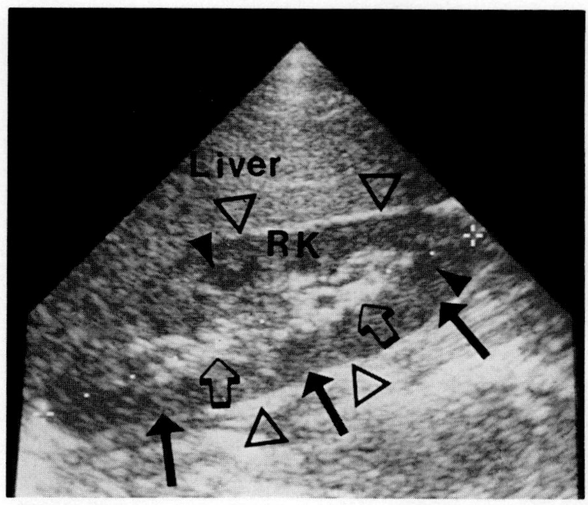

FIGURE 1-8. On a sagittal section of the right kidney (RK) measuring 9.9 cm the renal sinus *(open arrows)* and renal capsule *(open arrowheads)* are isoechoic, but the renal sinus is hyperechoic when compared to the hypoechoic renal cortex *(solid arrows)* and to the echopenic renal pyramids *(arrowheads)*. The renal pyramids become anechoic with increased diuresis.

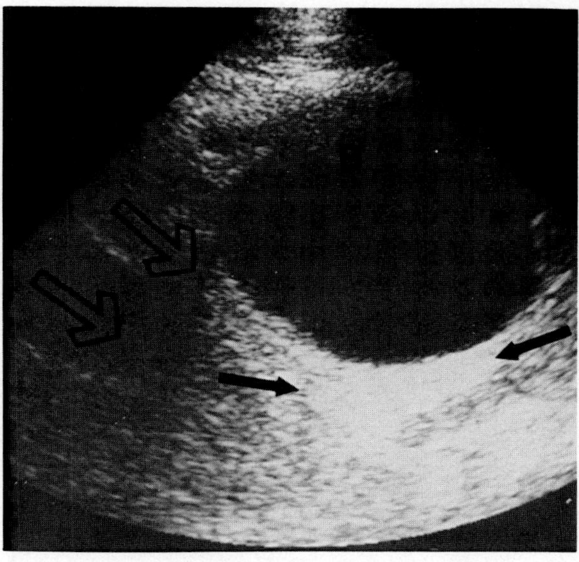

FIGURE 1-9. The cystic urinary bladder (B) retains an anechoic center even at high instrument gain settings, has smooth, well-defined walls and side wall or edge shadowing *(open arrows)*, as may be seen on this sagittal section. The echoes of structures distal to the cyst *(solid arrows)* demonstrate increased amplitudes beginning at the far wall and proceeding distally. This is the artifact known as acoustic enhancement.

ing from both fluid and soft tissue components within the mass. The relative echogenicity of a soft tissue mass is related to a variety of constituents, including collagen content, interstitial components, vascularity, and the degree and type of tissue degeneration (Fig. 1-11).

The amplitude of echoes distal to a mass, structure, or organ can be used to evaluate the attenuation properties of that mass. *Transonic* refers to masses, organs, or tissues that attenuate little of the acoustic beam and result in images with distal high-intensity echoes. An example is a cystic structure with the associated acoustic enhancement artifact. *Sonolucent* is also used for transonic but is a misnomer. Masses that attenuate large amounts of sound show a marked decrease in the amplitude of distal echoes. An example is calculi, with the associated shadow artifact.

Preparation

Before the patient is scanned it is important for the sonographer to obtain as much information as possible. The sonographer should be aware of the indications for the study and of any additional clinical information such as laboratory values, results of previous examinations, and related imaging examinations. The sonographic examination should be tailored to the clinical questions posed by the overall clinical assessment.

Patient apprehension is reduced when the examination is explained. Apprehension may be lessened further by providing a clean and neat examination room, extending common courtesies and a smile, and letting the patient know that she or he enjoys providing this diagnostic service. It is important that patients know they are the focus of the sonographer's attention.

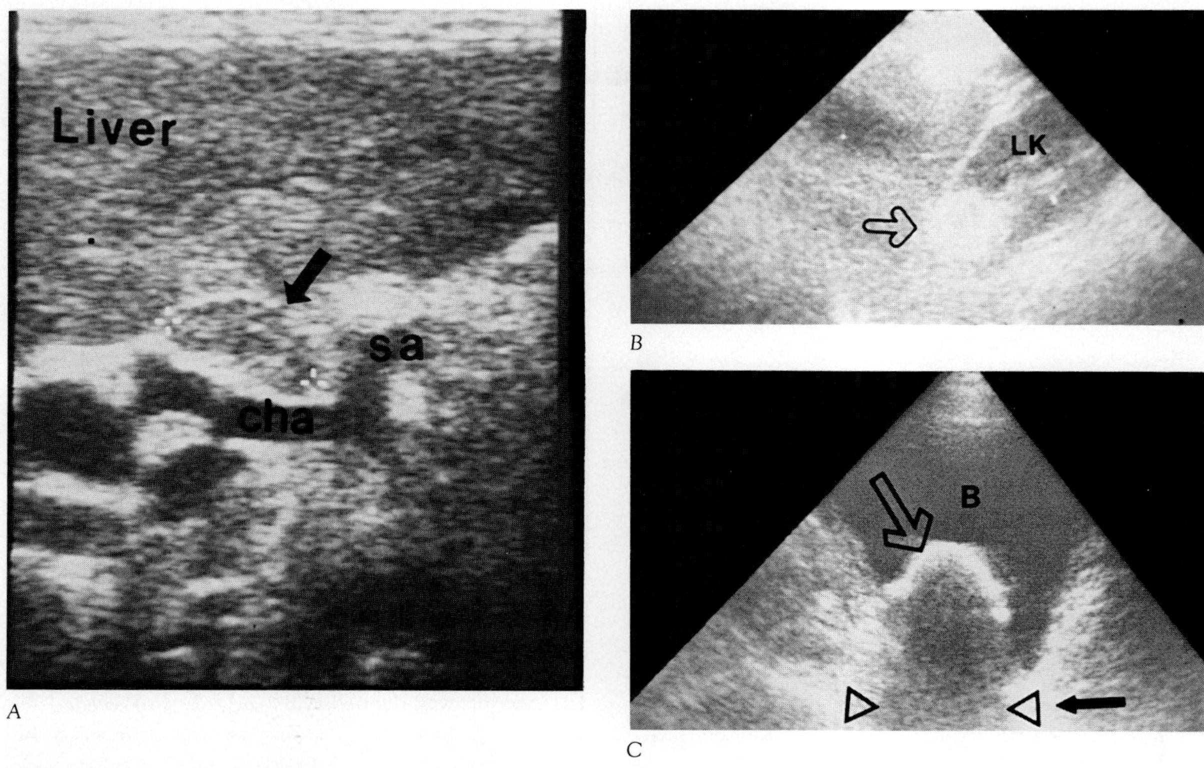

FIGURE 1-10. (*A*) A solid, homogeneous, hypoechoic tumor node *(cursors, arrow)* measuring 2.3 cm is identified anterior to where the common hepatic artery (cha) and splenic artery (sa) branch off of the celiac axis. (Courtesy Cathy Carr-Hoefer, Corvallis, OR.) (*B*) An angiomyolipoma *(arrow)* measuring 2.5 cm in diameter located on the upper pole of the left kidney (LK) is a solid tumor presenting with a heterogeneous echo texture because it is composed of fat cells intermixed with smooth muscle and aggregates of thick-walled blood vessels. (C) A urinary bladder (B) calculus *(open arrow)*, a solid mass, appears hyperechoic and attenuates sound energy, which casts a shadow artifact *(open arrowheads)*. Distal to the urinary bladder (B), an acoustic enhancement artifact *(arrow)* can also be identified.

The region of interest is visualized by planning the sonographic examination to image in multiple planes, two of which are perpendicular. Any abnormalities are imaged with differing degrees of transducer and patient obliquity to collect more information. The patient is released only after sufficient information is documented, as being called back for a repeat examination increases apprehension.

Conclusion

This reference chapter, like any good chapter, is never complete. It is provided to aid the communication skills within the profession. Paying close attention to the use of accurate and precise terminology enhances the quality of patient care.

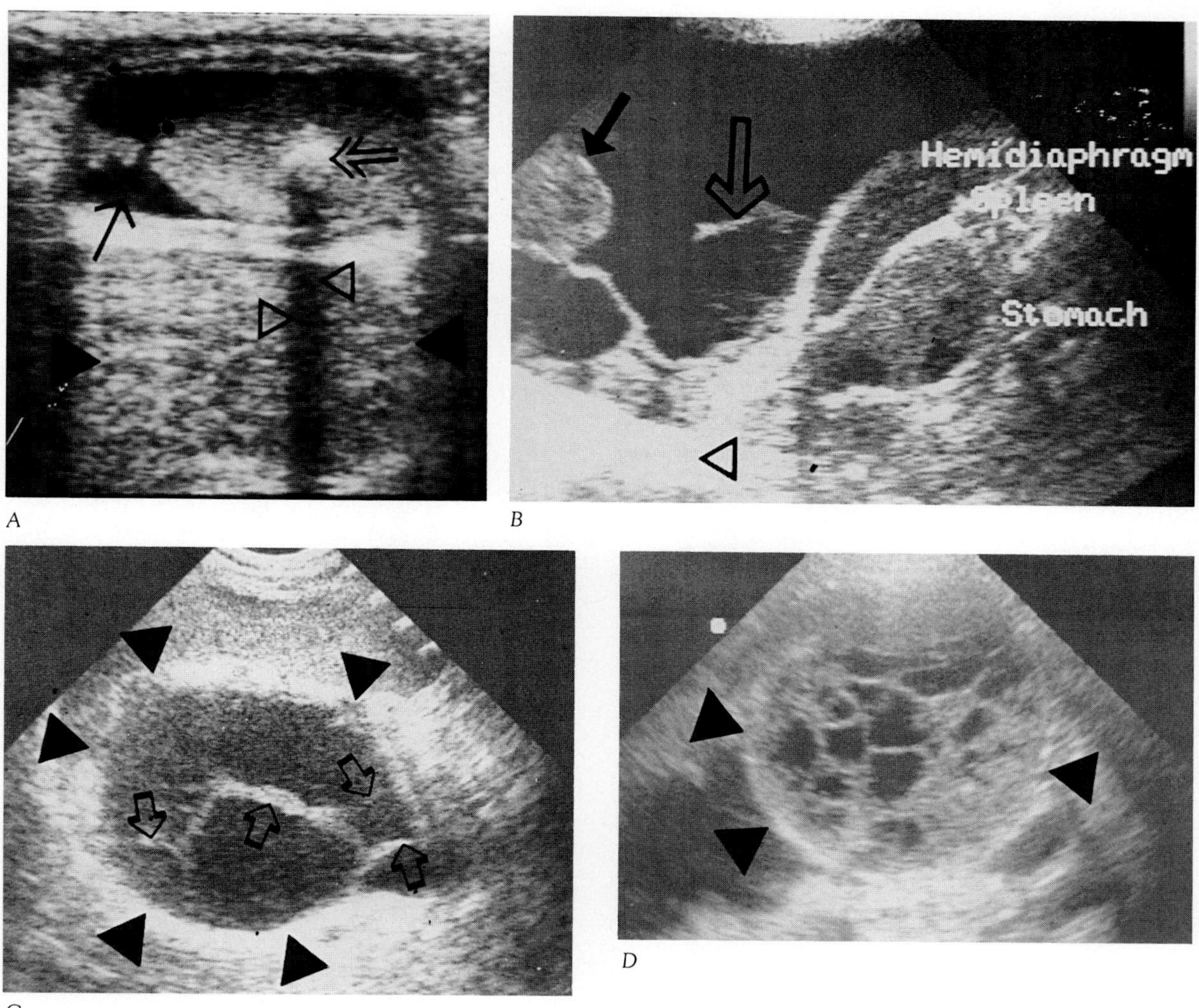

Figure 1-11. (*A*) With the patient in a left posterior oblique position, a transverse section of adenocarcinoma of the gallbladder presents as a complex mass displaying hypoechoic tissue *(dotted arrow)*, anechoic fluid *(solid arrow)* with acoustic enhancement *(solid arrowheads)*, and a hyperechoic calculus *(open arrow)*, which casts a shadow *(open arrowheads)*. (Courtesy Cathy Carr-Hoefer, Corvallis, OR.) (*B*) A complex tumor nodule *(open arrow)* presents with both anechoic and echogenic areas and is seen with a solid, homogeneous tumor nodule *(dark arrow)* within a pleural effusion. The pleural effusion is anechoic and there is acoustic enhancement (open arrowhead). (Courtesy Debra M. Joly, Kingston, TX.) (C) This leiomyosarcoma presents as a complex hypoechoic mass *(arrowheads)* with hyperechoic septa *(open arrows)*. (Courtesy Debra M. Joly, Kingston, TX.) (*D*) The encapsulated mass located in the lower pole of the right kidney measures 9.7 cm in diameter. It is a complex structure exhibiting septa between echogenic and anechoic areas. (Courtesy Lisa Schneiter, Ogden, UT.)

References

1. AIUM: Standard Presentation and Labeling of Ultrasound Images. Bethesda, MD 20814, American Institute of Ultrasound in Medicine, 1983.
2. Ballinger PH: Merrill's Atlas of Radiographic Position and Radiologic Procedures, 7th ed. St. Louis, CV Mosby, 1991.
3. Hagen-Ansert SL: The Anatomy Workbook. Philadelphia, JB Lippincott, 1986.
4. Marieb EN: Human Anatomy and Physiology. Redwood City, CA, Benjamin/Cummings, 1989.
5. Spence AP, Mason EB: Human Anatomy and Physiology. Menlo Park, CA, Benjamin/Cummings, 1987.
6. Thomas CL (ed): Taber's Cyclopedic Medical Dictionary, 16th ed. Philadelphia, FA Davis, 1989.
7. Tortora GJ, Anagnastakos NP: Principles of Anatomy and Physiology, 5th ed. New York, Harper and Row, 1987.

PART ONE
Abdominal Sonography

CHAPTER 2

Abdominal Wall and Peritoneal Cavity

MARVEEN CRAIG

The human body has several characteristic features: a backbone, bilateral symmetry, and two main cavities (ventral and dorsal), one situated on the anterior or ventral surface and the other on the posterior or dorsal surface. Each of these cavities, in turn, is divided into smaller cavities. The ventral cavity is separated by the muscular diaphragm into the thoracic cavity and the peritoneal cavity. The peritoneal cavity is subdivided into abdominal and pelvic portions. The abdominal wall and peritoneal cavity (particularly its abdominal subdivision) are the focus of this chapter.

Abdominal Cavity

EXTENT

As one of the two major sections of the peritoneal cavity, the abdominal cavity lies inferior to the diaphragm and is lined and divided by the peritoneum into many important fossae and spaces. It is continuous with the pelvic cavity inferiorly, through the pelvic inlet.[2,9,14,15,18]

DIVISIONS

Both abdominal and pelvic cavities are lined by a thin sheet of tissue called the peritoneal membrane. It is this structure that also divides the abdominal cavity into peritoneal and retroperitoneal compartments (Fig. 2-1). The portion of the peritoneum lining the cavity is called the parietal peritoneum; the visceral peritoneum covers the abdominal organs. One important function of these tissues is the secretion of serous fluid, which lubricates the surfaces of the peritoneum and facilitates free movement between the viscera. For clinical reasons, the abdomen is customarily divided by two vertical and two horizontal lines into nine regions (Fig. 2-2): (1) right hypochondrium, (2) epigastrium, (3) left hypochondrium, (4) right lumbar, (5) umbilical, (6) left lumbar, (7) right iliac fossa, (8) hypogastrium, and (9) left iliac fossa. Surface landmarks frequently used to describe scanning planes are the xiphoid process, costal margins, umbilicus, and iliac crest (Fig. 2-3).

CONTENTS

The contents of the abdominal cavity include the digestive organs (liver, gallbladder, stomach, pancreas, and intestines) plus the spleen, adrenal glands, kidneys, and ureters. Branches of the abdominal aorta send blood outward to supply each of these structures, and the inferior vena cava (IVC) and the main portal vein (MPV) receive and remove blood from them. The prevertebral vessels, all of the pancreas except its tail, and the kidneys and ureters lie behind the peritoneal membrane and are considered retroperitoneal rather than abdominal organs.

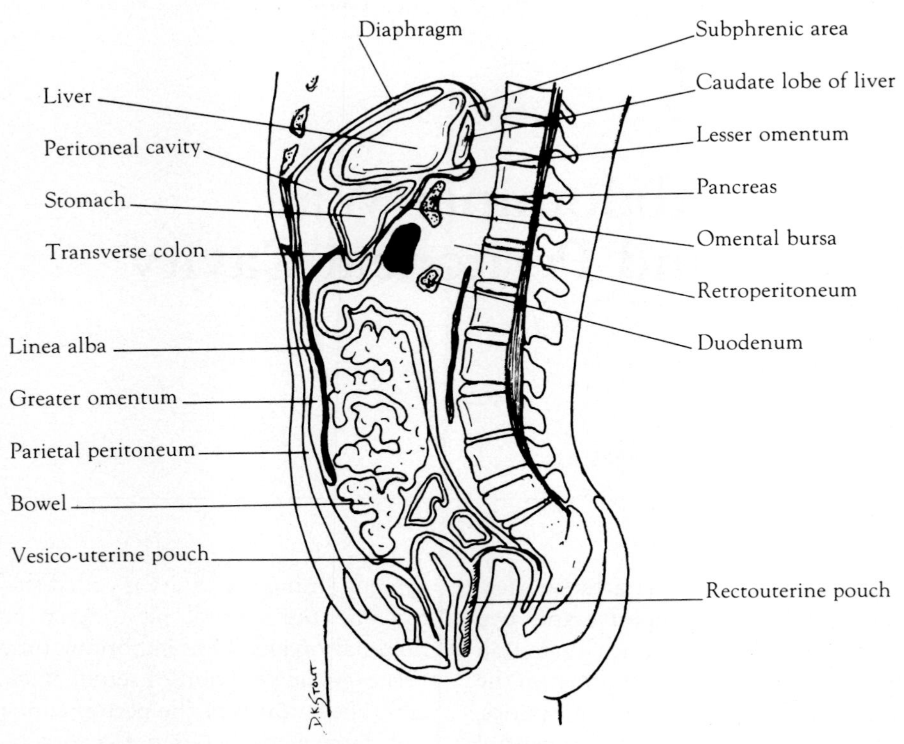

FIGURE 2-1. Sagittal view of the peritoneum.

Abdominal Wall

EXTENT

The anterior abdominal wall extends from the xiphoid process and lower costal cartilages to the upper anterior aspect of the pelvic bones. Deep beneath the subcutaneous tissue of the abdominal wall lies its musculature, which is divided into midline and anterolateral groups. Three muscles make up the anterolateral group (Fig. 2-4): the external oblique (most superficial), the middle and internal oblique (middle layer), and the transverse abdominis muscles and fasciae (deepest layer).

Posteriorly, the abdominal wall is formed in the midline by the five lumbar vertebrae and their intervertebral discs. Laterally, the abdominal wall is formed by the 12 ribs, the upper part of the bony pelvis, psoas muscles, the quadratus lumborum muscles, and the aponeurosis of the origin of the transverse abdominis muscles (Fig. 2-5).

SUBCUTANEOUS TISSUES

The skin of the abdominal wall is loosely attached to underlying structures except at the umbilicus. The linea alba is a fibrous seam, or line, that divides the abdomen symmetrically. Extending in the midline from the xiphoid process to the symphysis pubis, it is formed by the crossing strands of the three lateral abdominal wall muscles (see Fig. 2-4).

Subcutaneous tissue anterior to the muscle layers makes up the superficial fascia of the abdominal wall, which can be divided into two layers. The first is a fatty layer (Camper's fascia) containing small vessels and nerves. It is this layer that lies predominantly above the umbilicus and gives the body wall its rounded appearance. The second layer is a deep membranous layer (Scarpa's fascia), which is a combination of fat and fibrous tissue that blends with the deep fascia (Fig. 2-6).

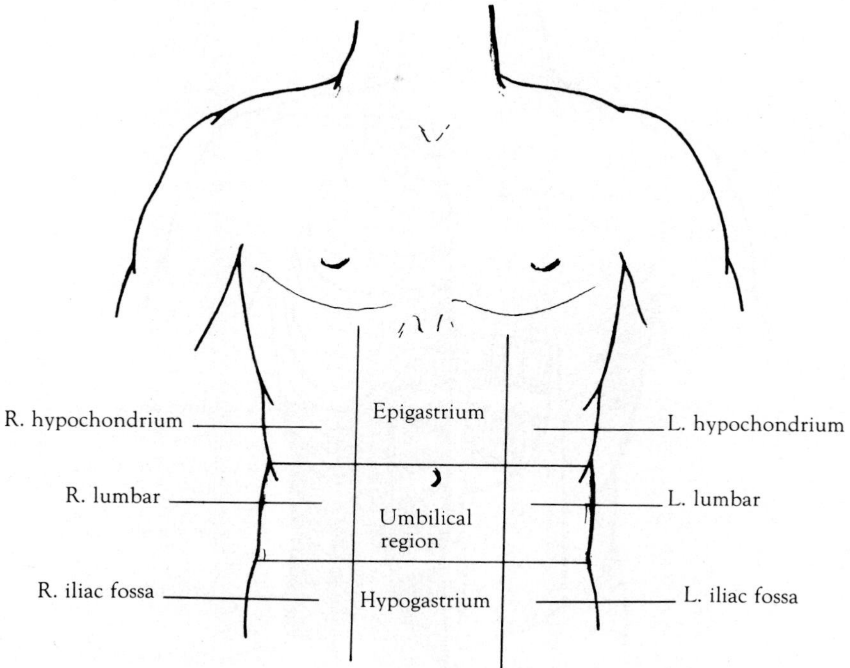

Figure 2-2.

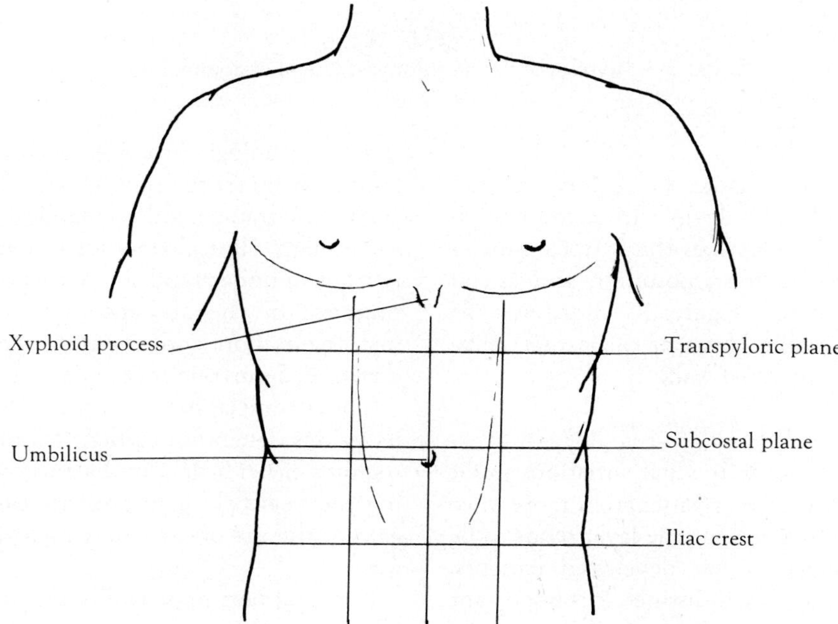

Figure 2-3.

Figure 2-2. Divisions of the abdominal wall.

Figure 2-3. Surface landmarks of the abdominal wall.

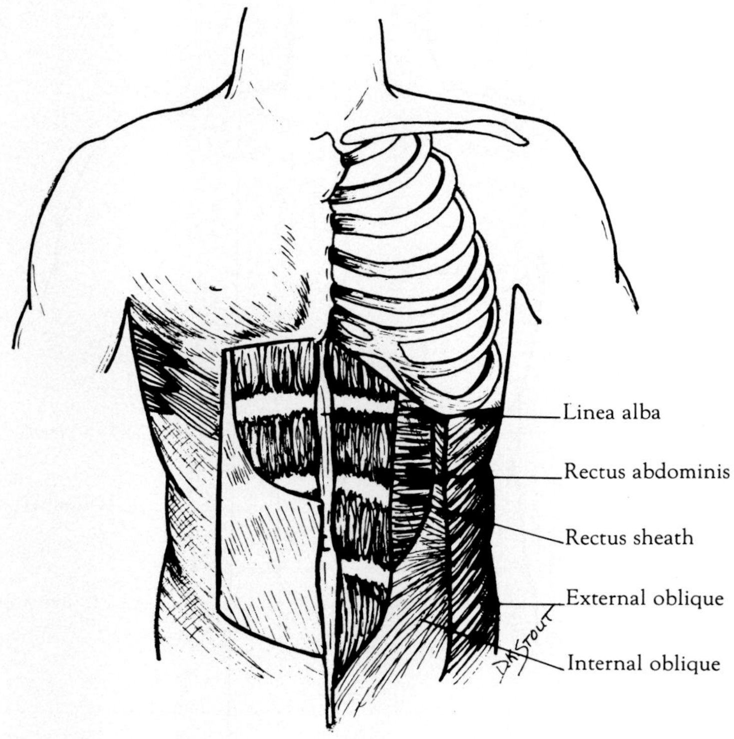

FIGURE 2-4. Muscles of the anterior and lateral abdominal wall.

MUSCLE LAYERS

Because subcutaneous tissues are principally fat, they are sonographically distinct from the muscular layers. Table 2-1 describes the various muscles that make up the anterior, posterior, and lateral walls of the abdomen. Figure 2-7 illustrates the sonographically visible layers of tissue that make up the anterior abdominal wall.

VARIANTS

Anatomic variants are individual variations in fat and muscle content among patients. In more muscular patients each lateral muscle layer tends to be identifiable, whereas in less developed patients, muscle groups tend to be indistinct. It is important to note that in obese patients the fat layer may be as thick as 8 cm.[18]

SONOGRAPHIC APPEARANCES AND TECHNIQUES

Sonography provides a valuable noninvasive method of imaging the normal abdomen and detecting pathologic processes, such as inflammatory lesions, hemorrhage, hernia, or masses. Its use in evaluating trauma and postsurgical patients can resolve many clinical questions. It is extremely important to understand the normal sonographic appearance of the abdomen and the appropriate instrumentation and scanning techniques necessary to demonstrate that appearance.

The superficial nature of the abdominal wall and its lesions demands excellent near-field imaging. It requires either a delicate balance between increasing the near-field gain and decreasing the system gain or the use of extremely high-resolution transducers.[13]

Sonographers must realize that the settings usually used to scan the contents of the abdominal cavity obliterate superficial wall structures. Excessive near-gain also produces a negative effect: obliteration of fine detail. Therefore, high-frequency, short-focal zone transducers are the optimal tools for scanning this area.

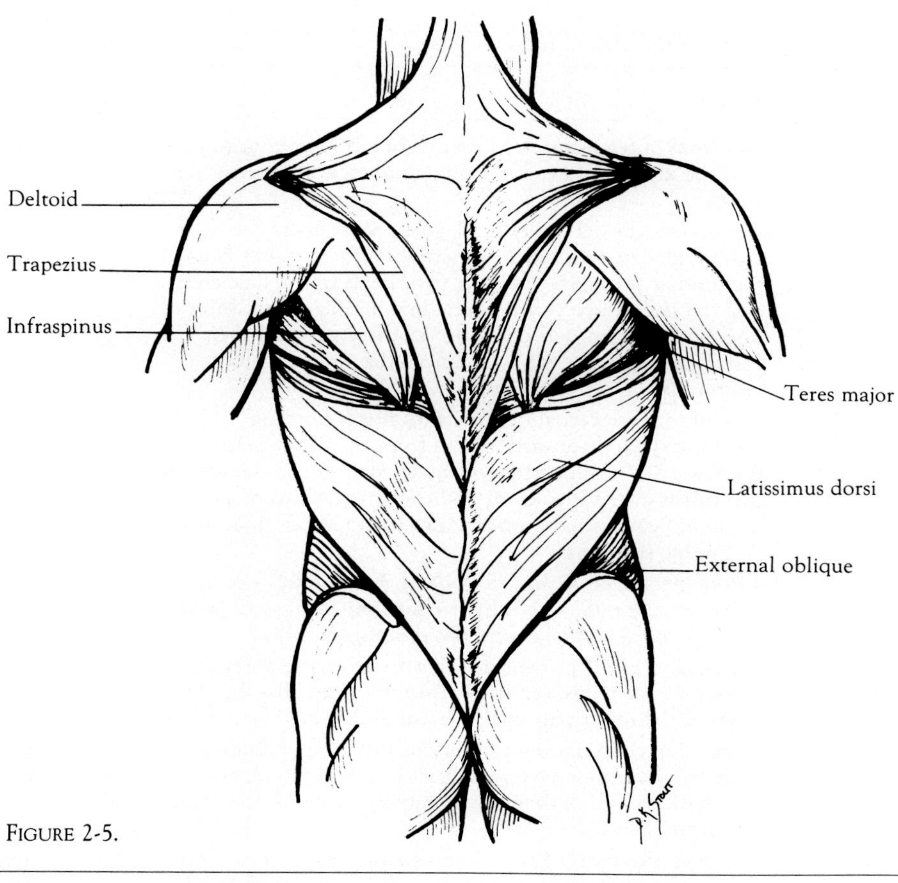

FIGURE 2-5.

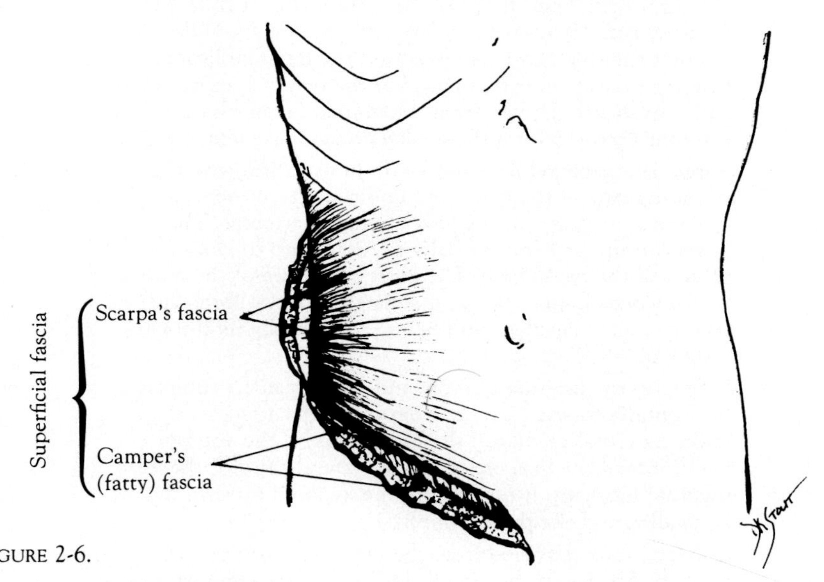

FIGURE 2-6.

FIGURE 2-5. Muscles of the posterior and lateral abdominal wall.

FIGURE 2-6. Superficial fascia(s): Scarpa's fascia (M) and Camper's (fatty) fascia (C).

Table 2-1. Muscular composition of the abdominal wall

Muscle Group	Location	Area Served
External oblique	Arises from outer surface of lower eight ribs. Fans out to insert into the xiphoid, linea alba, pubic bones, and anterior iliac crest.	Anterior abdominal wall
Internal oblique	Lies deep to external oblique. Majority of its fibers run at right angles to those of the external oblique. Arises from the lumbar fascia, the anterior two thirds of the iliac crest, and the lateral two thirds of the inguinal ligament. Inserts into the lower borders of the lower three ribs and their costal cartilages, the xiphoid, linea alba, and the pubic symphysis.	Anterior and lateral abdominal walls
Transverse	Lies deep to the internal oblique with fibers running horizontally and forward. Arises from the deep surface of the lower six costal cartilages, the lumbar fascia, the anterior two thirds of the iliac crest, and the lateral third of the inguinal ligament; also inserts into the xiphoid, linea alba, and pubic symphysis.	Lateral and anterior abdominal walls
Rectus abdominis	Arises by two heads from the front of the symphysis pubis and from the pubic crest. Inserts into the fifth, sixth, and seventh costal cartilages and the symphysis pubis.	Anterior abdominal wall
Pyramidalis	Often absent, but if present, it will arise from the anterior surface of the pubis and insert into the linea alba. Lies in front of the lower part of the rectus abdominis.	Anterior abdominal wall
Rectus sheath	Encloses the rectus abdominis muscle and the pyramidalis muscle (when present) and contains nerves, blood, and lymphatic vessels. Formed by the aponeuroses of the three lateral muscles.	Anterior abdominal wall
Psoas	Arises from the roots of the transverse processes, sides of the vertebral bodies and intervertebral discs, from T12 to L5. Its fibers run downward and laterally, leaving the abdomen to enter the thigh by passing behind the inguinal ligament. Inserts into the lesser trochanter of the femur. Is enclosed in a fibrous sheath derived from the lumbar fascia which thickens above to form the medial arcuate ligament.	Posterior abdominal wall
Quadratus lumborum	Flat muscle arising below from the iliolumbar ligament, the adjoining part of the iliac crest, and the tips of the transverse processes of the lower lumbar vertebrae. The fibers run upward and medially to insert into the lower border of the twelfth rib. The anterior surface of the muscle is covered by lumbar fascia, thickened above to form the lateral arcuate ligament and below, to form the iliolumbar ligament.	Posterior or lateral abdominal wall
Transversus abdominis	Lies deep to the internal oblique muscle, with fibers running horizontally forward. Arises from the deep surface of the lower six costal cartilages, the lumbar fascia, the anterior two-thirds of the iliac crest, and the lateral third of the inguinal ligament. It inserts into the xyphoid process, the linea alba, and the pubic symphysis.	Lateral or posterior abdominal wall
Iliacus	Fan-shaped muscle arising from the upper part of the iliac fossa. Its fibers join the lateral side of the psoas tendon to insert into the lesser trochanter of the femur. The combined muscles are often referred to as the iliopsoas. Lies in the posterior part of the diaphragm; also forms part of the posterior abdominal wall.	Posterior abdominal wall

(Data from Snell RS: Clinical Anatomy for Medical Students. Boston, Little, Brown, 1973.)

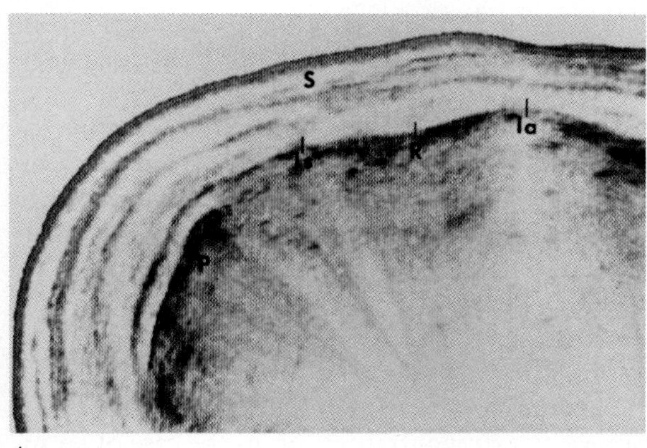

A

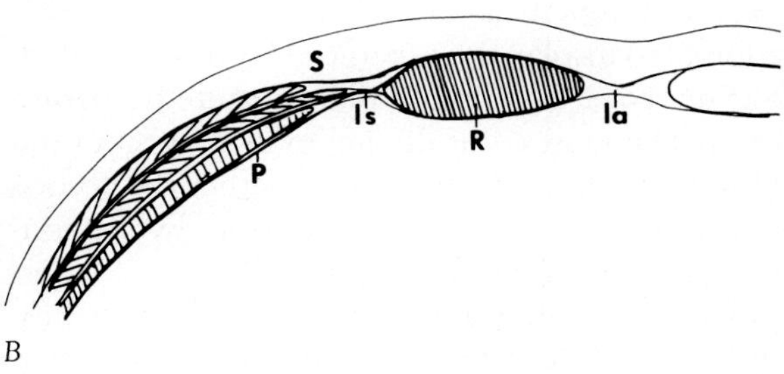

B

Figure 2-7. Normal Anatomy: (*A*) Transverse section and (*B*) line drawing of the upper abdominal wall. Subcutaneous tissue (S) lies anterior to muscle groups. The lateral muscle group (anterior external oblique, central internal oblique, and innermost transversalis) is separated from the rectus abdominis (R) by the linea semilunaris (ls), and the recti are separated by linea alba (la). The peritoneal-fascial interface (P) separates intraperitoneal structures from the anterior wall. (From Miller EI, Rogers A: Sonography of the anterior abdominal wall. Semin Ultrasound 1982, 3:278–287.)

If global views of the abdominal wall are desired, it is necessary to resort to the use of an articulated-arm imaging device. If such equipment is unavailable, sector or linear real-time devices can be used, though they present varying degrees of difficulty when scanning over areas that are curved or bony. In addition, the limited field of view of such scanning heads makes them less desirable for this application.

The use of excessive transducer pressure while scanning can cause distortion of the superficial layers.[13] In extreme cases of near-field artifact, it may be necessary to introduce a stand-off device between the transducer face and the body wall, to eliminate the artifact and to maximize the use of the transducer's focal zone.

The need to demonstrate the various layers of the abdominal wall should not be limited to patients with superficial lesions. The fine details of the abdominal wall should be an integral part of every proper abdominal study.

Clinical and Sonographic Findings of Pathology

Although this chapter focuses on the normal and atypical sonographic appearances of the abdominal and peritoneal cavity, a thorough understanding of the anatomy and sonographic appearances of the organs and compartments of the cavity is essential before pathologic changes can be fully appreciated. Three major categories of disease affect the abdominal wall, peritoneum, and abdominal spaces. Both the tissues of the abdominal wall and the membranes lining its spaces are affected by inflammatory, traumatic, and neoplastic changes.

Inflammation. The task of clinically oriented sonographers is to understand the clinical aspects of inflammation as well as its sonographic image. Inflammation can be acute or chronic. Acute inflammation frequently results because of cuts, scrapes, crushing injuries, or surgical trauma that produces tissue damage. Consequently, an inflammatory response can occur whenever bacterial infection damages the skin and underlying tissues.[4]

In most patients with acute inflammation, body responses permit a complete return to normal. This process, called resolution, can be hastened by the use of antiinflammatory drugs. Such drugs block the body's natural inflammatory reactions, thus allowing removal of debris and fluid exudates associated with the inflammation via the circulatory and lymphatic systems.

If resolution is slow to occur, other consequences may result. Fibrous tissue growth invades areas of long-standing cellular and fluid exudates, forming scar tissue. This process, called organization, is responsible for the development of adhesions following surgery. If sufficient necrosis of the involved tissues occurs, resolution does not take place and a cavity containing dead tissue and pus cells forms.

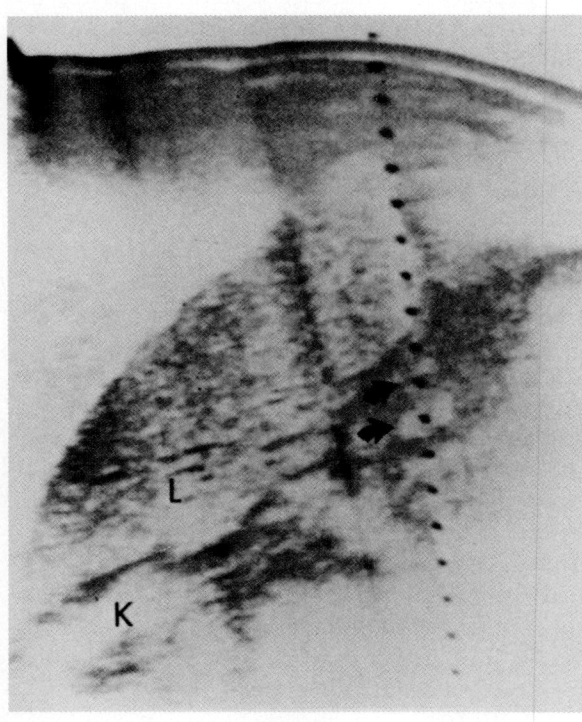

FIGURE 2-8. Large subphrenic abscess creates a mass effect by compressing and displacing the liver (L) medially and pushing the mesenteric vessels *(arrows)* leftward. The kidney (K) has been pushed inferiorly. (From Van Sonnenberg E: Abscess. Diagnostic Imaging. Clin Diagn Ultrasound 1984, 14:57–85.)

The liquid pus in such a cavity consists of living and dead microorganisms, necrotic tissue, exudate, and granulocytes. The cavity itself is called an abscess.[4]

Abscesses are space-occupying lesions whose fluid content allows them to assume varied shapes (usually spherical or elliptical). Because of their internal pressure, however, they can exert a mass effect on surrounding structures, causing compression or displacement (Fig. 2-8).

Wherever they occur, the usual treatment of abscesses involves antibiotic therapy, and sometimes drainage to facilitate resolution. Failure of an abscess to resolve can lead to thickening of the contents as a result of the reabsorption of water (inspissation), and eventually calcifications develop. If the cause of the acute inflammation is not eliminated, the processes of tissue injury and repair continue simultaneously; this is chronic inflammation.[4]

One variation is called chronic suppurative inflammation, in which an abscess is created as a result of persistent infection. "Suppurative" refers to this formation of pus. Body defenses may be poor because blood supply to the area is limited. If so, chronic suppurative inflammation can easily occur, requiring surgical drainage and the use of specific antibiotics to effect a cure.[4]

Superficial (abdominal wall) abscesses can be caused by external trauma, or, in the case of an incisional abscess, as a direct result of surgery. In evaluating superficial abscesses, precise scanning is required to display the superficial layers of the skin, subcutaneous fat, muscle planes, and the peritoneum. The most clinically important aspect of imaging abscesses is to determine whether the abscess is intraperitoneal or extraperitoneal by demonstrating the peritoneal line (Fig. 2-9).

In a study by Hey and Rabinowitz, superficial inflammatory lesions revealed variable echogenicity, but the abscesses were less echogenic than adjacent muscle walls.[20] The same study described the shape of various abscesses as flat, oval, or like a bonnet. Occasionally, large abscesses compress structures (such as the liver), making it difficult to differentiate extraperitoneal structures from intraperitoneal ones. The differential diagnosis of superficial abscesses includes rectus sheath hematomas and hernia, in addition to noninfected fluid collections.[6]

Superficial wound abscesses commonly result from intraoperative contamination (Fig. 2-10). In such cases sonography may have limited diagnostic use because the diagnosis can usually be made easily on physical examination. Most incisional abscesses are located superficially and are swollen and painful. However, if the abscess develops below the fascial plane, detection by physical examination alone can be difficult.[1]

SONOGRAPHIC APPEARANCES AND TECHNIQUES. Most abscesses appear as homogeneous fluid masses, but their internal patterns can range from uniformly echo free to mildly or even highly echogenic. Particulate debris or microbubbles floating in an abscess cavity is generally the cause of increased echogenicity. If the particulate matter is

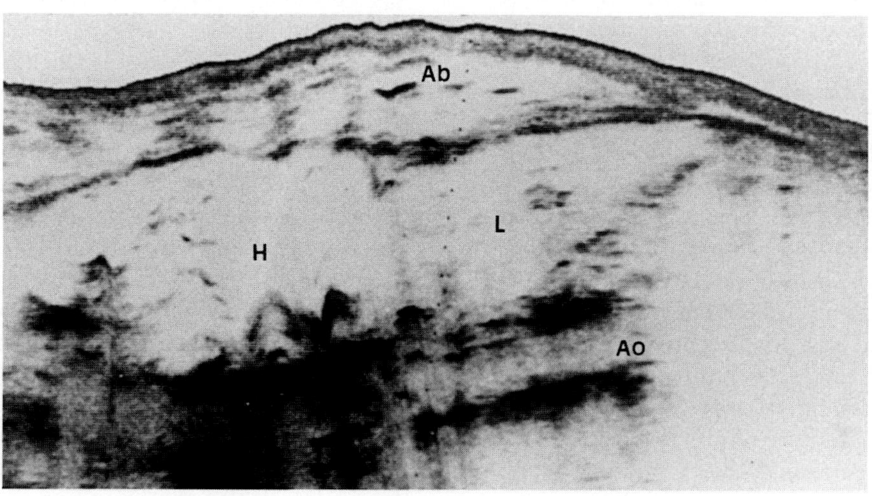

FIGURE 2-9. Superficial subcutaneous abscess (Ab) in a 20-year-old male struck in the chest by a car door. The patient complained of severe pain and swelling at the site of trauma. Anatomic landmarks seen in the scan are the left lobe of the liver (L), the heart (H), and the aorta (Ao). (Courtesy Laslie Mooney.)

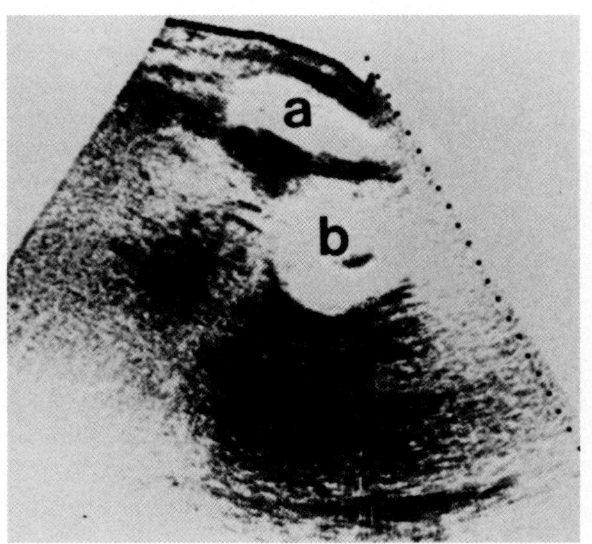

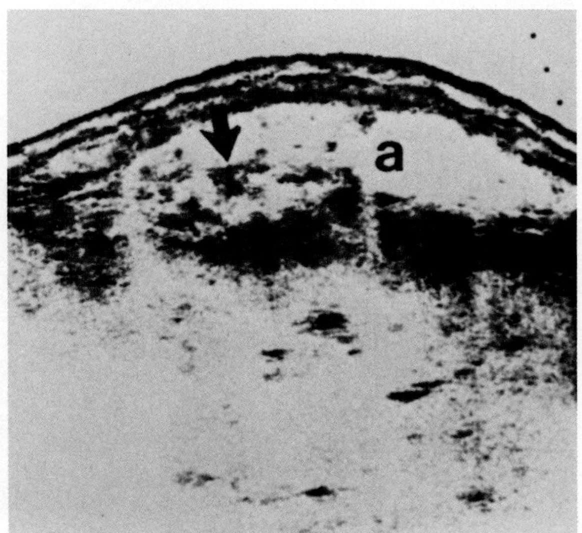

FIGURE 2-10. Postsurgical abscess involving the anterior abdominal wall. *(Left)* In the longitudinal scan the abscess (a) can be seen lying superior and anterior to the urinary bladder (b). (*Right*) In the transverse scan plane it is possible to identify both cystic and solid elements of the abscess (a). (From Anderhub B: Manual of Abdominal Sonography. Rockville MD, Aspen, 1983. Reprinted with permission of Aspen Publishers, Inc.)

distributed uniformly throughout the abscess, it may be difficult to recognize and differentiate it from surrounding structures (Fig. 2-11). Despite their variable internal textures, the majority of abscesses demonstrate posterior enhancement, so revealing their fluid contents.

Table 2-2 describes the common types of tissue changes associated with abscesses and their corresponding sonographic patterns. It is critical to appreciate how the effects of transducer frequency, focal length, beam profile, time gain compensation (TGC), output, and scan technique can alter the registration of echoes returning from an abscess. Occasionally, septations may be seen within abscesses. Such findings require documentation, since their presence contraindicates percutaneous drainage. Fortunately, septate abscesses are uncommon in the peritoneal cavity.

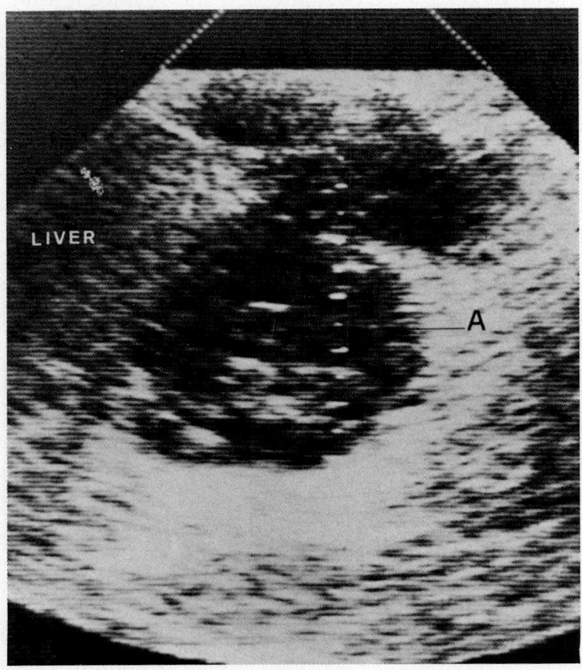

FIGURE 2-11. Longitudinal scan of a subhepatic abscess. Despite the presence of coarse and fine echoes within the round, hypoechoic, irregular-walled abscess (A), evidence of increased posterior sound transmission indicates the fluid nature of the mass. (From van Sonnenberg E: Abscess. Clin Diagn Ultrasound 1984, 14:57–85.)

To permit contact scanning, postoperative patients' surgical dressings must be removed. The face of the transducer should be washed in a sterilizing solution to avoid contamination. Caution must be taken not to damage the transducer's electrical connections when such a sterilizing process is used. The search for the abscess must be conducted in a systematic fashion, with special attention and care given to areas of swelling or tenderness. If there is an open wound, incision, drain site, or enterostomy it is important to use sterile gel and to scan around such sites by angling the transducer to view the area beneath.

As the survey of such areas is made, special techniques may be necessary to enhance the appearance of suspicious lesions. Because gain setting may affect the overall appearance of lesions, it is important to vary the gain. When gain settings are excessively high, small fluid collections may be overlooked because they "fill in." In contrast, when extremely low gain settings are used, there is a risk of making an homogeneously solid mass appear cystic. Moderate gain settings have their place in demonstrating the far wall of an abscess, but low gain may also be required to avoid the strong reverberation artifacts frequently seen at, or obscuring, the near walls. By creating several images using different gain settings and scanning planes, it will be possible to obtain maximum information about an abscess.

The shape of an abscess and its relationship to surrounding structures is valuable information if the clinician is planning percutaneous needle aspiration. Sonography not only aids in planning a safe aspiration route and monitoring such a procedure, but it also provides a means of evaluating the effectiveness of therapy on follow-up examinations.

Trauma. Among traumatic lesions that may involve the abdominal wall are hematomas, hernias, and foreign bodies. This discussion centers on hematomas and hernias, as they are the most common lesions.

Hematomas. Hematomas are generally associated with muscle trauma that results in hemorrhage. They can also result from infection, debilitating disease, collagen disorders, pregnancy, and child-

Table 2-2. Sonographic characteristics of fluid collections

Collection	Location	Shape	Acoustic Characteristics	Transonicity
Hematoma	Near wound or surgical site	Lenticular or shape of space	Change with stage of resolution: fresh blood is hypoechoic, as is clotted blood; fragmentation of clot creates internal echoes and anechoic areas with some scattered echoes; fluid-fluid level may be caused by cholesterol in breakdown of red blood cells; long-standing hematoma may have thick contours	Coincides with stage; good to slow or decreased; may increase due to fluid portion
Abscess	Near surgical site or painful area, subphrenic, subhepatic, paracolic gutters, and left perihepatic, perisplenic, and pelvis	Lenticular or shape of space	Anechoic with irregular or smooth borders, may have internal echoes, septations, fluid-fluid level; abscesses that contain gas are echogenic and might shadow	Usually good
Ascites	Most dependent areas of body: cul-de-sac, Morrison's pouch, paracolic gutter, pararenal areas, perihepatic midabdominal		Anechoic if benign, ascites if exudative, internal echoes if malignant; bowel and implants in anechoic ascitic fluid	Increased
Urinoma	Adjacent to kidneys		Usually anechoic unless infected	Increased
Lymphocele	Adjacent to renal transplant		Usually anechoic but may have septations	Increased

(Courtesy Mimi Berman.)

birth. Straining, coughing, and anticoagulant therapy can also be precipitating factors.[13]

Among the most common superficial abdominal wall hematomas are those within the rectus sheath (Fig. 2-12). Patients usually complain of pain and demonstrate a palpable abdominal mass that persists in both sitting and supine positions. Ecchymosis (discoloration) of the abdominal wall and a falling hematocrit value are often seen.

Hematomas of the rectus sheath tend to conform to its shape because it is a closed space. It is in patients whose bleeding is not confined to enclosed spaces that we find the most complaints of pain and ecchymosis. Another important finding is that hematomas in this region usually produce asymmetry of the abdominal wall (Fig. 2-13).

Postsurgical hematomas are usually intimately related to the incision site, frequently lying external to the anterior rectus fascia and presenting as a smooth-bordered, localized mass.

For any hematoma or thrombus, echogenicity varies, depending on the age of the lesion and the distribution of its cellular contents. An important reality is that hematomas are not limited to the anterior abdominal wall but can also involve the lateral or retroperitoneal muscles.

One of the frequent complications of anticoagulant therapy is hemorrhage. Ecchymosis at the needle site, exacerbation of existing lesions, and posttraumatic hematomas are its most common signs. Heparin therapy accounts for approximately a third of all retroperitoneal hematomas. Bleeding

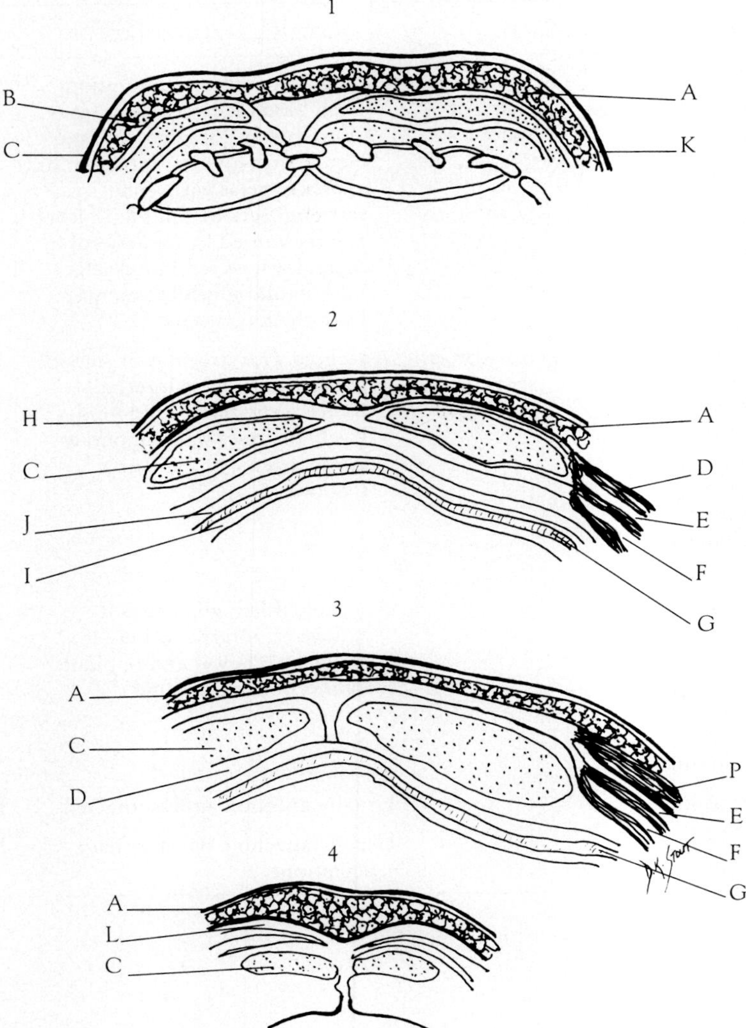

Figure 2-12. The rectus sheath: four sections of the rectus sheath muscle are presented from (*1*) above the costal margin, (*2*) between the costal margin and the anterior superior iliac spine, (*3*) between the level of the anterior superior iliac spine and the pubic symphysis, and (*4*) in front of the pubic symphysis. Key: A, superficial fascia; B, pectoralis major; C, rectus muscle; D, external oblique muscle; E, internal oblique muscle; F, transverse muscle; G, transverse fascia; H, linea alba; I, peritoneum; J, extraperitoneal fat; K, aponeurosis of the external oblique muscle.

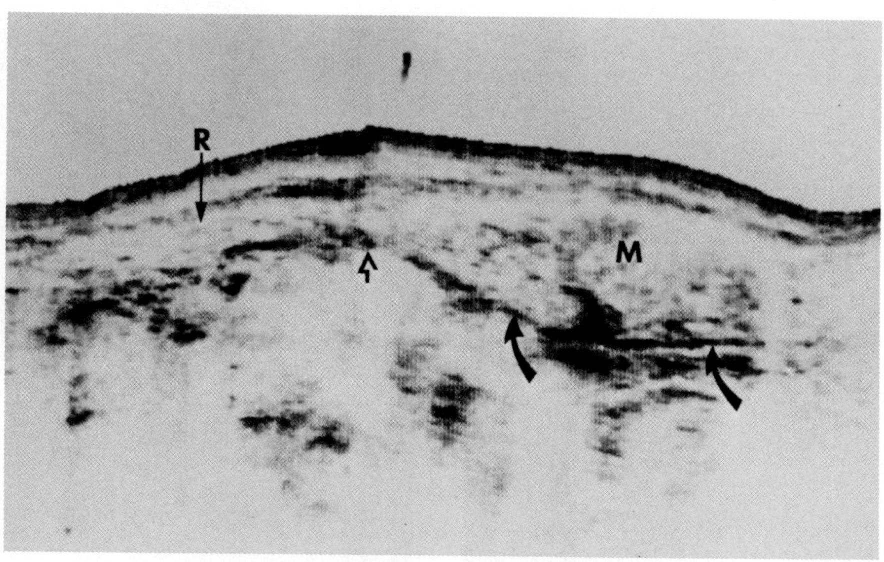

FIGURE 2-13. Progressive myositis. Transverse scan of a 30-year-old woman with a rapidly growing mass of 1 month's duration in the rectus sheath. Notice the limits of the mass (M) to the rectus sheath and its asymmetry compared to the normal rectus (R). The lineal alba *(open arrowhead)* and peritoneum *(curved arrows)* delineate the mass. Such lesions are self-limiting, but their occasional association with trauma can often lead to a clinical consideration of hematoma. (From Miller EI, Rogers A: Sonography of the anterior abdominal wall. Semin Ultrasound 1982, 3:278–287.)

usually occurs into the bulk of the retroperitoneal muscles, and while such hematomas can become large, they are usually self-limiting because of a tamponade effect. It is interesting to note that such hematomas can also result from mild, unnoticed trauma.[1]

SONOGRAPHIC APPEARANCES AND TECHNIQUES. Sonographic patterns closely follow the pathologic evolution of the hematoma. Recent blood collections tend to appear echo free and become more echogenic as they organize (Fig. 2-14), although the reverse may also occur. Hematomas and thrombi of the body behave differently, depending on their size and location. Wound hematomas that occur within the body generally resolve. The borders of such masses differ from their centers in echo reflection. In contrast, abdominal wall hematomas or those surrounded by a capsule show a gradual extinction of echoes.[8]

When bleeding is secondary to anticoagulant therapy, a wide range of sonographic appearances are possible. Although it is uncommon to scan such patients during active bleeding, the relative lack of coagulation would likely produce an echo-free or an unusual layered appearance, the latter due to the settling of moderately echogenic red blood cells to the bottom of the lesion. The fibrin content of the clot decreases its echogenicity. Movement of blood can sometimes be produced by changing the patient's position, but turbulent blood flow in any patient lying supine in a fixed position is diagnostic of active bleeding.[1] Sequential performance of modern high-resolution sonographic procedures that clearly delineate the muscle layers of the abdominal wall is a valuable way to study the response of such lesions to treatment.

Hernias. When abdominal wall muscles are extremely weak, the underlying viscera may protrude, producing a hernia (Fig. 2-15). Not surprisingly, the normally weaker areas of the abdominal wall,

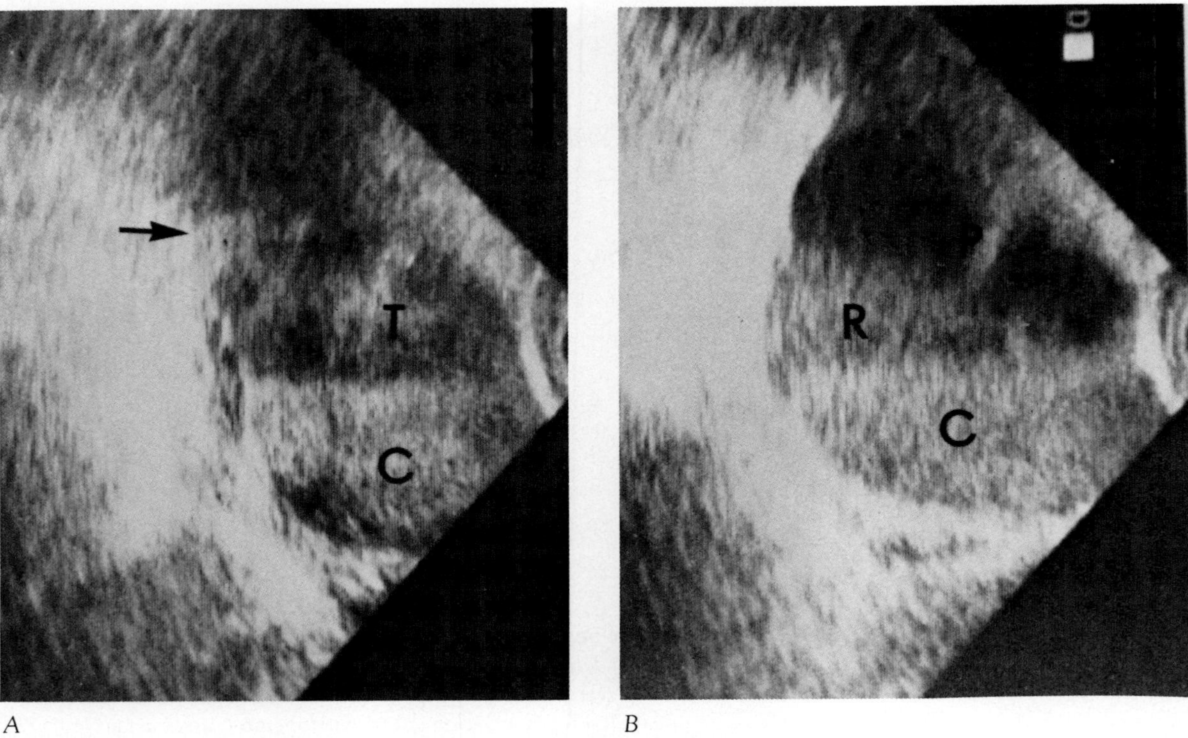

FIGURE 2-14. *(A)* In a longitudinal scan through a hematoma cavity a clot (C) lies in the dependent position, while turbulence (T) emanates from a point source *(arrow)* in the layer of unclotted blood. *(B)* In a delayed longitudinal scan through the same hematoma cavity, notice the layering of red cells (R) above the clotted layer (C). A layer of relatively echo-free plasma (P) lies above. (From Savage PD, Joseph AEA, Adam J: Massive abdominal wall hematoma: Real-time ultrasound localization of bleeding. J Ultrasound Med 1985, 4:157–158.)

the umbilical area and the femoral and inguinal rings, are the most common hernia sites. Surgery is generally indicated for hernias because uncorrected hernias are vulnerable to serious complications. An "incarcerated hernia" is one that cannot be reduced (pushed back into the abdominal cavity). Complicating factors, such as edema of the protruding structure and constriction of the opening through which intraabdominal contents have emerged, may make return to the abdominal cavity impossible. Strangulation of the bowel—interruption of its blood supply—can also occur in an incarcerated hernia that does not receive prompt surgical attention. The trapped bowel loop can ultimately become necrotic, requiring resection.[2]

Occasionally, hernias can develop after abdominal surgery. Elderly, obese, or malnourished patients are more prone to develop incisional hernias. Infection, which impairs wound healing, is also a predisposing factor.

Abdominal wall hernias consist of three parts: the sac, its contents, and its covering. Hernial contents may consist of any structure in the abdominal cavity and may vary from small pieces of omentum to the previously mentioned portions of bowel. Common locations for hernias are umbilical, epigastric, inguinal, femoral, and separation of the recti abdomini.[18]

Umbilical hernias can be either congenital (omphalocele) or acquired. Infants and small children

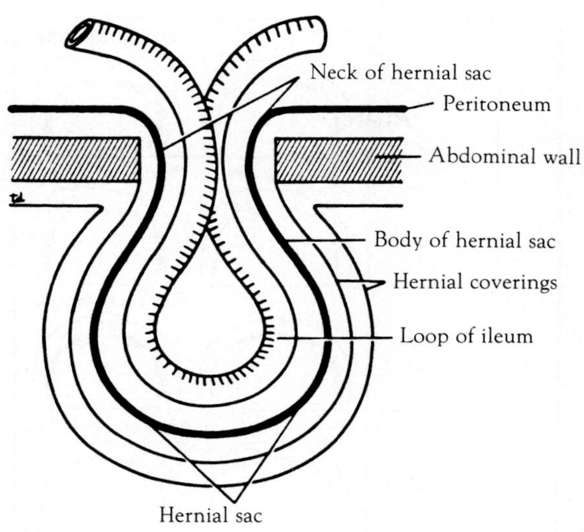

Figure 2-15. The components of a hernia. (From Snell RS: Clinical Anatomy for Medical Students. Boston, Little, Brown, 1973.)

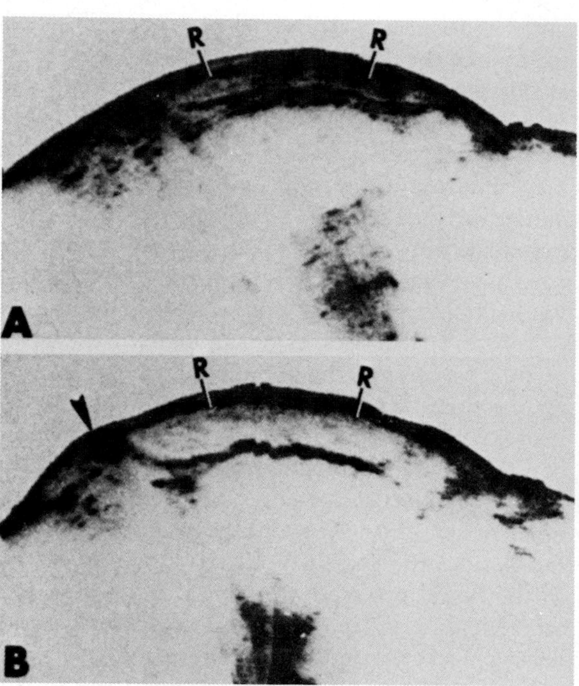

Figure 2-16. Speigelian hernia. (*A*) On transverse scan 7 cm above umbilicus no hernia is apparent. (R, rectus muscle.) (*B*) Repeat scanning during straining of abdominal muscle shows a small bulge *(arrowhead)* at the lateral edge of the right rectus muscle. Noted marked thickening and decreased echogenicity of the rectus muscle (R) due to contraction. (From Yeh HC, Lehr-Janus C, Cohen BA, et al: Ultrasonography and CT of abdominal and inguinal hernias. J Clin Ultrasound 1984, 14:479–486.)

often acquire hernias in this area due to the weakness in the linea alba at the umbilicus. In most cases, these hernias decrease in size and disappear without event or treatment as the child's abdominal cavity enlarges. In adults, acquired hernias are more commonly termed *paraumbilical hernias.* The major difference in adults is that their hernia protrudes through the linea alba in the regions of the umbilicus. In adults, paraumbilical hernias increase gradually in size and are the hernias that most often contain large intestine as well as omentum. Such hernias are more common in women than in men.[18]

Inguinal hernias (indirect) are one of the most common forms and are 20 times more common in males than in females. Nearly a third of inguinal hernias are bilateral, but unilateral ones more often are right sided. Boys and young men are commonly seen with these lesions of the inguinal canal, through which the testes descended. In contrast, direct inguinal hernias are a disease of elderly males with weak abdominal muscles, and are rarely found in women. They generally appear as nothing more than a generalized bulge.[18]

Epigastric hernias occur through the widest part of the linea alba, anywhere between the xiphoid process and the umbilicus. Usually, such hernias start out as small defects of protruding extraperitoneal fat. Over a period of months or years, that fat is forced through the linea alba, pulling behind it a small peritoneal sac, which often contains a small piece of the omentum.

A *spigelian hernia* is a variant of the ventral hernia and is found more laterally in the abdominal wall. Another type of ventral hernia associated with a previous incision is usually found in the midline and may be palpable intermittently (Fig. 2-16).

Sonographic appearances and techniques. Since abdominal wall hernias are generally palpable masses, the majority do not require sonographic evaluation. Some hernias, however, are occult and can mimic other lesions of the kidney, gastrointestinal tract, or pelvis. In obese patients, such hernias may mimic entities such as gallbladder disease, pancreatitis, or ulcers. In contrast, a simple localized weakening of the abdominal wall may simulate a hernia (pseudohernia). It is for these categories of lesions that sonography can be most helpful.[17]

Yeh and associates have summarized the sonographic features of the abdominal wall (Fig. 2-17). At the site of a hernia, interruption of the peritoneal line separating the muscles and abdominal contents is seen. Sonography can demonstrate the size of the defect and whether the hernia sac is fluid filled or contains peristaltic bowels or mesenteric fat. Besides the presence of peristaltic motion, gas in the bowel produces the typical shadowing artifact. Mesenteric fat, which also appears highly reflective, lacks peristalsis and shadowing.

If a hernia is not visible on the body, the patient can usually make it appear by lifting the head or straining the abdominal muscles (Fig. 2-18). All of this information is vital to a surgeon who must anticipate contingencies such as using prosthetic mesh or autogenous or heterogenous fascia and special suture techniques.[17]

Yeh also found that ascites can complicate the appearance of hernia by producing a clearly fluid-filled sac. At times, he was able to see this fluid evacuated out of the hernia sac and back into the peritoneal cavity when transducer pressure was applied to the area.[20]

The current sonographic criteria for abdominal wall hernia are (1) demonstration of an abdominal wall defect, (2) presence of bowel loops within a lesion, (3) exaggeration of the lesion on straining of the abdominal musculature, and (4) reducibility of the lesion by pressure.[7]

The use of linear-array or articulated-arm systems is advocated, since the limited field of view and small scanning surfaces provided by sector transducers makes them suboptimal for this type of study. In addition to diagnostic ultrasonography, computed tomography (CT) may also be used to make this diagnosis, but the noninvasiveness and rapid results provided by sonography are favored.[17]

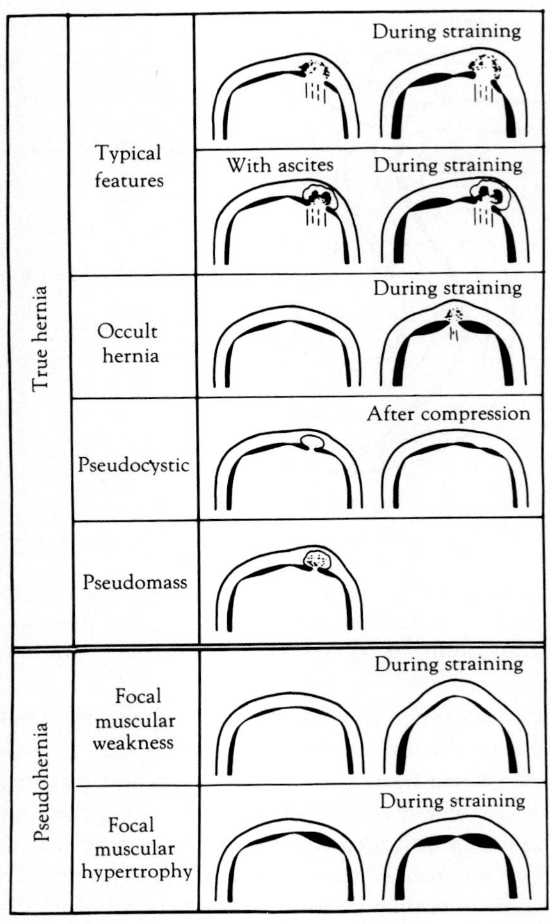

Figure 2-17. Sonographic features of abdominal hernias and pseudohernias. (From Yeh HC, Lehr-Janus C, Cohen BA, et al: Ultrasonography and CT of abdominal and inguinal hernias. J Clin Ultrasound 1984, 14:479–486.)

Neoplasms. Among the primary abdominal wall tumors are (1) lipomas, (2) areas of calcification in old surgical scars, (3) desmoid tumors, (4) metastatic carcinoma, and (5) soft tissue sarcomas. Most lesions are readily diagnosed by physical examination and clinical history. However, ultrasound, CT, magnetic resonance imaging (MRI), and fine-needle biopsy are all valuable tools when the distinction must be made between lipomas, hematomas, abscesses, and hernias and the more serious true neoplasm.

Lipomas (fatty tumors) are among the most common benign masses of the abdominal wall and subcutaneous tissues.[3] Desmoid tumors are benign, fibrous neoplasms commonly found in the anterior abdominal wall, most frequently in patients between the ages of 20 and 40 years. While these tumors can occur in either sex, they are three times more frequent in women. In fact, the tumor is often related to pregnancy. Childbirth, trauma, and hormonal changes during pregnancy are thought to be predisposing factors. There is also a marked increase in these tumors in patients with Gardner syndrome. Desmoid tumors often present as nontender, slowly enlarging masses. Their treatment includes radiation therapy and hormones, but surgical excision is the treatment of choice. Spontaneous regression of desmoid tumors has been recorded, and the estimated recurrence rate is 50%.[8]

Sarcomas arising from the abdominal wall include liposarcoma, rhabdomyosarcoma, and fibrosarcoma. These tumors can grow without evidence of clinical symptoms for a long time. As a result, they often attain large size and are difficult to differentiate from large pancreatic tumors, renal tumors, or splenomegaly.[9]

Metastatic carcinoma to the abdominal wall is frequently related to extension from a nearby primary carcinoma. For instance, in cases of primary ovarian carcinoma, there is a high incidence of clinically, unsuspected metastases to the aortic and pelvic lymph nodes, diaphragm, peritoneum, and omentum. Therefore metastases to the anterior abdominal wall can also be anticipated.

SONOGRAPHIC APPEARANCES AND TECHNIQUES. Lipomas appear as echogenic structures with unusually good through-transmission. They tend to be soft, and in some cases movable. The amount of transducer pressure applied must be moderate and consistent to avoid displacing the mass during scanning.

Desmoid tumors are relatively homogeneous, hypoechoic masses with only occasional internal echoes. Because they permit good through-transmission they are sometimes mistaken for cystic masses (Fig. 2-19). Strict documentation of the various sonographic criteria for a cystic mass is therefore the rule. Curiously, some desmoid tumors appear sonographically to be encapsulated, yet pathologic examination reveals no apparent capsule.[8]

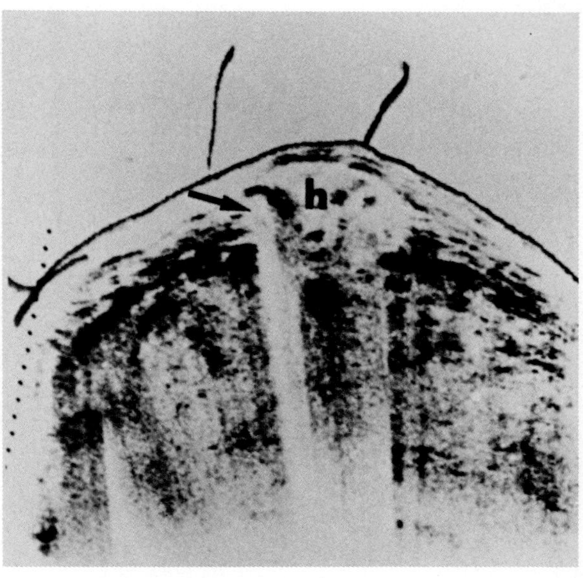

FIGURE 2-18. Transverse sonogram of the anterior abdominal wall containing a loop of herniated bowel (h). Note acoustic shadowing (*arrow*) behind gas in the hernia. (From Anderhub B: Manual of Abdominal Sonography. Rockville MD, Aspen, 1983.)

The broad spectrum of sonographic patterns seen in both primary and metastatic carcinomas makes it imperative that sonographers (1) perform gain studies on suspicious lesions, (2) take time to observe the boundaries of the mass and whether or not it encroaches into other areas, and (3) be prepared to relate the mass to its primary source, if at all possible. Some malignant masses are sonolucent, and their deposits or extensions appear very echogenic in contrast. Other masses, particularly rhabdomyosarcomas, are very echogenic. Tissue necrosis, of course, can produce echo-free areas within such masses. Once again, varying the gain during the studies and being alert to the most subtle changes that can be elicited are most desirable. Correlating what is seen on the sonogram with the physical appearance and clinical history of the patient is equally important.

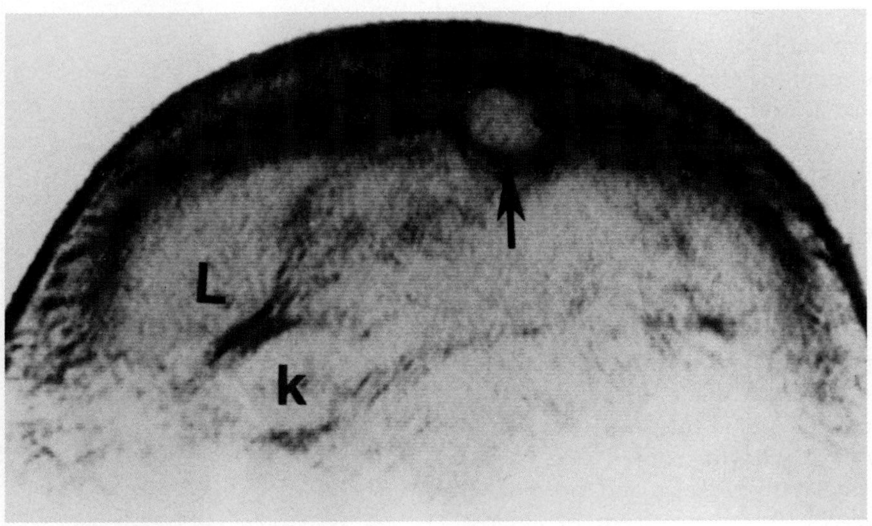

FIGURE 2-19. Desmoid tumor of the upper abdominal wall. Transverse scan of the paramedian upper abdomen show a well-demarcated solid mass *(arrow)* with pseudoencapsulation and a homogeneous internal structure. (L, Liver; k, kidney.) (From Hanson RD, Hunter TB, Haber K: Ultrasonographic appearance of anterior abdominal wall desmoid tumors. J Ultrasound Med 1983, 2:141–142.)

Peritoneal Cavity

Extent and Divisions

The largest of the body cavities is the peritoneal cavity, which encompasses the abdomen and pelvis. Its abdominal portion can further be divided into two compartments: the greater sac and the lesser sac. The greater sac, the larger of the two compartments, covers the entire width of the abdomen and also from the diaphragm to the pelvis. The smaller compartment, the lesser sac, lies behind the stomach and is created as a diverticulum from the greater sac (see Fig. 2-1).[2,9,14,15,18] The abdominal portion of the peritoneal cavity is further subdivided by many membranous reflections into important fossae and spaces. These are discussed later in the chapter.

Peritoneum

The peritoneum is a serous membrane resembling a thin sheet of tissue. Serous membranes like the peritoneum generally line body cavities that do not open to the exterior. Peritoneum also covers surfaces and divides organs. Two layers of the peritoneum make this possible: the parietal layer lines the cavity and the visceral layer covers the organs. Between the two layers is a potential space containing drops of serous fluid.

Complex by nature, the peritoneum is a structure that sonographers must thoroughly understand if they hope to correctly identify the sites of pathologic processes. To aid in that understanding, it may be helpful to compare the abdominal cavity to rooms of a house. The parietal layer of the peritoneum is comparable to the wallpaper in the rooms. Imagine that each room is filled with furniture (the organs), each piece of which is tightly wrapped in sheeting for protection (the visceral layer of the peritoneum). Next, think of all those articles of "furniture" being stacked close against each other and against the walls of the rooms. Obviously, there will be air circulating between the closely stacked pieces and between the pieces and the adjacent walls. This air is comparable to the small amount of lubricating serous fluid that lies in the space between the parietal and visceral layers of the peritoneum. Whenever an organ moves against the body wall, friction between the moving parts is prevented by the presence of the smooth, moist sheets of tissue lining the wall surfaces of the cavity and covering the organ surfaces within it. In this way the body carries out the simple mechanical principle that moving parts must have lubricated surfaces to avoid wear and tear and eventual breakdown.

Except in the area of the female reproductive organs, the peritoneum is essentially an empty sac. Not only does it line the walls of the abdominal cavity, it also projects from the lumbar region into the abdominal cavity to form the double-folded, fan-shaped structure called the mesentery.[2,9,14,15,18] By this means, the mesentery and most of the small intenstine are fastened to the posterior abdominal wall. Another double fold of peritoneum, the greater omentum, attaches at its upper border to the duodenum and to the lower edge of the stomach as the lesser omentum (Fig. 2-20).

The apron-shaped greater omentum hangs loosely over the intestines and should not be confused with the mesentery (Fig. 2-21). Varying amounts of fat deposited in the tissue layers of the greater omentum provide both protection and insulation to the structures that it covers. A final layer of parietal peritoneum presses the organs against the posterior body wall, giving rise to the term "retroperitoneal."[2]

Since serous membranes are very susceptible to bacterial invasion, their protective antifriction function is very significant. The peritoneum is an inviolable structure of critical importance that, if damaged can quickly become inflamed, resulting in peritonitis.

The presence of the peritoneum ensures that the contents of the abdomen will move smoothly past one another in the normal but often contorted movements of the body. If any of the organs were to become twisted or strapped down, however, its blood supply could be compromised, which could lead to serious consequences. Such problems are rare, except occasionally in newborns and with post-surgical adhesions.[2,18]

Lesser Sac. The lesser sac is an extensive peritoneal pouch located behind the lesser omentum of the stomach and in front of structures situated on the posterior abdominal wall (see Fig. 2-1).[2,9,14,15,18] It projects upward as far as the diaphragm and down-

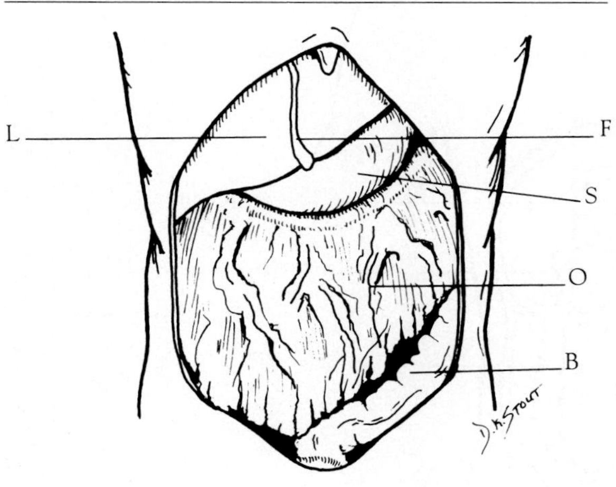

FIGURE 2-20. Omentum. The greater Omentum (O) attaches to the greater curvature of the stomach (S) and lies between the anterior abdominal wall and the small intestine. The lesser omentum attaches to the lesser curvature of the stomach and the undersurface of the liver (L). (F, falciform ligament; B, bowel.)

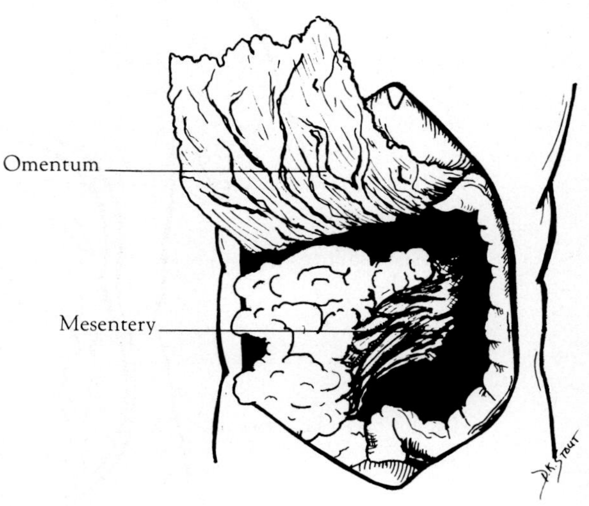

FIGURE 2-21. Mesentery. The mesentery is a supporting membrane formed from a double fold of the peritoneum, which enfolds most of the small intestine and attaches it to the spinal wall of the abdominal cavity.

ward between the layers of the greater omentum. The lower part of the lesser sac is often obliterated by the adherence of the anterior layers of the greater omentum to the posterior layers. Its left margin is formed by the spleen and the gastrosplenic omentum and the lienorenal ligaments. Below, it is formed by the left free border of the greater omentum. The right side of the sac opens into the greater sac, or main portion of the peritoneal cavity, through the opening of the lesser sac (epiploic foramen). Below the opening, the right margin is formed by the right free border of the greater omentum.[2,13,14,18] The opening into the lesser sac is bounded anteriorly by the free border of the lesser omentum, containing the common bile duct, the hepatic artery, and the portal vein; posteriorly by the inferior vena cava; superiorly by the caudate process of the caudate lobe of the liver; and inferiorly by the first part of the duodenum.

Fossae or Spaces. The complex arrangement of the peritoneum creates several important potential spaces in the abdominal and pelvic cavities. Space-occupying lesions, abscesses, and other types of free fluid often fill these spaces. Sonographers should be aware of the existence and location of such potential compartments and routinely examine them when a patient is suspected of harboring free fluid.[9]

The spaces that when filled with tissue or fluid can be imaged sonographically are depicted in Figure 2-22: (1) right and left subphrenic spaces, (2) subhepatic space (Morrison's pouch), (3) lesser sac, (4) perinephric space, (5) paracolic gutters, and (6) pelvic cul-de-sacs.

Right and left subphrenic spaces. The intraperitoneal subphrenic spaces are created by folding of the peritoneum in the hepatic region. Both right and left anterior subphrenic spaces lie between the diaphragm and the liver, one on each side of the

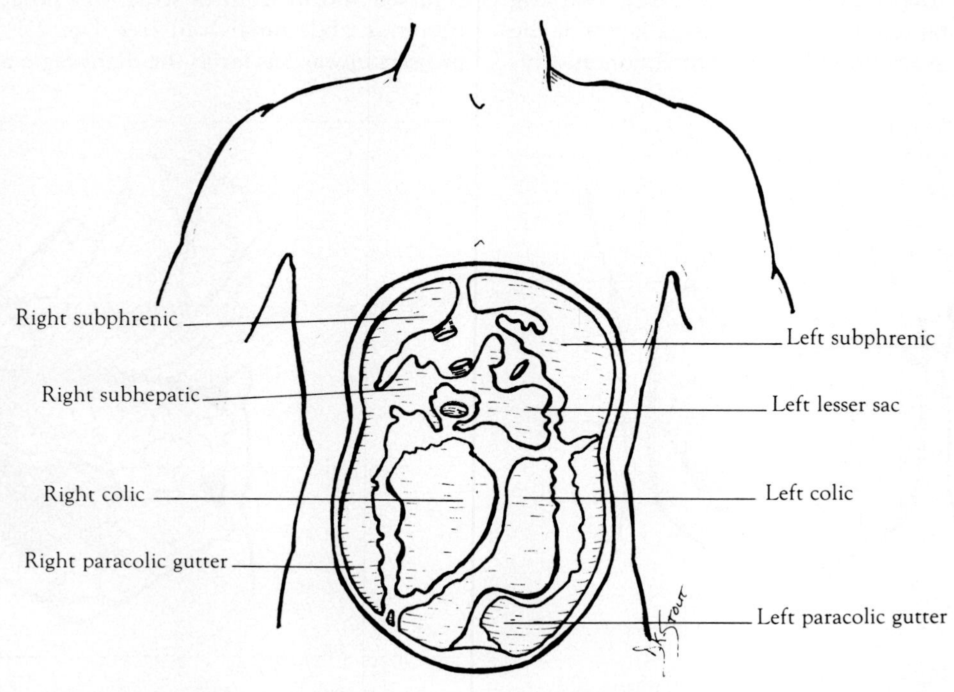

FIGURE 2-22. Anterior view of the peritoneum demonstrating its major divisions and spaces.

falciform ligament. The right posterior subphrenic space lies between the right lobe of the liver, the right kidney, and the right colic flexure. The right extraperitoneal space lies between the layers of the coronary ligament and is therefore situated between the liver and the diaphragm.[18]

Subhepatic space (Morrison's pouch). The right subhepatic space is located beneath the right lobe of the liver and includes Morrison's pouch, which lies between the posterior aspect of the right liver lobe and the upper pole of the right kidney.

Lesser sac. Located on the left side of the abdomen, behind the stomach, the lesser sac is an anatomically true subphrenic space because it occupies a part of the area between the diaphragm and the transverse colon.[13]

Perinephric space. Various spaces are situated retroperitoneally around the kidneys. The perinephric space, which lies within Gerota's fascia, opens inferiorly and encloses the kidney, fat, and adrenal glands.

Paracolic gutters. Four important paracolic gutters are formed by the arrangements of the ascending and descending colon and the posterior wall attachments of the transverse mesocolon and the mesentery and small intestine. These gutters lie on the lateral and medial sides of the ascending and descending colon, respectively. Note that the right medial paracolic gutter is closed off from the pelvic cavity inferiorly by the mesentery of the small intestine, whereas the others are in free communication with the pelvic cavity. The right lateral paracolic gutter is in communication with the right posterior subphrenic spaces, but the left lateral gutter is separated from the area around the spleen by the phrenicocolic ligament, a fold of peritoneum that passes from the left colic flexure to the diaphragm.[18]

Ligaments. Another important role of the peritoneum is the formation of folds or ligaments from which various organs are suspended within the peritoneal cavity. These ligaments also provide a means for conveying blood and lymphatic vessels and nerves to those organs. Large amounts of fat are stored in the peritoneal ligaments and mesenteries, and especially large amounts may be found in the greater omentum, providing both a cushioning and insulating effect.[2,15,18] The peritoneal ligaments are actually double-layered, thick folds of peritoneum. For example, the liver is attached by the falciform ligament to the anterior abdominal wall and to the undersurface of the diaphragm. The ligaments and their attachments are listed in Table 2-3.

Functions. A major function of the peritoneum is the secretion of peritoneal fluid. The serous fluid that it produces is a pale yellow, somewhat viscid liquid containing leukocytes. Owing to the movements of the diaphragm and abdominal muscles as well as the peristaltic motions of the intestinal tract, peritoneal fluid is not static. There appears to be continuous movement of fluid toward the diaphragm, where it is quickly absorbed into the superperitoneal lymphatic capillaries. Particulate matter introduced experimentally into the lower part of the peritoneal cavity is found to rapidly reach the subphrenic peritoneal spaces, regardless of the body's position.[18] This fact is important to remember when scanning patients with ascites or hemorrhage.

In the presence of infection, the peritoneal coverings of the intestines have a tendency to adhere to the adjacent organs. The greater omentum may also adhere to other peritoneal surfaces around the focus of infection. In this way, many intraperitoneal infections are sealed off and localized.[2,18]

SONOGRAPHIC APPEARANCES AND TECHNIQUES. Although layers of the abdominal wall are visible by sonography, they are frequently obscured by improper instrument settings or scanning technique. Figure 2-7 demonstrates the various layers of the abdominal wall, from the subcutaneous tissue through the muscle groups and peritoneal-fascial interface that separates the intraperitoneal structures from the abdominal wall. The most easily demonstrated section of peritoneal tissue lies on the lateral curvature of the abdominal wall rather than under its ventral surface. It appears sonographically as a band of transonic homogeneous tissue with strongly reflective anterior and posterior borders.[4] Sonographers scanning patients with any amount of intraperitoneal fat must not mistake a band of adipose tissue for the peritoneal structure or a neoplasm. Fat layers differ sono-

TABLE 2-3. The peritoneal ligaments and their attachments

LIGAMENT	ATTACHMENT
Falciform	Double-layered fold of peritoneum that ascends from the umbilicus to the liver. Contained within it is the ligamentum teres. The falciform ligament passes onto the anterior and then superior surface of the liver before splitting into two layers. The right layer forms the upper layer of the coronary ligament; the left layer forms the upper layer of the left triangular ligament.
Coronary	Formed by the right layer of the falciform ligament, its right extremity is known as the right triangular ligament. Because the layers of the peritoneum that form the coronary ligament are widely separated, there is a portion of the liver that is not covered by the peritoneum; this is known as the "bare" area of the liver.
Left triangular	Formed by the left layer of the falciform ligament.
Ligamentum teres	Remnant of the fetal umbilical vein, which is contained within the falciform ligament. It passes into a fissure on the visceral liver surface to join the left branch of the portal vein in the porta hepatis.
Ligamentum venosum	Exists as a fibrous band (remnant of the ductus venosus) attached to the left branch of the portal vein. It ascends in a fissure on the visceral liver surface to attach above the inferior vena cava. In fetal circulation, oxygenated blood flows to the liver via the umbilical vein (ligamentum teres). Most of the blood bypasses the liver in the ductus venosus (ligamentum venosum) and joins the inferior vena cava. The umbilical vein and ductus venosum close after birth to become the ligamentum teres and the ligamentum venosum, respectively.
Lesser omentum	Arising from the edges of the porta hepatis and the fissure for the ligamentum venosum, this fold of peritoneum passes down the lesser curvature of the stomach.

(Data from: Snell RS: Clinical Anatomy for Medical Students. Boston, Little Brown, 1973.)

graphically by failing to demonstrate the same reflective borders that the peritoneum does.

Another potential pitfall lies in confusing an engorged umbilical vein remnant (which lies in the area of the linea alba) with the peritoneum. Normally, this vascular remnant is not dilated. However, in patients with portal hypertension resulting in massive and extensive venous dilatation, this vestige of fetal circulation serves as the anastomosis between the main left portal vein and the epigastric veins that drain into the superficial veins and inferior vena cava.[4]

Pathologic Clinical and Sonographic Findings

INFLAMMATION

Abdominal pain arising from the parietal peritoneum is somatic and can be localized precisely to the site of origin. Despite the fact that the visceral peritoneum contains no pain-transmitting fibers, pain is usually severe because the root of the mesentery is extremely sensitive to stretching. In contrast, pain arising from the abdominal viscera is generally described as dull, is poorly localized, and is usually referred to the midline.[18]

Infection may enter the peritoneal cavity through a number of portals: the interior of the gastrointestinal tract, the abdominal walls, the fallopian tubes, or bloodstream. An inflamed parietal peritoneum is extremely sensitive to stretching, a fact that is clinically valuable in diagnosing peritonitis. Pressure applied to the abdominal wall over the site of the inflammation and suddenly released causes the abdominal wall to rebound, resulting in extreme local pain. This reflex is called rebound tenderness.[18]

The greater omentum is often referred to as the "abdominal policeman," since its lower right and left margins are free, and it can move about in the peritoneal cavity in response to peristaltic movements of the neighboring gut. Poorly developed in the first few years of life, it is less protective in young children. Later, however, in acute infections, such as an inflammed appendix, inflammatory exudates cause the omentum to adhere to the appendix and to wrap itself around the inflamed organ. The patient is saved from serious diffuse peritonitis by this phenomenon, which localizes the infection to a small area of the peritoneal cavity. The greater omentum has also been found to plug up the neck of hernia sacs, preventing the entrance and possible strangulation of coils of small intestine.[18]

Abscesses

When infected collections are not contained by the defenses of the peritoneal cavity the stage is set for the formation of an intraabdominal abscess. Generally caused by bacteria, necrotic tissue, and white blood cells, a purulent abscess may be located in any of the spaces of the peritoneal cavity or in any of the visceral organs, especially the liver and spleen. They usually result from trauma, surgery, or infection in other body areas. Intraabdominal abscesses can be seen as single or multiple entities and can also create new intraperitoneal cavities. There is no hard and fast rule about the development of abscesses: they may develop as quickly as a few days or as slowly as a year.[9]

Intraabdominal. Nearly half of all intraabdominal abscesses are the result of surgical disease and are located in the subphrenic spaces. In the past, they were often caused by a perforating ulcer or appendix. Modern medical advances have made possible earlier diagnosis and treatment and their prevalence has declined. Unfortunately, they are sometimes replaced by postsurgical infections.

Patients at particularly high risk for developing post-surgical infections are those undergoing immunosuppressive or steroid therapy and those with a debilitating disease such as chronic renal failure.[13] A 1970 study by Lehman and Archer found that fewer than a third of abscesses involved the left side of the abdomen.[11] Today, there is an increasing frequency of left-sided abscesses, probably as a result of the increase in colon surgery.[13] It is critically important, therefore, that sonographers perform complete survey scans of the peritoneal cavity in such high-risk patients and in any patient who presents with fever, pain, and elevated white blood cell count. Once the full extent of an abscess has been sonographically determined, the sonographer may also have the opportunity of assisting with the aspiration of purulent material for cytologic study.

The least common location for subdiaphragmatic infection is the lesser sac. Pancreatic disease, usually hemorrhagic or necrotizing pancreatitis, is the leading cause of infection in this area. In this situation clear-cut physical findings may be few, and delay in diagnosis may lead to the patient's death. Other causes of subdiaphragmatic infection are traumatic and inflammatory perforation of the gastrointestinal tract. Midabdominal infections characteristically follow perforation of the appendix or diverticulitis. Intermesenteric abscesses result, often involving the right and left gutters. Such abscesses tend to be multiple and quite small, and as such, can become the cause of ongoing sepsis and partial obstruction of the small intestine. Fortunately, because of the excellent blood supply to the mesenteric area, such abscesses often resolve spontaneously.[9]

Retroperitoneal Abscesses. Abscesses of the retroperitoneal spaces are among the most serious and carry high morbidity and mortality rates, principally because they are difficult to diagnose early. Only when such infections are suspected is early detection possible, even with all of the diagnostic modalities available today.[6] Although retroperitoneal abscesses generally arise from the organs lying in or adjacent to the retroperitoneum, occasionally idiopathic abscesses are encountered. Because of the arrangement of structures in the retroperitoneum, infection can spread upward into the thorax and downward into the thigh via the psoas muscles. Meticulous sonographic technique is required to visualize the fascial planes of the retroperitoneum, and knowledge of the compartmental anatomy is necessary to determine the location of lesions and possible causes.

Most infections of the retroperitoneal space tend to involve one side primarily; however, because the anterior and posterior divisions of the retroperitoneal space can communicate with the opposite side, it is wise to perform a complete study of the area, even when an obvious collection is found on one side of the body. Abscesses can collect in such a

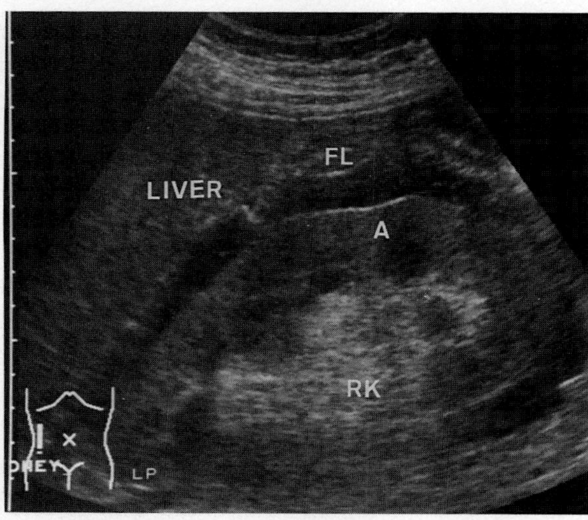

FIGURE 2-23. Perinephric abscess is demonstrated by a longitudinal scan of a 38-year-old woman who complained of right side upper quadrant pain. An abnormally echogenic right kidney (RK) surrounded by fluid (FL) suggests a renal abscess (A). Fluid is also present outside the renal fascia, beneath the liver margin, most likely representing reactive change. Intravenous pyelography confirmed the sonographic diagnosis of perinephric abscess.

way that they extend across the midline in a large horseshoe shape.

Perinephric Abscesses. The most common cause of retroperitoneal abscesses is perinephric infection (Fig. 2-23). Unfortunately, in at least half of patients, the correct diagnosis is not made before surgery. Among the misdiagnoses most frequently encountered are pyelonephritis, hydronephrosis, appendicitis, and diverticulitis. In 10 percent of patients, the origin of a retroperitoneal abscess remains unknown even at postmortem examination.[9] The retroperitoneum is discussed completely in Chapter 12.

Pelvic Abscesses. Pelvic abscesses are usually secondary to lower abdominal inflammation. In a recumbent patient the pelvis is the most dependent of all intraabdominal spaces. Pelvic inflammatory disease (PID) currently accounts for a large number of cases; perforated appendix and colonic diverticulitis are other causes. Because of the architecture of the peritoneal cavity, drainage from an upper abdominal infection could also pool in the pelvis. Once again, in patients found by sonography to have free fluid in the pelvic cavities, it is imperative that scans of the upper portion of the body be examined for concurrent involvement.[9] The pelvic structures are discussed in detail in Volume 1 of this book.

SONOGRAPHIC APPEARANCES AND TECHNIQUES. The sonographic range of appearances of abscesses is extremely variable. Depending on the site and duration of the infectious process, abscesses may be irregular-shaped, mild to moderately echogenic masses. In some cases an abscess may appear anechoic except for the presence of septations or of stringy tissue filaments. With resolution, most abscesses tend to develop more regular borders and an echo-free interior (see Table 2-2).

Abdominal abscesses containing air-fluid levels have been described by Kressel and Filly.[10] They have categorized the sonographic appearances of gas-filled abscesses as (1) densely echogenic with acoustic shadowing, (2) densely echogenic without shadowing, or (3) regions of acoustic shadowing only. Additional findings were described by Golding and coworkers: an echogenic line created by an air-fluid level.[7] Because air and gas are almost complete reflectors of ultrasound, abscesses may be missed if the patient is lying supine and the beam is directed posteriorly. The sound beam encounters a soft tissue-gas interface and is reflected almost completely back to the transducer, primarily producing an acoustic shadow. Reverberation artifacts may also be seen within such shadow zones. If the same patient is scanned with the beam directed anteromedially from the posterior flank, the fluid portion of such an abscess would be the first reflective material encountered. The image of a cystic mass containing fine, diffuse internal echoes (created by the presence of pus and necrotic debris) would result. When a gas-fluid level is encountered, again, the beam is almost totally reflected, producing a dense echogenic line. In difficult cases, air-fluid levels may also act as acoustic mirrors, causing duplication artifacts on the anterior, or air, side of the level (Fig. 2-24). Recognition of such an echo-

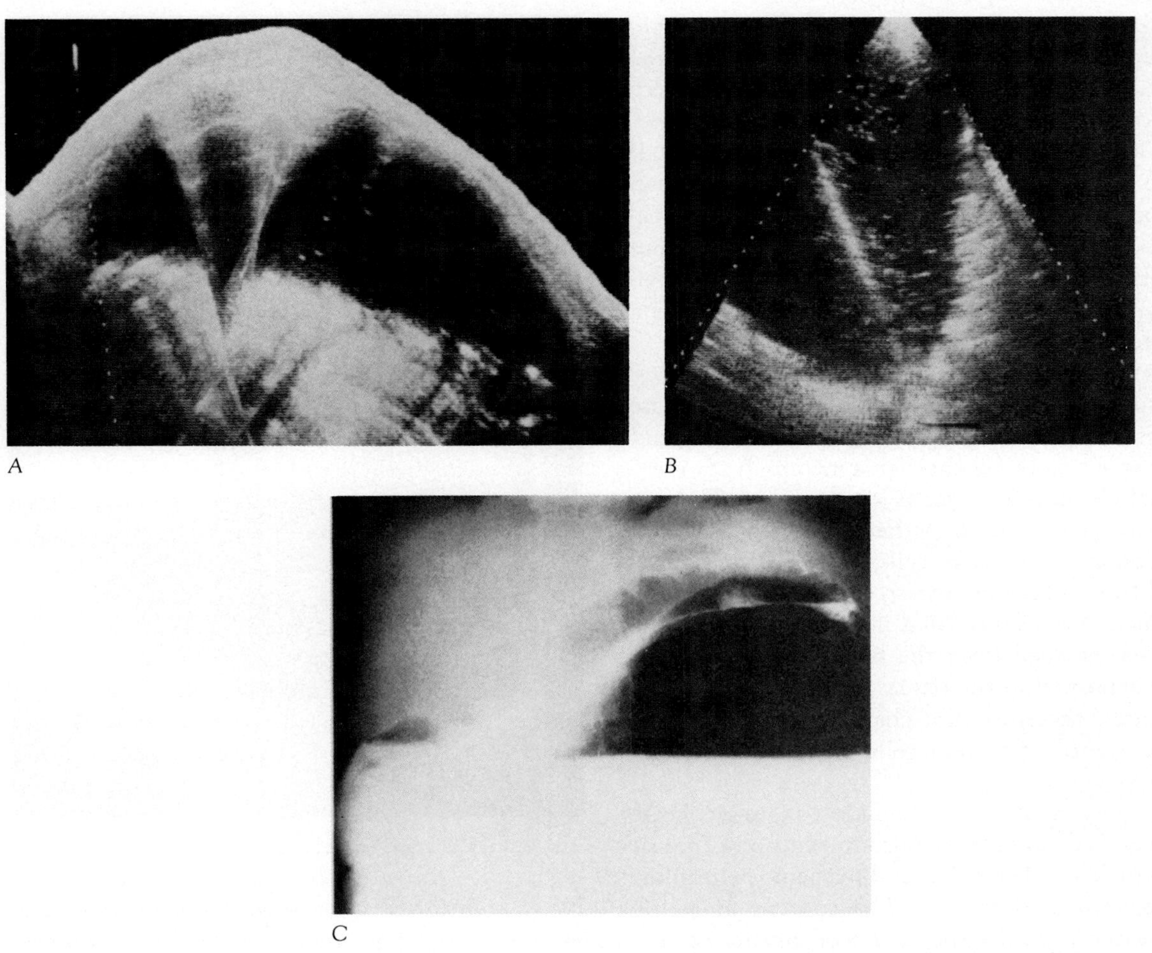

Figure 2-24. Abscess containing gas (*A*) Transverse "static" upper abdominal scan demonstrates a large fluid abscess collection containing ring-down artifacts from a gas collection in the anterior portion of the abscess. (*B*) Transverse real-time sector scan of the same patient with the beam aimed anteromedially from the posterior aspect of the left flank. (C) Upright radiograph from a barium enema study of the same patient reveals the extraluminal air-fluid level in the left upper quadrant. (From Golding RHR, Li DKB, Cooperberg PL: Sonographic demonstration of air-fluid levels in abdominal abscesses. J Ultrasound Med 1982, 1:151–155.)

genic line (the sonographic equivalent of an air-fluid level) is an indication for horizontal-beam radiographs to confirm the diagnosis. In positive cases, ultrasonography or CT can be very helpful in guiding percutaneous drainage of such abscesses.[7]

Ascites

The same forces that regulate fluid distribution between interstitial and intravascular compartments also control the fluid exchange between intraperitoneal fluid and blood plasma. Normally, the watery serum is filtered through the semi-permeable walls of arterial capillaries, where blood pressure is higher than oncotic pressure. This filtrate is reabsorbed as interstitial fluid by the blood within the venous capillaries, where oncotic pressure exceeds blood pressure.[15] If this mechanism is disturbed, fluid accumulates within the tissues (edema) and, if more fluid passes into the peritoneal cavity than the body can reabsorb, ascites develops. In thin patients, as much as 1500 ml of fluid has to accumulate before it can be clinically recognized. Obviously, in obese patients, detection would require a far greater amount.[6,14,18]

Ascites can be subdivided into two major types: transudative and exudative. The term transudate comes from the Latin word for sweating. Any fluid substance that passes through a membrane or is extruded through a tissue is a transudate. Transudates are characterized by their thin, clear fluid and low content of protein, cells, or solid material derived from cells. In contrast, an exudate is a material such as thickened fluid, cells, or cellular debris that has escaped from the blood vessels and has been deposited in the tissues or on tissue surfaces. Exudates, therefore, are characterized by a high concentration of protein, cells, or solid material derived from cells (Fig. 2-25).[6,18]

The causes of ascites include congestive heart failure, liver disease, nephrotic syndrome, infections such as tuberculosis and pyogenic peritonitis, malignancy, and trauma. The content of ascitic fluid often indicates the source of disease. For example, fatty or milky ascites appears when the cells in that fluid have undergone fatty degeneration. If bile is the main constituent of ascites the condition is termed choleperitoneum and is related to liver or gallbladder pathology. Bloody ascites suggests hemorrhage or trauma, as from a ruptured aneurysm. The presence of chyme (chylous ascites) points to anomaly, injury, or obstruction of the thoracic duct (Fig. 2-26). Both exudative and transudative types of ascites may be caused by infection or inflammation. Finally, ascites associated with or caused by severe malnutrition produces a watery quality in the blood called hydremic ascites.[9,13,14,18]

Patients with moderate to massive amounts of ascites usually appear to have an abnormally enlarged and swollen abdomen. Depending on the patient's body type, however, it may be difficult to determine whether the cause is ascites. Fortunately,

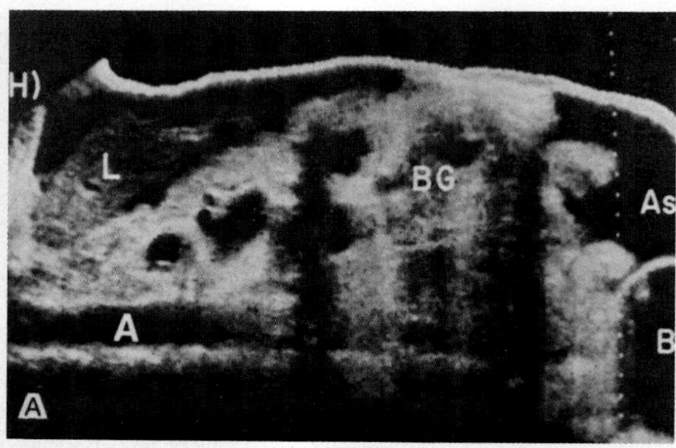

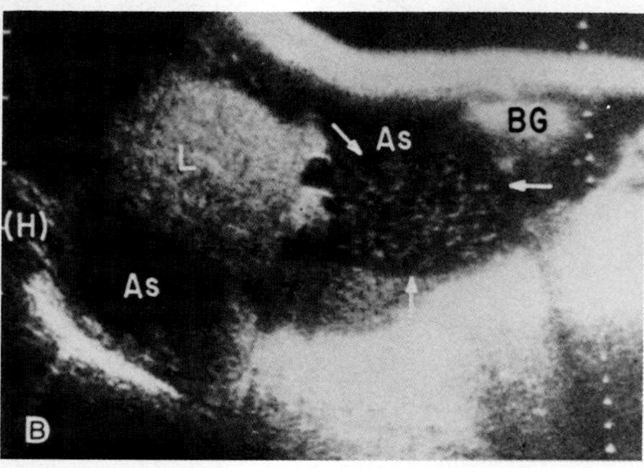

FIGURE 2-25. Ascites: comparison of a transudate and an infected exudate. (*A*) Longitudinal midline scan shows transudative echo-free ascites (As) with loops of gas-filled bowel (BG) floating within. (A, aorta; B, urinary bladder; L, liver.) (*B*) Longitudinal scan in another patient (5 cm right of midline) demonstrates infected exudative ascites (AS). Arrows indicate the echogenic fluid. (BG, gas-filled loop of bowel floating within the ascites; L, liver; H, toward patient's head.) (From Kurtz AB, Dubbins PA: The serosal membranes. Disease. Clin Diagn Ultrasound 1984, 11:55–77.)

with sonography it is very easy to make the diagnosis because of its sensitivity in differentiating fluid from solid materials (Fig. 2-27). Once the diagnosis is confirmed, ultrasound is further useful in guiding aspiration of the fluid and following patient management (Fig. 2-28).[2,16,18]

SONOGRAPHIC APPEARANCES AND TECHNIQUES. The demonstration of ascites varies with the amount of

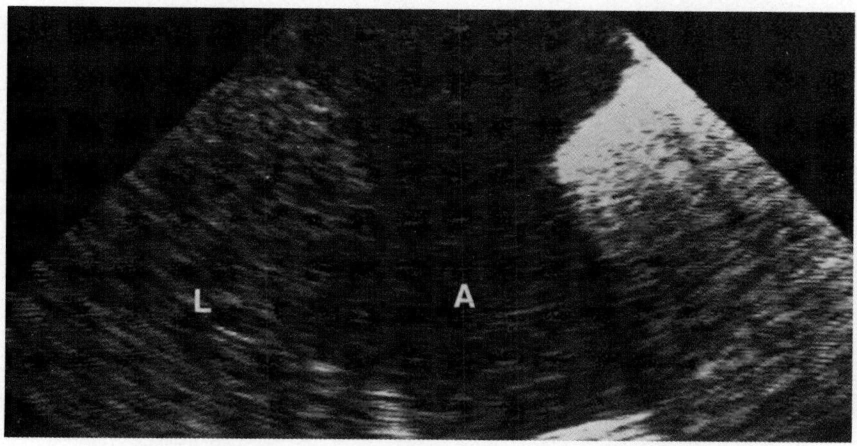

Figure 2-26. Longitudinal scan demonstrates chylous ascites (A) adjacent to the liver (L). Multiple high-amplitude echoes are present throughout the ascites fluid. (Reprinted from Franklin JT, Azose AA: Sonographic appearance of chylous ascites. Clin Ultrasound 1984, 12:239–240.)

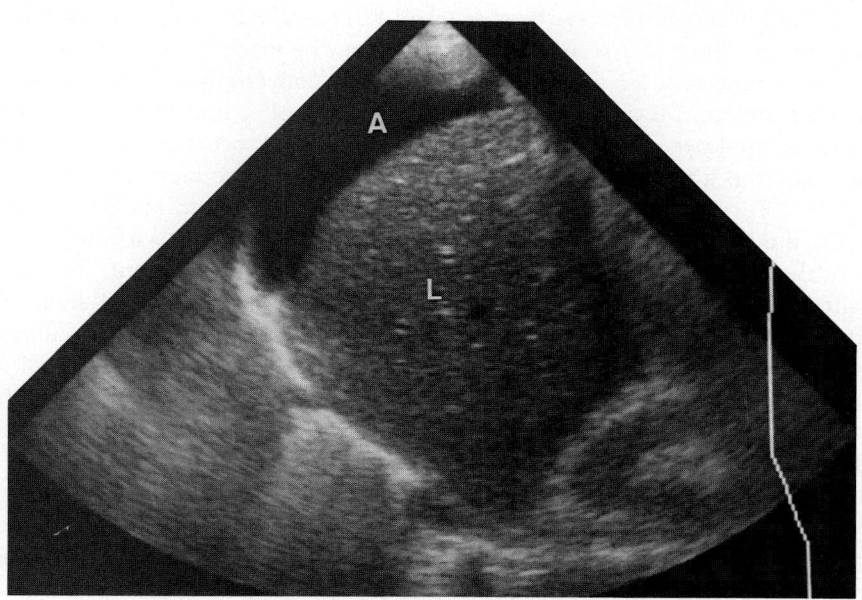

Figure 2-27. Moderate amount of ascites are visualized in a 73-year-old man admitted with possible sepsis. Liver appears normal; however, a moderate amount of ascites was seen in both right and left quadrants. Small pleural effusions were also demonstrated bilaterally.

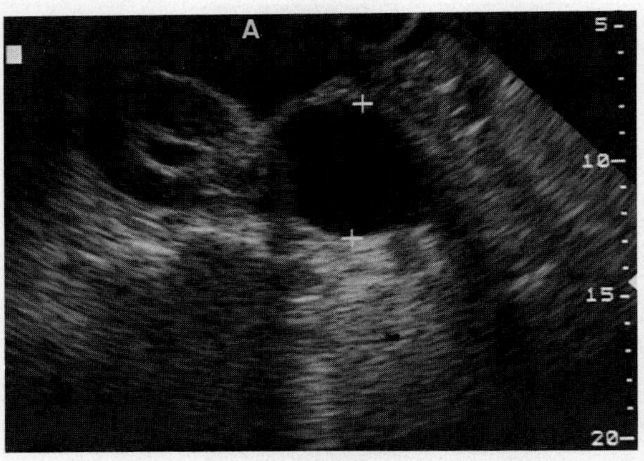

Figure 2-28. Transverse scan of a patient with multiple pancreatic pseudocysts and accompanying ascites (A). Cursors mark one of the pseudocysts. (Courtesy Helen Johnson, Salt Lake City, Utah.)

fluid present. In patients in whom the clinician suspects ascites or free fluid it may not always be possible to demonstrate the fluid if the patient is scanned only in the supine position. In cases in which free fluid is not obvious, it may be helpful to place the patient in the knee-chest position on the table and to scan the abdominal wall from below.[16]

In general, ascitic fluid collects in the most dependent portion of the body. The most obvious ascites collection sites are as follows: (1) inferior or posterior to the right liver lobe (Morrison's pouch), (2) the posterior pelvic cul-de-sac, (3) the paracolic gutter, and (4) anterior or lateral to the liver.

If a fluid collection appears to be loculated in one area, such as the subphrenic space, placing the patient in Trendelenburg or erect positions and scanning again should demonstrate whether the fluid remains isolated or drains into a new area. Lack of such flow would be consistent with an abscess or hematoma.[16] Inflammatory exudate, for example, may cause the omentum to adhere to the appendix and wrap itself around the infected organs, localizing the infection and preventing diffuse peritonitis.

A successful approach to imaging the patient with free fluid is to begin with the patient in the traditional supine position. Special attention should always be paid to the position of the bowel with respect to free fluid collections. Since bowel is filled with air, it should float to the top of the fluid collection (see Fig. 2-26A). Sometimes, especially in scans of the lower abdomen and pelvis, the superficially floating bowel inhibits the complete passage of the sound beam and the fluid collection is overlooked or minimized. Another valuable observation is the appearance of bowel that does not float in a fluid environment, implying that it may be trapped or held down by adhesions or metastatic implants. Such a finding should prompt a more extensive scan of the entire peritoneal cavity. The knowledge that free-floating fluid drains to the most dependent portion of the body prompts us to place patients left side down, especially when there is a question about free versus encysted fluid.

The almost universal use of real-time systems has created a potential diagnostic pitfall. Because of their limited field of view, it is possible to fail to realize the global nature of a large fluid collection and to mistake it for encysted fluid. Additional errors can be made by sonographers expecting transudative collections to be completely echo free and exudative collections to be associated with internal echoes. This is occasionally true, but it is not true consistently, since septa and debris can be found in both infective and malignant fluid collections.[6] One final admonition is to vary the gain settings of the ultrasound instrument. Too much gain may mask the appearance of small fluid collections; very low gain may be indicated to eliminate strong reverberation echoes at the near wall, but may inadvertently create the impression that uniformly solid masses are cystic.

Neoplasms

Mesenteric Cyst. Because of their variable size, location, and clinical presentations, primary cysts of the mesentery are frequently difficult to differentiate clinically from other cystic or solid abdominal masses. True mesenteric cysts are rare and are thought to be primarily lymphatic, arising from sequestered lymphatic tissue or developing spontaneously after trauma.[12] Such lesions may be unilocular or multilocular but are rarely multiple (Fig. 2-29). Secondary mesenteric cysts are not true mesenteric cysts but lesions resulting from pancreatic pseudocysts, other walled-off infections, or loculated, infected, or hemorrhagic ascites.

Omental Cysts. Cysts of the omentum, like those of the mesentery, are very uncommon and seldom are diagnosed except at surgery or autopsy. They are thin walled and filled with fluid, which may vary from clear liquid to a thick, cheesy substance. Since the omentum may migrate within the abdomen and pelvis, omental cysts may be found anywhere in the peritoneal cavity. They are usually single lesions, but multiple cysts can occur. Their size is variable, from small and unnoticeable to large, palpable masses. Omental cysts can occur in all age groups but are more often seen in young adults and children, and more frequently in females than in males. Both congenital and acquired causes have been proposed. Acquired causes include idiopathic ischemia and infarction, trauma, neoplasm, and infection of mycotic, parasitic, or tuberculous origin. The clinical picture is often variable and nonspecific, depending on the size of the cyst, its location, and its consistency.[5,19]

Mesenteric Lymphadenopathy. One type of lymphadenopathy involving the mesentery presents sonographically as a centrally located, isolated node in the abdomen. Unlike the mantle-shaped masses of paraaortic lymphadenopathy, the mesenteric variety extends to be more central and distinct, with mildly echogenic qualities and marginal convexities. In addition to appearing isolated, they are elliptical and relatively sonolucent.[5]

Peritoneal, Mesenteric, or Omental Implants. Such conditions suggest a malignant process and additional observation of ascites reinforces this concern. An extensive survey scan is indicated in such cases. Metastatic disease involving the omentum is common with ovarian carcinoma.[19]

Sonographic appearances and techniques. MESENTERIC CYST. The echo pattern of mesenteric cyst is that of a thin-walled, cystic mass with or without internal septations (see Fig. 2-29). Subjected to high-gain studies, true mesenteric cysts may demonstrate fine, diffuse, nonlayering echoes within.[12] Mesenteric cysts often have calcified walls. Sonographers should be alert to the fact that large mesenteric cysts can resemble a distended urinary bladder. Only by repeating the scan following partial or complete voiding may it be possible to determine the true nature of the mass.

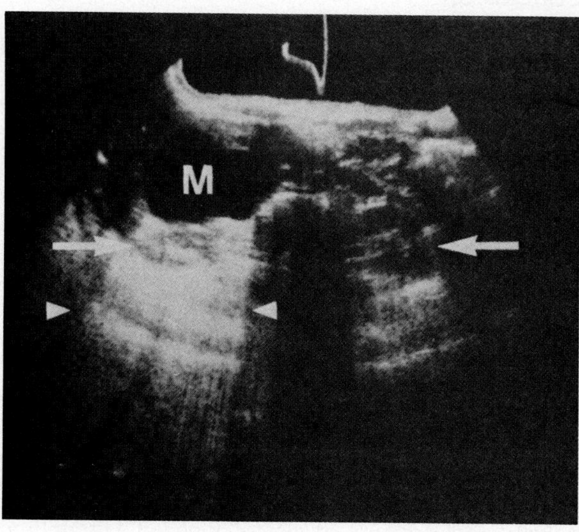

FIGURE 2-29. Mesenteric cyst. Transverse scan demonstrates an anechoic mass (M). Note the sharp posterior wall and strong through-transmission echoes (*arrowheads*) producing an asymmetric echo pattern of the kidneys (*arrows*). (From Longmaid HE, Tymkiw J, Rider EA: Sonographic diagnosis of a chylous mesenteric cyst. J Clin Ultrasound 1986, 14:458–460.)

OMENTAL CYSTS. Cysts are only one of many right side upper quadrant lesions that may yield a predominant cystic appearance on ultrasonography. Laboratory and other clinical findings may be of assistance in compiling a definitive diagnosis. In some cases, other modalities such as CT and an upper gastrointestinal radiograph may be needed for confirmation.

METASTATIC IMPLANTS. Metastatic involvement of the omentum can usually be recognized as a relatively anechoic band of tissue beneath the anterior abdominal wall. The omental band results from thickening of the omentum secondary to metastatic infiltration of neoplastic cells.

Conclusion

In earlier times, less emphasis was placed on imaging and recognizing the sometimes subtle details of the abdominal wall and the extensive and complex peritoneum. The expanded and improved capabilities of diagnostic ultrasonography available today demand a reassessment of the standard sonographic curriculum to include a fuller appreciation of the normal and abnormal appearances of this area. Only when these precepts are adopted and practiced will patients receive the complete and accurate benefits of abdominal ultrasound examination.

References

1. Alanen A, Kormano M: Correlation of the echogenicity and structure of clotted blood. J Ultrasound Med 1985, 4:421–425.
2. Burke SR: Human Anatomy and Physiology for the Health Sciences. New York, John Wiley, 1980.
3. Diakomakis EE, Weinberg B, Seife B: Unusual case studies of anterior abdominal wall mass as diagnosed by ultrasonography. J Clin Ultrasound 1984, 14:351–354.
4. Ferguson GG: Pathophysiology. Mechanisms and Expressions. Philadelphia, WB Saunders, 1984.
5. Fleischer AC, James AE: Introduction to Diagnostic Sonography. New York, John Wiley, 1980.
6. Gerzof SG: The role of ultrasound in the search for intraabdominal and retroperitoneal abscess. *In* Taylor KJW (ed): Ultrasound in Emergency Medicine. New York, Churchill Livingstone, 1981.
7. Golding RHR, Li DKB, Cooperberg PL: Sonographic demonstration of air-fluid levels in abdominal abscesses. J Ultrasound Med 1982, 1:151–155.
8. Hanson RD, Hunter TB, Haber K: Ultrasonographic appearance of anterior abdominal wall desmoid tumors. J Ultrasound Med 1983, 2:141–142.
9. Hiatt JR, Williams RA, Wilson SE: Intraabdominal abscess: Etiology and pathogenesis. Semin Ultrasound 1983, 2:71–79.
10. Kressel HY, Filly RA: Ultrasonographic appearance of gas-containing abscesses in the abdomen. Am J Roentgenol 1978, 130:71–73.
11. Lehman E, Archer VW: Suprahepatic (Subphrenic) abscesses. South Surg 1987, 6:407.
12. Longmaid HE, Tymkiw J, Rider EA: Sonographic diagnosis of a chylous mesenteric cyst. J Clin Ultrasound 1986, 14:458–460.
13. Miller EI, Rogers A: Sonography of the anterior abdominal wall. Semin Ultrasound 1982, 3:278–287.
14. Netter FH: Ciba Collection of Medical Illustrations, 2nd ed, Vol 3. New Jersey, Ciba Pharmaceutical Co, 1964.
15. Pansky B: Dynamic Anatomy and Physiology. New York, McMillan, 1975.
16. Sanders RC: Clinical Sonography. A Practical Guide. Boston, Little, Brown, 1973.
17. Savage PD, Joseph AEA, Adam J: Massive abdominal wall hematoma: Real-time ultrasound localization of bleeding. J Ultrasound Med 1985, 4:157–158.
18. Snell RS: Clinical Anatomy for Medical Students. Boston, Little, Brown, 1973.
19. Weill FW: Ultrasound of Digestive Diseases, 2nd ed. St. Louis, CV Mosby, 1982.
20. Yeh HC, Lehr-Janus C, Cohen BA, et al: Ultrasonography and CT of abdominal and inguinal hernias. J Clin Ultrasound 1984, 14:479–486.

CHAPTER 3

Vascular Structures

JOHN A. GUIDA

In the early days of diagnostic medical ultrasonography, one of its principal uses was in the detection of abdominal aortic aneurysms. With the advent of gray-scale ultrasound, smaller aortic branch vessels were more reliably visualized, along with their venous counterparts. Intraluminal abnormalities such as thrombi and tumors also became more visible.[28] Finally, owing to the development of pulsed Doppler and color-flow instrumentation, much more information is now obtainable about the abdominal vasculature in normal and abnormal states.

In this chapter I provide a comprehensive discussion of the use of diagnostic medical sonography in the assessment of various abdominal vascular abnormalities, with an introduction to Doppler and color-flow applications currently under investigation.

Also, because of the extended applications of ultrasonography beyond examination of the aorta and inferior vena cava (IVC) proper, more specific guidelines and scanning techniques will be interjected in each pertinent section in this chapter.

Patient Preparation

It is recommended that all patients fast prior to vascular scanning, as this tends to reduce the amount of air in the abdomen, which has the potential to obscure the anatomy under observation. In emergency situations, scanning can certainly be accomplished without any patient preparation.[52] If Doppler interrogation is desired, studies should be performed in a consistent manner, because flow characteristics in some of the abdominal vessels are different in a resting (fasting) state compared to an active postprandial state. In some instances it may be prudent to perform pre- and postprandial studies to determine correct or normal responses.

Equipment Considerations

Real-time imaging is preferred over static B-mode imaging because of the ease with which many of the main abdominal vessels can be identified. Also, the course of the various vessels is better appreciated with real-time monitoring than with static imaging.[28,52] The equipment in use should also provide duplex Doppler capability for further interrogation of the blood vessels as an aid in determining normal or abnormal blood flow, specifically in the evaluation of arterial stenoses and portal venous hypertension. Color-flow instrumentation may be beneficial, as it permits easier visualization of blood flow and reduces examination time.

Scanning Techniques

Most of the abdominal vasculature can be identified with the patient lying in the supine position. Scanning commences as the transducer is placed in the subxiphoid position with orientation in the transverse plane. Because of their proximity, the aorta and IVC can be demonstrated simultaneously, and once they are identified, gain settings should be adjusted to reveal their characteristic echo-free lumina. Some reverberation artifact may be present along the anterior aspect of each vessel, owing to the strong reflective interface at their walls; this is considered normal. Scanning continues inferiorly until the aortic bifurcation is reached. Images are recorded at 1- to 2-cm intervals along the course of the aorta and IVC, and additional sections are recorded in any area of disease. Once transverse scanning is completed, the aorta and IVC should be imaged in the longitudinal plane. Images are recorded in segments to demonstrate the entire length of each vessel.

If specific arterial branches or venous tributaries are being investigated, the examination should begin with the transducer positioned near the vessel's origin. Transducer manipulations are then carried out, in an attempt to follow the course of the vessel. Images are recorded to demonstrate vessel length as clearly as possible and any disease that may be present.

A sonographer who proposes to examine the many vascular branches and pathways in the abdomen must have a working knowledge of their general course throughout. Once their sites of origin are known and their general course through the abdomen learned, sonographic examination is made easier.

Circulatory Anatomy—Vascular Structure

Blood is distributed throughout the body by a vast network of arteries and veins. In the systemic circulation, arteries transport blood from the heart to the muscles and organs and veins transport blood from the muscles and organs back to the heart. Typically, blood vessels are composed of three distinct layers: tunica intima, tunica media, and tunica adventitia. The tunica intima, the innermost section of a vessel wall, consists of an endothelial lining and elastic tissue. Elastic fibers and smooth muscle constitute the second layer, the tunica media. The outer portion of the vessel wall, the tunica adventitia, is composed of elastic and collagen fibers.[82]

Although arteries and veins are histologically similar, there are differences in the distribution of each tissue within the walls that reflect pressure differences between the two systems. For example, arterial walls are thicker and contain more elastic and smooth muscle fibers than veins. This is true especially in the tunica media, which is the thickest layer of an artery and is largely responsible for its very elastic and contractile characteristics. Because of the thickness of arterial walls, they tend to maintain a constant shape and do not readily collapse in conjunction with low blood pressure.[47,82]

Since veins have less smooth muscle and elastic tissue, they are unable to contract to force through blood. Venous return to the heart therefore, is accomplished through the pressure gradient or difference between the arterial and venous network, breathing, and skeletal muscle contractions. Valves are also an important part of venous return, but they occur only in the veins of the extremities.[87] The circulatory network of blood vessels, the vasa vasorum, is located within their walls.[87]

Anatomy of the Aorta

The aorta is the main artery of the chest and abdomen from which all other branch vessels are derived. For reference purposes, the aorta is divided into various segments along its length (Fig. 3-1). The aorta originates from the left ventricle, and as it leaves the heart it courses rightward and superiorly to form the ascending aorta. It then curves toward the left and posteriorly to form the aortic arch. As the aorta completes its curve at the arch, it begins to descend inferiorly into the chest. This portion, the descending aorta, soon gives rise to the thoracic aorta. Once the aorta penetrates the diaphragm, it is termed the abdominal aorta, and it is this portion of the aorta that is most accessible to ultrasonographic examination.

As the abdominal aorta follows its course through the abdomen, it gives rise to several major vessels (Fig. 3-2). The first branch is the celiac axis. Originating from the anterior aspect of the aorta, it is usually found within the first 2 cm. The celiac axis is a short vessel, approximately 1 cm long, that divides into three others: the hepatic artery, the left gastric artery, and the splenic artery.[47,82]

The hepatic artery leaves the celiac axis at ap-

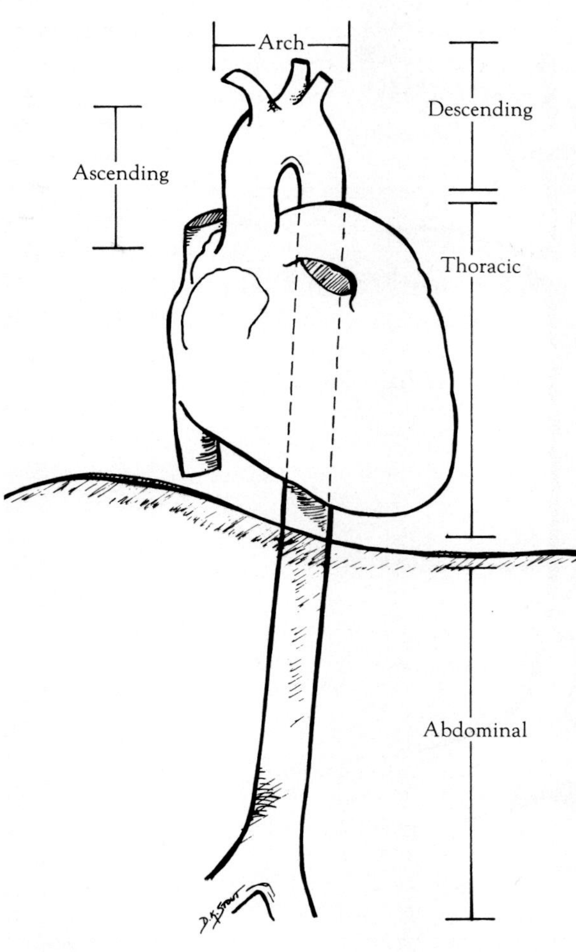

FIGURE 3-1. The segments of the aorta.

proximately a 90-degree angle and courses rightward, following the upper border of the pancreatic head. At the duodenum, the hepatic artery turns anteriorly to enter the liver hilum, following the course of the main portal vein. Intrahepatically, the artery then divides into left and right branches at the portal fissure to supply the left and right hepatic lobes, respectively.[28,33,47,82] The left gastric artery initially has an anterior and superior course from the celiac axis. It then turns leftward to supply the stomach and esophagus with blood.[28,33,47,82] The splenic artery takes a horizontal, leftward course from the celiac axis and follows the upper margin of the pancreatic body posteriorly. Along its route to the spleen it generates arterial branches to the stomach and pancreas.[28,33,47,82]

The second major branch vessel, the superior mesenteric artery, also originates from the anterior surface of the aorta approximately 1 to 2.5 cm below the celiac axis (although this distance varies). As it begins its caudad course, it travels posterior to the pancreatic body and anterior to the uncinate process. It then continues inferiorly, paralleling the aorta. Several branches arise along the length of the superior mesenteric artery and are responsible for supplying the small and large bowel with blood.

Just inferior to the superior mesenteric artery lie the renal arteries. The right renal artery tends to arise from the lateral aspect of the aorta, while the left renal artery tends to arise from the lateral or posterolateral aspect of the aorta. Both then course posterolaterally to enter the respective kidneys.[28,33,47,82]

The inferior mesenteric artery is the last major branch to arise from the abdominal aorta before it bifurcates. It originates from the anterior aspect of the aorta and runs slightly leftward and inferiorly into the abdomen. It is responsible for supplying the distal portion of the colon with blood. This vessel is not generally seen on ultrasound examination because of its small size and interference from overlying bowel.[28,33,47,82]

At about the level of the umbilicus, the aorta bifurcates into the right and left common iliac arteries. These vessels course inferiorly and posteriorly, holding a position fairly deep in the pelvis. As a result, the iliac arteries can be very difficult to image. Full bladder techniques may be necessary to visualize them.[28,33,47,82]

Sonographic Appearance of the Abdominal Arteries

Sonographically the lumina of the aorta and other vascular structures appear anechoic; so while scanning it is important to optimize gain settings to demonstrate them as anechoic structures. In the longitudinal plane, slightly to the left of midline, the proximal aorta can be seen as an anechoic tubular structure following a somewhat anterior and inferior course within the abdomen. The spine lies immediately posterior to it, providing a highly re-

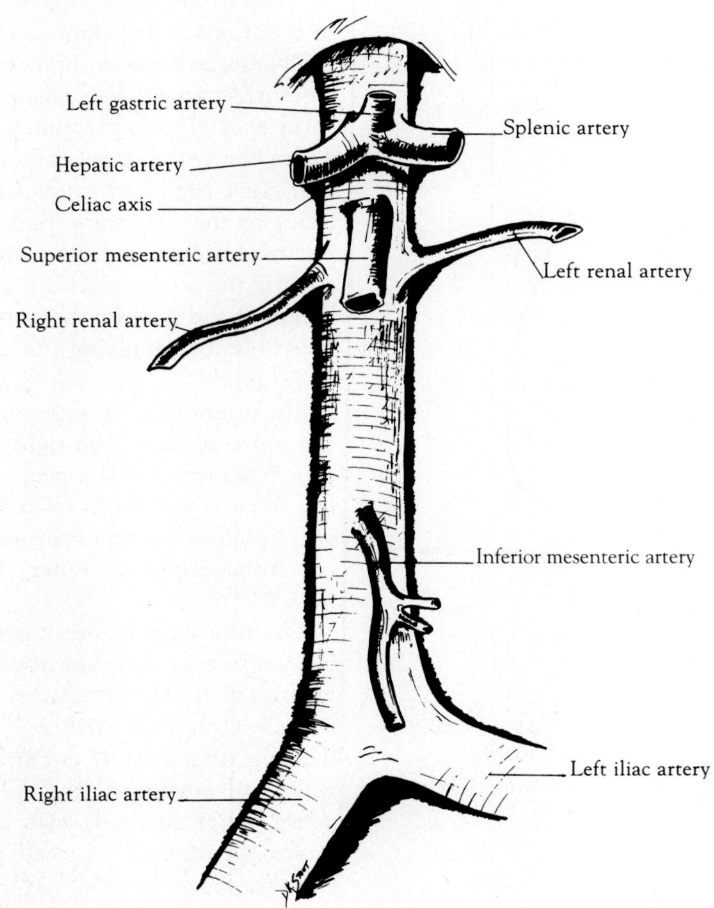

FIGURE 3-2. The abdominal aorta and its major branch vessels.

flective echo boundary (Fig. 3-3A, B). As the aorta courses inferiorly, it tapers, becoming smaller in caliber (Fig. 3-3C). In the proximal aspect of the aorta, both the celiac axis and the superior mesenteric artery can be seen as they arise anteriorly from the aorta (see Fig. 3-3A). A longitudinal scan provides the best plane of view of the proximity of the celiac axis and the superior mesenteric artery.

In transverse scan planes, the aorta takes on a more rounded appearance and again can be seen to lie atop the spine. As the transducer is moved inferiorly from the xiphoid process the first aortic branch to be encountered is the celiac axis. It appears as an anechoic tubular structure that divides into the hepatic artery and the splenic artery. Viewed in the appropriate plane, the image resembles a seagull (Fig. 3-4). The rightward branch of the celiac axis is the hepatic artery. It can be followed transversely and superiorly as it travels to enter the liver hilum. The splenic artery forms the leftward branch of the celiac axis and courses leftward to enter the splenic hilum. The splenic artery can be quite tortuous and is difficult to image in its entirety, especially in elderly patients.

The left gastric artery can occasionally be seen in its proximal aspect. This vessel, however, is usually smaller in caliber than the neighboring hepatic and splenic arteries and is more difficult to image consistently.

After moving the transducer inferiorly, the su-

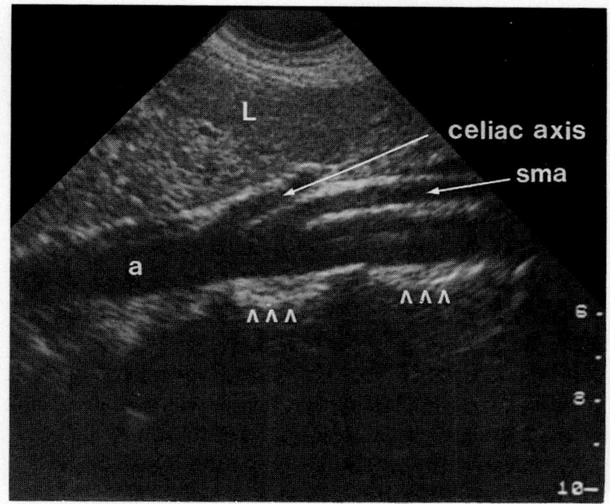

A

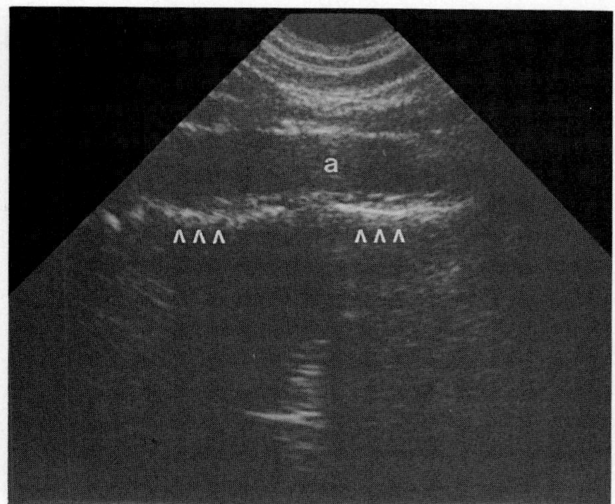

B

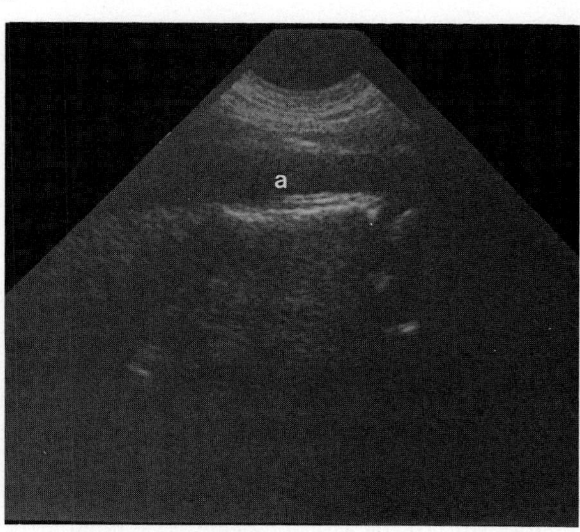

C

FIGURE 3-3. (*A*) Longitudinal sonogram through the proximal abdominal aorta (a) demonstrates the origins of the celiac axis and superior mesenteric artery (sma); (carets, anterior aspect of vertebral bodies; L, Liver). (*B*) Longitudinal sonogram through the middle portion of the abdominal aorta (a). (C) Longitudinal sonogram through the distal portion of the abdominal aorta (a). Note tapering of the vessel at this point.

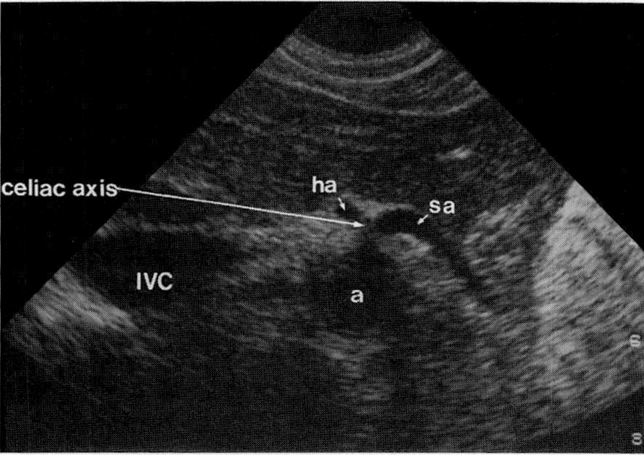

FIGURE 3-4. Transverse sonogram through the aorta (a) at the level of the celiac axis; (ha, hepatic artery; sa, splenic artery; IVC, inferior vena cava).

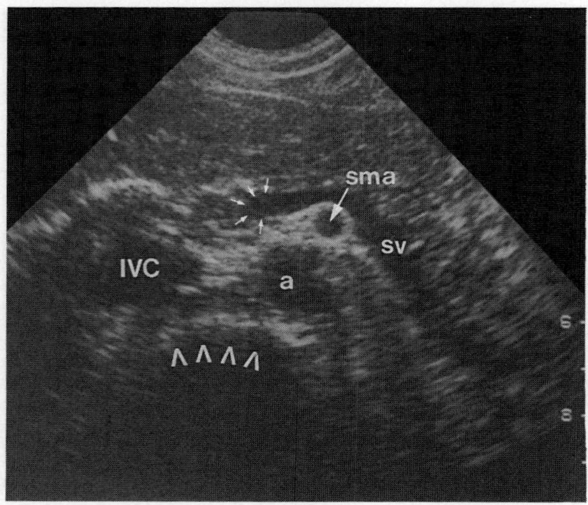

Figure 3-5. Transverse sonogram through the aorta (a) at a level just below the origin of the superior mesenteric artery (sma); (sv, splenic vein, IVC, inferior vena cava; carets, anterior aspect of a vertebral body).

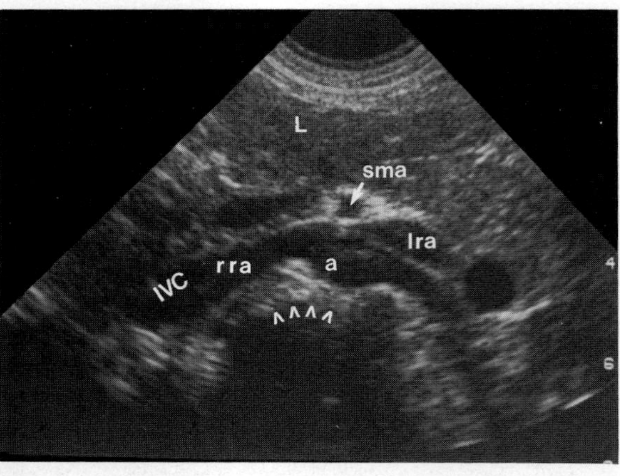

Figure 3-6. Transverse sonogram through the aorta (a) at the level of the renal artery origins (L, Liver; rra, right renal artery; lra, left renal artery; sma, superior mesenteric artery; IVC, inferior vena cava; carets, anterior aspect of a vertebral body).

perior mesenteric artery can be seen. It appears rounded and is surrounded by an echodense collar consisting of mesentery and fat (Fig. 3-5).

Immediately inferior to the level of origin of the superior mesenteric artery are the origins of the renal arteries. They are best appreciated in the transverse plane because of their perpendicular relationship to the acoustic beam. The renal arteries arise from the lateral aspect of the aorta and continue their course, respectively, to the right and left to enter the kidneys (Fig. 3-6).

At the level of the umbilicus, the right and left iliac arteries can be seen as they arise from the aortic terminus as rounded and anechoic vessels emerging from a common source (distal aorta) (Fig. 3-7). Further, more comprehensive imaging of the iliac arteries is accomplished by placing the transducer in the iliac fossa and angling medially with the scan plane oriented roughly 45 degrees from midline. Demonstration of the length of the iliac arteries is thus achieved. At times, successful imaging of the iliac arteries requires a distended urinary bladder. In this case, the transducer is placed in the midline of the pelvis and oriented 45 degrees from midline. Lateral angulation will result in visualization of the iliac vessels.

Anatomy of the Inferior Vena Cava

The IVC is the large vessel that returns blood to the heart from the lower portions of the body. Its origin is in the lower abdomen at about the level of the umbilicus, at the junction of the external iliac veins. The IVC travels superiorly in the abdomen and enters the right atrium of the heart. As the vena cava nears the heart, it courses somewhat anteriorly to form a hockey stick–like configuration before it terminates in the right atrium (Fig. 3-8).

There are many tributaries to the IVC, but most cannot be seen because of their small size. The renal and hepatic veins are the veins most consistently seen entering the IVC. The right renal vein is generally shorter than the left renal vein because of its close proximity to the IVC. The left renal vein traverses the abdomen, coursing anterior to the aorta and posterior to the superior mesenteric artery to finally enter the lateral aspect of the IVC.

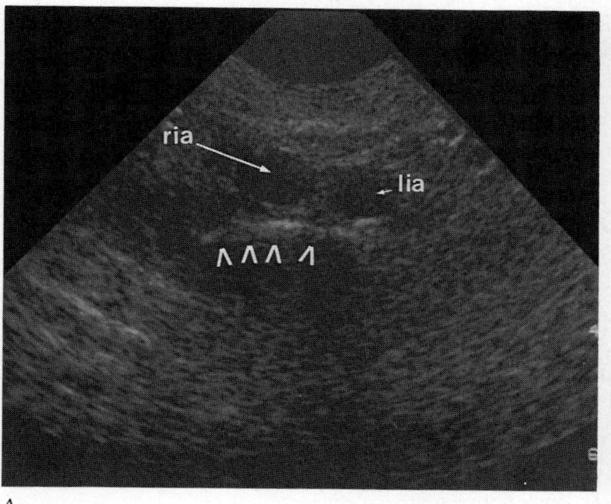

A

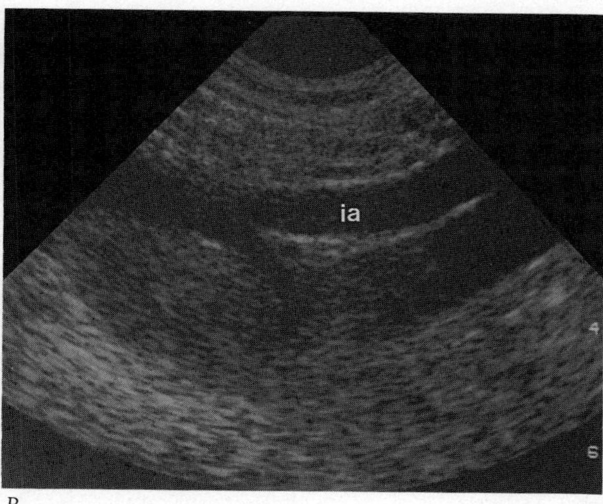

B

FIGURE 3-7. (*A*) Transverse sonogram through the distal aorta just beyond the bifurcation (ria, right iliac artery; lia, left iliac artery; carets, anterior aspect of a vertebral body). (*B*) Longitudinal sonogram through one of the iliac arteries (ia).

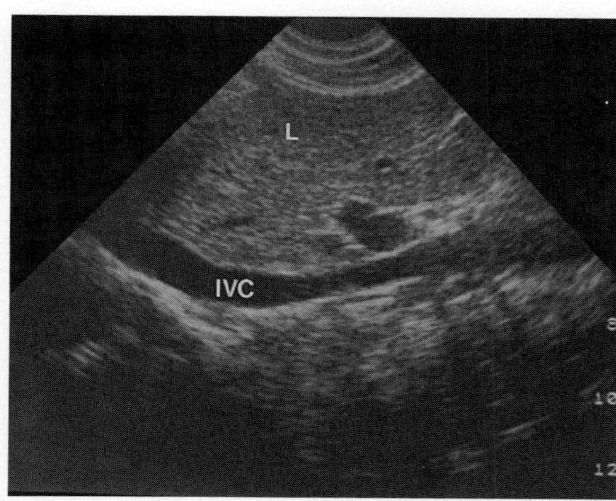

FIGURE 3-8. Longitudinal sonogram through the inferior vena cava (IVC) demonstrating the hockey stick configuration as the vessel nears the right atrium (L, liver).

The hepatic veins also drain directly into the IVC or right atrium. Normally, there are three hepatic veins: left, right, and middle (Fig. 3-9).

Sonographic Appearance of the Abdominal Veins

Sonographically, the IVC is an anechoic structure slightly to the right of midline. Unlike the aorta, which has a relatively constant diameter and a rounded appearance in the transverse plane, the IVC tends to have a more oval shape. It also responds to respiratory variations. During inspiration, the IVC should contract, owing to the decreased pressure within the thoracic cavity, allowing prompt blood flow from the IVC into the right atrium. The opposite is true for expiration, and the IVC expands during this maneuver. With suspended inspiration, the IVC expands due to increased intrathoracic pressure and decreased blood flow into the heart. During the Valsalva maneuver, the IVC collapses because of the increased abdominal pressure associated with this technique.[32]

The hepatic veins are best demonstrated in a transverse plane with the transducer just inferior to the xiphoid process and angled cephalad. Identifi-

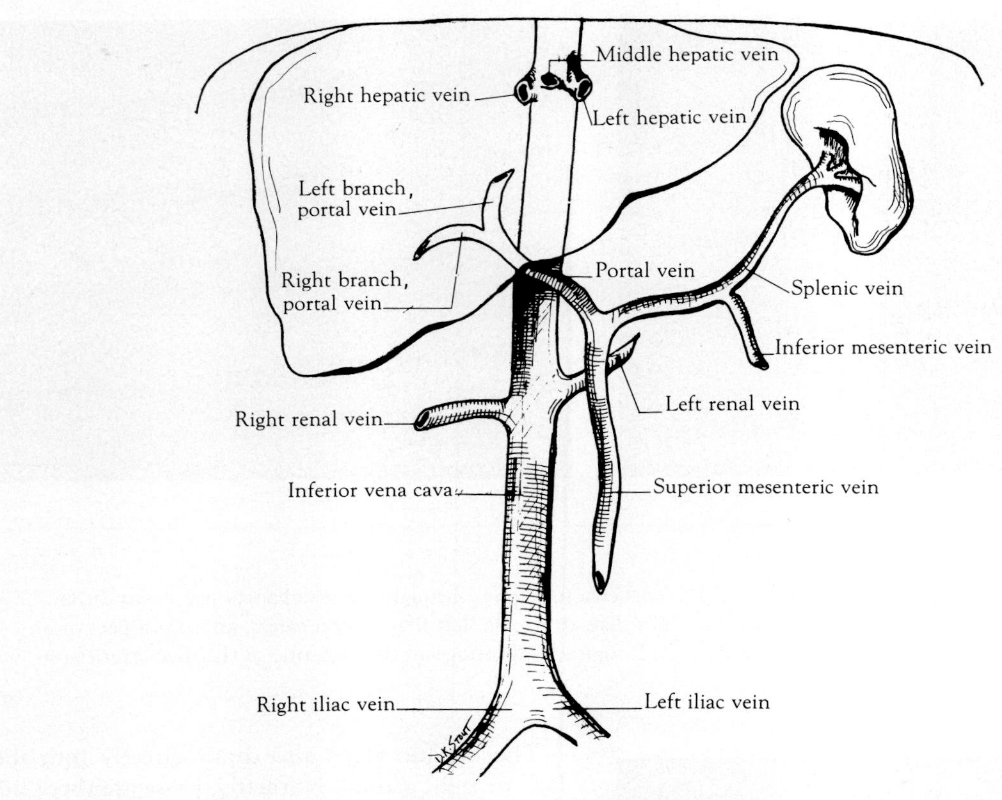

FIGURE 3-9. The inferior vena cava, the tributaries most often visualized sonographically, and the portal venous system and its relationship to the inferior vena cava.

cation of the right, middle, and left hepatic veins is relatively easy as they converge to empty into the IVC (Fig. 3-10). Partial imaging of the right hepatic vein with simultaneous imaging of the middle and left hepatic veins will result in the Playboy bunny or rabbit ear sign.

Optimal imaging of the renal veins is also accomplished using a transverse scanning approach. The renal veins should be visualized at about the same level as the renal arteries (just inferior to the origin of the superior mesenteric artery); (Fig. 3-11). The right renal vein is best imaged with the transducer placed in the right lateral abdomen over the right kidney and angled medially. The renal vein is identified as an echo-free tube exiting the renal hilus. When attempting to visualize the left renal vein, the transducer is placed (in a transverse orientation) in the midline of the abdomen just inferior to the superior mesenteric artery origin. The left renal vein is seen as an anechoic tubular structure coursing between the superior mesenteric artery and the aorta to enter the lateral aspect of the inferior vena cava.

Anatomy of the Portal Venous System

The portal venous system is comprised of the veins that drain blood from the bowel and spleen and is separate from the inferior vena cava.

The main portal vein is formed at the junction of the splenic vein and the superior mesenteric vein, which are easily seen by ultrasound tech-

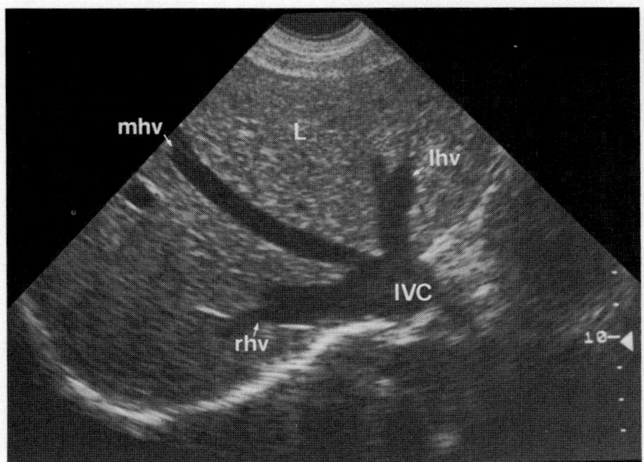

Figure 3-10. Transverse sonogram through the inferior vena cava (IVC) at a point just below the right atrium of the heart demonstrating the hepatic veins (rhv, right hepatic vein; mhv, middle hepatic vein; lhv, left hepatic vein; L, liver).

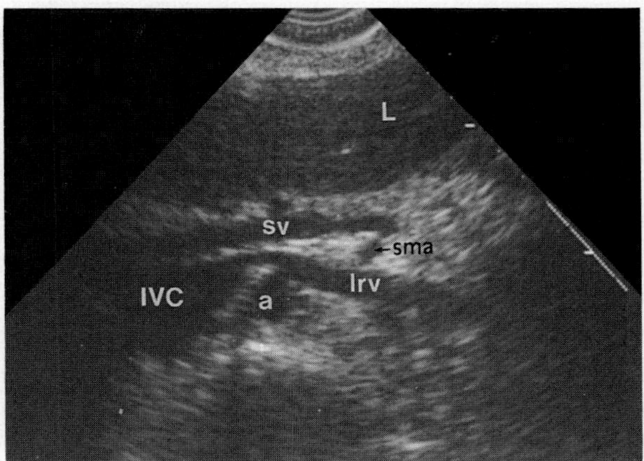

Figure 3-11. Transverse sonogram at the level of the left renal vein (a, aorta; IVC, inferior vena cava; lrv, left renal vein; sv, splenic vein; sma, superior mesenteric artery; L, liver).

niques in most patients (Fig. 3-9). To image the portal venous system it is easiest to begin by placing the transducer in the midline of the abdomen substernally with a transverse orientation. The splenic vein can be used as an initial reference point, as it is easily seen in this plane. The splenic vein emerges from the splenic hilus and courses medial and superiorly within the abdomen, bordering the posterior surface of the pancreatic body and tail. It is identified sonographically as a tubular structure with a superomedial course within the abdomen coursing anterior to the superior mesenteric artery as it nears the midline. At its termination, the splenic vein can be seen to increase in diameter. This is the point at which the splenic vein merges with the superior mesenteric vein to form the main portal vein (Fig. 3-12A). The junction of the superior mesenteric and the splenic vein is known as the portal confluence, and this confluence is immediately posterior to the neck of the pancreas. Visualization of the superior mesenteric vein is accomplished by placing the transducer over the portal confluence (transverse orientation) and rotating the transducer 90 degrees. The length of the superior mesenteric vein will be displayed having a longitudinal course within the abdomen that parallels that of the superior mesenteric artery to its left (Fig. 3-12B, C).

The main portal vein travels somewhat obliquely and anteriorly within the abdomen before it enters the liver hilus (Fig. 3-12D, E). Placement of the transducer over the portal confluence and subsequent clockwise rotation eventually demonstrates the portal vein in its long axis. It can then be followed into the liver, where it soon divides into left and right branches.

Other vessels contributing to portal venous circulation include the inferior mesenteric vein, coronary vein, pyloric vein, cystic vein, and paraumbilical veins. These generally are not seen on routine abdominal examinations but may be identified in abnormal states, which will be discussed later.

Relational Anatomy of the Arteries and Veins

Table 3-1 illustrates the relational anatomy of the abdominal arteries and veins. Because of the many vessels in the abdomen and their proximity to one another, it is useful to know their relationships to surrounding structures, especially for identification of the pancreas (see Table 3-1, Figs. 3-13, 3-14).[23]

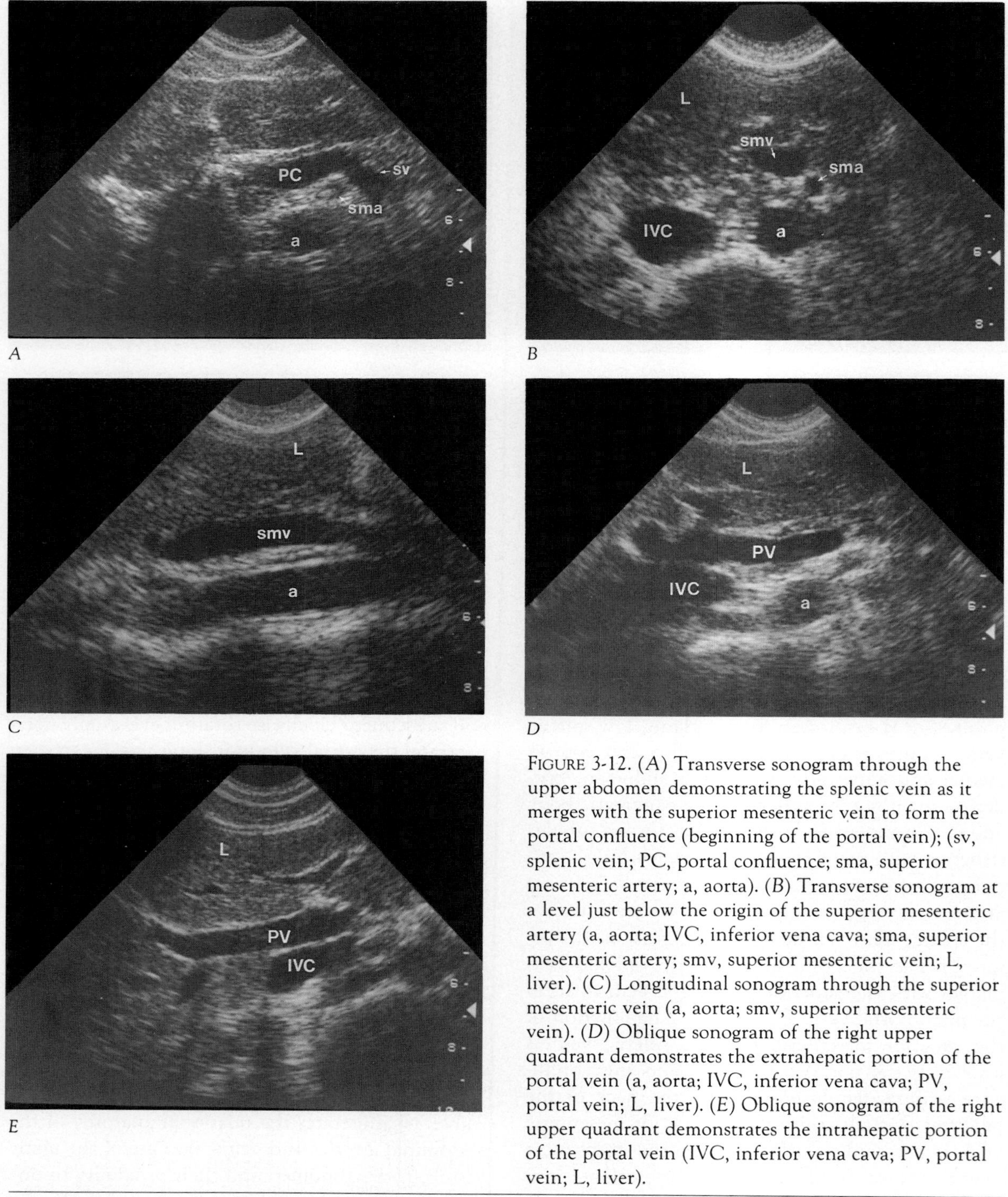

FIGURE 3-12. (*A*) Transverse sonogram through the upper abdomen demonstrating the splenic vein as it merges with the superior mesenteric vein to form the portal confluence (beginning of the portal vein); (sv, splenic vein; PC, portal confluence; sma, superior mesenteric artery; a, aorta). (*B*) Transverse sonogram at a level just below the origin of the superior mesenteric artery (a, aorta; IVC, inferior vena cava; sma, superior mesenteric artery; smv, superior mesenteric vein; L, liver). (*C*) Longitudinal sonogram through the superior mesenteric vein (a, aorta; smv, superior mesenteric vein). (*D*) Oblique sonogram of the right upper quadrant demonstrates the extrahepatic portion of the portal vein (a, aorta; IVC, inferior vena cava; PV, portal vein; L, liver). (*E*) Oblique sonogram of the right upper quadrant demonstrates the intrahepatic portion of the portal vein (IVC, inferior vena cava; PV, portal vein; L, liver).

Table 3-1. Relational anatomy of the abdominal arteries and veins

Vessel	Relational Anatomy	Figures
Aorta	Anterior to the spine, left of the inferior vena cava, more posterior proximally than distally	3-13A, B
Inferior vena cava	Anterior to the spine, right of the aorta, courses anteriorly to enter right atrium	3-13A, B
Hepatic artery	Anterior to the portal vein, left of the common bile duct, superior to the head of the pancreas	3-13A, 3-14B
Splenic artery	Superior to the body and tail of the pancreas	3-13A
Superior mesenteric artery	Posterior to the body of the pancreas and the splenic vein, anterior to the aorta	3-13A, B
Right renal artery	Posterior to the inferior vena cava	3-13A, 3-14A
Splenic vein	Posterior to the body and tail of the pancreas, inferior to the splenic artery	3-13A, 3-13B
Superior mesenteric vein	Right of and parallel to the superior mesenteric artery	3-12B, C, 3-13A
Left renal vein	Anterior to the aorta, posterior to the superior mesenteric artery, anterior to the left renal artery	3-11, 3-13A
Portal vein	Anterior to the inferior vena cava	3-13A, 3-14B
Common bile duct	Anterior to the portal vein, right of the hepatic artery	3-14B

Arterial Abnormalities

Atherosclerosis

Description. Atherosclerosis is a form of arteriosclerosis in which the intimal lining of the arteries is altered by the presence of any combination of the following: focal accumulation of lipids, complex carbohydrates, blood and blood products, fibrous tissue, and calcium deposits. The media of the arterial wall is also changed.[79]

Cause. The cause is not known, but several factors have been linked to the progression of atherosclerosis, and they include hyperlipidemia, hypertension, cigarette smoking, and diabetes mellitus.[41]

Clinical Signs and Symptoms. Generally, there are no symptoms of atherosclerosis until a significant stenosis develops. Then, symptoms vary and are related to the particular stenotic vessel. These are discussed later. Atherosclerotic disease also predisposes to development of aneurysms. There are generally no symptoms unless complications arise.

Sonographic Appearance. The sonographic findings of atherosclerosis include luminal irregularities (representative of the various changes of the intimal lining of the artery), tortuosity, and aortic wall calcification.

The wall irregularities detected by ultrasound can be seen as low-level echoes along the internal walls of the aorta with a propensity for development at the areas of bifurcation of the branch vessels.[28,92] In and of themselves, these areas of plaque

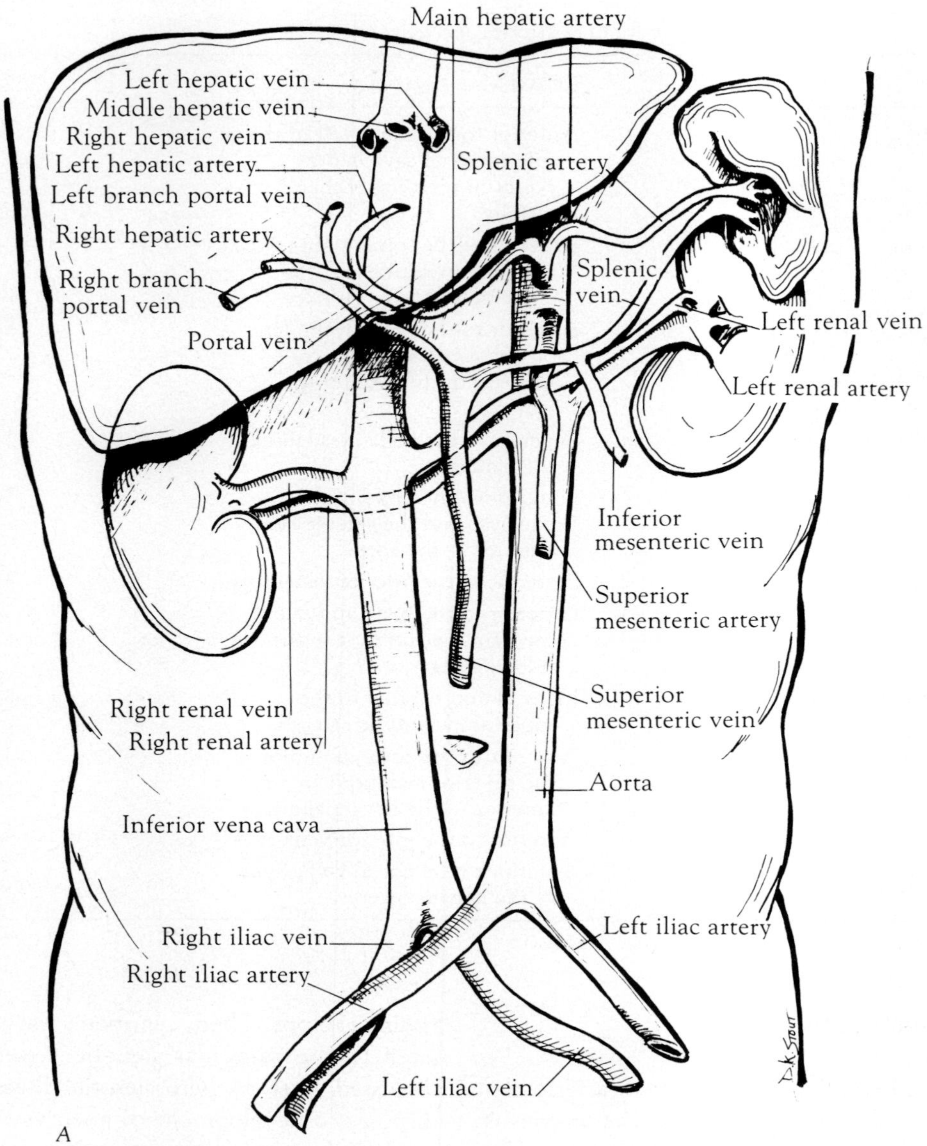

Main hepatic artery
Left hepatic vein
Middle hepatic vein
Right hepatic vein
Left hepatic artery
Left branch portal vein
Right hepatic artery
Right branch portal vein
Portal vein
Splenic artery
Splenic vein
Left renal vein
Left renal artery
Inferior mesenteric vein
Superior mesenteric artery
Superior mesenteric vein
Right renal vein
Right renal artery
Aorta
Inferior vena cava
Left iliac artery
Right iliac vein
Right iliac artery
Left iliac vein
D.K. Stout

A

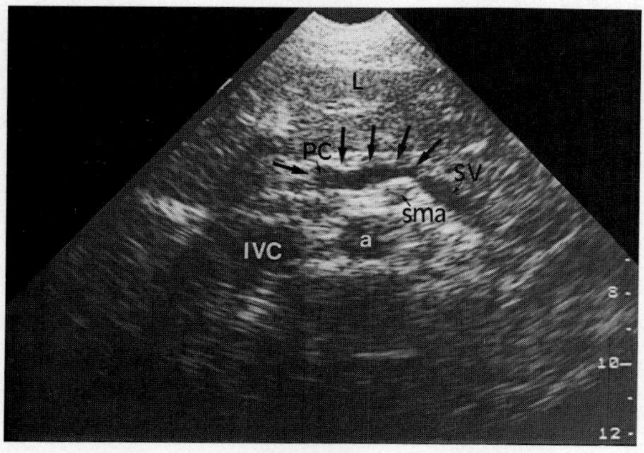

B

FIGURE 3-13. (*A*) The relationship of the major branches of the aorta, inferior vena cava, and the portal system. (*B*) Transverse sonogram through the splenic vein demonstrates relational anatomy of the surrounding vessels (a, aorta; IVC, inferior vena cava; sma, superior mesenteric artery; SV, splenic vein; PC, portal confluence; carets, pancreas; L, liver).

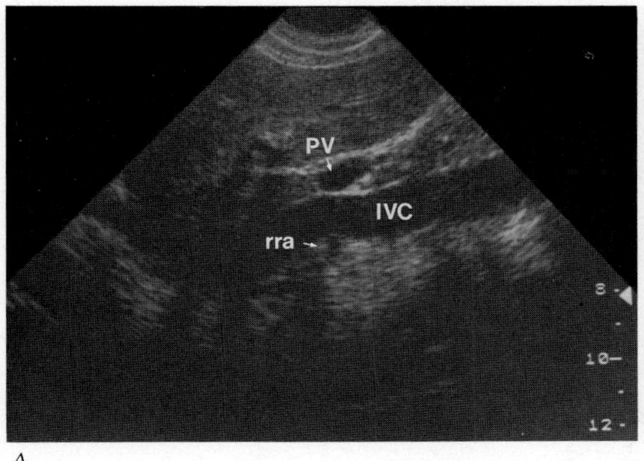

A

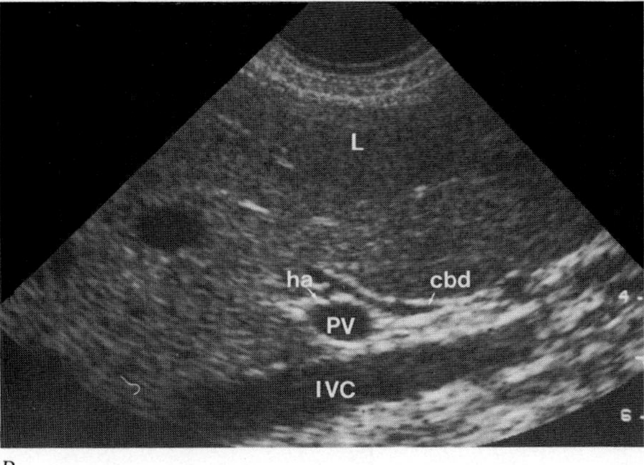

B

Figure 3-14. (*A*) Longitudinal sonogram through the inferior vena cava demonstrates the relational anatomy of the surrounding vessels (IVC, inferior vena cava; rra, right renal artery; PV, portal vein). (*B*) Longitudinal sonogram through the inferior vena cava demonstrates the relational anatomy of the surrounding vessels (L, liver; IVC, inferior vena cava; PV, portal vein; ha, hepatic artery; cbd, common bile duct).

formation are not terribly important unless they produce significant stenosis of a particular branch artery. Detection of a hemodynamically significant stenosis is discussed in detail later in this chapter.

In elderly persons, tortuosity of the aorta is often leftward but occasionally can be right sided.[28] Imaging of the vessel is best carried out in the transverse plane, as this affords a clearer picture of the course of a tortuous aorta.

Aortic wall calcification is easily detected as an echogenic focus in the arterial wall, which at times may produce acoustic shadows (Fig. 3-15).

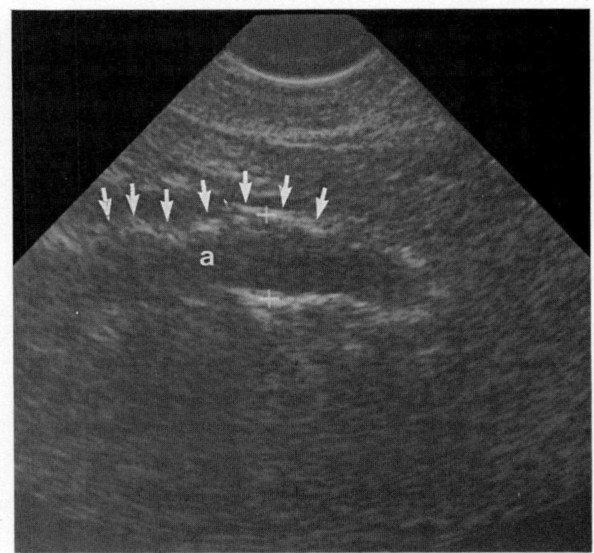

Figure 3-15. Longitudinal sonogram through the distal portion of an arteriosclerotic aorta (a, aorta; *arrows*, anterior aortic wall with the bright echoes representing calcification).

Aneurysms of the Abdominal Aorta

Description. An aneurysm is a focal dilatation of an artery caused by a structural weakness in its wall. A uniform dilatation is defined as a fusiform aneurysm, and a saccular aneurysm is one in which there is a saclike protrusion of the aorta toward one side or the other. In this configuration, a channel or opening connects the aorta to the aneurysmal sac; this orifice varies in size (Fig. 3-16). Most abdominal aortic aneurysms occur below the level of the renal arteries.[41]

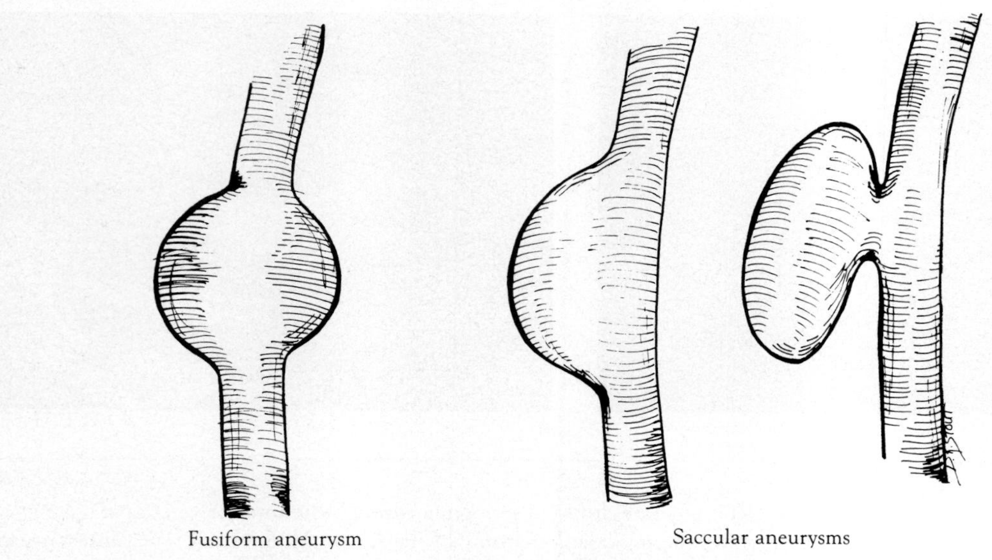

FIGURE 3-16. The types of aneurysms, fusiform and saccular.

Cause. Atherosclerosis is the most common cause of aneurysms in the United States. Syphilis and other diseases can cause aneurysms, although these are not very common causes.[41,52]

Clinical Signs and Symptoms. Generally, patients with aneurysms are asymptomatic, and the presence of an aneurysm is suspected during palpation of a pulsating mass in the area of the umbilicus, or by calcifications seen on plain film radiography of the abdomen. Patients with an expanding aneurysm may have vague lower back or abdominal pain.[52]

Sonographic Appearance. At the diaphragm, normal aortic diameters have been cited at approximately 2.5 cm.[28] During its course inferiorly the aorta tapers, reaching a diameter of about 1.5 to 2.0 cm at the level of the iliac arteries.[28] Ectasia of the aorta, as seen with atherosclerosis, is manifested by a slight widening of the normal aortic diameter up to 3.0 cm. There will also be aortic wall irregularities, owing to the calcific changes that take place in this disease process (Fig. 3-15). A true aneurysm is identified sonographically as a dilatation of the aorta 3.0 cm or greater near its bifurcation point, a focal dilatation along the course of the aorta, or lack of normal tapering of the aorta.[24,36,48]

Aneurysms vary in size and can range from 3 to 20 cm (Fig. 3-17). As a result of the abnormal blood flow patterns within an aneurysm, thrombus is formed. It can usually be detected by sonographic techniques, and is a common finding. Sonographically, thrombus typically produces a low-level echo pattern and tends to accumulate along the anterior and lateral walls of the aortic lumen (Fig. 3-18).[24,36] Adequate demonstration of the thrombus may require that gain settings be increased from initial settings to display the low-level echoes associated with thrombus. It may also be necessary to scan coronally or obliquely through the aorta to demonstrate thrombus. These maneuvers may help reduce confusion between reverberation artifacts and actual thrombus. Occasionally, there may be calcification within the thrombus. An interesting phenomenon that has been reported in association with aortic aneurysm thrombus is that of an anechoic crescent sign (Fig. 3-19).[43] In these instances, the anechoic area within the lumen of the aneurysm was found at surgery to be serosanguineous fluid or liquefying clot. In evaluating aortas for aneurysm formation it is important to distinguish this

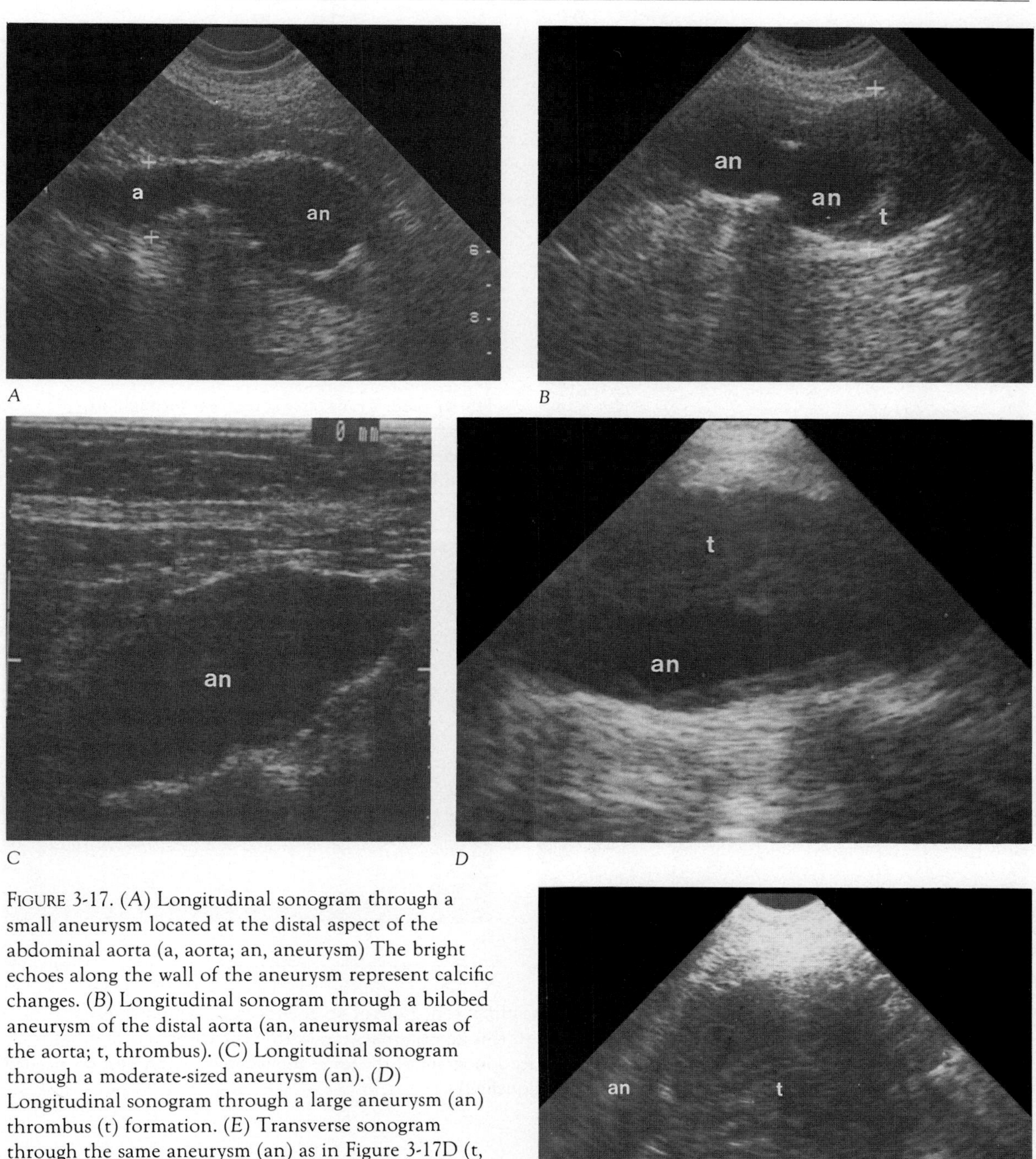

Figure 3-17. (*A*) Longitudinal sonogram through a small aneurysm located at the distal aspect of the abdominal aorta (a, aorta; an, aneurysm) The bright echoes along the wall of the aneurysm represent calcific changes. (*B*) Longitudinal sonogram through a bilobed aneurysm of the distal aorta (an, aneurysmal areas of the aorta; t, thrombus). (*C*) Longitudinal sonogram through a moderate-sized aneurysm (an). (*D*) Longitudinal sonogram through a large aneurysm (an) thrombus (t) formation. (*E*) Transverse sonogram through the same aneurysm (an) as in Figure 3-17D (t, thrombus). Note the relative smallness of the residual lumen, represented as the area between the cursors, as compared to the total size of the aneurysm.

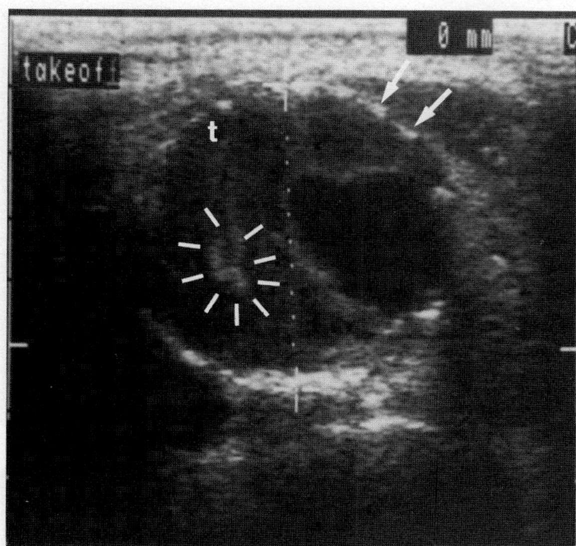

FIGURE 3-18. Transverse sonogram through an abdominal aortic aneurysm with thrombus and calcification *(area surrounded by lines)* within the thrombus (t).

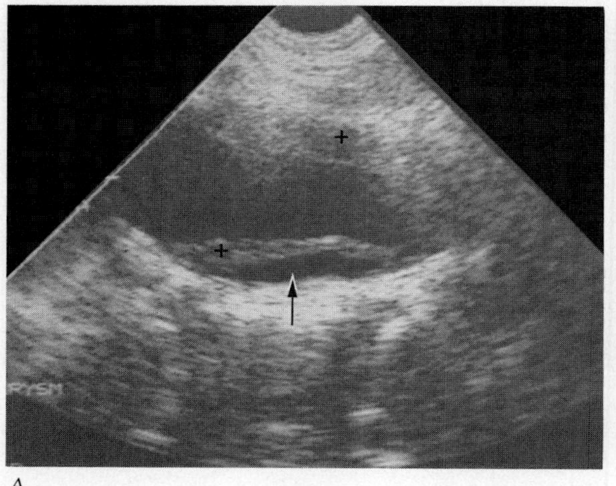

A

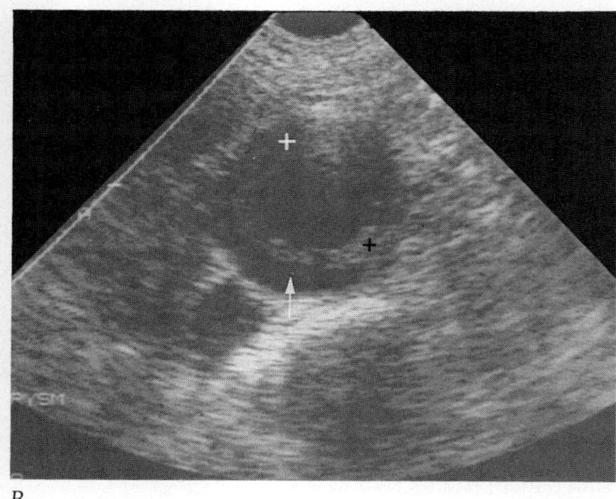

B

FIGURE 3-19. (*A*) Longitudinal sonogram of an aneurysm to demonstrate the anechoic crescent sign (t, thrombus; *arrow,* area within the thrombus that has liquefied). (*B*) Transverse sonogram of the same aneurysm (t, thrombus; *arrow,* area of thrombus that has liquefied).

finding from aortic dissection, as the surgical treatments are different.[43]

Thrombus within the aorta may be difficult at times to visualize, especially in an obese or gassy patient. Anterior reverberation artifacts from a calcific anterior aortic wall may obscure the clot as well. Instances have been reported in which an obstructing clot of the distal abdominal aorta was not detected sonographically[2]; however, these studies were performed without benefit of pulsed Doppler techniques. If obstructing clot is suspected on clinical grounds, Doppler examination of the aorta

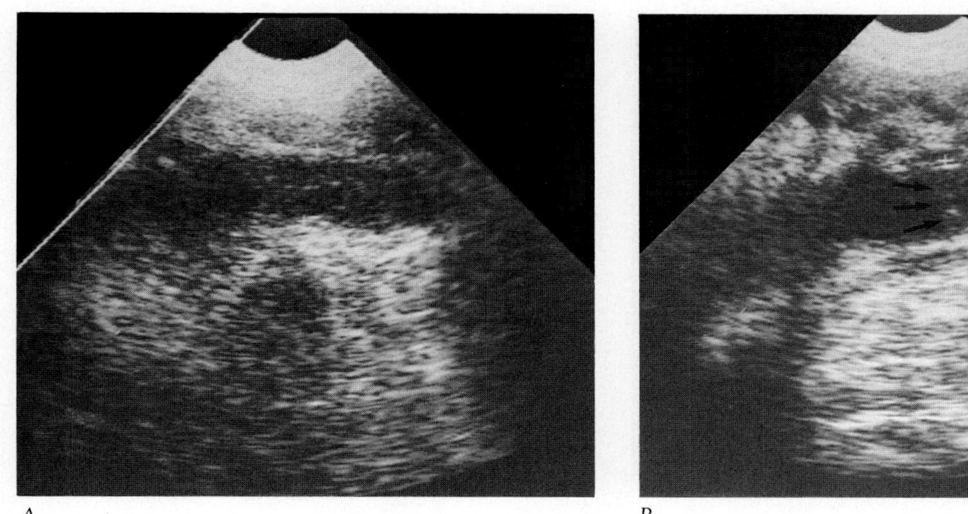

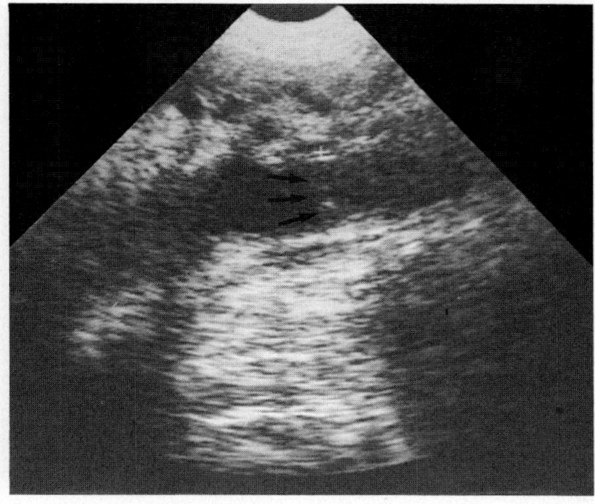

A B

FIGURE 3-20. (*A*) Longitudinal sonogram through the occluded portion of a normal-sized aorta. The very fine, faint echoes in the lumen of the vessel represent occlusive thrombus. On Doppler examination, no flow was detected in this portion of the aorta. (*B*) Longitudinal sonogram through the same aorta but toward the middle portion. The arrows identify the area where the clot begins. There is a subtle difference in the echogenicity of the clot-free lumen and the clot-filled lumen.

should confirm the presence or absence of flow within it, solving the problem (Fig. 3-20).

If an aneurysm is detected during sonographic examination, it is prudent to attempt to identify the origins of the renal arteries as well as to extend the examination into the iliac arteries to look for aneurysmal involvement in these areas.

Associated renal artery aneurysm in conjunction with abdominal aortic aneurysm has been reported to be 1% or less.[14] Nonetheless, it is important for the surgeon to know of this coexistence because of the difference in treatment procedures. When the renal arteries are involved in an aneurysm, renal artery enlargement generally coexists with aortic dilatation. Demonstration of this complication, however, can be quite difficult, since large aneurysms tend to displace surrounding bowel superiorly and subsequently cover the renal artery origins.[14] Because of the compounded bowel interference, diligent scanning techniques involving multiple patient positions and numerous transducer angulations may be necessary before adequate visualization of the renal artery origins is accomplished. If efforts to identify the renal arteries are unsuccessful, an attempt should be made to visualize the superior mesenteric artery. Because of the proximity of the renal arteries to the superior mesenteric artery, any aneurysm shown to involve the superior mesenteric artery also involves the renal arteries.

Abdominal aneurysms may also extend into the iliac arteries. In this instance, the iliac arteries will be abnormally dilated and thrombus may or may not be present in the dilated areas. Isolated iliac artery aneurysms are an occasional finding (Fig. 3-21).[52]

The accuracy rate for the detection of aortic aneurysms by ultrasonography approaches 100% in most reports.[1,11,49,57,87] Because of this, ultrasound is a very good screening tool as the first step in evaluation of suspected aortic aneurysm, but there are some important considerations to keep in mind to

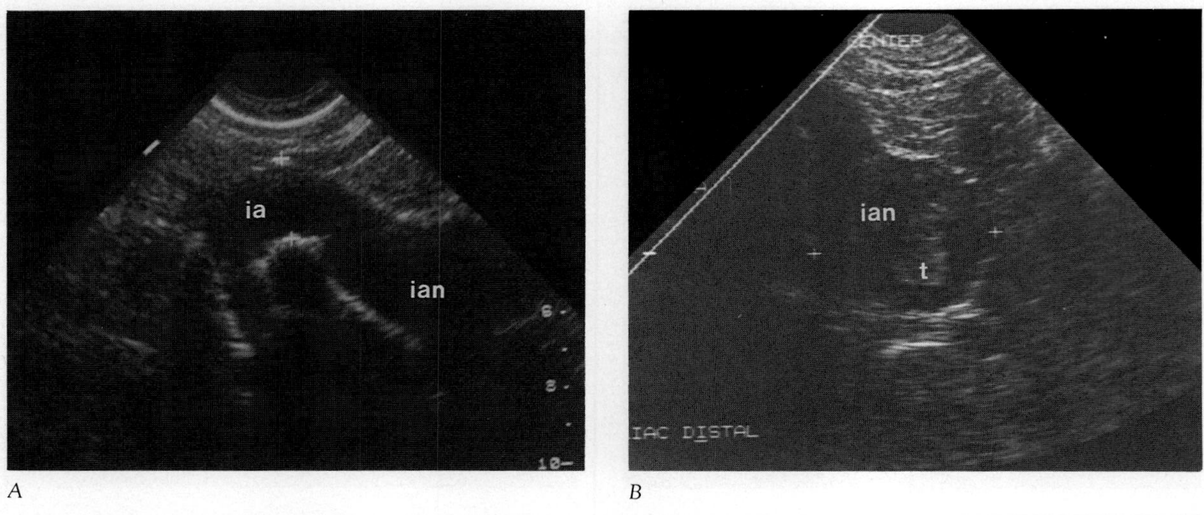

FIGURE 3-21. (*A*) Oblique sonogram of the pelvis through an ectatic iliac artery (ia, note its tortuosity) with associated aneurysm (ian, aneurysmal portion of the artery). (*B*) Transverse sonogram through the iliac artery aneurysm (ian) shown in Figure 3-21A (t, thrombus).

avoid misdiagnosis of an aneurysm. Tortuosity may make the aortic diameter appear larger than it is. This occurs when the plane of imaging is not truly perpendicular to the aortic walls. Therefore, careful observations should be made of the aortic curvature in these instances, to avoid misrepresentation of a tortuous aortic segment as an aortic aneurysm. Excessive air in the abdomen or obesity may obscure the distal aorta and iliac vessels and render some aneurysms invisible. Lymphadenopathy may also confound the picture.[11,49]

Normally, the abundant lymph nodes that are linked together chainlike along the anterior and lateral aspects of the aorta are invisible sonographically. When enlarged, however, their appearance can be dramatic—and initially confusing. Sonographically, enlarged lymph nodes are echo poor, but with increased gain settings, fine internal echoes may be appreciated. Several patterns of lymph node enlargement have been described: isolated large masses, which tend to develop along the aortic chain; mantlelike distributions of enlarged nodes draped atop the aorta and IVC; symmetric nodal enlargement along the aortic chain bilaterally; multiple spindle-shaped nodes dispersed in the mesentery; and large, confluent masses surrounding the aorta and IVC have been reported.[24] It is conceivable that the mantlelike configurations and the confluent mass effects may be confused with aortic aneurysm with thrombus. Close inspection of the area should reveal linear separations between lymph node masses. Also, the general appearance of extensive lymph node enlargement seems to be slightly more irregular, or "lumpy," than an aortic aneurysm.

The rates with which ultrasound can accurately detect renal artery involvement and other abnormalities (ruptured aneurysm) are, unfortunately, not as high as those for aneurysm detection. Therefore, other diagnostic imaging tests are necessary to further evaluate these complications if they are suspected.[1,20]

Recent literature has provided comparative analysis of computed tomography (CT), magnetic resonance imaging (MRI), and ultrasonography in the assessment of aortic aneurysms.[1] Although the study was small, some consistent observations were made. Ultrasonic imaging showed good correlation with CT and MRI assessment of aneurysm size in both AP and transverse diameters. Extension of an anuerysm into the iliac arteries was most consistently depicted with MRI, but good correlation of the ultrasound information existed when the iliac arteries could be imaged. MRI was also superior in evaluating the relationship of the renal arteries to the aneurysm. Even though MRI, and in some instances CT, provided more information, ultrasound was still considered the imaging technique of choice for screening patients suspected of having aortic aneurysms because of its low cost and noninvasive nature.

Aortic Dissection

Description. In aortic dissection, there is a separation of the layers of the arterial wall by blood or hemorrhage which generally begins in the proximal portion of the aorta. According to the DeBakey model there are three types of dissections (Fig. 3-22). Type I and type II involve the ascending aorta and the aortic arch; type III involves the descending aorta at a level below the left subclavian artery. There is a high incidence of mortality with type I and II dissections because of the propensity of the dissection to extend into the pericardium. A lower mortality rate, and a better prognosis, is associated with type III. Type I and III dissections are more common than type II, which are often associated with Marfan's syndrome. Once dissection has begun, it may extend for varying distances along the length of the aorta.[10,38]

Cause. The etiology of aortic dissection is not clear. Presumably the dissection results from a tear of the intimal lining of the aorta. It has been demonstrated, however, that this is not always the case, and postulation has been made that rupture of the

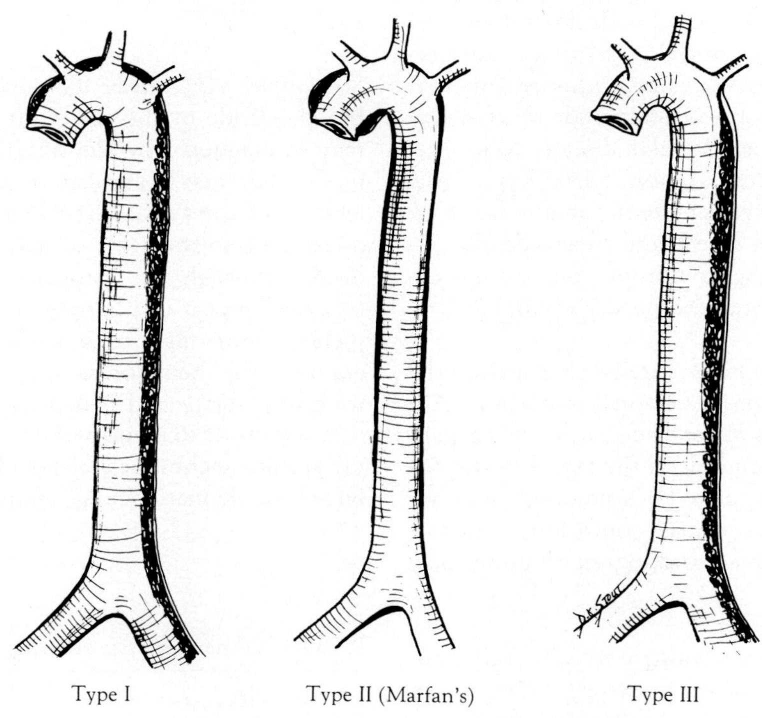

Figure 3-22. The types of aortic dissections as categorized by De Bakey. (Illustration concept from Breshnihan EF, Keates PG: Ultrasound and dissection of the abdominal aorta. Clin Radiol 1980, 31:108).

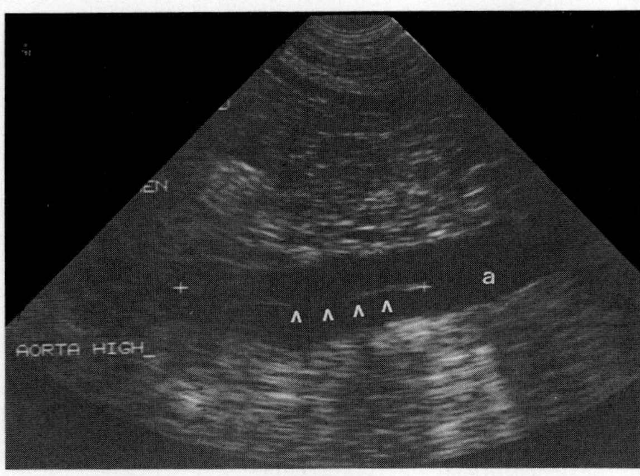

FIGURE 3-23. Longitudinal sonogram through the proximal portion of the abdominal aorta (a) in a patient with a dissection (carets, intimal flap).

vasa vasorum can initiate a dissection.[38,41] Hypertension is strongly associated with dissections, and cystic medial necrosis of the vessel is also well-recognized as an underlying cause. Other entities that contribute to aortic dissection include Marfan syndrome, pregnancy, aortic valve disease, congenital cardiac anomalies (coarctation, aortic hypoplasia, bicuspid aortic valve, persistent patent ductus arteriosus, atrial septal defect, and tricuspid valve abnormalities), Cushing's syndrome, pheochromocytoma, and catheter-induced needle wounds.[10,38,41,45]

Clinical Signs and Symptoms. Intense chest pain is the most common symptom of aortic dissection. Abdominal, as well as lower back, arm, or leg pain may also occur, depending on the extent of the dissection. There may also be vomiting, paralysis, transient blindness, coma, confusion, syncope, headache, and dyspnea, and extremity pulses may be absent.[10,38,41,45]

Sonographic Appearance. Sonographically, aortic dissection appears as a thin, linear echo flap within the arterial lumen (Fig. 3-23).[13] Because of the presence of blood flow along both sides of the dissection, there is usually motion of the flap with each cardiac cycle. Doppler interrogation is an additional diagnostic aid, providing demonstration of arterial blood flow on both sides of the flap. When evaluating a patient for aortic dissection, it is important to utilize both longitudinal and transverse imaging planes to carefully examine the aorta, as an intimal flap can be overlooked if it is located laterally in the artery.[10]

AORTIC RUPTURE

Description. Abdominal aortic aneurysms of any size may rupture, but the risk increases with aneurysms larger than 7 cm in diameter.[11,75,86] Table 3-2 illustrates the risk of aneurysm rupture in one study.[17] Most aneurysms rupture into the peritoneal space, with no predilection for a specific site. They may also rupture into the duodenum, left renal vein, IVC, or urinary tract. The mortality rate for untreated aortic rupture is virtually 100%; with surgery the mortality rate ranges between 40 and 60%.[17]

Clinical Signs and Symptoms. Typically, aortic rupture presents clinically as central back pain and hypotension.[28,41]

Sonographic Appearance. Because of the leakage of blood outside of the vessel lumen, aortic rupture may be diagnosed by identification of a hematoma in the abdomen in association with aneurysmal dilatation of the aorta. These hematomas may be located close to the aorta or may extend to varying degrees through the retroperitoneum. Aortic rupture may appear in a variety of stages, from a completely cystic mass to a complex mass. If large enough, the hematomas may also displace surrounding organs and structures.[79]

It is difficult to identify the actual rupture site by ultrasound techniques, although they may be inferred by hematoma "geography." CT, on the

TABLE 3-2. Aneurysm size and risk of rupture

SIZE (CM)	RISK (%)
<4	9.5
4.0–5.0	23.4
5.1–7.0	25.3
7.1–10.0	45.6
>10.0	60.5

other hand, is well-suited for detection of aortic rupture, as it allows for clear depiction of the extent and density of the hematoma as well as the site of rupture.[79] MRI has also shown potential in identifying early aortic aneurysm rupture sites.[1]

INFLAMMATORY ANEURYSMS

Description. Inflammatory aneurysms are enveloped by a dense, fibrotic reaction, generally including many inflammatory cell infiltrates and fatty tissue. This fibrotic reaction is also vascular in nature and involves the retroperitoneum to different degrees. The inflammatory reaction around the aneurysm may become adherent to the duodenum, sigmoid colon, small bowel, ureter, iliac vein, and inferior vena cava.[15,16,29,83]

Inflammatory aneurysms are an uncommon entity, reportedly between 5 and 20% of all aortic aneurysms.[16] They tend to occur in relatively younger persons than arteriosclerotic aneurysms. Even though the risk of rupture is less than that of a "normal" aneurysm, rupture is still a possible scenario.

Cause. The cause of inflammatory aneurysms is uncertain, but because they are always seen in the presence of an aneurysm, it has been postulated that the aneurysm itself may be the cause of the inflammatory reaction.[15,29]

Clinical Signs and Symptoms. Clinically, the symptoms of inflammatory aneurysms are similar to those of aortic aneurysm. Other symptoms may develop in accordance with the extent of inflammatory involvement to the neighboring areas. These may include leg edema, bothersome pulsations in the epigastrium, and constipation. Hydronephrosis with concomitant flank pain may develop in the presence of ureteral obstruction, and there may be anorexia, early satiety, and dyspepsia if bowel adheres to the aneurysmal inflammation.[6,29]

Sonographic Appearance. Typically, the ultrasonographic features of an inflammatory aneurysm include aneurysmal dilatation of the aorta with a hypoechoic mantle, usually seen anterior and lateral to a thickened aortic wall.[15,16,29] CT can also demonstrate this phenomenon, and it is actually better able to depict the extension of the inflammatory process to the surrounding structures in the retroperitoneum.[16]

It is important to distinguish inflammatory aneurysms from a condition known as retroperitoneal fibrosis.[15] Whereas inflammatory aneurysms are always associated with an aortic aneurysm, retroperitoneal fibrosis is not. Also, the makeup of the two fibrotic reactions is somewhat different. Symptoms of retroperitoneal fibrosis generally do not occur until there is vascular or ureteral compromise. Sonographically, it appears as an echo-free area around the anterior and lateral aspects of the aorta, similar to that seen in association with inflammatory aneurysms, although no aneurysm is present.[37]

Aortic Branch Vessel Aneurysms

SPLANCHNIC ARTERY ANEURYSMS

Splenic Artery Aneurysm.

Description. Splenic artery aneurysms are the most common type of splanchnic artery aneurysms. They are usually multiple and occur in the main splenic arterial trunk. There is apparently a female preponderance. Splenic artery aneurysms though not very common are life threatening.[6,31]

Cause. Causes of splenic artery aneurysm encompass fibromuscular disease of the renal arteries, pancreatic inflammation, peptic ulcer disease, primary arterial injury, and mycotic lesions. There is also a greater potential for patients with portal hypertension and multigravidas to develop splenic artery aneurysms.[6,18,31,86]

Clinical signs and symptoms. Symptoms vary and may range from none to nonspecific left side upper quadrant pain, nausea, vomiting, and a palpable mass if the aneurysm is large enough. There is about a 10% risk of rupture of a splenic artery aneurysm into the peritoneal cavity, with a lesser incidence of rupture into the gastrointestinal tract, spleen, or pancreas.[6]

Hepatic Artery Aneurysms.

Description. Hepatic artery aneurysms are the second most common type of splanchnic vessel aneurysms encountered. Seventy-five percent of all hepatic aneurysms are extrahepatic in origin. The remaining 25% occur intrahepatically, the right hepatic arterial branch being more often affected than the left.[65,71] Hepatic artery aneurysms are rare and tend to male preponderance.[6,31]

Cause. The most common causes of reported hepatic arterial aneurysms are systemic infection, arteriosclerosis, and blunt abdominal trauma. Other, less common causes include iatrogenic trauma, vasculitis due to pancreatitis, chronic cholecystitis, polyarteritis, and congenital abnormalities.[3,21,65,71,88]

Clinical signs and symptoms. Generally, hepatic artery aneurysms are silent or asymptomatic until the aneurysm attains large size or ruptures. When symptoms do occur, they are often vague and unclear and may include any of the following: epigastric pain (two-thirds of patients), gastrointestinal bleeding due to rupture of the aneurysm into the biliary tract and resulting hemobilia, and obstructive jaundice.[3,71] Because of the propensity of hepatic artery aneurysms to rupture, early detection is important so that prompt treatment can be obtained.

Superior Mesenteric Artery Aneurysm.

Description. Superior mesenteric aneurysms are the rarest of the splanchnic arterial aneurysms (reported incidence approximately 1 in 12,000). Branch superior mesenteric arterial aneurysms are also quite rare.[6,31]

Cause. The most common cause that has been cited in the pathogenesis of superior mesenteric artery aneurysms is cystic medial necrosis (mycotic aneurysm), which accounts for approximately 58% of the aneurysms detected. Arteriosclerosis, medial degeneration, and trauma have also been associated with superior mesenteric artery aneurysms.[31]

Clinical signs and symptoms. There may be intestinal angina and postprandial abdominal pain in association with a superior mesenteric artery aneurysm. General abdominal pain and fever (in association with the mycotic type aneurysms) may also be present.[6,31] Again, as with the other splanchnic vessel aneurysms, the symptoms are generally vague and nonspecific.

Sonographic Appearance of Splanchnic Artery Aneurysms. Sonographically, splanchnic artery aneurysms appear similar to one another. The distinguishing difference is location in the abdomen. All splanchnic aneurysms may appear as an anechoic or complex abdominal mass. Arterial pulsations or thrombus may or may not be discernible.[55] By demonstrating continuity of the mass with one of the splanchnic arteries, splanchnic artery aneurysms can be identified with a higher degree of confidence, but this is a difficult task to accomplish. Therefore in order to confirm or refute the vascular nature of the lesion, Doppler sonography should always be used to further investigate an anechoic or complex mass in the upper abdomen. In the case of a splanchnic artery aneurysm, the Doppler signal demonstrates turbulent arterial pulsations. Color-flow Doppler technology is also of benefit in this type of setting, as the blood flow patterns in these aneurysms are clearly recognized by their characteristic color patterns.

RENAL ARTERY ANEURYSMS

Description. Over the last two decades, renal artery aneurysms have been encountered with increasing frequency, although the overall incidence remains relatively low.[67] Most renal artery aneurysms tend to be extrarenal, but there are reports of intrarenal aneurysms. Generally, surgical intervention is required in the presence of aneurysms greater than 1.5 cm and associated pain, bleeding, or hypertension.[52] The prevalence of renal artery aneurysm rupture is about 20%.

Cause. Renal artery aneurysms are most commonly a result of atherosclerosis and polyarteritis, and represent true aneurysms; congenital abnormalities account for a relatively smaller portion of them. Aneurysms resulting from iatrogenic trauma, blunt trauma, or penetrating trauma are considered false aneurysms and tend to be among the least common types.[52]

Clinical Signs and Symptoms. Symptoms encountered with renal artery aneurysm may include a palpable mass, hypertension, and blood in the urine along with flank pain.[52]

Sonographic Appearance. A renal artery aneurysm appears as an anechoic mass along the extent of the renal artery, or occasionally intrarenally. Calcification of the wall may be present, and other findings may or may not include thrombus formation along the periphery of the mass and pulsations. Demonstrating continuity of the mass with the renal artery is a useful indicator of renal artery aneurysm. Doppler ultrasound interrogation is an excellent method of distinguishing the vascular nature of a suspicious mass in this area. The Doppler characteristics of a renal artery aneurysm include a turbulent arterial blood flow signal.

Care must be taken in the evaluation of renal artery aneurysms, since it is possible to mistake a normal left renal vein for a left renal artery aneurysm, especially in thin patients.[52] This is due to the fact that the left renal vein is prominent as it exits the renal hilus, but as it passes over the aorta to enter the IVC it narrows. At this point, part of the aortic wall may not be visualized owing to the angle of the incident ultrasound beam, and subsequently the renal vein may appear to arise from the aorta. In order to clarify this situation it may be helpful to study the area in question during suspended inspiration. If the structure is truly venous, the entire venous path should dilate, affording better visualization. If the vessel is arterial, inspiration techniques will not affect its size. Doppler investigation is probably the method of choice to determine the nature of the area in question. If the "mass" is found to have characteristic continuous low-velocity flow, it is most likely the renal vein. If arterial pulsations can be detected, the vessel is most likely the renal artery.

Iliac Artery Aneurysms

Description. Iliac artery aneurysms are most often associated with (continuations of) abdominal aortic aneurysms. Isolated iliac aneurysms are possible, however, and when they occur, tend to be bilateral. Isolated internal iliac artery aneurysms are rare. Half of all untreated iliac aneurysms rupture, making this the most common complication of iliac aneurysms.[52]

Cause. Most iliac aneurysms are arteriosclerotic in origin. Other, less common causes include external or surgical trauma, pregnancy, congenital abnormality, syphilis, and bacterial infection.[52]

Clinical Signs and Symptoms. Iliac artery aneurysms typically go unrecognized clinically and are often discovered unexpectedly. Because of compression on surrounding structures large iliac aneurysms may produce urologic, gastrointestinal, or neurologic symptoms. Pain may also be present, and a mass may be palpated on physical examination.[52]

Sonographic Appearance. An iliac artery aneurysm appears as a primarily anechoic mass in the pelvis. Smaller aneurysms may be difficult to identify in the presence of profuse bowel gas. Pulsations may be present. Thrombus may also be present along the periphery of the mass and calcific changes may be visualized within the wall. Continuity with the iliac artery is a strong indicator for iliac artery aneurysm, and Doppler ultrasonography reveals a turbulent arterial signal. Because of the strong tendency toward bilaterality, the contralateral iliac artery should also be examined carefully (see Fig. 3-21).[52]

Aortic Grafts and Associated Complications

Diagnostic medical ultrasound is useful not only for the detection of arterial abnormalities such as aneurysms but also for the assessment of aortic grafts and their related complications.

Description. An aortic graft or prosthesis is usually a manmade structure used to repair an aortic aneurysm. Grafts can be made of various materials including Teflon and Dacron. The graft is commonly attached by an end-to-end anastomosis to the normal portion of the aorta after the aneurysm is removed.[30] In some instances, the original aneurysm may be retained and actually sewn around the prosthesis as a stabilizer.[92] In aortofemoral bypass surgery the diseased segment of the aorta is left intact and an end-to-side anastomotic graft technique is used, resulting in graft placement anterior and adjacent to the native vessel.[30]

Sonographic Appearance. Sonographically, graft replacements are easily detected by their characteristic wall brightness, and at times it may also be possible to see their ribbing. The graft walls are also straighter than native vessel walls. At the level of the proximal anastomosis, the graft is usually seen to dive posteriorly and continue its course inferiorly with a slight angulation toward the anterior abdominal wall.[52] The graft then bifurcates, and a connection should be demonstrated at the iliac artery level or the common femoral artery level, depending on the extent of the prosthesis.

PSEUDOANEURYSMS

Of all aortic graft complications, pseudoaneurysms are perhaps the most common.[30,52,89] They occur at the site of anastomosis and result from bleeding at this site or from trauma. In essence, there is a pulsating hematoma connected to the lumen of the graft–native vessel interface. The presence of a pulsating mass is usually the first clinical evidence that a pseudoaneurysm may be forming. It may be demonstrated as a graft ending abruptly in an anechoic mass, but it is more often seen as a pulsating fluid collection near the site of anastomosis. Doppler interrogation of the mass reveals turbulent arterial signals, and color-flow Doppler affords a dramatic representation of the swirling blood flow patterns within pseudoaneurysms as well as their leakage site.

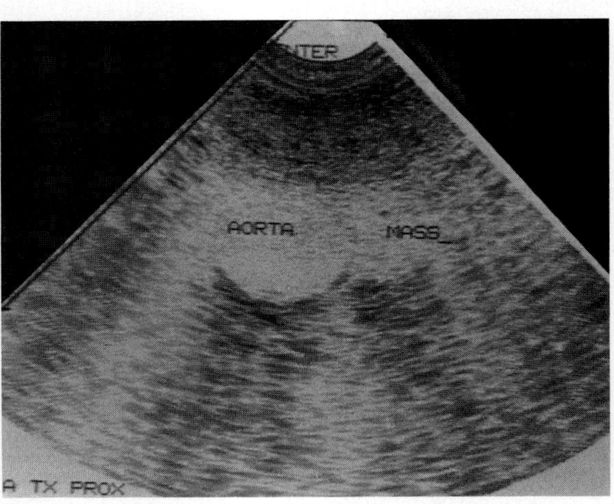

FIGURE 3-24. Transverse sonogram through an aortic graft with associated hematoma (mass).

GRAFT ANEURYSMS

Graft aneurysms result from degeneration of the graft material and appear sonographically as focal dilatations of the actual graft material. These are not common complications of aortic grafts.

HEMATOMAS

Hematomas are a normal part of the healing process of graft replacement surgery. Sonographically, they may present as an anechoic or complex mass in the area of the graft (Fig. 3-24).

ABSCESSES

Abscesses may also have a sonographic appearance consistent with an anechoic or a complex mass in the area of a graft. Consequently, it may be impossible to differentiate between abscesses and hematomas by sonographic appearance alone. In these instances, clinical signs such as tenderness in the area, history of fever, leukocytosis, and local erythema may be useful in differentiating an infectious process from a hematoma. If there is any question, aspiration of the fluid under ultrasonographic guidance will be diagnostic.

OCCLUSION

Graft occlusion was an elusive complication foı sonographers until the advent of Doppler techniques. Now, it is relatively simple to verify flow through a graft. Once the graft is located by real-time scanning, the Doppler sample volume cursor is moved into the graft lumen. If flow is present, it registers as arterial pulsations. Absence of flow denotes occlusion of the graft. Often, even though there is a complete occlusion, plain B-mode imaging cannot demonstrate the occluding clot.[30] Therefore, duplex Doppler is essential in this diagnosis. Color-flow Doppler dramatically represents flow within a graft, and can be used in conjunction with conventional Doppler to confirm graft patency.

Vascular Stenosis

Discussion of arterial abnormalities would not be complete if the subject of stenosis was not mentioned. Although there have not been many publications about this particular aspect of abdominal vascular diagnosis, currently there seems to be increasing interest. Recently published studies show encouraging results in the area of abdominal vascular stenosis.

Until recently, angiography, and no other method of medical imaging, was very successful in the actual investigation of abdominal visceral artery stenosis. With current Doppler technology capable of detecting blood flow at greater distances than was once possible, new interest has been generated in the possibility of a noninvasive means of evaluating suspected visceral artery stenosis.

Studies have shown that blood flow volumes through the visceral arteries can be assessed by Doppler techniques with a relative degree of accuracy when compared to more invasive methods.[4,50,54,61,63,69,72] Although promising, Doppler blood flow volumes studies are time consuming and their accuracy is limited by several inherent problems of the technique, such as underestimation of vessel diameter and overestimation of average blood flow velocity.

Even if Doppler techniques could precisely estimate flow volume, its routine use in the clinical setting would seem to be limited, as evidenced by prior investigations of significant peripheral occlusive arterial disease. It has been established that volume flows are not particularly helpful in the assessment of stenotic lesions because collateral pathways "normalize" flow volume beyond areas of stenosis. Therefore, investigators were led to identify significant stenoses qualitatively by recognition of the changes taking place in blood flow physiology.[92]

The commonly recognized two-dimensional and Doppler findings in association with vascular stenosis are as follows:[92]

1. Vessel lumen narrowed by atheromatous plaque or arteriosclerotic changes
2. Poststenotic dilatation
3. Increased velocities in the area of stenosis
4. Downstream changes: Turbulence (increases as the percentage of stenosis increases); decreased velocities; slowed acceleration during systole; and relative elevation of diastolic velocities

Because it may be difficult to visualize occlusive plaque in the visceral arteries, Doppler interrogation becomes very important in the assessment of visceral artery occlusive disease.

Before abnormal Doppler signals can be appreciated it is essential to be familiar with normal Doppler waveform patterns of the major abdominal visceral arteries (Fig. 3-25).

Renal Artery Stenosis

Description. Renal artery stenosis is a significant medical problem because of its association with uncontrollable hypertension. Other consequences of renal artery stenosis include decreased glomerular filtration rate and ischemic renal damage.[5,35]

Diagnostic Technique and Criteria. Several methods of blood flow analysis are useful in determining the presence of significant stenosis. These methods are based on the physiologic alterations that occur as a vessel is narrowed by occlusive plaques.

One team of investigators used direct visualization and Doppler interrogation of the renal arteries in an attempt to localize blood flow disturbances.[44,76] Examinations begin with a real-time search for the renal arteries and proceed with Doppler velocity recordings along the course of each artery. Multiple patient positions and scanning angles are required to facilitate complete visualization of the renal arteries. Some helpful suggestions include using the IVC as a window to the right renal artery and the left renal vein as a window to the left renal artery (Fig. 3-26). Diligence and innovative thinking are necessary to examine renal arteries thoroughly.

After real-time and Doppler evaluation of the renal artery, aortic blood flow velocity is also determined for comparison against the velocities of the renal arteries. The criteria used to determine the presence of a significant renal artery stenosis are shown on Table 3-3 (Fig. 3-27).

Of those arteries identified and adequately scanned, there was a sensitivity of 84%, specificity of 97%, and a positive predictive value of 94% for stenosis greater than 60%. There was overall agreement with angiography in 93% of the cases. The noninvasiveness of this procedure also lent itself to follow-up of postsurgical patients for the detection of recurrent stenosis, and results were encouraging.[44,76]

Because this technique relies heavily on the visualization and interrogation of the length of the renal arteries, it is a time-consuming and difficult procedure to master. Also, as a result of body habitus and excessive bowel air, inadequate examinations were reported in about 12.4% of patients.

A separate study conducted by Handa and colleagues used somewhat different criteria for the as-

(text continues on page 72)

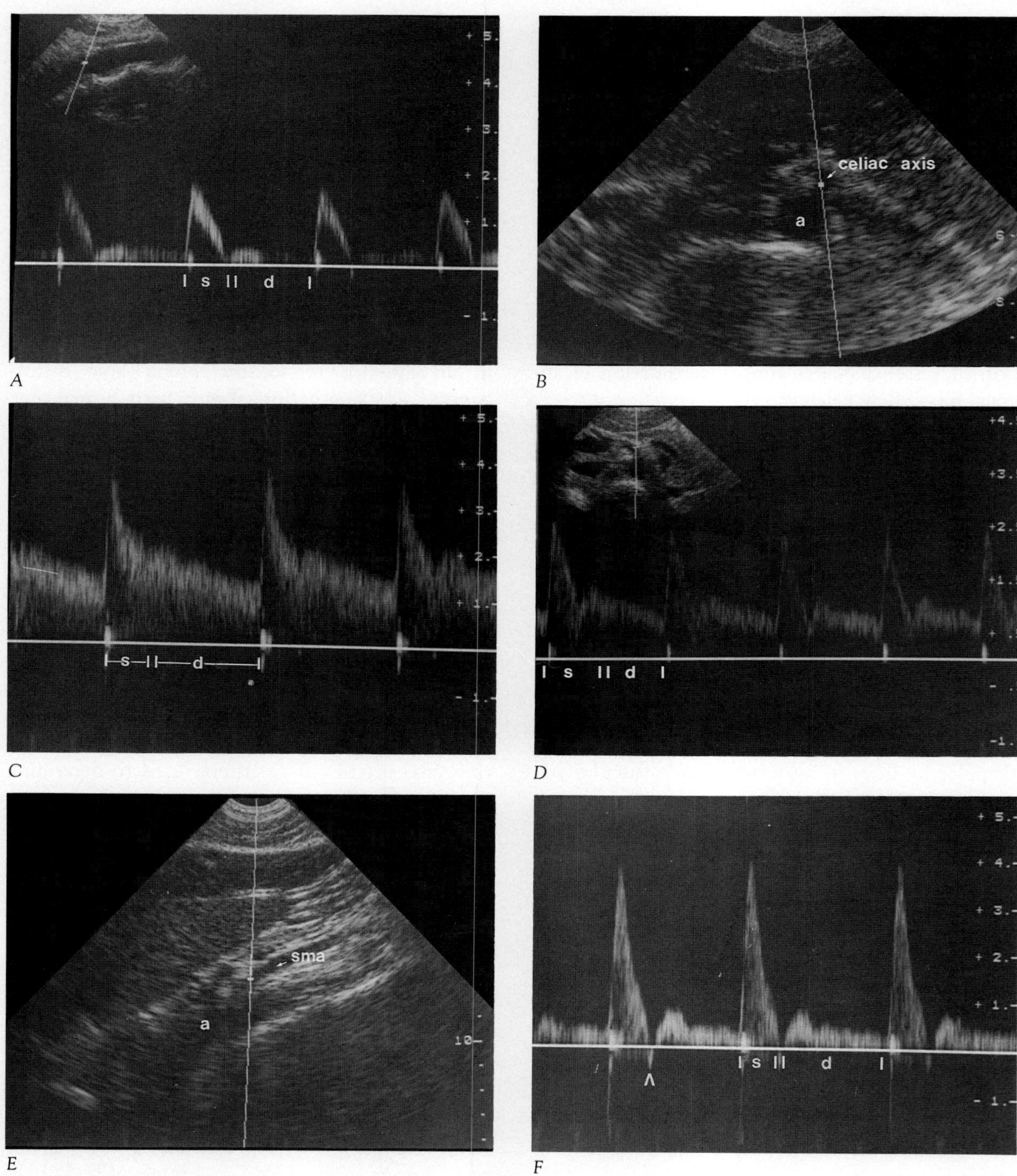

A B C D E F

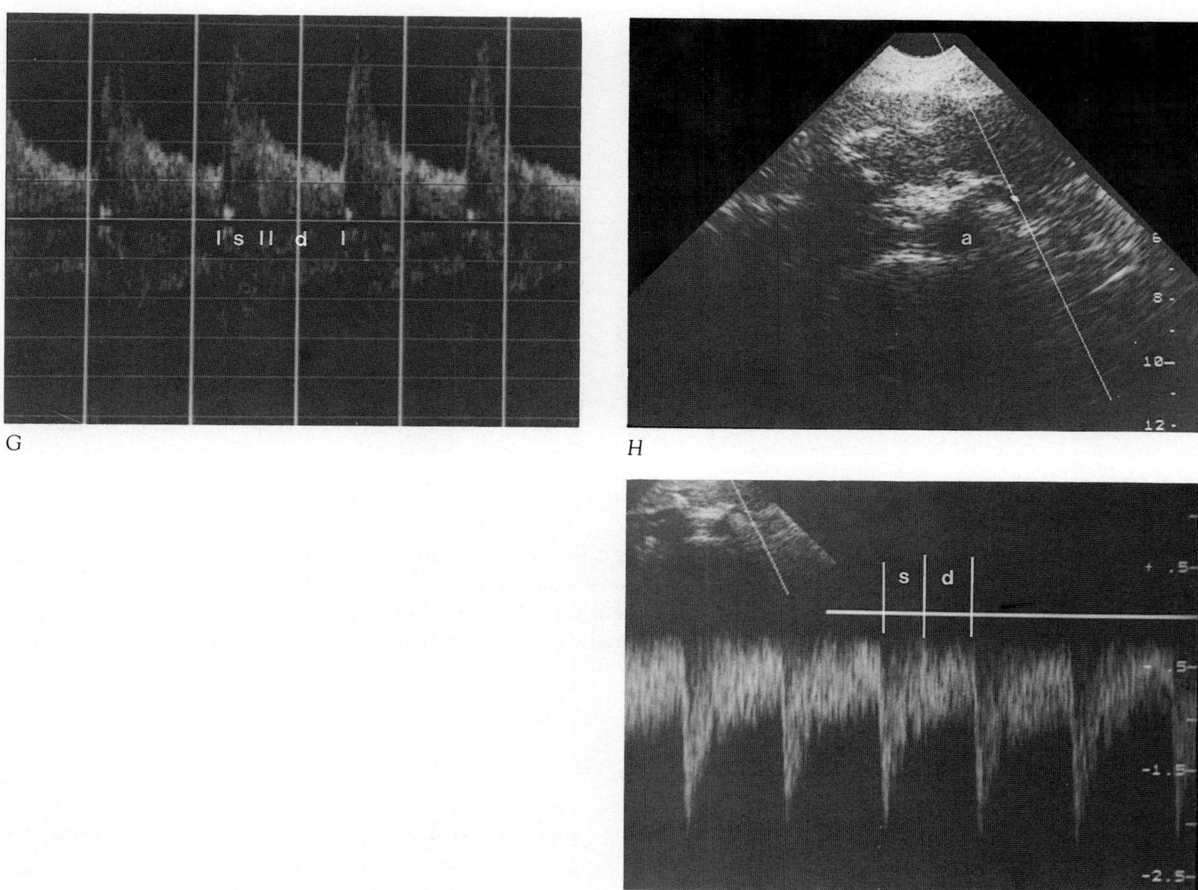

FIGURE 3-25. (*A*) Doppler tracing of the blood flow in the abdominal aorta. Note the low flow state of the blood in diastole represented as that part of the wave form closest to the 0 line (s, systole; d, diastole). (*B*) Transverse sonogram at the level of the celiac axis. Doppler sample placed in the celiac axis (a, aorta). (*C*) Doppler spectral tracing of the blood flow in the celiac axis. Note the high velocity of blood flow in diastole, which is representative of circulation to an area of low resistance (s, systole; d, diastole). In a low-resistance vascular bed flow through the arteries is relatively constant. (*D*) Doppler sample placed in the proximal hepatic artery and Doppler spectral tracing of the blood flow in the hepatic artery. Note the relatively rapid flow during diastole as compared with that in the aorta (s, systole; d, diastole). (*E*) Longitudinal sonogram of the aorta (a) made with the Doppler sample volume in the superior mesenteric artery (sma). (*F*) Doppler spectral tracing of the superior mesenteric artery in a fasting patient. Note the reversal of flow below the zero line in diastole (*arrowhead*) and the low-velocity flow throughout diastole. This is characteristic of blood flow to a highly resistant vascular bed (s, systole; d, diastole). (*G*) Doppler spectral tracing of blood flow through the renal artery. Note the relatively fast diastolic flow (s, systole; d, diastole). (*H*) Transverse sonogram through the aorta (a) with the Doppler sample volume placed in the splenic artery (sa). (*I*) Doppler spectral tracing of blood flow through the splenic artery. Note the relatively large diastolic flow component in the Doppler wave form (s, systole; d, diastole).

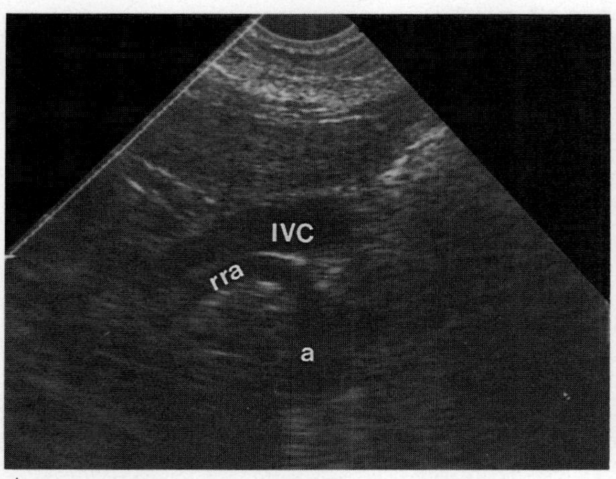

A

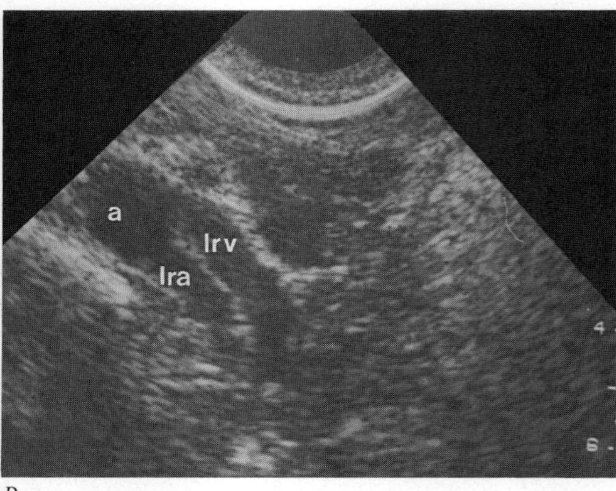

B

FIGURE 3-26. (*A*) Patient is in the left decubitus position, and the transducer is angled to use the inferior vena cava (IVC) as a window to see the right renal artery (rra); (a, aorta). (*B*) Patient is in the right decubitus position, and the transducer is angled to use the left renal vein (lrv) as a window to see the left renal artery (lra); (a, aorta).

TABLE 3-3. Criteria for renal artery stenosis

STENOSIS (%)	DUPLEX CRITERIA
0–59	RAR* <3.5, usually without localized velocity increase or poststenotic turbulence
60–90	RAR $\geq$ to 3.5, with localized increased velocity and poststenotic turbulence
Occlusion	No flow signal from renal artery, low-amplitude velocity signal from the renal parenchyma, and small kidney (length <9 cm) with an adequate examination

$$*RAR = \frac{\text{peak renal artery velocity}}{\text{peak aortic artery velocity}}$$

(Velocity measurements are angle corrected.)
(From Taylor DC, Kettler MD, Moneta GL, et al: J Vasc Surg 1988, 7:363–369.)

sessment and identification of significant renal artery stenosis. These studies claim higher success and accuracy rates than the method previously described.[34,35] This particular examination involved obtaining Doppler waveforms at the hilum of the kidney in the renal artery proper or its segmental branches and in the aorta at the level of the renal artery origins.[34,35] Characteristics of the Doppler signals were measured and calculated, then set against the norm. These diagnostic indices (Table 3-4) include acceleration index (AI), acceleration time (AT), and acceleration time ratio (ATR; Fig. 3-28).

The findings of this group have substantiated their earlier reports that the acceleration index decreases downstream from a significant stenosis and the acceleration time increases. The acceleration time ratio was used to offset the effects of dysfunction, however, it was less specific and sensitive than either AI or AT in the evaluation of renal artery stenosis.

According to the study, this method was 95% accurate in determining the presence of significant

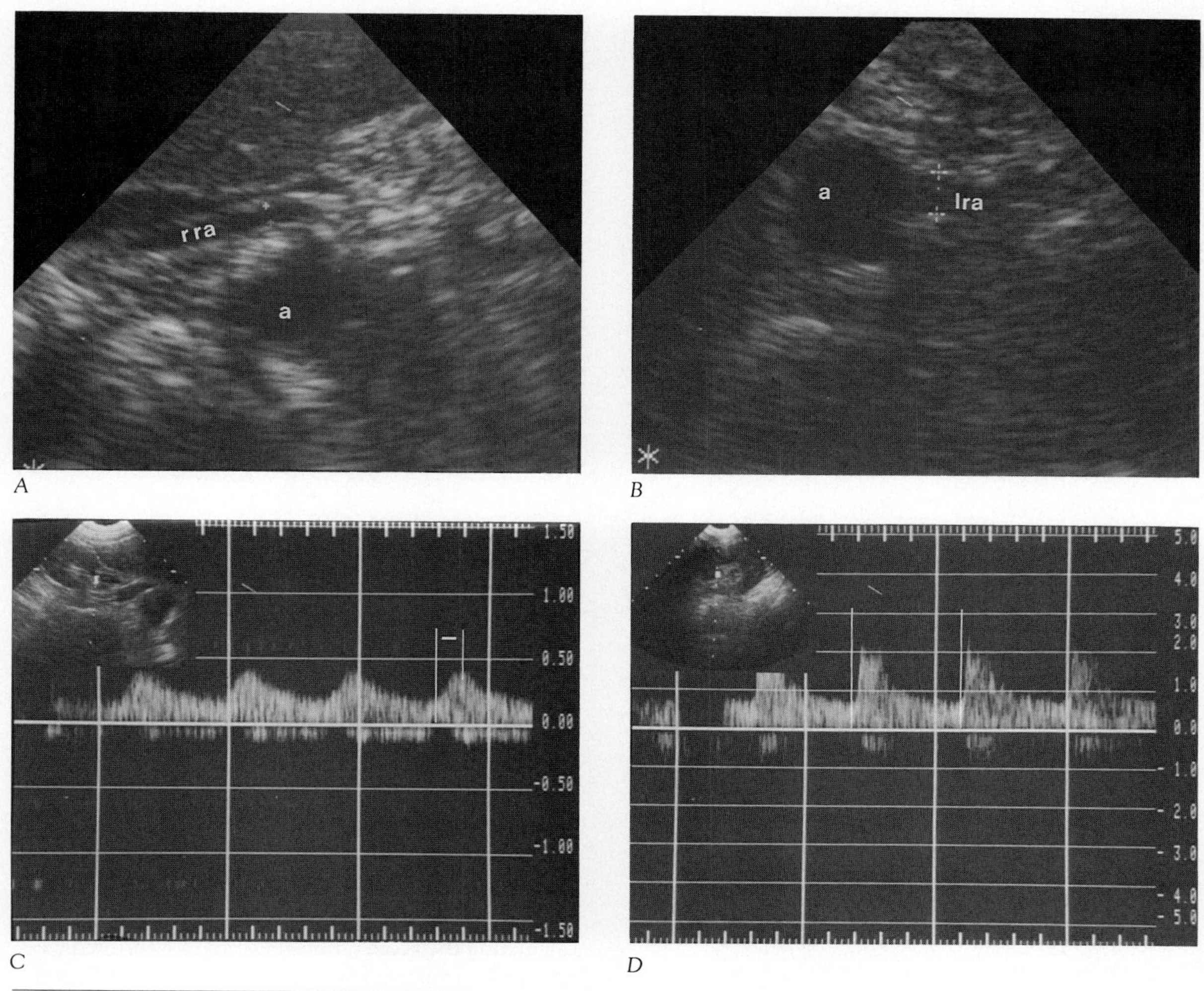

FIGURE 3-27. (*A*) Transverse sonogram through the aorta (a) at the level of the right renal artery in a patient with a total occlusion of the right renal artery (rra). No signal was detected by Doppler interrogation. (*B*) Transverse sonogram through the aorta (a) at the level of the left renal artery (lra) in the same patient. Note how much larger the left renal artery is than the right renal artery (cursors measure lra diameter). (C) Doppler spectral tracing in one of the right intrarenal arteries of the same patient. (*D*) Doppler spectral tracing in one of the left intrarenal arteries. Note the difference in the initial upsweep of the tracings between the affected kidney *(right)*, and the normal one *(left)*. Also, the amplitude (or velocity) of the signal from the affected kidney is much lower than that of the normal one.

stenosis. Specificity was 95%, and sensitivity was 100%. There were some false positive and false negative results, which were attributed to a kink in the abdominal aorta or the renal artery and to very stenotic vessels in which the acceleration times were relatively quick owing to the slow flow states downstream from the stenosis. Data showed that the acceleration index was probably the most sensitive measurement for identifying significant renal artery stenosis.[34,35]

TABLE 3-4. Normal ranges for Doppler analysis of renal artery

MEASUREMENT	EXPECTED VALUE
Acceleration index	>3.78
Acceleration time	<0.07
Acceleration time ratio	<1.35

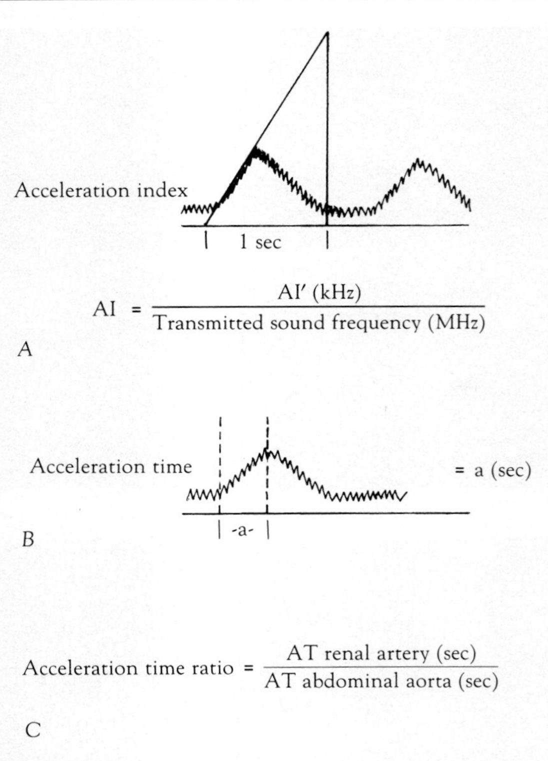

FIGURE 3-28. (*A*) The method of calculating acceleration index. The illustrations are representative of Doppler spectral tracings and the method of obtaining information from them. (*B*) The method of calculating the acceleration time. (C) The method of calculating the acceleration-time ratio. (Reprinted with permission from Handa N, Fukunaga R, Etani H, et al: Efficacy of echo-Doppler examination for the evaluation of renovascular disease. Ultrasound Med Biol 1988, 14:2. Copyright 1987 Pergamon Press.)

Mesenteric Insufficiency

Mesenteric insufficiency can be acute or chronic. Angiography is still considered the primary diagnostic tool to demonstrate acute occlusion of the vessels supplying the small bowel because expedient detection and intervention is necessary to prevent catastrophic consequences. On the other hand, Doppler ultrasonography may find a role in diagnosis of visceral artery stenosis in patients presenting with chronic mesenteric ischemia, a much less ominous disease.

Chronic mesenteric insufficiency has been established as an uncommon disease process whose vague symptoms make it difficult to diagnose; however, patients with chronic mesenteric insufficiency may suffer from intestinal angina 15 to 30 minutes after eating. Weight loss may also occur.[41,56]

A recent study indicates that combined stenosis and/or occlusion of the superior mesenteric and celiac arteries is associated with intestinal angina rather than an isolated stenosis of either vessel.[56] This is probably best explained by the abundance of collaterals available to the intestine when only one vessel is diseased.

In most cases, the cause of superior mesenteric and celiac artery stenosis is atherosclerosis. Arteriosclerotic or atherosclerotic changes in the coronary arteries and other aortic branches may be associated findings.[41]

DOPPLER FINDINGS IN SUPERIOR MESENTERIC ARTERY

The Doppler examination begins by placing the transducer just below the xiphoid process of a fasting patient to obtain a longitudinal section of the superior mesenteric artery. The Doppler sample volume is then moved to the vessel origin, and Doppler analysis is performed. At times, it may be necessary to use a transverse scanning plane to better visualize and interrogate the proximal portion of the superior mesenteric artery.

In a prepandial (fasting) state, Doppler spectral analysis of the normal superior mesenteric artery reveals a characteristic pattern that is associated with a highly resistant vascular bed. There is a sharp rise in flow during systole, and a rapid falloff during diastole with reversal of flow below the baseline (Figure 3-25f). In the postprandial state (after ingestion of a meal), the blood flow characteristics change and exhibit reduced or absent reversal of flow during the diastolic phase of the cardiac cycle concomitant with increased peak forward diastolic flow.[62]

With significant stenosis of the superior mesenteric artery, a loss of the reversed flow component,

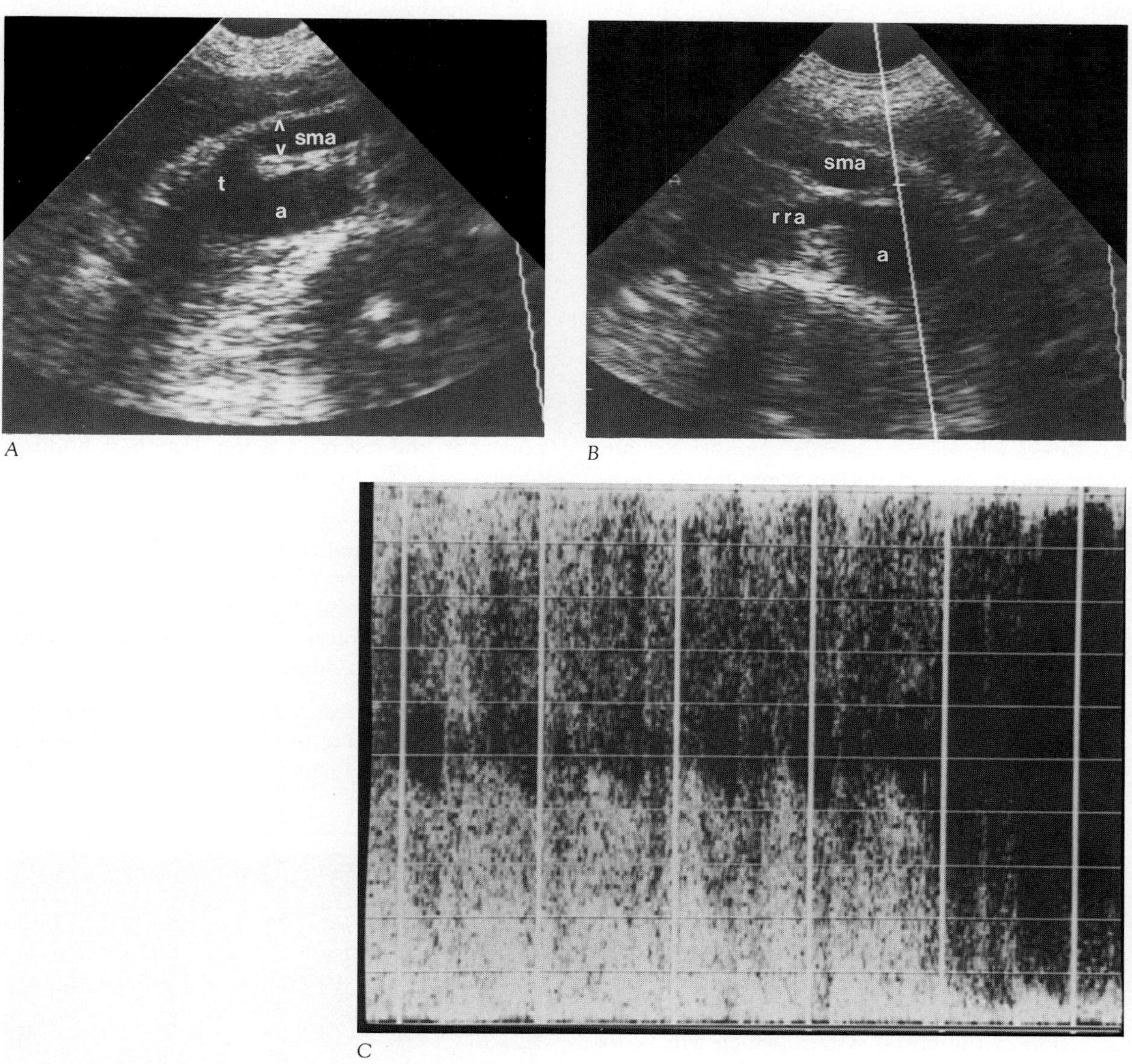

FIGURE 3-29. (*A*) Oblique sonogram through a stenotic superior mesenteric artery showing some poststenotic dilatation *(arrows)*; (a, aorta; sma, superior mesenteric artery; t, occluding thrombus or plaque near the origin of the vessel). (*B*) Oblique sonogram of the superior mesenteric artery with placement of the Doppler sample in the area of vessel narrowing (a, aorta; rra, right renal artery; sma, superior mesenteric artery). (C) Doppler spectral tracing of the stenotic portion of the superior mesenteric artery. Note the high amplitude of the signal. The normally decreased flow during diastole cannot be observed in this fasting patient. Instead, there is high-velocity diastolic flow with associated turbulence, as represented by the filled-in appearance beneath the outer edges of the spectral tracing.

even in the prepandial state, has been noted. Abnormally high velocities with associated poststenotic turbulence are also detected in the narrowed region of the vessel. Visually, poststenotic dilatation and arteriosclerotic plaque may be seen[56] (Figures 3-29A–C).

DOPPLER FINDINGS IN THE CELIAC ARTERY

Again, the transducer is placed in a subxyphoid position oriented to obtain a transverse view of the celiac artery. Doppler interrogation proceeds along the course of the vessel.

Doppler findings suggesting significant celiac artery stenosis include: a localized area of high velocity, post-stenotic turbulence, and blunted flow downstream from a highgrade stenosis. Visually, poststenotic vessel dilatation may also be recognized (Figures 3-30A–C).

Although these general guidelines can be used to suggest superior mesenteric and celiac artery stenosis, specific velocity criteria have not yet been published. Therefore, extreme care must be taken in the Doppler evaluation of patients with suspected mesenteric artery stenosis. Further investigation into this area may produce more objective diagnostic criteria for the detection of significant superior mesenteric and celiac artery stenosis.

HEPATIC ARTERY WITH A HEPATIC TRANSPLANT

Description. The area of hepatic artery Doppler examination is becoming very popular, especially in the investigation of liver transplant recipients. The portable nature of the technique makes it a very good tool for the detection of postsurgical complications such as occlusion of the hepatic artery or occlusion of the portal system (which will be discussed in the following section, Venous Abnormalities).

Technique. Initially, the transducer is placed intercostally to identify the portal vein. After the portal vein is visualized, the transducer is maneuvered to identify the hepatic artery, usually located anterior to the portal vein. The Doppler sample volume is electronically moved into the area of interest to identify blood flow. Color-flow Doppler instrumentation is very helpful for hepatic artery localization and subsequent placement of the sample volume. In a normal examination, the Doppler flow pattern is pulsatile and has a high diastolic flow component owing to the low resistance of the blood bed in the liver. Absent or very blunted flow is almost always indicative of hepatic arterial obstruction and is most critical in the immediate postoperative period. If hepatic arterial occlusion occurs in the later period of transplant recovery, its significance is not as profound because of the collateral circulation that has had a chance to develop.[78]

Originally it was hoped that liver transplant rejection could be reliably detected using hepatic artery duplex scanning techniques as well. In these instances, the hepatic arterial Doppler signal was expected to show evidence of increased vascular resistance, depicted as a decreased diastolic flow component in the spectral tracing, but these findings turned out to be inconsistent.[78]

Venous Abnormalities

VENA CAVAL OBSTRUCTION

In order to assess the IVC for the presence of obstruction it is important to remember the effects of normal respiration on it:

1. IVC caliber decreases during initial inspiration.
2. After suspended respiration, the IVC enlarges to its maximum diameter.

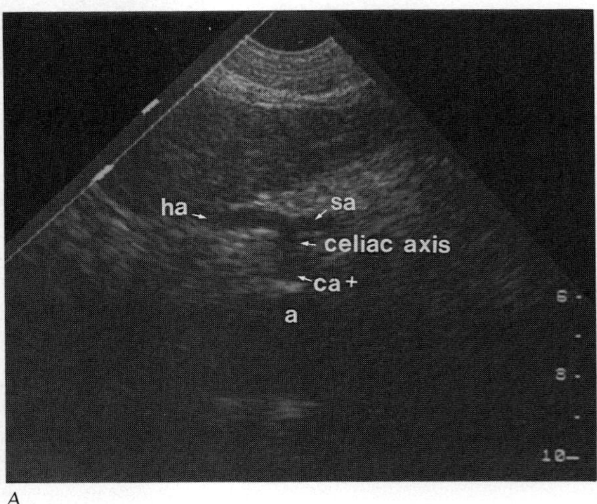

FIGURE 3-30. (*A*) Transverse sonogram through the aorta at the level of the celiac axis demonstrates calcification (ca^+) at the origin of the celiac axis (a, aorta; ha, hepatic artery; sa, splenic artery).

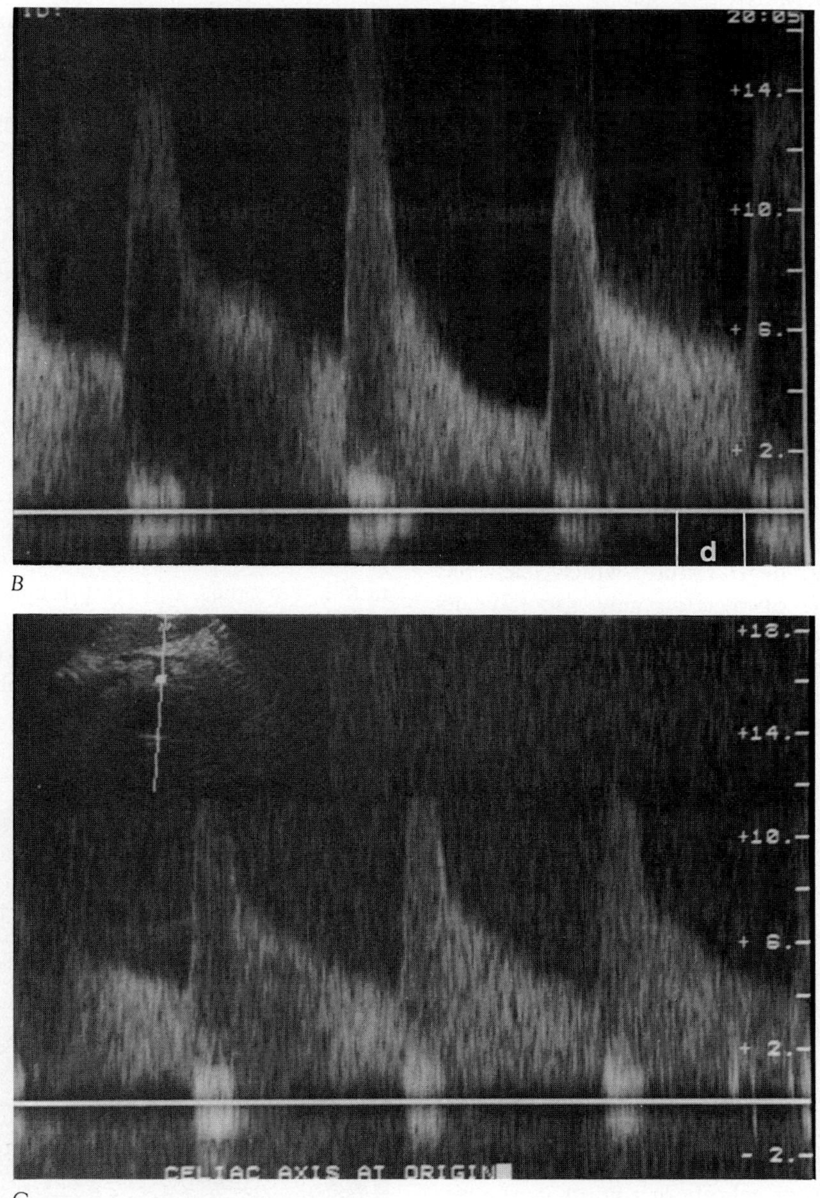

Figure 3-30 (*continued*). (*B*) In this Doppler tracing of the blood flow in the celiac axis at the level of the calcification note the high amplitude of the signal and the broadening of the spectral trace during diastole (d). (C) Doppler tracing of the blood flow farther from the calcification in the celiac axis. Note the filled-in appearance of the entire spectrum, which is indicative of turbulent flow.

3. IVC caliber enlarges during expiration.
4. IVC caliber diminishes, nearly obliterating the lumen, during the Valsalva maneuver, owing to the increased abdominal pressure created by this technique.

Because of the variations in the caliber of the IVC during respiration it is imperative that IVC examinations be done in a consistent manner. This is usually best accomplished by examining while the patient suspends inspiration.[32]

Description. When blood flow in the IVC is obstructed, the normal response of the vessel is to increase in caliber below the point of obstruction. Because of the elastic capacity of the veins, the expansion of the IVC can be quite dramatic.

Etiology. The most common cause of IVC obstruction is right-sided heart failure, which itself has many causes. IVC obstruction may also have its origins with an enlarged liver, para-aortic lymph node enlargement, retroperitoneal masses or tumors, and pancreatic tumors. A congenital IVC valve may also obstruct the lumen of the IVC.[41]

Clinical Signs and Symptoms. Signs and symptoms may include abdominal pain, ascites, or tender hepatomegaly. Lower extremity edema may also be present in the more severe forms of IVC blockage.[41]

Sonographic Appearance. In the presence of obstruction, the IVC tends to dilate below the level of obstruction. Respiratory changes are decreased or absent below the obstructed segment.[77]

In right-sided heart failure, the proximal IVC and hepatic veins become congested, resulting in a concurrent increase in diameter (Fig. 3-31). Respiratory changes are markedly decreased or absent.

Solid, complex, or echo-poor tumors in the retroperitoneum or pancreas may be seen to impinge on the IVC. If large enough, they can obstruct the vessel, and dilatation below the impingement would be recognized. Intravenous tumors, primary or metastatic, also obstruct flow within the IVC. Again, dilatation of the vein below the tumor mass will be identified.

In the superior vena cava obstruction syndrome, collateral vein formation and enlargement may develop involving the epigastric veins, the ligamentum teres, and the caudate lobe veins.[77]

Tumors of the Inferior Vena Cava

Tumors of the IVC may be primary, metastatic, or an extension from a primary.

Primary Tumors. Primary tumors of the IVC, most of which are leiomyomas or leiomyosarcomas, tend to be uncommon (vascular incidence only 2%). These types of tumors tend to develop in women and the median age of detection is 61 years. With leiomyosarcomas, metastasis to the liver and lung has been reported in 40% to 50% of cases. A 36% recurrence rate is also reported, and prognosis is poor.[8,12]

Metastasis or Extension of Tumors. Malignant invasion of the IVC may occur from renal carcinoma (the most commonly reported incidence at 9 to 33%), secreting and nonsecreting adrenal tumors, retroperitoneal sarcomas, hepatocellular carcinoma, teratomas, and lymphomas.[19]

Clinical Signs and Symptoms. Symptoms are generally unremarkable, but this depends on tumor size and

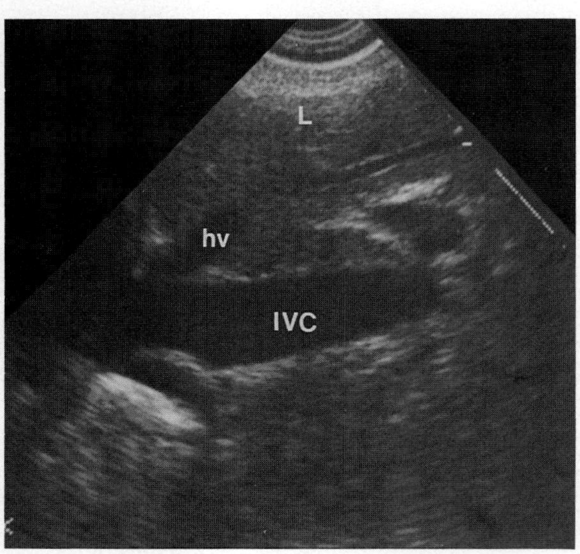

Figure 3-31. On a longitudinal sonogram through the inferior vena cava of a patient with increased right-sided heart pressures, note the large caliber of the vessel. No respiratory changes were noted (IVC, inferior vena cava; hv, hepatic vein; L, liver).

the degree of obstruction they present to the IVC. With tumors of large proportions, leg edema as well as ascites and abdominal pain may develop.[77] This is true for the primary tumors of the IVC as well as those that are metastatic.

Sonographic Appearance. Tumors within the IVC tend to appear as echogenic foci. Occasionally, they may be isodense with the blood in the lumen, in which case they are more difficult to visualize. Tumors, especially the larger primary types, may be heterogeneous, with areas of necrosis.

Depending upon tumor size, there may be normal or increased IVC caliber as well as loss of respiratory changes. Because of the similarity in echographic appearance of vascular tumor masses the differential diagnosis is large: primary vascular neoplasm, malignant IVC mass, thrombus (chronic), and large primary tumors outside the vessel.[19] The latter differential is important, since large tumors distort their surroundings making normal anatomy difficult to identify.

Recently, Doppler and color-flow instrumentation have aided in the diagnosis of vena caval obstruction by tumors. Normally, blood flow in the inferior vena cava is steady. Near the heart, effects of cardiac pulsations cause some reversal of flow. When the cava is partially obstructed, the blood flow patterns are changed and the velocity at the narrowed segment increases. Color-flow can demonstrate the increased velocities and compromised lumen quite nicely. With pulsed Doppler technique it is necessary to move the sample volume along the length of the IVC to look for increased flow velocity. Abnormal flow velocity findings may be useful in suggesting vena caval obstruction when the obstructing lesion is echopoor. Complete occlusion of the IVC results in absence of detectable blood flow by Doppler interrogation.

When an IVC mass is identified during sonography, it is important to attempt to identify (1) the presence of a primary tumor and its site; (2) the cranial extent of the tumor mass (does it involve the hepatic veins or the right atrium?); and (3) Possible tumor involvement or invasion of the wall of the vessel (CT is better able to show this type of involvement than ultrasound).[19] To localize a lesion in the IVC, it should be placed into one of three (or a combination) designated segments, as surgical management depends on its cranial extent. The upper IVC is that part of the vessel that is seen between the right atrium and the hepatic veins. The middle IVC includes the part between the hepatic veins and the renal veins, and the lower IVC is the portion that lies below the renal veins (Fig. 3-32).[12]

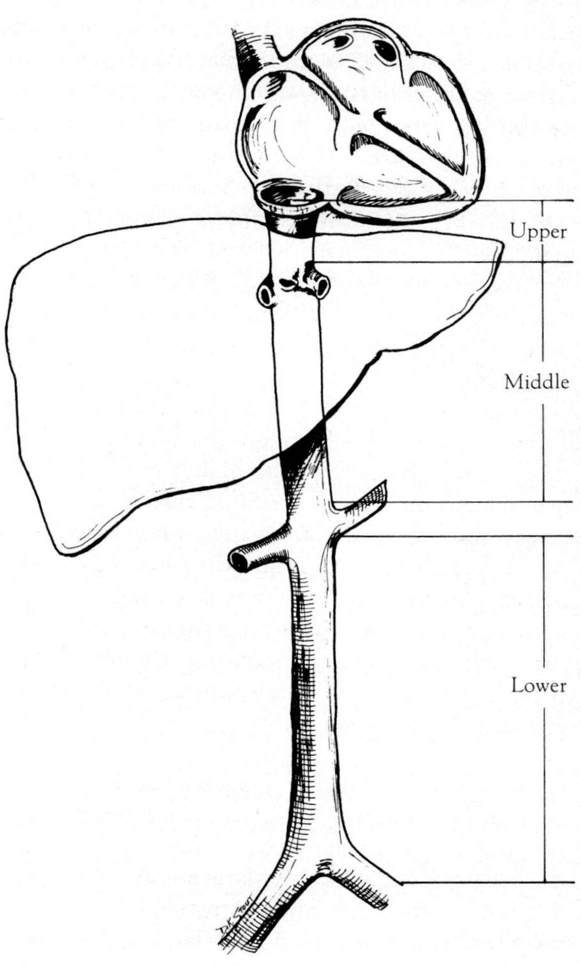

FIGURE 3-32. Segmentation of the inferior vena cava for the localization of masses.

Renal Vein Enlargement

Discussion and Cause. There are several reasons why renal veins enlarge: increased flow due to a splenorenal or gastrorenal shunt in patients with portal hypertension or portal thrombosis, tumor involvement from a renal cell carcinoma, and increased flow from an arteriovenous malformation in the kidney are the most common.[9,80,81]

In portal hypertension, several collateral pathways are apt to develop as the pressure in the portal system increases. Consequently, blood flow is diverted to the collaterals, which may in turn fistulize to the left renal vein as a means of relieving the increased pressure.[40] The same mechanism can take place in a patient with portal venous thrombosis.

It has been determined that the prevalence of renal vein involvement in renal cell carcinoma is approximately 21% to 55%.[80] When invasion occurs, obstruction to the renal vein results in dilatation. Expansion may also be the direct result of tumor growth.

In arteriovenous malformation there is an abnormal connection between the arterial and venous vessels. Because of the higher pressure in the arterial system, blood is routed directly from the artery into the vein, thus increasing blood flow through the veins. A natural response for the vein under increased blood volume is to dilate. Arteriovenous fistulas may occur for a number of reasons, including blunt or penetrating trauma, biopsy complications, tumor involvement, nephrectomy, and idiopathic causes.[81]

Clinical Signs and Symptoms. Symptoms, in the presence of an enlarged renal vein are generally associated with the initial disease process and are not the result of the venous enlargement. With portal venous hypertension and gastrorenal or splenorenal shunting, there may be no obvious distinguishing clinical features.

Tumor involvement of the renal veins usually produces no specific symptoms that would lead to suspicion of tumor extension. Such findings are generally made during the routine work-up of patients with known renal cell carcinoma.

In patients with small arteriovenous malformations generally no clinically significant symptoms are recognized. With larger malformations, however, there may be hematuria, abdominal pain, abdominal bruit, congestive heart failure, and cardiomegaly with possible systolic hypertension, diastolic hypertension, and renal ischemia.[52,81]

Sonographic Appearance. Evaluation of symmetry between the renal veins is useful in differentiating the types of disease processes that may cause venous enlargement.[80]

If enlargement of the renal veins is bilateral or symmetric, the disease process most likely involves the IVC at a level above the insertion of the renal veins. Such may include congestive heart failure and tumor involvement or thrombosis of the IVC.

Unilateral renal vein enlargement may indicate tumor involvement, portal venous hypertension with renal vein collateral anastomosis, or arteriovenous fistula. In portal venous hypertension, there is isolated left renal vein involvement, whereas either the left or the right renal vein may be involved by tumor invasion or arteriovenous fistula.

Sonographically, an enlarged renal vein is defined as one with a diameter in excess of 1.5 cm. Another sonographic finding suggestive of increased flow volume into the renal vein is abrupt IVC dilatation at the level of the renal insertion point.[80]

Blood flow patterns can be determined with Doppler ultrasound techniques and may be useful in differentiating the various types of renal vein enlargement. For instance, in the presence of a gastrorenal or splenorenal shunt associated with portal hypertension or in the presence of an arteriovenous malformation disturbed or turbulent venous flow signals are evident in the enlarged renal vein. Velocities may also be abnormally rapid.

With tumor involvement, an echogenic focus is usually present in the vessel lumen. If this is a finding during ultrasound examination, the IVC should be searched carefully to identify the extension of the tumor beyond the renal veins.

There are pitfalls: In a tumor-free vessel, reverberation artifact may mimic a tumor or possibly a thrombus. It is also possible that some metastatic tumors may appear isoechoic with the surrounding blood, making them very difficult to identify.

The left renal vein may appear enlarged at the point where it crosses over the aorta before entering the IVC. It should be noted that this is a normal finding in many persons. Dilatation should be suspected only if the entire length of the renal vein is enlarged, especially in conjunction with any of the other findings associated with renal vein enlargement.

Although duplication of the inferior vena cava is not common, it is possible that a duplicated inferior vena cava could be misinterpreted as left renal vein enlargement. To avoid this confusion, it is wise to follow the vessel in question to its origin, if possible.[80]

Renal Vein Thrombosis

Cause. Renal vein thrombosis may occur in any of the following disorders: nephrotic syndrome, renal tumors, renal transplantation, trauma, infant dehydration, and compression of the renal vein secondary to extrinsic tumor.[9]

Clinical Signs and Symptoms. Symptoms of acute renal venous thrombosis may include loin or flank pain, leg swelling, proteinuria, and hematuria.[9]

Sonographic Appearance. With renal vein thrombosis, the renal vein is dilated at a point proximal to the occlusion. In many cases, the thrombus is visible in the vessel lumen. Thrombus generally appears as an echogenic focus, especially in long-standing cases. In the more acute phase, however, thrombus may not appear echogenic but isoechoic to the surrounding blood. In these instances, Doppler interrogation may be helpful (no venous signal is heard in the presence of renal vein occlusion). The acute phase of renal vein thrombosis causes enlargement of the kidney and loss of normal renal architecture.[9]

Venous Aneurysms

Description. Venous aneurysms are very rare, tending to occur principally in the neck or lower extremity veins. The next most common area of venous aneurysm formation is the portal vein, often in the extrahepatic portion and among younger persons. Other venous aneurysms such as splenic vein aneurysms, superior mesenteric vein aneurysms, and cystic vein aneurysms have been reported sporadically.[69]

Cause. Several theories have been developed to explain the cause of venous aneurysms. They include weakening of the vessel wall by pancreatitis, portal hypertension, and embryonic malformations (congenital anomalies). Most of the literature reviewers seem to believe that the cause is embryonic and that portal hypertension is a result of portal vein aneurysm and not vice versa.[22,69]

Clinical Signs and Symptoms. Usually, no symptoms are associated with small aneurysms of the portal venous system. When an aneurysm enlarges, it may cause any of the following commonly reported symptoms: duodenal compression, common bile duct obstruction, chronic portal hypertension, jaundice, recurrent crampy abdominal pain, upper gastrointestinal bleeding, obstruction of the portal vein due to thrombus, and rupture of the aneurysm.[41]

Sonographic Appearance. Sonographically, portal venous aneurysms can be recognized as anechoic areas in the porta hepatis. There may or may not be thrombus, and a communication with the portal vein may be seen. Pulsed Doppler techniques can be used to verify the venous nature of the echo-free structure by detecting a turbulent venous signal in the lesion. Included in the differential diagnosis (especially in the absence of Doppler data) are neoplastic cysts and visceral arterial aneurysms.

Other venous aneurysms are rare, but it stands to reason that they all resemble a portal vein aneurysm, except for their location in the abdomen. Doppler investigation should be used to help define the vascular nature of any suspicious lesion within the abdomen.

Portal Venous Abnormalities

Portal Venous Thrombosis

Description and Cause. Portal venous thrombosis can be caused by a variety of pathologic states: portal hypertension, inflammatory abdominal processes (appendicitis, peritonitis, pancreatitis, colon diverticulum), trauma, postsurgical complications, hypercoagulability states (oral contraceptives, pregnancy, migratory thrombophlebitis, antithrombin III deficiency, polycythemia vera, thrombocytosis), abdominal neoplasms (hepatocellular, colonic, pancreatic), renal transplant, and benign ulcer disease.[25,27,42,53,60,66,70] It can also be idiopathic. A potential complication of portal vein thrombosis is bowel ischemia and perforation.[25]

Clinical Signs and Symptoms. A patient with portal vein thrombosis may exhibit any of the following symptoms: abdominal pain, low-grade fever, leukocytosis, hypovolemia, and shock, which is unlikely unless there is an associated bowel infarction. Abdominal rigidity, elevated liver function test results, nausea, and vomiting may also be present. Changes in bowel habit, hematemesis, and melena can occur.[42,60]

Sonographic Appearance. Portal venous thrombosis goes through several stages, and its sonographic appearance varies at different stages of the disease process.[42] In the first stage there is echogenic thrombus in the vessel lumen; then thrombus and smaller collaterals are visible in the immediate area. Finally larger collaterals (cavernomatous transformation of the portal vein) are observed in the absence of an identifiable portal vein. The latter two stages are usually seen in benign processes and are due to chronic disease.

Direct signs of portal venous thrombosis include visualization of a clot in the lumen of the portal vein (Fig. 3-33).[53] Clot appears more echogenic than the surrounding blood, however, in the acute process, when thrombus is fresh, it may be very difficult to identify. A localized bulge of the vein at the clot level may also be recognized. Doppler evaluation of the portal vein may be useful. Total occlusion would produce an absence of venous signals in the portal vein. A partially occlusive portal thrombus may exhibit normal venous flow characteristics, or decreased flow through the vein, depending on the extent of the clot.

The normal caliber of the portal vein has been established to be smaller than 13 mm.[84] In the event of an acute thrombotic episode, the caliber is likely to exceed 13 mm, but in a more chronic process, it may indeed be less than 13 mm.[53]

Indirect evidence of portal vein thrombus includes lack of normal portal vein landmarks, collateral vessel formation in the area of the portal vein, and increased caliber of the superior mesenteric vein and splenic veins.[42] It has been demonstrated that in some cases of complete obliteration of the portal vein by thrombus the thrombus actually appeared isodense with the liver parenchyma. The only indication of portal involvement was echoic margins surrounding the clot, which were generated from the portal vein walls.[27]

In cavernous transformation of the portal vein, multiple worm-like, serpiginous vessels can be seen in the region of the portal vein. This particular process is the result of longstanding thrombus and subsequent collateral vessel formation.[85]

Ultrasound techniques can also be used to detect superior mesenteric– and splenic vein thrombosis (Fig. 3-34).[25,42] Sonographically, signs of thrombosis appear similar to those seen in portal thrombosis. Echogenic material may be visualized directly inside the vessel lumen and the caliber of the superior mesenteric and splenic veins may be increased, especially in the acute phase. Absence of flow is detectable by Doppler techniques in the presence of total obstruction of the vein, while flow characteristics may be normal or diminished when thrombus is partially occlusive.

It is difficult to differentiate between thrombus and tumor by ultrasonography alone. Other findings, such as primary tumor or lymphadenopathy, may be useful in pinpointing the correct diagnosis. Because improper gain settings and reverberation artifact may appear as clot within the lumen of the portal vein, careful attention to technique is critical.

PORTAL VENOUS HYPERTENSION

Description. Portal hypertension is an increase in the portal venous pressure. Normally, pressure in

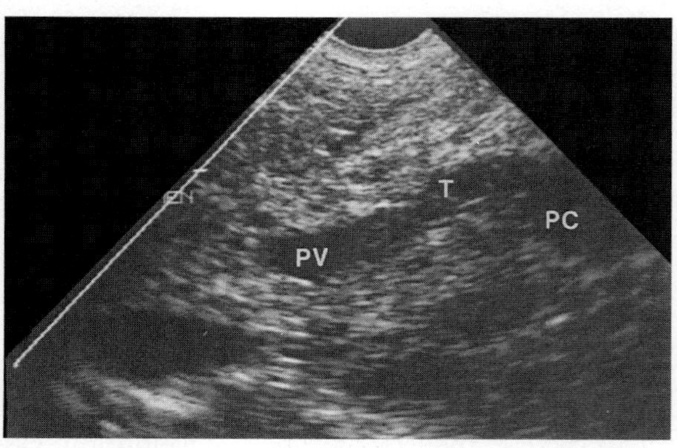

FIGURE 3-33. On this oblique sonogram through the portal vein of a patient with portal hypertension notice the normal caliber of the vein and the clot within it, near the junction of the superior mesenteric vein and the splenic vein (portal confluence); (PV, extrahepatic portal vein; T, thrombus; PC, portal confluence).

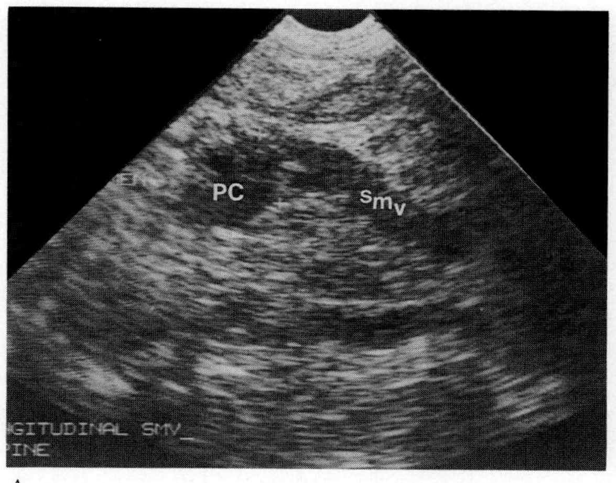

A

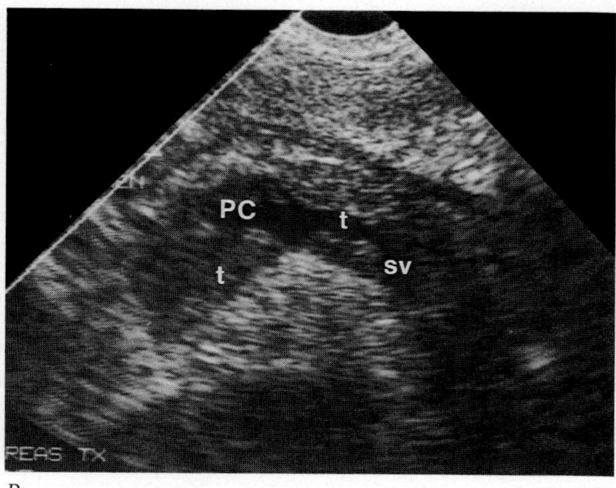

B

FIGURE 3-34. (*A*) Longitudinal sonogram through the superior mesenteric vein demonstrating obstructive clot within that fills the entire lumen of the vein (smv, superior mesenteric vein filled with clot; PC, portal confluence). (*B*) Transverse sonogram through the splenic vein demonstrates thrombus (t) within the portal confluence (PC) and the splenic vein (sv) in a patient with portal hypertension.

the portal venous system is sustained between 0 and 5 mm Hg. In the pathologic state of portal hypertension, it increases to 10 to 12 mm Hg or more.[41]

Cause. Portal hypertension may be induced by an increase in the splanchnic blood flow or by increased hepatic vascular resistance.[41] Conditions associated with increased splanchnic blood flow include splenic, hepatic, and mesenteric arteriovenous fistulas resulting from either trauma or rupture of an aneurysm into the splanchnic vessel circulation. These particular mechanisms are not common causes in the United States.[41]

Conditions associated with increased resistance to hepatic vascular flow include extrahepatic obstruction of the portal vein, such as thrombosis and presinusoidal obstruction of portal vein radicles in which there is fibrosis of the portal triads. These can be idiopathic or associated with schistosomiasis, chronic arsenic or vinyl chloride toxicity, congenital hepatic fibrosis, granulomatous disease, or neoplastic infiltration. Perhaps the most common cause of portal hypertension in the United States is sinusoidal and postsinusoidal obstruction, as is seen with fatty infiltration and inflammation of the liver in patients with acute alcoholic hepatitis and cirrhosis. The Budd-Chiari syndrome or hepatic venous obstruction may also be a mechanism of portal hypertension. In these instances hepatic venous occlusion results from congenital webs, thrombosis, or neoplasia.[41]

Clinical Signs and Symptoms. In more advanced cases of portal hypertension there may be ascites and gastrointestinal bleeding. Other complications include poor renal function and impaired coagulation[6,74,80] but these symptoms are nonspecific, and the total clinical picture must be correlated with physical and ultrasonographic findings to arrive at the correct diagnosis.

Sonographic Appearance. In healthy persons the portal vein diameter is usually less than 13 mm. It has been proposed that the presence of a larger portal vein is suggestive of portal venous hypertension, but this is not a consistent finding. Interestingly, in persons with known portal hypertension portal vein caliber was frequently reported to be normal or small compared to that of normal persons. This is probably due to the development of collateral circulation pathways in patients with more severe portal hypertension. Increased portal vein caliber is not regarded as a reliable indicator of portal venous hypertension.[46]

In order to diagnose portal venous hypertension, it is important to look for the secondary effects of increased pressure within the venous system, which can include such things as collateral channel development and abnormal respiratory responses. More recently, Doppler techniques have been investigated in the hope they might allow the physician to more confidently diagnose portal venous hypertension, especially in the absence of visible collateral pathways or other changes associated with portal hypertension.

The collateral network associated with portal hypertension can be extensive and can involve many areas—coronary vein, gastroesophageal veins, umbilical vein, pancreatic duodenal veins, gastrorenal, and splenorenal veins.

It has been noted that a dilated coronary vein (vein of the stomach located in the midepigastric area and visualized as a tortuous anechoic structure measuring more than 5 mm and following the lesser omentum) was detected in a majority of patients with portal hypertension (Fig. 3-35A, B). This, along with the identification of esophageal varices, is a good indicator of portal hypertension. Because esophageal varices and coronary vein enlargement seem to be involved quite frequently in association with portal hypertension (80 to 90%),[73] it would be prudent to search the midepigastric region thoroughly to identify any of these collateral pathways (Fig. 3-35C, D). Of course, visualization of the collaterals depends on their size, larger ones being much more readily visible than smaller ones. Esophageal varices are also the most clinically significant of the collateral pathways because of their propensity to bleed, and a positive correlation between increasing size of the coronary vein and risk of variceal bleeding has been established.[59] Other collaterals are seen, but not to the extent of the coronary vein and esophageal varices.

Ten to twenty percent of patients with portal hypertension may also have a patent umbilical vein. This structure is seen in the falciform ligament as a tubular area of 3 mm or greater (Fig. 3-36).[26]

Pancreatic and duodenal collaterals may also be present. They would be located in the region of the descending duodenum, lateral to the pancreatic head. Depending on the amount of air in the duodenum at the time of study as well as the size of the collateral vessels, they may be easy or difficult to identify.[74]

Splenorenal and gastrorenal venous involvement is detected in the area of the splenic hilum, renal hilum, and the greater curvature of the stomach, respectively (Fig. 3-37). Their proximity may make it difficult to distinguish them from one another.[39] With this particular type of collateral, blood may also be shunted to the left renal vein to relieve the high pressure in the system, in which case, the caliber of the left renal vein also increases. If unilateral left renal vein enlargement is present, portal venous hypertension with gastrorenal or splenorenal shunting may be a cause.[73] Other causes could include arteriovenous fistula of the kidney or tumor involvement.

Retroperitoneal and paravertebral collateral vessels as well as omental collaterals may be detected, although their position in the abdomen makes it difficult.[73] Investigators have reported imaging dilated cystic veins of the gallbladder in patients with portal hypertension. The technique utilizes a high-frequency transducer and pulsed-wave Doppler.[51] Other related sonographic findings in the presence of portal hypertension may include a comma-shaped portal trunk, increased periportal echogenicity, increased caliber of the splenic and superior mesenteric veins, ascites, and an enlarged spleen.[7]

Respiratory effects on the portal system have been studied in an attempt to diagnose portal hypertension by abnormal findings. It has been stated that portal venous caliber does not change much with respiration[7]; therefore, repiratory dynamics of the superior mesenteric vein and the splenic vein have been investigated for usefulness in detecting portal venous hypertension.

It was found that in normal subjects, the caliber of both the superior mesenteric and splenic vein was less than 1 cm. During suspended inspiration, the diameters increased by 14% to 100% in the majority of normal subjects. In persons who developed

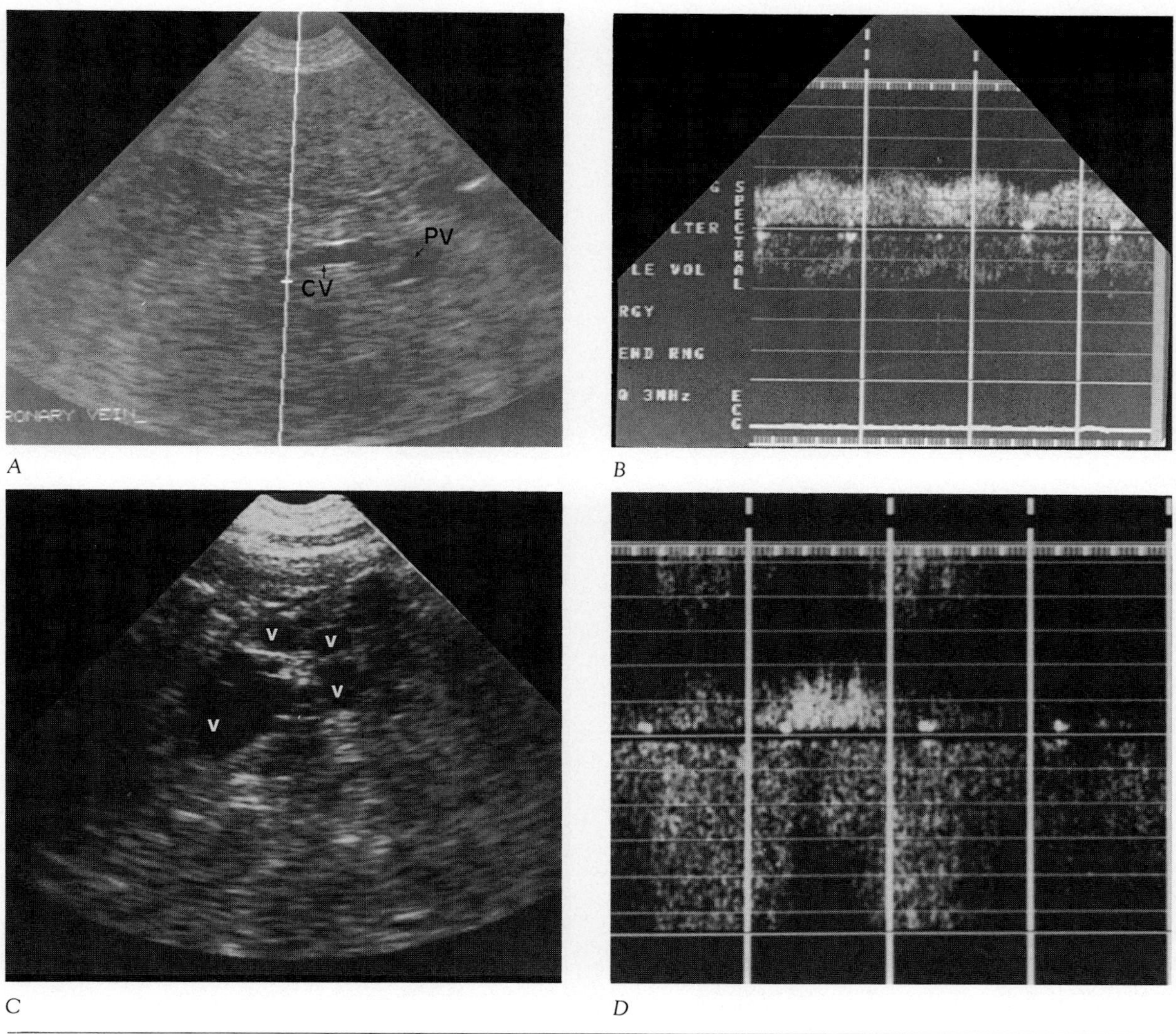

FIGURE 3-35. (*A*) Longitudinal sonogram through the midepigastric area in a patient with cirrhosis of the liver demonstrates a dilated (7 mm) coronary vein (CV) suggestive of portal venous (PV) hypertension. (*B*) Doppler tracing reveals that the vessel is a vein (the coronary vein in fact). (C) Longitudinal sonogram through the midepigastric region of a patient with portal hypertension and esophageal varices (v). (*D*) Doppler spectral tracing of blood flow in the varices. Note the turbulence.

portal hypertension as a result of cirrhosis, vessel diameters were usually 1 cm or greater and the inspiration-induced caliber changes were less than 10%.[64]

Early work with Doppler techniques is promising. Opinions differ on whether or not Doppler estimation of flow rates and volumes is useful and accurate for the study of portal hypertension. While some authors have reported a positive correlation between standard methods of measurement and

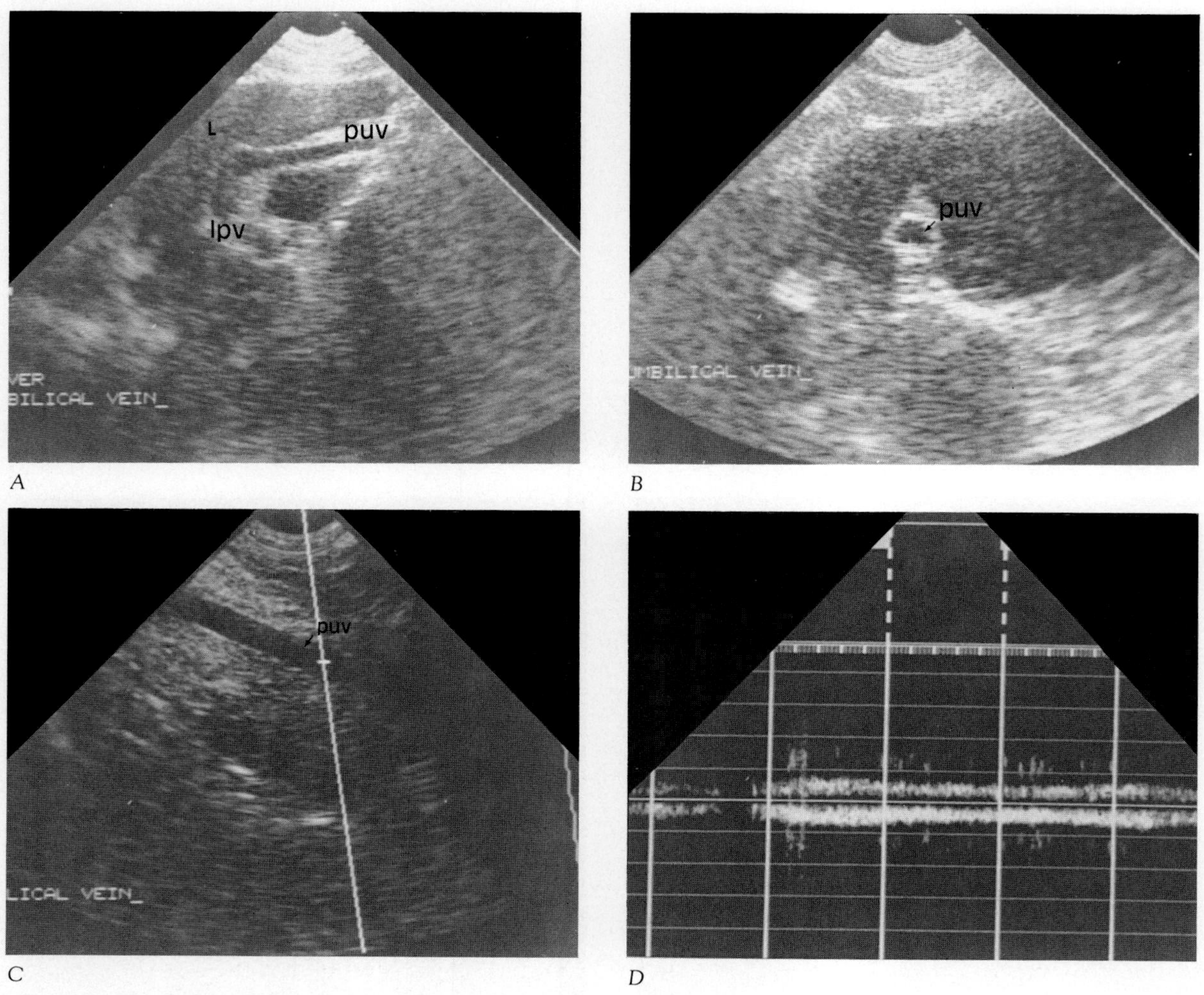

FIGURE 3-36. (*A*) Longitudinal sonogram through the left lobe of the liver (L) in a patient with cirrhosis and portal hypertension demonstrates a patent umbilical vein (puv); (lpv, left portal vein). The bright echogenic margins around the patent umbilical vein represent the falciform ligament. (*B*) Transverse sonogram of the patent umbilical vein (puv). (C) Longitudinal sonogram of the patent umbilical vein (puv) after it has exited the liver. (*D*) Doppler signal in the patent umbilical vein demonstrates that the vessel is a vein.

Doppler methods, they are quick to realize the problems inherent in using Doppler techniques for flow rate determinations.[54,72]

In any event, investigators continue to explore the usefulness of Doppler technology in the assessment of portal venous hypertension. Because of the inherent inaccuracies with Doppler-derived flow estimates, a more qualitative assessment of flow characteristics is being investigated, which it is hoped will point toward a diagnosis of portal venous hypertension.

The qualitative Doppler examination begins

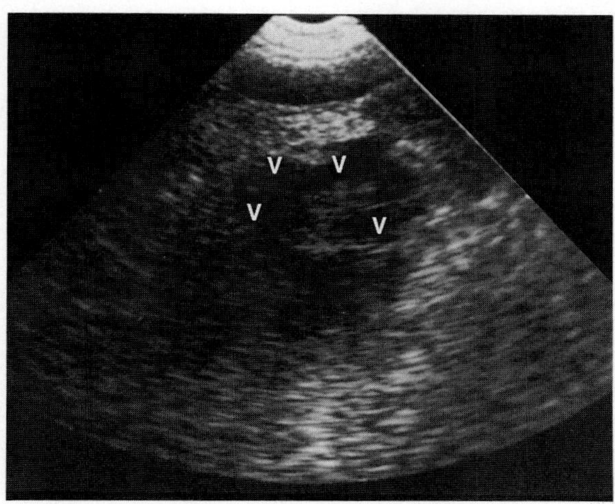

FIGURE 3-37. Longitudinal sonogram through the left side upper quadrant in a patient with portal hypertension and splenorenal and/or gastrorenal varices (v).

with visualization of the portal vein and its branches, by placing the transducer at the right intercostal spaces overlying the liver. This intercostal approach generally affords better detection of Doppler signals by virtue of better Doppler angles. Doppler interrogation is then carried out in the right, left, and main portal veins.[58,59] Once accomplished, flow is assessed in the superior mesenteric vein and along the splenic vein. Transducer positions for the latter examination are determined by the position of the vessel and the angle necessary to obtain Doppler data.

In normal subjects, the velocity of blood flow in the portal vein has been measured at 16.0 ± 0.5 cm per second. In fasting adults, portal blood flow velocity ranged from 8 to 18 cm per second. After ingestion of a meal, velocities increased by 50 to 100%. The flow characteristics in the majority of the normal subjects were a wavy continuous pattern (70%)[91] and traveled toward the liver (hepatopetally). Flow in the superior mesenteric and splenic veins was also orthograde.[59]

Several blood flow abnormalities were detected in patients with portal hypertension. Flow was reversed (hepatofugal) in the portal veins, and in some cases, this reversal of flow was detected only when the patient was asked to suspend inspiration. Reversed flow in the superior mesenteric vein suggested mesentericocaval shunting and prompted the examiner to look for collaterals in the pelvis. Reversed flow in the splenic vein and an associated increase in left renal vein caliber along with high-velocity, turbulent blood flow suggested splenorenal shunting. This prompted the examiner to look closely for collateral flow in the splenic and renal hilar areas. Hepatofugal flow was also detected in the left gastric (coronary), paraduodenal, periportal, and paraumbilical veins. The flow observed by Doppler techniques in the collateral vessels tended to be fast and turbulent.[59]

It was also noted that the venous flow pattern in the portal system was continuous in approximately 72% of persons who had portal hypertension and associated cirrhosis. Blood flow velocity tended to be slower than in normal control subjects.[91]

To date, it would seem that most authors agree that portal venous volume flow measurements and quantification of the portal flow are time-consuming studies, rather difficult, and not as accurate as people once hoped they would be. It appears that Doppler ultrasound findings that suggest abnormal portal hemodynamics should prompt the examiner to look more carefully for collateral vessels to establish the diagnosis of portal hypertension.

As more studies are carried out and findings reported, a clearer picture of the usefulness of Doppler in the assessment and detection of portal venous hypertension may emerge.

References

1. Amparo EG, Hoddick WK, Hricak H, et al: Comparison of magnetic resonance imaging and ultrasonography in the evaluation of abdominal aortic aneurysms. Radiology 1985, 154:451–456.
2. Anderson JC, Baltaxe HA, Wolf GL: Inability to show clot: One limitation of ultrasonography of the abdominal aorta. Radiology 1979, 132:693–696.
3. Athey PA, Sax S, Lamki N, Cadavid G: Sonography in the diagnosis of hepatic artery aneurysms. AJR 1986, 147:725–727.
4. Avasthi PS, Greene ER, Voyles WF, et al: A comparison of echo-Doppler and electromagnetic renal blood flow measurements. J Ultrasound Med 1984, 3:213–218.

5. Avasthi PS, Voyles WF, Greene ER: Noninvasive diagnosis of renal artery stenosis by echo-Doppler velocimetry. Kidney Int 1984, 25:824–829.
6. Baker KS, Tisnado J, Cho SR, et al: Splanchnic artery aneurysms and pseudoaneurysms: Transcatheter embolization. Radiology 1987, 163:135–139.
7. Bolondi L, Gandolfi L, Arienti V, et al: Ultrasonography in the diagnosis of portal hypertension: Diminished response of portal vessels to respiration. Radiology 1982, 142:167–172.
8. Bousquet JC, Goze A, Hassan M, et al: Leiomyosarcoma of the inferior vena cava:Ultrasonographic appearance. J Ultrasound Med 1987, 6:7–12.
9. Braun B, Weilemann LS, Weigand W: Ultrasonographic demonstration of renal vein thrombosis. Radiology 1981, 138:157–158.
10. Breshnihan ER, Keates PG: Ultrasound and dissection of the abdominal aorta. Clin Radiol 1980, 31:105–108.
11. Brewster DC, Darling RC, Raines JK, et al: Assessment of abdominal aortic aneurysm size. Circulation 1977, 56(suppl 2):II-164–II-169.
12. Cederlund CG, Edin R: Asymptomatic leiomyosarcoma of the inferior vena cava: incidental finding at ultrasonography. Acta Radiol 1987, 28:181–183.
13. Conrad MR, Davis GM, Green CE, et al: Real-time ultrasound in the diagnosis of acute dissecting aneurysm of the abdominal aorta. AJR 1979, 132:115–116.
14. Crawford ES, Beckett WC, Greer MS: Juxtarenal infrarenal abdominal aortic aneurysm: special diagnostic and therapeutic considerations. Ann Surg 1986, 203:661–670.
15. Crawford JL, Stowe CL, Safi HJ, et al: Inflammatory aneurysms of the aorta. J Vasc Surg 1985, 2:113–122.
16. Cullenward MJ, Scanlan KA, Pozniak MA, et al: Inflammatory aortic aneurysm (periaortic fibrosis): Radiologic imaging. Radiology 1986, 159:75–82.
17. Darling RC, Messina CR, Brewster DC, et al: Autopsy study of unoperated abdominal aortic aneurysms: A case for early resection. Circulation 1977, 56(suppl 2):II-161–II-164.
18. Derchi LE, Biggi E, Cicio GR, et al: Aneurysms of the splenic artery: Noninvasive diagnosis by pulsed Doppler sonography. J Ultrasound Med 1984, 3:41–44.
19. Didier D, Racle A, Etievent JP, et al: Tumor thrombus of the inferior vena cava secondary to malignant abdominal neoplasms: US and CT evaluation. Radiology 1987; 162:83–89.
20. Eriksson I, Hemmingsson A, Lindgren PG: Diagnosis of abdominal aortic aneurysms by aortography, computed tomography and ultrasound. Acta Radiol Diagn 1980, 21:209–214.
21. Falkoff GE, Taylor KJW, Morse S: Hepatic artery pseudoaneurysm: Diagnosis with real-time pulsed Doppler US. Radiology 1986, 158:55–56.
22. Fanney D, Castillo M, Montalvo B, et al: Sonographic diagnosis of aneurysm of the right portal vein. J Ultrasound Med 1987, 6:605–607.
23. Filly RA, Carlsen EN: New ultrasonographic anatomy in the upper abdomen: II. The major systemic veins and arteries with a special note on localization of the pancreas. J Clin Ultrasound 1985, 4:91–96.
24. Freimanis AK: Echographic diagnosis of lesions of the abdominal aorta and lymph nodes. Radiol Clin North Am 1975, 13:557–571.
25. Freling NJM, Schuur KH, Haagsma EB, et al: Ultrasound as first imaging modality in superior mesenteric and portal vein thrombosis. J Clin Ultrasound 1986, 14:554–557.
26. Funston MR, Goudie E, Richter IA, et al: Ultrasound diagnosis of the recanalized umbilical vein in portal hypertension. J Clin Ultrasound 1980, 8:244–246.
27. Gansbeke DV, Avni EF, Delcour CJ, et al: Sonographic features of portal vein thrombosis. AJR 1985, 144:749–752.
28. Goldberg BB: Abdominal Ultrasonography, 2nd ed. New York, John Wiley, 1977.
29. Goldstone J, Malone JM, Moore WS: Inflammatory aneurysms of the abdominal aorta. Surgery 1978, 83:425–430.
30. Gooding RAW, Herzog KA, Hegdcock MW, et al: B-Mode ultrasonography of prosthetic vascular grafts. Radiology 1978, 127:763–766.
31. Graham JM, McCollum CH, DeBakey ME: Aneurysms of the splanchnic arteries. Am J Surg 1980, 140:797–801.
32. Grant E, Rendano F, Sevinc E, et al: Normal inferior vena cava: Caliber changes observed by dynamic ultrasound. AJR 1980, 135:335–338.
33. Hagen-Ansert SL: Textbook of Diagnostic Ultrasonography, 3rd ed. St. Louis, C V Mosby, 1989.
34. Handa N, Fukunaga R, Etani H, et al: Efficacy of echo-Doppler examination for the evaluation of renovascular disease. Ultrasound Med Biol 1988, 14:1–5.
35. Handa N, Fukunaga R, Uehara A, et al: Echo-Doppler velocimeter in the diagnosis of hypertensive patients: The renal artery Doppler technique. Ultrasound Med Biol 1986, 12:945–952.
36. Harter LP, Gross BH, Callen PW, et al: Ultrasonic evaluation of abdominal aortic thrombus. J Ultrasound Med 1982, 1:315–318.
37. Henry LG, Doust B, Korns ME, et al: Abdominal aortic aneurysm and retroperitoneal fibrosis: Ultra-

sonographic diagnosis and treatment. Arch Surg 1978, 113:1456–1460.
38. Hume DM, Porter RR: Acute dissecting aortic aneurysms. Surgery 1963, 53:122–150.
39. Juttner HU, Jenney JM, Ralls PW, et al: Ultrasound demonstration of portosystemic collaterals in cirrhosis and portal hypertension. Radiology 1982, 142:459–463.
40. Kane RA, Katz SG: The spectrum of sonographic findings in portal hypertension: A subject review and observations. Radiology 1982, 142:453–458.
41. Kaye D, Rose LF: Fundamentals of Internal Medicine. St. Louis, C V Mosby, 1983.
42. Kidambi H, Herbert R, Kidambi A: Ultrasonic demonstration of superior mesenteric and splenoportal venous thrombosis. J Clin Ultrasound 1986, 14:199–201.
43. King PS, Cooperberg PL, Madigan SM: The anechoic crescent in abdominal aortic aneurysms: Not a sign of dissection. AJR 1986, 146:345–348.
44. Kohler TR, Zierler E, Martin RL, et al: Noninvasive diagnosis of renal artery stenosis by ultrasonic duplex scanning. J Vasc Surg 1986, 4:456.
45. Kumari SS, Pillari G, Mandon V, et al: Case reports: Occult aortic dissection: Diagnosis by ultrasound. Br J Radiol 1980, 53:1093–1095.
46. Lafortune M, Marleau D, Breton G, et al: Portal venous system measurements in portal hypertension. Radiology 1984, 151:27–30.
47. Langley LL, Telford IR, Christensen JB: Dynamic Anatomy and Physiology, 5th ed. New York, McGraw-Hill, 1980.
48. Leopold GR, Goldberger LE, Bernstein EF: Ultrasonic detection and evaluation of abdominal aortic aneurysms. Surgery 1972, 72:939–945.
49. Maloney JD, Pairolero PC, Smith B, et al: Ultrasound evaluation of abdominal aortic aneurysms. Circulation 1977, 56(suppl 2):II-80–II-85.
50. Manoharan A, Gill RW, Griffiths KA: Splenic blood flow measurements by Doppler ultrasound: A preliminary report. Cardiovasc Res 1987, 21:779–782.
51. Marchal GJF, Holsbeeck MV, Tshibwabwa-Ntumba E, et al: Dilatation of the cystic veins in portal hypertension: Sonographic demonstration. Radiology 1985, 154:187–189.
52. Mittelstaedt CA: Abdominal Ultrasound. New York, Churchill Livingstone, 1987.
53. Miller VE, Berland LL: Pulsed-Doppler duplex sonography and CT of portal vein thrombosis. AJR 1985, 145:73–76.
54. Moriyasu F, Ban N, Nishida O, et al: Clinical application of an ultrasonic duplex system in the quantitative measurement of portal blood flow. J Clin Ultrasound 1986, 14:579–588.
55. Mourad K, Guggiana P, Minasian H: Superior mesenteric artery aneurysm diagnosed by ultrasound. Br J Radiol 1987, 60:287–288.
56. Strandness ED: Duplex scanning in vascular disorders. New York, Raven Press, 1990.
57. Nusbaum JW, Freimanis AK, Thomford NR: Echography in the diagnosis of abdominal aortic aneurysm. Arch Surg 1971, 102:385–388.
58. Ozaki CF, Anderson JC, Liebermann RP, et al: Duplex ultrasonography as a noninvasive technique for assessing portal hemodynamics. Am J Surg 1988, 155:70–75.
59. Patriquin H, Lafortune M, Burns PN, et al: Duplex Doppler examination in portal hypertension: Technique and anatomy. AJR 1987, 149:71–76.
60. Phillips G, Dimitrieva Z: Sonographic diagnosis of thrombosis of the superior mesenteric vein and small bowel infarction. J Ultrasound Med 1985, 4:565–566.
61. Qamar MI, Read AE, Skidmore R, et al: Transcutaneous Doppler ultrasound measurement of superior mesenteric artery blood flow in man. Gut 1986, 27:100–105.
62. Qamar MI, Read AE, Skidmore R, et al: Pulsatility index of superior mesenteric artery blood velocity waveforms. Ultrasound Med Biol 1986, 12:772–776.
63. Qamar MI, Read AE, Skidmore R, et al: Transcutaneous Doppler ultrasound measurement of coeliac axis blood flow in man. Br J Surg 1985, 72:392–393.
64. Rector WG, Campra J, Ralls PW, et al: Utility and limitations of splanchnic venous ultrasonography in diagnosis of portal hypertension. J Clin Ultrasound 1986, 14:689–696.
65. Rigaux A, Vossen P, Baarle AV, et al: Hepatic artery aneurysm: Ultrasound diagnosis. J Clin Ultrasound 1986, 14:401–403.
66. Rosen A, Korobkin M, Silverman PM, et al: Mesenteric vein thrombosis: CT identification. AJR 1984, 143:83–86.
67. Rutherford RB: Vascular Surgery, 2nd ed. Philadelphia, W B Saunders, 1984.
68. Sato S, Ohnishi K, Sugita S, et al: Splenic artery and superior mesenteric artery blood flow: Nonsurgical Doppler US measurement in healthy subjects and patients with chronic liver disease. Radiology 1987, 164:347–352.
69. Schild H, Schweden F, Braun B, et al: Aneurysm of the superior mesenteric vein. Radiology 1982, 145:641–642.
70. Shaw PJ, Saunders AJ, Drake DP: Case report: Ultrasonographic demonstration of portal vein thrombosis in the acute abdomen. Clin Radiol 1986, 37(1):101–102.

71. Shultz S, Druy EM, Friedman AC: Common hepatic artery aneurysm: Psuedopseudocyst of the pancreas. AJR 1985, 144:1287–1288.
72. Smith HJ, Grottum P, Simonsen S: Ultrasonic assessment of abdominal venous return II. Volume blood flow in the inferior vena cava and portal vein. Acta Radiol Diagn 1986, 27:23–27.
73. Subramanyam BR, Balthazar EJ, Madamba MR, et al: Sonography of portosystemic venous collaterals in portal hypertension. Radiology 1983, 146:161–166.
74. Subramanyam BR, Balthazar EJ, Raghavendra BN, et al: Sonographic evaluation of patients with portal hypertension. Am J Gastroenterol 1983, 78:369–373.
75. Szilagyi DE, Elliott JP, Smith RF: Clinical fate of the patient with asymptomatic abdominal aortic aneurysm and unfit for surgical treatment. Arch Surg 1972, 104:600–606.
76. Taylor DC, Kettler MD, Moneta GL, et al: Duplex ultrasound scanning in the diagnosis of renal artery stenosis: A prospective evaluation. J Vasc Surg 1988, 7:363–369.
77. Taylor KJW: Ultrasonic investigation of inferior vena caval obstruction. Br J Radiol 1975, 48:1024–1026.
78. Taylor KJW, Morse SJ, Weltin GG, et al: Liver transplant recipients: Portable duplex US with correlative angiography. Radiology 1986, 159:357–363.
79. Thomas CL (ed): Taber's Cyclopedic Medical Dictionary, 15th ed. Philadelphia, F A Davis, 1985.
80. Thomas JL, Bernardino ME: Neoplastid-induced renal vein enlargement: Sonographic detection. AJR 1981, 136:75–79.
81. Thomas JL, Lymberis MEB, Hunt TH: Ultrasonic features of acquired renal arteriovenous fistula. AJR 1979, 132:653–655.
82. Tortora GJ, Anagnostakos NP: Principles of Anatomy and Physiology, 56th ed. New York, Harper and Row, 1987.
83. Walker DI, Bloor K, Williams G, et al: Inflammatory aneurysms of the abdominal aorta. Br J Surg 1972, 59:609–614.
84. Weinreb J, Kumari S, Phillips G, et al: Portal vein measurements by real-time sonography. AJR 1982, 139:497–499.
85. Weltin G, Taylor KJW, Carter AR, et al: Duplex Doppler: Identification of cavernous transformation of the portal vein. AJR 1985, 144:999–1001.
86. Wheeler WE, Beachley MC, Ranninger K: Angiography and ultrasonography: A comparative study of abdominal aortic aneurysms. Surgery 1976, 126:95–100.
87. Winsberg F, Cole-Beuglet C, Mulder DS: Continuous ultrasound "B" scanning of abdominal aortic aneurysms. Surgery 1974, 121:626–633.
88. Wolinski AP, Gall WJ, Dubbins PA: Hepatic artery aneurysm following pancreatitis diagnosed by ultrasound. Br J Radiol 1985, 58:768–770.
89. Wolson AH, Kaupp HA, MCDonald K: Ultrasound of arterial graft surgery complications. AJR 1979, 133:869–875.
90. Zoli M, Dondi C, Marchesini G, et al: Splanchnic vein measurements in patients with liver cirrhosis: A case-control study. J Ultrasound Med 1985, 4:641–646.
91. Zoli M, Marchesini G, Cordiani MR, et al: Echo-Doppler measurement of splanchnic blood flow in control and cirrhotic subjects. J Clin Ultrasound 1986, 14:429–435.
92. Zwiebel WJ: Introduction to Vascular Ultrasonography. Orlando, FL, Grune and Stratton, 1986.

CHAPTER 4

Liver

DIANE M. KAWAMURA, KATHY GILL, SUE ELLEN BEAVERS

Anatomy

EMBRYOLOGY

Early in the fourth week of fetal development, the liver, gallbladder, and bile duct system develop from an endodermal outgrowth, or hepatic diverticulum.[34,94] During week five, the diverticulum differentiates into the origin of the cystic duct and the gallbladder in the caudad portion; and in the cephalad portion, two endodermal cellular buds begin forming the right and the left hepatic lobes.[34,49,94] These solid cell buds grow into columns or cylinders that branch and form anastomoses, form networks, and invade the vitelline and the umbilical veins.[49] The capillary-like vessels of the plexus eventually differentiate into the liver sinusoids.[34,49] The endothelial cells of the plexus become the Kupffer cells.[94] The columns of endodermal cells and the liver parenchyma grow out into the surrounding mesoderm.[49] The mesoderm provides the hemopoietic tissue and the connective tissue for the fibrous liver capsule (Glisson's capsule) and the portal tracts.[34,94] As the terminal branches of the right and left hepatic lobes canalize, the bile duct system is formed.[94]

Both lobes are equal in size until the beginning of the sixth week, at which time, the right lobe becomes larger, the caudate and quadrate lobes develop from the right lobe,[34] and the left lobe actually undergoes some degeneration.[49] At week six, the liver fills most of the abdominal cavity and the relative development of the liver becomes less active.[34,49]

The yolk sac regresses as the liver enlarges. Hemopoiesis takes place in the liver at week six, peaks at 12 to 24 weeks, and ceases at birth.[34,52] At week 10, lymphocyte formation occurs in the liver, which also ceases at birth.[34] Coagulation factors are manufactured at 10 to 12 weeks and bile is produced by 13 to 16 weeks,[34] but the fetal liver does not function in digestion until after birth.[145]

Oxygenated blood and nutrients are delivered to the fetus through the umbilical vein, which ascends and divides into two branches.[81,124] The left branch joins the portal vein and enters the liver, and the right branch, the ductus venosus, flows directly into the inferior vena cava (IVC), bypassing the liver.[81,95,145] Normally, both of these vessels deteriorate into fibrous cords sometime after birth.[145] The left umbilical vein becomes the ligamentum teres, or round ligament, and the ductus venosus becomes the ligamentum venosum.[94,145] In some persons, the left umbilical vein persists, and both the ligamentum teres and the ligamentum venosum can become recanalized as collateral vessels with certain disease processes such as portal hypertension.[43,95]

LOCATION AND SIZE

The liver fills the right side and part of the left side of the upper abdomen, displaces gas-filled structures, and provides an acoustic window through which may be imaged the upper abdomen and retroperitoneum (Fig. 4-1A).[105] Sonographically, it has a relatively homogeneous parenchymal back-

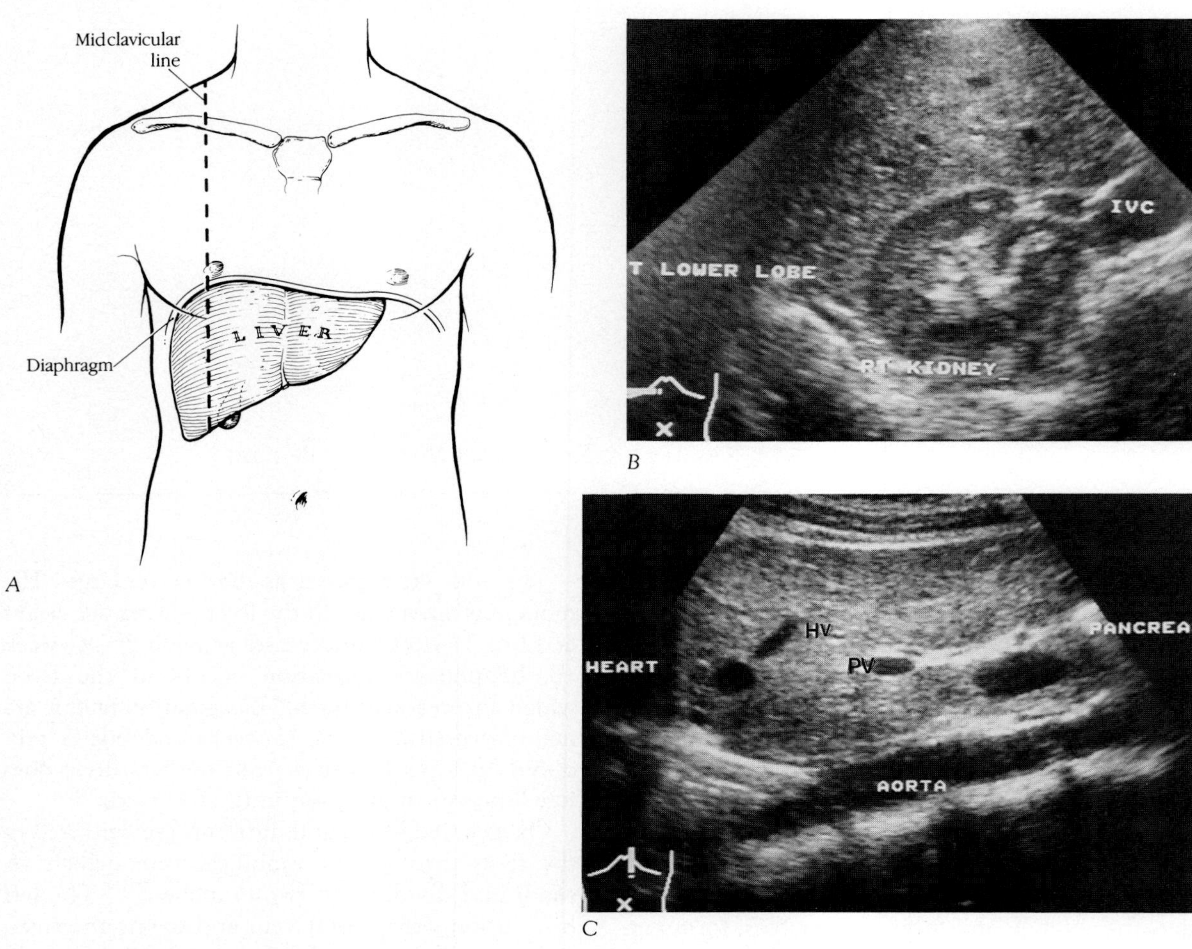

Figure 4-1. (*A*) Located in the upper part of the abdomen, the liver occupies the right hypochondrium, the greater part of the epigastric region, and extends in varying degrees into the left hypochondrium as far as the mammary line.[94] The lateral segment of the left lobe and the length of the right lobe determine the contour and shape of the liver. Overall, it can be described as irregular, hemispheric,[49] or wedge shaped.[94] (*B*) A transverse section of a normal right lower liver lobe demonstrates the relatively homogeneous hepatic parenchymal echo pattern as isoechoic or slightly more echogenic than the renal parenchyma. Rounded echogenic areas represent fibrofatty tissue surrounding ducts and vessels too small to be imaged. Incidental to the liver scan is the notation that this thin woman has very little perinephric fat around the right kidney (IVC, inferior vena cava). (*C*) A sagittal section demonstrates the relatively homogeneous liver echo pattern as isoechoic or slightly less echogenic than the pancreas. Portal veins (PV) and hepatic veins (HV) can be identified interspersed within normal hepatic parenchyma. (*B*, C Courtesy Doug Amussen, Logan, UT.)

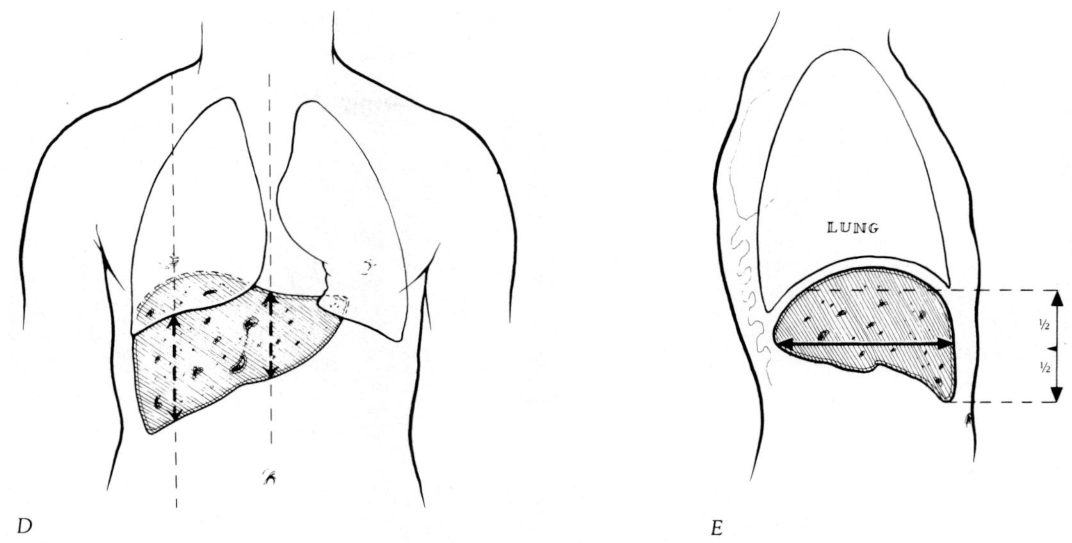

FIGURE 4-1 (*continued*). (*D*) The liver's length is measured from above downward from the margin of the lung, since the upper border is located in the diaphragm dome and hidden by air. At the 95th percentile the normal liver measurement obtained at the midline was 10.9 cm for the longitudinal length (mean 8.3 ± 1.7 SD). The 95th percentile for the AP dimension was 8.2 (mean 5.7 ± 1.5 SD).[97] The normal measurement at the midclavicular line at the 95th percentile was 12.6 cm for the longitudinal diameter (mean 10.5 ± 1.5 SD). The 95th percentile for the AP dimension was 11.3 (mean 8.1 ± 1.9 SD).[97] (*E*) The AP dimension is measured at the midpoint of the longitudinal measurement, and the cross section area of the liver is calculated from the longitudinal and AP diameters using the equation (longitudinal diameter × AP diameter)/2 = cross-sectional area. [97] (Adapted with permission from Niederau C, Sonnenberg A, Muller JE, et al: Sonographic measurements of the normal liver, spleen, pancreas, and portal vein. Radiology 1983, 149:537–540.)

ground. The medium-level echo pattern is believed to be due primarily to nonspecular reflections, thought to be the lobules and their surrounding stroma.[105] The homogeneous parenchymal background may be isoechoic or slightly more echogenic than the renal parenchyma and is isoechoic or slightly less echogenic than the pancreas.[66,88] Interspersed within are tubular, fluid-filled structures representing branches of the portal and hepatic veins,[66] and small, rounded echogenic areas representing periportal, fibrofatty tissue, where the hepatic artery, bile duct, and portal vein lumina are too small to be imaged (Fig. 4-1B, C).[105]

The largest internal organ of the body,[124] the liver varies somewhat in shape, topography, and vascular disposition, depending on a subject's morphotype.[101] It constitutes approximately one eighteenth of an infant's total body weight and one thirty-sixth of an adult's.[19] The exact weight varies, but usually ranges from 1200 g in adult females to 1600 g in males.[5,94,124]

There is also a range of normal measurements. The greatest transverse portion ranges from 20 to 22.5 cm; the greatest anteroposterior (AP) measurement, from 10 to 12.5 cm,[49] and the greatest length on the right surface, from 15 to 17 cm.[65,66] Routinely taking liver measurements in sagittal section views will help detect hepatomegaly. Liver length and AP dimensions are obtained from sagittal and parasagittal sections obtained at the midline and

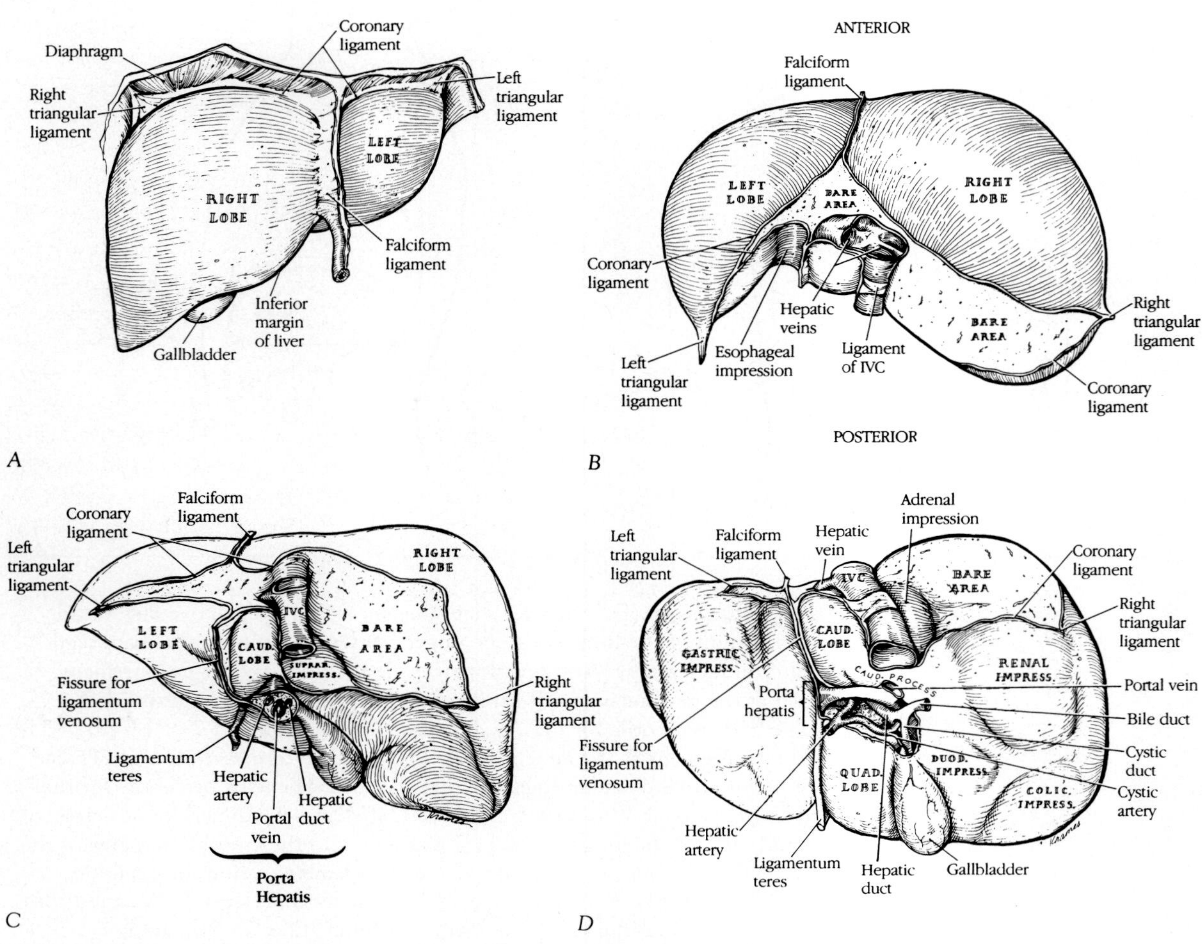

FIGURE 4-2. (*A*) The anterior surface is described as thin and sharp. It is separated from the diaphragm from the sixth to tenth ribs and their costal cartilages on the right side, from the seventh and eighth cartilages on the left side, and it lies posterior to the xiphoid process in the midline.[49] The border between the anterior surface and the visceral surface is the inferior margin.[94] Opposite the attachment of the falciform ligament, the anterior surface is marked by a deep notch, the umbilical notch, where the ligamentum teres, the obliterated fetal umbilical vein, reaches from the umbilicus to the underside of the liver. Opposite the cartilage of the ninth rib is the notch for the fundus of the gallbladder.[94] (*B*) The dome of the diaphragm separates the superior portion from the pleura and lungs on the right and the pericardium and heart on the left.[49] The surface is covered by peritoneum except along its posterior part, where it attaches to the diaphragm by the superior reflection of the coronary ligament. The coronary ligament separates the part covered with peritoneum from the bare area.[94] (*C*) The posterior portion is round and broad on the right but narrow on the left.[49] The central part presents a deep concavity as it is molded over the vertebral column and crus of the diaphragm. To the right of this concavity, the IVC lies almost buried in its fossa and forms part of the posterior boundary of the porta.[49,94] Approximately 2 to 3 cm to the left of the IVC is the narrow fossa for the ligamentum venosus. The caudate lobe lies between

the midclavicular line, which runs parallel to the spine midway between it and the right side of the body.[135,154]

Niederau and coworkers[97] did an extensive measurement study on 915 healthy subjects. Their technique allows for accurate follow-up examinations (Fig. 4-1D, E). Their results indicated that the diameters were smaller in women than in men. They demonstrated a positive correlation between body height and liver surface area and provided evidence that with age, liver diameter decreases and portal vein diameter increases.[97]

PERIHEPATIC RELATIONSHIPS

The liver is an intraperitoneal organ, almost completely covered by peritoneum and completely covered by a dense, fibroelastic, connective tissue layer[145] referred to as Glisson's capsule.[59,143] A rather delicate structure,[94] Glisson's capsule contains blood and lymphatic vessels and nerves. Distention of the capsule by liver disease or swelling causes pain, and the lymphatics may ooze fluid into the peritoneal space.[59] The areas not covered by peritoneum are along the line of attachment for the falciform ligament, the gallbladder fossa, the porta, areas surrounding the IVC, and a "bare area."[94]

The smooth diaphragmatic surface is convex and is divided into anterior, superior, and posterior portions (Fig. 4-2A–C).[49,94] The abdominal visceral surface is concave (Fig. 4-2D).[49]

LIGAMENTS

The liver is tethered to the undersurface of the diaphragm, the anterior wall of the abdomen, the lesser curvature of the stomach, and the retroperitoneum by seven ligaments, six of which are either parietal or visceral peritoneal folds and one of which is a round, fibrous cord.[94,131] These are the coronary, falciform, round (ligamentum teres), right and left triangular (lateral), gastrohepatic, and hepatoduodenal ligaments. An understanding of the liver's ligamentous attachments and the caudate lobe's relational anatomy to the lesser sac is important for accurate localization of some lobar demarcations and perihepatic fluid collections.[111] They are described in Table 4-1 and can be identified on Figures 4-2D and 4-3.

LOBES

Lobular divisions of the liver can be described as anatomic, based on external landmarks, or segmental, based on hepatic function. Since some investigators may combine these methods or may not

FIGURE 4-2 (*continued*) these two fossae.[49,94] To the right of the IVC and partly on the visceral surface is the suprarenal impression, a small triangular depressed area for the right adrenal gland. The posterior surface is in direct contact with the diaphragm and is attached by loose connective tissue, and most of it is not covered by peritoneum.[131] This uncovered bare area is bounded by the superior and inferior reflections of the coronary ligament, which connect the liver to the diaphragm.[94] (*D*) The visceral surface is concave, facing posterior, caudad, and to the left, and contains several fossae and impressions.[49] The left central part has a prominent marking, the porta hepatis, a fissure for the passage of the blood vessels and bile duct.[49] Peritoneum covers the visceral surface except at the gallbladder attachment and at the porta.[49,94] Lying to the right of the gallbladder, the right lobe has three impressions.[49] From lateral to medial, the colic impression is a flattened or shallow area for the hepatic flexure; more posterior is the larger and deeper impression for the right kidney; and lying along the neck of the gallbladder, the duodenal impression is a narrow and poorly marked area.[49] The quadrate lobe, located between the gallbladder and fossa for the umbilical vein, is in relationship with the stomach's pyloric end, the duodenum's superior portion, and the transverse colon.[49] On the left, the gastric impression for the ventral surface of the stomach is a large hollow extending out to the margin. The caudate process is just anterior to the IVC and connects the right inferior angle of the caudate lobe to the right lobe.[49] The peritoneal covering of the caudate process forms the ventral boundary of the epiploic foramen.[49]

Table 4-1. Ligament attachments to the liver

Ligament	Description
Coronary	The coronary ligament connects the posterior liver surface to the diaphragm and consists of an anterior and a posterior layer. The anterior layer is formed by the reflection of the parietal peritoneum, and the posterior layer is reflected from the caudal margin of the bare area onto the right adrenal gland and right kidney (hepatorenal ligament).[49,111,131] These two layers are continuous on each side with the right and left triangular ligaments and in front with the falciform ligament.[94,105,131]
Falciform	The falciform ligament is a broad, thin anteroposterior fold of the parietal peritoneum.[131] It originates from the midportion of the coronary ligament; inserts itself in a parasagittal plane anteriorly and shifts obliquely to its posterior surface; separates the right and left liver lobes at the diaphragmatic surface; and extends from the liver to the abdominal wall between the diaphragm and umbilicus.[49,94,105,131] At its base or free edge, the ligamentum teres is released from between its layers.[131]
Ligamentum teres	The ligamentum teres (round ligament) is the fibrous cord resulting from the obliterated left umbilical vein.[94,131] It ascends from the umbilicus in the free margin of the falciform ligament to the notch in the anterior border of the liver. Here it courses along a fissure on the visceral surface and continues as the ligamentum venosum, the obliterated ductus venosus, as far back as the IVC.[94]
Triangular	The right and left triangular ligaments are so named because of their triangular shape. They are formed by the apposition of the upper and lower ends of the coronary ligament and extend from the diaphragm of the liver.[94] The right ligament is attached to the border at the right extremity of the bare area and passes to the diaphragm.[49] The left ligament is the larger of the two and attaches to the upper surface of the left lobe, where it lies anterior to the esophageal opening in the diaphragm.[94] Its anterior layer is continuous with the left layer of the falciform ligament.[49]
Gastrohepatic	The gastrohepatic ligament, also known as the lesser omentum, is composed of two folds of visceral peritoneum.[145] It originates on the undersurface of the liver, is continuous with the ligamentum venosum, and it courses caudad to attach to the lesser curvature of the stomach and first portion of the duodenum.[105,111] Pathologies, such as varices and enlarged lymphatic nodes, may be imaged in this region.[105]
Hepatoduodenal	The hepatoduodenal ligament surrounds the portal triad (the portal vein, the hepatic artery, and the common duct) prior to entering the porta hepatis. It is located on the right free edge of the gastrohepatic ligament, forming the anterior boundary of the epiploic foramen (foramen of Winslow), a potential space representing the only communication of the lesser peritoneal sac with the rest of the peritoneal cavity.[94] The IVC and caudate lobe form the posterior wall of the lesser sac.[94] The size of the caudate process in part determines the length of the hepatoduodenal ligament and its proximity to the IVC.[105] Below the caudate process, the portal vein, within the hepatoduodenal ligament, is contiguous with the posteriorly located IVC.[105]

specify which method is being described, the literature can be confusing and appear contradictory. In the next section we discuss each division separately.

Anatomic Division. The anatomic division of the liver is based on external markings. A broad division that uses the falciform ligament to divide the liver into the right and left hepatic lobes classifies the quadrate and caudate lobes as part of the right lobe. A more accurate anatomic approach is to divide the liver into right, quadrate, caudate, and left hepatic lobes. This system uses the falciform ligament and a simulated "H" configuration on the visceral surface (Fig. 4-4A).[65,66]

Right lobe. The right lobe, six times larger than the left,[49] occupies the right hypochondrium and, when used as a scanning window, determines the

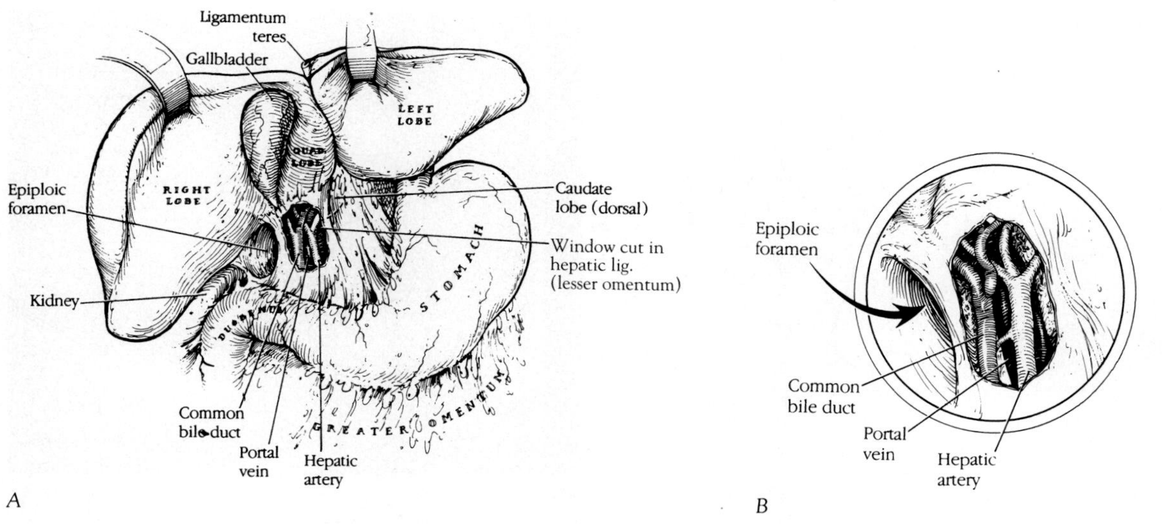

FIGURE 4-3. (*A*) The gastrohepatic ligament originates on the undersurface of the liver and courses caudad to attach to the lesser curvature of the stomach and the first portion of the duodenum. The hepatic ligament is located on the right free edge of the gastrohepatic ligament, surrounds the portal triad, and forms the anterior boundary of the epiploic foramen (of Winslow). (*B*) Enlarged cutaway view of the hepatic ligament reveals the portal triad.

sonographic detail of the entire right upper quadrant. It is separated from the left lobe by the falciform ligament on its diaphragmatic surface and by the left sagittal fossa or the left intersegmental fissure on its visceral surface (see Fig. 4-4A). It is somewhat quadrilateral. The anterior surface is marked by the falciform ligament, and its visceral and posterior surfaces by the three fossae: the porta, the gallbladder, and the IVC (Fig. 4-B, C).[4,49,53]

Caudate lobe. The caudate lobe, anatomically distinct from the left and right liver lobes, is interposed between the IVC posteriorly, the left liver lobe anteriorly and superiorly, and the main portal vein inferiorly.[21] It has been mistaken for a tumor arising from the head of the pancreas.[116] Although it is in close relation to the head of the pancreas, its echo pattern is that of liver tissue and it is located anterior to the tenth and eleventh thoracic vertebrae. Sonographically, there are three major identifiable anatomic landmarks: (1) The fissure for the ligament venosum on the left sharply separates it from the left lobe and appears hyperechoic due to its fat content, (2) The anechoic IVC appears on the right, (3) The left portal vein courses over the anterior margin of the inferior caudate lobe, separating it from the more anterior left hepatic lobe (Fig. 4-4D, E).[21,87] The left margin forms the hepatic boundary of the superior recess of the lesser sac.[105]

The caudate process is a small elevation extending obliquely and laterally off the caudate lobe's right margin, as a tonguelike projection, coursing between the IVC and the portal vein and extending to the visceral surface of the right lobe.[33] Situated dorsal to the porta hepatis it separates the gallbladder fossa from the commencement of the IVC fossa.[49] The shorter the caudate process, the longer is the association between the IVC and portal vein (see Fig. 4-4A).[21,88,105]

Quadrate lobe. The quadrate lobe is described by anatomists as a distinct lobe, but it is distinguished physiologically and sonographically as the medial segment of the left lobe. Situated on the visceral surface, it is bounded posteriorly by the porta hepatis, anteriorly by the inferior margin of the liver, and laterally by the gallbladder fossa on the right

(text continues on page 100)

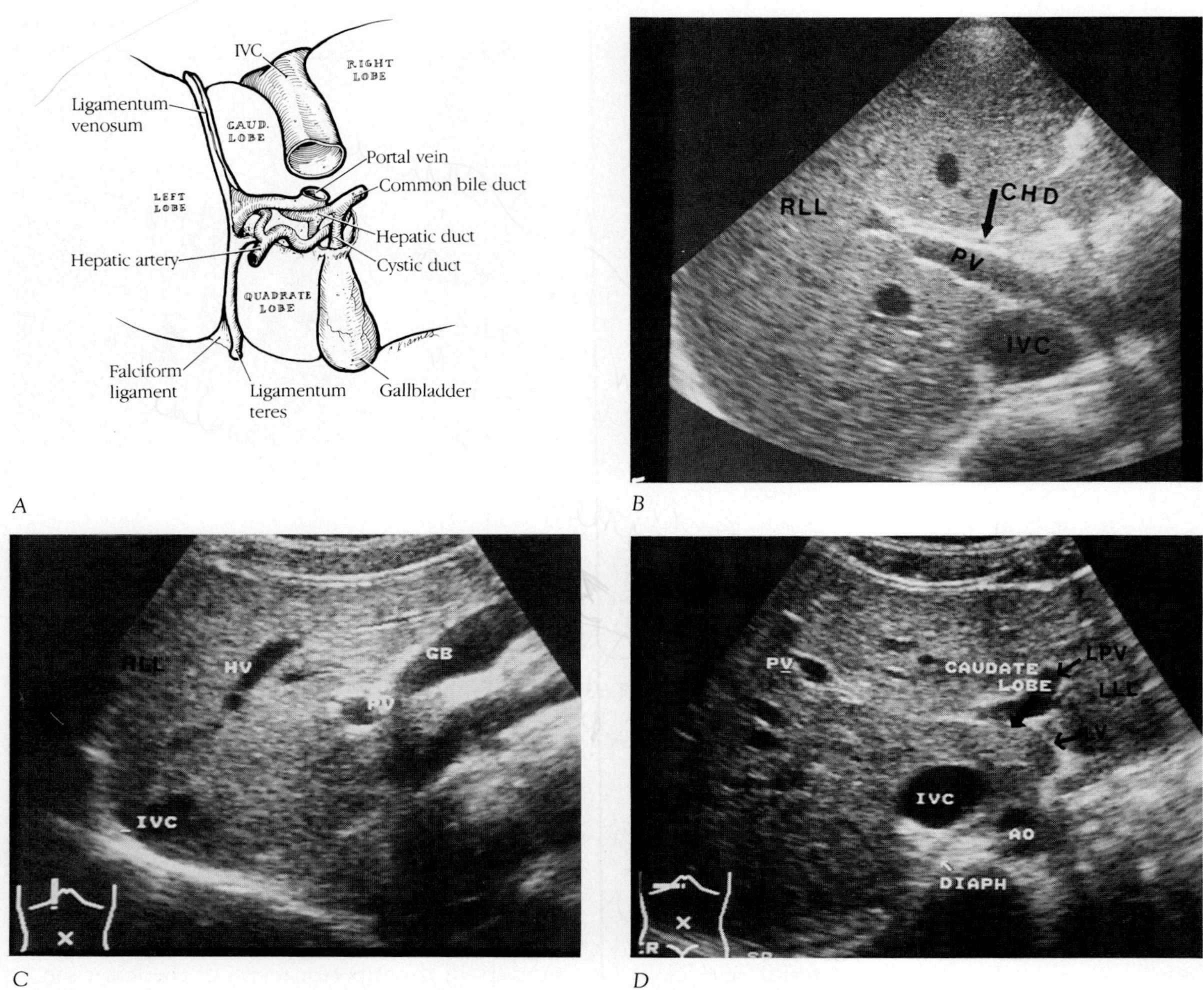

FIGURE 4-4. (*A*) The gallbladder and IVC fossas form the right vertical limb of the H.[65,66] The gallbladder fossa, shallow and oblong, extends from the inferior free margin of the liver to the right extremity of the porta.[49] The IVC fossa is a short, deep depression on the posterior surface between the caudate lobe and the bare area.[49] It is separated from the porta by the caudate process.[49] The left vertical limb of the H is formed by the left intersegmental fissure (left sagittal fossa), a deep groove in the visceral surface that extends from the notch on the inferior margin to the cranial border.[49] The porta joins it at right angles (representing the crossbar of the H) and divides it into cephalad and caudad parts.[49] The caudad part separates the quadrate lobe and the left lobe of the liver and is partially bridged by the pons hepatis, an extension of hepatic substance.[49,94] It provides the fissure for the ligamentum teres.[49] The cephalad part lies between the left lobe and the caudate lobe and provides the fissure for the ligamentum venosum and the gastrohepatic ligament.[49,65,66] The porta fossa, containing the porta hepatis and hepatoduodenal ligament, form the crossbar of the H.[65,66,94] The porta fossa is short, about 5 cm, but deep.[49] It extends transversely across the visceral surface of the left portion of the right lobe.[49] It joins the left intersegmental fissure (left sagittal fossa) at nearly a right angle and separates the quadrate lobe in front from the caudate lobe and caudate process behind.[49] It transmits the portal triad, nerves, and lymphatics.[49]

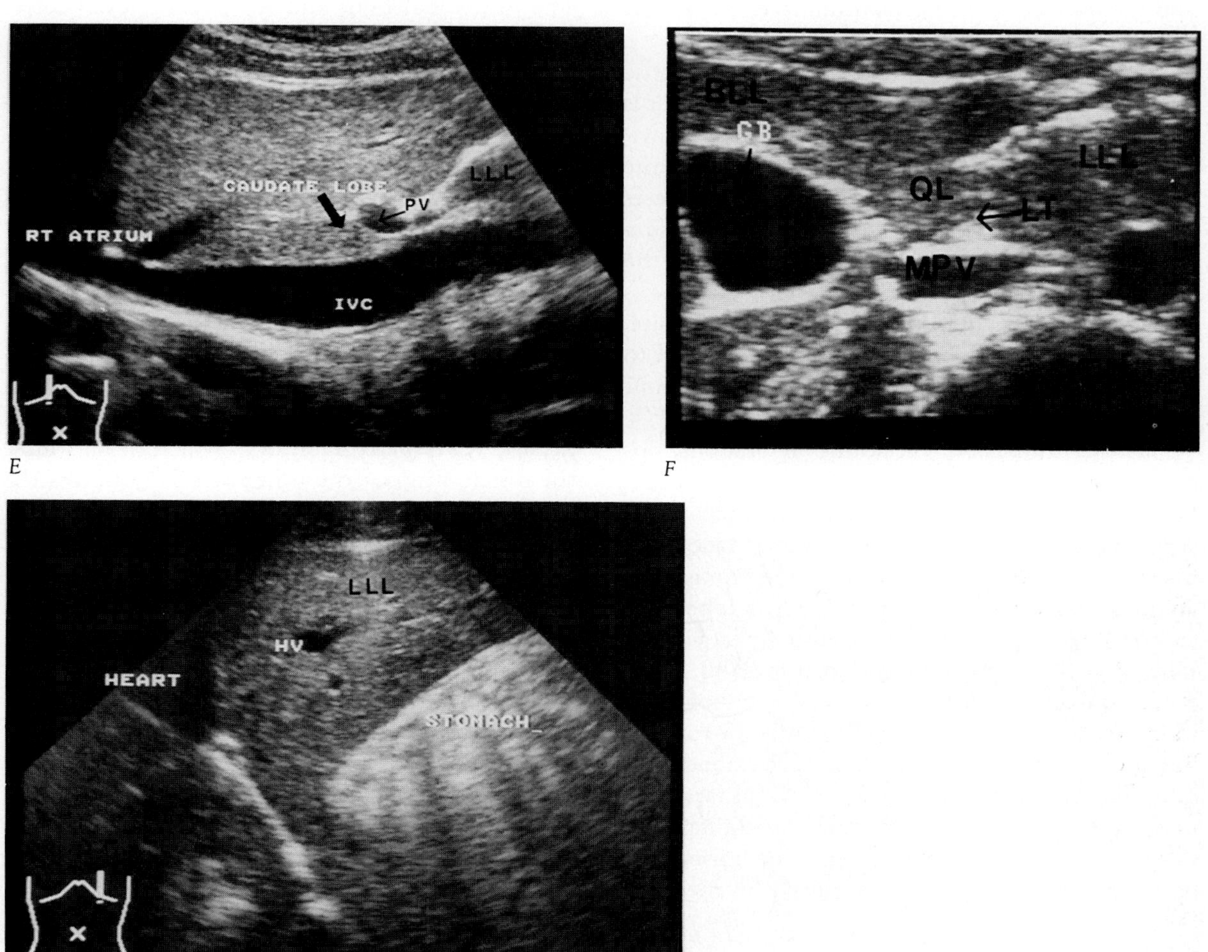

FIGURE 4-4 (*continued*). (*B*) The IVC within the IVC fossa and the main portal vein (PV) and common hepatic duct (CHD) within the porta fossa are seen on this transverse section of the right liver lobe (RLL). (C) A sagittal section of the right liver lobe (RLL) visualizes the area of the gallbladder fossa (GB, gallbladder; PV, portal vein; HV, hepatic vein). (*D*) The caudate lobe *(large arrow)* is bounded on the right by the IVC, on the left by the fissure for the ligamentum venosum (LV) separating it from the left liver lobe (LLL), and on the anterior inferior margin by the left portal vein (LPV). This transverse section demonstrates the normal sonographic appearance of hepatic parenchyma (AO, aorta; PV, right portal vein; DIAPH, crus of the diaphragm). (*E*) The caudate lobe's *(large arrow)* relationship with the IVC, left portal vein (PV) *(small arrow)*, and left liver lobe (LLL) can be identified on this sagittal section. (C–*E* Courtesy Doug Amussen, Logan, UT.) (*F*) The anatomic quadrate lobe (QL) can be identified anterior to the porta hepatis (MPV, main portal vein), posterior to the inferior margin of the liver, to the left of the gallbladder (GB) fossa and to the right of the fissure for the ligamentum teres (LT); (RLL, right liver lobe; LLL, left liver lobe). (Courtesy Cathy Carr-Hoefer, Corvallis, OR.) (G) The left liver lobe (LLL) tapers off at about the left mammary line and can be identified in the epigastric and left hypochondrium regions (HV, hepatic vein). (Courtesy Doug Amussen, Logan, UT.)

and the fissure for the ligamentum teres on the left (see Fig. 4-4A, F).

Left lobe. The left lobe is situated in the epigastric and left hypochondriac regions. Anatomically, it is separated from the right hepatic lobe by the falciform ligament on its diaphragmatic surface. On the visceral surface, the fissure for the ligamentum teres separates it from the quadrate lobe and the fissure for the ligamentum venosum separates it from the caudate lobe (Fig. 4-4A, D, E, F). The left lobe is flatter and smaller than the right but varies in size. Its superior surface is slightly convex, is molded to the diaphragm, and tapers off to the left at about the left mammary line (Fig. 4-4G).

Anatomic variations. Variations in anatomy include situs inversus, normal variations in shape, variations in lobe size,[6] high posterior hepatodiaphragmatic interposition of the colon,[10] accessory fissures,[11,153] thinning of the left lobe, congenital absence of the left lobe,[15] and Reidel's lobe[94] (an anatomic variant in which an unusually large right lobe gives the impression of hepatomegaly).[39] It is more common in women than in men. Sonographically, it is identified as a small handle, or tongue-like projection, on the right lobe that extends distally. The caudal extension may extend as far as the iliac crest. To distinguish it from a pathologic lesion, the sonographer must observe the normal hepatic echo pattern and its contiguity with the right lobe.[148]

Segmental Division. Segmental division is based on two of the liver's greater functions, as a gland with bile ducts and as a vascular and storage organ supplied by blood from the portal veins and the hepatic arteries.[49,65,66] The internal lobar divisions do not coincide completely with those established by external markings and the liver does not display surface lobulations, as the lungs do.[94] The functional lobar divisions are very important for sonographers to understand and they can be defined by demonstrating various ligaments and planes in the parenchyma. This is clinically important in determining the segmental confinement of neoplasms, lesions, and other nonmalignant (and some malignant) abnormalities in preparation for surgical resection.[65,66,88]

The primary branching of the portal vein and hepatic artery at the porta establishes two right segments, two left segments, and the caudate lobe.[148] The functional right and left hepatic lobes correspond to an oblique plane extending from the IVC fossa to the gallbladder fossa (Fig. 4-4A, 4-5A). This plane can be identified sonographically because it corresponds in part to the incomplete main lobar fissure,[65,66] which extends over a variable but short distance between the gallbladder neck and right portal vein.[39,116] It is echogenic because it contains fat (Fig. 4-5B, C).[125] On a transverse section, it has a comet-tail appearance that can be used to help locate the gallbladder.[114] If the main lobar fissure is not identified clearly the right and left intrahepatic lobes' location can be closely approximated.[105] Through this fissure extends the middle hepatic vein, the tributaries of which never follow the distribution of the other vessels but cross the portal vein branches in an interdigitated fashion (Fig. 4-5B, D).[94] Remember that segmental divisions are a functional description, whereas the hepatic veins pursue an independent course within the liver substance that does not completely conform to the vascular supply and bile passages.[65,66]

Right lobe. The right intrahepatic lobe is subdivided into posterior and anterior segments based on the branching patterns of the portal vein passing centrally within these intrahepatic segments and by the short intersegmental fissure, which is frequently indistinguishable from the porta hepatis structures.[137] The anterior segment is located farther superior and is somewhat larger than the posterior segment. Sonographically, a high transverse section demonstrating the right hepatic vein identifies this intrasegmental division (see Fig. 4-5A, E, F).[125] More inferior, the division is not readily as discernible and the portal vein branches are used to make arbitrary distinctions on sonographic images.[125] Both segments are also divided into superior and inferior portions.[94]

Left lobe. The left intrahepatic lobe is comprised of the medial and lateral segments. The medial segment corresponds to the traditional quadrate lobe (see Fig 4-4F). The lateral segment comprises the left lobe in the traditional anatomic description. Sonographically, the left intrahepatic segments are not as easily defined. The left hepatic vein, separating the segments cranially, is not always imaged.[105] Furthermore, it is difficult to image the vertical, dorsal-to-ventral branching pattern of the left portal vein.[105] The hyperechoic ligamentum teres is usually imaged and can be used to identify

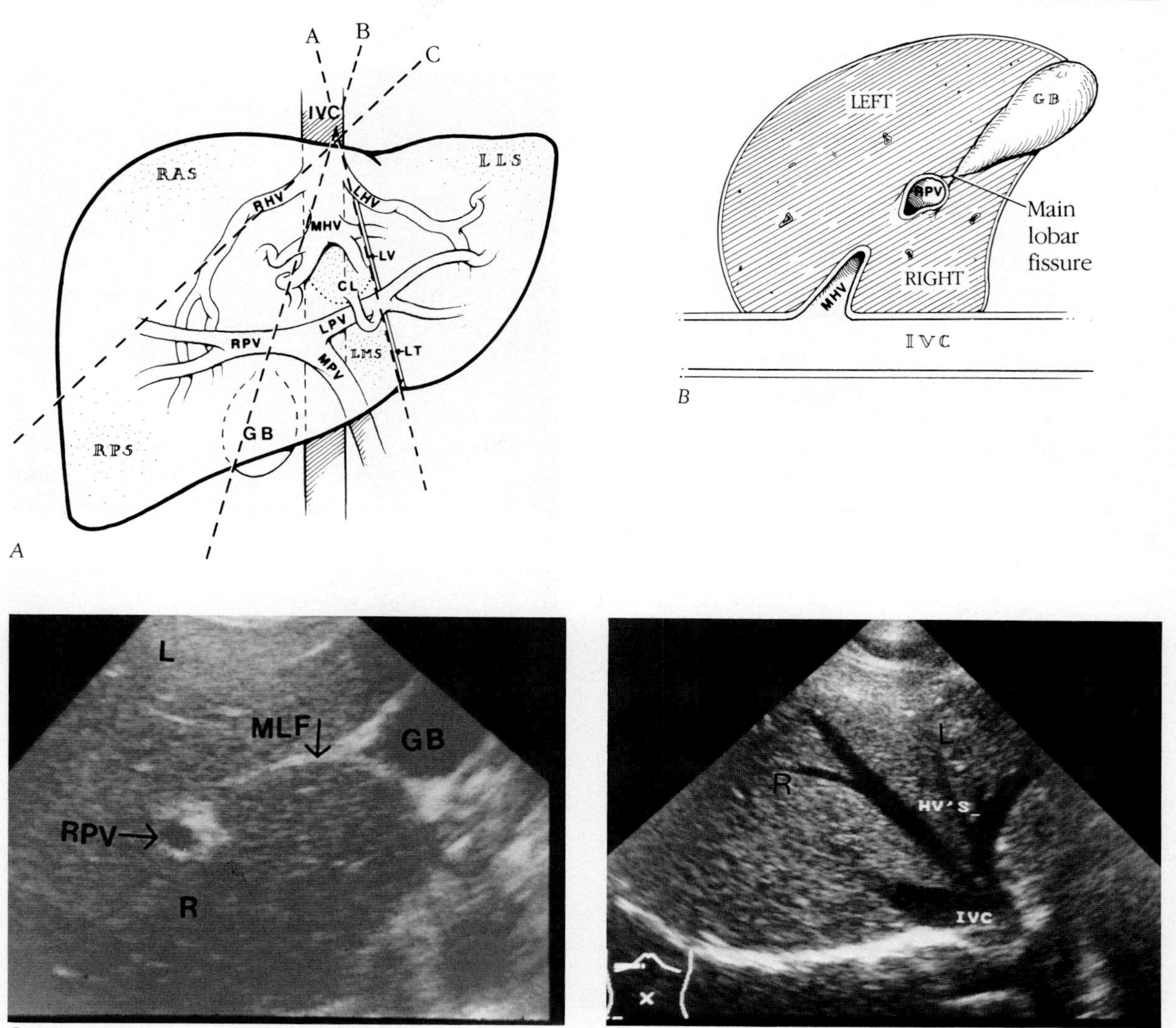

FIGURE 4-5. (*A*) A "see-through" anterior-posterior profile. The lettered lines are scanning levels, which are referred to in subsequent illustrations and sonograms. Line B depicts the separation between the intrahepatic right and left lobes. (RAS, right anterior segment; RPS, right posterior segment; LMS, left medial segment; LLS, left lateral segment; CL, caudate lobe; IVC, inferior vena cava; RHV, right hepatic vein; MHV, middle hepatic vein; LHV, left hepatic vein; MPV, main portal vein; RPV, right portal vein; LPV, left portal vein; GB, gallbladder; LV, ligamentum venosum; LT, ligamentum teres.) (*B*) Scanning through line B (Fig. 4-5A), the main lobar fissure, located between the gallbladder neck and the right portal vein, divides the liver into the intrahepatic right and left lobes. (C) The main lobar fissure (MLF) can be identified by its hyperechoic appearance, coursing between the right portal vein (RPV) and the gallbladder (GB), separating the intrahepatic right (R) and left (L) lobes. (*D*) The middle hepatic vein (MHV) extends through the main lobar fissure and delineates the right (R) and left (L) intrahepatic lobes. The right hepatic (RHV) and left hepatic (LHV) veins drain into the IVC and are identified on this transverse section made in the liver's superior portion. (Courtesy Doug Amussen, Logan, UT.)

(continued on next page)

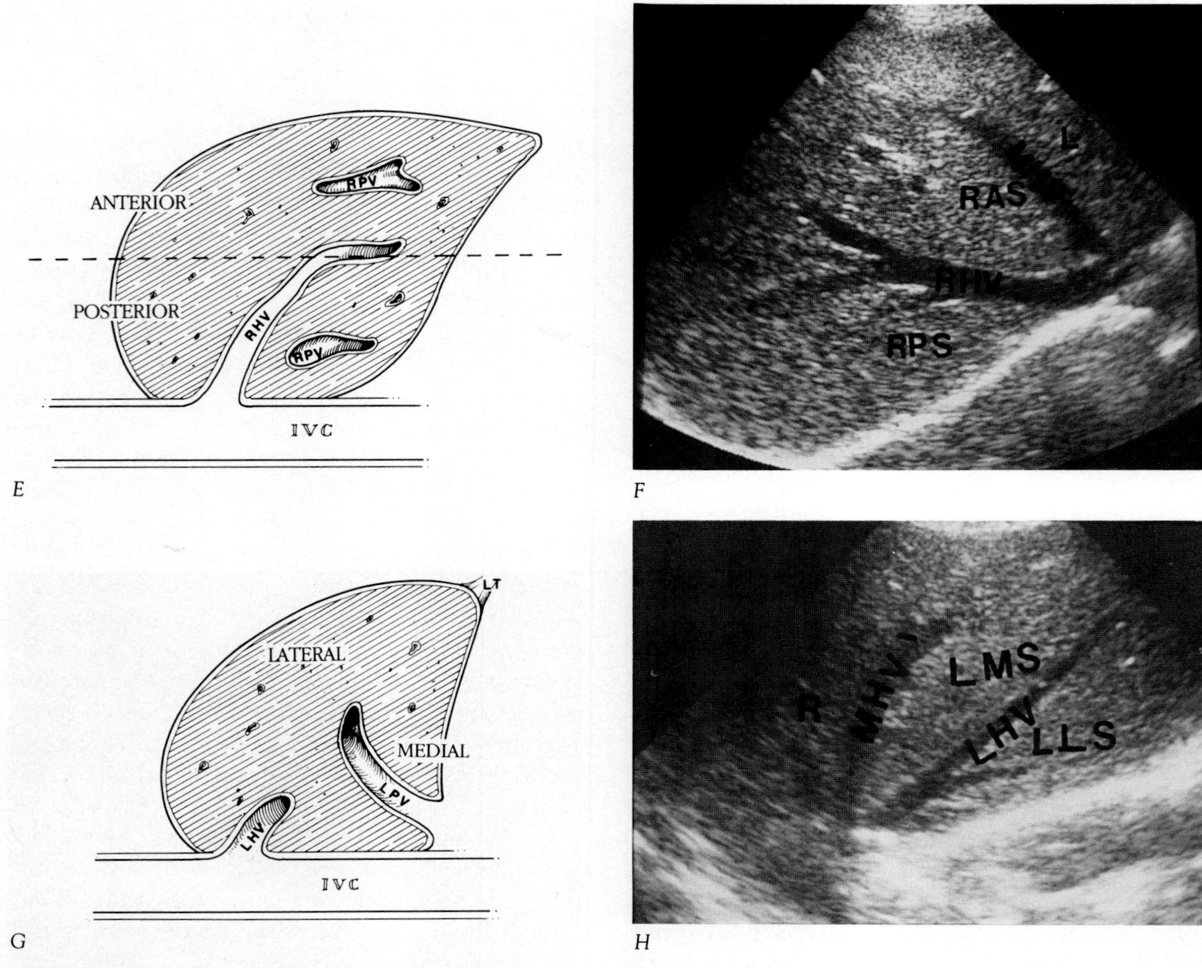

Figure 4-5 (*continued*). (*E*) Scanning through line C (Fig. 4-5A), the right hepatic vein courses between the right anterior and right posterior branches of the portal vein, which supplies blood to the right intrahepatic lobe and divides it into an anterior and a posterior segment. (*F*) An oblique transverse image demonstrates the right hepatic vein (RHV) dividing the right anterior (RAS) and right posterior (RPS) segments of the right intrahepatic lobe. The middle hepatic vein (MHV) is also visualized dividing the left and right intrahepatic lobes. (*G*) Scanning through line A (Fig. 4-5A), the left hepatic vein divides the left intrahepatic lobe into a lateral and a medial segment. The scanning plane sections through the hyperechoic ligamentum teres. (*H*) An oblique transverse image demonstrates the left hepatic vein (LHV) dividing the left medial (LMS) and left lateral (LLS) segments of the left intrahepatic lobe. The middle hepatic vein (MHV) is also visualized dividing the left and right (R) intrahepatic lobes.

the left intrahepatic division (see Fig. 4-5A, G, H).[105,125] Both segments are also divided into superior and inferior portions.[94]

Caudate lobe. The caudate lobe corresponds to the anatomic division (see Fig 4-4D, E). It is functionally distinct and is not considered a right or a left lobe, as it receives its blood supply from both right and left portal radicles and from the hepatic arterial branches[65,66] and has its own bile ducts.[21,88] It is drained by short venous channels that extend directly from the posterior aspect into the IVC.[21] This independent blood supply has significant clinical implications that produce changes in cirrhosis as well as in Budd-Chiari syndrome.[21] The afferent vessels, portal veins, and hepatic arteries have a short intrahepatic course which is not as readily affected by hepatic fibrosis. Caudate lobe enlargement and right lobe shrinkage seen in cirrhosis patients may be attributed to the discrepancy between blood perfusion in the two lobes.[21,88] Caudate lobe enlargement with associated compression of the underlying IVC is implicated in various cirrhotic complications such as, IVC hypertension, ascites, portacaval shunt failure, and, possibly, hepatorenal syndrome (renal failure sometimes seen during the terminal stages of cirrhosis and ascites).[21]

VASCULAR SYSTEM

The liver is unique in that it receives a double supply of blood. The hepatic arterial blood is oxygen rich and the portal venous blood is nutrient rich after it traverses the walls of the gastrointestinal tract. The blood from the portal vein and hepatic arteries mingles in the liver sinusoids and is drained by the hepatic veins (Fig. 4-6A).

Hepatic Arteries. The common hepatic artery branches off the celiac axis and passes forward and to the right to enter the right margin of the gastrohepatic ligament. Here it ascends, lying to the left of the common bile duct and anterior to the portal vein. As it turns cephalad, it gives origin to the gastroduodenal artery, the supraduodenal artery, and the right gastric artery. The hepatic artery proper is the continuation of the hepatic artery beyond the bifurcation of these vessels. It ascends and divides into several branches, most commonly into a right and a left ramus, which supply the right and left segmental lobes, respectively. The cystic artery arises off the right ramus and the middle hepatic artery usually arises from the left one (Fig. 4-6B–D).

Portal Veins. The main portal vein (MPV) originates just to the right of the midline at the junction of the splenic vein and superior mesenteric vein and then courses cephalad and to the right into the porta hepatis.[66,98] At this point, the MPV normally measures 11 $\pm$2 mm (range 6 to 15 mm),[149] is anterior to the IVC, and is cephalad to the head of the pancreas (see Fig. 4-6C). The MPV divides into a smaller left portal vein (LPV) somewhat to the right of the midline, more anterior, and more craniad and into a larger right portal vein (RPV) located more posterior and more caudad.[82] The porta hepatis can be identified as the elongated portion of the MPV at the origin of the LPV (Fig. 4-6E).[82]

The LPV courses craniad along the anterior surface of the caudate lobe, then arches, curving toward the left and anteriorly prior to its major bifurcation, giving a branch that courses back to the right to supply the left medial intrahepatic lobar segment (quadrate lobe)[66] and a branch for the left lateral intrahepatic lobar segment. Both are intersegmental in their course.[82,98] Prior to the bifurcation is the umbilical portion, so named because in utero the umbilical vein attached at this point.[66] The umbilical portion provides a portion of the caudate lobe's blood supply through small branches that are not visualized sonographically.[66] The size of the LPV and its angle of bifurcation with the MPV vary, depending largely on the size and configuration of the left lobe.[53] It is visualized in 61% of patients (Fig. 4-6F).[82]

The main segment of the RPV is larger than the LPV, bifurcates from the MPV farther posterior, and has a long horizontal course.[88] It can be identified sonographically as a round or ovoid vessel positioned centrally in the right hepatic lobe.[37] It bifurcates at various distances from the MPV to supply the right anterior and right posterior intrahepatic lobar segments (Fig. 4-6G).[94]

The common hepatic and intrahepatic ducts and the portal veins normally course parallel to each other[75]; however, venous blood and bile flow in opposite directions. Intrahepatic ducts are not visualized routinely. If biliary radicles and portal ve-

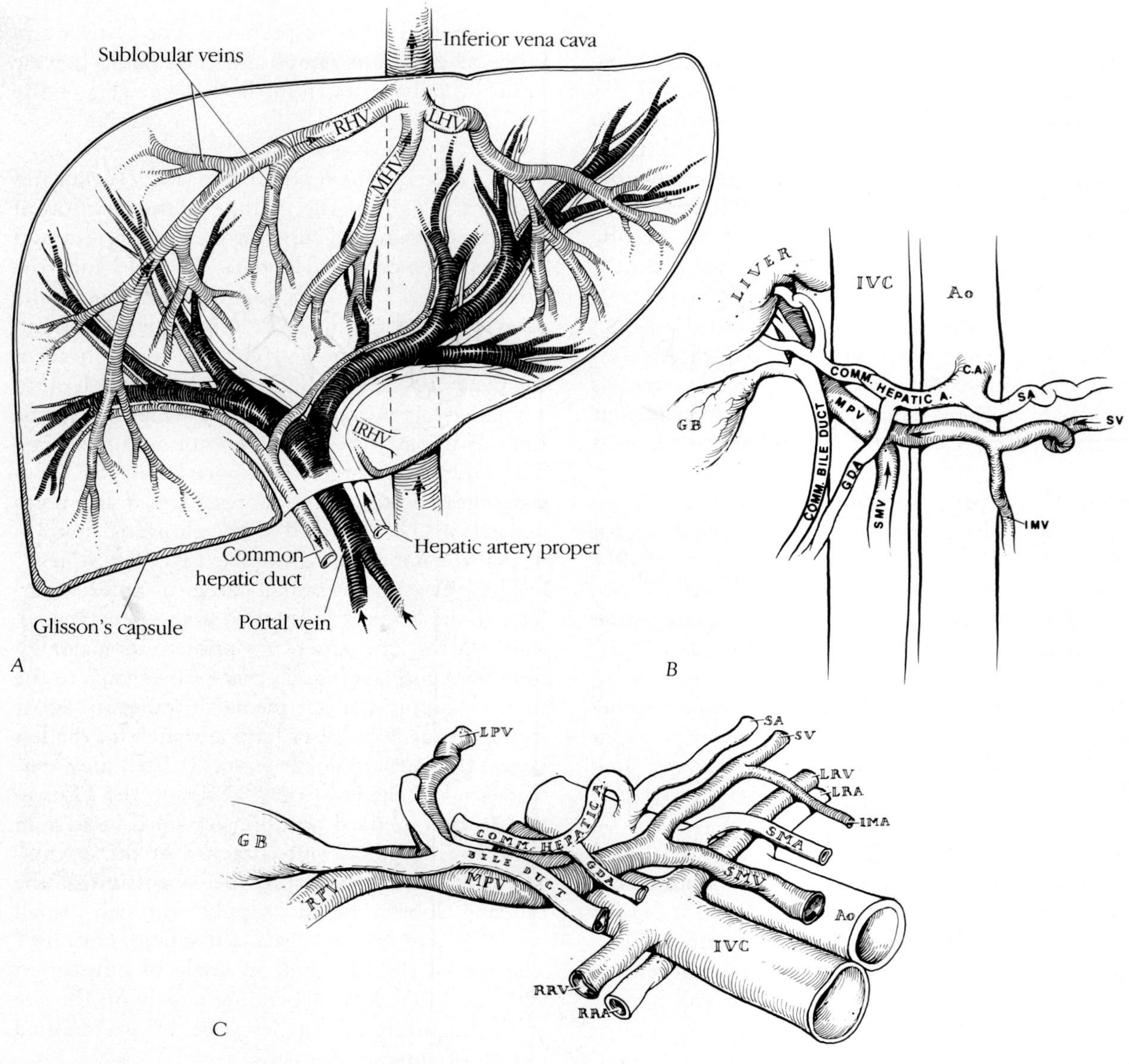

FIGURE 4-6. (*A*) Intrahepatic distribution of the hepatic arteries, hepatic veins, portal veins, and biliary ducts. An accessory right hepatic vein draining directly into the IVC is a variant identified in some patients. (RHV, right hepatic vein; MHV, middle hepatic vein; LHV, left hepatic vein; IRHV, inferior right hepatic vein.) (*B*) The vessels and ducts of the upper abdomen. (IVC, inferior vena cava; AO, aorta; GB, gallbladder; MPV, middle hepatic vein; SMV, superior mesenteric vein; GDA, gastroduodenal artery; CA, celiac axis; SA, splenic artery; COMM. HEPATIC A, common hepatic artery; SV, splenic vein; IMV, inferior mesenteric vein.) (*C*) The relationship between the vessels and ducts of the upper abdomen. (GB, gallbladder; LPV, left portal vein; RPV, right portal vein; MPV, middle portal vein; GDA, gastroduodenal artery; COMM. HEPATIC A, common hepatic artery; SA, splenic artery; LRV, left renal vein; LRA, left renal artery; IMA, inferior mesenteric artery; SMA, superior mesenteric artery; SMV, superior mesenteric vein; AO, aorta; IVC, inferior vena cava; RRA, right renal artery; RRV, right renal vein.)

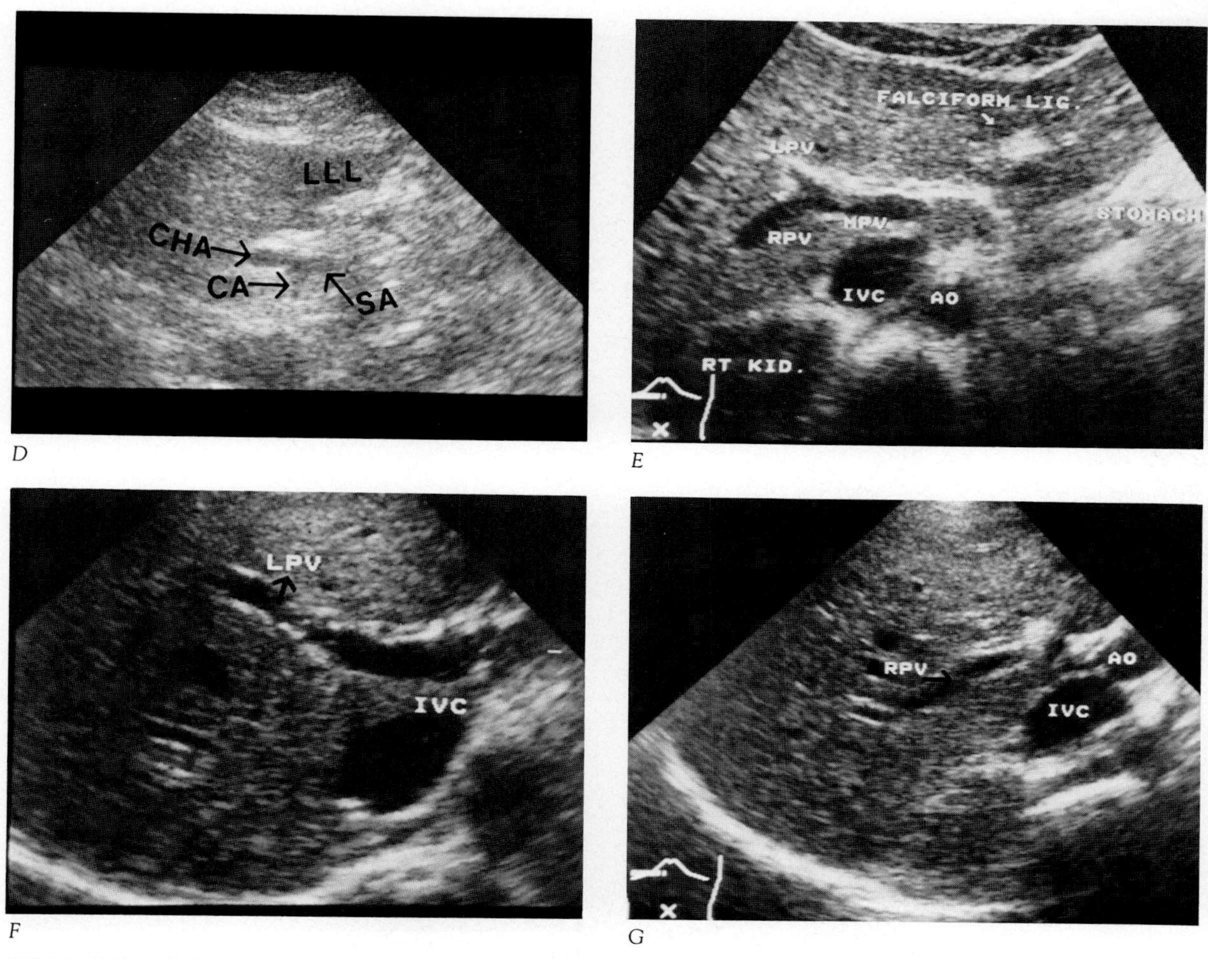

FIGURE 4-6 (*continued*).(*D*) A transverse section demonstrates the left liver lobe (LLL), the common hepatic artery (CHA), and the splenic artery (SA) branching off the celiac axis (CA). (*E*) On a transverse section, the anterior location of the main portal vein (MPV) location to the IVC and the left portal vein (LPV) and right portal vein (RPV) branches are identified (AO, aorta). (*F*) The left portal vein (LPV) (*arrow*) is identified prior to the point of bifurcation anterior to the IVC on this transverse section. (G) A transverse section demonstrates the right portal vein (RPV), the IVC, and the aorta (AO). (E–G Courtesy Doug Amussen, Logan, UT.)

(*continued on next page*)

nous radicles are imaged simultaneously side by side, the appearance, referred to as the parallel-channel sign, is used to diagnose obstruction (Fig. 4-6H, I).[14,26,68,74,150] A corollary is the rule of three: two structures could represent two limbs of a bifurcating vein, whereas a third round structure seen side by side in the liver implies abnormal dilatation of the biliary tract.[14,75]

Hepatic Veins. Hepatic veins are best visualized on transverse scans made in the cephalad portion of the liver. They drain directly into the superior aspect of the IVC. Three should be demonstrated routinely: the right hepatic vein (RHV), the middle hepatic vein (MHV), and the left hepatic vein (LHV); (Fig. 4-5D, 4-6J).

The RHV is the largest.[137] It courses between the

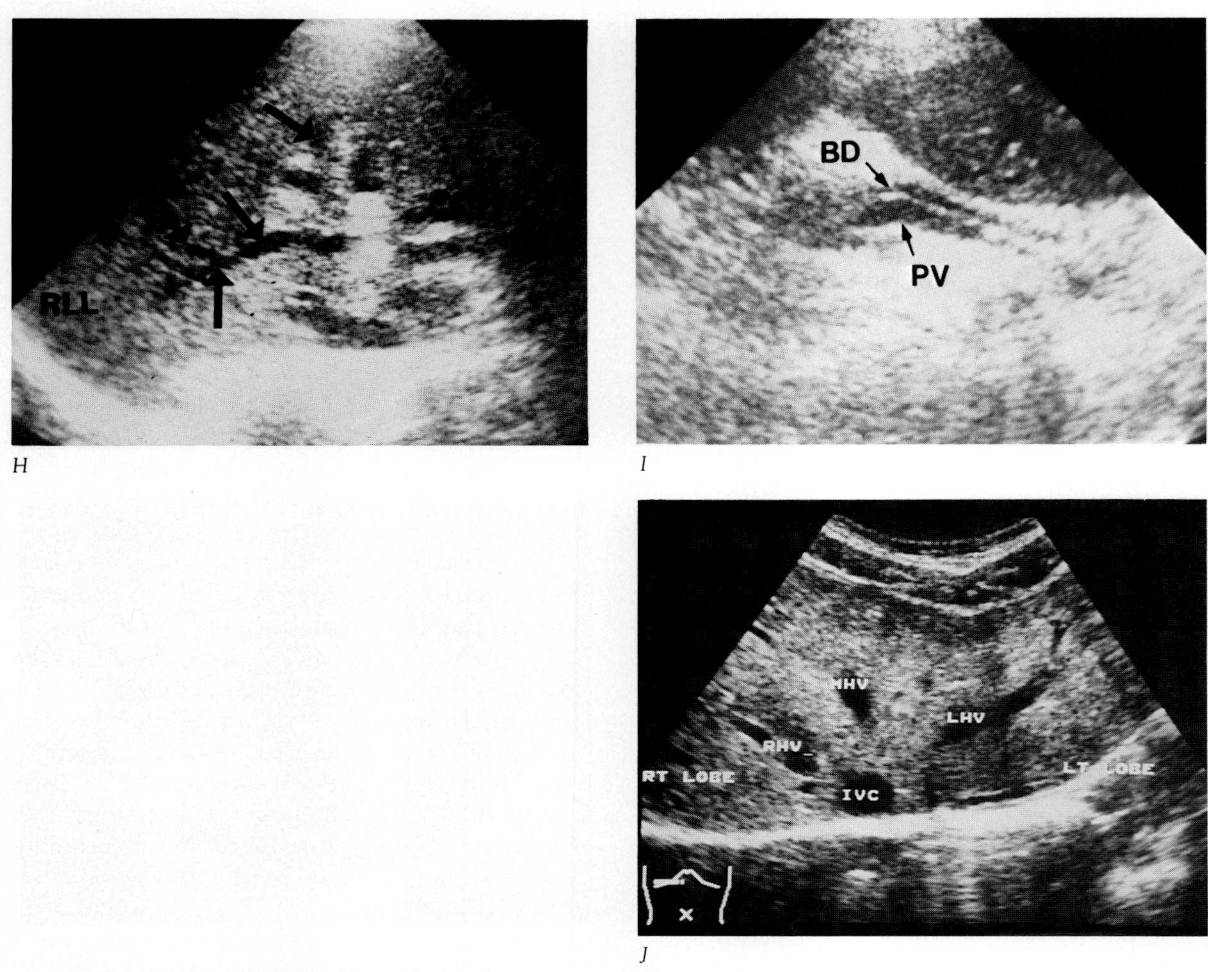

H

I

J

FIGURE 4-6 (*continued*). On a transverse section scan (*H*) of a 76-year-old woman with ill-defined upper abdominal pain and jaundice, prominent dilated bile ducts (*arrows*) create an irregular branching pattern in the right liver lobe (RLL). The parallel-channel sign (*I*) represents a dilated bile duct (BD, *arrow*) and the portal vein (PV, *arrow*). A mass, most likely representing adenopathy, located in the porta hepatis was believed the cause of the obstruction. (Courtesy Mary Davies, American Fork, UT.) (*J*) The middle hepatic vein (MHV) extends through the main lobar fissure and delineates the right and left intrahepatic lobes. The right hepatic vein (RHV) and left hepatic vein (LHV) delineate the intrahepatic segments. (Courtesy Doug Amussen, Logan, UT.)

anterior and posterior branches of the right portal vein,[56,82] is located in the right intersegmental fissure, and divides the cephalic aspect of the anterior and posterior segments of the right hepatic lobe.[98,125,137] The MHV is located in the main lobar fissure corresponding to the anatomic and segmental division between the right and left lobes.[82,125,137] The smaller LHV is located in the cranial portion of the left segmental fissure, dividing the left lobe into lateral and medial intrahepatic segments.[56,82,137]

The inferior right hepatic vein (IRHV) is a variant and can be difficult to visualize. It was identified in only 10% of the cases by Makuuchi and coworkers[80] and Doehner[32] but in 15.5% of liver examinations in a recent study by Sunder.[137] When it can be identified it is visualized on a transverse section at the level of the porta hepatis, on a longitudinal section situated behind the right portal venous branch,[80,137] or in a right intercostal coronal section; it measures 3 to 8 mm in diameter (Fig. 4-6A).[137] When identified, it may present as a "pseudo-parallel-channel sign" as it crosses the liver posteriorly and parallel to the right portal venous branch in the posteroinferior segment of the right lobe.[80] Attempting to identify an IRHV variant is clinically important for several reasons: (1) The entire main RHV is resected during hepatectomy because the right lobe can be preserved along with the hypertrophic IRHV, (2) Thrombus has been identified in the IRHV in patients with hepatocellular carcinoma, (3) The right lobe's main drainage vein is the IRHV, as seen in primary Budd-Chiari syndrome, (4) Obstruction of the bile ducts presents a real parallel-channel sign, which needs to be differentiated from a false one.[80]

Sonographic Distinction. The portal and hepatic vascular system is extremely important to identify sonographically.[24] With ligaments, fissures, and fossas, it provides an important map for localizing specific abnormalities, affords the ability to distinguish dilated portions of the biliary tree,[37] and can be used to successfully perform follow-up examinations. The five criteria used to distinguish hepatic veins and portal veins are described in Table 4-2 and can be identified by comparing Figures 4-2E and 4-2H.

Porta Hepatis

The porta (gate) hepatis (liver) is a fissure where the portal vein and hepatic artery enter the liver and the hepatic duct (common hepatic duct) leaves it.[49,53,94] In the normal relationship of these three structures within the hepatoduodenal ligament the common hepatic duct is ventral and to the left, the hepatic artery is ventral and to the right, and the portal vein is dorsal, located between artery and duct (Fig. 4-6C).[49]

It is important to evaluate these structures and measure the common hepatic duct in either a transverse or longitudinal section. To do this, the sonographer locates the splenic vein on a transverse section and follows it to the right, where it is joined by the superior mesenteric vein and becomes the main portal vein (Fig. 4-7A). The main portal vein courses toward the liver and appears round. The transducer is angled approximately 45 degrees until the hepatic duct and hepatic artery are identified. A transverse section through the portal triad has a Mickey Mouse silhouette (Fig. 4-7B).[14] The duct is measured in either a transverse or longitudinal section. Care must be taken to avoid an off-axis longitudinal section, leading to underestimating the measurement (Fig. 4-7C).[14] Published values for the normal internal diameter vary from 4 to 8 mm,[99,100,112,150,151] and it has been recommended that 4 to 5 mm be used as a maximum and that an internal diameter greater than 6 mm suggests dilatation caused by partial obstruction or loss of elasticity due to preexisting obstruction.[27,47,117,155]

The common duct and hepatic artery may be confused[26,112,154] because of their proximity, similar internal diameter (maximum internal diameter of the hepatic artery is reported to be 2 to 6 mm),[17] and the common anatomic variations of the triad structures.[63,74,107] The literature addresses accurate criteria for measuring bile ducts,[47,68,117,155] including comparisons with findings of intravenous cholangiography[117] and comparisons before and after cholecystectomy.[47,90,117] Berland and colleagues[17] found several reliable sonographic signs to differentiate the common duct and hepatic artery, including evaluating the porta hepatis with duplex scanning:

1. Only intrinsic pulsations should be exhibited by an artery or a vein.
2. A crossing artery can sharply indent a duct or a vein, whereas the reverse is not true, probably owing to the lower venous and ductal pressure and a thicker, less easily deformed arterial wall.
3. The duct can occasionally decrease several millimeters in caliber during an examination and can have various calibers along its course, whereas arteries are uniform in caliber.
4. The artery may not parallel the vein or do so only for a short distance, whereas the duct parallels the vein closely.

TABLE 4-2. Sonographic criteria for differentiating the portal and hepatic veins

Origin and drainage	Observe the point of origin and drainage of the vessels. Portal vein branches can be traced back to the portal vein, distinguishing them from the hepatic veins draining into the IVC.[66]
Collagen content	Encased in a collagenous sheath and running in common with the hepatic artery and bile duct, the margins of portal veins are highly reflective, making them appear thicker and hyperechoic in contrast to the parenchymal background.[66,88] By contrast, the hepatic veins are surrounded by parenchymal tissue and have rather imperceptible margins owing to a minimal amount of collagen.[66] This is the simplest of the criteria, but it is also the least reliable.[24] A specular reflection may occur if the sound beam strikes the hepatic wall at right angles, which results in a rather high-amplitude echogenic margin[24] similar in appearance to the portal vein branches.[66]
Branching patterns	An angle formed by the limbs of a branched systemic venous structure points in the direction of flow.[24] For the portal vein, branching is horizontal and the angle's apex is oriented toward the porta hepatis.[24,88,97] Hepatic vein branching is longitudinal, and the angle's apex formed at the communication points superiorly or supermedially toward the IVC.[24,97]
Caliber changes	The direction of blood flow also dictates the caliber of the venous radicles. The caliber of the hepatic veins becomes greater as they course toward the diaphragm and the IVC,[88] and the caliber of the portal veins decreases further from their point of origin, the porta hepatis.
Segmental location	Hepatic veins are interlobar and intersegmental, coursing between lobes and segments,[105] and portal veins are intrasegmental, coursing within lobar segments.[88]

5. Arteries may be tortuous and loop in and out of the scanning plane.
6. Arteries produce pulsatile Doppler signals; veins produce continuous Doppler signals; and ducts produce no signal.[17]

MICROSCOPIC STRUCTURES

Hepatic lobes are made up of the basic functional unit, the liver lobule.[81,145] The liver parenchyma is made up of 50,000 to 100,000 individual lobules (Fig. 4-8A, B).[49,102] Within each lobule, small bile canaliculi lie adjacent to the cellular plates, receive the bile produced by the hepatocytes,[51,59] and carry it toward the bile duct branches in the triad regions (Fig. 4-8C).[81,130] These open into the interlobular bile ducts accompanying the hepatic artery and portal vein system, except that bile flows in the direction opposite that of blood in these vessels.[49,81,131] Bile ducts join other bile ducts and form two main trunks, the right and left hepatic ducts, which eventually drain into the common hepatic duct.[81,124,131] The biliary duct walls consist of a connective tissue coat composed of muscle cells arranged both concentrically and longitudinally and an epithelial layer consisting of short columnar cells resting on a distinct basement membrane.[49,94]

Physiology

In ancient Babylonian time, the liver was thought to have mystic powers. Priest-physicians often would dissect and examine the liver of sacrificial animals for omens from the gods. The liver was chosen for this purpose because it contains the most blood. Since life and blood were synonymous, the liver was considered the seat of the soul.

The liver is an organ most essential to life, as it performs more than 500 separate activities.[104] A single liver cell is so diversified in its activities that it is analogous to a factory for many chemical compounds; to a warehouse with short- and long-term storage capabilities; to a power plant producing heat; to a waste disposal plant excreting waste; and to a chemist regenerating tissue that has not been too severely damaged. These functions are carried out by three types of cells in the parenchyma: the hepatocyte, which carries out most metabolic func-

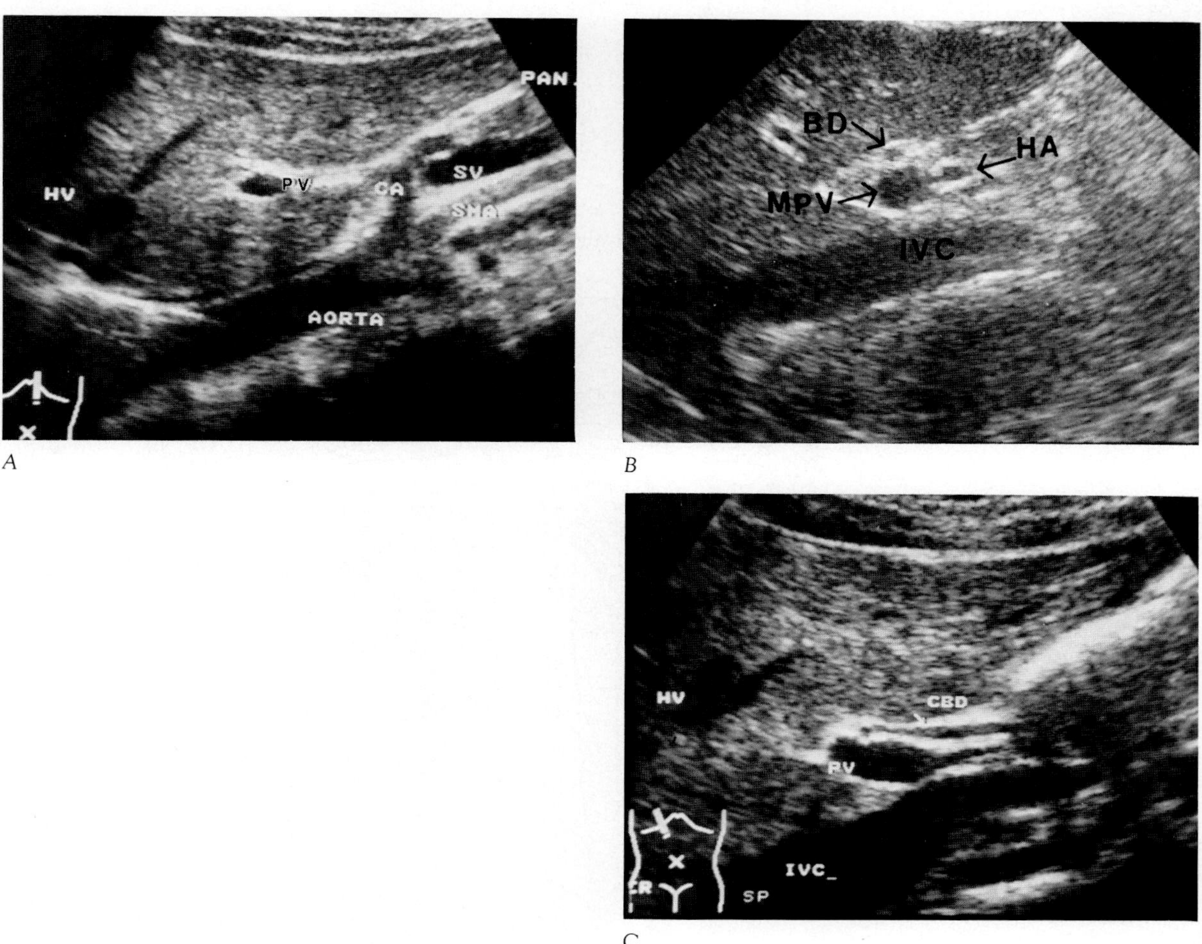

FIGURE 4-7. (*A*) A sagittal section visualizes the splenic vein (SV) to the right of the celiac axis (CA). Locating the confluence of the splenic and superior mesenteric veins helps identify the formation of the main portal vein (PV); (HV, hepatic vein; SMA, superior mesenteric artery; PAN, pancreas). (*B*) A transverse oblique section of the portal triad has a Mickey Mouse silhouette: the main portal vein (MPV) represents the face, the common hepatic duct (BD) the right ear, and the hepatic artery (HA) the left ear. (C) The portal vein (PV) and common hepatic duct (CBD) are identified anterior to the IVC on an oblique sagittal section (HV, hepatic vein). (A,C Courtesy Doug Amussen, Logan, UT.)

tions; the biliary epithelial cells, which line the biliary system, bile ducts, canaliculi, and the gallbladder; and the Kupffer cells, which are phagocytic and belong to the reticuloendothelial system.[52]

It is not necessary to know all of these liver functions in great detail to obtain quality sonograms; however, since hepatic diseases alter these functions and produce identifiable clinical manifestations it is important to have a basic understanding of some normal functions (Table 4-3).

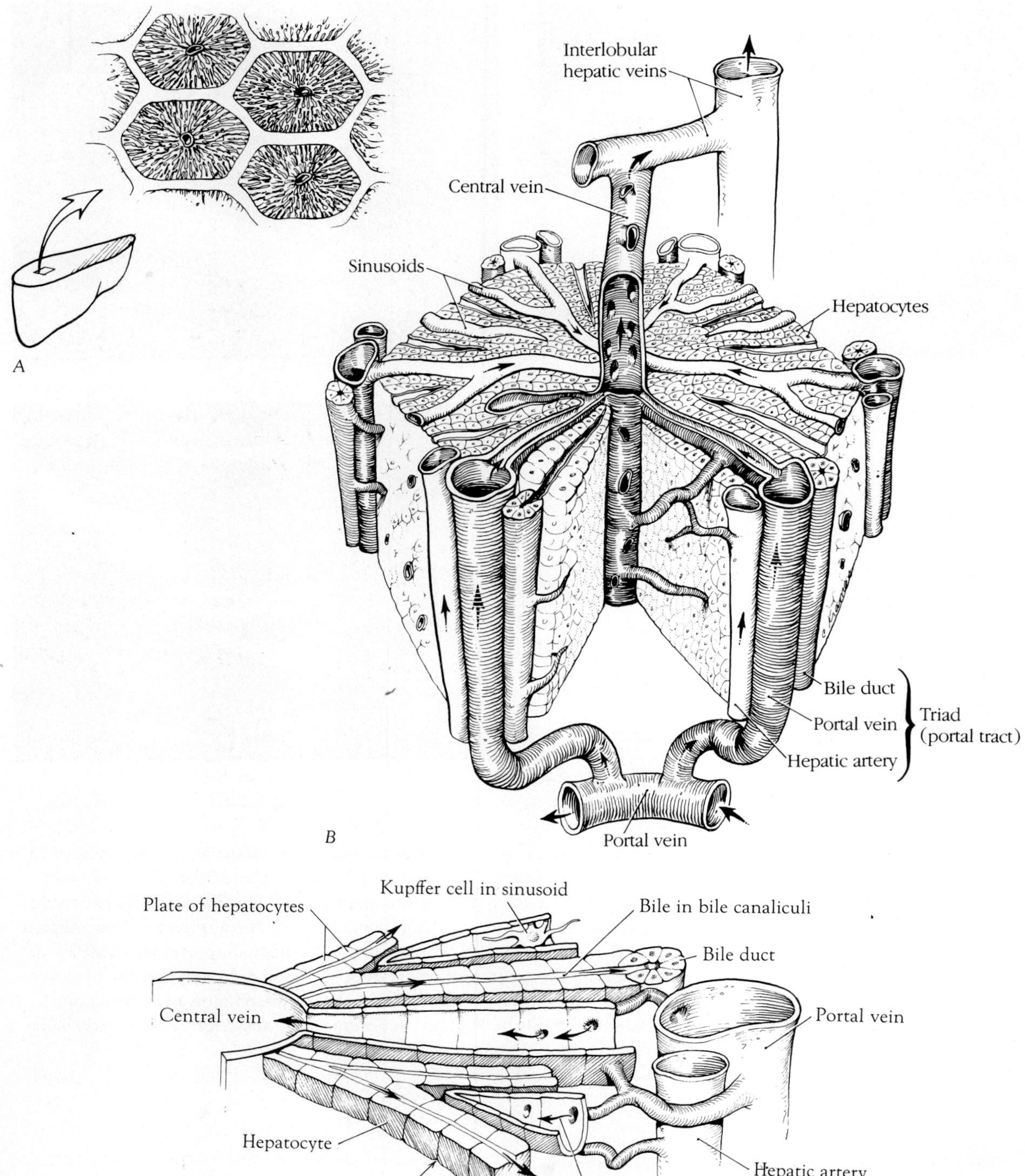
Interlobular
hepatic veins
Central vein
Sinusoids
Hepatocytes
A
Bile duct
Portal vein
Hepatic artery
Triad
(portal tract)
Portal vein
B
Plate of hepatocytes
Kupffer cell in sinusoid
Bile in bile canaliculi
Bile duct
Central vein
Portal vein
Hepatocyte
Disse's space
Hepatic artery
Blood flowing in sinusoids
(lined by endothelial cells)
C

Liver Function Tests

Enzyme names can generally be recognized because they normally end in *-ase,* but laboratory function tests are sometimes named with initials. Thus ALP may not be immediately recognized as an enzyme test for alkaline phosphatase. Adding to the confusion, the transaminases often referred to in the literature have new names that are more chemically correct. Serum glutamic-pyruvic transaminase (SGPT) is now called alanine aminotransferase (ALT) and serum glutamic-oxaloacetic transaminase (SGOT) is now called asparate aminotransferase (AST). In the remainder of the chapter we present the current terminology followed by the former designations in parentheses.

Alterations in any of the normal liver functions can produce a spectrum of disorders that can severely impair some liver functions and leave others entirely unaffected. Obstruction to the intra- or extrahepatic biliary system or damage to the hepatocyte or Kupffer cells can alter the plasma chemistry. Understanding the major tests performed to evaluate liver function helps correlate the clinical history and presenting symptoms (especially distinguishing obstructive from nonobstructive jaundice) with the sonographic visualization of hepatobiliary structures. The more common laboratory examinations are listed in Table 4-4. Because normal ranges vary by sex, age, and geographic region they are not represented; usually they appear in parentheses on a laboratory report.

Scanning Procedure

PATIENT PREPARATION

Most of the liver can be visualized without special patient preparation, but since initial liver examinations should include a comprehensive study of all upper abdominal organs, the patient should fast (taking nothing by mouth) 6 to 8 hours before the study.[53,148] Patients who fast for longer periods may take sips of water to avoid dehydration. Patients should abstain from smoking, chewing gum, and talking, activities that increase the amount of intestinal gas.[30]

PATIENT INSTRUCTIONS

Breathing Techniques. Normal and deep suspended inspiration techniques are used as well as a belly-out technique that is accomplished by pushing out

(text continues on page 116)

FIGURE 4-8. (*A*) An enlarged sectional cut of the liver shows the hexagonal or cylindric shape of its lobules. Each lobule measures several millimeters in length and 0.8 to 2 mm in diameter.[49,51,52] (*B*) The arrows indicate the direction of blood flow on this schematic representation of one liver lobule. Constructed around a central vein, each lobule is composed principally of many cellular plates, or hepatocytes, the functional cells of the liver. The cellular plates radiate centrifugally from the central vein like wheel spokes.[51,59] Hepatocytes are capable of regenerating which allows damaged or resected liver tissue to regrow.[59] A lobule has six corners. At each is a triad (portal tract), so named because three basic structures are always present: a branch of the hepatic artery, a branch of the portal vein, and a bile duct.[81,124] (*C*) An enlarged schematic view of a small portion of one liver lobule illustrates the sinusoids and portal triad. Sinusoids are small capillaries that have a highly permeable endothelial lining located between the cellular plates. They receive a mixture of portal venous and hepatic arterial blood.[51,52,59] The blood drains into the central vein in the middle of each lobule and flows into the hepatic veins.[51,59] Unlike other capillaries, they are also lined with phagocytic cells known as Kupffer cells.[59,81,145] Kupffer cells belong to the reticuloendothelial system and function to remove foreign substances from the blood, such as bacteria and worn out white and red blood cells.[81,104,145] Disse's space, located between the endothelial lining and the hepatocyte, drains interstitial fluid into the hepatic lymph system.[51,59] Small bile canaliculi are adjacent to the cellular plates and receive the bile produced by the hepatocytes.[51,59]

Table 4-3. Hepatic functions

Bile formation and secretion	Bilirubin, or bile pigment, is a major end-product resulting from the breakdown of hemoglobin by Kupffer cells[59] and other reticuloendothelial cells.[52] Bilirubin bound to plasma protein travels via the bloodstream to the liver, where it is conjugated (that is, made water soluble) and excreted into bile. Bile is produced continuously by the hepatic cells at a rate of 700 to 1200 ml per day.[59] Bile salts are formed from cholesterol in the hepatic cells and emulsify fats and assist in the absorption of fatty acids from the intestinal tract.[52] Calculus formation occurs if the bile salt content is abnormally high due to cholesterol precipitation. A metabolic deficit occurs when bile salts are not present in the intestinal tract and the fat-soluble vitamins, A, D, E, and K, are poorly absorbed. No bile secretion after a few days produces a vitamin K deficiency, leading to impairment of blood coagulation.[52]
Carbohydrate metabolism	The liver acts as a glucose buffer. It removes excess glucose from the blood, stores it, and returns it to the blood when the glucose concentration begins to fall.[59] Functions of carbohydrate metabolism include: (1) glycogenesis, the conversion of glucose to glycogen for storage;[52] (2) glycogenolysis, the reduction of glycogen to glucose;[51] and (3) gluconeogenesis, formation of glycogen from noncarbohydrates such as protein, amino acids, and fatty acids which maintains a relatively normal blood glucose concentration.[52,59]
Fat metabolism	(1) β-Oxidation of fatty acids and formation of acetoacetic acid, a soluble acid that passes from the liver cells into the extracellular fluids[52]; (2) formation of lipoprotein by synthesis of fat from glucose and amino acids[51]; (3) formation of cholesterol, which forms bile salts and phospholipids[52]; and (4) conversion of proteins and carbohydrates to fat to be transported as lipoprotein for storage in adipose tissue.[59] Fatty acids are a source of metabolic energy.[59] Approximately 60% of all preliminary breakdown of fatty acids occurs in the liver.
Protein metabolism	(1) Deamination of amino acids, which is necessary before they can be used for energy or converted into carbohydrates or fats[59]; (2) formation of urea by the liver removes ammonia from body fluids[52]; (3) formation of approximately 85% of the plasma proteins (except approximately 45% of the γ-globulins) at a maximum rate of 50 to 100 g/day[51,52]; (4) interconversions or synthesis of amino acids and other compounds vital to metabolism.[52] The reticuloendothelial tissue performs an essential role in protein anabolism by synthesizing various blood proteins—prothrombin, bilinogen, albumins, accelerator globulin, factor VII—and other less important coagulation factors.[72,124,145] Blood proteins are essential for normal circulation, as they maintain water balance, contributing to the blood's viscosity.[81] In addition, the liver manufactures the anticoagulant heparin.[124]
Reticuloendothelial tissue activity	The activity of the reticuloendothelial tissue in the liver starts before birth with the production of blood cells, a process called hemopoiesis.[34,124] By birth, this function is carried out by the bone marrow.[59] Plasma has three major types of protein, albumin, globulin, and fibrinogen.[52] All of the albumin and fibrinogen and 50% or more of the globulins are formed in the liver.[59] The rest of the globulins are formed by the lymphatic and other reticuloendothelial systems. The function of albumins is to provide colloid osmotic pressure, which prevents plasma loss from the capillaries. Fibrinogen polymerizes into long fibrin threads during blood coagulation, forming blood clots to help repair leaks in the circulatory system. Globulins perform a number of enzymatic functions in the plasma. The principal function of globulins is to provide natural and acquired immunity against invading organisms.[52,59]

TABLE 4-3. (*continued*)

Reticuloendothelial tissue activity (continued)	After a circulation time of approximately 120 days, red blood cells die.[51,59] It is assumed that they simply wear out with age and rupture during passage through a tight spot in the circulatory system.[81] The reticuloendothelial tissue of the spleen and the liver digests the hemoglobin released from ruptured red blood cells.[145] In this process, the iron from destroyed red cells is released back into the blood, bone marrow, or to the other tissues.[51,52] The bile pigment bilirubin is recovered by the reticuloendothelial cells from the heme portion of the hemoglobin molecule and released into the blood, where it is later secreted by the liver.[52,59] Large numbers of bacteria invade the body through the intestinal tract, passing through the mucosa into the portal blood.[52] The sinuses of the liver through which the blood passes are lined with Kupffer cells, which are tissue macrophages.[59] Kupffer cells form an effective particulate filtration system.[51,52] Almost all the bacteria from the gastrointestinal tract undergo phagocytosis.[59,145]
Storage depot	The liver has the capacity to store enough vitamin A to prevent a deficiency for as long as 1 or 2 years[52] and enough vitamin D and vitamin B_{12} to prevent deficiency for 1 to 4 months.[52] The liver also stores glycogen, fats, and amino acids and can metabolize them into glucose or vice versa, depending on the bodies needs.[59] Aside from the iron in the hemoglobin by far the greatest proportion of iron is stored in the liver in the form of ferritin. When extra iron is available in the body fluids it combines with apoferritin, a protein in hepatic cells capable of combining with iron. Apoferritin synthesizes with ferritin for iron storage. When the body becomes iron-deficient, the ferritin releases the iron.[52] The liver is also the storage depot for copper and some poisons that cannot be broken down or detoxified and excreted, such as DDT.
Blood reservoir	Approximately 1000 to 1100 ml of blood flows from the portal vein through the liver sinusoids each minute, and another 350 to 400 ml flows through the hepatic artery.[52] As a blood reservoir, the liver has the capacity to enlarge and store 200 to 400 ml of blood with a rise of only 4 to 8 mm Hg in hepatic venous pressure. If there is hemorrhage and large amounts of blood are being lost in the circulatory system, the liver releases its blood from that stored in the sinusoids to help compensate for this loss in blood volume.[59] Liver cirrhosis is a common cause of increased vascular resistance because the sinusoids become blocked. Cardiac congestion causes an increase in hepatic venous pressure of 10 to 15 mm Hg.[109]
Heat production	The liver, a significant metabolizer, produces heat as a result of its chemical reactions. On average, 55% of the energy of food ingested becomes heat during adenosine triphosphate (ATP) formation. Even more heat is produced during the ATP cell formation process.[59]
Detoxification	To a great degree the liver is a detoxifier, converting exogenous and endogenous chemicals, foreign molecules, and hormones to compounds that are not as toxic or biologically active.[59] When amino acids are burned for energy, they leave behind toxic nitrogenous wastes that are converted to urea by the liver cells. These moderate amounts of urea are then easily removed by the kidneys or sweat glands.[52]
Lymph formation	Under resting conditions the liver produces between a third and half of all the body's lymph.

Table 4-4. Liver function tests[29,61,73,144]

Test	Explanation	Result	Clinical Indication
Bilirubin	Formed in large part from heme of destroyed erythrocytes or from breakdown of developing red blood cells in bone marrow or other hemoproteins. Heme is converted to biliverdin in the spleen, kidney, and liver. Unconjugated bilirubin, formed from biliverdin, is not water soluble and is not excreted in urine. Unconjugated, or indirect, bilirubin is bound to albumin and transported to liver cells. Bilirubin is conjugated by liver enzymes, becomes water soluble, is not protein bound, and is excreted in urine. Most laboratories report the total value and the direct (conjugated) value. The indirect (unconjugated) value is calculated by subtracting the direct value from the total.	Indirect increase	Diseases that cause hemolysis, such as hemolytic jaundice; diseases that affect liver's ability to conjugate, such as Gilbert or Crigler-Najjar syndrome.
		Direct increase	Hepatocellular jaundice from hepatitis or cirrhosis; with decreased albumin and increased enzymes, parenchymal or obstructive liver disease; intrahepatic cholestasis from hepatic drug reactions, alcoholic hepatitis, primary biliary cirrhosis, or gram-negative septicemia; posthepatic jaundice from lower biliary tract obstruction.
Alanine aminotransferase (ALT), formerly serum glutamic pyruvic transaminase (SGPT)	Necessary enzyme in Krebs cycle essential for tissue energy production; largest amounts in the liver, smaller amounts in kidney, heart, and skeletal muscle. When damage to these tissues occurs, ALT increases. ALT is a rather specific indicator of hepatocellular damage. It is used in conjunction with AST to help distinguish between cardiac and hepatic damage. AST levels are very high and ALT levels are only mildly elevated with cardiac damage. ALT can differentiate between hemolytic jaundice when there is no rise in ALT and jaundice due to liver disease with high ALT levels. Hepatitis, cirrhosis, Reye's syndrome, and toxic drug treatment can be monitored with ALT.	Increase	Liver cell damage due to hepatitis, cirrhosis, liver tumors, Reye's syndrome, or biliary tract obstruction; other disease involving liver, heart failure, alcohol or drug abuse; elevated with some renal diseases, some musculoskeletal diseases, systemic lupus erythematosus, other conditions that cause trauma or hypoxia, and hemolysis. Ratio of AST to ALT can be meaningful. AST levels are greater in cirrhosis and metastatic carcinoma of the liver. ALT levels are usually greater with acute hepatitis and nonmalignant hepatic obstruction.

TABLE 4-4. (*continued*)

TEST	EXPLANATION	RESULT	CLINICAL INDICATION
Aspartate aminotransferase (AST), formerly serum glutamic oxaloacetic transaminase (SGOT)	Enzyme in all tissues, but largest amounts in cells that use the most energy, such as liver, heart, and skeletal muscles. AST is released with injury to cells.	Increase	In hepatitis, elevated before jaundice appears; Cirrhosis, shock, or trauma may cause lesser elevation; other conditions include Reye's syndrome and pulmonary infarction. Damaged cardiac cells have other correlating examinations. Ratio of AST to ALT is significant (see ALT).
Alkaline phosphatase (ALP)	Enzyme in the tissues of liver, bone, intestine, kidney, placenta; higher levels are normal with new bone formation, in children, and in pregnancy; normally excreted in bile	Increase	Biliary obstruction from tumors or space-occupying lesions, hepatitis, metastatic liver carcinoma, pancreatic head carcinoma, cholelithiasis, or biliary atresia; elevation may also occur from bone or kidney origin and congestive heart failure due to hepatic blood flow obstruction
Lactic dehydrogenase (LDH)	An enzyme in all tissues, LDH normally is not used for liver evaluation because other enzyme values are more specific. LDH is evaluated as separate isoenzymes. LDH_4 and LDH_5 make up only 10% of the total and are found in liver, skeletal, kidney, placenta, and striated muscle tissue.	Increase LDH_4, LDH_5	Liver damage due to cirrhosis, chronic viral hepatitis, etc.
γ-Glutamyl transpeptidase (GGTP or GGT)	Responsible for transport of amino acid and peptide across cell membranes, it is found chiefly in liver, kidney, and pancreas, with smaller amounts in other tissues. The test is the most sensitive indicator of alcoholism and is also sensitive to other liver diseases.	Increase	Marked elevations in liver disease and posthepatic obstruction; moderate elevations with liver damage from alcohol, drugs, chemotherapy; elevation may also occur from pancreas, kidney, prostate, heart, lung, or spleen disease.
Prothrombin time (PT)	Test used to determine pathologic deficiency of clotting factors due either to liver dysfunction or absence of vitamin K	Increase	Correlated with obstructive disease PT can be corrected with parenteral vitamin K; when correlated with parenchymal disease, scarred nonfunctioning liver tissue does not produce prothrombin.

TABLE 4-4. Liver function tests[29,61,73,144] (*continued*)

TEST	EXPLANATION	RESULT	CLINICAL INDICATION
Albumin	The smallest protein molecule, it makes up the largest portion of total serum protein. It is almost totally synthesized by the liver and is catabolized and excreted as an end-product of protein metabolism. Albumin plays an important role in total water distribution or colloid osmotic pressure because of its high molecular weight. With dehydration, albumin levels increase. A lack of albumin in the serum allows fluid to leak out into the interstitial spaces and into the peritoneal cavity. Globulin, the other serum protein, is also measured with a total protein test, and more extensive tests can be carried out on the five types of globulin if necessary.	Decrease	Chronic liver disease, especially cirrhosis; ascites from cirrhosis, right-sided heart failure, cancer, or peritonitis; other conditions related to the gastrointestinal tract, inflammation, pregnancy, and aging
		Increase	Hemolysis, other conditions related to dehydration, exercise, anxiety, depression
α-Fetoprotein (AFP)	A globulin formed in yolk sac and fetal liver. It is normally present only in trace amounts after birth; produced with primary carcinoma of the liver (hepatoblastoma) and certain types of testicular cancer.	Increase	In nonpregnant adults carcinoma of the liver, as in hepatoblastoma

the anterior abdomen by contracting the diaphragm.[128] One maneuver may be more effective than another for a given patient.[150] During deep inspiration some patients' rib cage can expand considerably, actually causing the diaphragm to elevate and obscure some of the liver as it moves superiorly.[127] For them, the belly-out technique allows the liver to descend below the ribs between the abdominal wall and the pancreas, displaces bowel gas inferiorly, and provides better visualization of both organs.[127]

Supine Position. The study begins with the patient in a supine position. Using either an articulated-arm or a real-time unit, the liver is systematically evaluated in both sagittal and transverse planes. Additional oblique scanning planes are imaged, as necessary, with the patient supine, until the entire liver parenchyma, ligaments, fissures, vessels, biliary elements, and retroperitoneal spaces are adequately evaluated. Initial examinations should include evaluation of diaphragm motion, the integrity of the gallbladder, abdominal aorta, IVC, and adequate visualization of other abdominal organs for the purpose of comparing the echogenicity of the liver to the pancreas, spleen, and kidneys.

Oblique and Erect Positions. Additional planes are imaged with the patient in the left posterior oblique and right posterior oblique position. Usually, as the patient gradually shifts from the left posterior oblique position up to the left lateral decubitus position, the right lobe of the liver descends inferiorly and rotates medially to expose more of the upper portion.[128] With intercostal probe placement, the oblique or erect position affords good visualization of the portal vein and common hepatic duct.[127] The IVC also moves in position and can be identified anterior to the aorta. Patients with hepatomegaly should be examined in the oblique or erect position, because in the supine position, the large liver normally compresses the IVC.[127]

The lower liver segment is better visualized with the patient in the right posterior oblique position. This allows the liver to displace the duodenum and transverse colon inferiorly.[53] Owing to the effects of gravity, an erect or semierect position may expose even more liver tissue.[128]

SCANNING TECHNIQUE

Sagittal Sections. With an articulated-arm instrument, a midline scanning plane is selected between the xiphoid tip and umbilicus. Parasagittal sections are obtained moving left and right in 0.5- to 1-cm increments in the midsagittal region. Farther from the midline area, 1- to 2-cm increments are imaged until the series is completed.[53] Using a continuous sweeping motion, the transducer is angled cephalad, swept under the patient's costal margin, perpendicular to the diaphragm and the dome of the liver to demonstrate the juxtadiaphragmatic portion of the liver,[67] and then it is slowly angled caudad to record the lower liver segment.[53]

Using a real-time system, it is important to maintain a scanning plane perpendicular to the scanning surface. As the scanning plane moves laterad, the plane of section changes from sagittal to coronal with the normal abdominal wall curvature.[128] The liver dome is best visualized by manipulating and angling the transducer cephalad.[148] Scanning begins in the midsagittal plane and proceeds to the left lobe and then the right lobe. Because of the smaller field of view, a complete parasagittal section of the right liver lobe is obtained by moving through a series of superior to inferior sliding and arching motions as the examiner mentally integrates partial images of each section to obtain a complete image of that plane.[128] To complete the sagittal sections, each intercostal space is scanned in superior-to-inferior direction. The dome of the liver is documented by including portions of the heart located just superior to the liver (Figs. 4-4G, 4-9).

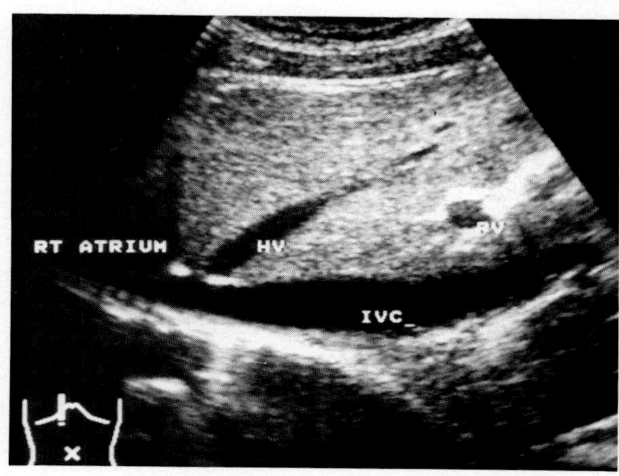

FIGURE 4-9. A sagittal section through the right liver lobe documents that the dome of the liver was examined by including the IVC emptying into the right atrium (HV, hepatic vein; PV, portal vein). (Courtesy Doug Amussen, Logan, UT.)

Transverse Sections. With an articulated-arm instrument, scanning starts at the xiphoid process and moves in 1-cm increments caudad until the lower margin of the right lobe is documented.[53] After the initial pie sweep, the space between the intercostal spaces is filled in bilaterally, keeping the beam angles directed posteriorly to avoid excessive overwriting.[67] This provides a global section of the entire upper abdomen. The dome of the liver is visualized by angling the transducer 10 to 15 degrees cephalad.[53]

Using real-time the transducer is swept from above downward. To obtain complete transverse sections of the larger right lobe with the smaller field of view, the transducer is moved through a series of superior-to-inferior sliding and arching motions, integrating partial images of each section to obtain a complete image of that plane.[128] The transverse sections are completed by obtaining intercostal images through at least the last four interspaces. The examination field is expanded by using superior-to-inferior rocking motions,[148] and the dome of the liver is documented by moving the transducer in a cephalad angle to see portions of the heart located just superior to the diaphragm.

Oblique Sections. To document all hepatic segments, oblique sections are necessary, which are easier to obtain with real-time instruments. Both the patient's position and the transducer orientation are often oblique for completion of the evaluation. With the patient in a 30- to 60-degree right posterior oblique position, the transducer is placed parallel to and below the costal margin. A downward sliding and arching motion is used until the right lobe is completely visualized. The procedure can be repeated for the left lobe with the patient in a right posterior oblique position.

TECHNICAL CONSIDERATIONS

Real-time scanning has several advantages over static imaging, the greatest of which is observing the study as it is performed and assessing the motion of structures.[105] The highest-frequency transducer to obtain the best resolution should be selected.[88] For optimal imaging, a multifocus transducer is ideal because it has a focus range for several depths.[127] If a multifocus transducer is not available, the liver must be imaged with several different transducers of different focal ranges. Convex transducers are more effective than linear transducers for outlining the anatomic boundaries of the liver but their ability to image deep tissue structures is poor.[91]

The near and far gain settings or time gain compensation (TGC), and the system gain settings should be adjusted to give a uniform representation of the hepatic parenchyma from the anterior to the posterior of the liver.[2,67] Careful attention to proper TGC settings helps evaluate deep hepatic pathology or subdiaphragmatic fluid collections (Fig. 4-10).

PITFALLS

Normal anatomy sometimes can have misleading sonographic characteristics. Anatomic variants and artifacts can simulate pathologic conditions.[86,103] An echogenic ligamentum teres, fat anterior to the liver or between the liver and right kidney, acoustic shadowing from vascular and biliary structures, air in the biliary tree, and the heart have all been cited as causes of pseudolesions.[86] The posterior portion of the left liver lobe may be mistaken for the pancreas because of the echogenic line around the left portal vein (Fig. 4-6F).[50] On a transverse section or right costal margin view, perinephric fat may appear echopenic, rather than echogenic, and mimic metastases. A sagittal section through the suspicious area that images the kidney should clarify whether it is perirenal fat or a metastatic lesion (see Fig. 4-1B).[133] Another normal structure that can mimic metastases is the ligamentum teres. This fibrous structure surrounded by fat may appear as an echogenic lesion in the left liver lobe[133] or cause the caudate lobe to appear as a hypoechoic pseudolesion in patients with more than the usual amount of fat or fibrous tissue (Fig. 4-4F).[87]

Echogenic areas adjacent to the anterior gallbladder wall may be due to reverberation artifacts and may be extremely pronounced if the gallbladder is very superficial.[30,132] These can be minimized by increasing the distance of the gallbladder from the transducer with either a water path or a standoff[30] or by placing the patient in an oblique, decubitus, or erect position.[130]

A solitary focal lesion may be observed adjacent to the gallbladder and the portal vein. The lesion is homogeneous and hypoechoic compared to normal hepatic parenchyma, may present with various shapes and a well-defined border, and is usually less than 4 cm in diameter.[16] When such a pseudolesion presents and there is no evidence of significant liver disease, metastatic malignancy, or subsequent evidence of developing liver masses, it may be dismissed or followed.[16] The incidence of this anomaly is not known. Another type of hepatic pseudolesion can be caused by the convex shape of rib cartilage.[19]

The ribs can cause shadows. When shadowing is seen within the liver substance, intraductal calculi should be considered, although they are not the only possible cause (Fig. 4-11A, B). Others are air in the biliary ducts, calcified hematoma, infarct, granulomatous deposits, the calcified rim of an echinococcal cyst, or a recent surgical procedure that forced air into the ductal system or used surgical metal clips (Fig. 4-11C–E).[77] An attempt should be made to distinguish reverberation and shadowing artifacts caused by gas from surgical clips. Gas foci may be long or short but usually cast

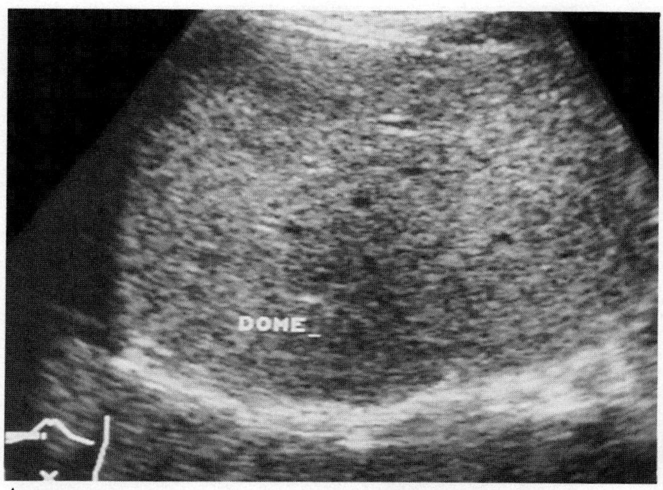

A

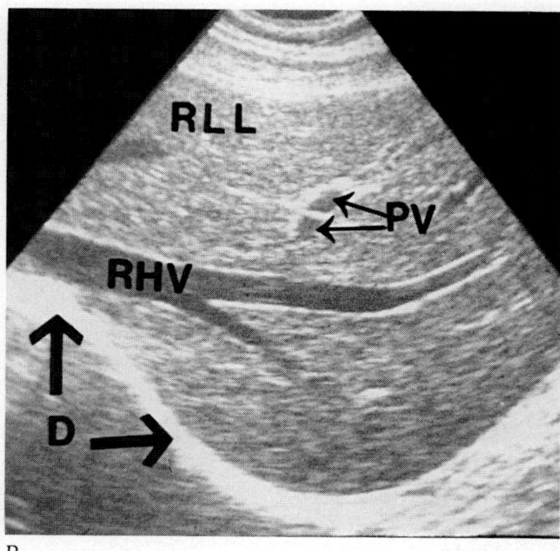

B

FIGURE 4-10. (*A*) A transverse section of the right liver dome demonstrates the proper time gain compensation and system gain settings so that the homogeneous, medium-level echo pattern is as uniform as possible from the anterior to the posterior liver margins. (Courtesy Doug Amussen, Logan, UT.) (*B*) A sagittal section demonstrates the use of proper gain settings, showing uniform texture from anterior to the diaphragm (D, *arrows*) and the normal echo pattern of the hepatic parenchyma in the right liver lobe (RLL) interrupted by the longitudinal orientation of the right hepatic vein (RHV) and the horizontal orientation of the right portal vein bifurcation (PV, *arrows*). (Courtesy Debra M. Joly, Kingston, TX.)

an acoustic shadow masked by intermittent reverberation artifacts; surgical clips are short, echogenic foci that persist and are easily followed with real-time scanning.[77]

A common scanning pitfall is stomach and bowel gas. Gas reflects sound and is always a problem as it interferes with transmission; thus visualization of the liver substance can be especially difficult if bowel loops are not located in the usual inferior and posterior positions.[4] Patient motion, especially with static scanning, produces extraneous, indiscernible echo patterns.

Necrotic tumors can also be mistaken for cystic lesions. When a thick-walled cyst is observed, cystic degeneration of a solid mass must be ruled out.

Normal structures can appear as bile duct obstruction in three different situations. After the right portal vein bifurcates into two branches, they continue to run parallel for a short distance. Sonographically, this can appear as a normal portal vein and a dilated duct (Fig. 4-10B).[134] The normal hepatic artery can reach a size of more than 6 mm and mimic a dilated duct because it lies anterior to the portal vein and is close to the common bile duct.[134] The gallbladder neck can appear sonographically separate from the body and sometimes lies anterior to the common bile duct; it can also mimic a dilated duct.[134]

In two other situations, bile duct enlargement results from a pathologic process that has been relieved. Large bile ducts can develop as a sequela of longstanding biliary obstruction. Although the obstruction has been relieved, the condition causes the duct walls to lose elasticity. Since the common hepatic duct serves as a reservoir for bile, it appears larger than expected after cholecystectomy.

It may be difficult to differentiate extrahepatic and intrahepatic masses, especially near the diaphragm. One area of confusion may be caused by the superimposition of a prominent left liver lobe

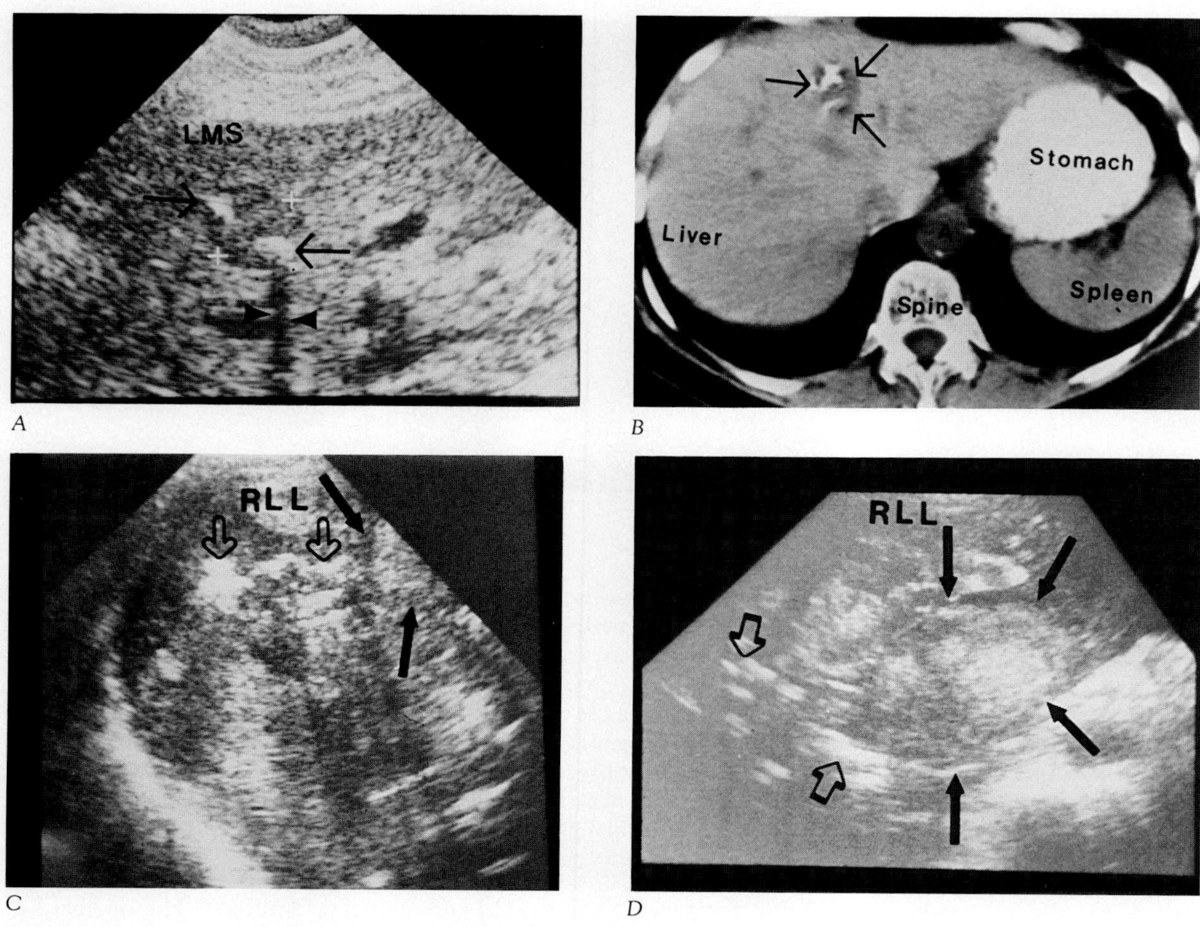

Figure 4-11. (*A*) A sagittal section through the left medial segment in a 58-year-old woman suspected of having a stomach mass demonstrates an ovoid hypoechoic lesion *(cursors)* with two hyperechoic calculi *(arrows)*, one of which is casting a distinct shadow *(arrowheads)*. (*B*) A CT section demonstrates the same 2 × 2.5 cm lesion *(arrows)* in the left medial segment, with coarse-looking calcifications. Included in the differential diagnosis was a quiescent lesion representing an infection such as an amebic abscess or hematoma (A, aorta). (Courtesy Valerie Sowers, Ogden, UT.) *(C,D)* Following post surgical embolization of hepatic arteries for liver cancer in a 60-year-old woman, embolized arteries *(open arrows)* are hyperechoic due to air in the vessels and cast acoustic shadows. On both sagittal (C) and transverse (*D*) sections a mass *(arrows)* is also identified in the right liver lobe (RLL). (Courtesy James Hansen, Vernal, UT.)

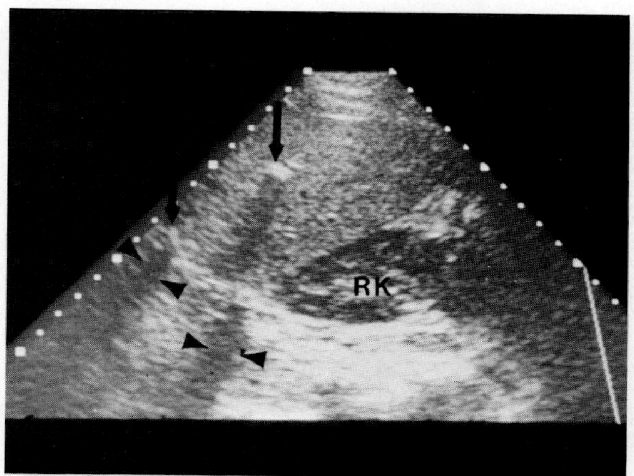

E

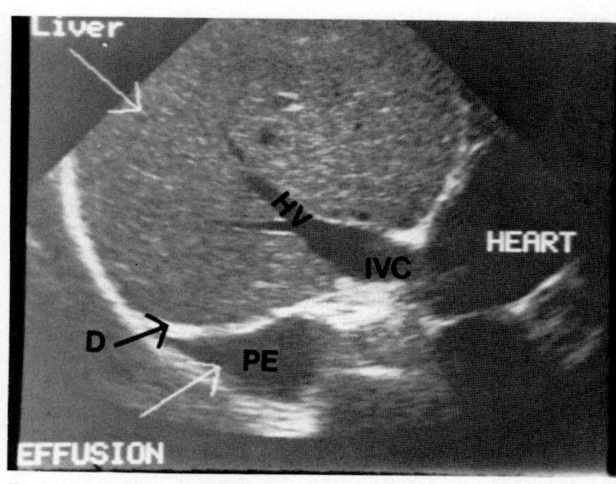

F

FIGURE 4-11 (*continued*) (E) A sagittal scan of a woman in her early twenties demonstrates echogenic spots representing calcifications (*arrows*) with associated shadowing (*arrowheads*) in the lower liver over the 11th rib. The calcifications were felt to be intrahepatic, secondary to previous infection, probably parasitic (RK, right kidney). (Courtesy Helen Johnson, Salt Lake City, UT.) (*F*) On a transverse oblique section, an extrahepatic pleural effusion (PE) is identified by the fact that it displaces the liver capsule internally, causes some discontinuity of the liver capsule, and shifts the IVC anteromedially (D, diaphragm; HV, hepatic vein). (Courtesy Debra M. Joly, Kingston, TX.)

between the spleen and diaphragm or chest wall.[6,31,78] Careful scanning in the transverse plane should demonstrate the continuity of a prominent left hepatic lobe before a diagnosis of subcapsular hematoma or subdiaphragmatic abscess is rendered.[6,31,78] The sonographic features most often observed in an extrahepatic mass include internal displacement of the liver capsule, capsule discontinuity, a triangular fat wedge anteromedial, shift of the IVC, and anterior displacement of the right kidney (Fig. 4-11F).[44,48] The most often observed sonographic features of an intrahepatic mass are displaced hepatic vascular radicles, external bulging of the liver capsule, and posterior shifting of the IVC.[48] The intrahepatic mass criteria can be noted on the sonograms in this chapter that demonstrate hepatic cysts, hepatic abscesses, benign neoplasms, and malignant neoplasms. These criteria should help define the anatomic origin and location of right upper quadrant masses.

Diffuse Hepatocellular Disease

Hepatocellular disease, dysfunction of the hepatocytes, interferes with normal liver function.[88] The effect of the disease process on the whole liver ranges from simple fatty changes to more severe hepatitis or progressive cirrhosis. The parenchymal disease process produces changes that can decrease but more commonly increase the normal echo density and often affects the liver's size. As the disease progresses, the liver is generally more difficult to penetrate owing to increased sound attenuation. Sonography detects diffuse hepatocellular changes but cannot provide quantitative estimates of the severity of parenchymal damage.

FATTY INFILTRATION

Fatty (lipid) infiltration of the hepatocytes, by itself, usually does not significantly disrupt physiologic processes in the cells. Over time, however, fibrous material surrounds fatty cells which causes

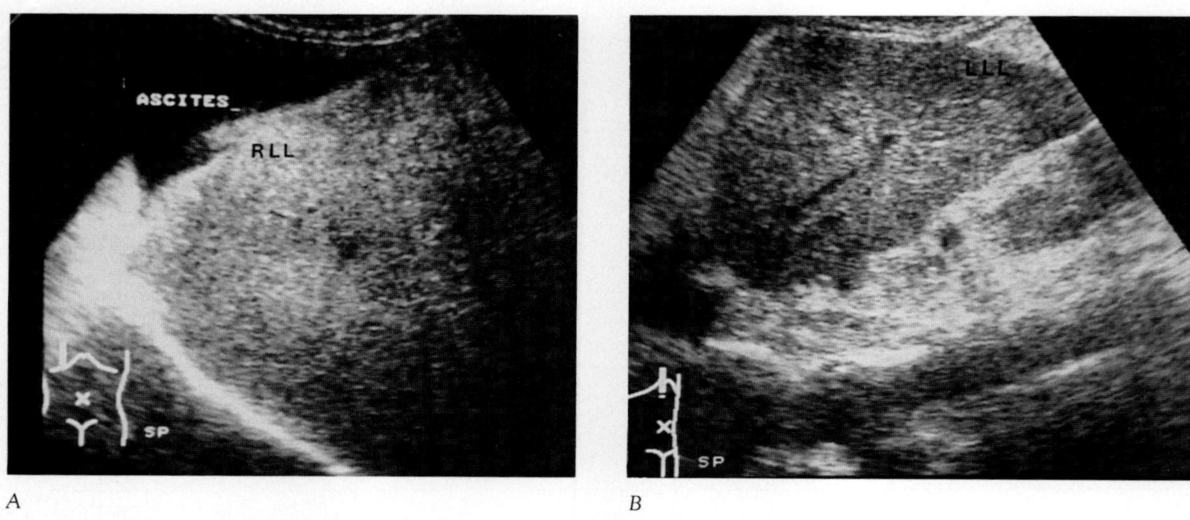

FIGURE 4-12. Fatty infiltration of the liver is sonographically similar to cirrhotic changes. Sagittal sections of (*A*) the right (RLL) and (*B*) left liver lobe (LLL) demonstrate hepatomegaly; a diffuse hyperechoic, granular, and homogeneous texture; poor penetration; difficulty visualizing hepatic vessels; and ascites, all findings that are consistent with this male patient's diagnosis of fatty infiltrative disease. (Courtesy Tally Call, Logan, UT.) (C) Sagittal and (*D*) transverse section views of a 27-year-old woman with acute toxemia demonstrate a diffuse hyperechoic pattern that was particularly evident in the right hepatic lobe though there are a number of scattered densities throughout the remainder of the liver. In addition to the diffuse pattern characteristic of fatty infiltrative disease caused by the patient's toxic state, there is a focal, fatty infiltrative, hyperechoic area mimicking a tumor (*arrows* and *cursors*). The portal system was also prominent, and the patient may have had some portal hypertension. (Courtesy Lisa Schneiter, Ogden, UT.) (*E*) A section through the left lateral segment (LLL) view of a 78-year-old woman demonstrates a bandlike area of decreased echoes (*arrows*), which represents an area of focal sparing. The remainder of the liver has a diffuse pattern of brightly reflective echoes with a granular texture seen with fatty infiltrative disease. (Courtesy Julee Ballingham, Ogden, UT.)

the liver lobules to separate and increases the organ's weight.[22] Factors that influence the deposition of fat include a diet high in fat or too low in protein, starvation, obesity, excessive overeating, alcoholism, metabolic disorders, diabetes mellitus, cystic fibrosis, tuberculosis, corticosteroid therapy, hyperlipidemia, Reye syndrome, severe hepatitis, glycogen storage disease, and jejunoileal bypass surgery for obesity.[121] In the more advanced stages, abnormalities of liver function tests are more pronounced.

Sonographically, the echo pattern features depend on the severity of the condition. The majority of patients have a diffuse pattern of brightly reflective echo with a granular texture within the liver. Hepatomegaly, obscure portal vein walls, difficulty visualizing the course of the hepatic vessels, and poor penetration are all characteristic of fatty infiltrative disease (Fig. 4-12A, B).[92] Although the process is usually diffuse, fatty infiltration may be focal, looking like a hyperechoic mass mimicking a tumor (Fig. 4-12C, D).[122,123] Another sonographic

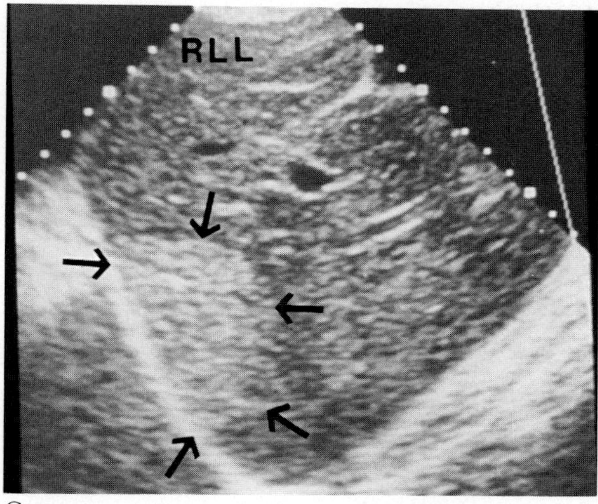

C

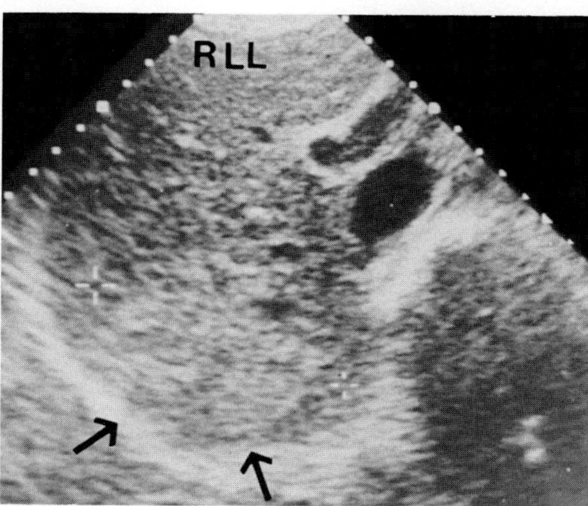

D

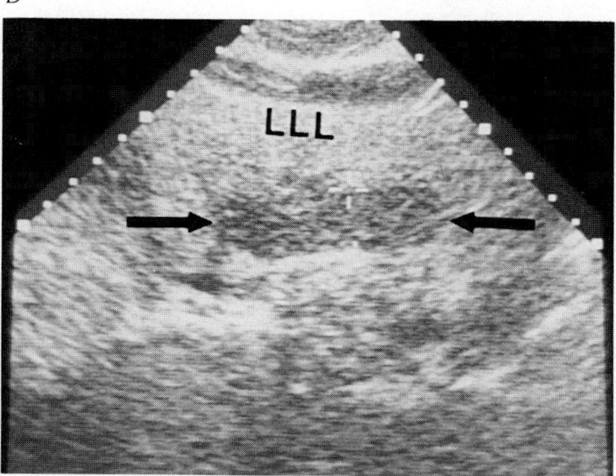

E

appearance is that of focal sparing, which may occur in an otherwise diffuse process, making the normal tissue appear as hypoechoic defects.[122,123] Usually it is the left medial segment or caudate lobe that is spared (Fig. 4-12E).[118]

HEPATITIS

Hepatitis is broadly defined as inflammation of the liver. It can be caused by a reaction to viruses, drugs, or alcohol (Table 4-5).[22] Viral hepatitis may be mild or extensive, with three distinct pathologic features: liver cell injury, necrosis, and scarring; regeneration of hepatic cells within 48 hours of injury, sometimes resulting in crowded, disorganized cells; and Kupffer cell hyperplasia with swelling and reduplication resulting from a mononuclear phagocyte reaction.[22,60] The clinical features of the various viral hepatitides are difficult to distinguish, but those of clinical syndromes resulting from fulminating viral hepatitis, toxic reactions to drugs, and congenital metabolic disorders are fairly distinctive.[22,60] For fulminant hepatitis, liver transplantation may be life saving, as hepatic necrosis is irreversible and 60% to 90% of affected children die.[60]

The ALT (SGPT) and AST (SGOT) values are usually elevated. During the icteric phase (Table 4-5) both the conjugated and unconjugated fractions of the serum bilirubin are elevated and prothrombin time increases with the severity of disease. Health care workers should avoid transmission of viral hepatitis by wearing gloves and washing hands after examining patients with hepatitis A.[60] Direct contact with blood and body fluids must be avoided in case of hepatitis B, non-A–non-B hepatitis, or δ hepatitis.[60,102]

The role of ultrasonography in hepatitis is to evaluate parenchymal changes; in patients with jaundice suspected of having hepatitis, it is to rule out biliary duct obstruction (Fig. 4-13A). Sonographic patterns have been reported to correlate with histologic changes.[72] In the acute phase, the appearance ranges from normal to hypoechoic due to parenchymal enlargement caused by the inflammatory process. The portal vein walls appear much more hyperechoic against the background of hypoechoic parenchyma. On the other hand, fibrosis resulting from chronic hepatitis produces a hyperechoic texture and the portal vein walls appear less echogenic than usual (Fig.4-13B, C).

(text continues on page 126)

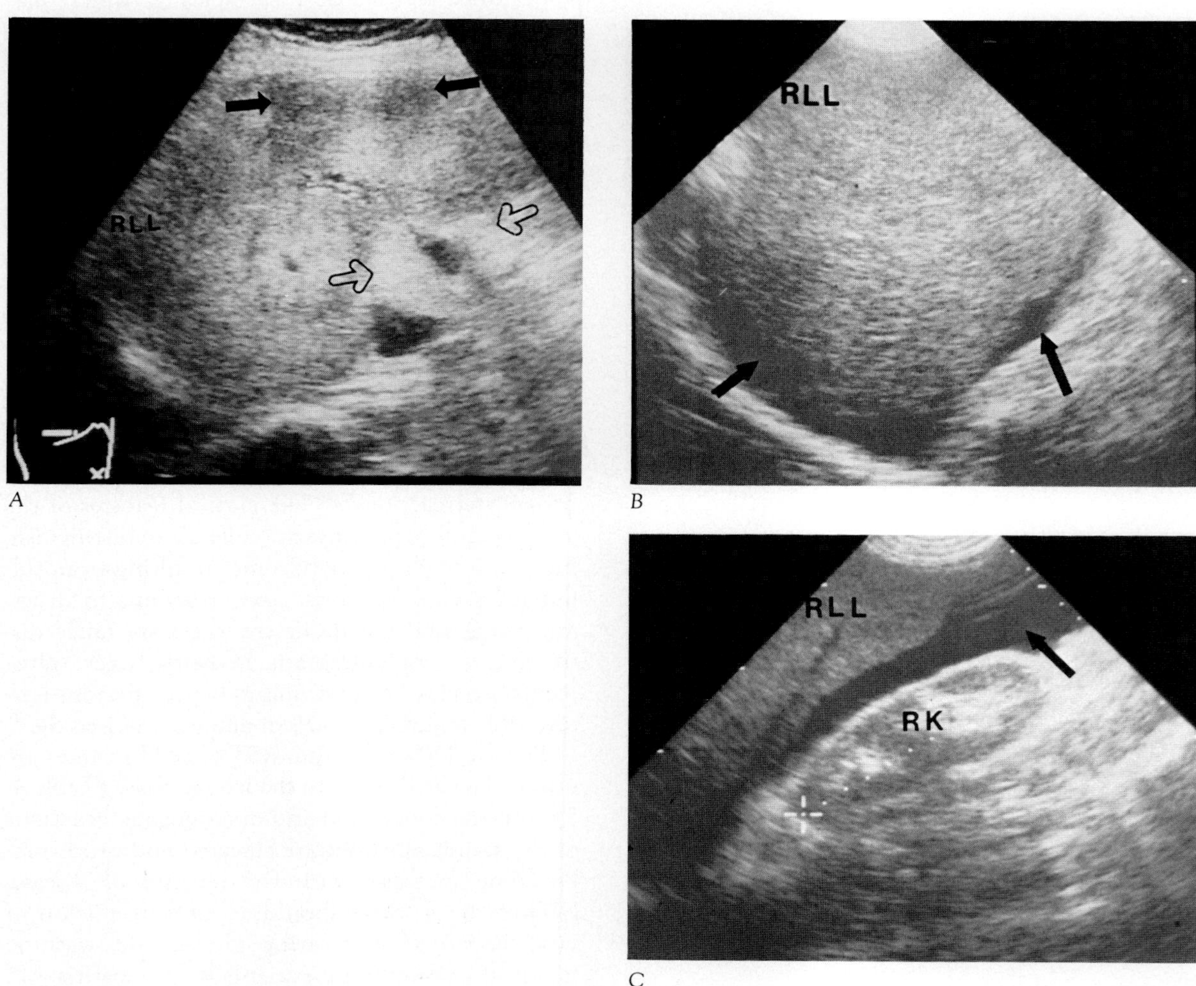

Figure 4-13. (*A*) Without a good patient history, it is impossible to diagnose hepatitis sonographically with confidence. This patient's history was alcohol abuse. With the patient in a left lateral oblique position, this sagittal section demonstrates an irregular echo pattern in the right liver lobe (RLL) consisting of both hypoechoic *(dark arrows)* and hyperechoic *(open arrows)* areas. The sonographic findings of the complete examination included the irregular echo pattern in the liver, more prominent in the periportal region; the normal caliber of the common bile duct; marked gallbladder contraction and wall thickening; and ascites, principally in the right gutter and pelvis. These findings are consistent with a differential diagnosis of hepatitis, cholangitis, or psoriasis. The patient also had a small right kidney. (Courtesy Tally Call, Logan, UT.) (*B*,*C*) A 48-year-old man had a history of chronic hepatitis for 2 years. Sagittal sections of the right liver lobe (RLL) demonstrate a hyperechoic texture with loss of visible portal veins due to fibrosis. Moderate perihepatic ascites fluid can be identified *(arrows)* separating the liver from the right kidney (RK).

Table 4-5. Pathophysiology of hepatitis[22,60,88]

Type	Cause	Route of Transmission	Persons at Risk	Incubation Period (days)	Common Manifestations	Sonographic Appearance
Hepatitis A	Virus (HAV)	Parenteral (fecal-oral), contaminated water, milk, shellfish	Children, young adults	15–40	*Incubation Period:* Headache, nausea, vomiting *Prodromal phase* (begins 2 weeks after exposure, lasts 3–12 days, ends with jaundice): Fatigue, anorexia, malaise, nausea with food odors, changes in taste suppresses desire to smoke or drink alcohol, vomiting, headache, hyperalgia, cough, and low-grade fever; elevations of AST (SGOT), ALT, (SGPT), LDH_1, LDH_2. *Icteric phase* (jaundice, lasts 2–6 weeks): Abdominal pain and tenderness; elevated total bilirubin, dark urine, clay-colored stools, prothrombin time may be prolonged, may have pruritus if severe. *Recovery phase* (resolution of jaundice 6–8 weeks after exposure): Symptoms diminish but hepatomegaly may persist; liver function tests return to normal within 2–12 weeks.	Normal at first. Acute phase: Hyperechoic portal vein radicles; hypoechoic parenchyma due to swelling of liver. Chronic phase: Periportal, perilobular, and portal changes (increased amount of fibrous tissue and inflammatory cells surrounding hepatic lobules) produce coarse echo pattern.
Hepatitis B	Virus (HBV)	Parenteral, sexual, mother-to-infant	IV drug abusers, people on dialysis, health care workers	14–180		
Hepatitis non-A–non-B	Unidentified virus (HNANBV)	Parenteral	IV drug abusers, health care workers	35–60		
δ Hepatitis	RNA virus	Parenteral, sexual	IV drug abusers, health care workers	Unknown		
Fulminant hepatitis	Viral, toxic reactions; metabolic disorders	Complication of HNANBV, HBV, δ virus infection	Same as HNANBV, HBV, δ virus	Not applicable		

Cirrhosis

Cirrhosis is a general term for a diffuse process that destroys the normal architecture of the liver lobules. The parenchyma are destroyed, fibrous tissue resulting from inflammation separates the liver lobules, and regenerative nodules are formed.[22,92] The distorted parenchymal changes alter or obstruct biliary channels, producing jaundice; obstruction can cause portal hypertension;[89] new vascular channels can form shunts causing portal venous blood to bypass the liver;[89] and vascular changes compromise liver function, producing hypoxia, necrosis, and atrophy that ultimately lead to liver failure.[60] Although alcoholism is usually associated with cirrhosis and 75% of deaths attributable to alcoholism are caused by cirrhosis,[102] in actuality, the prevalence of cirrhosis among alcoholics is relatively low (approximately 25 percent).[60] Cirrhosis also develops in the course of other disorders, such as viral hepatitis, toxic drug and chemical reactions, biliary obstruction, and cardiac disease.[102] Cirrhosis is also associated with metabolic defects and storage diseases that cause minerals to be deposited in the liver—glycogen storage disease, hemochromatosis (iron deposition), Wilson's disease (copper deposition), galactosemia.[22,102] No matter what the cause, cirrhosis can take one of four forms; alcoholic (Laennec's, portal, or fatty), biliary (primary or secondary), postnecrotic, or metabolic (Table 4-6).[60]

Liver function test abnormalities depend on the stage and extent of disease. AST (SGOT), ALT (SGPT), lactate dehydragenase (LDH_4, and LDH_5), and serum and urine conjugated bilirubin values are elevated. Serum alkaline phosphatase may also be elevated, whereas, serum albumin is decreased and γ-globulin proteins are increased.[144] No symptoms may appear for a long time.

When clinical manifestations do occur, patients may present with fatigue, weight loss, diarrhea, and hepatomegaly (large, palpable liver). Hepatomegaly causes stretching of Glisson's capsule and patients may complain of a dull and aching pain in the epigastric region or right upper quadrant, with a feeling of fullness. Sonographically, the liver is enlarged but the examination is insensitive and unreliable for detecting the early histologic changes of cirrhosis.[140] If diffuse changes are present, they may appear as increased anterior echoes and decreased posterior echoes, more echogenic liver parenchyma than renal parenchyma, and clearly identifiable small portal and venous vessels that are even smaller in the peripheral liver. The diagnosis is often hepatocellular disease.[46,88]

As the disease continues to progress, the liver returns to normal, the right lobe begins to shrink and atrophy, whereas, the caudate lobe is usually spared or will hypertrophy, probably because of its blood supply.[88] The chronic effects of cirrhosis—alterations in normal liver function, portal hypertension, and hepatic cell failure—are detailed in Table 4-7.

Sonographically, the cirrhotic liver typically appears atrophic, with irregular contour secondary to nodular regeneration.[18] The hyperechoic liver parenchyma presents with a fine, heterogeneous texture, and the usually echogenic portal veins are not as readily apparent (Fig.4-14A–C).[18,92] The appearance of coarse echoes represents fibrosis and an irregular contour represents nodular regeneration. A lower-frequency transducer may be necessary to compensate for the increased sound attenuation. It is useful to determine the caudate lobe width and divide it by the width of the right lobe on a transverse section.[54,55] Cirrhosis is diagnosed with 99% confidence if the ratio is greater than 0.73 and if the ratio is less than 0.60, cirrhosis is unlikely.[54] Hess and colleagues[55] found the most reliable index to be the product of the caudate lobe's longitudinal transverse, and AP diameter divided by the width of the right lobe. For patients with fatty liver, liver metastases, lymphomatous liver involvement, and cirrhosis and for a healthy control group the three-dimensional measurement (cutoff point of 5.4 cm^2) was 94.7% sensitive.[55]

Vascular Abnormalities

The sonographic examination for portal venous hypertension and portal vein thrombosis is described in Chapter 3.

Hepatic Venous Outflow Obstruction

Obstruction to the hepatic venous outflow tract by thrombus or tumor and the associated clinical features of abdominal pain, jaundice, hematemesis, ascites, hepatomegaly, and liver function abnormalities indicative of hepatocellular dysfunction are

TABLE 4-6. Cirrhosis[22,60,88]

TYPE	CAUSE	PATHOPHYSIOLOGY	SONOGRAPHIC APPEARANCE
Alcoholic	Toxic effects of chronic, excessive alcohol intake (alcohol is a hepatotoxin that induces metabolic changes that damage hepatocytes).	Fat accumulation, inflammation (alcoholic hepatitis), and derangement of the lobular architecture by necrosis and fibrosis (cirrhosis)	In early stages, hepatomegaly; liver may appear hyperechoic compared to normal renal parenchyma; diffuse parenchymal changes lead to a diagnosis of hepatocellular disease. As cirrhosis progresses, hepatic tissue begins to atrophy and attenuates more sound, fibrosis appears more coarse, vascular structures are not as readily visualized and may present an irregular contour due to nodular regeneration. With portal hypertension, splenomegaly and ascites may be seen.
Biliary	Primary, unknown, possible autoimmune mechanism; secondary, obstruction by cholelithiasis, stricture, or neoplasm	Primary, lobular bile ducts become inflamed and scarred; secondary, bile ducts become inflamed and scarred proximal to the obstruction	
Postnecrotic	Viral hepatitis (HAV or HNANBV), drugs, toxins, autoimmune destruction	Necrotic tissue is replaced with cirrhotic tissue, specifically fibrous, nodular scar tissue	
Metabolic	Metabolic defects and storage disease (glycogen storage disease, Wilson's disease, hemochromatosis, galactosemia	Morphologic changes resulting in inflammation and scarring related to cause	

TABLE 4-7. Chronic effects of hepatic cirrhosis[22,60,102]

ALTERATIONS IN FUNCTION	SYMPTOMS AND SIGNS
Portal Hypertension	
Collateral vessel development	Esophageal varices often lead to GI bleeding and possible hemorrhage; hemorrhoids; caput medusae (a radiating plexus of dilated periumbilical subcutaneous veins secondary to increased flow in the paraumbilical veins)
Increased portal vein pressure	Recanilization of the ligamentum teres (umbilical vein)
Increased portal vein pressure and decreased serum albumin level	Ascites, peripheral edema
Splenomegaly	Hematopoietic disorders: anemia, leukopenia, thrombocytopenia
Hepatorenal syndrome	Elevated serum creatinine, azotemia, oliguria; precursor of hepatic coma
Portsystemic shunting of blood	Hepatic-systemic encephalopathy (precursor of confusion, coma, and convulsions)
Hepatocellular Dysfunction	
Inability to remove conjugated bilirubin	Jaundice
Impaired bile synthesis	Malabsorption of fats and fat-soluble vitamins
Impaired plasma protein synthesis	Decreased levels of albumin (precursor to edema and ascites)
Decreased synthesis of blood-clotting factors	Tendency to bleed
Impaired drug metabolism	Drug reactions and toxicity
Impaired gluconeogenesis	Glucose intolerance
Capillary congestion	Spider angiomas and palmar erythema
Decreased ability to convert ammonia to urea	Elevated blood ammonia levels
Depressed metabolism of sex hormones	Females, menstrual disorders; males, testicular atrophy, gynecomastia, decrease in secondary sex characteristics

known collectively as Budd-Chiari syndrome. Distended superficial veins and lower extremity edema may be present if the IVC is also involved. The possible causes are varied. Although in a majority of cases the cause is never determined,[88] thrombosis of the hepatic veins has been linked with several causes, such as oral contraceptives; invasion of tumors into the hepatic veins from hepatocellular carcinoma, renal carcinoma, and adrenal carcinoma; and radiation to the liver with obliteration of small hepatic veins.[108,109]

The sonographic findings of Budd-Chiari syndrome depend on the degree of venous obstruction and the underlying cause. The hepatic veins may not be visible or may appear thick walled. In longstanding cases, the right lobe atrophies and there is hypertrophy of the left lateral segment and of the caudate lobe,[18] the latter owing to its multiple, small, direct connections to the patent portion of the IVC.[88] As the disease progresses, sonographic appearances include hyperechoic areas from fibrosis and periportal regenerative nodules within infarcted areas, ascites, splenomegaly, pleural effusion, and an hourglass configuration of the IVC if there is coarctation.[18] Since blood flows to unobstructed vessels, flow may be to interlobular hepatic veins, to subcapsular arcades, or retrograde (hepatofugal), through branches of the portal veins. Vascular Doppler assessment is useful in demonstrating altered hemodynamics in the IVC, hepatic veins, and portal veins and the level of obstruction (Fig. 4-15).[58,136]

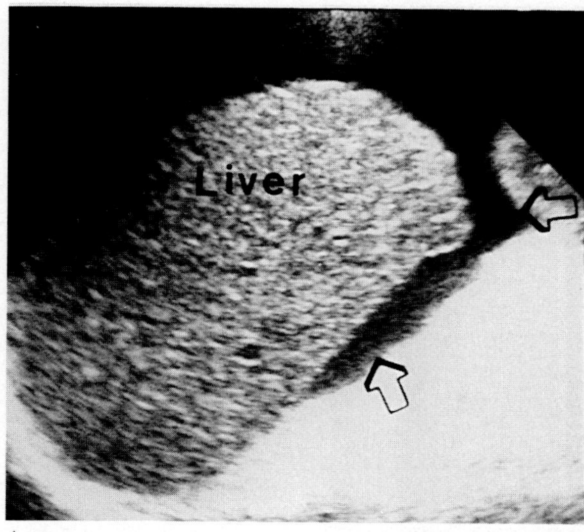

A

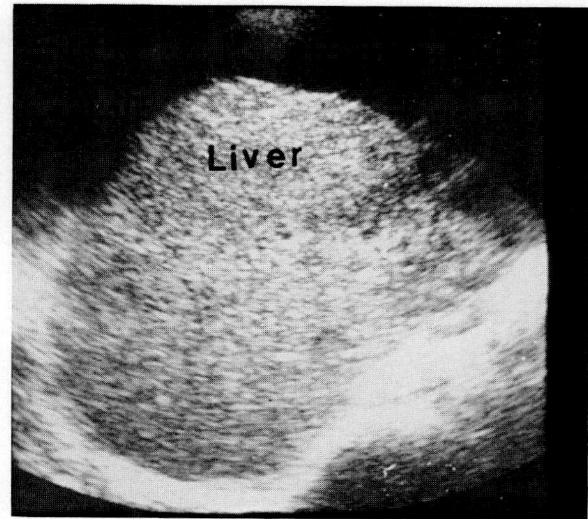

B

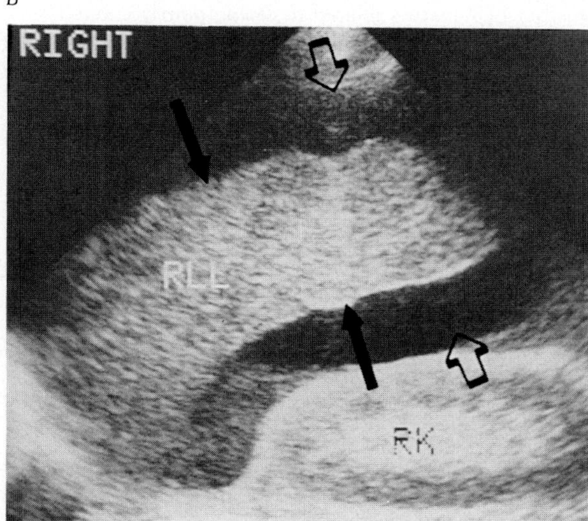

C

FIGURE 4-14. With advanced cirrhosis, nodularity of the liver and perihepatic ascitic fluid *(arrows)* are identified on sagittal (*A*) and transverse (*B*) sections. The liver texture is hyperechoic and homogenous, with visual loss of hepatic vasculature. (C) With progressive cirrhosis the sagittal section demonstrates an atrophic right nodular liver lobe and perihepatic ascitic fluid *(arrows)*. The liver texture is hyperechoic and homogenous, appearing more echogenic than the renal parenchyma, with visual loss of hepatic vasculature. (RK, right kidney.) (Courtesy Cathy Carr-Hoefer, Corvallis, OR.)

Hepatic Cysts

Hepatic cysts may be classified as congenital or acquired. The incidence on abdominal laparotomy is 17 in 10,000 although it may be somewhat higher, as small cysts are not always recorded.[115] Most hepatic cysts are congenital, and 82 of 150 are solitary. They are more common in females[115] and are discovered in the fifth through seventh decade of life.[147] Hepatic cysts may also be multiple (49 of 150 incidence) and may be acquired due to trauma, parasites, or inflammatory reaction.[113,115]

The imaging modality of choice for hepatic cysts is ultrasound.[113] Sonographically, they can be characterized, measured, and localized precisely for fine needle aspiration. The histologic nature of the cysts is determined only in certain situations with correlation to patient history. Sonographically they present these characteristic cystic appearances:

1. They are anechoic even at high gain settings, which indicates the lack of internal echoes.
2. They appear as well-defined masses with a

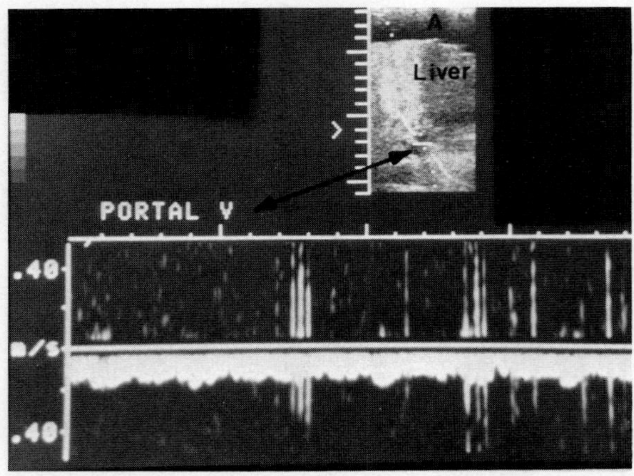

FIGURE 4-15. A young female patient presented with a history of hepatitis related to eating poorly cooked shellfish several years earlier. The liver appears to have hepatocellular disease, and Budd-Chiari syndrome was diagnosed, with hepatitis, cirrhosis, and associated ascites (A). Vascular Doppler assessment demonstrated retrograde (hepatofugal) portal venous flow through collateral channels and retrograde flow in the superior mesenteric vein. (Courtesy KayLynn Schmidt, Rock Springs, WY.)

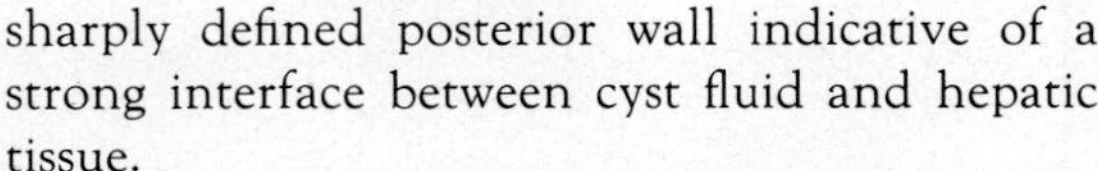

sharply defined posterior wall indicative of a strong interface between cyst fluid and hepatic tissue.

3. There is increased amplitude of echoes compared to surrounding tissue beginning at the far wall and proceeding distally (acoustic enhancement or through-transmission).
4. Reverberation artifacts are identified at the near wall if the cyst is located close to the transducer.
5. Edge-shadowing artifacts caused by refraction and reflection may occur, depending on the incident angle.

CONGENITAL

Congenital cysts are developmental defects of bile ducts[113] that are usually asymptomatic and are discovered incidentally (Fig. 4-16A, B). Solitary lesions are more common than multiple cysts, and the right lobe is affected twice as often as the left.[88] The cysts range in size from millimeters to 20 cm.

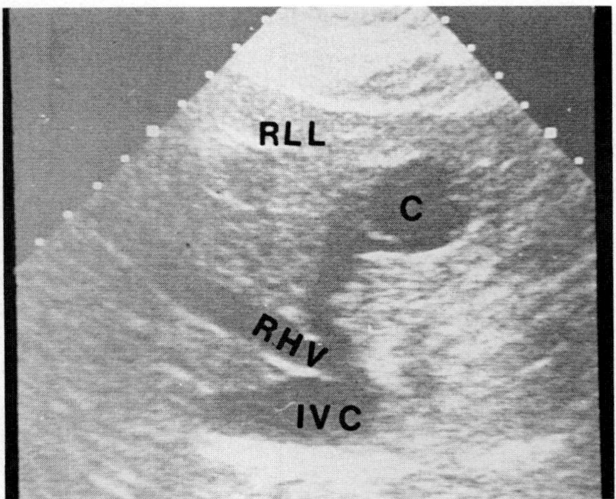

FIGURE 4-16*A*

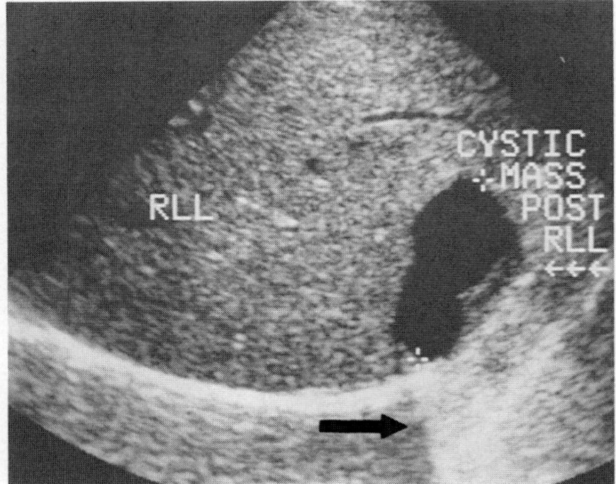

B

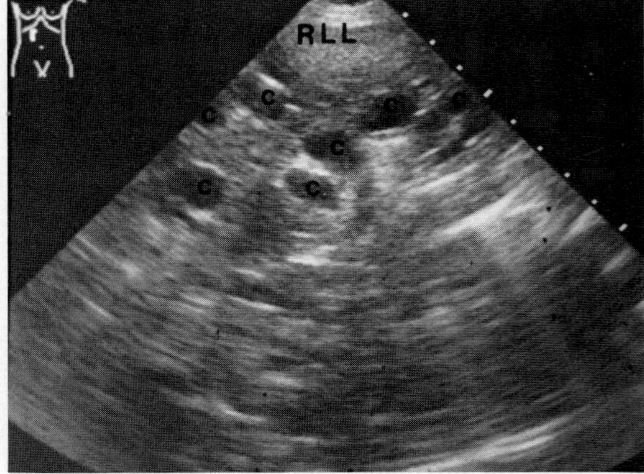

C

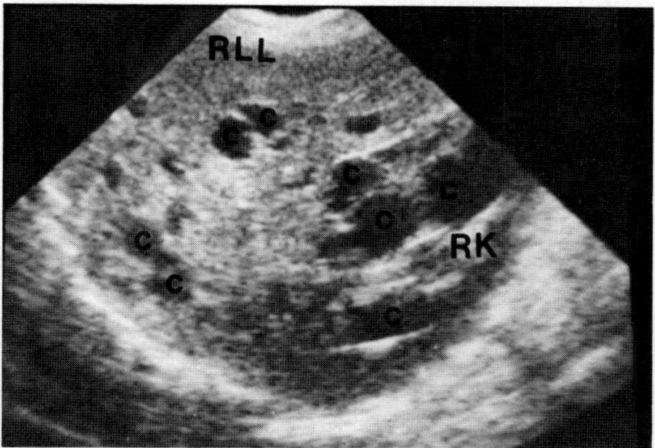

D

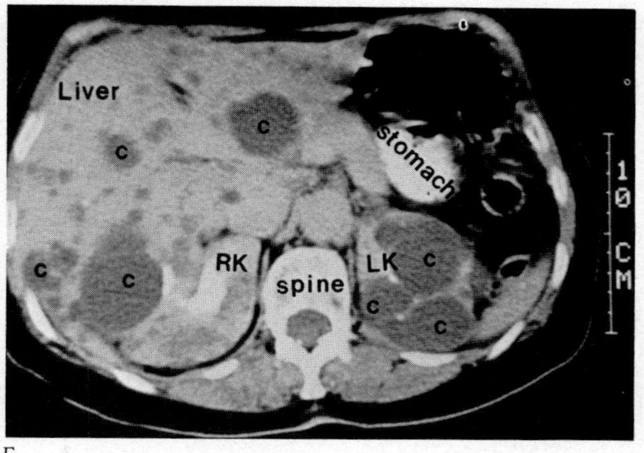

E

FIGURE 4-16. (*A*) A solitary 2.5 cm cyst (c) is identified in the right liver lobe (RLL) on a transverse section. This was an incidental finding on cardiac sonography of a 32-year-old woman with palpitations and arrythmia who had no liver symptoms. (RHV, right hepatic vein.) (*B*) On a sagittal section of the right liver lobe (RLL) 8 cm from midline, a solitary 3.96 mm cyst is identified. It nicely demonstrates the increased echo amplitude in comparison to surrounding tissue, beginning at the far wall and proceeding distally *(arrow)*. (C) A 59-year-old woman had right side upper quadrant pain. Multiple cysts (c) of varying sizes in both the right (RLL) and left liver lobes suggested polycystic disease, which was confirmed with further investigation and a follow-up intravenous pyelographic examination. The gallbladder could not be distinguished from the other cystic structures, but no calcifications or thick cystic walls could be identified in the region of the gallbladder fossa. In another case, polycystic kidney disease was diagnosed in a 62-year-old woman with abdominal pain and discomfort. (*D*) A sagittal section demonstrates multiple cysts (c) in the right liver lobe (RLL) and right kidney (RK). These cysts were identified on follow-up CT (*E*) in both the right and left hepatic lobes and the right (RK) and left (LK) kidneys. (Courtesy Janet Hubert, Worland, WY.)

It is rare that a solitary cyst grows large enough to cause hepatomegaly, to be palpated, to compress intrahepatic ducts causing jaundice,[146] or to cause abnormal elevation in liver enzymes.[129]

Polycystic disease of the liver is caused by a developmental defect in the formation of bile ducts. Histologically, the cysts are lined with cuboidal epithelium and are scattered randomly throughout the liver, causing disruption of the normal echo appearance. A quarter to a half of all persons who have autosomal dominant polycystic kidney disease also have a polycystic liver[71,142]; renal cysts are found in 60% of patients with polycystic liver (Fig. 4-16C–E).[71] The kidneys should be carefully evaluated when multiple cysts are discovered in the liver because of this association.

Ultrasonographic diagnosis of a hepatic cyst is 95% to 100% accurate, but the differential diagnosis includes necrotic metastasis, echinococcal cyst, hematoma, hepatic cystadenoma, and abscess.[88]

ACQUIRED

Acquired cysts can be categorized as traumatic (hematoma, biloma), parasitic (echinococcal), or inflammatory (abscess).[98] They are often suspected prior to scanning because patients usually have symptoms. The sonographic appearance ranges from the standard cyst features to complex masses.

In addition to localizing and measuring these masses, it is important to characterize the appearance of acquired cysts and correlate the sonographic representation to the clinical setting.

Hematoma. The liver's abundant vascular supply makes it highly susceptible to hemorrhage when a hard blow to the abdomen ruptures or tears hepatic tissue. Symptomatically it is tender. With a significant bleed the patient shows signs of collapse and shock. The blood pressure and pulse rate decrease and the hematocrit value drops.

Sonographically, the appearance of a hematoma depends on the age of the bleed. Very fresh blood is anechoic, but early in its evolution acoustic enhancement may not be exhibited as in a typical cyst. Although posttraumatic intrahepatic biloma is a rare lesion, it may be suspected if there is acoustic enhancement. A radionuclide-enhanced cholescintigraphic examination may be necessary to distinguish a hematoma from a biloma.[35] Gradually, as a hematoma becomes organized and develops a clot, it reveals internal echoes, presenting a complex pattern that is both hyperechoic and hypoechoic. Eventually, it undergoes complete liquefaction and becomes a seroma, which again has an anechoic cystic pattern. Chronic hematomas may become calcified and produce characteristic acoustic shadows. Frequently, hepatic hematomas are contained by the liver capsule. A subcapsular hematoma produces a striking appearance as it displaces the liver medially.

Echinococcal Cyst. The *Taenia* echinococcus or *Echinococcus granulosus* is a parasitic tapeworm. When a dog eats infested animal organs the tapeworms mature in the dog's intestine and the ova are passed in the feces. Cattle, sheep, hogs, and humans serve as intermediate hosts. The parasites were once confined to specific geographic areas, but world travel and world markets for foodstuffs (that have been fertilized with infected manure) increase their transmission. Sanitary measures reduce the incidence.[94] Larvae ingested by humans hatch in the intestine and migrate most often to the right hepatic lobe (and less frequently to lungs, brain, or another organ).[94] The cysts may deform the organ, leading to unusual findings on palpation. Clinical symptoms range from the extreme of anaphylactic shock if the cyst ruptures and the hydatid fluid enters the circulation to slight elevation of alkaline phosphatase and jaundice if the daughter cysts obstruct bile ducts.[94]

If the larvae are successful in invaginating and developing they become encysted and generations of daughter cysts develop.[22] The original uniloculr-looking cyst is enventually filled in by hundreds of cysts of varying size. When it grows to approximately 20 cm the patient experiences discomfort and pain. The daughter cysts float in a protein-free, highly irritating hydatid fluid, which also contains hydatid sand.[94]

The sonographic appearance depends on the course of larval maturation. The possibilities include (1) solitary cyst with or without mural (shell-like) calcification obscuring internal cystic nature or without calcification; (2) multiple cysts with dense daughter cells; (3) fluid collections with septa presenting a honeycomb appearance; and (4) solid-looking cysts, with or without calcification (Fig. 4-17A, B).[13,40,76,88106]

Hepatic Abscesses

The cause of an hepatic abscess is usually bacterial infection or amebiasis. Sonographic examination can noninvasively locate, measure, and characterize such hepatic masses. Hepatic abscesses have been located in the intrahepatic, subhepatic, and subphrenic areas.[53]

Pyogenic Abscess

A pyogenic abscess develops when the reticuloendothelial system is compromised by altered immune function or when there is overwhelming sepsis. Bacterial infection reaches the liver from the biliary tree, portal vein, or hepatic artery, by direct extension from a contiguous infection,[113] or as an operative sequela. For instance, hepatic artery thrombosis or occlusion following transplantation compromises the arterial supply of the liver, which can produce tissue hypoxia and may lead to infection and abscess formation.[119]

Pyogenic abscesses produce varying symptoms, depending on the severity and extent of the process. Clinical symptoms may include fever, leukocytosis, elevated liver function test values, rightside upper quadrant pain, pleuritic pain, and hepato-

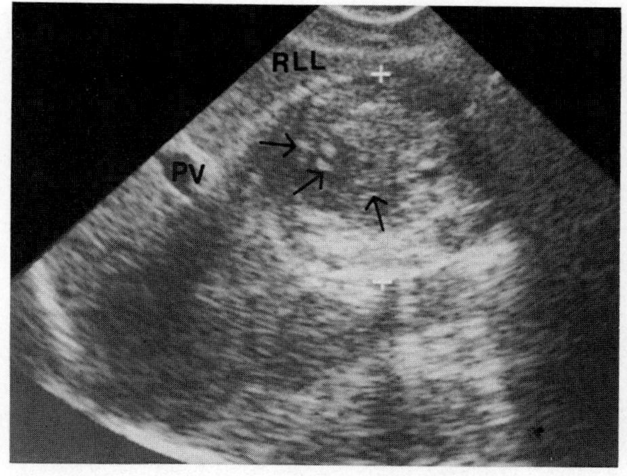

A

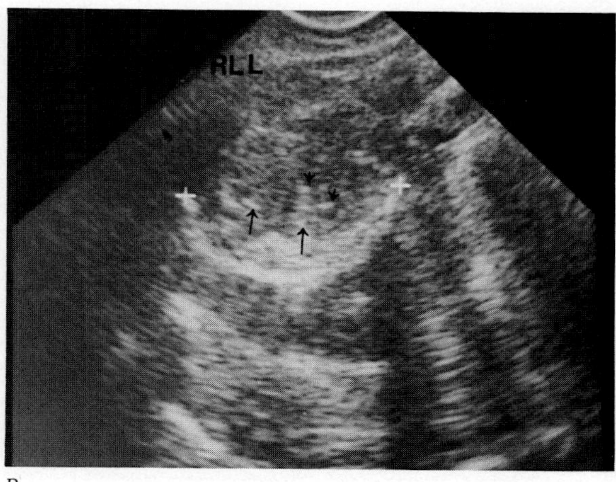

B

FIGURE 4-17. A 31-year-old man presented with right upper quadrant pain and nausea. Two mobile gallbladder calculi were discovered. (*A,B*) A 7 × 8 cm echinococcal cyst *(cursors)* in the right liver lobe (RLL) is identified and has not changed in sonographic appearance since it was diagnosed 5 years earlier. It is heterogeneous, with proteinaceous material within *(arrows)* and encapsulated in a calcified wall. The fact that its appearance has not changed in 5 years and the calcified wall are indicative of an inactive cyst and disintegration of the daughter cysts. (Courtesy Bonnie Kennington, Bountiful, UT.)

megaly. An abscess in the subhepatic or subphrenic region is more likely the result of bacterial infection. A pyogenic abscess in the subhepatic region may result from cholecystectomy and is found in the gallbladder bed or Morrison's pouch. In the subphrenic region, abscess formation results from bacteria spilling into the peritoneum at surgery, bowel rupture, perforated peptic ulcer, or trauma.[53] The mortality rate can be 100% in untreated cases.[109]

Several sonographic features have been described: single or multiple (10%) masses, measuring 1 cm or larger, 80% in the right lobe. The shape is variable but pyogenic abscesses may be round or ovoid, with walls that are usually irregular (90%) and poorly defined. The internal character is anechoic to hyperechoic, (if it contains debris, adhesions, or air or microbubbles) but it is less echogenic than hepatic parenchyma. Acoustic enhancement at the far wall and distal to the mass occurs in 50% of cases. The clinical setting and echo enhancement are important considerations in the differential diagnosis, which includes cyst, hematoma, necrotic tumor, echinococcal cyst, and primary or metastatic cystadenocarcinoma (Fig. 4-18).[45,69,70,96]

AMEBIC ABSCESS

An amebic abscess occurs when parasites, usually from the colon, reach the liver through the portal vein. Once confined to specific geographic areas, amebic diseases are now transmitted to many developed countries. Humans serve as an intermediate host and are usually asymptomatic, as the organism is confined to the gastrointestinal tract.[88] Patients may present with right upper quadrant pain, hepatomegaly, diarrhea, elevated values on liver function tests, diarrhea, and melena.[88]

In 40% of amebic abscesses, the sonographic features included a round or ovoid homogeneous mass that was less echogenic than the normal liver parenchyma and lacked signifcant wall echoes. They are located contiguous to the liver capsule and have acoustic enhancement beginning at the far wall and distal to the mass.[88]

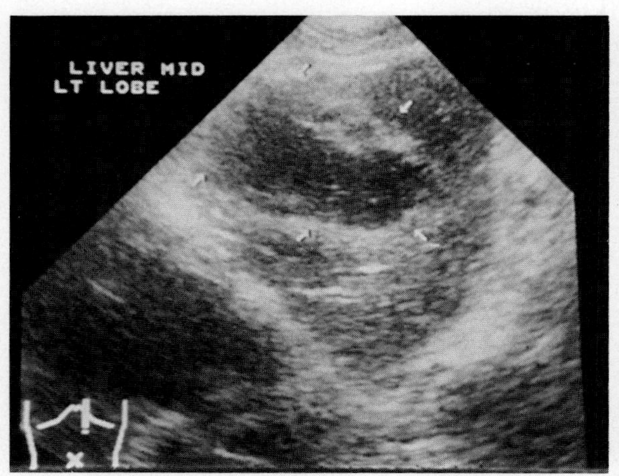

A

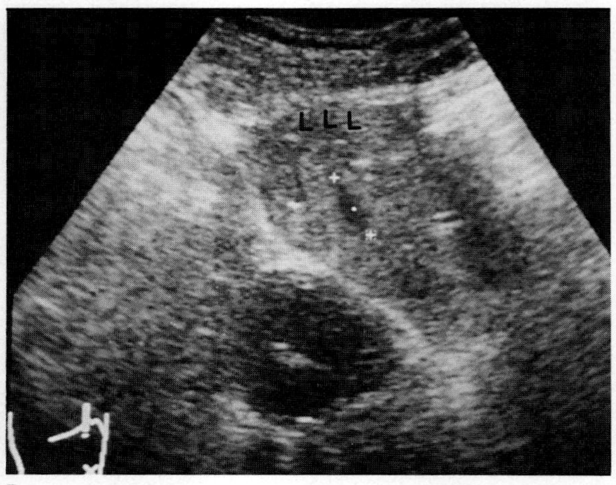

B

FIGURE 4-18. A man presented with right and left upper quadrant pain, leukocytosis, night sweats, and fatigue. (*A*) On a sagittal section a large, irregular, hypoechoic 6 × 4 cm mass (*white arrows*) was identified in the left liver lobe. Air in the bile duct was noted on another image. (*B*) Follow-up examination was performed 2 months after aspiration of the abscess and antibiotic therapy demonstrates the remaining abscess (*cursors*) in the left liver lobe (LLL) measuring 1.8 cm. Air was again noted in the bile duct. It is believed that bacteria entered the liver through the dilated bile duct and that the liver provided a conducive environment for formation of a pyogenic abscess. (Courtesy Tally Call, Logan, UT.)

Benign Neoplasm

In neonates and infants, benign hepatic tumors are more common than malignant ones[18]; in older children and adults, they are rarer than malignant ones, whether primary or metastatic.[88] Primary liver tumors may originate from the parenchymal cells or bile duct epithelium or represent a mixture of the two.[109] Ultrasound is an excellent imaging modality for liver tumors, although it lacks the necessary histologic specificity.

Cavernous Hemangioma

Cavernous hemangioma is the most common benign hepatic tumor (frequency at autopsy up to 7.3%).[93] They are not true neoplasms, as histologically they are arteriovenous malformations, being composed of a large network of vascular endothelium–lined spaces filled with red blood cells.[109] Hemangiomas are most common in women (70% to 95%)[1] and can occur at any age but increase in frequency with age.[113] The spaces are separated by fibrous septa which commonly proliferate centrally and extend peripherally to varying degrees.[85]

Most hemangiomas are incidental findings as they cause no symptoms.[93,109] They may enlarge during pregnancy or enlarge slowly, resulting in hepatomegaly and abdominal discomfort[93] with degeneration and fibrosis.[113] Occasionally calcifications are identified, but phleboliths are rare.[12]

Cavernous hemangiomas smaller than 1.5 cm are found more reliably with ultrasound than with computed tomography (CT).[62] The classic sonographic appearance is a homogeneous (58% to 73%),[20,138] hyperechoic (67% to 70%)[62] mass with sharp, well-defined margins[20,38,138,152] and posterior acoustic enhancement,[93,138] located in the posterior right liver lobe (Table 4-8, Fig. 4-19).[20] It has been reported that when hemangiomas are smaller than

TABLE 4-8. Benign liver neoplasms

NEOPLASM	HISTOLOGIC APPEARANCE	CLINICAL SIGNS	SONOGRAPHIC APPEARANCE
Cavernous hemangioma	Large network of vascular endothelium-lined spaces filled with red blood cells	No symptoms; 70%–95% are in women; frequency increases with age	Usually homogeneous, hyperechoic mass, sharp well-defined margins; may have posterior acoustic enhancement, usually in the posterior right segment
Focal nodular hyperplasia	Hepatocytes, Kupffer cells, bile duct elements, and fibrous connective tissue; central fibrous band with radiating septa separates mass into nodules; no known malignant potential	Usually asymptomatic, usually an incidental finding	May be hypoechoic, hyperechoic, or isoechoic with normal tissue; 0.5 to 20 cm, well-circumscribed mass
Liver cell adenoma	Encapsulated, slightly atypical hepatocytes, often with areas of bile stasis, focal hemorrhage, and necrosis; malignant potential of a hepatoma; susceptible to hemorrhage	Usually symptomatic; incidence increases in women of child-bearing age and is associated with oral contraceptives	Usually hyperechoic relative to normal tissue; well-circumscribed mass; with hemorrhage, internal pattern ranges from anechoic to hyperechoic, depending on age of bleed

2.5 cm in diameter, acoustic enhancement is not seen in 87.5% of cases.[138] Larger lesions present with more variable echo patterns—hypoechoic, isoechoic, heterogeneous[93]—as they become necrotic from outgrowing their blood supply. Gibney and coworkers[41] reported that 82% of the hemangiomas studied over a period of 1 to 6 years demonstrated no change in sonographic appearance. Three lesions became isoechoic and could not be found, seven lesions became less echoic, one lesion shrank from 2.8 to 2.0 cm and one grew from 5.0 to 7.0 cm.[41]

Hepatic scintigraphy, using single-photon-emission CT (SPECT) and technectium-99m-labeled red blood cells, is very sensitive and specific for diagnosing hepatic cavernous hemangiomas.[83] This procedure is recommended over CT and angiography if a hypoechoic or mixed echogenic hepatic lesion is found in a symptomatic patient who has abnormal liver function test values or a known primary tumor.[83] A 6-month follow-up ultrasound examination is recommended if a hyperechoic hepatic lesion is discovered incidentally in an asymptomatic patient with normal liver function tests and no known primary tumor.[83]

FOCAL NODULAR HYPERPLASIA

Focal nodular hyperplasia is a rare benign tumor, a hyperplastic nodule that contains all the normal cellular elements of liver tissue (hepatocytes, Kupffer cells, bile duct elements, fibrous connective tissue) but lacks the normal hepatic architecture and so functions poorly.[18,23] This benign condition may occur at any age, although it is rare in children.[18] It is more common in females before age 40 years,[88] and there is some controversial evidence of a relationship to the use of oral contraceptives.[114] Other findings suggest that the risk of hemorrhage is greater for patients with either focal nodular hyperplasia or liver cell adenoma who also take oral contraceptives.[25,36] Patients with either liver cell adenoma or focal nodular hyperplasia commonly present with a palpable abdominal mass or pain in the right upper quadrant, which may be sudden and severe due to hemorrhage within the lesion.[114] Focal nodular hyperplasia usually causes no symptoms whereas adenomas do.[114]

Even though the mass is not encapsulated and multinodular, it is well-circumscribed, with a characteristic depressed central or eccentric stellate scar composed of dense fibrous connective tissue, pro-

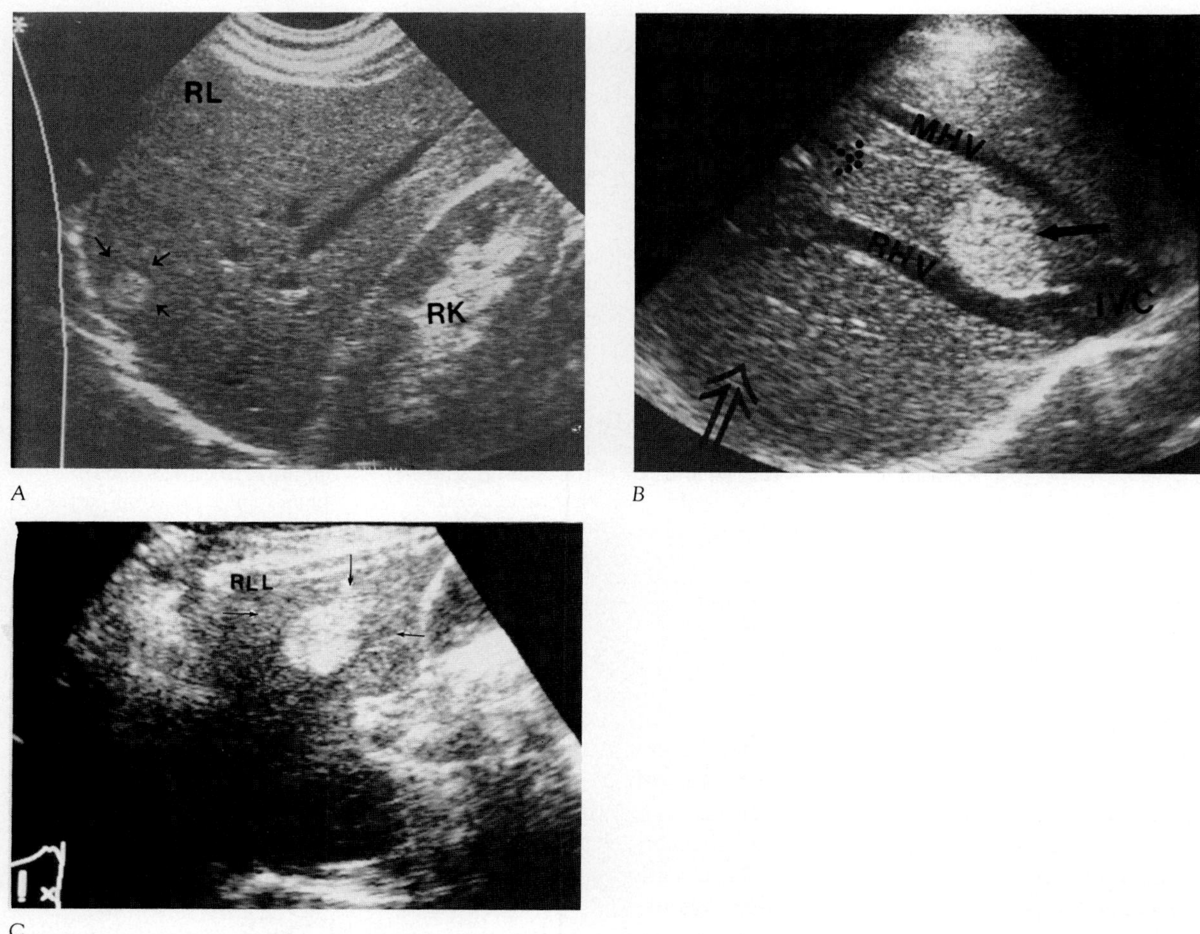

Figure 4-19. A sagittal section demonstrates the classic homogeneous, hyperechoic sonographic appearance of a cavernous hemangioma *(arrows)* with well-defined margins located in the posterior right liver lobe (RL); (RK, right kidney.) (Courtesy Debra M. Joly, Kingston, TX.) (*B*) A cavernous hemangioma *(black arrow)* is located in the right anterior hepatic segment *(dotted arrow)* rather than the more typical right posterior segment *(open arrow)*. The hemangioma is impinging on the right hepatic vein (RHV). (MHV, middle hepatic vein; IVC, inferior vena cava.) (Courtesy Cathy Carr-Hoefer, Corvallis, OR.) (C) This sagittal section of the right liver lobe (RLL) of a 64-year-old woman demonstrates a lesion measuring 17 × 23 mm *(arrows)*, most likely a cavernous hemangioma although its appearance is somewhat mottled rather than homogeneous. CT examination with dynamic contrast was recommended as follow-up to determine if enhancement of the lesion would typify cavernous hemangioma. (Courtesy Tally Call, Logan, UT.)

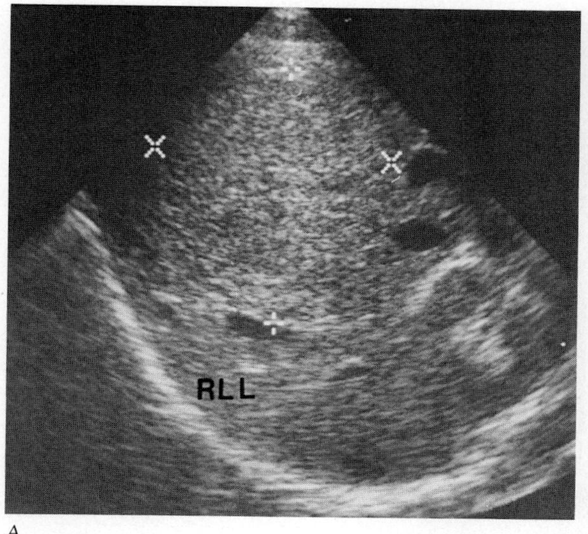

A

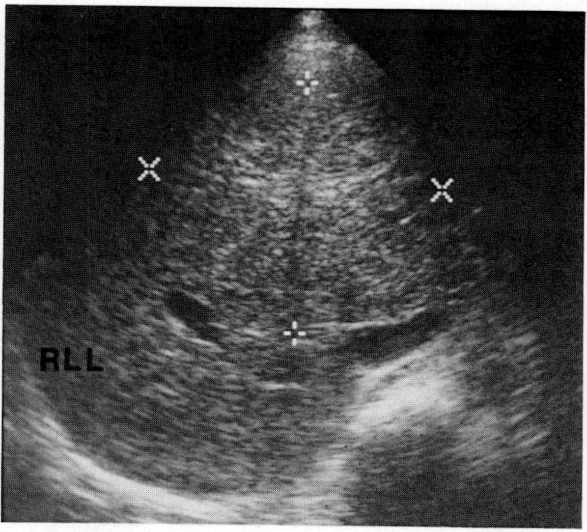

B

Figure 4-20. A solid 7 × 8 cm mass *(cursors)* contained within the right liver lobe (RLL) distorting the adjacent vascular structures is identified on (*A*) sagittal and (*B*) transverse sections. A female patient presented with epigastric pain, and focal nodular hyperplasia was the primary diagnostic consideration, given her history. Follow-up imaging studies were suggested.

liferating bile ducts, and thin-walled blood vessels, which may or may not appear on images.[110,120] Sonographically it has been described as a cirrhosis-like mass in normal tissue (see Table 4-8).[120] The mass ranges in size from 0.5 to 20 cm and can appear hypoechoic, hyperechoic, or isoechoic relative to normal liver.[8,110,120] It is usually located in the right lobe or left lateral segment.[8,110] In 13% of cases they are multiple (Fig. 4-20).[18] The reported sensitivity of various imaging modalities for focal nodular hyperplasia is as follows: ultrasonography, 100%; CT, 78%; angiography, 82%; radionuclide scanning, 55%.[110] Since these masses contain Kupffer cells that accumulate injected technetium-99m–sulphur colloid and liver cell adenomas do not, colloid uptake by a focal hepatic mass is virtually diagnostic of focal nodular hyperplasia.[110,114]

Liver Cell Adenoma

Liver cell adenomas differ from focal nodular hyperplasia in that they contain no bile duct or Kupffer cells, but they are true hepatic encapsulated neoplasms, consisting of normal to slightly atypical hepatocytes, often with areas of bile stasis, focal hemorrhage, and necrosis.[23] A liver cell adenoma is usually solitary with identifiable margins. It is rare but most common in women of child-bearing age,[114] and the frequency is increased among those who use oral contraceptives.[36] It produces no significant laboratory anomalies and is sometimes an incidental finding. Usually adenomas cause symptoms, ranging from a palpable mass and abdominal pressure to acute and severe right upper quandrant pain due to rupture and sudden intraperitoneal hemorrhage.[113]

The sonographic features are variable and may not be specific for liver cell adenoma, focal nodular hyperplasia, metastatic disease, hepatoma, or even some hemangiomas (see Table 4-8).[38,152] Close correlation with the clinical setting, radionuclide studies, and in some cases angiography may be necessary to make a definitive diagnosis.[114] The usual appearance is of an encapsulated, well-circumscribed hyperechoic mass; but, it may appear hy-

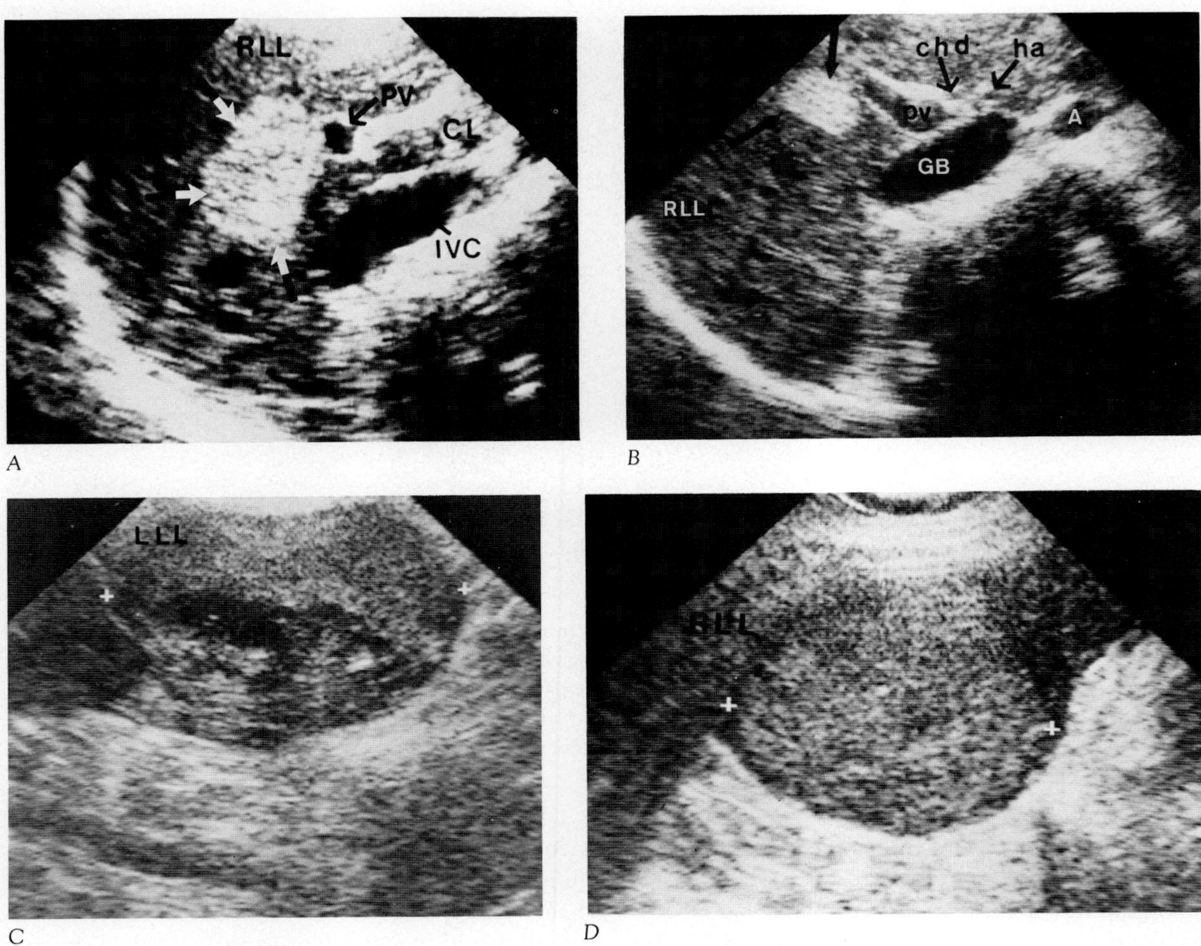

FIGURE 4-21. (*A*) On oblique and (*B*) transverse sections, a homogeneous, hyperechoic 4.5 cm mass *(arrows)* was identified superior to the porta hepatis region in the right liver lobe (RLL). The female patient's clinical history favored a benign liver cell adenoma, which was confirmed with follow-up scintigraphy and CT. Other possibilities included focal nodular hyperplasia and primary carcinoma such as hepatoma or cholangiocarcinoma (PV, portal vein; chd, common hepatic duct; ha, hepatic artery; CL, caudate lobe; IVC, inferior vena cava; A, aorta; GB, gallbladder). Another patient, a 34-year-old woman with a history of oral contraceptive use, presented with abdominal distension. A 10 × 12 cm complex mass *(cursors)* involving the inferior aspect of the left liver lobe (LLL) is identified in a sagittal section (C). In a transverse section (*D*), a second 8 × 10 cm homogeneous mass *(cursors)* involving the posterior aspect of the right liver lobe (RLL) was also identified.

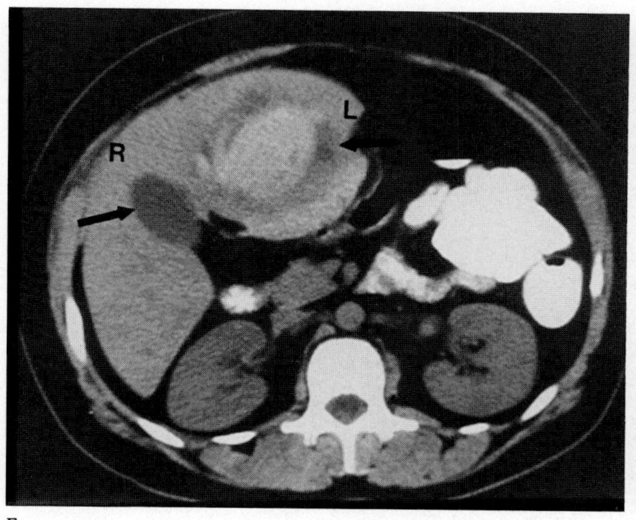

E

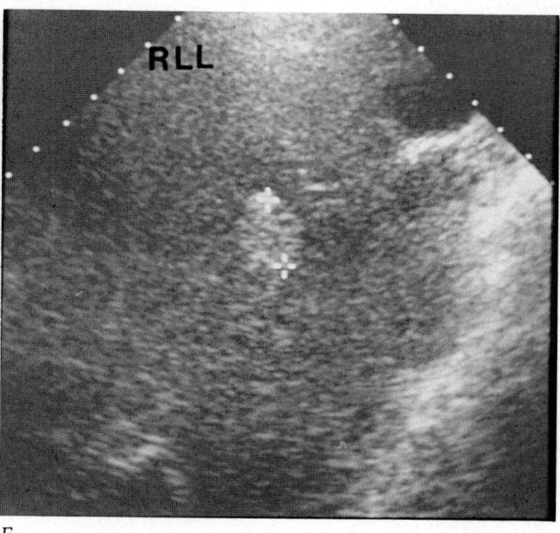

F

FIGURE 4-21. (*continued*). The clinical history and follow-up radionuclide and CT examinations (*E*) favored the diagnosis of benign liver cell adenoma. The CT section demonstrates a complex mass indicating fresh hemorrhage as well as necrosis located in the left lobe (L). The arrow is pointing to the homogeneous gallbladder. The patient underwent surgical resection of the adenoma and a large portion of the left lobe. Approximately a year later, she returned for a sonographic pregnancy evaluation at 15.1 weeks. The liver had regenerated successfully; however, at the 30.8th week of gestation, a new lesion measuring 1.8 cm (*cursors*) was identified on a sagittal section (*F*; RLL, right liver lobe). This is most likely a new liver cell adenoma. (Courtesy KayLynñ Schmidt, Rock Springs, WY.)

poechoic or isoechoic relative to normal liver parenchyma (Fig. 4-21A, B). If there has been hemorrhage, the appearance varies with the age and extent, from anechoic to hyperechoic (Fig. 4-21C–F).[113]

Malignant Neoplasm

PRIMARY MALIGNANT TUMORS

Primary liver cancer is relatively rare in the United States (less than 3%)[22] but is common in densely populated parts of the Far East, Southern Africa, China, and Greece.[60] In the United States, it is unusual before age 40 years and most common in the sixth decade. Males are more often affected than females, and blacks more than caucasians (2 to 10 per 100,000 per annum).[60] A epidemiologic study of primary liver carcinomas indicates they may be related to exposure to carcinogens such as mycotoxins in the diet; chronic liver disease, especially cirrhosis; viral infections, especially hepatitis B; and parasitic liver infections.[22,102] Histologically, tumors are either hepatocellular carcinoma (80% to 90%), which develops in the hepatocytes (hepatocarcinoma or hepatoma), or cholangiocellular carcinoma (cholangiocarcinoma), which develops in the bile ducts (see Chapter 5).

Hepatocellular Carcinoma. Morphologically, hepatocellular carcinoma may be limited to one area (focal) or it can occur in numerous nodules (multiple) or as infiltrates on the surface of the liver (diffuse).[22,102] Physiologically, hepatocellular carcinoma interferes with normal hepatocyte function, causing biliary obstruction with juandice, portal hypertension with ascites, portal vein thrombosis, and different metabolic disturbances. Liver function tests demonstrate increased levels of alkaline phosphatase, AST (SGOT), and ALT (SGPT).[60,109] The most significant liver function anomaly is the presence of α-fetoprotein in 70% of cases.[88] Erythrocytosis is secondary to erythropoietin production.[60] The pathophysiology may include invasion of the hepatic veins (producing Budd-Chiari syndrome)[109] and the portal veins,[105] resulting in metastasis to the heart and lungs and to other sites such as brain, kidney, and spleen.[102] Patients usually present with right upper quadrant pain, sudden deterioration of hepatic function in an already compromised liver, a palpable mass, rapid liver enlargement, and fever of unknown origin. By the time it is discovered, hepatocellular carcinoma is usually in an advanced stage and patients survive only 3 to 4 months. The 5-year survival rate is about 1%.[60,102] The diagnosis is based on clinical manifestations, laboratory function variances especially the presence of α-fetoprotein, imaging modalities, and exploratory laparotomy.

Sonographically, hepatocellular carcinoma has a range of appearances, evolving from progressively hypoechoic to isoechoic. As they grow, they become unevenly hyperechoic. A few are diffusely hyperechoic from the beginning and retain the same features thereafter.[126] The principal role of ultrasonography is its ability to localize, measure, and characterize the presentation of the disease, and it is the most cost-effective imaging technique for screening patients at high risk.[105] Portal vein thrombosis is reported in 26% to 33% of hepatocellular carcinoma cases and is recognized by the presence of echogenic intraluminal material.[9] Tanaka and colleagues[139] correlated sonographic findings with histology and found that hypoechoic lesions correspond to solid tumors without necrosis; complex masses are seen in tumors with some necrotic areas; and hyperechoic lesions were seen in two types of tumor, those with fatty metamorphosis and those with marked sinusoidal dilatation (Fig. 4-22).

METASTASES

Metastatic lesions arising from other areas of the body, especially from gastrointestinal (particularly the colon), breast or pulmonary carcinoma, are the most common forms of neoplastic liver disease.[109]

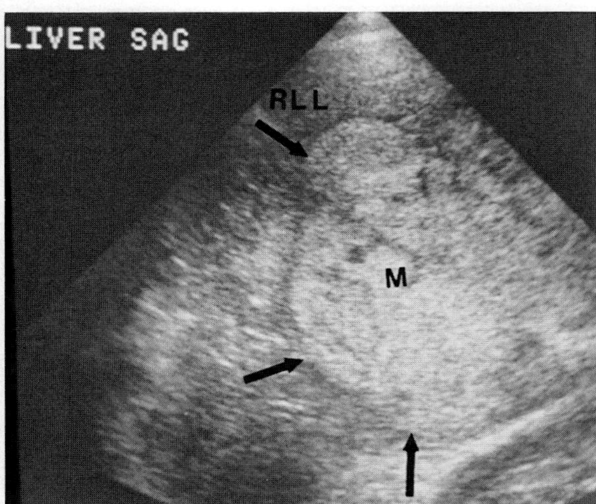

FIGURE 4-22 A

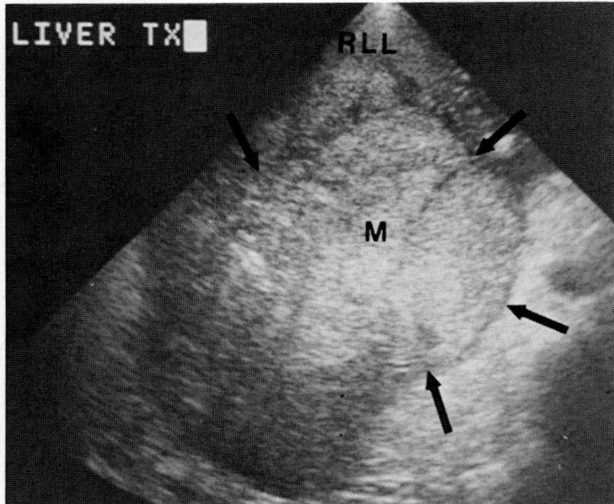

B

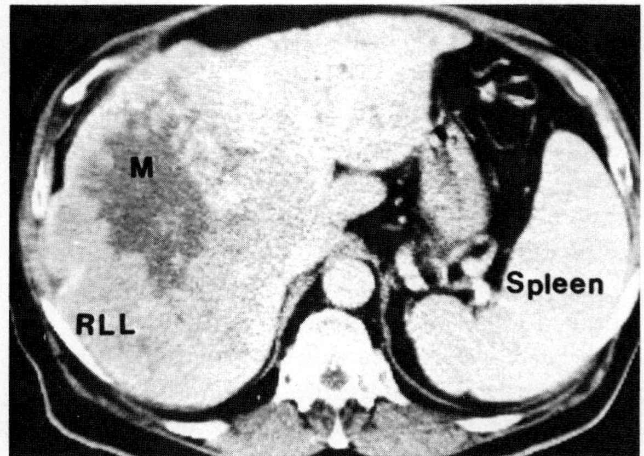

C

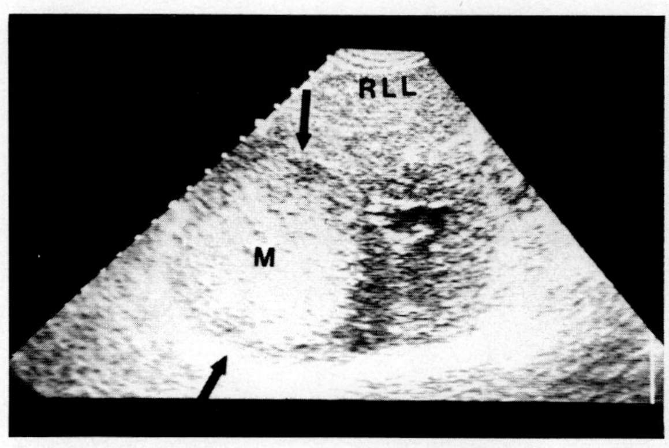

D

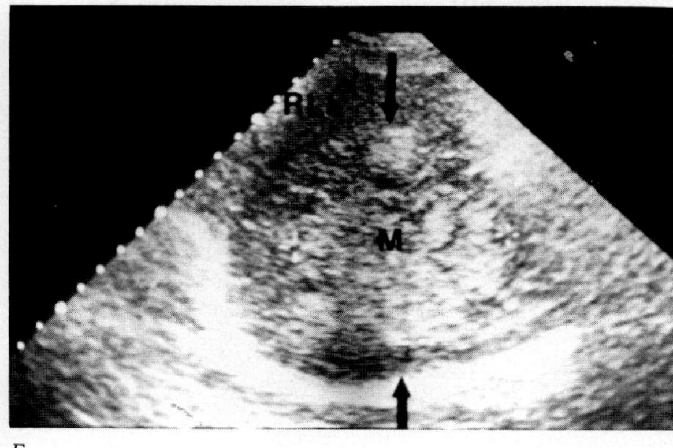

E

FIGURE 4-22. On both (*A*) sagittal and (*B*) transverse sections through the right liver lobe (RLL), a 7 × 9 cm heterogeneous, well-circumscribed mass (M, *arrows*) is demonstrated, which accounts for this 77-year-old man's enlarged, palpable liver. It was not possible to measure the entire mass longitudinally, as it began near the upper margin and extended caudad. Given the patient's history, it was strongly suspected to be hepatocellular carcinoma. CT examination afforded a better appreciation of the liver anatomy and adjacent structures in continuity. A CT section (C) demonstrates the mass (M) involving the right lobe (RLL), with mixed areas of enhancement and nonenhancement and a large central area of nonenhancement, necrotic breakdown, and calcifications. These findings augmented the suspicion of hepatocellular carcinoma, and biopsy examination of the lesion confirmed the diagnosis. On both sagittal (*D*) and transverse (*E*) sections through the right liver lobe (RLL), an abnormal hyperechoic lobulated mass (M, *cursors, arrows*) measuring 8 cm in diameter was demonstrated on a 68-year-old man whose laboratory values indicated altered liver function. A follow-up CT examination demonstrated three masses, the largest appearing in the dome of the liver. In light of the clinical history, primary malignant tumors such as hepatocellular carcinoma (hepatoma) with multifocal lesions or an uncommon form of multifocal cholangiocarcinoma were strong diagnostic possibilities.

Physiologically, the liver is vulnerable to metastatic carcinoma because of the large volume of blood it receives each minute, the high nutrient level of the blood, and the large reserve of lymphatic drainage.[22] In one report, approximately 40% of patients with carcinoma had liver metastasis.[105] Clinically, metastases are frequently silent and cause symptoms in only half of affected patients.[105] The clinical course relates to the growth of the metastatic lesion and the site of the primary malignancy.[22] Symptoms may include hepatomegaly, jaundice, pain, nutritional wasting, and muscle wasting; other dysfunctions depend on the amount of hepatocellular involvement.[22] Liver function test values are frequently abnormal, especially alkaline phosphatase, AST (SGOT), and ALT (SGPT), and α-fetoprotein is increased in many cases of liver metastasis. Multiple metastases give rise to multiple masses in the liver, suggesting that tumor seeding has occurred in episodes.[18] The prognosis is poor because of poor response to treatment, the impossibility of resecting the tumor surgically, and reseeding of the liver. The 5-year survival rate has been reported to be less than 5%.[22]

Sonographically, metastases can present a wide variety of appearances, reflecting the spectrum of tumor types[18]: (1) hypoechoic, (2) hyperechoic, (3) isoechoic, (4) anechoic, (5) mixed (hyperechoic and

(text continues on page 144)

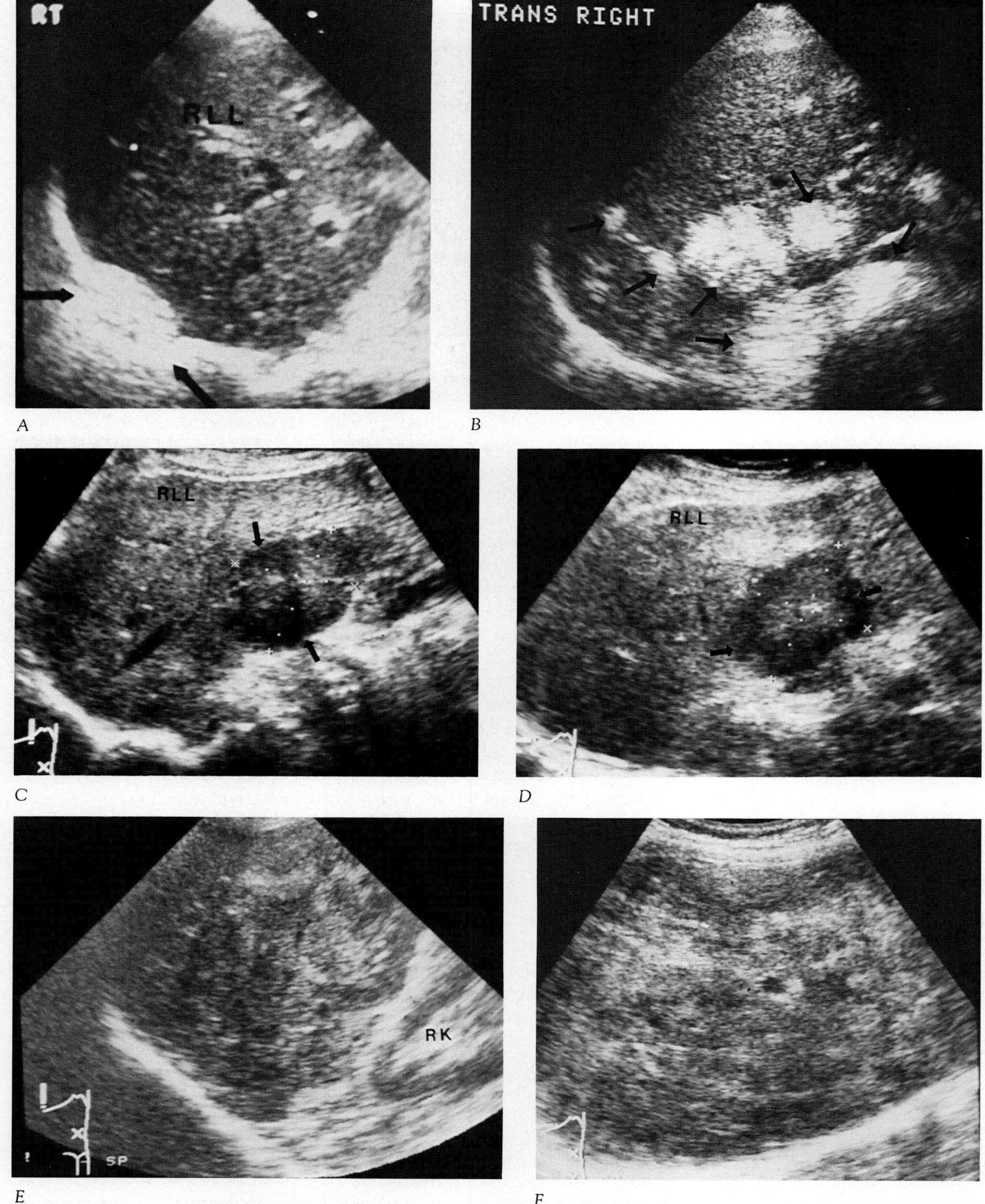
RT
RLL
A
TRANS RIGHT
B
RLL
C
RLL
D
RK
SP
E
F

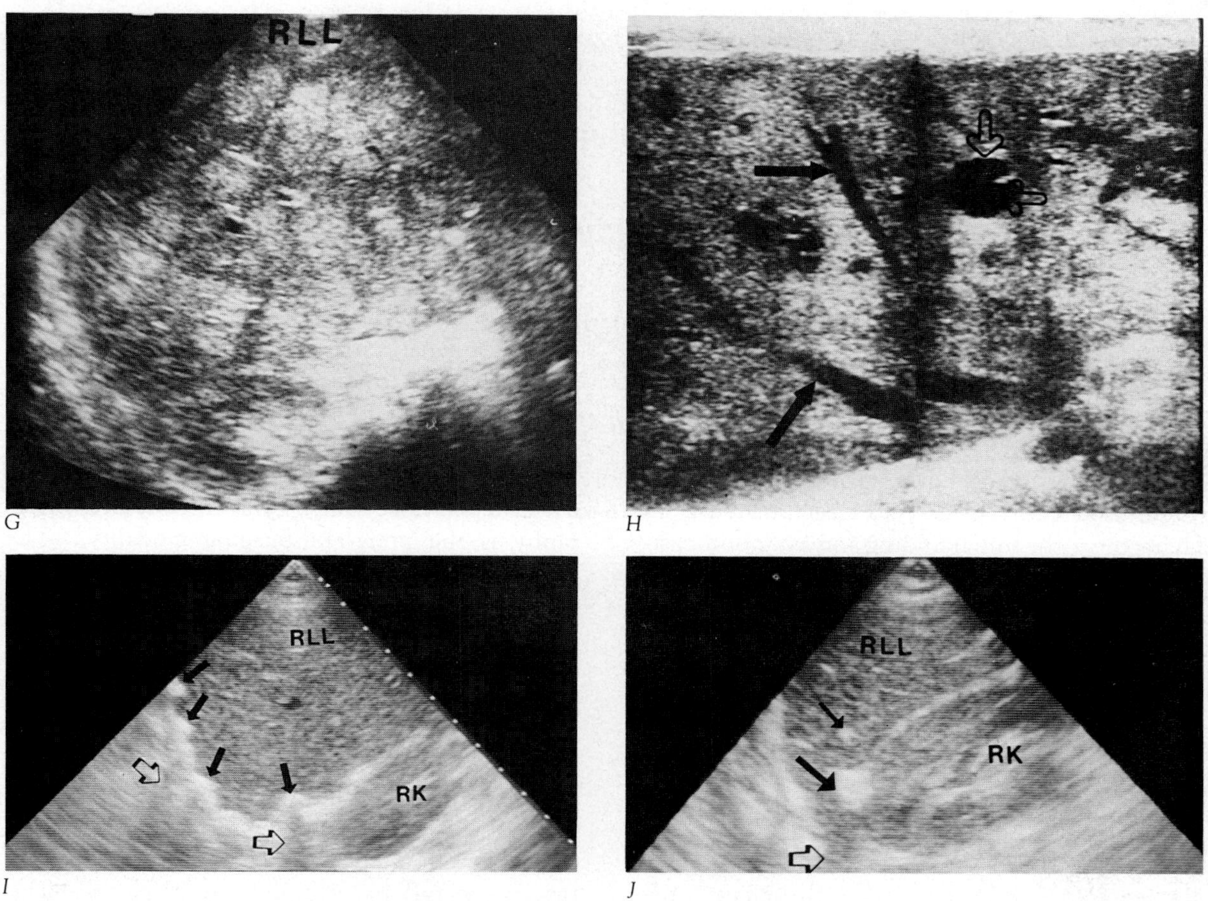

FIGURE 4-23. On a sagittal section, a hyperechoic subdiaphragmatic metastatic lesion *(arrows)* in the right liver lobe (RLL) is demonstrated displacing the usually smooth diaphragmatic contour. The primary tumor is ovarian carcinoma. (*B*) Irregularly contoured, focal, hyperechoic metastatic tumors *(arrows)* are identified on a transverse section of the right liver lobe. The primary lesion was breast carcinoma. (*A,B* Courtesy Cathy Carr-Hoefer, Corvallis, OR.) In another case, an irregular metastatic mass *(arrows, cursors)* measuring 5.5 × 4.5 cm is identified with an isoechoic, hyperechoic, and hypoechoic mixed pattern and an anechoic periphery on (C) sagittal and (*D*) transverse sections within the right liver lobe (RLL) of a 73-year-old woman. A third case of diffuse, irregular, echo pattern of metastases is identified throughout the liver as presented in (*E*) sagittal and (*F*) transverse sections of the right lobe of a 74-year-old man. The primary site is not known (RK, right kidney). (*C-F* Courtesy Tally Call, Logan, UT.) (G) A diffuse hepatic malignancy seen in a transverse section of the right lobe (RLL) gives the liver a motheaten or mottled appearance. The patient has a history of breast carcinoma. (Courtesy Cathy Carr-Hoefer, Corvallis, OR.) (*H*) A transverse section demonstrates dilated ducts *(black arrows)* and a heterogeneous liver texture representing metastasis from pancreatic carcinoma. A liver cyst *(open arrows)* was an incidental finding. (*G, H* Courtesy Cathy Carr-Hoefer, Corvallis, OR.) (*I, J*) Multiple calcified nodules *(arrows)* are identified outlining the dome of the diaphragm (*I*) and in the right liver lobe (RLL, *J*) casting acoustic shadows (*open arrows*; RK, right kidney). With this 37-year-old woman's history of ovarian carcinoma, this finding is very suggestive of metastatic liver involvement. (Courtesy Marsha McIntosh, Salt Lake City, UT.)

hypoechoic), (6) bullseye or target (the center of the lesion may be hyperechoic or hypoechoic with a halo), (7) complex (both cystic and solid).[18,84,88,105] Ultrasonography lacks specificity for correlating the sonographic appearance of hepatic metastases with the organ or cell type of origin.[57,88,105] The tendencies noted are that a majority of hyperechoic masses are from a primary colon tumor (54%),[141] cystic necrosis is associated with leiomyosarcomas[156] and hypoechoic masses with lymphoma.[18,42] Additional findings include calcification in tumors that are partially involuting.[88] As with all tumors in the liver, an important finding is that hypervascular metastatic lesions are hyperechoic and hypovascular lesions are hypoechoic (Fig. 4-23).[88]

Ultrasound can be used to locate, measure, and characterize the initial finding and as a noninvasive follow-up procedure to assess metastases for increased or decreased size or extent and other changes.[88] It is a very valuable modality for distinguishing obstructive from nonobstructive jaundice in patients suspected of having underlying malignant disease.[7]

Other Imaging Procedures

ARTERIOGRAPHY

Radiographic procedures, once the mainstay for imaging diffuse, obstructive, or focal liver pathology, have been replaced by newer technologies and techniques. Hepatic arteriography is occasionally indicated to evaluate tumor resectability and to define hepatic arterial and venous anatomy before resection.[83]

NUCLEAR MEDICINE

Radionuclide imaging is infrequently used to determine the cause and location of obstruction in patients with jaundice. It is primarily a back-up procedure used when other modalities fail to solve the diagnostic problem.[64] Hepatic scintigraphy and SPECT are very useful for detecting masses as small as 1 cm in diameter, either as "cold" lesions representing filling defects or as "hot" lesions such as cavernous hemangiomas, which accumulate more radionuclide than the surrounding parenchyma.[83]

COMPUTED TOMOGRAPHY

CT is very accurate (90 to 95%) in demonstrating a dilated biliary system in patients with obstructive jaundice and demonstrates the lesion causing the obstruction in approximately 75% of patients.[64] CT also demonstrates differences of attenuation between the mass and the surrounding normal hepatic parenchyma. Particularly helpful to surgeons in the operating room and to nonradiologists, CT images are easier to understand than many diagnostic images and they clearly demonstrate organ-mass and organ-organ relationships.[28,79] In obese or gaseous patients, where ultrasonography cannot resolve intrahepatic anatomy, CT is the preferred imaging modality. In one study, CT performed better than sonography for evaluation of the liver for metastases, especially in patients with breast carcinoma.[3] On the other hand, for patients who are emaciated or have little perivisceral fat, ultrasonography is the preferred imaging modality.[64] The major disadvantages of CT are the higher cost of the examination, the exposure to ionizing radiation, and the possibility of allergic reaction to the contrast material.

MAGNETIC RESONANCE

Magnetic resonance imaging (MRI) is at present of limited value.[64] In the upper abdomen its major limitations are relatively poor resolution due to respiratory motion and prolonged scanning time.[83] In future generations of equipment these problems may be resolved.

Summary

Sonography is easily performed and offers a noninvasive and cost-effective means of evaluating the liver. As a result, a sonographic examination provides valuable information on the appearance of the hepatic parenchymal, normal and abnormal, and on the location, measurements and character of hepatic lesions. When correlated with clinical findings, the examination plays a significant role in the diagnosis and health care management of patients with liver disease.

References

1. Abrams RM, Bernbaum, ER, Santos JS, et al: Angiographic features of cavernous hemangioma of the liver. Radiology 1969, 92:308–312.
2. Albarelli JN, Springer GE: A technical approach to evaluating the jaundiced patient. Semin Ultrasound 1980, 1:96–101.

3. Alderson PO, Adams DF, McNeil BJ, et al: Computed tomography, ultrasound, and scintigraphy of the liver in patients with colon or breast carcinoma: A prospective comparison. Radiology 1983, 149: 225–230.
4. Anderhub B: Manual of Abdominal Sonography. Baltimore, University Park Press, 1983.
5. Anthony CP, Thibodeau GA: Textbook of Anatomy and Physiology, 10th ed. St. Louis, CV Mosby, 1979.
6. Arenson AM, McKee JD: Left upper quadrant pseudolesion secondary to normal variants in liver and spleen. J Clin Ultrasound 1986, 14:558–561.
7. Arger PH: Obstructive jaundice of malignant origin. Semin Ultrasound 1980, 1:113–117.
8. Atkinson GO, Kodroff M, Sones PJ, et al: Focal nodular hyperplasia of the liver in children: A report of three new cases. Radiology 1980, 137:171–174.
9. Atri M, de Stempel J, Bret PM, et al: Incidence of portal vein thrombosis complicating liver metastasis as detected by duplex ultrasound. J Ultrasound Med 1990, 9:285–289.
10. Auh YH, Pardes JG, Chung KB, et al: Posterior hepatodiaphragmatic interposition of the colon: Ultrasonographic and computed tomographic appearance. J Ultrasound Med 1985, 4:113–117.
11. Auh YH, Rubenstein WA, Zirinsky K, et al: Accessory fissure of the liver: CT and sonographic appearance. AJR 1984, 143:565–572.
12. Barnett PH, Zerhouni EA, White RI, et al: Computed tomography in the diagnosis of cavernous hemangioma of the liver. AJR 1987, 134:439–447.
13. Barriga P, Cruz F, Lepe V, et al: An ultrasonographically solid tumor-like appearance of echinococcal cysts in the liver. J Ultrasound Med 1983, 2:123–125.
14. Bartrum RJ, Crow HC: Inflammatory diseases of the biliary system. Semin Ultrasound 1980, 1:102–111.
15. Belton RL, VanZandt TF: Congenital absence of the left lobe of the liver: A radiologic diagnosis. Radiology 1983, 147:184.
16. Berland LL: Focal areas of decreased echogenicity in the liver at the porta hepatis. J Ultrasound Med 1986, 5:157–159.
17. Berland LL, Lawson TL, Foley WD: Porta hepatis: Sonographic discrimination of bile ducts from arteries with pulsed Doppler with new anatomic criteria. AJR 1982, 138:833–840.
18. Bissett RAL, Khan AN: Differential Diagnosis in Abdominal Ultrasound. London, Bailliere–Tindall, 1990.
19. Bonhof JA, Linhart P: A pseudolesion of the liver caused by rib cartilage in B-mode ultrasonography. J Ultrasound Med 1985, 4:135–137.
20. Bree RL, Schuab RE, Neiman HL: Solitary echogenic spot in the liver: Is it diagnostic of a hemangioma? AJR 1983, 140:41–45.
21. Brown BM, Filly RA, Callen PW: Ultrasonographic anatomy of the caudate lobe. J Ultrasound Med 1982, 1:189–192.
22. Bullock BL, Rosendahl PP: Pathophysiology: Adaptations and Alterations in Function, 2nd ed. Glenview, IL, Scott, Foresman, 1988.
23. Casarella WJ, Knowles DM, Wolff M, et al: Focal nodular hyperplasia and liver cell adenoma: Radiologic and pathologic differentiation. AJR 1978, 131:393–402.
24. Chafetz N, Filly RA: Portal and hepatic veins: Accuracy of margin echoes for distinguishing intrahepatic vessels. Radiology 1979, 130:725–728.
25. Cimmino CV, Scott DW: Case report: Benign liver tumor with central necrosis. J Clin Ultrasound 1978, 6:119–120.
26. Conrad MR, Landay MJ, Janes JO: Sonographic "parallel channel" sign of biliary tree enlargement in mild to moderate obstructive jaundice. AJR 1978, 130:279–286.
27. Cooperberg PL, Li D, Wong P, et al: Accuracy of common hepatic duct size in the evaluation of extrahepatic biliary obstruction. Radiology 1980, 135:141–144.
28. Copeland EM: Screening for diffuse and focal liver disease: A surgeon's viewpoint. J Clin Ultrasound 1984, 12:91–92.
29. Corbet JV: Laboratory Tests and Diagnostic Procedures with Nursing Diagnosis, 2nd ed. Norwalk, CT, Appleton and Lange, 1987.
30. Craig M: Pocket Guide to Ultrasound Measurements. Philadelphia, JB Lippincott, 1988.
31. Crivello MS, Peterson IM, Austin RM: Left lobe of the liver mimicking perisplenic collection. J Clin Ultrasound 1986, 14:697–701.
32. Doehner GA: The hepatic venous system, its normal roentgen anatomy. Radiology 1968, 90:1119–1123.
33. Donoso L, Martinez-Noguera A, Zidan A, et al: Papillary process of the caudate lobe of the liver: Sonographic appearance. Radiology 1989, 173:631–633.
34. England MA: Color Atlas of Life Before Birth: Normal Fetal Development. Chicago, Year Book Medical Publishers, 1983.
35. Esensten M, Ralls PW, Colletti P, et al: Posttraumatic intrahepatic biloma: Sonographic diagnosis. AJR 1983, 140:303–305.
36. Fechner RE: Benign hepatic lesions and orally administered contraceptives. Human Pathol 1977, 8:255–268.
37. Filly RA, Laing FC: Anatomic variation of portal

venous anatomy in the porta hepatis: Ultrasonographic evaluation. J Clin Ultrasound 1978, 6:83–88.
38. Freeny PC, Vimont TR, Barnett DC: Cavernous hemangioma of the liver: Ultrasonography, arteriography, and computed tomography. Radiology 1979, 132:143–148.
39. Fried AM, Kreel L, Cosgrove DO: The hepatic interlobar fissure: Combined in vitro and in vivo study. AJR 1984, 143:561–564.
40. Gharbi HA, Hassine JW, Braunner MW, et al: Ultrasound examination of hydatid liver. Radiology 1981, 139:459–463.
41. Gibney RG, Hendlin AP, Cooperberg PL: Sonographically detected hepatic hemangiomas: Absence of change over time. AJR 1987, 149:953–957.
42. Ginaldi S, Bernardino ME, Jing BS, et al: Ultrasonographic patterns of hepatic lymphoma. Radiology 1980, 136:427–431.
43. Glazer GM, Laing FC, Brown TW, et al: Sonographic demonstration of portal hypertension: The patient umbilical vein. Radiology 1980, 136:161–163.
44. Gore RM, Callen PW, Filly RA: Displaced retroperitoneal fat: Sonographic guide to right upper quadrant mass localization. Radiology 1982, 142:701–705.
45. Gosink B: Intrahepatic gas: Differential diagnosis. AJR 1981, 137:763–767.
46. Gosink BB, Lemon SK, Scheible W, et al: Accuracy of ultrasonography in diagnosis of hepatocellular disease. AJR 1979, 133:19–23.
47. Graham MF, Cooperberg PL, Cohen MM, et al: The size of the normal common hepatic duct following cholecystectomy: An ultrasonographic study. Radiology 1980: 135:137–139.
48. Graif M, Manor A, Itzchak Y: Sonographic differentiation of extra- and intrahepatic masses. AJR 1983, 141:553–556.
49. Gray H: Gray's Anatomy: Anatomy of the Human Body, 29th ed (American Edition, Edited by Charles Mayo Goss). Philadelphia, Lea & Febiger, 1973.
50. Guidi SM, Sanders RC: Epigastric pain (upper abdominal pain). *In* Sanders RC (ed): Clinical Sonography: A Practical Guide. Boston, Little, Brown, 1984.
51. Guyton AC: Human Physiology and Mechanisms of Disease, 4th ed. Philadelphia, WB Saunders, 1987.
52. Guyton AC: Textbook of Medical Physiology, 6th ed. Philadelphia, WB Saunders, 1981.
53. Hagen-Ansert SL: Textbook of Diagnostic Ultrasonography, 3rd ed. St. Louis, CV Mosby, 1989.
54. Harbin WP, Robert NJ, Ferruci JT: Diagnosis of cirrhosis based on regional changes in hepatic morphology. Radiology 1980, 135:273–282.
55. Hess CF, Schmiedl U, Koelbel G, et al: Diagnosis of liver cirrhosis with US: Receiver-operating characteristic analysis of multidimensional caudate lobe indexes. Radiology 1989, 171:349–351.
56. Hill MC, Sanders RC: Sonography of the upper abdominal venous system. *In* Sanders RC, Hill MC (eds): Ultrasound Annual. New York, Raven Press, 1983.
57. Hillman BJ, Smith EH, Gammelgaard J, et al: Ultrasonographic pathologic correlation of malignant hepatic masses. Gastrointest Radiol 1979, 4:361–365.
58. Hosoki T, Kuroda C, Tokunaga K, et al: Hepatic venous outflow obstruction: Evaluation with pulsed duplex sonography. Radiology 1989, 170:733–737.
59. Huether SE: Structure and function of the digestive system. *In* McCance KL, Huether SE (eds): Pathophysiology: The Biologic Basis for Disease in Adults and Children. St. Louis, CV Mosby, 1990.
60. Huether SE, McCance KL, Tarmina MS: Alterations of digestive function. *In* McCance KL, Huether SE (eds): Pathophysiology: The Biologic Basis for Disease in Adults and Children. St. Louis, CV Mosby, 1990.
61. Ingis DA: Pathophysiology of jaundice—a primer. Semin Ultrasound 1980, 1:143–147.
62. Itai Y, Ohtomo K, Araki T, et al: Computed tomography and sonography of cavernous hemangiomas of the liver. AJR 1983, 141:315–320.
63. Jacobson JB, Brody PA: The transverse common duct. AJR 1981, 136:91–95.
64. Janes JO, Nelson JA: Jaundice. *In* Eisenberg RL (ed): Diagnostic Imaging: An Algorithmic Approach. Philadelphia, JB Lippincott, 1988.
65. Kane RA: Ultrasonographic anatomy of the liver and biliary tree. Semin Ultrasound 1980, 1:87–95.
66. Kane RA: Sonographic anatomy of the liver. Semin Ultrasound 1981, 2:190–197.
67. Kane RA, Lavery M: Techniques of liver examination. Semin Ultrasound 1981, 2:198–201.
68. Koenigsberg M, Weiner SN, Walzer A: The accuracy of sonography in the differential diagnosis of obstructive jaundice: A comparison with cholangiography. Radiology 1979, 133:157–165.
69. Kuligowska E, Noble J: Sonography of hepatic abscesses. Semin Ultrasound 1983, 4:102–116.
70. Kuligowska E, Conners SK, Shapiro JH: Liver abscess: Sonography in diagnosis and treatment. AJR 1982, 138:253–257.
71. Kuni CC, Johnson ML, Holmes JH: Polycystic liver disease. J Clin Ultrasound 1978, 6:332–333.
72. Kurtz AB, Rubin CS, Cooper HS, et al: Ultrasound

findings in hepatitis. Radiology 1980, 136:717–723.
73. Lamb JA: Laboratory Tests for Clinical Nursing. Bowie, MD, RJ Brady, 1984.
74. Laing FC, Jeffrey RB: The pseudodilated common bile duct: Ultrasonographic appearance created by the gallbladder neck. Radiology 1980, 135:405–407.
75. Laing FC, London LA, Filly RA: Ultrasonographic identification of dilated intrahepatic bile ducts and their differentiation from portal venous structures. J Clin Ultrasound 1978, 6:90–94.
76. Lewall DB, McCorkell SJ: Hepatic echinococcal cysts: Sonographic appearance and classification. Radiology 1985, 155:773–775.
77. Lewandowski B, French G, Winsberg F: The normal postcholecystectomy sonogram: Gas vs. clips. J Ultrasound Med 1985, 4:7–12.
78. Li DK, Cooperberg PL, Graham MF, et al: Pseudoperisplenic "fluid collections": A clue to normal liver and spleen echogenic texture. J Ultrasound Med 1986, 5:397–400.
79. Lightdale CJ: Screening for diffuse and focal liver disease: A gastroenterologist's viewpoint. J Clin Ultrasound 1984, 12:93–94.
80. Makuuchi M, Hasegawa H, Yamazaki S, et al: The inferior right hepatic vein: Ultrasonic demonstration. Radiology 1983, 148:213–217.
81. Marieb EN: Human Anatomy and Physiology. Redwood City, CA, Benjamin/Cummings, 1989.
82. Marks WM, Filly RA, Callen PW: Ultrasonic anatomy of the liver: A review with new applications. J Clin Ultrasound 1979, 7:137–146.
83. Marks WM, Freeny PC: Hepatic masses. *In* Eisenberg RL, (ed): Diagnostic Imaging: An Algorithmic Approach. Philadelphia, JB Lippincott, 1988.
84. Mayes GB, Bernardino ME: The role of ultrasound in the evaluation of hepatic neoplasms. Semin Ultrasound 1981, 2:212–218.
85. McLoughlin MJ: Angiography in cavernous hemangioma of the liver. AJR 1971, 113:50–55.
86. Melson GL, Stanley RJ: Ultrasound and computed tomography of the liver. *In* Alavi A, Arger PH (eds): Abdomen. New York, Grune & Stratton, 1980.
87. Mitchell SE, Gross BH, Spitz HB: The hypoechoic caudate lobe: An ultrasonic pseudolesion. Radiology, 1982, 144:569–572.
88. Mittelstaedt CA: Abdominal Ultrasound. New York, Churchill Livingstone, 1987.
89. Mostbeck GH, Wittich GR, Herold C, et al: Hemodynamic significance of the paraumbilical vein in portal hypertension: Assessment with duplex US. Radiology 1989, 170:339–342.
90. Mueller PR, Ferrucci JT, Simeone JF, et al: Postcholecystectomy bile duct dilatation: Myth or reality? AJR 1981, 136:355–358.
91. Nakanishi T, Ogawa H, Kawamura T, et al: Comparison of convex and linear transducers for sonographic assessment of the liver, spleen, and pancreas. AJR 1984, 143:1110–1112.
92. Neiman HL: Hepatocellular causes of jaundice. Semin Ultrasound 1980, 1:118–122.
93. Nelson RC, Chezmar JL: Diagnostic approach to hepatic hemangiomas. Radiology 1990, 176:11–13.
94. Netter FH: The CIBA Collection of Medical Illustrations. "Digestive System," volume 3, part III. Rochester, The Case-Hoyt Corporation, 1964.
95. Neumaier CE, Cicio GR, Derchi LE, et al: The patent ductus venosus: An additional ultrasonic finding in portal hypertension. J Clin Ultrasound 1983, 11:231–233.
96. Newlin N, Silver TM, Stuck KJ, et al: Ultrasonic features of pyogenic liver abscesses. Radiology 1981, 139:155–159.
97. Niederau C, Sonnenberg A, Muller JE, et al: Sonographic measurements of the normal liver, spleen, pancreas, and portal vein. Radiology 1983, 149:537–540.
98. Odwin CS, Dubinsky T, Fleischer AC: Ultrasonography Examination Review and Study Guide. Norwalk, CT, Appleton and Lange, 1987.
99. Parulekar SG: Ligaments and fissures of the liver: Sonographic anatomy. Radiology 1979, 130:409–411.
100. Parulekar SG: Ultrasound evaluation of common bile duct size. Radiology 1979, 133:703–707.
101. Pietri H, Boscaini M, Berthezene P, et al: Hepatic morphotypes: Their statistical individualization using ultrasonography. J Ultrasound Med 1988, 7:189–196.
102. Porth CM: Alterations in function of the hepatobiliary system and exocrine pancreas. *In* Porth CM: Pathophysiology: Concepts of Altered Health States. Philadelphia, JB Lippincott, 1986.
103. Prando A, Goldstein HM, Bernardino ME, et al: Ultrasonic pseudolesions of the liver. Radiology 1979, 130:403–407.
104. Price SA, Wilson LM: Pathophysiology: Clinical Concepts of Disease Processes, 2nd ed. New York, McGraw-Hill, 1982.
105. Ralls PW: Hepatic section. *In* Sarti DA (ed): Diagnostic Ultrasound: Text and Cases, 2nd ed. Chicago, Year Book Medical Publishers, 1987.
106. Ralls PW, Quinn MF, Bowswell WD, et al: Patterns of resolution in successfully treated hepatic amebic abscess: Sonographic evaluation. Radiology 1983, 149:541–543.
107. Ralls PW, Quinn MF, Rogers W, et al: Sonographic anatomy of the hepatic artery. AJR 1981, 136:1059–1063.

108. Redel D, Fehske W, Kirchhoff PG: Budd-Chiari syndrome in child with posttraumatic obstruction of inferior vena cava. Radiology 1981, 139:151–154.
109. Robbins SL, Cotran RS: Pathologic Basis of Disease, 2nd ed. Philadelphia, WB Saunders, 1979.
110. Rogers JV, Mack LA, Freeny PC, et al: Hepatic focal nodular hyperplasia: Angiography, CT, sonography, and scintigraphy. AJR 1981, 137:983–990.
111. Rubenstein WA, Auh YH, Whalen JP, et al: The perihepatic spaces: Computed tomographic and ultrasound imaging. Radiology 1983, 149:231–239.
112. Sample WF, Sarti DA, Goldstein LI, et al: Grayscale ultrasonography of the jaundiced patient. Radiology 1978, 128:719–725.
113. Sandler MA, Marks DS, Hricak H, et al: Benign focal diseases of the liver. Semin Ultrasound 1981, 2:202–211.
114. Sandler MA, Petrocelli RD, Marks DS, et al: Ultrasonic features and radionuclide correlation in liver cell adenoma and focal nodular hyperplasia. Radiology 1980, 135:393–397.
115. Sanfelippo PM, Beahers OH, Weiland LH: Cystic disease of the liver. Ann Surg 1974, 179:922–925.
116. Sarti DA: Diagnostic Ultrasound: Text and Cases, 2nd ed. Chicago, Year Book Medical Publishers, 1987.
117. Sauerbrei EE, Cooperberg PL, Gordon P, et al: The discrepancy between radiographic and sonographic bile duct measurements. Radiology 1980, 137:751–755.
118. Sauerbrei EE, Lopez M: Pseudotumor of the quadrate lobe in hepatic sonography: Sign of generalized fatty infiltration. AJR 1986, 147:923–927.
119. Savastano KJ, Ehlers DW: Intrahepatic abscess in liver transplant rejection. J Diagnost Med Sonog 1989, 5:62–64.
120. Scatarige JC, Fishman EK, Sanders RC: The sonographic "scar sign" in focal nodular hyperplasia of the liver. J Ultrasound Med 1982, 1:275–278.
121. Scatarige JC, Scott WW, Donovan PJ, et al: Fatty infiltration of the liver: Ultrasonographic and computed tomographic correlation. J Ultrasound Med 1984, 3:9–14.
122. Scott WW, Donovan PJ, Sanders RC: The sonography of diffuse liver disease. Semin Ultrasound 1981, 2:219–225.
123. Scott WW, Sanders RC, Siegelman SS: Irregular fatty infiltration of the liver: Diagnostic dilemmas. AJR, 1980, 135:67–71.
124. Seeley RR, Stephens TD, Tate P: Anatomy and Physiology. St. Louis, Mosby College Publishing, 1989.
125. Sexton CC, Zeman RK: Correlation of computed tomography, sonography, and gross anatomy of the liver. AJR 1983, 141:711–718.
126. Sheu J-C, Chen D-S, Sung J-L, et al: Hepatocellular carcinoma: US evolution in the early stage. Radiology 1985, 155:463–467.
127. Skolnick ML: Guide to the Ultrasound Examination of the Abdomen. New York, Springer-Verlag, 1986.
128. Skolnick ML: Real-Time Ultrasound Imaging in the Abdomen. New York, Springer-Verlag, 1981.
129. Spiegel RM, King DL, Gream WM: Ultrasonography of primary cysts of the liver. AJR 1978, 131:235–238.
130. Sommer FG, Gregory PB, Fellingham LL, et al: Measurement of attenuation and scatterer spacing in human liver tissue: Preliminary results. J Ultrasound Med 1984, 3:557–561.
131. Spence AP, Mason EB: Human Anatomy and Physiology. Menlo Park, CA, Benjamin/Cummings, 1987.
132. Smith NA: Right upper quadrant pain. *In* Sanders RC: Clinical Sonography: A Practical Guide. Boston, Little, Brown, 1984.
133. Smith NA, Sanders, RC: Cold defects on liver scan: Possible metastases to liver. *In* Sanders RC: Clinical Sonography: A Practical Guide. Boston, Little, Brown, 1984.
134. Smith NA, Sanders RC: Jaundice. *In* Sanders RC: Clinical Sonography: A Practical Guide. Boston, Little, Brown, 1984.
135. Smith NA, Sanders RC: Right upper quadrant mass. *In* Sanders RC: Clinical Sonography: A Practical Guide. Boston, Little, Brown, 1984.
136. Stanley P: Budd-Chiari syndrome. Radiology 1989, 170:625–627.
137. Sunder T: Hepatic venous sonography: Some variations and their implications on surgical anatomy. J Diagnost Med Sonog, 1988, 4:185–188.
138. Taboury J, Porcel A, Tubiana J-M, et al: Cavernous hemangiomas of the liver studied by ultrasound: Enhancement posterior to a hyperechoic mass as a sign of hypervascularity. Radiology 1983, 149:781–785.
139. Tanaka S, Kitamura T, Imaoka S, et al: Hepatocellular carcinoma: Sonographic and histologic correlation. AJR 1983, 140:701–707.
140. Taylor KJW, Gorelick FS, Rosenfield AT, et al: Ultrasonography of alcoholic liver disease with histological correlation. Radiology 1981, 141:157–161.
141. Taylor KJW, Richman TS: Diseases of the liver. Semin Roentgenol 1983, 18:94–101.
142. Taylor KJW, Viscomi GN: Ultrasound diagnosis of cystic disease of the liver. J Clin Gastroenterol 1980, 2:197.

143. Thomas CL (ed): Taber's Cyclopedic Medical Dictionary, 16th ed. Philadelphia, FA Davis, 1989.
144. Tilkian SO, Conover MB, Tilkian AG: Clinical Implications of Laboratory Tests, 3rd ed. St. Louis, CV Mosby, 1983.
145. Tortora GJ, Anagnastakos NP: Principles of Anatomy and Physiology, 5th ed. New York, Harper and Row, 1987.
146. Walt AJ: Cysts and benign tumors of the liver. Surg Clin North Am 1977, 57:449–464.
147. Weaver RM, Goldstein HM, Green B, et al: Gray scale ultrasonographic evaluation of hepatic cystic disease. AJR 1978, 130:849–852.
148. Weill FS: Ultrasonography of Digestive Diseases, 2nd ed. St. Louis, CV Mosby, 1982.
149. Weinreb J, Kumari S, Phillips G, et al: Portal vein measurements by real-time sonography. AJR 1982, 139:497–499.
150. Weinstein BJ, Weinstein DP: Biliary tract dilatation in the nonjaundiced patient. AJR 1980, 134:899–906.
151. Weinstein DP, Weinstein BJ, Brodmerkel GJ: Ultrasonography of biliary tract dilatation without jaundice. AJR 1979, 132:729–734.
152. Wiener SN, Parulekar SG: Scintigraphy and ultrasonography of hepatic hemangioma. Radiology 1979, 132:149–153.
153. Wilbur AC, Schmit DJ, Ryva JC, et al: Accessory hepatic fissure mimicking an acoustically shadowing lesion. J Ultrasound Med 1986, 5:341–342.
154. Willi UV, Teele RL: Hepatic arteries and the parallel-channel sign. J Clin Ultrasound 1979, 7:125–127.
154. Wolson AH: Liver. *In* Goldberg JBB, Kurtz AB (eds): Atlas of Ultrasound Measurements. Chicago, Year Book Medical Publishers, 1990.
155. Wolson AH: Common bile duct measurements. *In* Goldberg BB, Kurtz AB (eds): Atlas of Ultrasound Measurements. Chicago, Year Book Medical Publishers, 1990.
156. Wooten WB, Green B, Goldstein HM: Ultrasonography of necrotic hepatic metastases. Radiology 1978, 128:447–450.

CHAPTER 5

Gallbladder and Biliary Tree

ROSEMARIE P. CANN

Sonography plays a key role in the evaluation of suspected gallbladder and biliary disease. Since the quality of sonographic examinations is strongly operator dependent, it is crucial to understand the anatomy, physiology, pathology, techniques, and pitfalls of scanning these organs. The more motivation and experience a sonographer has, the more accurate the findings tend to be.[1] This is especially true of the gallbladder and biliary tree as scanning may require extra patience, skill, and a trick or two to demonstrate a small gallstone or thoroughly interrogate a common bile duct.

Anatomy

The normal distended gallbladder is usually 7 to 10 cm long and not more than 3 cm in diameter.[62] It is a pear-or teardrop-shaped sac the walls of which are not more than 3 mm thick (usually 1 to 2 mm).[18,37,54,81] The gallbladder is located in the major interlobar fissure between the right and left hepatic lobes. It lies under the visceral surface of the liver, lateral to the second part of the duodenum and anterior to the right kidney and transverse colon (Fig. 5-1).[2]

The gallbladder is divided into neck, body, and fundus (see Fig. 5-1). The narrow neck lies to the right of the porta hepatis and occasionally contains a small posterior infundibulum, Hartman's pouch, where stones can collect. The body is the central or main portion. The position of the fundus can vary considerably. Normally the most inferolateral portion of the gallbladder, it extends caudally to the inferior border of the liver,[2] but it can extend as low as the right lower quadrant and as far left as the left anterior axillary line.[17]

Histologically, the gallbladder consists of an inner epithelial mucosa with folds, a muscular layer, a subserous layer, and an outer serosal surface. Mucous glands are found only in the neck. Aberrant vestigial bile ducts of the liver may enter the adventitia (outermost covering) of the gallbladder and serve as a path for infection from the liver to enter it (see Fig. 5-1).[59]

The normal gallbladder has a bile capacity of 30 to 60 ml.[2] Bile contains bile pigments (chiefly bilirubin), bile acids, cholesterol, lecithin, mucin, and other organic and inorganic substances.[59] The cystic duct, 2 to 6 cm long, arises from the superior aspect of the gallbladder neck. Its lumen contains a series of mucosal folds, the spiral valves of Heister, which prevent collapse or over-distention because of sudden position changes.[2]

The intrahepatic bile ducts run along side portal veins and hepatic arteries in portal triads, surrounded by connective tissue and radiating through the lobes and segments of the liver. The fibrous connective tissue makes the walls of the portal vein branches appear very echogenic. The intrahepatic ducts join to form the right and left main hepatic ducts. The right and left main ducts join near the porta hepatis to form the com-

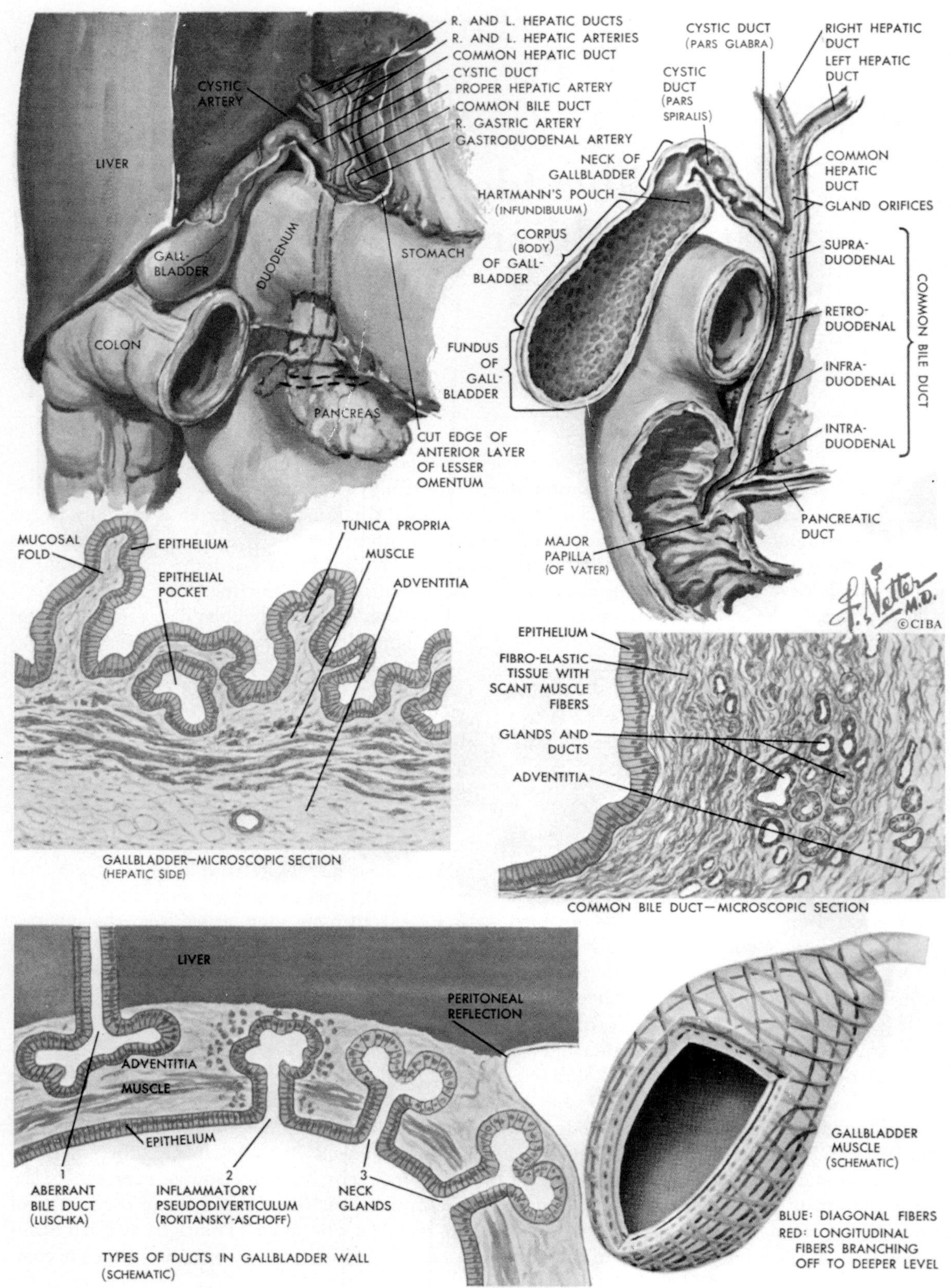

GALLBLADDER—MICROSCOPIC SECTION (HEPATIC SIDE)

COMMON BILE DUCT—MICROSCOPIC SECTION

TYPES OF DUCTS IN GALLBLADDER WALL (SCHEMATIC)

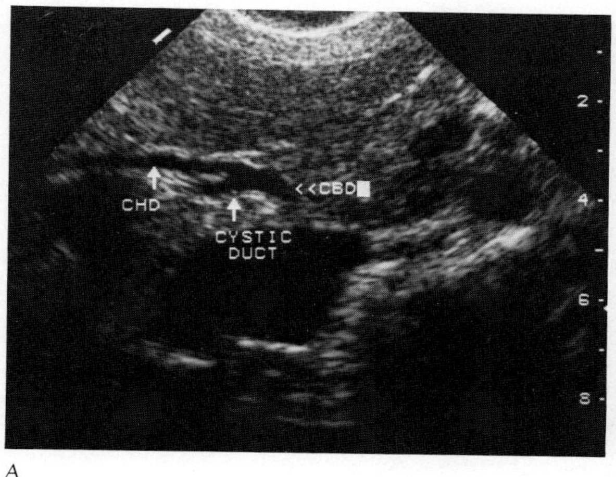

A

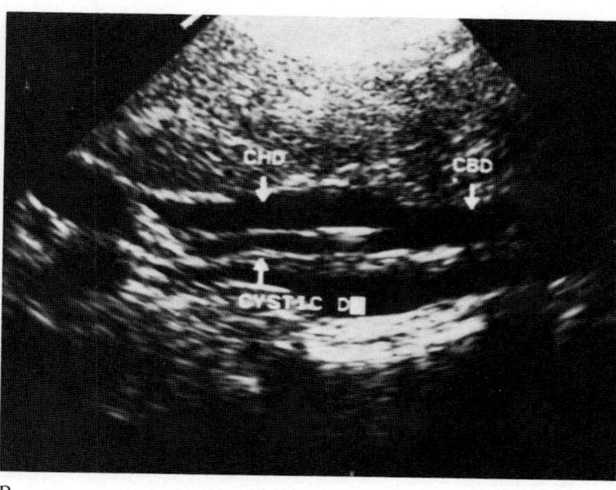

B

FIGURE 5-2. Views of the cystic duct joining the common hepatic duct (CHD) to form the common bile duct (CBD).

mon hepatic duct (CHD). The cystic duct joins the CHD to form the common bile duct (CBD; Fig. 5-2). The CBD courses inferiorly along the right border of the lesser omentum, then along the hepatoduodenal ligament and posterior to the first part of the duodenum, into a groove near the posterolateral aspect of the head of the pancreas just anterior to the inferior vena cava (IVC; see Fig. 5-1). In some cases, it is surrounded by pancreatic tissue. The CBD then narrows and enters the posteromedial aspect of the descending portion of the duodenum. It is joined by the main pancreatic duct, and together they empty through the papilla of Vater, a protrusion of mucosal lining, into the duodenal lumen at the sphincter of Oddi. All bile ducts run anterior to the portal vein and to the right of the hepatic artery in the portal triads (Fig. 5-3). Ducts can vary in their course and length; for example, the CBD can be straight, curved, or angled.[2]

The extrahepatic bile ducts are lined with epithelium. The subepithelial connective tissue is rich in elastic fibers but contains only few scattered smooth muscle fibers (see Fig. 5-1).[59,87]

Normal ducts are thin walled, with a normal luminal diameter (excluding the walls) of no more than 0.5 cm for the CHD or no more than 0.7 to 0.8 cm for the CBD (Fig. 5-4).[2,31] Bile duct diameter tends to remain constant throughout the day, as adequate relaxation of the sphincter of Oddi compensates for increased bile flow.[68] During pregnancy, the largest normal CHD diameter has also been found to be 0.5 cm.[57] In elderly patients, the normal recoil of the elastic fibers of the duct may be lost, resulting in an ectatic "floppy duct."[88] All the major extrahepatic ducts can vary in length, general course, and site of anastomosis. There can also be accessory hepatic ducts.[2,59] Sonography can be performed repeatedly to assess dynamic physiologic or pathologic changes in duct size.[68]

FIGURE 5-1. Gallbladder anatomy and histology. Overall anatomy *(top left, top right)*, histology *(middle left)*, CBD histology *(middle right)*. Types of gallbladder ducts *(bottom left)*; gallbladder musculature *(bottom right)*. (Copyright 1957. Ciba-Geigy Corporation. Reproduced with permission from The Ciba Collection of Medical Illustrations, by Frank H. Netter, M.D. Also by courtesy of Ciba-Geigy Limited, Basle, Switzerland. All rights reserved).

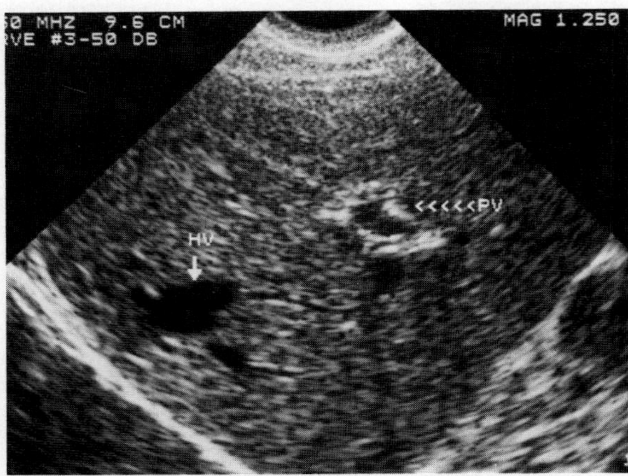

FIGURE 5-3. The walls of the portal veins (PV) appear more echogenic than the thin-walled hepatic veins (HV) because the portal veins run in portal triads surrounded by fibrous tissue accompanied by the intrahepatic bile ducts and hepatic arteries.

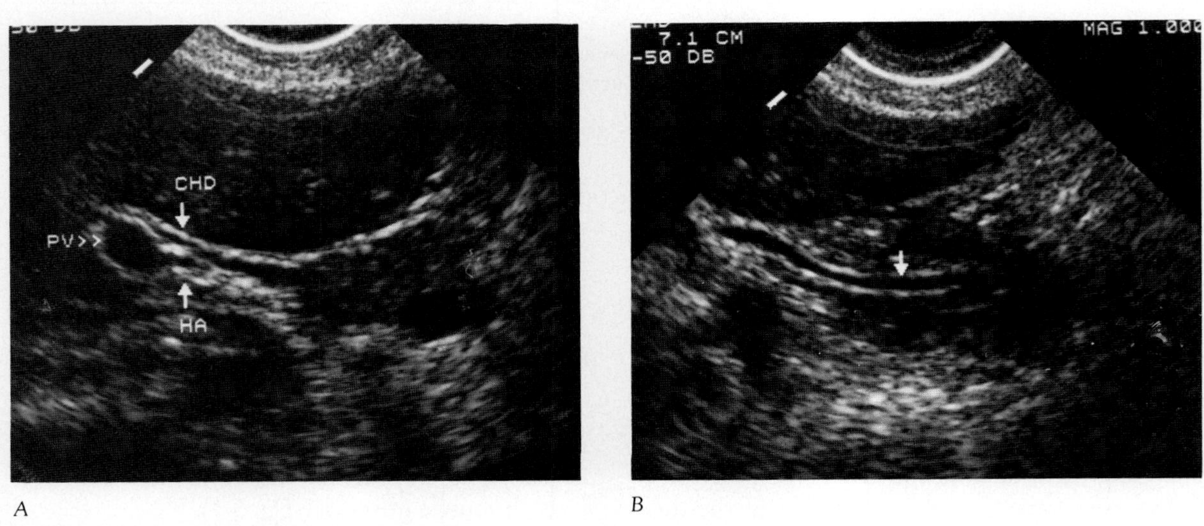

FIGURE 5-4. Sonographic views of the extrahepatic biliary tree. (*A*) Portal triad showing CHD, portal vein (PV), and hepatic artery (HA). (*B*) Long axis view of distal CBD *(arrow)*.

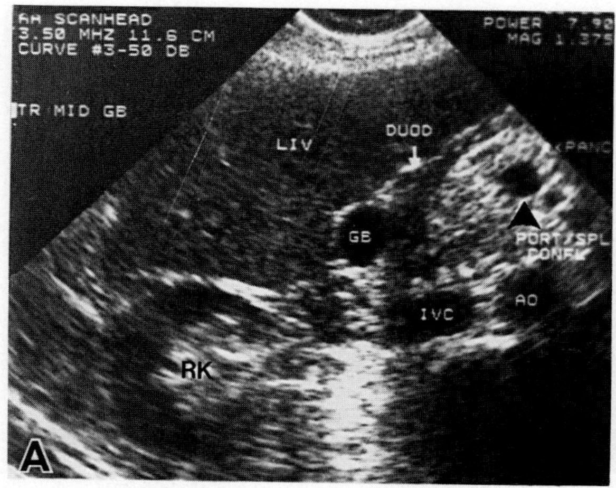

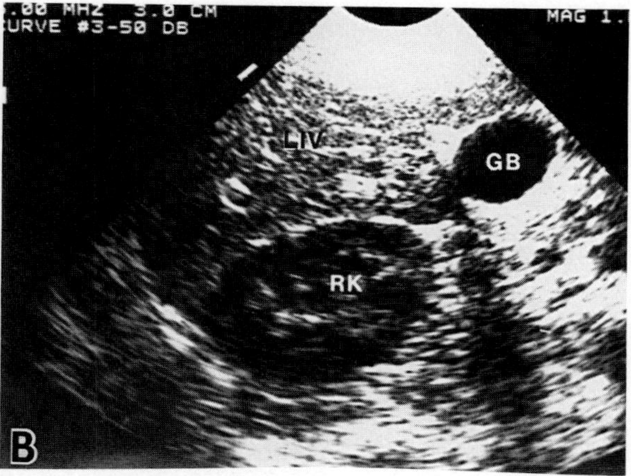

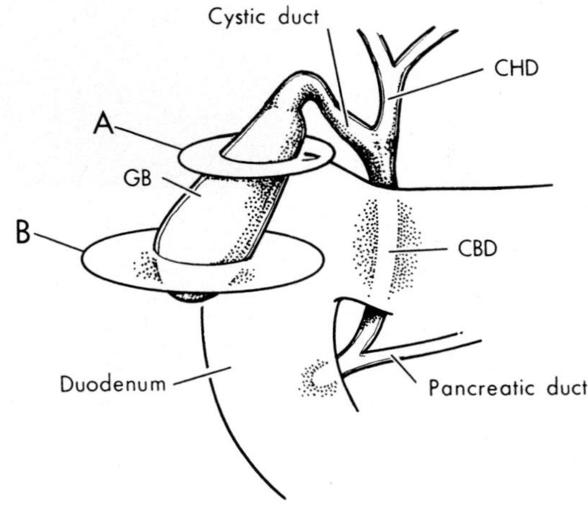

PLATE I

Key: AO, aorta; CBD, common bile duct; CHD, common hepatic duct; cy (or cystic d), cystic duct; DUOD, duodenum; GB, gallbladder; gda, gastroduodenal artery; HA, hepatic artery; IVC, inferior vena cava; LIV, liver; L Main Hep Duct, left main hepatic duct; lrv, left renal vein; P (or panc), pancreas; PSC (or Port/Spl Confl), portal-splenic confluence; PV, portal vein; RK, right kidney; R Main Hep Duct, right main hepatic duct; sma, superior mesenteric artery; spl v, splenic vein.

Sectional Views

The plates on this and the following pages consist of schematic views of the gallbladder and extrahepatic biliary tree along with corresponding sonographic sectional images that demonstrate the relationship of surrounding organs.

(text continues on page 158)

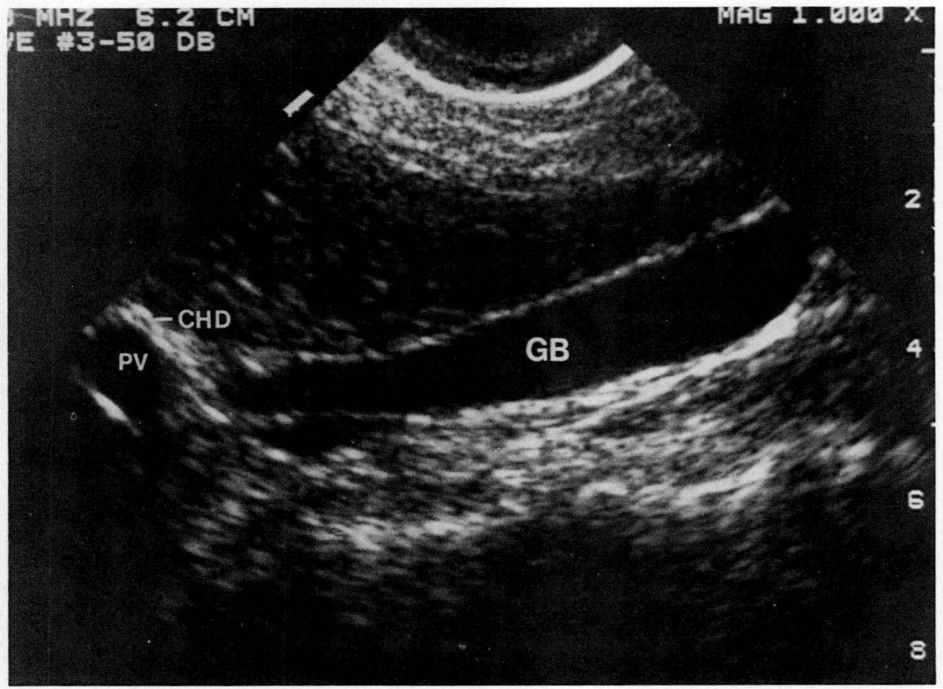

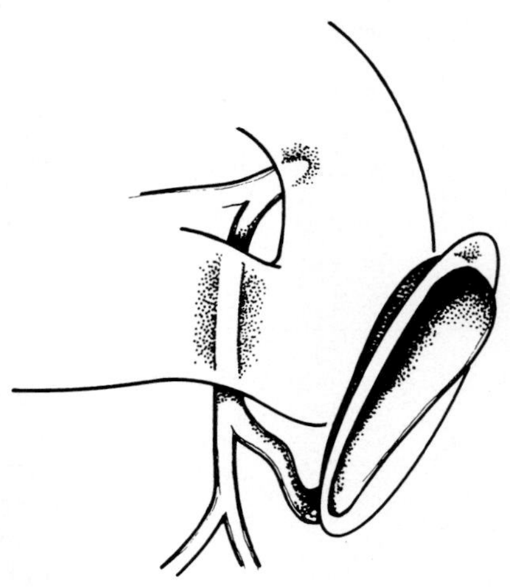

PLATE II

Key: AO, aorta; CBD, common bile duct; CHD, common hepatic duct; cy (or cystic d), cystic duct; DUOD, duodenum; GB, gallbladder; gda, gastroduodenal artery; HA, hepatic artery; IVC, inferior vena cava; LIV, liver; L Main Hep Duct, left main hepatic duct; lrv, left renal vein; P (or panc), pancreas; PSC (or Port/Spl Confl), portal-splenic confluence; PV, portal vein; RK, right kidney; R Main Hep Duct, right main hepatic duct; sma, superior mesenteric artery; spl v, splenic vein.

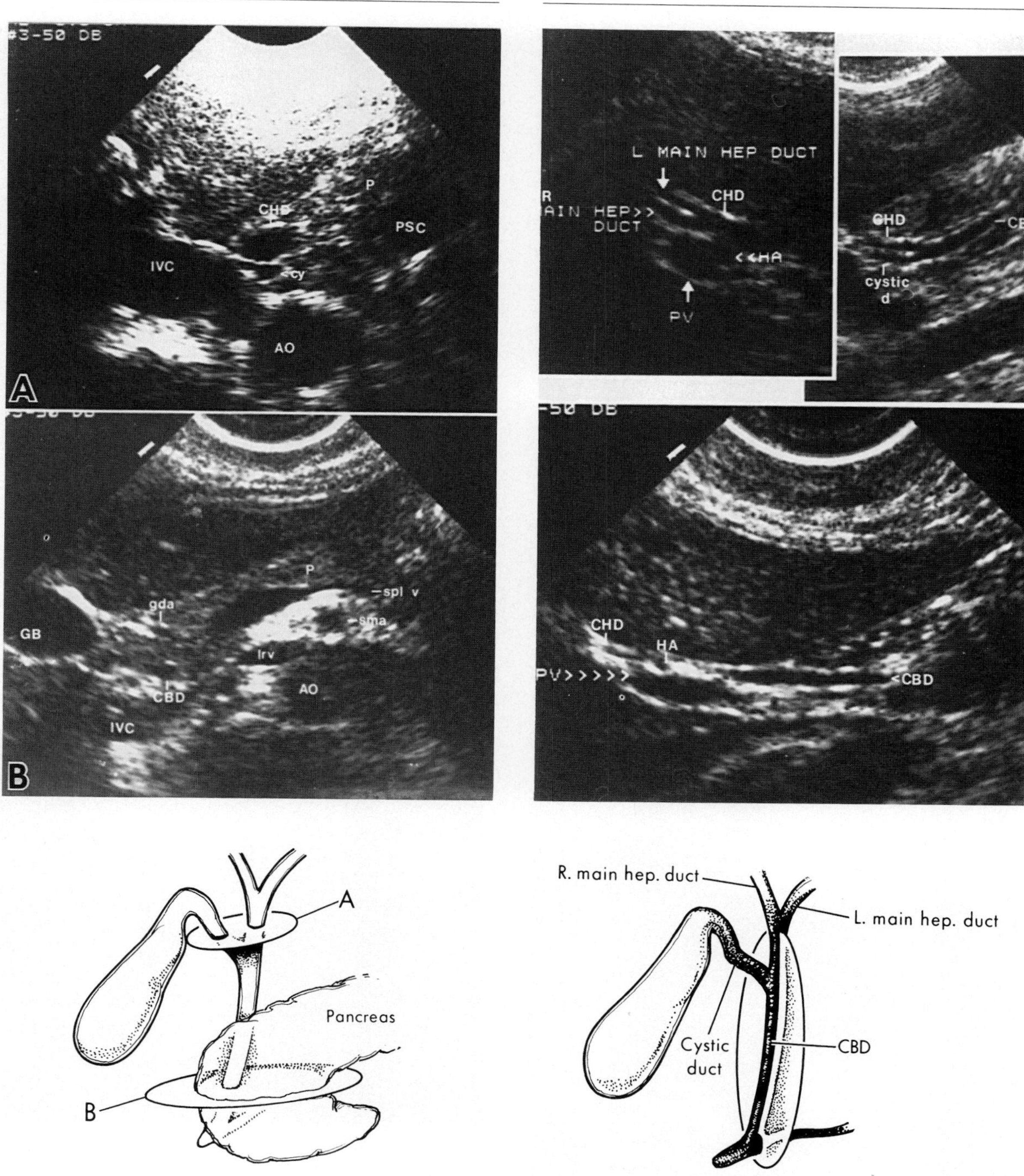

PLATE III

PLATE IV

Variants

There are many common gallbladder variations, including different shapes (e.g., hourglass), junctional folds, or septations (Fig. 5-5). The phrygian cap is a common variant that forms when the fundus kinks or folds back on the body (Fig. 5-6). The gallbladder can be excessively mobile, ectopic (on the left, in the midline, positioned transversely, situs inversus, or ptotic), or low lying in the right lower quadrant (RLQ; Fig 5-7). It can also be partially or totally embedded in the liver parenchyma, completely surrounded by peritoneum, in the abdominal wall or falciform ligament, in the retroperitoneum, or above the liver (rare, may be associated with right hepatic lobe hypoplasia).[2,59,82]

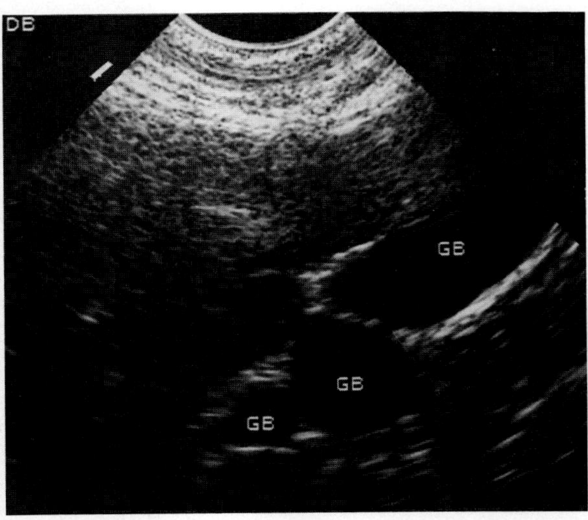

FIGURE 5-5. Junctional folds seem to create three compartments within this gallbladder (GB).

Physiology

The biliary system transports bile, which is produced continually by hepatic parenchymal cells, to the duodenum, where it aids in digestion. Bile helps to emulsify and promote the absorption of fats. It also facilitates the actions of lipase, a pancreatic enzyme. The gallbladder concentrates and stores bile until needed and regulates biliary pressure.[2,59]

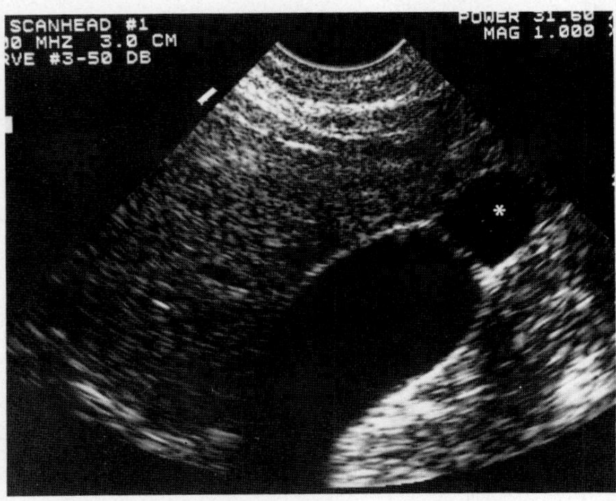

FIGURE 5-6. Longitudinal sonogram of phrygian cap (*asterisk*) extending from fundus of gallbladder.

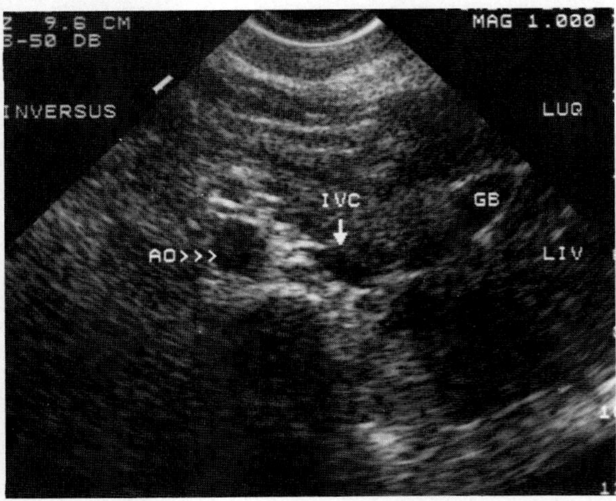

FIGURE 5-7. Transverse view of left upper quadrant (LUQ) in patient with situs inversus shows gallbladder (GB), liver (LIV), and IVC on the left and the aorta (AO) on the right.

When food, especially fats, enter the small intestine, cholecystokinin (CCK) is secreted by the proximal small intestine, causing the gallbladder to contract and the sphincter of Oddi to relax. Bile is then released into the cystic duct, flows through the CBD, and enters the duodenum.[2,59] Gallbladder contraction can also be induced by commercially available "fatty meals" or by intravenous injections of CCK.[36] Gallbladder emptying may be diminished in some patients with gallstones. Residual gallbladder volume is known to increase during pregnancy. Sonography can monitor such gallbladder kinetics by measuring the gallbladder volume in various fasting and postprandial states. A complex sum-of-cylinders calculation can be used, but the ellipsoid method is much simpler:

$$V = 0.52\,(l \times w \times h).$$[21]

Several laboratory tests can be helpful in evaluating pathophysiology of the biliary tract. An increased white blood cell count (WBC) indicates infection. Aspartate aminotransferase (AST), formerly serum glutamic-oxaloacetic transaminase (SGOT), and alanine aminotransferase (ALT), formerly serum glutamic pyruvic transaminase (SGPT), are enzymes produced by tissues of high metabolic activity, including the liver. Both values, but particularly the latter can be mildly to moderately elevated in biliary obstruction. Lactic dehydrogenase (LDH), another enzyme, can be mildly elevated in obstructive jaundice. Alkaline phosphatase, another liver enzyme, markedly increases in obstructive jaundice. Bilirubin results from the breakdown of hemoglobin in red blood cells. Direct, or conjugated, bilirubin tends to elevate in obstructive (surgical) jaundice, whereas the indirect, or unconjugated, bilirubin level rises in hepatocellular disease and hemolytic anemias.[2] Although helpful, the results of liver function tests can be nonspecific and must be considered with the clinical presentation and the findings of diagnostic imaging. Trends can be seen over time, however, so it is important not to look at just one day's laboratory results but to review and compare changes day to day to determine if function is improving or deteriorating.

Sonographic Examination Techniques

PREPARATION AND PROTOCOL

Ideally, patients should not eat or drink anything for 6 to 8 hours before sonographic examination of the gallbladder and biliary tree. Fasting distends the gallbladder and reduces bowel gas for optimal visualization and scrutiny. In emergency situations, however, this may not always be possible; and the diagnosis of cholelithiasis may be made in a partially contracted nonfasting gallbladder.[18] Also, although it is preferable not to have barium contrast examinations for 24 hours prior to sonography of the gallbladder, this is not necessarily an insurmountable problem in an emergency.

Meticulous real-time examination should be performed in all standard planes (sagittal, transverse, coronal) and any necessary oblique planes. The presence or absence of pathology in the gallbladder, porta hepatis, and intra- and extrahepatic biliary system should be documented.

PROCEDURE AND TECHNICAL HINTS

To mimimize the patient's anxiety, the examiner briefly explains the procedure in simple terms—safe, reliable, easy, painless—and asks whether the patient has properly prepared by taking nothing to *eat* or *drink* since midnight. It is a mistake to just assume this. When a patient has not received or followed instructions, rescheduling saves time and trouble and avoids confusing findings.

The sonographer briefly interviews the patient about the chief complaint and pertinent medical or surgical history including type, frequency, and duration of symptoms, location of pain, what aggravates or alleviates symptoms, prior similar episodes, and previous surgery or medical illnessess. Specifics are important: the patient who reports "gallbladder surgery" has not necessarily had a cholecystectomy; it could have been a cholecystostomy for removal of stones, in which case new stones could since have formed. The examiner does well to gather as many clues as possible before scanning the patient—from inpatients' charts, admission notes, attending physician's history and physical examination, specialists' consultations, nurses' notes, doctors' progress notes, laboratory reports, diagnostic test results, and any other areas of the chart that might have useful information. This is especially important with patients who are poor historians.

The examiner next *looks* at the patient, noticing jaundice and looking for surgical scars not accounted for in the history. Any palpable masses should be palpated to determine if they are hard, soft, mobile, fixed, tender. Sonographers need to get acquainted with the look and feel of an abdomen filled with ascites and to observe such details as protuberance, distention, or the feel of an abdomen that is "doughy" or tense. These preliminaries may take time, but they are an essential part of a thorough, high-quality, and complete sonographic examination. This initial information must be correlated with the sonographic findings to help formulate accurate preliminary impressions and the differential diagnosis.

Scanning begins with proper setting of the overall (system) gain and the time gain compensation (TGC). The normal gallbladder has an anechoic lumen with posterior enhancement. The bile duct lumen should also appear anechoic, so the gains may have to be decreased from those used during hepatic imaging to avoid artifactual filling in of these structures.[2] The gallbladder is located in the major interlobar fissure to the right of the ligamentum teres. Although its position can vary, the neck has a constant relationship to the region of the porta hepatis (Fig. 5-8).[18] The CHD is identified anterior to the portal vein and hepatic artery near the porta hepatis and followed distally as far as possible toward the pancreatic head. Evidence of dilated intrahepatic biliary radicles is sought along the intrahepatic portal vein branches. The gallbladder and ducts are carefully evaluated for size, wall thickness, contents, course, and caliber (is it displaced by a mass, does the duct taper distally, etc.?). Small but significant lesions can be missed if they are scanned over too quickly.

Techniques for identifying, confirming, or excluding disease need to be varied with each individual patient. A few suggestions follow:

1. Start with supine and left lateral decubitus (LLD) patient positions. If necessary, change to the right lateral decubitus (RLD) position, sitting or standing positions, or even a prone position scanning through the right lateral intercostal space. The erect positions demonstrate gravity dependence. A prone position (1) demonstrates the mobility of stones; (2) avoids reverberation artifacts from the abdominal wall or bowel; (3) allows the liver to fall anteriorly providing an acoustic window and displacing bowel; (4) brings the gallbladder more into the focal zone in some cases; and (5) permits unfolding of the gallbladder, allowing better visualization of the neck.[64] For the decubitus positions, even small changes in the patient's angle, from 45 degrees to 60 to 90 degrees or more, can improve the visibility of some structures.
2. A 3.5- and a 5-MHz transducer are used routinely; a 7.5- MHz or greater scanhead is useful on a thin patient with a superficial gallbladder (Fig. 5-9).
3. Choose a transducer with an adequate focal zone. Calculi smaller than the width of the ultrasound beam may not shadow because they do not totally block the sound beam. The focal zone is the narrowest segment of the beam, and the suspected calculi should lie within this zone to demonstrate shadowing. Even then, many small calculi may not shadow.[2,18] Try adjusting

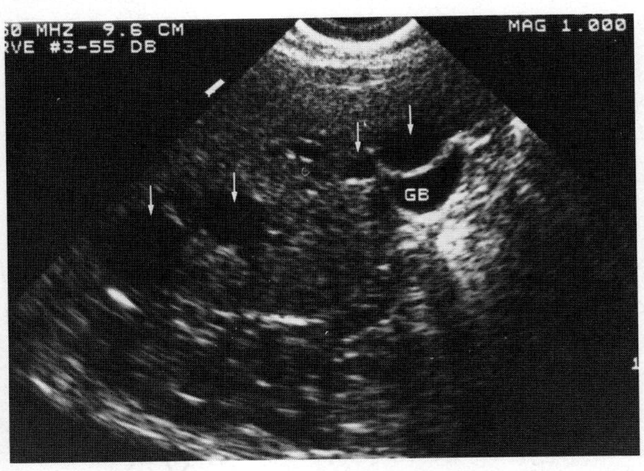

FIGURE 5-8. Transverse view of the gallbladder (GB) in a patient with polycystic liver disease. This gallbladder could easily be confused with one of the cysts *(arrows)*; however, sagittal scanning and a careful search for landmarks of the porta hepatis confirmed it to be gallbladder.

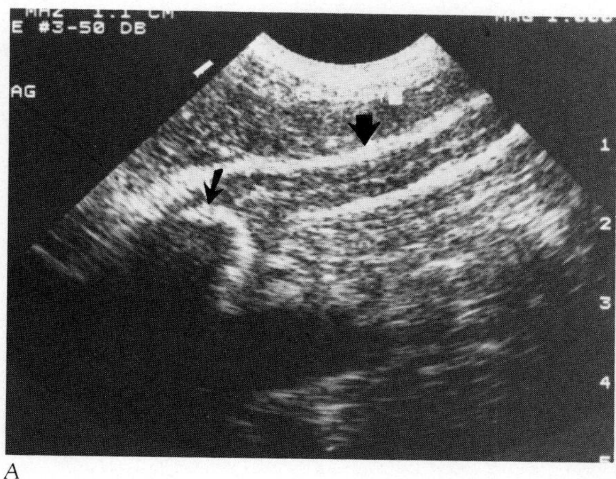

A

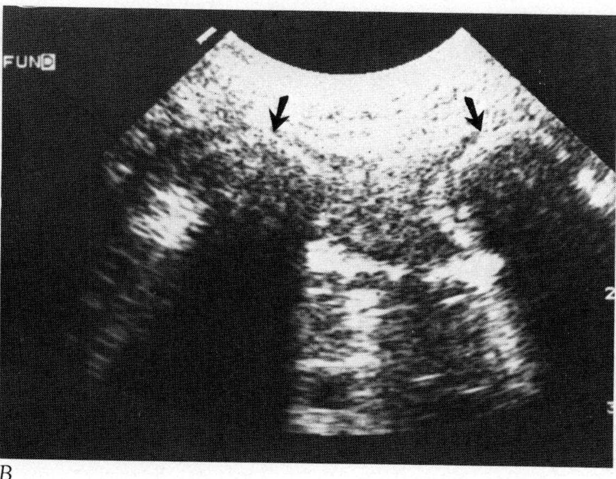

B

FIGURE 5-9. Sagittal scans in a very thin 18-year-old female using a 10-MHz transducer. (*A*) Thick-walled body of the gallbladder (*wide arrow*) with stone in neck (*thin arrow*). (*B*) Two more stones (*arrows*) are demonstrated in the fundus.

the focal zone if dynamic focusing is available (Fig. 5-10). If the focal zone of the transducer cannot be adjusted, change the transducer's position or angle to bring the gallbladder into the focal zone.

4. Employ patient breathing techniques. Suspended, full inspiration is often best, but sometimes varying degrees of inspiration or expiration may be better, depending on the patient's body habitus and ability to cooperate. "Diaphragmatic breathing" is helpful in moving organs inferiorly for improved subcostal access, but many patients have difficulty complying.
5. Vary the scanning approaches. Scan subcostally, following the rib cage contour closely and angling superiorly to avoid bowel (deep inspiration is often necessary). Scan intercostally to avoid gas (normal shallow breathing is often sufficient for this approach, making it useful for patients who are unable to take or hold a deep breath). Ask the patient to raise both arms overhead during decubitus and supine positioning to widen the intercostal spaces and elongate the subcostal area of access (Fig. 5-11). Evaluate structures by sweeping through from many different angles to achieve perpendicular-

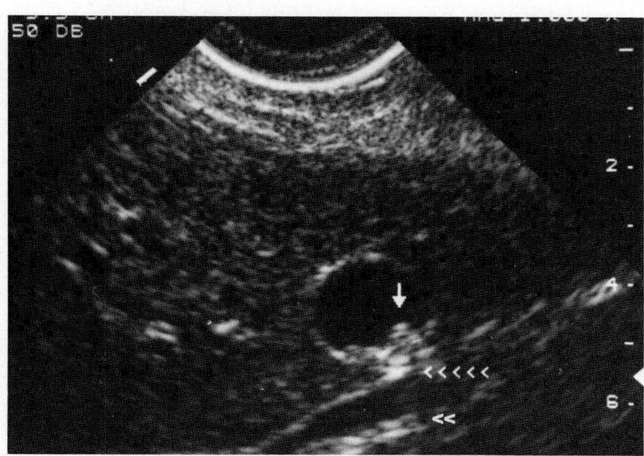

FIGURE 5-10. Transverse view of the gallbladder. Good technique was required to display shadowing from this stone. The dynamic focusing was adjusted to bring the stone (*arrow*) into the focal zone to optimally show acoustic shadowing (*arrowheads*).

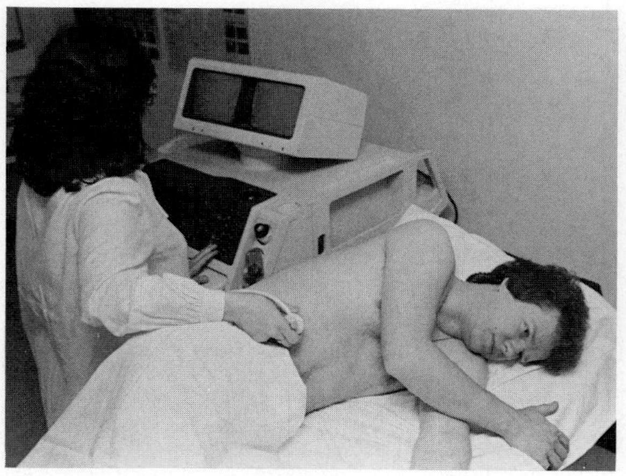

A

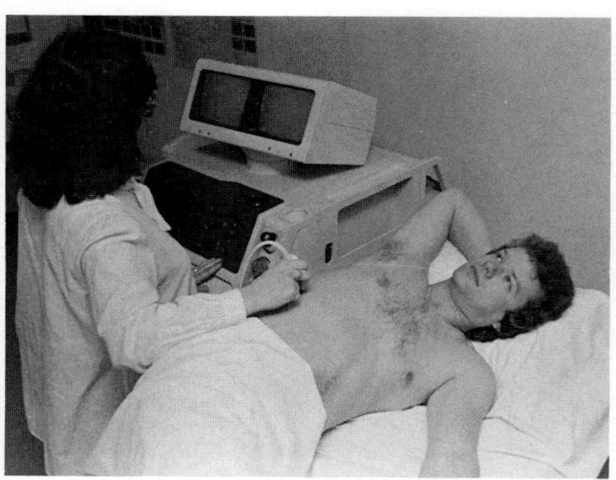

B

Figure 5-11. (*A*) Patient presented in a typical side-lying position. (*B*) By changing the patient's position (raising the arm overhead and leaning the patient slightly back at the shoulder) intercostal and subcostal access to RUQ organs is improved and the liver and gallbladder are moved up and away from potentially overlying bowel.

ity to as many areas of interest as possible (angle medial to lateral, lateral to medial, superior to inferior, and angle around gas pockets). Try slight rotations of the transducer or small changes in scanning angles; since some structures are only several millimeters wide, often only subtle movements are needed.

6. Do gain studies. Do not use only one setting, but vary the gain during scanning to obtain better definition of structures and to distinguish artifacts from pathology. Excessive gain can mask shadows[2] whereas too little gain can delete important information. Vary pre- and postprocessing curves to enhance the image.
7. Use gentle transducer pressure to move bowel gas out of the way.
8. Try gently shaking the patient to prompt movement of stones.
9. It may help to give the patient water to drink. Water can fill the duodenum to distinguish it from the gallbladder or it can also displace overlying gas and act as an acoustic window to better examine the distal CBD and pancreatic head. Give the patient 6 to 12 ounces of tap water to drink through a straw, to minimize swallowed air. Then place him or her in the RLD position for 2 or 3 minutes before repeating scan with the patient semierect.[42]
10. A fatty meal may be needed to assess changes in duct size during confirmation of obstruction or to evaluate gallbladder contractility and emptying. Patients with gallstones have exhibited higher resting gallbladder volumes, less fractional emptying after a fatty meal, and higher postprandial residual volumes.[40]

Scanning is a dynamic, interactive process. One or several of the above maneuvers may be needed for any given examination. Since there are no hard-and-fast rules that work for every patient, the sonographer should be creative and learn to improvise. Refinements in technique and an intuitive sense of what will be successful in which situation will come with experience. Meticulous scanning technique is crucial and can decrease or eliminate the need for other diagnostic tests.[42]

Congenital Anomalies

Embryonic development of the liver, gallbladder, and biliary duct system arise from the hepatic diverticulum of the foregut in the fourth week of gestation. This diverticulum divides into two parts, a larger cranial part, which gives rise to the liver, and a smaller caudal part, which develops into the gallbladder and cystic duct. At the beginning of the fifth week, the hepatic ducts, extrahepatic duct system, gallbladder, cystic duct, and pancreatic duct are demarcated as a solid cord of cells. Ductal lumina begin establishing during the sixth week in the common duct and slowly progress distally. The lumen extends into the cystic duct by the seventh week, but the gallbladder remains solid until the 12th week. Therefore, most gallbladder anomalies probably occur between the fourth and 12th week (Fig. 5-12).[35,76]

Agenesis and duplication of the gallbladder are rare.[2] Anomalies of the gallbladder alone do not generally give rise to any characteristic symptoms. While some of the defects predispose to bile stasis and attacks of cholecystitis, the attacks themselves have no unusual aspects. The symptoms only call attention to the anomaly.[35]

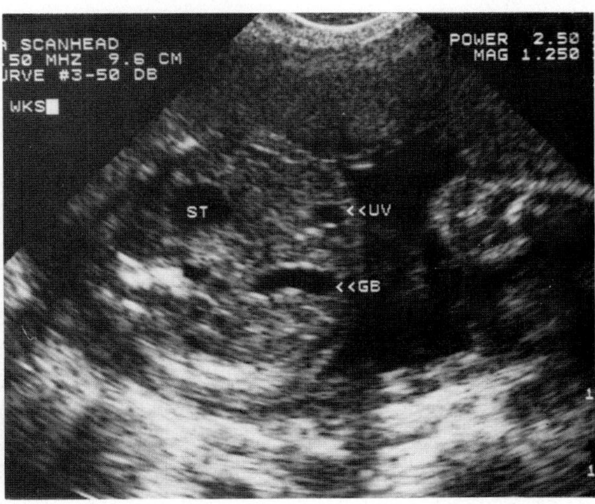

FIGURE 5-12. Transverse view of fetal abdomen at 30 weeks shows normal gallbladder (GB), stomach (ST), and umbilical vein (UV). The fetal gallbladder can often be identified after 20 weeks. Duplication, deformation, abnormal position, and fetal cholelithiasis can be detected antenatally with sonography.[35]

Biliary Atresia

Biliary atresia is the most common type of obstructive biliary disease in infants and young children.[70] Previously thought to be a congenital anomaly, it is now thought by many to evolve after birth, possibly owing to a viral infection. Progressive obliteration of the extrahepatic ducts, and in many instances the gallbladder as well, takes place. This obliteration extends into the proximal intrahepatic duct system, which usually remains patent in the first few weeks of life; the severity varies with the duration of involvement. Fibrosis and obliteration of the biliary tree progress distal to proximal.[34]

More than 50% of neonates have transient jaundice characterized by mild elevation of serum bilirubin which resolves spontaneously. Persistent or sudden onset jaundice after the first and second week of life may indicate a more serious abnormality, most commonly biliary atresia or neonatal hepatitis. Less common causes include choledochal cysts, inspissated bile syndrome, enzyme deficiencies, metabolic abnormalities, hemolysis, hyperalimentation, and other congenital biliary anomalies.[34,76]

Biliary atresia is twice as common in males and neonatal hepatitis four times as common in females. It is important to distinguish biliary atresia from neonatal hepatitis, since atresia may be treated surgically with a liver transplant or the Kasai procedure. The outcome is better with early surgical intervention[34]; indeed, if surgical correction is not possible, death usually occurs within months, although a few children survive several years.[59] Complications of untreated biliary atresia are cirrhosis, cholangitis, portal hypertension, malabsorption, and failure of biliary drainage.[34]

In normal neonates, the CHD is generally visible sonographically and measures no more than 1 mm. Intrahepatic duct dilatation combined with inability to visualize the CHD is suggestive of biliary atresia.[34] If only the cystic duct is obstructed, gallbladder hydrops develops.[59] Detection of both intra- and extrahepatic dilatation excludes atresia and indicates obstruction (choledochal cyst, inspissated bile, biliary calculi). Also, if the gallbladder shrinks (length decreases more than 2 mm and transverse diameter decreases) within 30 minutes of feeding, biliary atresia is unlikely.[34] Large kidneys with increased echogenicity have been associated with some cases of biliary atresia. The mechanism for this is not known, and it should be recognized as a transitory phenomenon.[8]

CHOLEDOCHAL CYSTS

There are three types of choledochal cysts, the most common being the cystic dilatation of the entire length of the CHD and CBD with the cystic duct entering the cyst. It can occur anywhere along the biliary tree.[2] Different causes have been cited: (1) congential weakness of the duct wall, which results in the formation of a cystic structure, and (2) angulation of the CBD, causing partial obstruction, which leads to dilatation and cyst formation.[2,59] Clinically, the signs and symptoms include intermittent jaundice associated with colicky pain and sometimes a palpable subhepatic mass displacing the stomach to the left and the duodenum downward.[59]

Choledochal cyst is four times more common in females than males. More than 30 percent of these cases are diagnosed during the first 10 years of life, and surgery is generally indicated.[2]

Sonographically, choledochal cysts appear as a localized cystic mass, separate from the gallbladder, in the region of the porta hepatis (Fig. 5-13). To avoid being fooled by a fluid-filled bowel loop in

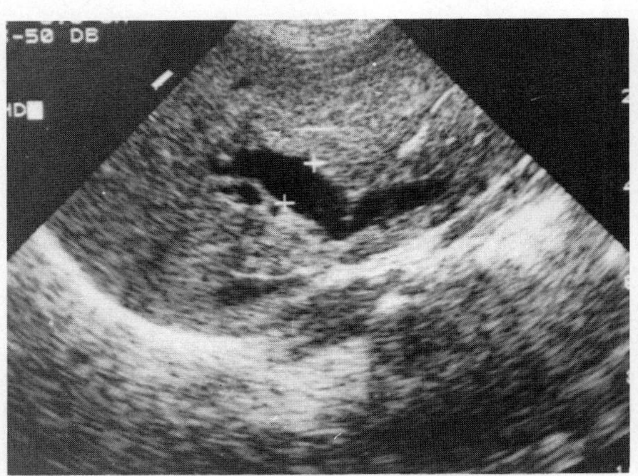

A

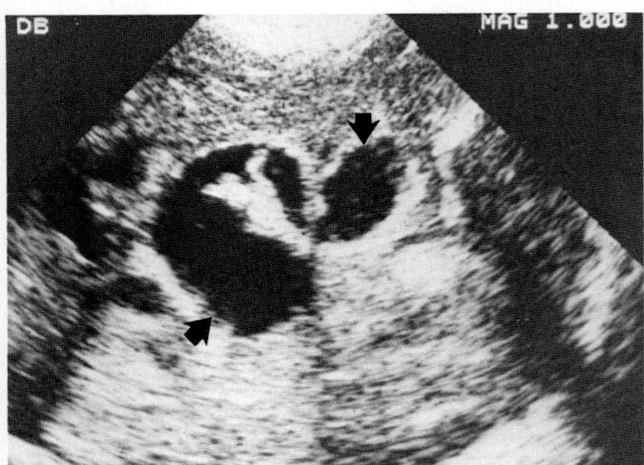

B

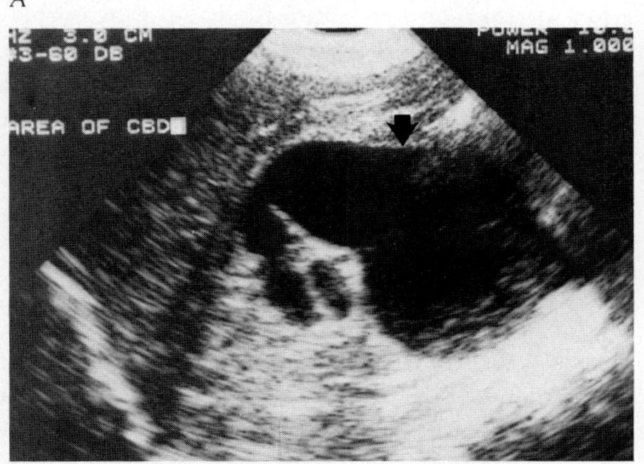

C

FIGURE 5-13. The presence of a choledochal cyst is sonographically signalled by a fluid collection or cystic mass near the porta (separate from the gallbladder) and/or dilated extrahepatic ducts. The classic triad of symptoms is jaundice, pain, and a RUQ mass. (*A*) Forme fruste variant of choledochal cyst in a 3-year-old who also had dilated intrahepatic ducts. The dilated common duct *(between caliper markers)* measures 1.04 cm. (*B*, *C*) Dilated tortuous cystic mass *(arrows)* represents choledochal cyst in a 4-year-old girl.

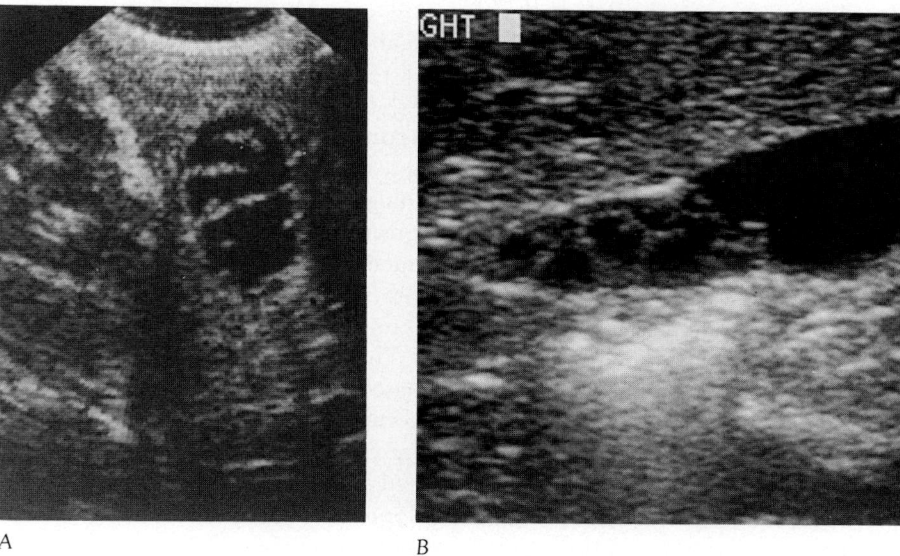

Figure 5-14. Multiseptate gallbladder. (*A*) Fine linear septa bridging the gallbladder lumen. (*B*) "Honeycomb" pattern of septations near the gallbladder neck. (From Lev-Toaff AS, Friedman AC, Rindsberg SN, et al: Multiseptate gallbladder: Incidental diagnosis on sonography. AJR 1987, 148:1119–1120. Copyright 1987 by American Roentgen Ray Society.)

the area the examiner should observe for peristalsis.

Septate Gallbladder

A gallbladder septum may result from a congenital mucosal diaphragm, adenomyomatosis, or a combination of the two. Since the gallbladder develops by cannulation of a blind sac, a septum will form if cannulation is incomplete. Although a gallbladder septum may be an incidental finding during an otherwise normal examination, stasis of bile in the distal segment predisposes to calculus formation.[22] A single septum appears as a thin linear echo separating the gallbladder into compartments. Simple junctional folds may mimic a septum.

The multiseptate gallbladder is one of the rarest congenital gallbladder malformations. There are two theories about its origin: incomplete vacuolization of the developing gallbladder bud and persistent wrinkling of the gallbladder wall. The septa consist of two epithelial layers with a muscular layer interposed. This anomaly may be associated with biliary colic or cholelithiasis or may be entirely asymptomatic without associated cholelithiasis.[47]

A multiseptate gallbladder can have variable sonographic appearances. There can be fine linear septa or a honeycomb pattern of clustered septations resulting in multiple communicating cyst-like compartments (Fig. 5-14). Septa may cluster in the neck and body region of the gallbladder. Differential diagnoses include desquamated gallbladder mucosa (an unusual finding in acute cholecystitis) and hyperplastic cholecystoses (such as polypoid cholesterolosis or adenomyomatosis). Desquamated gallbladder mucosa appears as multiple, haphazardly arranged, linear, nonshadowing densities within the gallbladder lumen which do not consistently arise from the gallbladder wall as they do in multiseptate gallbladder. Polypoid cholesterolosis may more resemble multiseptate gallbladder, although the nonshadowing polypoid densities are more bulbous and there is no bridging of the lumen by septa as in the multiseptate gallbladder.

In adenomyomatosis, Rokitansky-Aschoff sinuses could be confused with the honeycomb pattern, but cyst-like Rokitansky-Aschoff sinuses are smaller and are actually within the thickened gallbladder wall; there is no bridging of the lumen itself to form cystlike compartments.[47]

INTERPOSITION OF THE GALLBLADDER

Childhood jaundice is not unusual. Although interposition of the gallbladder (absence of the CHD and cystic duct) is a rare anomaly, its diagnosis is important because it is surgically correctable. Normally, the right and left main hepatic ducts join to form the CHD, which is entered by the cystic duct to form the CBD. In interposition, the main hepatic ducts drain, separately or together, directly into the gallbladder. The gallbladder then drains directly into the CBD, although variants can also occur (Fig. 5-15). The cause of interposition of the gallbladder is unknown.[76]

The patient presents with jaundice, which may be intermittent, abdominal pain, and sometimes an enlarged gallbladder. Sonography may show enlarged intrahepatic ducts with a normal CBD, mimicking Caroli's disease, or the ducts may appear to enter a cystic mass in the porta hepatis, mimicking choledochal cyst. Although sonography may be difficult to interpret in this situation, it is still a good first step, indicating that jaundice is due to an anatomic biliary abnormality.[76]

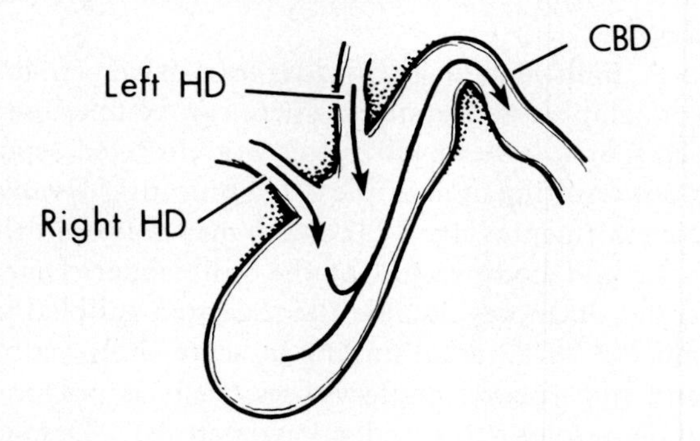

FIGURE 5-15. Schematic diagram of bile flow pattern (*arrows*) in interposition of the gallbladder. The sonographic appearance reveals dilated intrahepatic ducts adjacent to a normal or enlarged gallbladder with no dilatation of the CBD. Differential diagnosis includes choledochal cyst, gallbladder hydrops, and Caroli's disease.[76] (Right HD, right hepatic duct; Left HD, left hepatic duct.)

Acquired Diseases

BILIARY SLUDGE

Sludge represents precipitates formed in the bile. It consists of a collection of calcium bilirubinate, mucus, and lesser amounts of cholesterol crystals within viscous bile that contains high concentrations of mucus and other proteins.[24,45]

The pathogenesis, clinical significance, and ultimate prognosis of sludge remains uncertain. Sludge alone can produce biliary symptoms—and even the classic pain of gallstones—and can be associated with other complications. Therefore sludge alone as a finding associated with biliary pain is not necessarily insignificant. Recent studies could not detect sludge in healthy persons after simple fasting. The presence of sludge implies the formation of a precipitate and should not be regarded as normal. Sludge is sometimes a precursor to gallstone disease.[45]

Sludge could be caused by bile composition abnormalities (due to total parenteral nutrition [TPN] or underlying disease), bile stasis (from lack of gallbladder contractions), or both.[10] It frequently occurs in compromised postoperative patients and in patients who require TPN.[10,45] Since gallbladder emptying is significantly reduced in patients fed parenterally, sequential CCK injections may help to induce gallbladder contraction.[10]

Sludge produces a homogenous, low-amplitude echo pattern that tends to layer dependently (Fig. 5-16); it does not produce acoustic shadowing.[45] True sludge often forms a straight horizontal line that remains at a constant level in sagittal and transverse images. This fluid-fluid level moves slowly with changes in patient position.[24] Scattered brighter echoes within sludge may represent larger cholesterol crystals. If sludge completely fills the gallbladder (total bile sludging or hepatinization of bile), it may be difficult to distinguish the echo-filled gallbladder from adjacent liver parenchyma (Fig. 5-17).[18] Tumefactive sludge from longstanding biliary obstruction frequently does not layer but often appears "fluffy," resembling a polypoid mass or pseudotumor that can mimic a gallbladder neo-

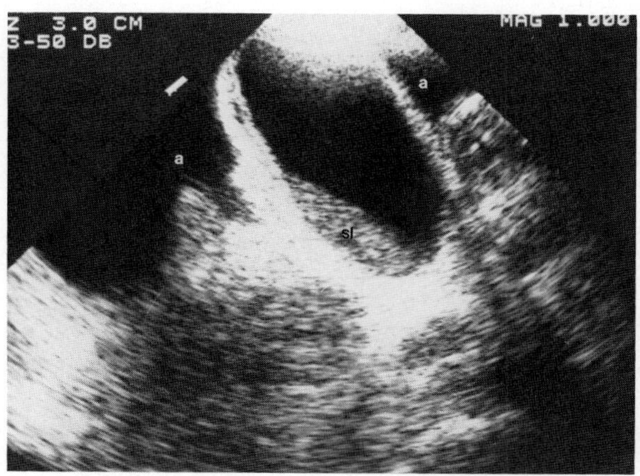

Figure 5-16. Sludge (sl) in thick-walled gallbladder. The low-amplitude echo pattern of sludge is produced by particulate matter. Simply increasing the thickness of bile does not change its echogenicity (a, ascites around gallbladder).[45]

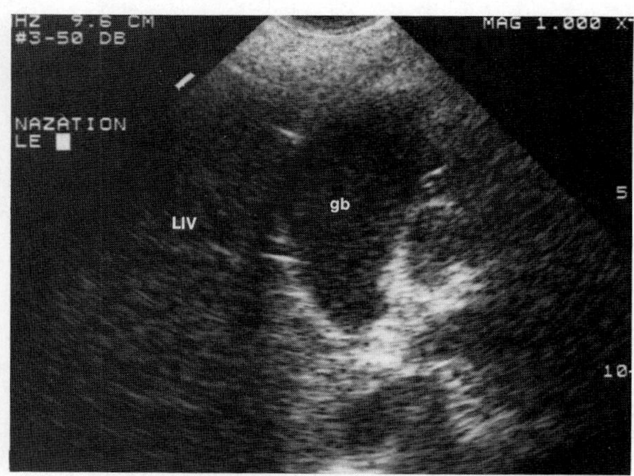

Figure 5-17. Hepatinization of bile (total bile sludging). Bile in the gallbladder (gb) has same echo texture as liver (LIV).

plasm (Fig. 5-18).[17,24] Occasionally, mobile, round, echogenic, nonshadowing masses known as sludge balls are seen within the gallbladder.[17,18]

Using excessively high gain settings fills the gallbladder with artifactual echoes, giving a false appearance of sludge. This artifactual pattern has a snowflake appearance, whereas true sludge has a better-defined, low-level pattern. Increased echogenicity of surrounding organs is another clue to too much gain.[2] It is also important to distinguish sludge from the "false debris" echo pattern of slice thickness artifacts.[24]

Cholelithiasis (Gallstones)

Gallstones can be large or small, single or multiple, symptomatic or silent. The majority of stones contain a mixture of cholesterol, bilirubin, and calcium. Pure cholesterol or bilirubin stones are rare.[59]

Many factors are associated with gallstone formation (Fig. 5-19). Hypercholesteremia (elevated serum cholesterol) may increase the cholesterol level in the bile and the cholesterol may precipitate out of the supersaturated bile to form stones. Hypercholesteremia is a metabolic phenomenon observed in obese, diabetic, and pregnant patients,

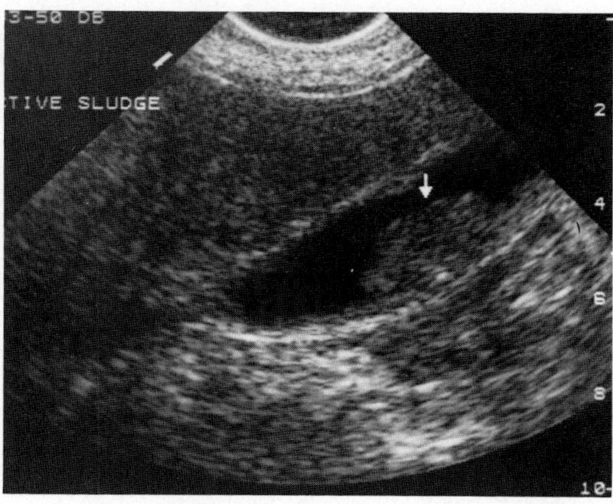

Figure 5-18. Sonogram shows a "clump" of sludge (*arrow*) within the thick-walled gallbladder of a 54-year-old alcoholic with cirrhosis and ascites. The cluster of sludge moved from the gallbladder neck to the body as the patient changed position.

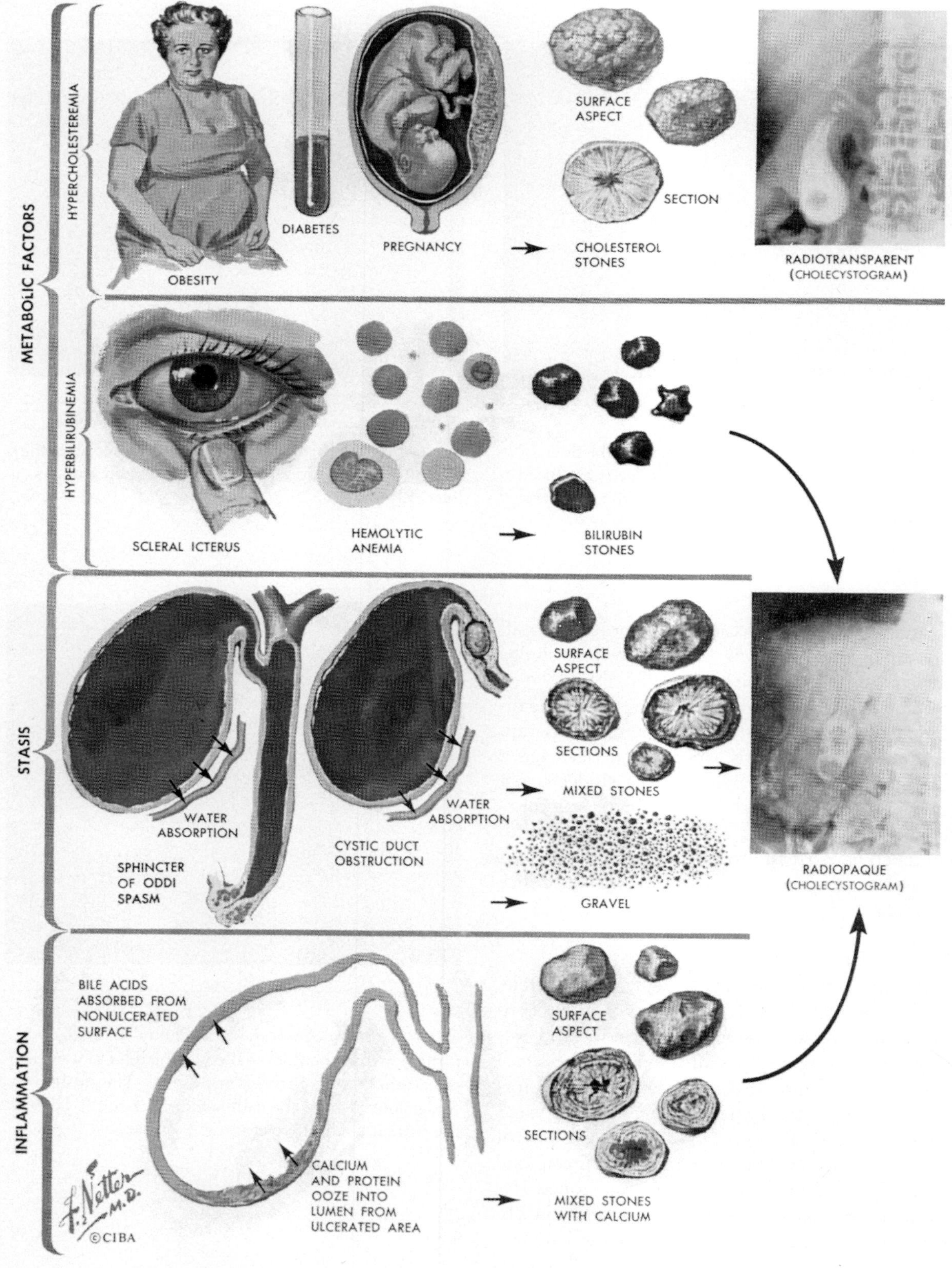
METABOLIC FACTORS
HYPERCHOLESTEREMIA
OBESITY
DIABETES
PREGNANCY
SURFACE ASPECT
SECTION
CHOLESTEROL STONES
RADIOTRANSPARENT (CHOLECYSTOGRAM)
HYPERBILIRUBINEMIA
SCLERAL ICTERUS
HEMOLYTIC ANEMIA
BILIRUBIN STONES
STASIS
WATER ABSORPTION
SPHINCTER OF ODDI SPASM
CYSTIC DUCT OBSTRUCTION
WATER ABSORPTION
SURFACE ASPECT
SECTIONS
MIXED STONES
GRAVEL
RADIOPAQUE (CHOLECYSTOGRAM)
INFLAMMATION
BILE ACIDS ABSORBED FROM NONULCERATED SURFACE
CALCIUM AND PROTEIN OOZE INTO LUMEN FROM ULCERATED AREA
SURFACE ASPECT
SECTIONS
MIXED STONES WITH CALCIUM
F. Netter M.D.
©CIBA

three groups in whom gallstones are commonly found.[59] During pregnancy, bile stasis (from hormonal changes that decrease gallbladder contractility) and changes in the physicochemical nature of bile salts also contribute to stone formation.[14,86] The gallbladder may also modify bile so that cholesterol crystals can precipitate out more readily.[45] Another general mechanism in the development or proliferation of gallstones may be abnormal gallbladder motor function. Decreased gallbladder contractility may be the result of delayed gastric emptying, impaired release of CCK, impaired gallbladder innervation, abnormal gallbladder smooth muscle, fibrosis of the gallbladder wall, or any combination of these. It is questionable, however, whether abnormal gallbladder emptying antedates the stones and contributes to their development or whether it occurs secondary to the presence of stones and the possible inflammatory changes they may create in the gallbladder.[40] Gallbladder motor disorders during TPN can cause cholelithiasis. An increased tendency to form stones can also be observed in hemolytic anemias (from hyperbilirubinemia), in children with cystic fibrosis (which is associated with microgallbladder, inspissated gallbladder mucus, abnormal bile salt metabolism, abnormal gallbladder function), and in short bowel syndromes.[10,32,59,70]

Although gallstones can be asymptomatic, patients generally present with right-side upper quadrant (RUQ) pain that may radiate to the right shoulder or epigastrium, nausea, vomiting, and excessive belching.[2] Because gallbladder disease can mimic the pain of ischemic heart disease sonography of the biliary tree often plays a role in the work-up of chest pain as well.[25] Pertinent laboratory values may include an elevated alkaline phosphatase and mildly elevated AST and ALT levels.[2]

Cholelithiasis affects 15 to 20 million Americans and approximately 1 million new cases develop annually.[14,86] It is not uncommon in children.[70] Early in adult life, cholelithiasis is predominantly a disease of women (2:1 over males). The prime candidates for cholelithiasis are "fair, fat, forty, and fertile." Age, obesity, and parity are associated factors, as are the use of oral contraceptives and exogenous estrogen replacement therapy.[14,86] Gallstones also occur more frequently in Caucasians than in blacks and in patients with regional enteritis and diabetes mellitus.[2] During pregnancy, the prevalence of cholelithiasis increases to 3.5 to 11.3%.[86] Gestational diabetes may contribute to development of stones.[14]

Prognosis and treatment of cholelithiasis can vary, depending on the size of stones (small calculi may be more troublesome as they may roll out of the gallbladder and cause CBD obstruction) and the frequency and severity of the attacks (some people have more frequent attacks of colic, or eventually cholecystitis). A low-fat diet may be sufficient treatment in some cases, but elective or emergency cholecystectomy may be necessary in others. Experts still disagree about whether it is best to remove incidental, asymptomatic gallstones to reduce the chance of future morbidity. A new appreciation of the benign course of asymptomatic stones suggests that they should be left alone.[69] Percutaneous cholecystostomy may assume a limited role in elderly patients and patients at high risk. Surgical cholecystotomy to remove stones is done occasionally but cholecystectomy is often necessary subsequently because of the high recurrence rate. Percutaneous lithotripsy has been used to break up large gallstones so that the fragments could be extracted.[41] Several agents, such as methyl tert-butyl ether (MTBE) and ursodeoxycholic acid (UDCA) are being investigated for their effectiveness in dissolving cholesterol gallstones.[44–46] In the future it may be important to try to sonographically distinguish cholesterol gallstones from other types, since they might be amenable to medical dissolution.[19,63]

The classic sonographic appearance of a gallstone is that of an echogenic structure in the gallbladder lumen that casts a posterior acoustic shadow (Fig. 5-20).[18] If the proper technique and transducer are used, virtually all calculi cast a shadow, owing to sound absorption, regardless of

FIGURE 5-19. Pathogenesis of gallstone formation. (Copyright 1957. Ciba-Geigy Corporation. Reproduced with permission from The Ciba Collection of Medical Illustrations, by Frank H. Netter, M.D. Also by courtesy of Ciba-Geigy Limited, Basle, Switzerland. All rights reserved.)

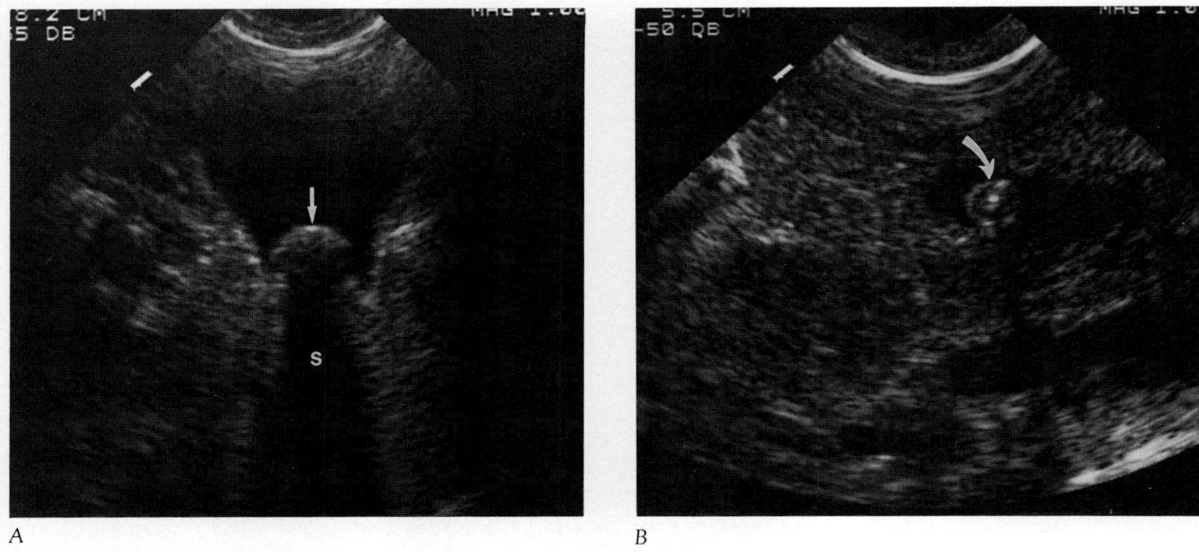

FIGURE 5-20. (*A*) Classic sonographic appearance of a gallstone *(arrow)* (S, acoustic shadow). (*B*) Unusual varied appearance of a gallstone *(curved arrow)*. Stone has a bullseye appearance with shadowing from the central portion only.

their size, shape, surface characteristics, or composition (including calcium content).[6,17,18,70] The strength of the shadow depends on the intrinsic attenuation properties of the stone. Attenuation is increased by a more rigid stone structure, a larger percentage of crystalline material, and larger crystal size.[80] The majority of gallstones produce "clean" shadows with distinct margins because only 20% to 30% of the incident beam is usually reflected. Calcified gallstones reflect a much larger percentage of the incident beam, but they produce reverberations within the shadow: the denser the calcification, the stronger the reverberations.[63] The visualization of reverberations and scattered echoes in the shadow are very dependent on gain settings, transducer positioning, and focusing.[63,80] Studies have also shown cholesterol stones or polyps to demonstrate reverberations and comet tail artifacts as well, though they do so because of the rigidity and other physical characteristics of cholesterol.[19] Other causes of echogenic foci with associated reverberations and comet-tail artifacts include air in the biliary tree, surgical clips in the gallbladder bed, gas in an intrahepatic abscess, drainage catheters, emphysematous cholecystitis, lead pellets, focal hepatic calcifications, scars, and weak comet tails emanating from a normal gallbladder wall if the beam is perpendicular.[19,80]

Gallstones should also demonstrate mobility to the most dependent portion of the gallbladder as the patient changes postion (the "rolling stone" sign Fig. 5-21).[17] The examiner must be aware of which wall is truly gravity dependent, especially when the patient is in the decubitus position, since the image orientation may be skewed (Fig. 5-22). Some stones are adherent, but others may float for a variety of reasons: (1) after a long fast, the specific gravity of bile may increase (stones sink when eating is resumed); (2) the calculus may contain enough gas to reduce its specific gravity (this may produce reverberations in the shadow); and (3) oral contrast material from cholecystography (OCG) may increase the specific gravity of bile and cause stones to float.[6,89] Mimickers of floating stones include "stacked" stones and obscuring of the posterior aspect of the stone by shadowing.[89]

Many of the other possible technical, anatomic, and diagnostic pitfalls with identifying cholelithi-

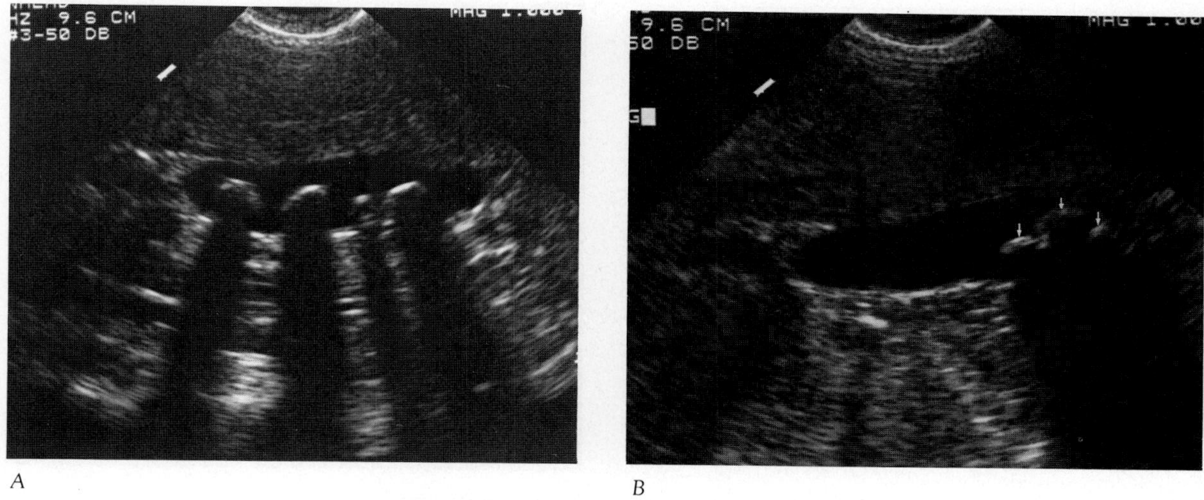

FIGURE 5-21. Rolling stone sign. (*A*) With the patient supine, four distinct stones are seen along the posterior gallbladder wall. (*B*) When the patient sat up, all of the stones (*arrows*) rolled to the fundus.

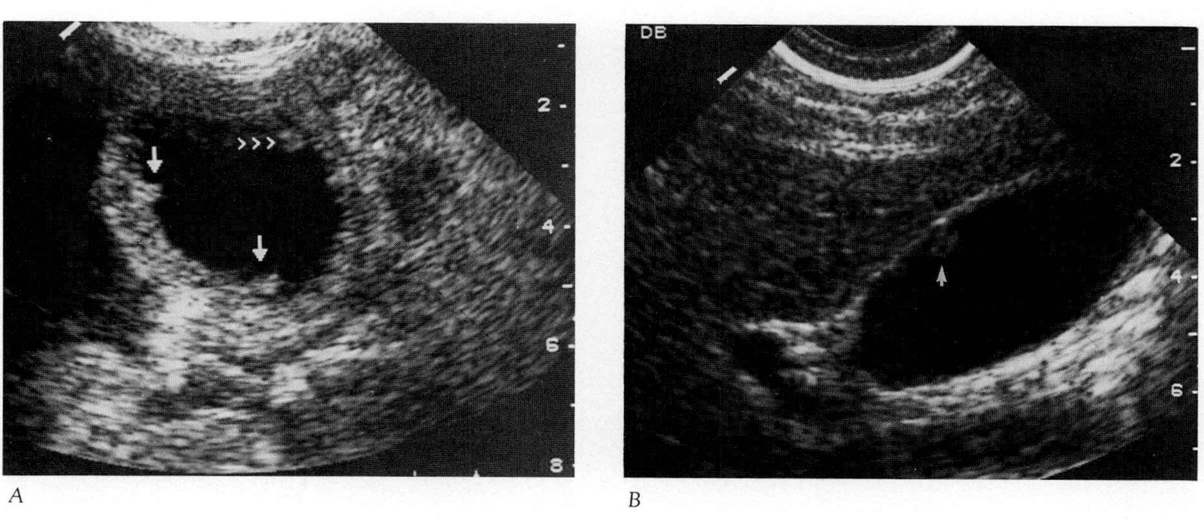

FIGURE 5-22. (*A*) Transverse view of thick-walled gallbladder with three polyps (*arrows, carets*) protruding into lumen. As the patient changes position, any one of the polyps may appear to be gravity dependent, but the attached polyps do not actually move away from their respective walls. (*B*) Hypoechoic gallbladder polyp (*arrow*) hangs from nondependent wall. Scanning from different planes, angles, and with patient in different positions assists in confirming which wall is gravity dependent.

Table 5-1. Pitfalls in identifying cholelithiasis

Mistaking bowel gas, the ligamentum teres, hepatic granulomas, a calcified aorta, or a migrating dermoid for gallstones
Using the wrong technique: not moving the patient, or using the incorrect transducer, focal zone, or gain settings
Junctional folds or the valves of Heister mimicking an echogenic focus with distal shadowing (Fig. 5-23)
Gallbladder edge shadowing mimicking shadowing from a stone
Not noticing stones in the fundus, phrygian cap, or Hartman's pouch
Missing very small stones or a very thin layer of stones (Fig. 5-24A, B)
Mistaking the IVC for the gallbladder in a very thin patient
Food or gas mimicking stones after cholecystoenterostomy
Postcholecystectomy scarring or clips mimicking stones
Bouveret's syndrome (gallstone ileus) mistaken for a stone-filled gallbladder
Gallbladder agenesis or ectopia
Pseudocalculi created by side lobe artifacts
Asymptomatic gallstones erroneously assumed to be the cause of the patient's complaint[27]

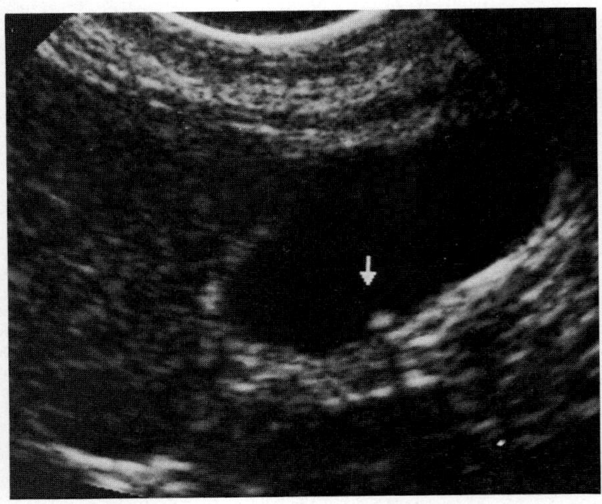

Figure 5-23. Initially, there was some question about whether this was a small stone or a fold in the neck. As the patient moved to left lateral decubitus and then to a sitting position, this small stone (*arrow*) easily rolled out of the neck and into the body, thus eliminating the possibility that the shadowing came from a fold.

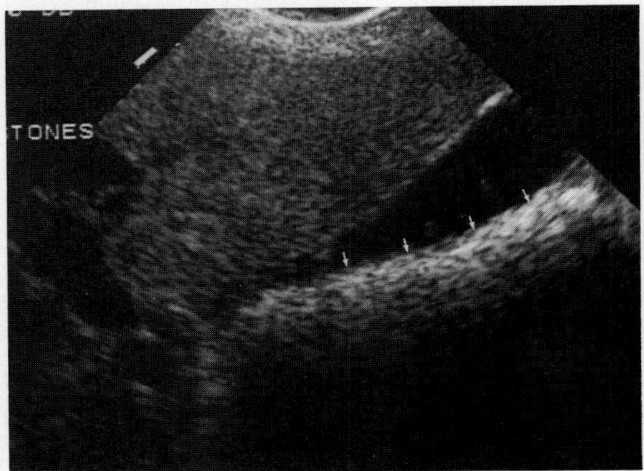

A

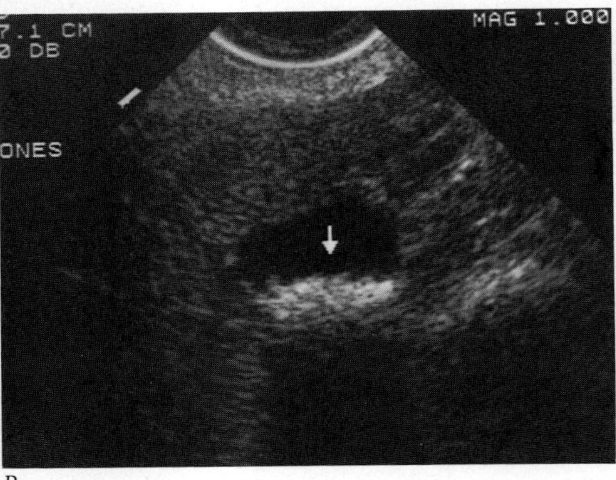

B

Figure 5-24. (*A*) The thin layer of numerous small stones (*arrows*) in this sagittal view of the gallbladder could be mistaken for bowel gas with shadowing just behind the gallbladder, but the small stones were observed to move within the gallbladder lumen. (*B*) Transverse view of the same gallbladder shows relationship of stones (*arrow*) to lumen wall and confirms their echoes are within the confines of the gallbladder and not outside, adjacent to it.

asis are presented in Table 5-1 (Figs. 5-23, 5-24). Once again, meticulous scanning in multiple planes using a variety of techniques and transducers is crucial to accurate diagnosis for proper patient management.

ACUTE CHOLECYSTITIS (CALCULOUS AND ACALCULOUS)

In 85% to 95% of cases acute cholecystitis, inflammation of the gallbladder, originates from impacted stones obstructing the cystic duct.[49,84] Inflammation occurs behind the obstruction, resulting in necrosis, ulceration, swelling, and edema (Fig. 5-25).[2] Acute acalculous cholecystitis (AAC) occurs (1) in the setting of trauma; (2) as a postsurgical complication (following surgery for nonbiliary disease); (3) after massive transfusions; (4) with severe burns, sepsis, shock, or long-term parenteral nutrition; (5) in children with congenital biliary malformations; (6) in patients with ileal disorders such as Crohn's disease; or (7) in any condition involving dehydration, prolonged fasting, reflux of pancreatic juices, excessive hemolysis, or overwhelming systemic infection.[7,49,58,84]

A combination of two factors may be responsible for AAC: stagnant bile and direct vascular changes. High concentrations of stagnant bile can be directly toxic and cause overdistension of the gallbladder leading to vascular compromise. Viscous stagnant bile can also act as a functional obstruction to gallbladder outflow, providing an excellent milieu for secondary bacterial invasion. Direct vascular changes can occur because the clotting cascade is activated by factors common to most causes of AAC, such as severe burns and trauma. This leads to selective thrombosis of vessels supplying the gallbladder, followed by ischemia, necrosis, secondary bacterial involvement, infection, and possibly perforation through the gallbladder wall.[7,49,58]

Clinically, the signs and symptoms of calculous and acalculous cholecystitis are indistinguishable and somewhat nonspecific; both can present with RUQ pain and tenderness, nausea, vomiting, distention, fever, and a palpable RUQ mass.[2,49] Twenty-five percent of cases of calculous cholecystitis also present with jaundice.[2] These symptoms could be confused with acute pancreatitis, perforated peptic ulcer, liver abscess, or hepatitis.[2] Symptoms of AAC can occur 24 hours to 50 days after the inciting event, but usually occur within 2 weeks.[7] Laboratory results can also be vague, possibly showing leukocytosis, hyperbilirubinemia, elevated alkaline phosphatase, and mildy elevated AST and ALT levels.[2,7]

Calculous cholecystitis is more prevalent in females, and AAC has a male predominance of 3.5:1.[3,7] The incidence of AAC varies greatly with age, race, and geographic location but is influenced directly by such predisposing factors as congenital biliary malformations, vascular disorders, trauma, sepsis, extensive burns, and dehydration.[58]

The prognosis for acute cholecystitis depends on whether prompt treatment is instituted. Treatment for both forms of cholecystitis is the same: early surgical removal of the inflamed gallbladder.[49] In very ill or elderly patients with severe acute cholecystitis, who are poor surgical risks, sonographically guided aspiration and percutaneous drainage of the gallbladder followed by antibiotic therapy is an alternative, albeit a risky one. It can decompress the gallbladder and relieve pain, but it can also be associated with serious vasovagal complications (i.e., hypotension) and bile peritonitis.[50]

Possible complications of acute cholecystitis include cholangitis, intraluminal hemorrhage, empyema (pus in the gallbladder), gangrenous cholecystitis (necrosis), emphysematous cholecystitis (air in the gallbladder wall), perforation of the gallbladder, and pericholecystic abscess.[2,3,49] Mortality rates from AAC far exceed those from acute calculous cholecystitis. This could be due to several factors, such as the lack of clinical and laboratory specificity in the diagnosis of AAC, which may contribute to delay in making the proper diagnosis, or because gangrene and rupture of the gallbladder occur with greater severity and frequency in AAC.[6,49] Again, early surgical treatment is the best way to avoid or minimize complications.

The pathophysiologic events of acute cholecystitis represent a dynamic process. Time is needed for these changes to occur. As a result, the clinical onset may precede the appearance of sonographic signs by 12 to 24 hours.[84] Except for the absence of calculi, the sonographic criteria for AAC are virtually the same as for acute calculous cholecystitis:

(text continues on page 176)

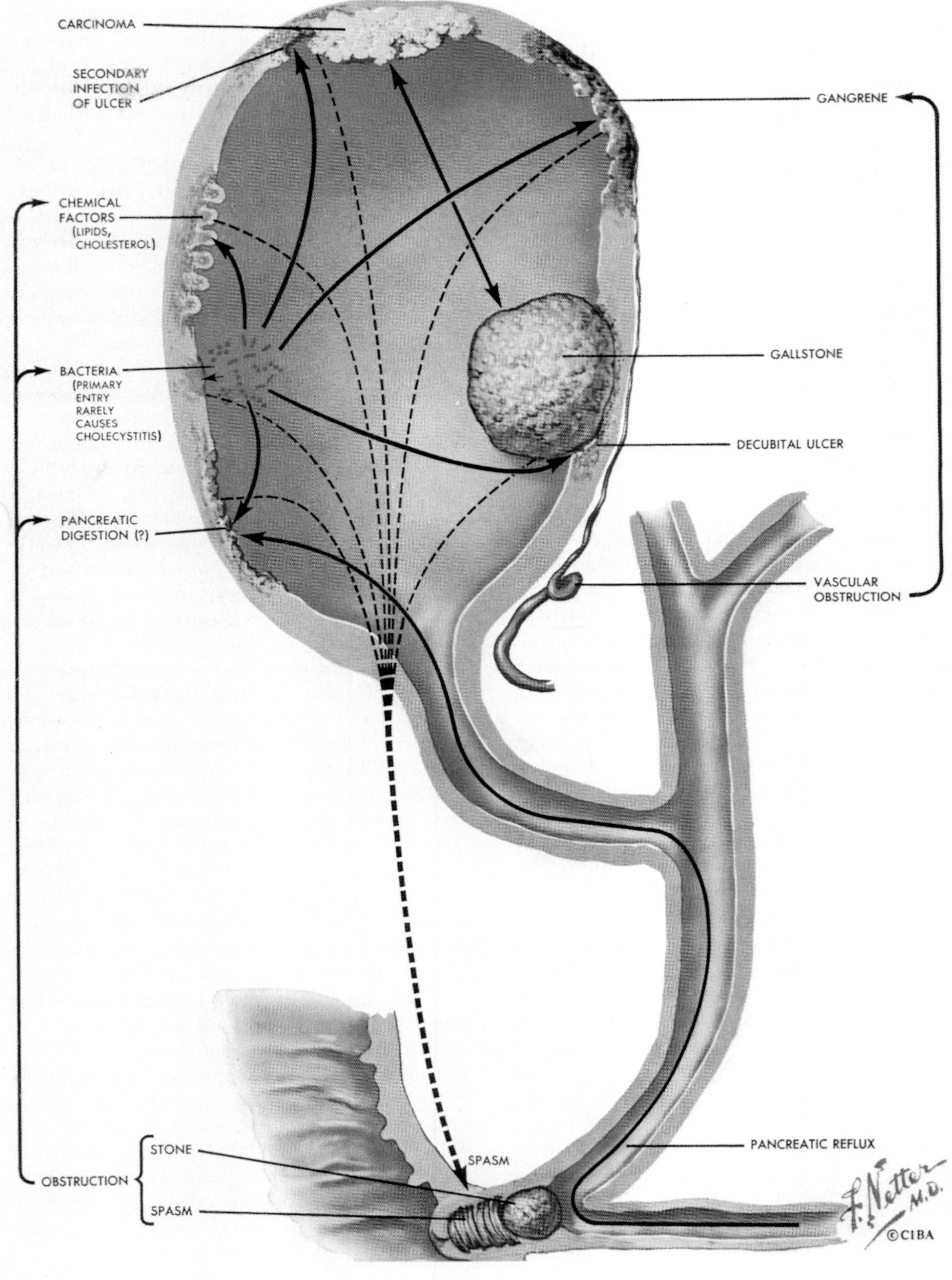

CARCINOMA
SECONDARY INFECTION OF ULCER
GANGRENE
CHEMICAL FACTORS (LIPIDS, CHOLESTEROL)
BACTERIA (PRIMARY ENTRY RARELY CAUSES CHOLECYSTITIS)
GALLSTONE
DECUBITAL ULCER
PANCREATIC DIGESTION (?)
VASCULAR OBSTRUCTION
STONE
SPASM
OBSTRUCTION
SPASM
PANCREATIC REFLUX
F. Netter M.D.
©CIBA

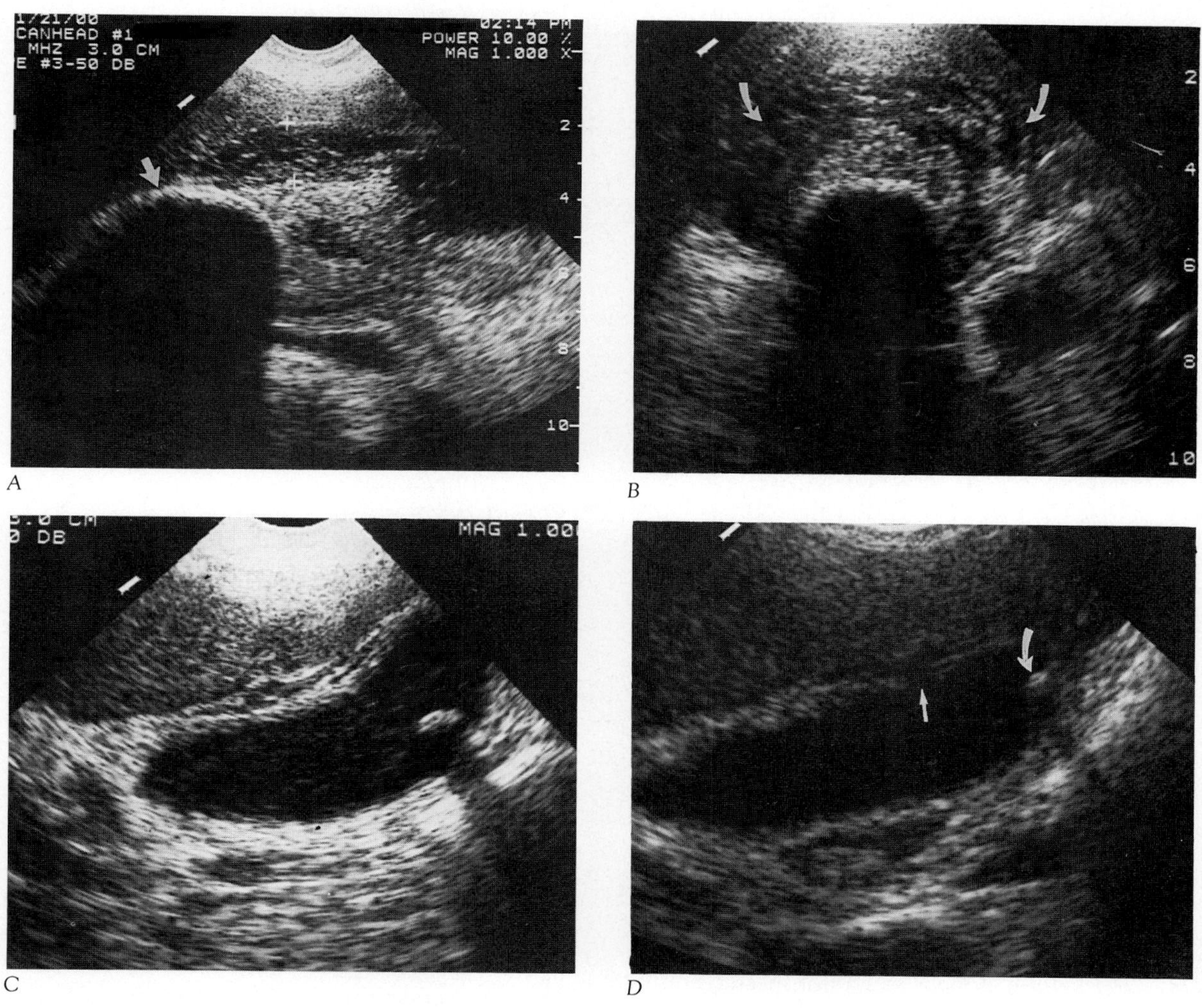

FIGURE 5-26. Acute cholecystitis. (*A*) Sagittal view showing large gallstone *(arrow)* within a very thick, swollen-walled gallbladder *(between caliper markers)*. Sludge and debris are seen inferior to the stone. (*B*) On a transverse view of the same patient, again, a thick, edematous, hypoechoic gallbladder wall *(curved arrows)* is demonstrated. (C) In a different patient (with positive Murphy's sign), this sagittal view shows a thick wall, halo, and cholelithiasis. (*D*) On the patient in C there is a possible perforation *(straight arrow)* in the gallbladder wall and a stone in the distal fundus *(curved arrow)*.

FIGURE 5-25. Interrelation of gallbladder diseases. (Copyright 1957. Ciba-Geigy Corporation. Reproduced with permission from The Ciba Collection of Medical Illustrations, by Frank H. Netter, M.D. Also by courtesy of Ciba-Geigy Limited, Basle, Switzerland. All rights reserved.)

1. gallbladder distention greater than 5 cm in the anteroposterior (AP) or transverse diameter;
2. gallbladder wall thickness greater than 5 mm;
3. cholelithiasis (in calculous cholecystitis);
4. Murphy's sign (maximum tenderness when transducer pressure is directly over the sonographically localized gallbladder);
5. halo sign (a sonolucent double-outline halo in gallbladder wall suggesting subserosal edema);
6. pericholecystic fluid or abscess, which may represent gallbladder perforation;
7. bizarre gallbladder wall echoes suggesting necrosis or gangrene;
8. nonshadowing, mobile, intraluminal echoes, which may represent blood, pus, or sloughed gallbladder mucosa in this clinical setting; and
9. a tense, rounded shape to the gallbladder as opposed to the normal pear or teardrop shape (Fig. 5-26).[3,7,48,55,62,75]

Although the *number* of criteria detected seems to correlate better than the presence of any single sign alone with the presence of acute cholecystitis,[75] when signs such as an enlarged gallbladder or a thick gallbladder wall are observed, an active search must be made for other causes of these findings, to exclude other possible diagnoses (Tables 5-2 and 5-3, Fig. 5-27). Some investigators even suggest that the cause of gallbladder wall thickening can be determined by the pattern of wall thickening (i.e. striated versus three-layer thickening). Wall thickening alone is still a nonspecific finding, and further research is needed to determine whether analysis of specific morphologic features will help differentiate acute cholecystitis.[15]

TABLE 5-2. Causes of gallbladder enlargement[62]

Prolonged fasting
IV hyperalimentation
Cystic duct obstruction (gallbladder hydrops)
CBD obstruction
Courvoisier's gallbladder (from tumor in head of pancreas, distal CBD tumor, duodenal or periampullary carcinoma)
Diabetes (longstanding insulin dependency)
Vagotomy

(Data from Odwin CS, Dubinsky T, Fleischer AC: General Abdominal Sonography Examination. Ultrasonography Examination Review and Study Guide. Norwalk, CT, Appleton & Lange, 1987.)

TABLE 5-3. Causes of gallbladder wall thickening[15,26,37,48,52,54,62,66,72,81,84]

Intrinsic causes
Acute cholecystitis
Chronic cholecystitis
Adenomyomatosis
Gallbladder carcinoma (primary or metastatic)
Gallbladder torsion
Extrinsic causes
Right-sided heart failure
Alcoholic liver disease
Hepatitis (adjacent liver infection can affect gallbladder)
AIDS (possibly from opportunistic gallbladder infection, AAC)
Hypoalbuminemia
Renal failure
Ascites
Multiple myeloma
Portal node lymphatic obstruction
Systemic venous hypertension
Gallbladder wall varices (dilated cystic veins from portal hypertension)
Physiologic cause
Contracted gallbladder after eating
Technical cause
Inappropriate TGC or gain

CHRONIC CHOLECYSTITIS

Chronic cholecystitis, the most common form of symptomatic gallbladder disease is virtually always associated with stones.[2,62] Repeated acute attacks generally herald this condition and produce a series of inflammatory changes that result in thickening and fibrosis of the gallbladder wall (Fig. 5-28).[2,51]

Clinically, the patient tends to have a history of intolerance to fatty or fried foods, possibly associated with intermittent nausea and vomiting. There is often moderate, intermittent RUQ and epigastric pain, which may radiate to the scapula. Alkaline phosphatase, AST, and ALT levels may be elevated. If jaundice is present, the direct bilirubin value is also elevated. It is possible for an attack of acute cholecystitis to be superimposed on underlying chronic disease, in which case some clinical and sonographic features of both entities could be present.[2]

Without cholecystectomy, complications some-

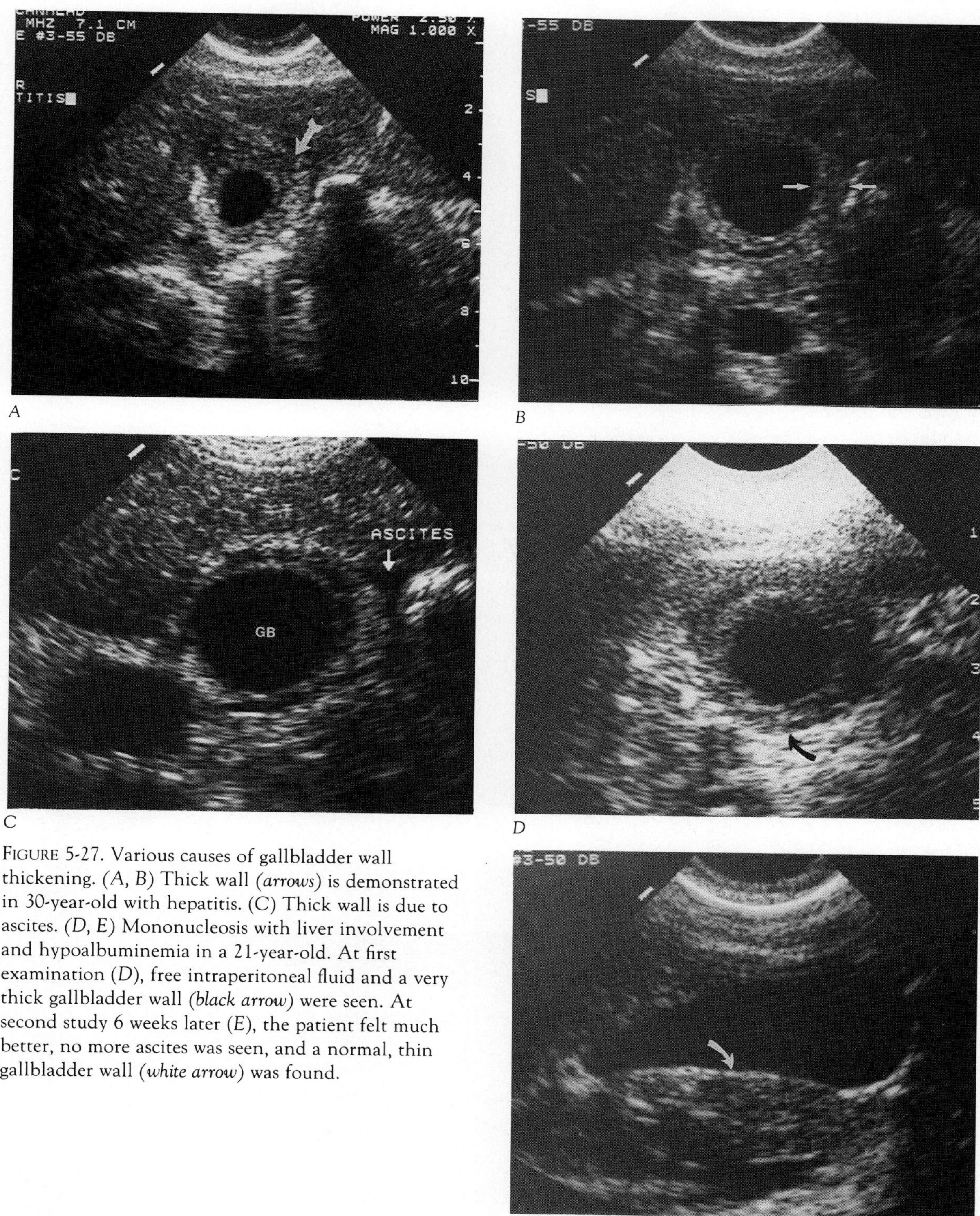

FIGURE 5-27. Various causes of gallbladder wall thickening. *(A, B)* Thick wall *(arrows)* is demonstrated in 30-year-old with hepatitis. (C) Thick wall is due to ascites. *(D, E)* Mononucleosis with liver involvement and hypoalbuminemia in a 21-year-old. At first examination *(D)*, free intraperitoneal fluid and a very thick gallbladder wall *(black arrow)* were seen. At second study 6 weeks later *(E)*, the patient felt much better, no more ascites was seen, and a normal, thin gallbladder wall *(white arrow)* was found.

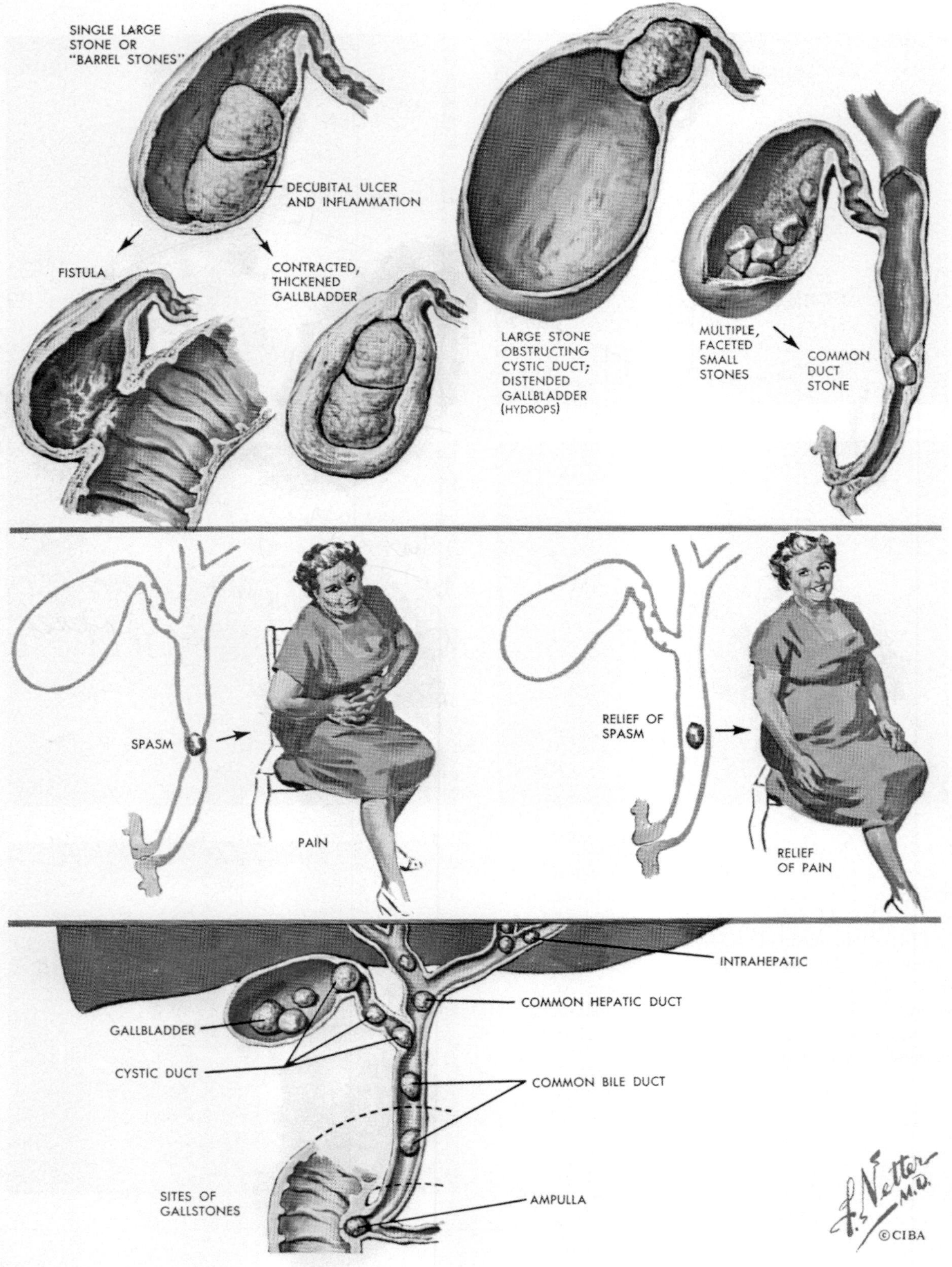
SINGLE LARGE STONE OR "BARREL STONES"
DECUBITAL ULCER AND INFLAMMATION
FISTULA
CONTRACTED, THICKENED GALLBLADDER
LARGE STONE OBSTRUCTING CYSTIC DUCT; DISTENDED GALLBLADDER (HYDROPS)
MULTIPLE, FACETED SMALL STONES
COMMON DUCT STONE
SPASM
PAIN
RELIEF OF SPASM
RELIEF OF PAIN
INTRAHEPATIC
COMMON HEPATIC DUCT
GALLBLADDER
CYSTIC DUCT
COMMON BILE DUCT
SITES OF GALLSTONES
AMPULLA
F. Netter M.D.
©CIBA

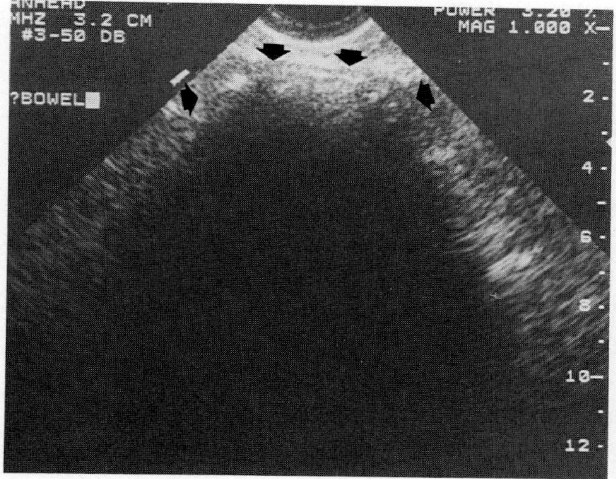

A

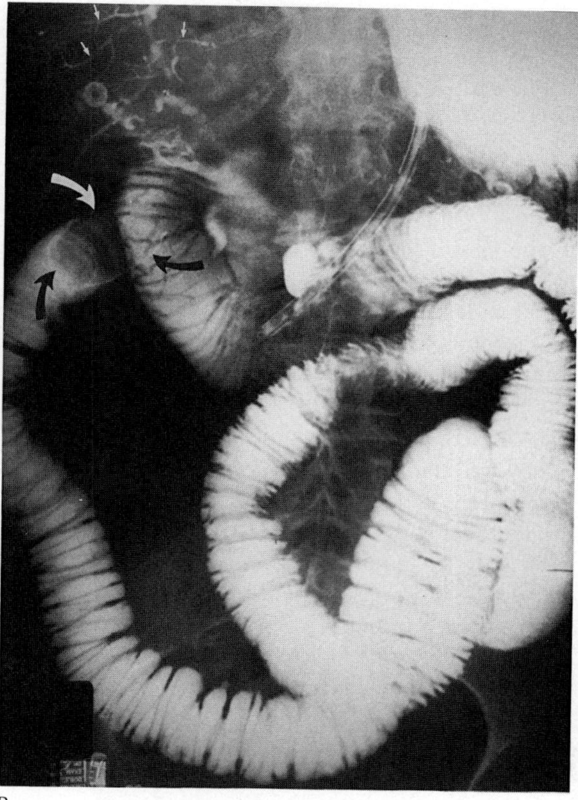

B

FIGURE 5-29. Gallstone ileus in a 90-year-old woman. (*A*) Sonogram of RUQ shows bowel wall *(outlined by arrows)* and large stone with shadowing filling bowel lumen. This was seen separate from a shrunken gallbladder. (*B*) Small bowel series shows a fistula between duodenal bulb and gallbladder which allowed radiographic contrast medium to reflux into the intrahepatic biliary tree *(small arrows)*. Large gallstone *(larger black and white curved arrows)* is seen in the jejunum causing small bowel obstruction.

FIGURE 5-28. Possible progressions and outcomes with cholelithiasis. (Copyright 1957. Ciba-Geigy Corporation. Reproduced with permission from The Ciba Collection of Medical Illustrations, by Frank H. Netter, M.D. Also by courtesy of Ciba-Geigy Limited, Basle, Switzerland. All rights reserved.)

times arise from untreated chronic cholecystitis. Among these is Bouveret's syndrome, or gallstone ileus (Fig. 5-29). This is the most common form of biliary-enteric fistulization and occurs between the gallbladder and duodenum. Inflammatory changes in the gallbladder lead to the formation of adhesions between the gallbladder and duodenum. Eventually, large stones can erode through the gallbladder wall and into the duodenal bulb, where they become impacted in the duodenal lumen. There, the stone may cause gastric outlet obstruction (gastric dilatation) or distal bowel obstruction

TABLE 5-4. Causes of small gallbladder[26,54,62]

Chronic cholecystitis
Hepatitis (decreased gallbladder volume from decreased bile production due to hepatocyte injury)
Congenital hypoplasia (rare)
CHD obstruction (gallbladder does not fill with bile)
Failure of patient to fast

in the ileum, colon, or rectum, or it may be passed spontaneously. Although rare, this syndrome must be considered, especially in women older than 60 years who complain of upper intestinal obstruction in addition to gallbladder symptoms.[27,51] Another possible complication of untreated cholecystitis is the Mirizzi syndrome in which a gallstone impacted in the gallbladder neck or cystic duct exerts pressure on the adjacent common duct. This leads to inflammatory strictures, and the pressure necrosis eventually erodes the wall of the common duct, allowing the stone to pass into the lumen and cause obstructive jaundice.[5]

The sonographic features of chronic cholecystitis are a small contracted gallbladder with stones and a thick, fibrous echogenic wall (Tables 5-3, 5-4, Fig. 5-30). With careful technique, wall-echo-shadow (WES) triad or double arc shadow sign may be seen. The first arc or curved echogenic line represents the thickened gallbladder wall; the second arc is from the surface of the stone followed by posterior acoustic shadowing.[2,17,62] With chronic disease, the gallbladder may be so contracted that it is not sonographically visible, although a diligent search often reveals it (Table 5-5). The WES sign or just strong, broad acoustic shadowing from or near the gallbladder fossa can be mimicked by residual barium, a porcelain gallbladder, or Bouveret's syndrome. With Bouveret's, though, pneumobilia (air in the biliary tree) and gastric or intestinal dilatation may be present and one may even be able to sonographically establish the actual presence of the calculus within the bowel lumen, separate from the gallbladder or gallbladder fossa.[18,27,51] Air-filled bowel loops in the RUQ may create shadowing, which can be mistaken for a contracted gallbladder with stones, but if evidence of peristalsis is sought or the area is scanned again later, the bowel gas pattern generally will have changed.

TABLE 5-5. Causes of failure to visualize gallbladder

Gallbladder contracted with stones
Gallbladder filled with tumor
Agenesis (rare)
Ectopic gallbladder
Absence (cholecystectomy)
Porcelain gallbladder (calcified wall)
Gallstone ileus or Mirizzi syndrome (contents of gallbladder erode out causing it to shrink so visualization becomes difficult)
Air in gallbladder wall
Air in gallbladder lumen
Failure of patient to fast
Overlying bowel
Residual barium in nearby bowel from recent x-ray examination

GALLBLADDER NEOPLASMS

Primary gallbladder carcinoma, the fifth most common cancer of the gastrointestinal tract, represents 4% of all cancers.[2,85] It predominantly affects women older than 60 years.[2] Gallstones are present in as many as 98% of cases and porcelain gallbladders in as many as 25% of gallbladder cancers.[85] The incidence of gallbladder cancer is also increased among automotive, rubber, textile, and metal-fabricating workers.[11] Eighty percent of gallbladder carcinomas are adenocarcinomas, and 20% are undifferentiated or squamous cell types. Gallbladder carcinoma can spread through the lymphatics to local nodes, through the venous system of the gallbladder, or by direct extension to the liver.[2] Intraductal spread occurs in at least 4% of cases and can clinically mimic pancreatic or bile duct tumors.[85] Gallbladder cancer is often difficult to detect in its early stages, as it may be asymptomatic or present with the signs and symptoms of cholelithiasis or cholecystitis.[2,85] About 50% of patients have jaundice and approximately 65% a palpable RUQ mass. The laboratory findings are nonspecific and do little to differentiate it from benign gallbladder pathology. Fewer than 20% of gallbladder carcinomas are diagnosed preoperatively but they are often found incidentally at routine cholecystectomy.[2] Cholecystectomy should be performed if metastasis has not yet occurred. The 5-year survival rate for primary gallbladder carcinoma is only 4% to 12% though.[85]

Gallbladder metastases are not as rare as was once thought and are often found incidentally at

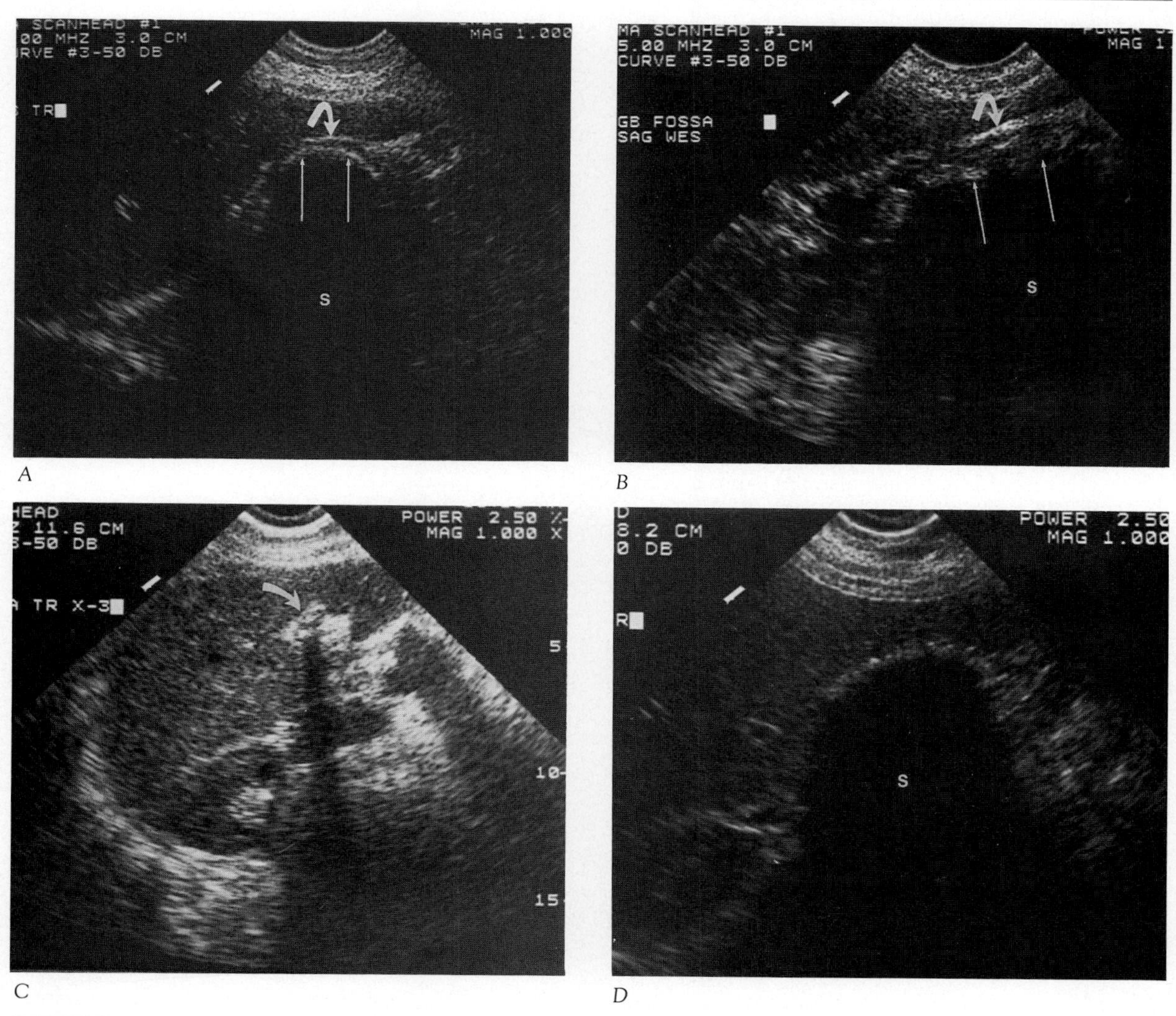

FIGURE 5-30. Chronic cholecystitis and lithiasis. (*A, B*) WES sign. (*curved arrow*, gallbladder wall; *long, thin arrows*, echo from stone; S, shadow). (C) Small, contracted gallbladder with stones (transverse). (*D*) Broad acoustic shadowing (S) from gallbladder fossa represents chronic cholecystitis and cholelithiasis.

surgery or autopsy.[65] Malignant melanoma is the most common tumor to metastasize to the gallbladder, usually by embolic hematogenous spread.[17,65] Other bloodborne metastases can occur from the lungs, kidneys, and esophagus. Metastases from the stomach, pancreas, and bile ducts can reach the gallbladder by direct invasion. Cancer of the liver, ovary, and colon can also metastasize to the gallbladder.[65] Primary gallbladder cancer is strongly associated with stones and inflammatory gallbladder disease, but metastatic disease is completely independent of cholelithiasis and cholecystitis. The clinical presentation can mimic acute or chronic gallbladder inflammation. It is important to consider the overall clinical picture; if the patient presents with pain and fever the physician may think "inflammation," but if the patient presents with pain, jaundice, malaise, weight loss, or increased abdominal girth the possibility of a neoplasm should be entertained.[65] Treatment and prognosis depend on the location and extent of the primary tumor and other metastases.

Sonographically, primary gallbladder carcinoma and gallbladder metastases can share a similar appearance; the presence of stones may be the deciding factor.[65] The earliest sonographic sign is irregular wall thickening. It may also appear as a poorly defined polypoid mass protruding into the lumen that is larger than would be expected for a cholesterol polyp (more than 1 cm; Fig. 5-31). More advanced disease may fill or replace the gallbladder, causing a large RUQ mass that is indistinguishable from a liver or hepatic flexure lesion.[17,18,65] The ultrasonographic findings depend on the stage of involvement. Diffuse circumferential thickening can be associated with tumor, but more common causes include cholecystitis, hemorrhage, abscess formation, edema, scarring, ascites, hypoproteinemia, or a normal gallbladder that is slightly contracted. The differential diagnosis for stationary, nonshadowing, intraluminal soft tissue masses and focal wall thickening includes the following more common and benign entities: cholesterol polyps, benign adenomas, hyperplastic cholecystoses, inflammatory polyps, small nonshadowing stones adherent to the gallbladder wall, empyema, atypical viscous sludge (usually less echogenic than tumor), or even artifactual echoes from too much gain.[65] If a gallbladder malignancy is suspected, it is imperative to search the entire abdomen for other signs of malignancy such as liver metastases, porta hepatis nodes, retroperitoneal adenopathy, ascites, or signs of a primary tumor in another organ.[65,85]

Hyperplastic Cholecystoses

Hyperplastic cholecystoses are a group of benign, noninflammatory conditions that are both degenerative and proliferative[2,67]: adenomyomatosis, cholesterosis, neuromatosis, fibromatosis, and lipomatosis.[2]

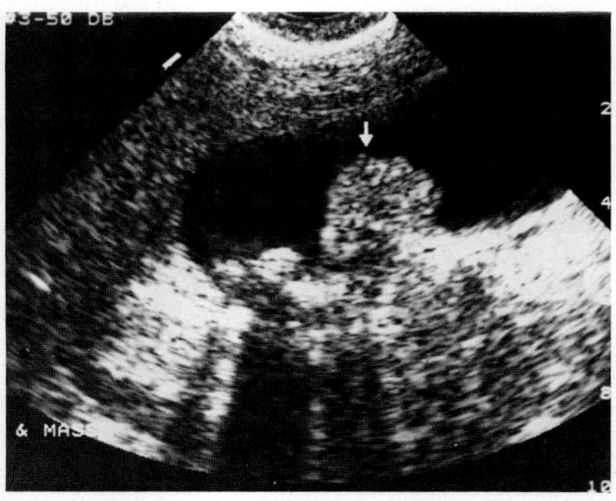

Figure 5-31. Mass in gallbladder lumen *(arrow)* was confirmed to be a primary gallbladder carcinoma. Stones are seen to the left of the mass. When the patient sat up, neither the stones nor the mass moved. Differential diagnosis includes large polyp, sludge ball, and metastatic lesion.

Adenomyomatosis is characterized by excessive proliferation of the surface epithelium with glandlike formations and outpouchings of the mucosa into or through a thickened muscle layer. These pouches, or diverticula, are called Rokitansky-Aschoff sinuses.[2,67] There are three forms of adenomyomatosis: (1) diffuse, involving the entire gallbladder; (2) segmental, in which the proximal, middle, or distal one-third is involved circumferentially; and (3) localized, the most common type, confined almost exclusively to the fundus. The incidence of adenomyomatosis is difficult to determine, although Rokitansky-Aschoff sinuses have been found in 60% to 86% of cholecystectomy specimens.[67] It is more common in women, and the incidence increases after age 40 years.[2] The ability to diagnose it sonographically depends on the degree and nature of wall thickening, a nonspecific finding, and on the identification of intramural diverticula, an essential to confirming the ultrasound diagnosis (Fig. 5-32). The appearance of the diverticula varies, depending on their size, content, and whether papillary projections are present. Sinuses that contain bile often appear as small, round, anechoic spaces in the gallbladder wall. Those that are small or contain sludge, stones, or papillary projections appear as echogenic foci spaced at varying intervals in the gallbladder wall. The echogenic focus can be associated with acoustic shadowing or comet-tail reverberation artifacts, possibly produced by frondlike projections in the diverticulum.[67]

Cholesterosis, or "strawberry gallbladder," is characterized by abnormal cholesterol deposits in the gallbladder wall and can be associated with cholelithiasis.[2] It occurs far more frequently in women than in men.[59] The lesions may be diffuse, with no impairment of gallbladder function, or localized single or multiple polypoid lesions, which may be pedunculated and can interfere with function.[2]

Neuromatosis and fibromatosis are rare proliferations of nerve and fibrous tissue, respectively. Lipomatosis is an excessive build-up of fat layers in the gallbladder wall. These three processes may or may not interfere with gallbladder function.[2]

The hyperplastic cholecystoses are often asymptomatic, but when symptoms do occur they often mimic those of cholelithiasis, even though stones often are not present. Laboratory values are usually normal unless function is impaired. Then, the alkaline phosphatase value may be elevated. The risk of malignancy is low. Surgery may be performed if there is intractable pain.[2]

Often these lesions are not detected sonographically, but when they are visible their appearance can vary. Fixed polypoid lesions or a small, misshapen gallbladder may be seen. The contractility of the gallbladder can also be checked by comparing scans made 30 minutes after a fatty meal and in the fasting state.[2]

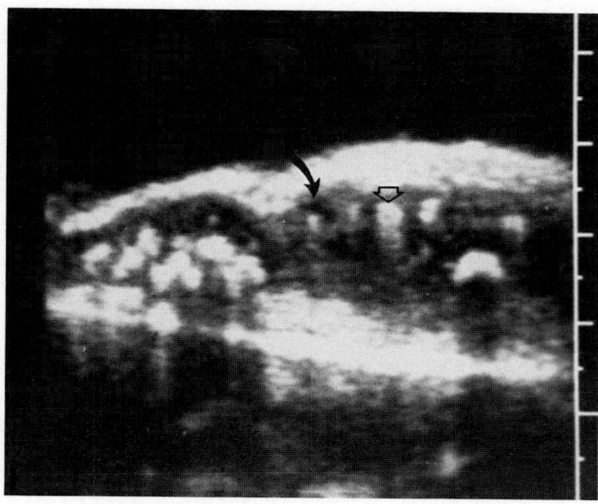

FIGURE 5-32. Adenomyomatosis. Stones are demonstrated within the gallbladder lumen and thickened wall. Some of the Rokitansky-Aschoff sinuses are filled with bile and appear cystic *(curved arrow)* while others are filled with stones *(open arrow)*. (Reprinted with permission from Kidney M, Goiney R, Cooperberg PL: Adenomyomatosis of the gallbladder: A pictorial exhibit. J Ultrasound Med 1986, 5:331–333. Copyright 1986 by the American Institute of Ultrasound in Medicine.)

MISCELLANEOUS GALLBLADDER PATHOLOGY

Torsion, or volvulus, of the gallbladder is rare, but its incidence may be increasing, possibly because today people live longer. It can occur at all ages but is more common in elderly patients. It is three times more frequent in women. The cause is uncertain but is thought to be lengthening of the gallbladder mesentery in old age that allows the gallbladder to be free floating on a pedicle. Vigorous bowel peristalsis, a mobile gallbladder fundus, gallstones, atherosclerosis of the cystic artery, and kyphosis have all been implicated as predisposing or contributing factors. Pathologically, the walls of the twisted gallbladder become thickened, edematous, and hemorrhagic. Gangrene may be present. Stones are unusual. An elongated mesenteric attachment generally is seen. The diagnosis of torsion is seldom made preoperatively. The treatment is immediate cholecystectomy. The sonographic features include gross wall thickening, a spherical distended gallbladder, and often absence of calculi, although this appearance is nonspecific.[66]

Calcification of all or part of the gallbladder wall is called porcelain gallbladder (Fig. 5-33). It is a relatively rare manifestation of chronic cholecystitis and is frequently asymptomatic. It is associated with a high incidence of gallbladder carcinoma. Three sonographic patterns can be seen: (1) a hyperechoic semilunar structure with posterior acoustic shadowing simulating a stone-filled gallbladder; (2) a biconvex curvilinear echogenic structure with

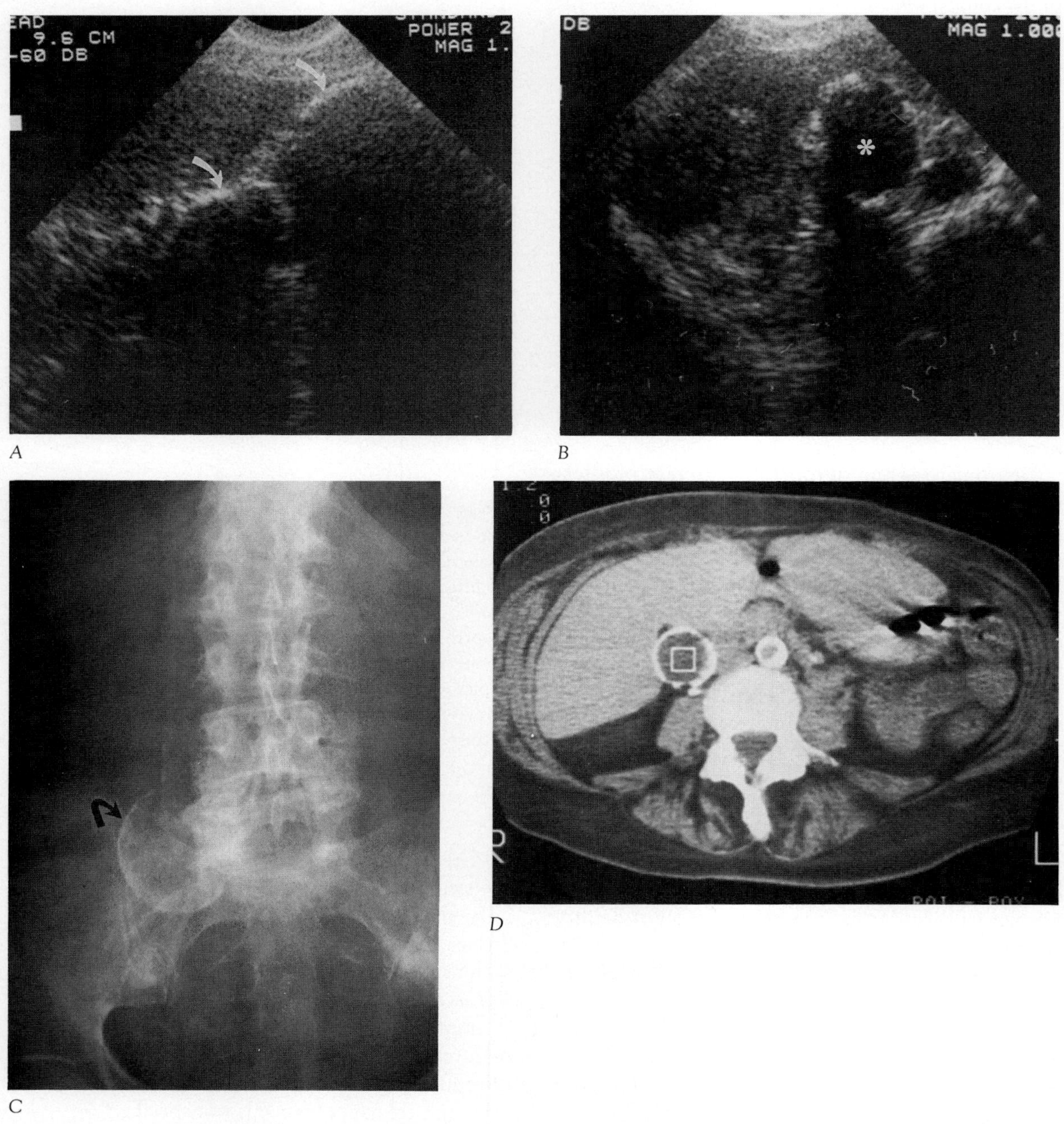

FIGURE 5-33. Imaging series of porcelain gallbladder. (*A*) Sagittal sonogram of calcified gallbladder wall *(curved arrows)*, which could mimic two large stones. Shadowing posterior to calcified areas is noted. (*B*) On a transverse sonogram, the gallbladder is not completely calcified, since the back wall can be partially imaged (*asterisk*, gallbladder lumen). (C) An abdominal radiograph shows low-lying calcified gallbladder *(curved arrow)*. (*D*) CT study demonstrates thickened, calcified wall of the gallbladder. The marker box represents gallbladder lumen.

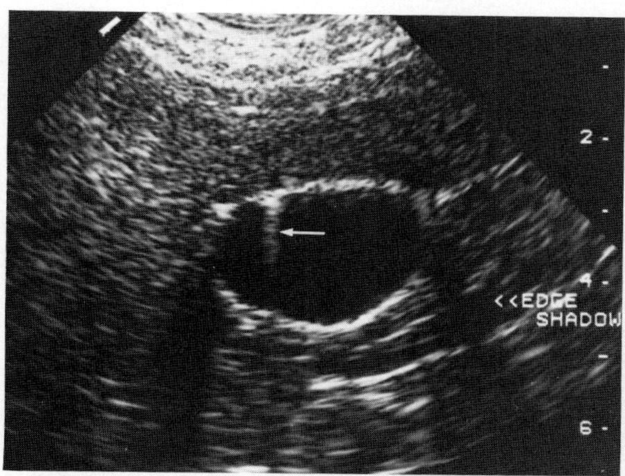

Figure 5-34. Comet-tail artifact *(arrow)* emanates from possible cholesterol crystals in the wall of this gallbladder (transverse view). The edge shadow artifact should not be mistaken for shadowing from a stone. This could be confirmed by scanning from several different angles.

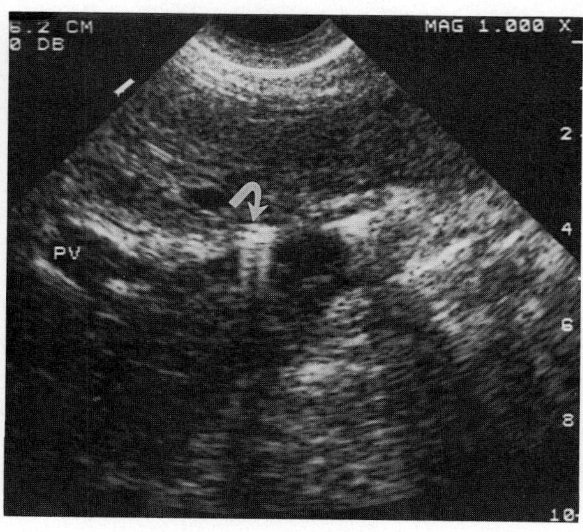

Figure 5-35. Echogenic foci *(curved stone)* with reverberations in the gallbladder fossa of this postcholecystectomy patient represent surgical clips (PV, portal vein).

variable acoustic shadowing; or (3) an irregular clump of echoes with posterior shadowing.[38]

An enlarged and distended Courvoisier gallbladder occurs when there is obstruction distal to the cystic duct due to malignancy (e.g., pancreatic head carcinoma, periportal adenopathy).[2] With any distal mass, the gallbladder dilates first, followed by the common duct (CD), and finally the intrahepatic tree dilates. Upon removal of the obstructing mass, the gallbladder decompresses actively (because of its contractile muscle), while the ducts passively return to normal in reverse order.[82]

Adenomas represent 28% of all benign gallbladder neoplasms. The majority are pedunculated. They can be associated with carcinoma in situ.[11]

Microabscesses in the gallbladder wall may be seen as hyperechoic foci in the wall, which may produce comet-tail reverberations. Intramural diverticula filled with inspissated bile, small stones, or cholesterol crystals can have the same appearance (Fig. 5-34).[33]

The Postcholecystectomy Patient

The appearance of the postcholecystectomy gallbladder fossa can be (1) a postoperative abscess or fluid collection, (2) echogenic foci with associated reverberations and/or shadows representing surgical clips, or (3) more commonly, bowel loops filling the empty fossa (Fig. 5-35).

Controversy exists over whether the size of the common duct should increase after the gallbladder is removed (Fig. 5-36). Some say the duct may increase in caliber because it becomes a floppy, passive tube from previous episodes of inflammation, or as the result of surgical exploration of the duct at the time of cholecystectomy, or because in the absence of the gallbladder the duct may act as a reservoir for bile.[87] While some studies say that a normal postcholecystectomy common duct can measure up to 11 mm, others claim it should be considered dilated if it exceeds 6 mm in maximum intraluminal AP diameter.[42,60,74] Rescanning 30 to 45 minutes after a fatty meal may help determine

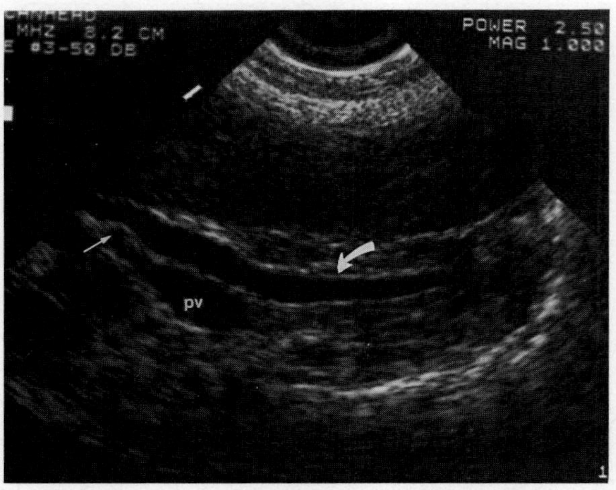

FIGURE 5-36. The maximum diameter of the common duct in this post-cholecystectomy patient measured 0.85 cm. The distal CBD *(curved arrow)* is clearly seen. Also noted are the portal vein (pv) and hepatic artery *(straight arrow)*, which complete the portal triad.

whether obstruction truly exists. Fatty meals stimulate biliary flow and relax the sphincter of Oddi. If a normal or slightly dilated duct enlarges after a fatty meal or an abnormally large duct fails to shrink, CBD obstruction is strongly indicated. After a fatty meal, healthy nondilated, patent ducts should decrease slightly in caliber if they change at all. A slight decrease in diameter virtually excludes obstruction.[74,87] Fatty meals are especially useful to confirm that an asymptomatic patient with equivocal or midly prominent ducts has normal function.[74]

Postcholecystectomy syndrome refers to recurrence of pre-operative symptoms, particularly biliary colic, 2 months or longer after cholecystectomy. Retained common duct stones are the most frequent cause. Other causes include an excessive cystic duct stump, sphincter of Oddi spasms, CBD strictures, biliary tract carcinomas, pancreatitis, an amputation neuroma, and adhesions constricting the CBD.[59]

CHOLANGITIS

Cholangitis is an inflammation or infection of the biliary system. Signs and symptoms can include intermittent fever, upper abdominal pain, pruritus, and jaundice. Laboratory tests may reveal an increased alkaline phosphatase value, mildly elevated AST and ALT levels, increased WBC, and an increased direct bilirubin value (if jaundice is present). Although it is most often associated with choledocholithiasis, it can also be caused by choledochal cysts, bile duct carcinoma, acquired immunodeficiency syndrome (AIDS), or it may ascend from the gastrointestinal tract.[2,72] The inflammation can ultimately extend into the intrahepatic biliary system and cause hepatic abscesses also.[2]

Cholangitis does not have a characteristic ultrasonographic appearance. Findings may include thickened and edematous duct walls, dilated ducts (if obstructed), or air in the biliary tree (which could be from an anaerobic cholangitis or from other causes such as a surgical or pathologic fistula between bowel and the biliary tree).[2]

BENIGN STRICTURES OF THE EXTRAHEPATIC BILIARY TREE

Surgical trauma is the culprit in 95% of benign strictures. The remaining cases are usually due to blunt abdominal trauma or erosion of the duct wall by a gallstone, the Mirizzi syndrome. The symptoms usually resemble those of cholangitis; jaundice is associated with complete occlusion. Alkaline phosphatase levels are frequently elevated. Sonographically, strictures can mimic the appearance of cholangitis. Dilated ducts and signs of obstruction will be evident if the duct is significantly occluded.[2]

OBSTRUCTIVE JAUNDICE

Obstructive jaundice results from direct interference with the flow of bile along the biliary tract (Fig. 5-37). It is important to distinguish it from nonobstructive jaundice (Table 5-6). When something inside or outside the bile duct causes a blockage, the ducts proximal to the site of obstruction dilate,[62] but a dilated common duct is not necessarily pathognomonic for obstruction. It could be due to previous episodes of obstruction or inflammation with loss of elasticity, or it could result from ampullary dysfunction.[87] Patients can have enlarged ducts without obstruction or obstruction without enlarged ducts. A duct can also appear normal despite abnormal laboratory values, or the duct can be abnormal even though laboratory val-

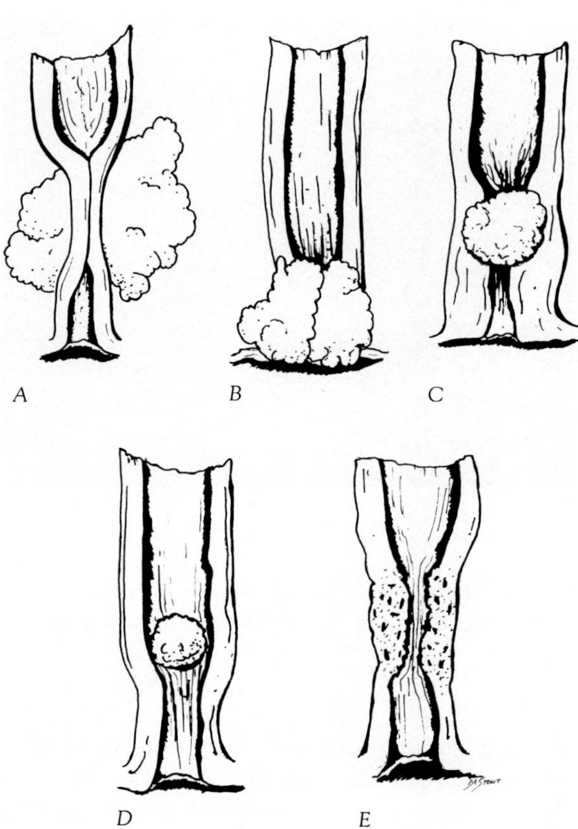

Figure 5-37. Types of extrahepatic biliary obstruction: (*A, B, C*) complete CBD obstructions, (*D, E*) incomplete obstruction. (*A*) Extrinsic cancer fixing and compressing duct, (*B*) intrinsic cancer, (C) impacted stone with edema of duct, (*D*) ball-in-valve stone causing intermittent obstruction, (*E*) stricture of duct.

Table 5-6. Causes of jaundice[42,62]

Surgical jaundice (obstructive)
Choledocholithiasis
Pancreatitis
Pancreatic pseudocyst
Neoplasm of pancreatic head or ampulla of Vater
Hepatoma
Metastatic carcinoma (usually of gastrointestinal origin)
Cholangiocarcinoma
Porta hepatis mass (i.e., adenopathy)
Klatskin tumor
Medical jaundice (nonobstructive)
Hepatocellular disease (interferes with excretion of bilirubin):
Hepatitis
Drug-induced cholestasis
Fatty liver
Cirrhosis
Hemolytic disease (hepatocytes cannot keep up with increased red blood cell destruction causing elevated indirect bilirubin):
Sickle-cell anemia
Cooley's anemia

Table 5-7. Defining the level and cause of intrahepatic biliary dilatation[42,62,87]

With intrahepatic dilation and normal CBD look for:
Proximal bile duct tumors
Proximal CHD stone
Right or left main hepatic duct obstruction (especially if only segmental dilatation in one lobe)
Sclerosing cholangitis
Porta hepatis metastases or adenopathy
With intrahepatic dilatation and dilated CBD look for:
CBD stone
Pseudocyst obstructing CBD
Acute pancreatitis (swollen pancreatic head may obstruct bile flow)
Chronic pancreatitis (periductal fibrosis and stenosis may obstruct bile flow)
Carcinoma of head of pancreas
Choledochal cyst

ues are normal.[74] Significant biliary pathology can be present with sonographically dilated ducts in the absence of clinical jaundice and without serum bilirubin elevation.[31] Duct size can also change spontaneously, since it is part of a dynamic system that responds as obstructions occur and resolve.[60]

Sonography is an important tool for locating the level and cause of biliary obstruction (Table 5-7, Fig. 5-38). The findings depend on the type and location of the obstruction (dilatation may be intrahepatic, extrahepatic, or both) and on when the scan is performed (ducts may not yet have dilated if obstruction occurred just 12 to 24 hours earlier, they may be decompressing if the obstruction has passed, or intermittent or partial obstruction may allow enough bile to pass without causing dilatation).[62] The extrahepatic ducts tend to dilate before the intrahepatic ones, and ducts can return rapidly to normal if the obstruction passes.[17] With real-time scanning it is easier to trace the extent of duc-

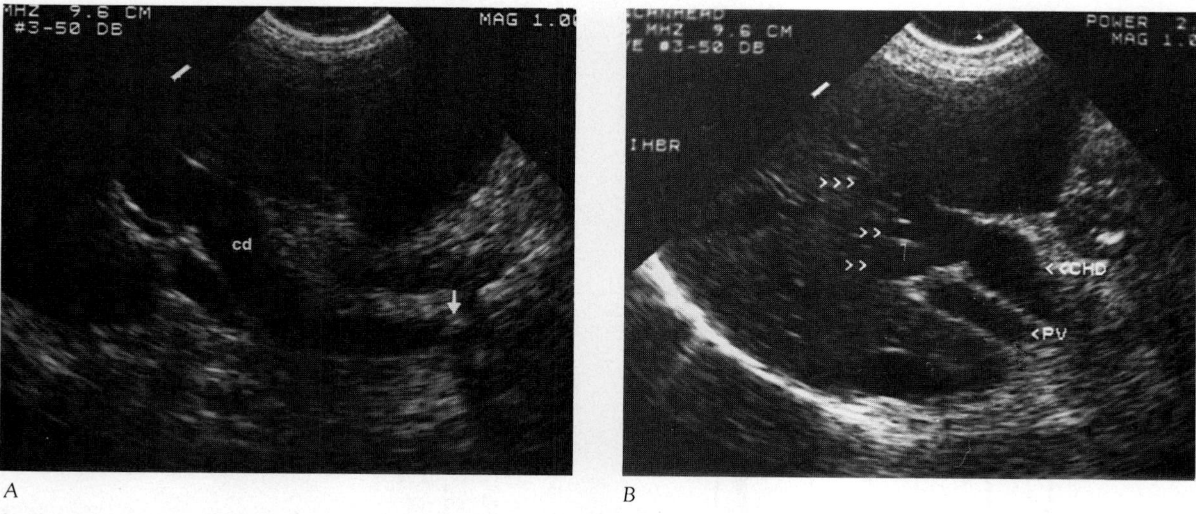

FIGURE 5-38. (*A*) Stone (*arrow*) in distal portion of dilated common duct (cd) is demonstrated. (*B*) On the same patient, dilatation extends into the intrahepatic ducts (*arrowheads*; PV, portal vein).

tal dilatation, and it is also important to note whether obstruction is focal or diffuse. The entire course and caliber of the duct must be examined to see whether it tapers distally. One isolated measurement is not enough.

With newer electronically focused equipment and careful scanning, structures representing normal intrahepatic bile ducts may be seen measuring from less than 1 to 3 mm in diameter. The mere observation of intrahepatic ducts no longer implies intrahepatic biliary dilatation.[9] The sonographic criteria for intrahepatic dilatation include (1) the parallel-channel sign (double-barreled shotgun sign, "too many tubes" sign), representing the dilated duct running anterior to its accompanying portal vein; (2) irregular, jagged walls and branching patterns of the ducts (compared to smooth walls and smooth bifurcations of the portal venous system); (3) stellate confluence of dilated ducts converging toward the porta hepatis; and (4) acoustic enhancement posterior to the dilated ducts occurring because bile attenuates less than the blood in the portal veins (Fig. 5-39).[13,17,62,88]

All of these signs are more obvious with more extreme dilatation.[88] Other conditions that can mimic dilated intrahepatic biliary radicles are Caroli's disease (communicating cavernous ectasia of the intrahepatic ducts), enlarged hepatic arteries (to provide increased blood flow to the liver in patients with cirrhosis or portal hypertension), and cavernous transformation of the portal vein (wormlike network of extensive collateral venous channels that form if the portal vein becomes occluded).[17,73,88]

The sonographic criteria for dilation of extrahepatic ducts are CHD internal diameter greater than 6 mm or CBD internal diameter greater than 6 to 8 mm.[2,16,31] The signs may be subtle in an early, partial, or mild obstruction. Again, a fatty meal may help clarify a borderline situation.

Once intra- or extrahepatic dilatation has been established, the next step is to diligently search for the cause.

Choledocholithiasis. Common duct stones are usually formed in the gallbladder and then pass into the CBD, where they may lodge (Fig. 5-40). After cholecystectomy, stones in the duct may have been missed at surgery and be retained or they may form spontaneously in the duct.[2] Cystic duct stones re-

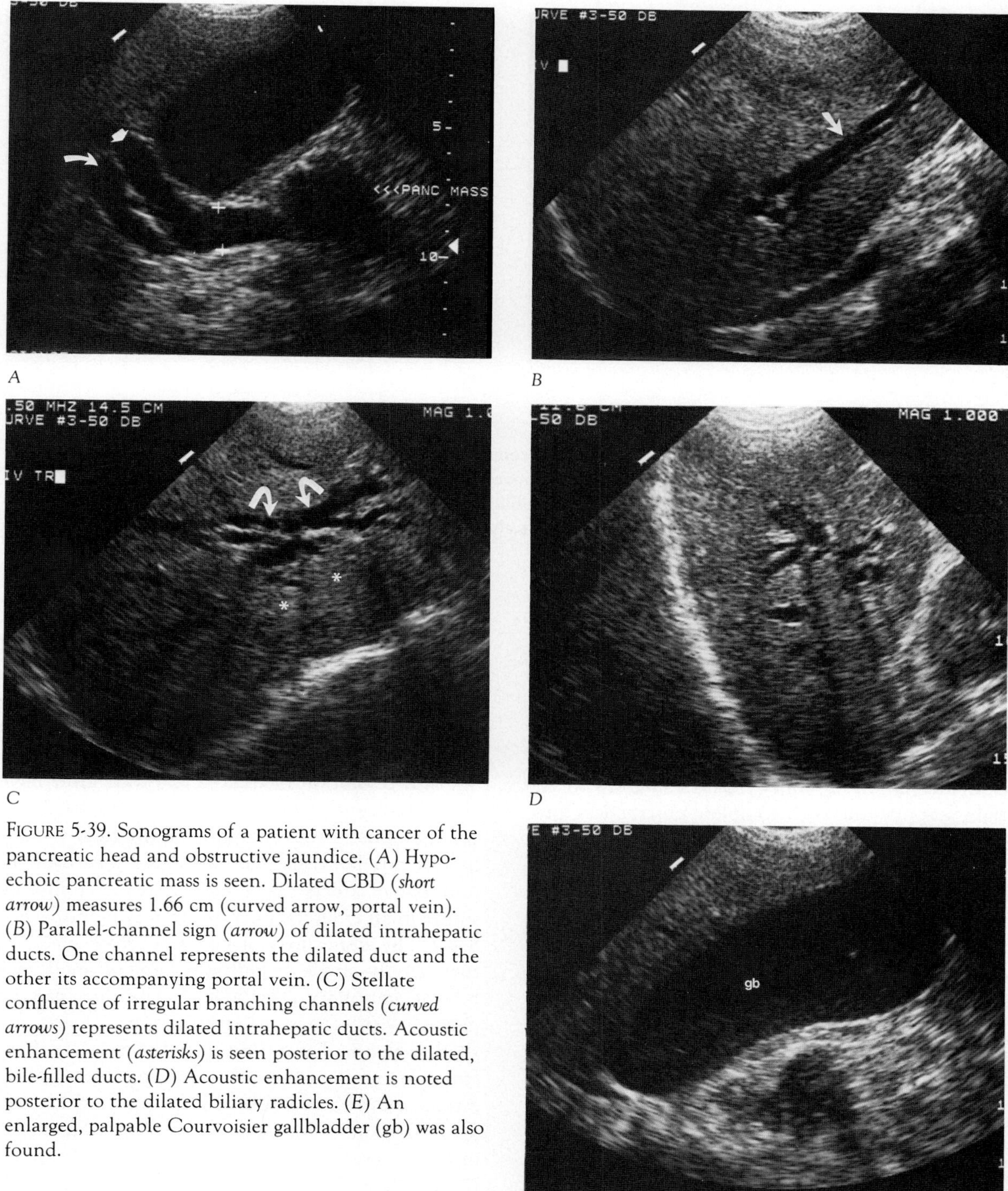

Figure 5-39. Sonograms of a patient with cancer of the pancreatic head and obstructive jaundice. (*A*) Hypoechoic pancreatic mass is seen. Dilated CBD (*short arrow*) measures 1.66 cm (curved arrow, portal vein). (*B*) Parallel-channel sign (*arrow*) of dilated intrahepatic ducts. One channel represents the dilated duct and the other its accompanying portal vein. (C) Stellate confluence of irregular branching channels (*curved arrows*) represents dilated intrahepatic ducts. Acoustic enhancement (*asterisks*) is seen posterior to the dilated, bile-filled ducts. (*D*) Acoustic enhancement is noted posterior to the dilated biliary radicles. (*E*) An enlarged, palpable Courvoisier gallbladder (gb) was also found.

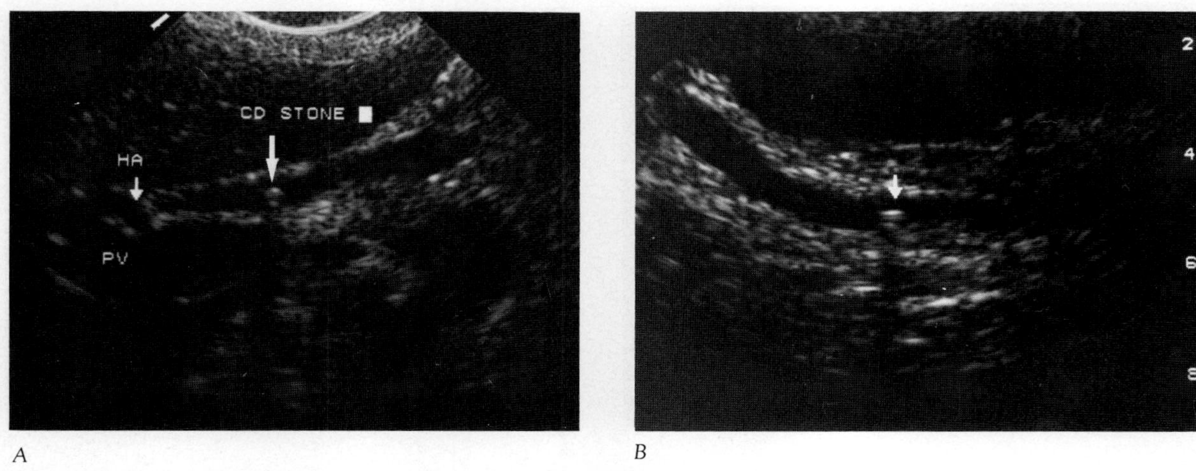

FIGURE 5-40. (*A*) Small common duct stone rolled from proximal to distal portion of duct as the patient moved (HA, hepatic artery, PV, portal vein). (*B*) Distal CBD shows another small mobile stone *(arrow)* in same patient. The duct measured 0.75 cm and there was no intrahepatic dilatation.

tained after cholecystectomy cause recurrent biliary pain.[4]

Choledocholithiasis is the most common cause of obstructive jaundice.[2,74] Patients are generally asymptomatic unless obstruction occurs. Small stones may not obstruct, but symptoms of obstruction include RUQ colicky pain radiating to the right scapula and, with complete obstruction, progressive jaundice. The obstruction can be complete or intermittent (ball-in-valve type).[2,61] With obstruction, direct bilirubin, alkaline phosphatase, AST, and ALT values increase.[2]

Common duct stones are found in 7% to 15% of patients undergoing gallstone surgery[2,16] and even more often in the elderly patient.[2] Common duct stones are often treated surgically. With recent developments in the nonsurgical therapy of gallbladder and common duct calculi, though, this trend may change. Such developments include endoscopic retrograde sphincterotomy (endoscopically guided cutting or enlarging of the sphincter of Oddi so the stone can pass easily into the duodenum), biliary tract extracorporeal shock wave lithotripsy (ESWL fragments stones for easier passage or extraction), percutaneous or endoscopic retrieval with a wire basket, electrohydraulic fragmentation, dissolution with MTBE, and physical fragmentation and extraction.[4,28,41]

Meticulous scanning of the duct in multiple planes and sonographer persistence are required in pursuing this diagnosis.[16,20] The improved technology and resolution of today's real-time units have also significantly improved our ability to detect common duct stones compared to the early 1980s.[20] Stones can be visualized in dilated and even in nondilated ducts (although bile surrounding stones in an enlarged duct is certainly helpful; (Fig. 5-41). The stones may or may not create shadows; they may be single or multiple, large or small, mobile or stationary (Fig. 5-42).[20] The duct can be packed with stones, producing a broad acoustic shadow that makes it difficult to differentiate them from surrounding bowel or resulting in an underestimation of the number of stones in the duct (Fig. 5-43). If visualization of the CBD down to the head of the pancreas is obscured by gas, "water loading" the duodenum may help displace the gas and improve visualization.[20,61] Shadowing from nearby bowel must not be mistaken for shadowing from a stone (Fig. 5-44). The hepatic artery wall and other

Figure 5-41. Choledocholithiasis. Bile surrounding the stone (arrowheads) makes visualization easier (pv, portal vein).

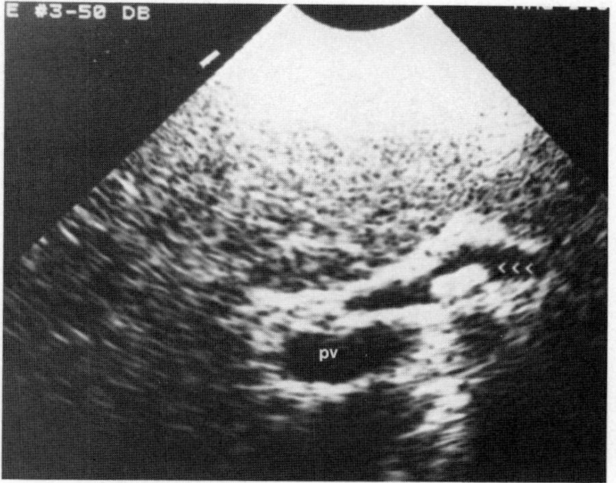

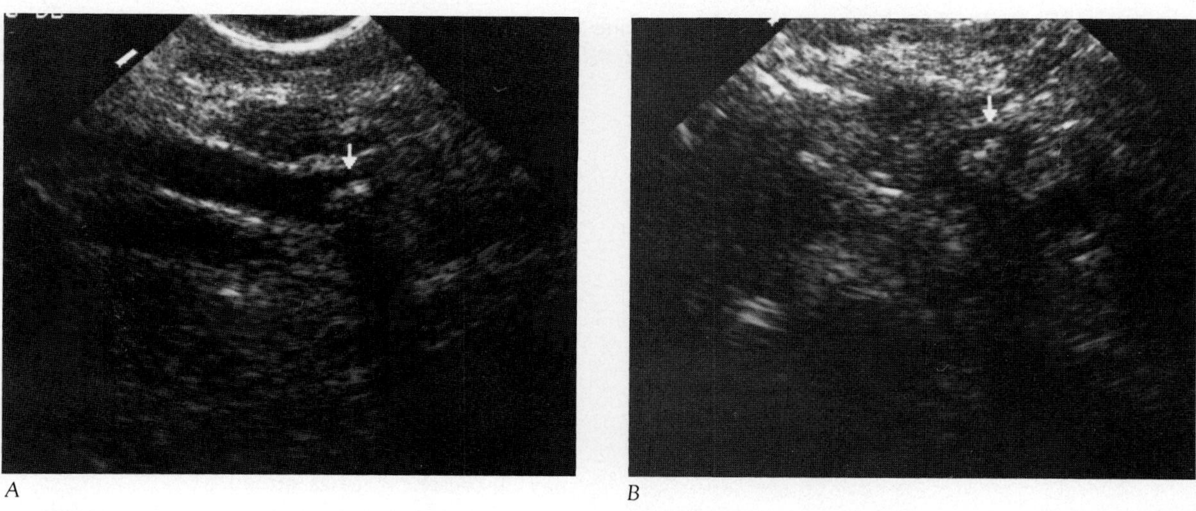

Figure 5-42. Choledocholithiasis. (*A*) Sagittal view of stone (*arrow*) in duct. (*B*) Transverse view of stone (*arrow*) filling lumen of duct. Shadowing can be seen posterior to the stone in both views.

periductal structures may also mimic a stone at first glance. A pseudocalculi effect may also be caused by surgical clips or postoperative scar tissue at the site of the gallbladder bed.[61] Obviously, if stones are found the presence and extent of obstruction must be documented.

Cholangiocarcinoma. Cholangiocarcinoma is a primary malignancy of the duct.[2] Most of these tumors are annular infiltrating scirrhous carcinomas that grow slowly and usually extend along the length of the ducts. A minority of cases have papillary or polypoid tumors.[78] Cholangiocarcinomas

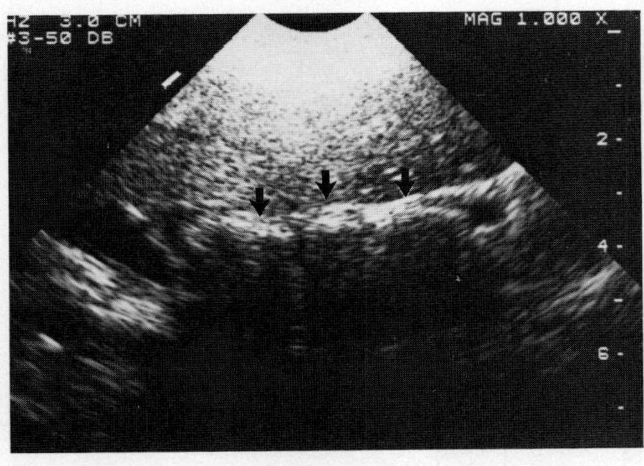

A

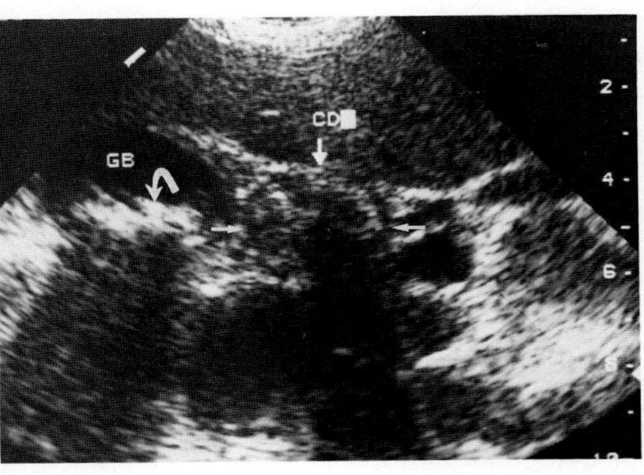

B

Figure 5-43. (*A*) Sagittal view of common duct packed with large stones *(arrows)*, which could mimic a stone-filled gallbladder. (*B*) Transverse view of large common duct stone *(outlined by straight white arrows)* and gallstones *(curved arrow)* in the same patient.

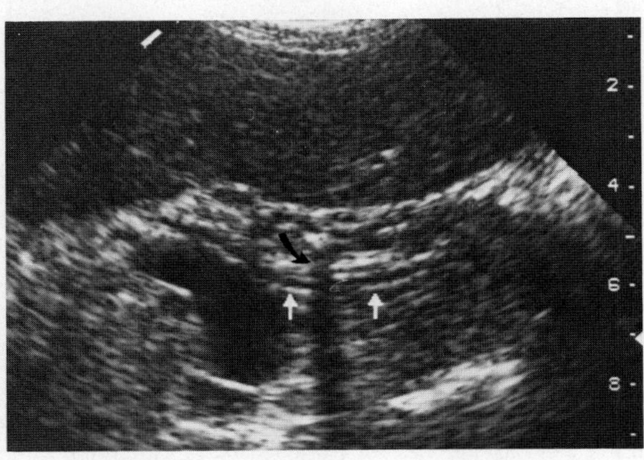

Figure 5-44. In this longitudinal view of the CBD *(white arrows)*, shadowing *(curved black arrow)* comes from the duodenum anterior to the CBD and not from anything in the CBD itself.

usually arise in the larger bile ducts: a third occur in the CBD and only a minority in the intrahepatic ducts. Those that arise high in the CHD near the confluence of the right and left main hepatic ducts are called Klatskin tumors.[2,78] Ampullary carcinomas may also include the distal portion of the CBD.[71]

Signs and symptoms include marked jaundice and a palpable gallbladder if the obstruction is distal to the cystic duct. Hepatomegaly and ascites may be present if it has spread.[2]

A laboratory work-up often reveals markedly elevated direct bilirubin, elevated alkaline phosphatase, and normal to mildly elevated AST and ALT levels.[2]

Cholangiocarcinoma occurs equally in men and women, usually between 50 and 70 years of age. It represents 3% of all cancer deaths in the United States.[2] Nonsurgical percutaneous biliary drainage, which can be selectively guided by ultrasound, can effectively decompress obstructed bile ducts, but this treatment is only palliative. A stent, an endoprosthesis, may be placed to keep the duct patent longer.[43,82] Ultrasound can be used to monitor the effectiveness of such stents by monitoring biliary dilatation.[82] Unfortunately though, death usually occurs in several months.[2]

The tumor itself may be sonographically invisible, since obstruction often occurs when the tumor is quite small. Tumors that are visible may appear as persistent intraluminal soft tissue echoes similar to those of liver parenchyma or as echogenic bands extending across the lumen.[2,52,78] Such intraductal masses may cause local bulging of the walls and enlargement of the lumen. The walls may look intact or the mass may have invaded through with extension to local periductal tissues.[52] Signs of biliary obstruction proximal to the tumor will be seen as well, for example, the "too many tubes" sign. Other signs of malignancy should also be sought: liver metastases, ascites, adenopathy.

The list of differential diagnoses is extensive. Other possible malignant intraductal tumors include hepatocellular carcinoma invading the bile duct, cystadenocarcinoma, metastases of melanoma to the bile ducts, lymphoma or other metastases in the porta hepatis simulating Klatskin tumors, and rhabdomyosarcomas.[29,52,71,78] Benign intraluminal tumors are very rare, but they include cystadenoma (may appear as small cystic structures within the mass), papilloma, adenoma, granular cell myoblastoma, fibroma, neurinoma, leiomyoma, hamartoma, and lipoma.[52,71,78] Other causes of nonshadowing solid intraductal masses include material from a ruptured hydatid cyst, biliary sludge, blood clots, nonshadowing calculi, and congenital bile duct diaphragm (can produce an echogenic intraluminal band).[71,78]

Miscellaneous Pathology of the Biliary Tree

Air in the biliary tree (pneumobilia) can result from surgical causes, such as anastomosis of the biliary tree to bowel, or non-surgical causes, such as gallstone ileus or a patulous sphincter of Oddi in an elderly person allowing air from bowel to reflux into the biliary tree.[51] Sonographically, the air produces "dirty" shadows which move and follow the branching of the portal venous tree (Fig. 5-45). The air moves and rises as the patient changes position. Another possible diagnosis is air in the portal venous system, which can result from necrotic bowel.

Intra- or extrahepatic bile duct dilatation can be found in AIDS patients (despite the absence of stones), possibly indicating an opportunistic biliary tract infection.[72]

Bilomas, collections of bile, can appear as upper abdominal fluid collections.[17]

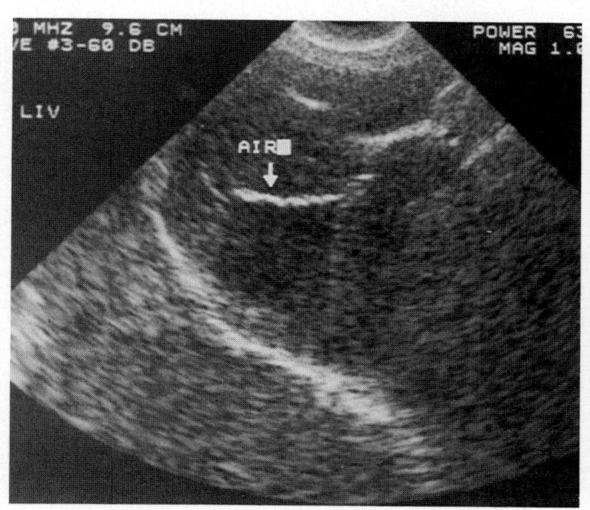

A

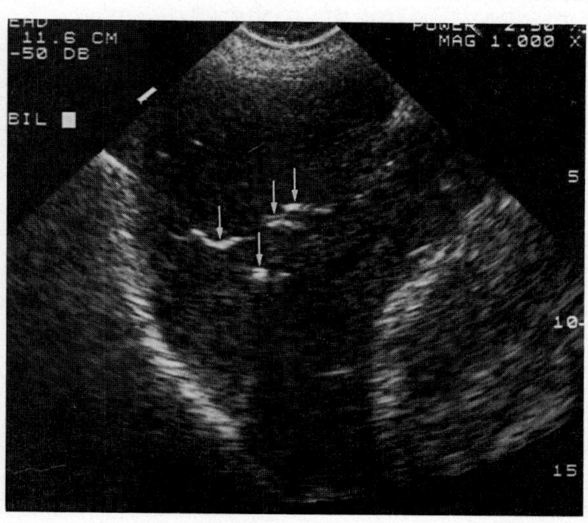

B

Figure 5-45. Air in the biliary tree is demonstrated. (*A*) Highly echogenic air and dirty shadowing posterior to it are seen. (*B*) Air in the intrahepatic ducts *(arrows)* follows the branching pattern of the ducts and portal venous tree. The air moves under real-time observation.

Caroli's disease, communicating cavernous ectasia of the intrahepatic ducts, can appear as segmental tubular fluid collections in the liver.[17]

Sclerosing cholangitis is an inflammation and fibrosis of the bile duct. Intrahepatic calculi are a common complication.[62] Recurrent pyogenic cholangitis, common in Hong Kong, may also be associated with intrahepatic calculi.[13] In general, though, intrahepatic calculi are extremely rare in Western countries.[56]

In some areas of the world, roundworms (Ascaris) may infest the bile ducts and gallbladder and may or may not cause obstruction. Sonographically, the worms appear as long, thin, echogenic, linear structures that move within the bile ducts or gallbladder.[12]

Correlation of Other Diagnostic Imaging Procedures

Plain abdominal radiographs can reveal calcified gallstones (but only 10% to 15% contain sufficient calcium to be visualized), air in the biliary tree, porcelain gallbladder, gas-containing calculi (characteristic stellate appearance of gas collections), and mass effects distorting the abdominal organs.[2,6,18]

Oral cholecystography (OCG) requires the patient to ingest iodinated contrast medium 12 to 14 hours before the examination. A normally functioning gallbladder should opacify on the radiograph, although this study does have limitations. If the gallbladder is poorly visualized or not visualized at all, the OCG is generally repeated the next day.[2] Some feel that a combination of ultrasonography and OCG is superior to either test alone.[69]

Barium-contrast radiographic examinations such as a gastrointestinal (GI) series may confirm the presence of biliary-enteric fistulas (i.e., gallstone ileus), because the barium refluxes into the biliary tree.[51]

Radionuclide scintillation examinations, such as the HIDA scan, are commonly done and require injection of a radioactive tracer such as technetium^{99m}. It is a functional test that can tell if the cystic duct is patent, thus ruling out acute cholecystitis. It will also demonstrate the major bile ducts and excretion of the tracer into the duodenum. Consequently, obstructive choledocholithiasis can also be diagnosed. For investigation of the gallbladder and biliary tree nuclear medicine is better than 90% accurate, but it can generate false positive results[2,16,23] and provides only an isolated view of what is happening in the patient with acute RUQ pain. Ultrasound affords a more global view of the surrounding anatomic structures.

Percutaneous transhepatic cholangiography (PTC) is an invasive procedure performed under x-ray guidance. A small needle is inserted through the liver into the biliary tree. Iodinated contrast medium is used to opacify the bile ducts and evaluate the location and cause of obstructions. Congenital biliary anomalies can also be assessed. While it provides excellent detail, the morbidity and mortality rates are higher than with noninvasive tests.[2,30,76]

Endoscopic retrograde cholangiopancreatography (ERCP) requires the insertion of an endoscope through the esophagus and stomach and then into the duodenum. At that point, radiopaque contrast material can be injected retrograde through the ampulla of Vater to opacify the pancreatic and biliary ducts for radiographic visualization. Common duct stones can be effectively removed endoscopically via sphincterotomy, so ERCP can be therapeutic as well as diagnostic. Although it is a very accurate imaging procedure for biliary disorders, ERCP has definite risks, contraindications, and complications.[13,28,30,61]

Computed tomography (CT) is another ionizing radiation imaging modality that can provide useful information on the biliary system. Dilated bile ducts, intra- and extrahepatic masses, large gallstones, thickened gallbladder wall, and porcelain gallbladder may be detected by CT. CT generally does not produce good images of very thin patients; some intraabdominal fat is necessary to produce optimal images.[2,30]

Conclusion

Ultrasound imaging of the gallbladder and biliary tree is accurate, easy, quick, painless, noninvasive, and carries no risk of ionizing radiation.[18] It has many obvious advantages, but results are very operator dependent: it takes a skilled, educated, well-trained sonographer to produce a high-quality study. Each sonogram depends on the interaction of three elements: sonographer, patient, and equipment. Much diagnostic information can be gained if this interaction is optimal.

Scanning the gallbladder and biliary tree requires perseverance and thorough, meticulous technique. The reward is the ability to detect not only a lot of biliary lesions but many incidental abdominal findings—renal tumors and cysts; hepatic cysts, hemangiomas, and metastases; pancreatic, gastric, and intestinal neoplasms; ascites, aortic aneurysms, pleural effusions, and hydronephrosis.[79] It is counter productive to narrow-mindedly focus on the gallbladder when other chance and pertinent findings may lie nearby.

The future of gallbladder and biliary sonography is an exciting prospect. Manufacturers are constantly introducing more sophisticated equipment with better resolution and greater versatility. Some researchers are even investigating endoscopic biliary sonography using even higher-frequency transducers at close proximity for superior resolution.[77] There is much to look forward to, and ultrasonography will continue to have an important role in the diagnostic evaluation and management of gallbladder and biliary disease.

Acknowledgments

I want especially to thank Stephanie M. Kawamura for her assistance in preparing this manuscript. I also want to thank Jeff Cann for his patience and support, Linda Chase, Mimi Berman, and Ron Panetta for their assistance, and Kathy Gebhart for her meticulous artwork.

References

1. Allen-Mersh TG, Motson RW, Hately W: Does it matter who does ultrasound examination of the GB? Br Med J 1985, 291:389–390.
2. Anderhub B: Manual of Abdominal Sonography. Baltimore, University Park Press, 1983.
3. Becker CD, Burkhardt B, Terrier F: Ultrasound in postoperative acalculous cholecystitis. Gastrointest Radiol 1986, 11:47–50.
4. Becker CD, Fache JS, Gibney RG, et al: Treatment of retained cystic duct stones using extracorporeal shockwave lithotripsy. AJR 1987, 148:1121–1122.
5. Becker CD, Hassler H, Terrier F: Preoperative diagnosis of the Mirizzi syndrome: Limitations of sonography and computed tomography. AJR 1984, 143:591–596.
6. Becker CD, Vock P: Appearance of gas-containing gallstones on sonography and computed tomography. Gastrointest Radiol 1984, 9:323–328.
7. Beckman I, Dash N, Sefczek RJ, et al: Ultrasonographic findings in acute acalculous cholecystitis. Gastrointest Radiol 1985, 10:387–389.
8. Boechat MI, Querfeld U, Dietrich RB, et al: Large echogenic kidneys in biliary atresia. Ann Radiol 1986, 29:660–662.
9. Bressler EL, Rubin JM, McCracken S: Sonographic parallel channel sign: A reappraisal. Radiology 1987, 164:343–346.
10. Cano N, Cicero F, Ranieri F, et al: Ultrasonographic study of gallbladder motility during total parenteral nutrition. Gastroenterology 1986, 91:313–317.
11. Carter, SJ, Rutledge J, Hirsch JH, et al: Papillary adenoma of the gallbladder: Ultrasonic demonstration. J Clin Ultrasound 1978, 6:433–435.
12. Cerri GG, Leite GJ, Simoes JB, et al: Ultrasonographic evaluation of *Ascaris* in the biliary tree. Radiology 1983, 146:753–754.
13. Chau EM, Leong LL, Chan FL: Recurrent pyogenic cholangitis: Ultrasound evaluation compared with endoscopic retrograde cholangiopancreatography. Clin Radiol 1987, 38:79–85.
14. Chesson RR, Gallup DG, Gibbs RL, et al: Ultrasonographic diagnosis of asymptomatic cholelithiasis in pregnancy. J Reprod Med 1985, 30:920–922.
15. Cohan RH, Mahony BS, Bowie JD, et al: Striated intramural gallbladder lucencies on US studies: Predictors of acute cholecystitis. Radiology 1987, 164:31–35.
16. Coletti PM, Ralls PW, Lapin SA, et al: Hepatobiliary imaging in choledocholithiasis. A comparison with ultrasound. Clin Nucl Med 1986, 11:482–486.
17. Cooperberg PL: Gallbladder and Bile Ducts. *In* Goldberg BB (ed): Abdominal Ultrasonography, 2nd ed. New York, John Wiley & Sons, 1984.
18. Cooperberg PL, Gibney RC: Imaging of the gallbladder, 1987. Radiology 1987, 163:605–613.
19. Cover KL, Slasky BS, Skolnick ML: Sonography of cholesterol in the biliary system. J Ultrsound Med 1985, 4:647–653.
20. Cronan JJ: US diagnosis of choledocholithiasis: A reappraisal. Radiology 1986, 161:133–134.
21. Dodds WJ, Groh WJ, Darweesh RM, et al: Sonographic measurement of gallbladder volume. AJR 1985, 145:1009–1011.
22. Doyle TC: Flattened fundus sign of the septate gallbladder. Gastrointest Radiol 1984, 9:345–347.
23. Dykes EH, Wilson N, Gray HW, et al: The role of

^{99m}Tc HIDA cholescintigraphy in the diagnosis of acute gallbladder disease: Comparison with oral cholecystography and ultrasonography. Scott Med J 1986, 31:170–173.
24. Fakhry J: Sonography of tumefactive biliary sludge. AJR 1982, 139:717–719.
25. Fein AB, Rauch RF, Bowie JD, et al: Value of sonographic screening in patients with chest pain and normal coronary arteries. AJR 1986, 146:337–339.
26. Ferin P, Lerner RM: Contracted gallbladder: a finding in hepatic dysfunction. Radiology 1985, 154:769–770.
27. Fitzgerald EJ, Toi A: Pitfalls in the ultrasonographic diagnosis of gallbladder diseases. Postgrad Med J 1987, 63:525–532.
28. Gelfand DW, McCullough DL, Meyers RT, et al: Choledocholithiasis: Successful treatment with extracorporeal lithotripsy. AJR 1987, 148:1114–1116.
29. Geoffray A, Couanet D, Montagne JP, et al: Ultrasonography and computed tomography for diagnosis and follow-up of biliary duct rhabdomyosarcomas in children. Pediatr Radiol 1987, 17:127–131.
30. Gibney RG, Cooperberg PL, Scudamore CH, et al: Segmental biliary obstruction: False negative diagnosis with direct cholangiography without US guidance. Radiology 1987, 164:27–30.
31. Gilbert F, Calder JF, Bayliss AP: Biliary tract dilatation without jaundice demonstrated by ultrasound. Clin Radiol 1985, 36:197–198.
32. Graham N, Manhire AR, Stead RJ, et al: Cystic fibrosis: Ultrasonographic findings in the pancreas and hepatobiliary system correlated with clinical data and pathology. Clin radiol 1985, 36:199–203.
33. Graif M, Horovitz A, Itzchak Y, et al: Hyperechoic foci in the gallbladder wall as a sign of microabscess formation or diverticula. Radiology 1984, 152:781–784.
34. Green D, Carrol BA: Ultrasonography in the jaundiced infant: A new approach. J Ultrasound Med 1986, 5:323–329.
35. Hata K, Aoki S, Hata T, et al: Ultrasonographic identification of the human fetal gallbladder in utero. Gynecol Obstet Invest 1987, 23:79–83.
36. Hopman WP, Rosenbusch G, Jansen JB, et al: Gallbladder contraction: Effects of fatty meals and cholecystokinin. Radiology 1985, 157:37–39.
37. Kaftori JK, Pery M, Green J, et al: Thickness of the gallbladder wall in patients with hypoalbuminemia: A sonographic study of patients on peritoneal dialysis. AJR 1987, 148:1117–1118.
38. Kane RA, Jacobs R, Katz J, et al: Porcelain gallbladder: Ultrasound and CT appearance. Radiology 1984, 152:137–141.
39. Kidney M, Goiney R, Cooperberg PL: Adenomyomatosis of the gallbladder: A pictorial exhibit. J Ultrasound Med 1986, 5:331–333.
40. Kishk Sm, Darweesh RM, Dodds WJ, et al: Sonographic evaluation of resting gallbladder volume and postprandial emptying in patients with gallstones. AJR 1987, 148:875–879.
41. Laffey KJ, Martin EC: Percutaneous removal of large gallstones. Gastrointest Radiol 1986, 11:165–168.
42. Laing FC, Jeffrey RB, Wing VW, et al: Biliary dilatation: Defining the level and cause by real-time US. Radiology 1986, 160:39–42.
43. Lameris JS, Obertop H, Jeekel J: Biliary drainage by ultrsound-guided puncture of the left hepatic duct. Clin Radiol 1985, 36:269–274.
44. Lee LL, McGahan JP: Dissolution of cholesterol gallstones: Comparison of solvents. Gastrointest Radiol 1986, 11:169–171.
45. Lee SP, Maher K, Nicholls JF: Origin and fate of biliary sludge. Gastroenterology 1988, 94:170–176.
46. Lefkof IR, Frenkiel PG, Lee DW, et al: Effect of diet on dissolution of gallstones by ursodeoxycholic acid, including a comparison between ultrasonography and cholecystography. Mt Sinai J Med 1986, 53:241–249.
47. Lev-Toaff AS, Friedman AC, Rindsberg SN, et al: Multiseptate gallbladder: Incidental diagnosis on sonography. AJR 1987, 148:1119–1120.
48. Lim HJ, Ko YT, Kim SY: Ultrasound changes of the gallbladder wall in cholecystitis: A sonographic-pathological correlation. Clin Radiol 1987, 38:389–393.
49. Lin KY: Acute acalculous cholecystitis: A limited review of the literature. Mt Sinai J Med 1986, 53:305–309.
50. Lohela P, Soiva M, Suramo I, et al: Ultrasonic guidance for percutaneous puncture and drainage in acute cholecystitis. Acta Radiol (Diagn) 1986, 27:543–546.
51. Maglinte DD, Lappas JC, Ng AC: Sonography of Bouveret's syndrome. J Ultrasound Med 1987, 6:675–677.
52. Marchal G, Gelin J, Van Steenbergen W, et al: Sonographic diagnosis of intraluminal bile duct neoplasm: A report of three cases. Gastrointest radiol 1984, 9:329–333.
53. Marchal GJ, VanHolsbeeck M, Tshibwabwa-Ntumba E, et al: Dilatation of the cystic veins in portal hypertension: Sonographic demonstration. Radiology 1985, 154:187–189.
54. Maresca G, DeGaetano Am, Mirk P, et al: Sonographic patterns of the gallbladder in acute viral hepatitis. J Clin Ultrasound 1984, 12:141–146.
55. Martinez A, Bona X, Velasco M, et al: Diagnostic ac-

curacy of ultrasound in acute cholecystitis. Gastrointest Radiol 1986, 11:334–338.

56. Menu Y, Lorphelin JM, Scherrer A, et al: Sonographic and computed tomographic evaluation of intrahepatic calculi. AJR 1985, 145:579–583.
57. Mintz MC, Grumbach K, Arger PH, et al: Sonographic evaluation of bile duct size during pregnancy. AJR 1985, 145:575–578.
58. Munster AM, Goodwin MN, Pruitt BA: Acalculous cholecystitis in burned patients. Am J Surg 1971, 122:591–593.
59. Netter FH: The CIBA Collection of Medical Illustrations, 2nd ed. vol 3 (Digestive System), part III (Liver, Biliary Tract, and Pancreas). Summit, NJ, CIBA Pharmaceutical Company, 1964.
60. O'Connor HJ, Bartlett RJ, Hamilton I, et al: Bile duct calibre: The discrepancy between ultrasonic and retrograde cholangiographic measurement in the postcholecystectomy patient. Clin Radiol 1985, 36:507–510.
61. O'Connor HJ, Hamilton I, Ellis WR, et al: Ultrasound detection of choledocholithiasis: Prospective comparison with ERCP in the postcholecystectomy patient. Gastrointest Radiol 1986, 11:161–164.
62. Odwin CS, Dubinsky T, Fleischer AC: General Abdominal Sonography Examination. Ultrasonography Examination Review and Study Guide. Norwalk, CT, Appleton & Lange, 1987.
63. Parulekar SG: Ultrasonic detection of calcification in gallstones: "The reverberation shadow." J Ultrasound Med 1984, 3:123–129.
64. Parulekar SG: Evaluation of the prone view for cholecystosonography. J Ultrsound Med 1986, 5:617–624.
65. Phillips G, Pochaczevsky R, Goodman J, et al: Ultrasound patterns of metastatic tumors in the gallbladder. J Clin Ultrasound 1982, 10:379–383.
66. Quinn SF, Fazzio F, Jones E: Torsion of the gallbladder: Findings on CT and sonography and role of percutaneous cholecystectomy. AJR 1987, 148:881–882.
67. Raghavendra BN, Subramanyam BR, Balthazar EJ, et al: Sonography of adenomyomatosis of the gallbladder: Radiologic-pathologic correlation. Radiology 1983, 146:747–752.
68. Raptopoulos V, Smith EH, Karellas A, et al: Daytime constancy of bile duct diameter. AJR 1987, 148:557–558.
69. Richter JM, Christensen MR, Simeone JF, et al: Chronic cholecystitis. An analysis of diagnostic strategies. Invest Radiol 1987, 22:111–117.
70. Riddlesberger MM: Diagnostic imaging of the hepatobiliary system in infants and children. J Pediatr Gastroenterol Nutr 1984, 3:653–664.
71. Robledo R, Prieto ML, Perez M, et al: Carcinoma of the hepaticopancreatic ampullar region: Role of US. Radiology 1988, 166:409–412.
72. Romano AJ, vanSonnenberg E, Casola G, et al: Gallbladder and bile duct abnormalities in AIDS: Sonographic findings in eight patients. AJR 1988, 150:123–127.
73. Ros PR, Viamonte M, Soila K, et al: Demonstration of cavernomatous transformation of the portal vein by magnetic resonance imaging. Gastrointest Radiol 1986, 11:90–92.
74. Simeone JF, Butch RJ, Mueller PR, et al: The bile ducts after a fatty meal: Further sonographic observations. Radiology 1985, 154:763–768.
75. Soiva M, Suramo I, Taavitsainen M: Ultrasonography of the gallbladder in patients with a clinical suspicion of acute cholecystitis. Diagn Imaging Clin Med 1986, 55:337–342.
76. Stringer DA, Dobranowski J, Ein SH, et al: Interposition of the gallbladder—or the absent common hepatic duct and cystic duct. Pediatr Radiol 1987, 17:151–153.
77. Strohm WD, Kurtz W, Classen M: Detection of biliary stones by means of endosonography. Scand J. Gastroenterol 1984, 19 (suppl 94):60–64.
78. Subramanyam BR, Raghavendra BN, Balthazar EJ, et al: Ultrasonic features of cholangiocarcinoma. J Ultrasound Med 1984, 3:405–408.
79. Suramo I, Paivansalo M, Pamilo M: Chance findings in ultrasonography of the gallbladder and the abdominal organs. Ann Clin Res 1984, 16 (suppl 40):55–57.
80. Suramo I, Paivansalo M, Vuoria P: Shadowing and reverberation artifacts in abdominal ultrasonography. Eur J Radiol 1985, 5:147–151.
81. Tsujimoto F, Miyamoto Y, Tada S: Differentiation of benign from malignant ascites by sonographic evaluation of gallbladder wall. Radiology 1985, 157:503–504.
82. VanGansbeke D, de Toeuf J, Cremer M, et al: Suprahepatic gallbladder: A rare congenital anomaly. Gastrointest Radiol 1984, 9:341–343.
83. VanGansbeke D, Van Gossum A, Schils J, et al: Sonographic monitoring of biliary endoprostheses. Gastrointest Radiol 1984, 9:335–339.
84. van Weedle BJ, Oudkerk M, Koch CW: Ultrasonography of acute cholecystitis: Clinical and histological correlation. Diagn Imaging Clin Med 1986, 55:190–195.
85. Weiner SN, Koenigsberg M, Morehouse H, et al: Sonography and computed tomography in the diagnosis of carcinoma of the gallbladder. AJR 1984, 142:735–739.
86. Williamson SL, Williamson MR: Cholecystosonog-

raphy in pregnancy. J Ultrasound Med 1984, 3:329–331.

87. Willson SA, Gosink BB, vanSonnenberg E: Unchanged size of dilated common bile duct after a fatty meal: Results and significance. Radiology 1986, 160:29–31.
88. Wing VW, Laing FC, Jeffrey RB, et al: Sonographic differentiation of enlarged hepatic arteries from dilated intrahepatic bile ducts. AJR 1985, 145:57–61.
89. Yeh HC, Goodman J, Rabinowitz JG: Floating gallstones in bile without added contrast material. AJR 1986, 146:49–50.

CHAPTER 6

Pancreas

JIM BAUN

Anatomy

The pancreas, both an endocrine and exocrine gland, is pinkish yellow and situated obliquely in the anterior portion of the retroperitoneum. It consists of three main portions, head, body, and tail. The head is situated to the right and is inferior to the body and tail, a fact that must be borne in mind when attempting transverse sonographic imaging. The head has the greatest anteroposterior (AP) diameter of any portion of the gland and is tucked into the duodenal sweep. Extending posterior and medial from the head is a beaklike projection of pancreatic tissue, the uncinate process. The uncinate process may be seen just behind the portal confluence in transverse sections. The body and tail of the pancreas are bounded anteriorly and superiorly by portions of the stomach, duodenum, and left lobe of the liver. The pancreatic body sits in front of the epigastric prevertebral vessels, which provide identifying landmarks during upper abdominal sonography. The tail of the pancreas extends into the left anterior pararenal space and lies anterior to the left kidney and medial to the splenic hilus. The pancreas is a nonencapsulated retroperitoneal structure with the peritoneal membrane traversing the anterior aspect of the organ (Fig. 6-1).

Successful cross-sectional sonographic imaging of the pancreatic bed requires a detailed understanding of the surrounding prevertebral vasculature. Blood supply to the pancreas itself is provided by branches of the gastroduodenal, splenic, and superior mesenteric arteries, all of which should be identified during the examination process (Fig. 6-2). The gastroduodenal artery is a branch of the common hepatic artery, which perforates the pancreatic parenchyma along the superior aspect of the head. Branches of the splenic and superior mesenteric arteries enter the pancreas at numerous points along the body and provide necessary perfusion.[54] In cross-section the head of the pancreas is seen anterior to the inferior vena cava, with the gastroduodenal artery within the head just anterior to the common bile duct (Fig. 6-3).

The body of the pancreas is seen anterior to the aorta and superior mesenteric artery. Between these structures and the pancreatic parenchyma, the splenic vein may be identified as it courses toward its confluence with the inferior mesenteric vein. The constricted pancreatic neck may be seen just anterior to this confluence, where the vessels merge to form the portal vein. In many patients the left lobe of the liver lies between the body and the anterior abdominal wall. Branches of the celiac axis, namely the hepatic, left gastric, and splenic arteries, course along the superior border of the body.

The tail of the pancreas extends from the body into the left upper quadrant. Bordered posteriorly by the splenic vein, it frequently is found extending in the region of the splenic hilus. The tail is bordered anteriorly by the stomach and laterally by the left kidney. Because of its proximity to the

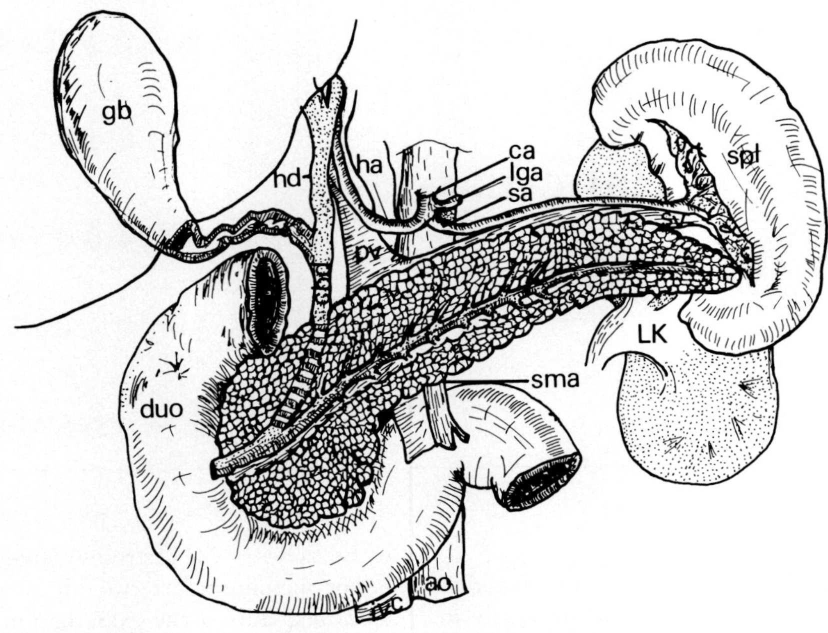

Figure 6-1. Gross anatomy of the peripancreatic area, demonstrating the relationship of the various prevertebral vessels and surrounding upper abdominal organs (gb, gallbladder; hd, common hepatic duct; cbd, common bile duct; duo, duodenum; ha, hepatic artery; pv, portal vein; ca, celiac axis; lga, left gastric artery; sa, splenic artery; sma, superior mesenteric artery; ao, aorta; ivc, inferior vena cava; spl, spleen; LK, left kidney).

stomach, care should be taken when imaging to avoid mistaking a pancreatic tail mass for fluid in the stomach.

The largest mass of pancreatic parenchyma consists of small groups of acini, which secrete digestive enzymes, clustered in multiple lobules, each surrounding a tributary duct. The smaller ducts merge into increasingly larger ducts, subsequently emptying into the main pancreatic duct, or duct of Wirsung. Exocrine secretions, or pancreatic juice, is carried by the main pancreatic duct into the alimentary tract via the ampulla of Vater. Near the ampulla, the main pancreatic duct merges with the distal common bile duct to produce a single perforating channel into the duodenum (Fig. 6-4). A normal variation of this configuration exists in which an accessory duct, the duct of Santorini, branches from the main pancreatic duct and perforates into the duodenum separately from the ampulla.[11]

Wedged within the acinar lobules, like islands, are groups of endocrine cells known as the islets of Langerhans. These clusters contain various types of cells that release their products directly into the blood and lymph. This internal, or endocrine, secretion of hormones permits them to be distributed throughout the body, where they stimulate other organs or functional tissues. The principal endocrine secretions of the pancreas are insulin and glucagon.

Physiology

The physiologic functions of the pancreas can be categorized as either endocrine or exocrine. Insulin and glucagon are the primary endocrine secretions.

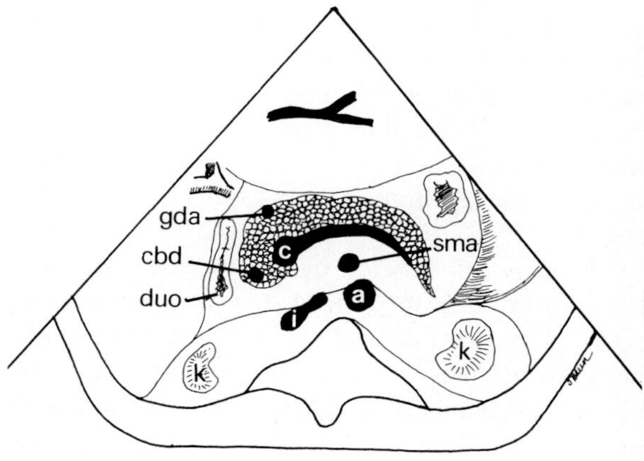

A

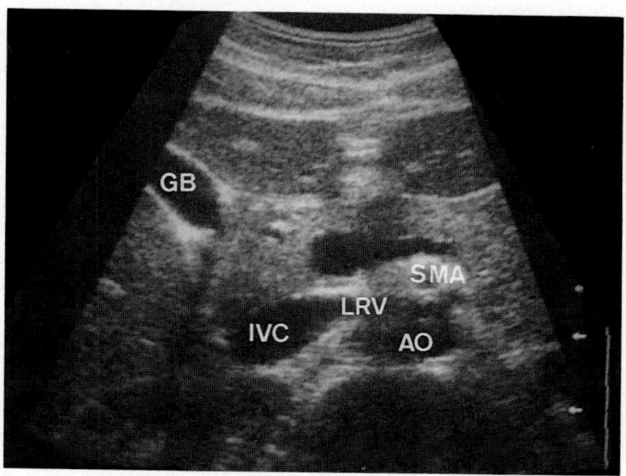

B

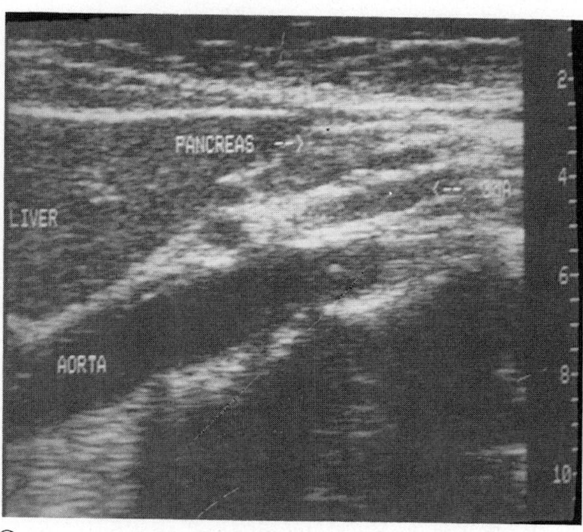

C

Figure 6-2. (*A*) Transverse view demonstrates the relationship between the pancreas and other upper abdominal organs (gda, gastroduodenal artery; cbd, common bile duct; duo, duodenum; sma, superior mesenteric artery; i, inferior vena cava; a, aorta; c, portal confluence; k, kidney). (*B*) Transverse sonogram demonstrates the prevertebral vasculature normally seen during pancreatic sonography (SMA, superior mesenteric artery; AO, aorta; IVC, inferior vena cava; GB, gallbladder, LRV, left renal vein). (C) Sagittal sonogram through the pancreas demonstrates adjacent anatomic structures.

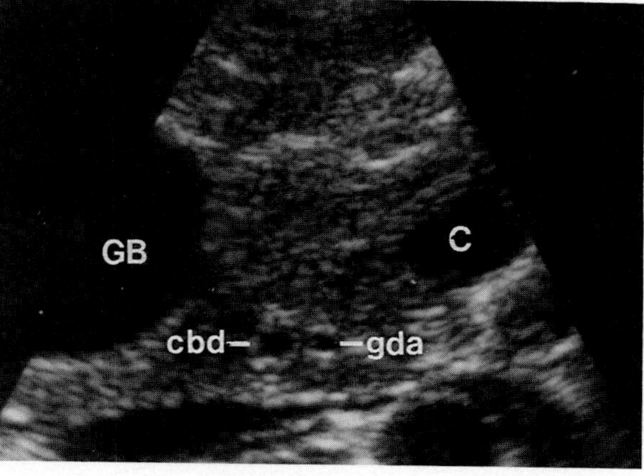

Figure 6-3. Transverse sonogram demonstrates the gastroduodenal artery (gda) and common bile duct (cbd) as they course into the pancreas (GB, gallbladder; C, portal venous confluence).

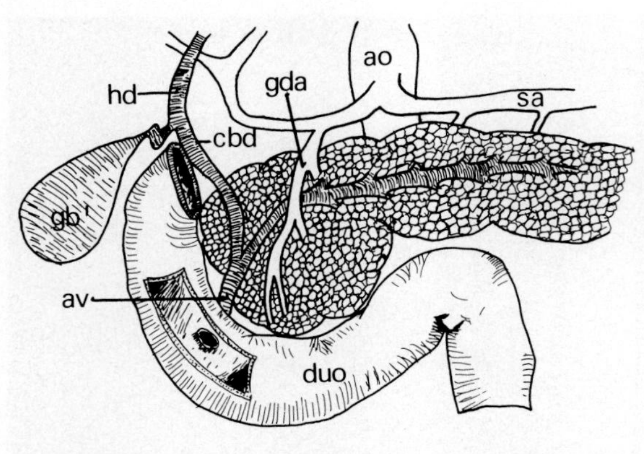

FIGURE 6-4. Line drawing demonstrates common bile duct (cbd) and pancreatic duct as they merge and enter the ampulla of Vater (av; duo, duodenum; gda, gastroduodenal artery; hd, hepatic duct; ao, aorta; sa, splenic artery; gb, gallbladder).

Insulin is a necessary element in the metabolism of carbohydrates, a process that provides energy for the body's many and varied functions. By facilitating the transport of glucose across cell membranes, insulin increases the energy available for normal physiologic functions. It also influences the metabolism of proteins and fats. It is released by the pancreas as a direct result of a negative feedback mechanism. When the blood glucose level rises above a certain level, believed to be 100 mg/dl, the beta cells in the islets of Langerhans immediately exude insulin.[60] When the blood glucose level falls, insulin secretion decreases. Many other factors—autonomic nervous system responses, the release of other endocrine hormones, certain drugs—also affect the secretion of insulin.[11] Abnormalities of insulin secretion result in impairment of metabolic functions throughout the body. Diabetes results from an imbalance between insulin secretion and the metabolic needs of the body.

Glucagon, secreted by alpha cells in the islets of Langerhans, is another potent endocrine pancreatic enzyme. It functions primarily in the liver and aids in conversion of glycogen into glucose, or usable energy. As with insulin, blood glucose levels initiate the release of the hormone.

Exocrine function may be defined as the external secretions of a gland. These secretions generally accumulate in small ductules or intercellular spaces and eventually leave the gland through a larger duct. The primary pancreatic exocrine secretion, pancreatic juice, is essential to the digestion of foodstuffs. Chemical analysis of pancreatic juice shows that it consists of water, inorganic salts such as potassium, sodium, and calcium, and digestive enzymes.

The enzymes secreted by the pancreas are amylase, lipase, trypsinogen, and chymotrypsinogen, all of which are essential to the digestion and ultimate absorption of essential nutrients. Amylase breaks down complex carbohydrates into usable sugars; lipase is an enzyme that breaks down fats; and trypsinogen and chymotrypsinogen are preproteolytic enzymes that reduce proteins to their component amino acids. Additionally, some of these substances play an important role in the pathogenesis of pancreatic disease, especially in pancreatitis. The preproteolytic enzymes in the normal pancreas are inert. It is postulated that an inhibiting factor is secreted by the same cells that secrete exocrine enzymes. This inhibiting factor prevents trypsinogen and chymotrypsin from autodigesting the protein in the cell walls of the pancreas. With injury or disease the inhibiting factor is unable to prevent the activation of proteolytic enzymes, which spill out into the surrounding parenchyma. Once the process begins, it can advance rapidly, each bursting cell releasing yet more digestive juice, reducing normal tissue to amorphous fluid.[30] Another component of pancreatic juice is the alkaline substance bicarbonate, which neutralizes the acidic gastric enzymes and triggers the action of the otherwise inert pancreatic enzymes in the duodenum. The pancreas is capable of secreting up to 4 liters of exocrine fluid per day.[60]

Sectional Views with Sonographic Correlations

TRANSVERSE

Transverse sonograms through the pancreas should demonstrate the prevertebral vascular landmarks as well as the gland itself. The pancreas may be identified as a crescent-shaped structure draping over the prevertebral vessels (Fig. 6-5A). It has been described variously as horseshoe-, dumbbell-, and comma shaped.[55] Normally, its echogenicity is

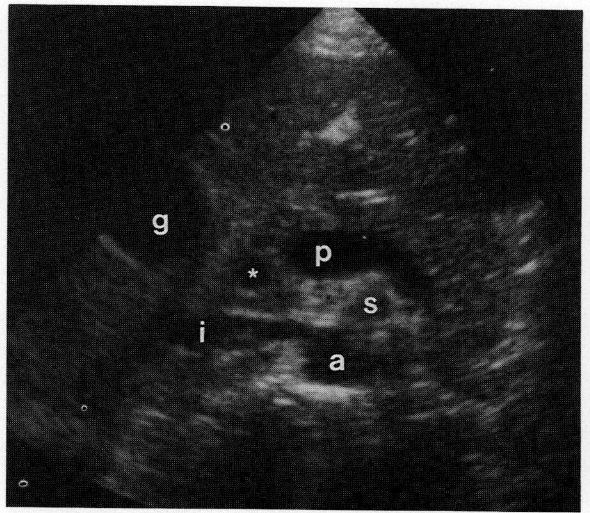

A

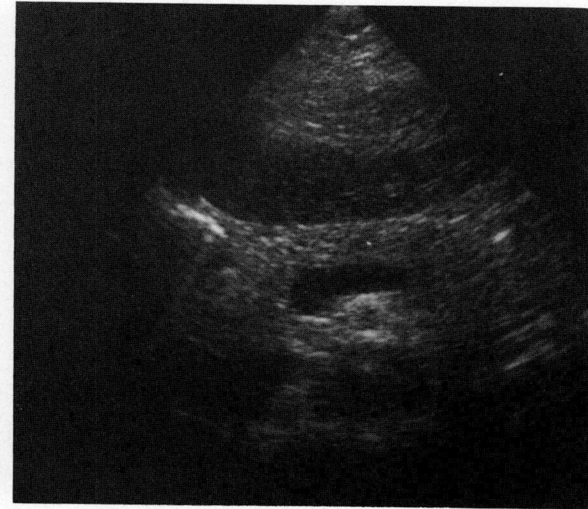

B

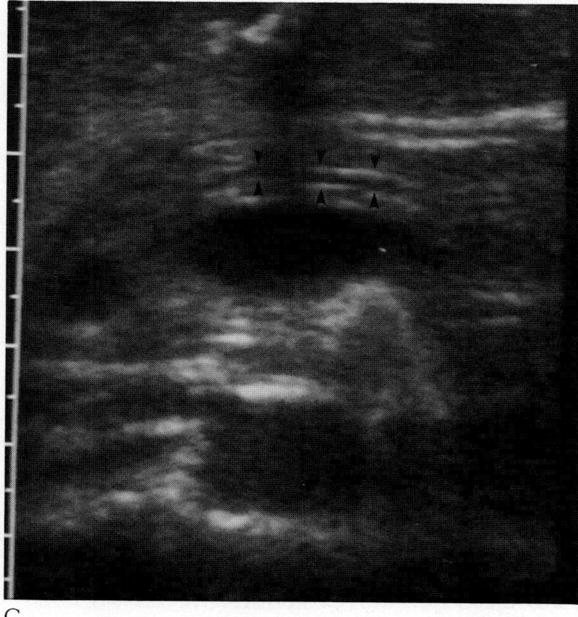

C

FIGURE 6-5. (*A*) Transverse sonogram through upper abdomen demonstrates the normal pancreas and adjacent structures (g, gallbladder; i, inferior vena cava; a, aorta; s, superior mesenteric artery; p, portal venous confluence; *, common bile duct). (*B*) Transverse sonogram demonstrates increased pancreatic echogenicity due to increased fat deposition. (C) Visualization of a normal pancreatic duct is indicated between arrowheads.

equal to or greater than that of the liver, but this depends on the patient's age and body habitus.[21] Fat deposition in the interlobular areas is the most likely explanation for the varying degrees of pancreatic echogenicity and may, in fact, cause contour alterations (Fig. 6-5B).[53] Children have less fat than adults, so the hypoechoic character noted in pediatric patients is a normal finding (see Chapter 15).[34] While varying degrees of echogenicity may be found in normal organs, most authors agree that a hypoechoic pancreas represents an abnormal finding.[21] With high-resolution real-time scanners, the pancreatic duct is frequently seen in normal patients (Fig. 6-5C),[18,70] most commonly in the body of the pancreas, as two parallel linear echoes surrounding an anechoic lumen.[57] The AP diameter of a normal duct should not exceed 2 mm, and the contour of the walls should be smooth without any areas of focal dilatation.[10]

The dimensions of the pancreas are best assessed using a true transverse plane of section. It is important to align the transducer so that the incident beam intersects the pancreas perpendicular to its transverse axis. The head is the widest portion of the gland, the AP dimension measuring no more than 2.5 cm. The body is thinner than the head and normally measures not more than about 1.2 cm.[55] The tail may be difficult to image from a projection that provides a true AP measurement, but in the normal gland it usually does not exceed 2.0 cm (Fig. 6-6).[59] A child's pancreas is smaller than an adults (Table 6-1) but relative to other upper abdominal organs such as the liver and kidneys, it may appear larger.

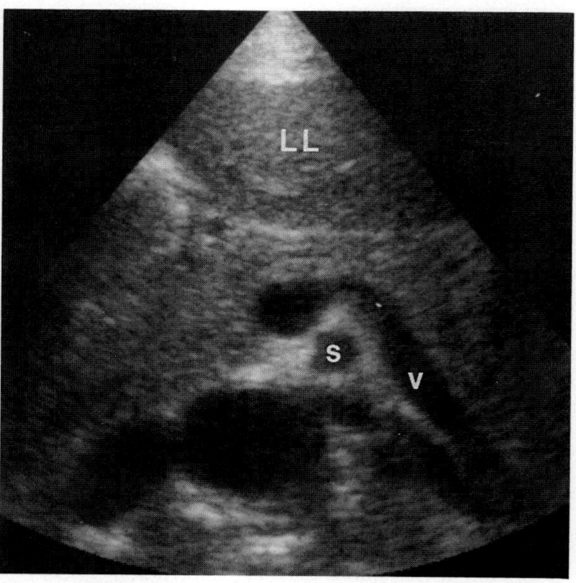

Figure 6-6. Transverse sonogram demonstrates the body of the pancreas and adjacent structures (LL, left lobe of liver; S, superior mesenteric artery; V, splenic vein).

Sagittal

Sagittally, the pancreas may be identified as an ovoid or circular structure lying anterior to the prevertebral vessels (Fig. 6-7). Its AP thickness varies considerably with the level of section, the head being the thickest and usually the most easily demonstrable. From a slightly oblique sagittal section, the common bile duct may be seen traversing the head and joining the pancreatic duct. Anterior to the bile duct the gastroduodenal artery may be seen (Fig. 6-8A). The neck appears as a narrow structure just anterior to the anastomosis of the superior mesenteric and the splenic veins (Fig. 6-8B). The body can be seen anterior to the superior mesenteric artery (SMA) and posterior to the left lobe of the liver. In a true sagittal section through the left anterior pararenal space, the tail appears thicker than the other portions because it is being transsected as it dips posteriorly.

Sonographic Examination Technique

Preparation

Preparation for pancreatic sonography attempts to minimize the amount of gas in the stomach and duodenum by having the patient refrain from eating or drinking anything for 8 to 12 hours before the examination. The patient should also avoid smoking or chewing gum, since both activities increase the amount of swallowed air. Small sips of water or ice chips may be allowed, especially for patients

Table 6-1. Normal pancreatic measurements[12,56,61,67]

Patient's Age (yr)	Head (cm) Standard (Range)	Body (cm) Standard (Range)	Tail (cm) Standard (Range)
0–6	1.6 (1.0–1.9)	0.7 (0.4–1.0)	1.2 (0.8–1.6)
7–12	1.9 (1.7–2.0)	0.9 (0.6–1.0)	1.4 (1.3–1.6)
13–18	2.0 (1.8–2.2)	1.0 (0.7–1.0)	1.6 (1.3–1.8)
> 18	≦ 2.5	≦ 1.25	≦ 2.0

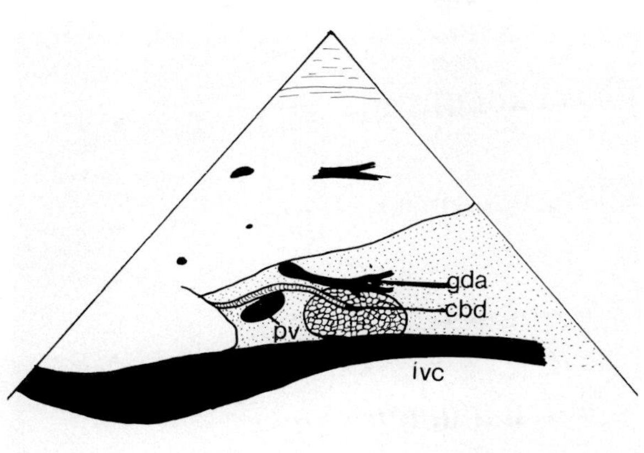

FIGURE 6-7. Sagittal line drawing of the pancreas and related upper abdominal organs (pv, portal vein; cbd, common bile duct; gda, gastroduodenal artery; ivc, inferior vena cava).

who dehydrate easily: decreased water content in the tissues also inhibits transmission of the acoustic beam. Additionally, the examination should be performed in the morning, before air ingested during normal swallowing and talking accumulates in the stomach and duodenum. Pancreatic sonography is contraindicated for patients who have undergone gastroscopic examination within 6 hours because large amounts of air are introduced into the stomach during this procedure. Since the head of the pancreas is intimately related to the duodenum, gas present here as well as in the transverse colon, which overlies the pancreas, may easily obscure visualization.

INDICATIQNS

Pancreatic sonography is indicated for suspected inflammatory diseases such as acute or chronic pan-

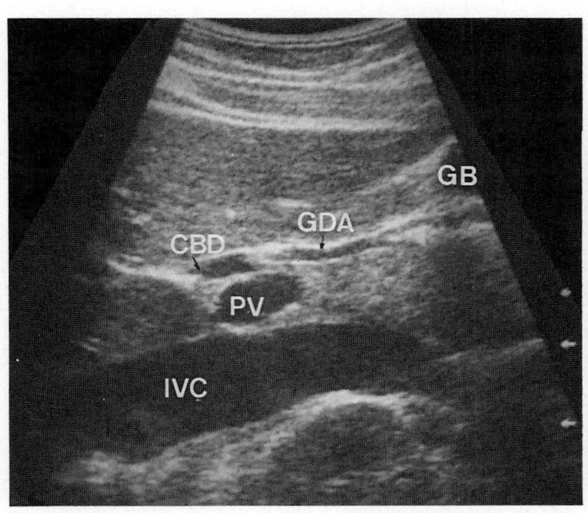

A

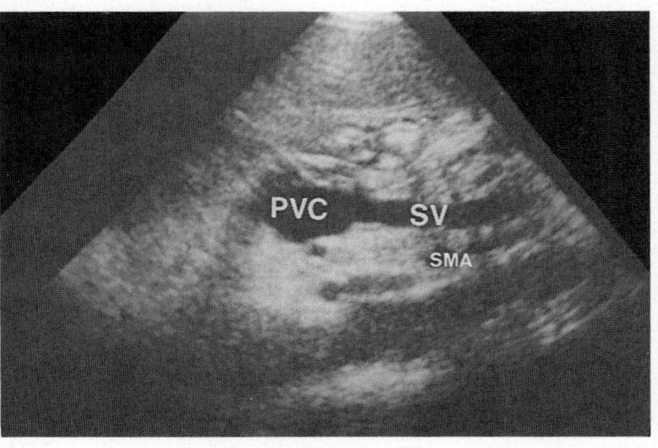

B

FIGURE 6-8. (*A*) Sagittal section through head of pancreas demonstrates common bile duct (CBD) and gastroduodenal artery (GDA; GB, gallbladder; PV, portal vein; IVC, inferior vena cava). (*B*) Sagittal section through pancreatic neck demonstrates the superior mesenteric vein anastomosing with the splenic vein at the portal venous confluence (SV, splenic vein; SMA, superior mesenteric artery).

creatitis or neoplastic disease of the pancreas.[5] Neoplastic diseases, which are discussed in detail later, include acinar cell adenocarcinoma, benign adenomas and cystadenomas, squamous cell carcinomas, adenocanthomas, insulinomas, gastrinomas, and glucagonomas. Because of the pitfalls associated with the presence of gas in the alimentary tract, computed tomography (CT) is generally the method of choice for adult pancreatic imaging. Sonography is useful, however, as a primary screening procedure in cases where suspicion of pancreatic disease is low or as a follow-up procedure in patients who have had a successful previous examination.[8,31,33,36,43,68] Because of the relative cost effectiveness of ultrasound over other imaging modalities it should be the first examination technique when pancreatic disease is suspected. In patients with known neoplastic disease, staging and follow-up is best accomplished with CT.

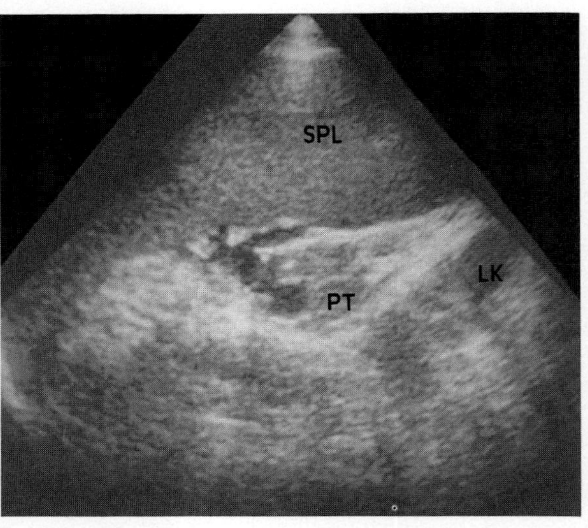

FIGURE 6-9. Coronal section through the tail of the pancreas (SPL, spleen; PT, tail of pancreas; LK, upper pole of left kidney).

PROCEDURE AND PROTOCOL

The initial examination begins with the patient supine. Using the left lobe of the liver as a window, the transducer is aligned in a tranverse position, just below the xiphoid process. A slight caudal angulation is applied, and the transducer position is adjusted so that the prevertebral vessels are identified. Instructing the patient to take a deep breath usually enhances the liver's usefulness as an acoustic window. During deep inspiration the liver and diaphragm move inferiorly and over the pancreas. Since the head of the pancreas usually sits below the body and tail, rotating the probe counterclockwise a few degrees may permit visualization of the entire organ in a single image; however, this is not normally the case, and additional acoustic windows must be found to image the various portions of the pancreas. The head and body are imaged most frequently and can be seen to good advantage 77% and 70% of the time, respectively.[17,59]

The pancreatic tail can present a difficult imaging challenge. Bordered anteriorly by the stomach and splenic flexure of the colon, it is frequently obscured by air that has accumulated in the lumen of one or both of these organs. The tail of the pancreas is demonstrated in only 37% of patients on routine sonographic examination.[59] There are alternative approaches to imaging the tail using various acoustic windows. By rotating the patient into the right lateral decubitus or prone position the examiner can attempt to image through the left lateral or posterior intercostal spaces. In using the lateral approach, it should be remembered that the plane of section is now coronal with the near field representing lateral and the far field representing medial (Fig. 6-9).[45] With the patient prone, the tail of the pancreas may be seen anterior to the left kidney. Although this approach produces limited results, it may be useful when other approaches have failed.[27]

Another technique, imaging the pancreas in patients with small left lobes or excessive gas, involves having the patient drink approximately 150 ml of water through a straw. The patient can be examined either upright or in the left lateral decubitus position, depending on which position provides the best acoustic window (Fig. 6-10). Most examiners prefer to begin with the upright position, since air in the stomach rises above the water to lodge in the fundus. Pitfalls to this approach include the swallowing of even more air and subsequent annihilation of partially useful acoustic windows.

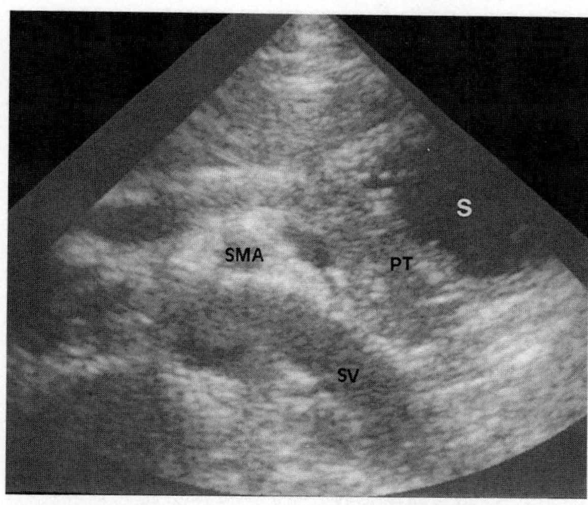

Figure 6-10. Transverse section through the tail (PT) using the water-filled stomach(s) technique (SMA, superior mesenteric artery; SV, splenic vein).

Pathology

Laboratory Examinations

Amylase, an enzyme essential in the digestion of fats, is one of the most useful laboratory values for the diagnosis of pancreatic disease. In a diseased pancreas, disintegrating acinar cells release their digestive enzymes into the organ's parenchyma, and ultimately into the capillaries that supply the diseased area. Normal serum amylase values vary with the method used to measure them. Generally, 80 to 180 units per deciliter of serum is considered normal. With acute pancreatitis, the amylase level largely increases, starting 3 to 6 hours after the first signs of clinical symptoms. The elevated level persists for approximately 24 hours after the acute episode and then begins to decrease.[22] Amylase elevation also occurs in chronic pancreatitis (acute attack), partial gastrectomy, obstruction of pancreatic duct, perforated peptic ulcer, alcohol poisoning, acute cholecystitis, and intestinal obstruction and strangulation.

Amylase is excreted in the urine and may be found in nonpathologic states. Normal urinary amylase values range between 40 and 250 units. In pancreatitis, it remains elevated for up to 7 days after serum values have returned to normal. Elevation of the serum amylase without concurrent elevation of the urinary amylase value may represent a pathologic process not related to pancreatic disease.[63] A decreased amylase value is associated with hepatitis and cirrhosis of the liver.[13] Because the amylase test is not specific for acute pancreatitis, some authorities recommend that the diagnosis of acute pancreatitis be based on clinical symptoms.[64]

Lipase is a fat-splitting enzyme excreted by the pancreas. It is released into the bloodstream in increased quantities in the presence of inflammatory (and occasionally neoplastic) pancreatic disease. Normal serum lipase values range from 0.2 to 1.5 units. Elevation indicates pancreatitis or pancreatic duct obstruction.[63] The lipase level remains elevated longer (up to 14 days) than amylase level, which is particularly helpful when patients wait to seek medical attention until days after the onset of clinical symptoms. Lipase elevation also occurs in patients with obstruction of the pancreatic duct, pancreatic carcinoma, acute cholecystitis, cirrhosis, and severe renal disease.[4]

Fecal fat values reveal the amount of undigested fat molecules passing through the alimentary tract. In normal physiologic states, the fat content of human feces should be less than 30% of the dry weight of the specimen. An increase indicates that pancreatic enzyme function is altered, as it may be in both acute and chronic pancreatitis. Excess of fat in the feces (steatorrhea) is symptomatic of pancreatitis.

Important to understanding the significance of other laboratory tests in the evaluation of pancreatic function is an appreciation of the anatomic relationship of structures surrounding the pancreas, especially the relationship between the pancreatic head and the common bile duct. This explains the elevation of bilirubin and other liver function values that are frequently associated with pancreatic disease. Pathologic processes in one structure may cause disease in the other. Neoplasia or inflammatory enlargement of the head of the pancreas frequently causes stenosis or complete obstruction of the distal common bile duct. In such cases, total serum bilirubin values are above the normal 1.1 to 1.2 mg/dl. Conversely, biliary duct disease, such as calculi and subsequent inflammation, may spread into the pancreas. Altered biliary and hepatic function values may suggest an underlying pancreatic process.

Inflammatory Diseases

Acute Pancreatitis. In acute pancreatitis, all or part of the pancreas is inflamed. Most often it is caused by excessive intake of alcohol or concomitant biliary tract disease, acute pancreatitis is characterized by an edematous, enlarged gland; subsequently there is a breakdown of the pancreatic architecture. It is believed that blockage of the pancreatic ductules leads to a release of digestive enzymes, which lyse cell walls.[11] Duct obstruction can be caused by biliary or duodenal reflux or hypersecretion of pancreatic enzymes. As the cell walls are destroyed by proteolytic digestive enzymes, more enzymes are released into the interstitial spaces, precipitating further destruction. Lipolytic enzymes, which break down fat, also effect changes in the internal morphology of the pancreas. Necrosis of blood vessel walls may cause hemorrhage into or around the pancreas. An inflammatory reaction occurs and the gland becomes edematous.[62] While alcohol and biliary tract pathology, especially gallstones, are the most common predisposing factors, abdominal trauma, drugs, viral infections, and many other causes exist.[26]

Although acute pancreatitis is frequently a self-limiting disease lasting about 5 days, a number of complications can occur. Pancreatic abscess results from a localized suppurative process that results in pus collecting in or around the gland. Fluid collections in the pancreatic parenchyma break through the thin-walled connective tissue layer surrounding the organ and spill into the surrounding area. Most frequently this fluid accumulates in the anterior pararenal space, although it may extend posteriorly to a potential space behind the renal fascia (Fig. 6-11).[19,61] Pancreatic abscess is frequently associated with a left side pleural effusion and splenomegaly resulting from splenic vein thrombosis.[74] In phlegmonous pancreatitis, the inflammatory reaction spreads to the soft tissues surrounding the pancreas. (A phlegmon is an inflammatory process that spreads along fascial pathways, producing edema and swelling.[19]) Other complications of acute pancreatitis include dehydration resulting from fluid loss, subsequent renal failure, pulmonary edema, and the development of chronic pancreatitis. Death may occur in a small percentage of patients from accompanying shock.[62] Complications of acute pancreatitis are varied. The course and prognosis of the disease depend on the severity of the complications and the underlying cause.

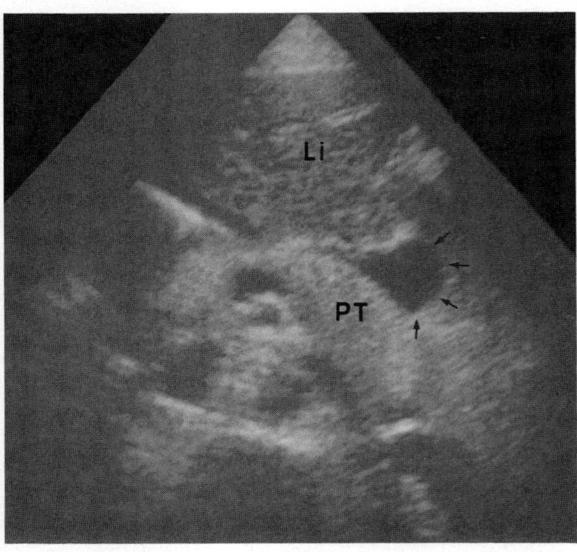

Figure 6-11. Fluid collection (*arrows*) in the anterior pararenal space as a complication of acute pancreatitis (Li, liver; PT, pancreatic tail).

Clinically, the patient presents with sudden onset of severe abdominal pain, usually localized in the epigastrium or upper quadrants, often radiating to the back. The pain reaches a maximum within minutes or a few hours after onset of the disease and continues steadily, diminishing only as the inflammation subsides. Characteristic of the pain associated with pancreatitis is the relief obtained by sitting up or bending at the waist. Nausea and vomiting are frequently present, and a mild fever may develop within the first few days. Serum amylase concentration increases to its maximum value within 24 hours after onset and gradually returns to normal over 3 to 10 days. An elevated white blood cell count (leukocytosis), proteinuria, and elevated bilirubin value may be present. Serum lipase concentration also increases and remains elevated longer than that of serum amylase.

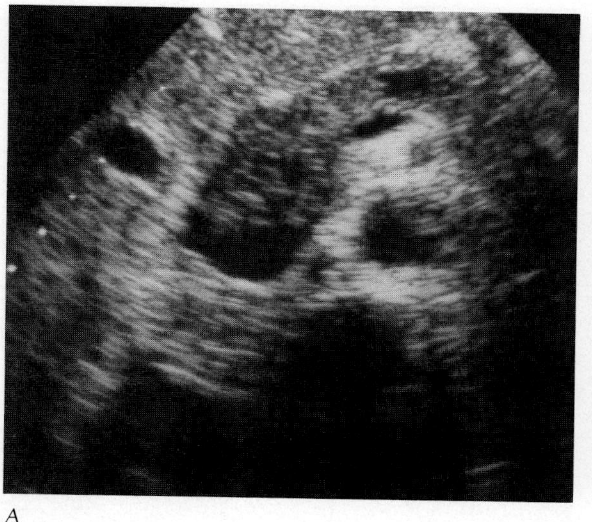

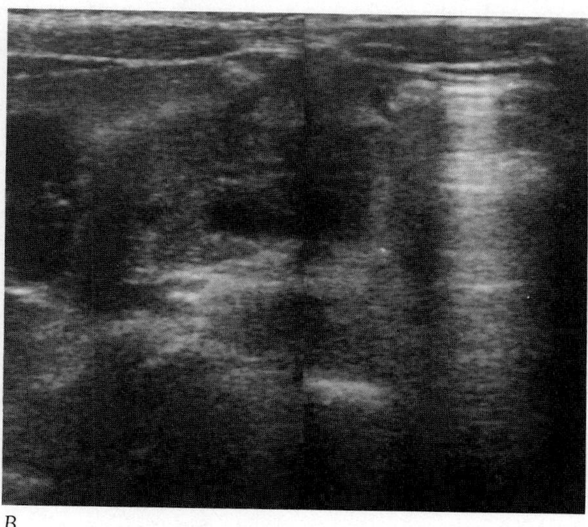

FIGURE 6-12. (*A*) Sonogram of acute pancreatitis demonstrates enlargement and decreased echogenicity. (*B*) Sonogram of acute pancreatitis demonstrates an enlarged, irregularly marginated gland with decreased echogenicity.

Sonographically, an inflamed pancreas appears enlarged and hypoechoic, although in some cases it may appear normal (Fig. 6-12).[34] The pancreatic duct may be enlarged beyond the normal 2 mm AP diameter (Fig. 6-13).[20] Since echogenicity is assessed by comparing the pancreas to the liver, transverse sections must be obtained with the gain curve properly adjusted. Additionally, care must be taken in young patients whose pancreas may normally appear less echogenic to differentiate it from a diseased organ. In children, acute pancreatitis presents a similar sonographic appearance, with decreased echogenicity and increased AP diameter.[23] In children, diffuse or focal enlargement of the pancreas is generally a more reliable indicator of disease than altered echogenicity.[13] Occasionally, when biliary calculi are the precipitating factor in acute pancreatitis, small stones may make their way through the ductal system and into the pancreatic duct. These may be seen sonographically as highly echogenic foci within a dilated duct (Fig. 6-14).

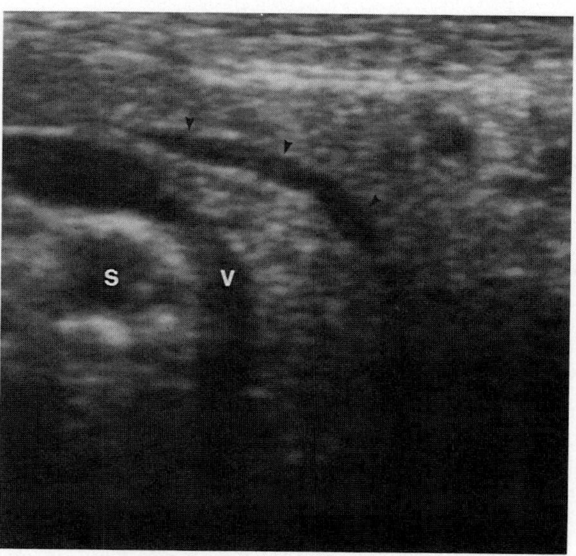

FIGURE 6-13. Enlarged pancreatic duct (*arrowheads*) in a patient with acute pancreatitis (V, splenic vein; s, superior mesenteric artery).

Pancreatic pseudocysts, encapsulated collections of the by-products of tissue destruction, arise in about half of patients with severe disease.[28] Ultrasound may be used to follow pseudocyst maturation and, when necessary, to guide drainage. Although they can occur anywhere in the abdominal cavity, they are most frequently found in or around the pancreas itself, especially in the area of the tail. Hemorrhage of a pseudocyst may occur as a result of tissue necrosis, and if blood loss is massive emergency surgical intervention may be indicated. Secondary infection of a pseudocyst may necessitate drainage.[44] The composition of the fluid component in a pseudocyst varies: pancreatic juice, blood, pus, and/or inflammatory by-products.[19]

Since pseudocysts are a frequent complication of acute pancreatitis, any cystic-looking structures in the region of the pancreas should be carefully evaluated. They may have any of a wide spectrum of sonographic appearances, from smooth-bordered and entirely cystic to poorly marginated, seemingly solid masses with no posterior acoustic enhancement.[41] Septa or debris may be seen within and free fluid may be found in the retroperitoneal compartments (Fig. 6-15).[38,61] The walls may be thin, smooth, and membranous or thick and irregular. Ultrasound is an excellent modality for detecting and following pseudocysts; its reported accuracy is 96%, owing to displacement of gas-containing bowel by the mass.[59]

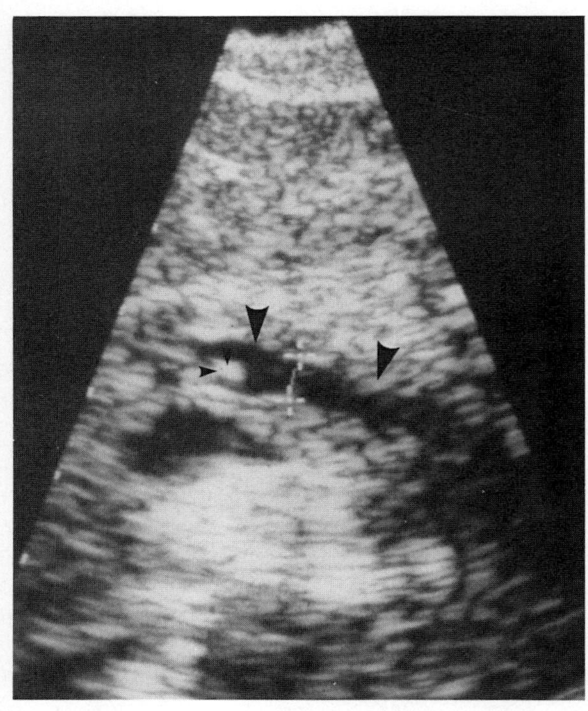

FIGURE 6-14. Acute pancreatitis with intraductal stones. (*large arrowheads,* dilated pancreatic duct; *small arowheads,* calculus).

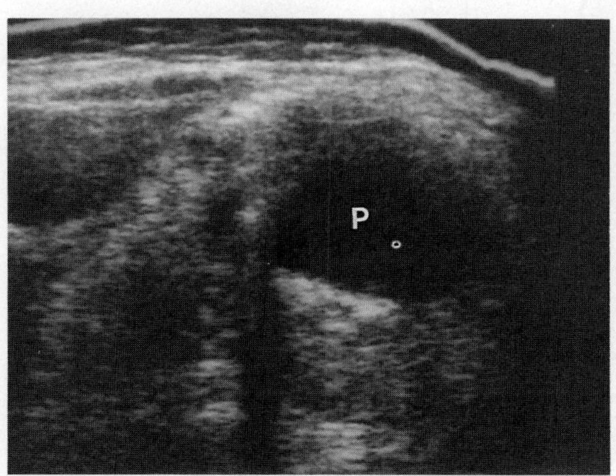

FIGURE 6-15A

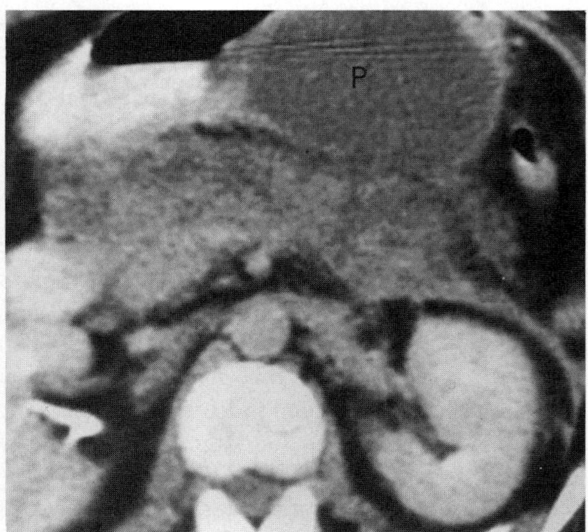

B

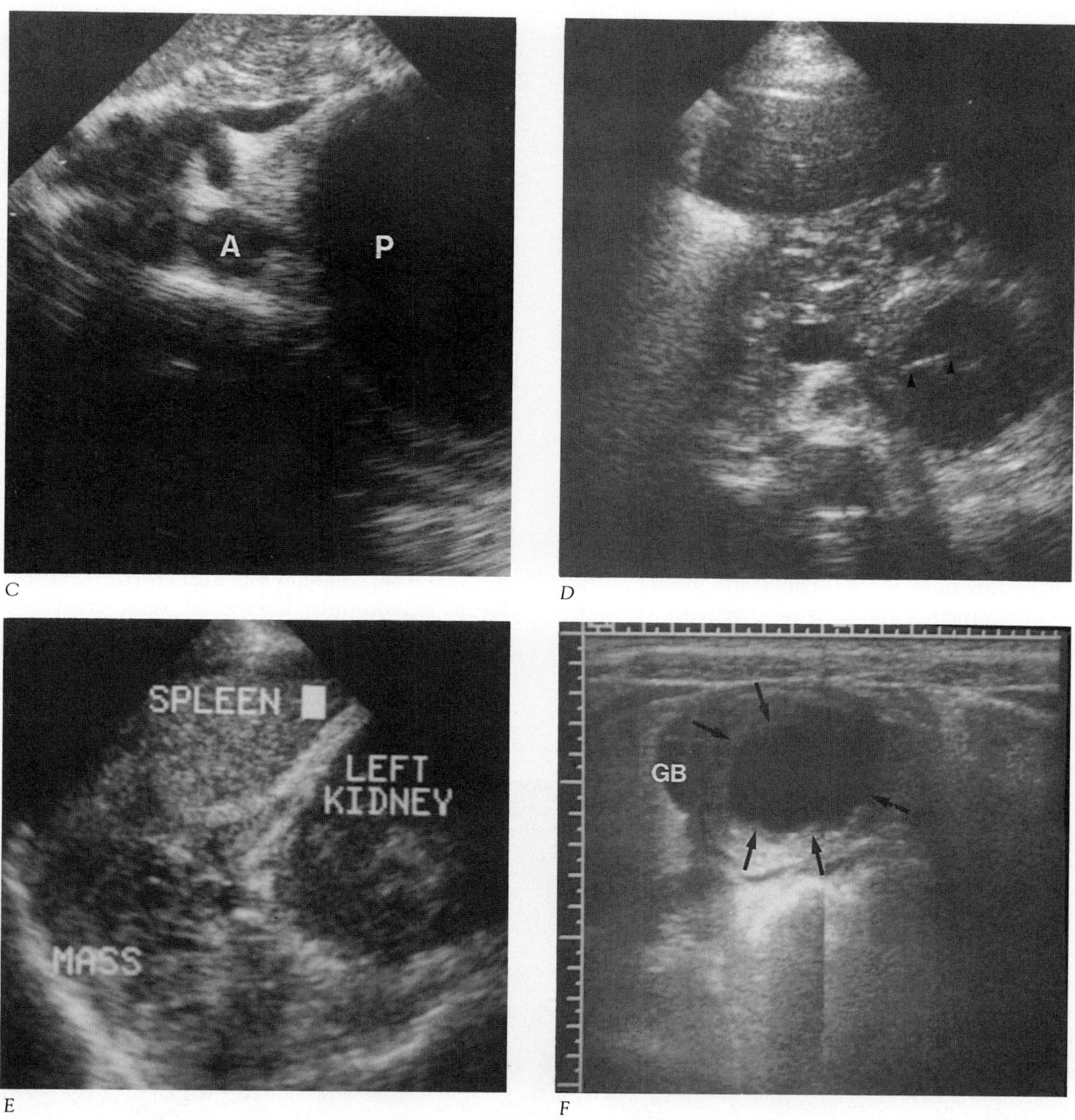

Figure 6-15. (*A*) Sonogram demonstrates large pancreatic pseudocyst (P) in pancreatic tail with low-level internal echoes. (*B*) CT of the same patient (P, pseudocyst). (C) Large anechoic pancreatic pseudocyst (A, aorta; P, pseudocyst). (*D*) Septate pseudocyst in pancreatic tail (*small arrowheads,* septation). (*E*) Mature pancreatic pseudocyst with well-organized, middle to high-level internal echoes. Sagittal sonogram through left upper quadrant. (*F*) Pseudocyst (*arrows*) in the head of the pancreas. Note thickness of walls (GB, gallbladder).

Chronic Pancreatitis. Chronic pancreatitis is characterized by histologic changes in the pancreas. Protein plugs develop within the ducts, blocking the release of digestive enzymes. Progressive interlobular fibrosis and destruction and atrophy of functioning tissue results. In the early stages, gross anatomic changes may be absent. The pancreas may become enlarged and edematous, with increasing dilatation of the main pancreatic duct. As the disease progresses, the gland becomes small and atrophic. Interparenchymal fluid collections are frequently seen.[11] Calculi may be found within the pancreatic duct system, and cystic formations are common.

The prognosis of chronic pancreatitis is best when the causative agent can be removed, as it can in chronic cholecystitis, hyperparathyroidism, or alcohol-induced disease. Unfortunately, the prognosis is worse in cases where the cause is not clearly defined, because the disease process progresses until the pancreas is unable to carry out normal physiologic functions. This is pancreatic insufficiency.[3,7]

The patient complains of persistent epigastric pain radiating to the left lumbar region, nausea, vomiting, flatulence, and weight loss. Paralytic ileus is a common complication. During exacerbation of acute inflammatory disease, which frequently occurs in chronic relapsing pancreatitis, serum amylase and bilirubin levels may be elevated.

The sonographic findings in chronic pancreatitis are varied. Since gross anatomic changes may not occur in the course of this disease, sonography may not detect abnormalities. In cases where anatomic changes have occurred, however, sonographic evaluation most frequently reveals inhomogenously increased echogenicity with coarse, focally dense echoes. The organ may be enlarged with irregular borders, and the pancreatic duct may be dilated. A radiographic hallmark of chronic pancreatitis is the presence of calcifications in the epigastrium, which appear sonographically as bright reflections that cast a posterior acoustic shadow (Fig. 6-16).[1,59] Reported complications associated with chronic relapsing pancreatitis include a dilated biliary system resulting from common bile duct strictures,[51] pseudocyst erosion into the portal vein, and focal masses.[47]

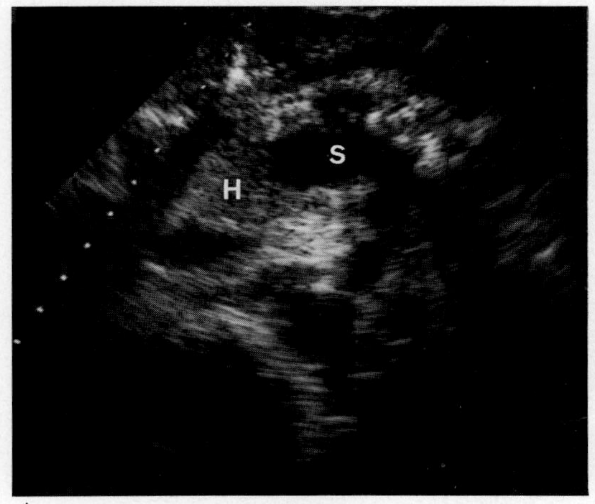

A

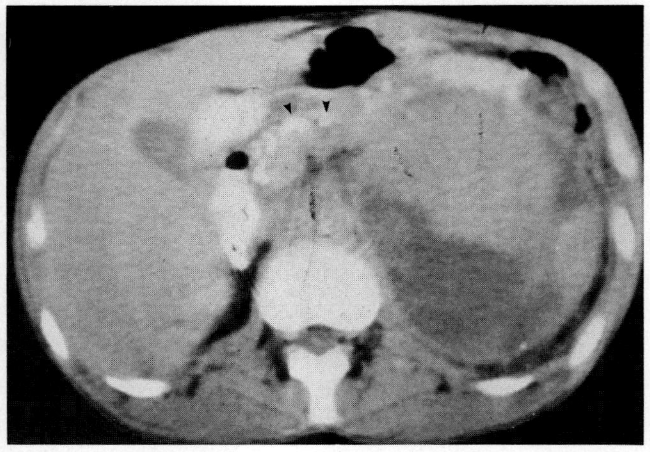

B

Figure 6-16 (*A*) Chronic pancreatitis is demonstrated sonographically with intrapancreatic calcifications (H, pancreatic head; S, splenic vein). (*B*) CT of same patient demonstrates a large, well-circumscribed pseudocyst in the left upper quadrant (*arrowheads,* calcifications).

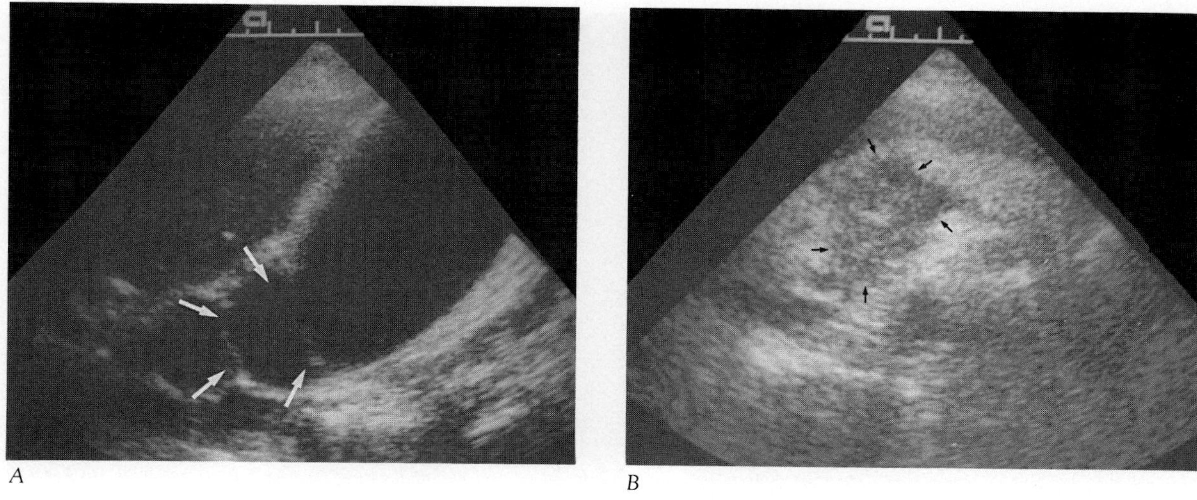

FIGURE 6-17. (*A*) Courvoisier gallbladder is demonstrated sonographically. Note dilated valves of Heister. (*B*) Mass *(arrows)* in head of pancreas compresses biliary outflow tract in the same patient.

NEOPLASTIC DISEASE

Malignant tumors of the pancreas rank as the fifth leading cancer killer in the United States.[2] Early diagnosis is associated with a slightly better prognosis, but since many pancreatic malignancies do not produce symptoms until late in the disease, early detection is rare. Tumors are most common in men older than 30 years and about 50% more common in black men.[46] Risk factors may include smoking, high-fat diet, chronic pancreatitis, diabetes, and cirrhosis, although no causal relationship has been proved conclusively.

Because of its dual role as an exocrine and endocrine gland, the pancreas is unique in cellular structure and physiologic function. Tumors may be classified according to the cell of origin.[16,42] Neoplasms of exocrine origin comprise the largest group of pancreatic tumors and include the single most common malignant lesion, acinar cell adenocarcinoma.[6,29,32,40,69] Slightly more than 70% of these lesions occur in the head of the pancreas. The remainder occur equally in the body or tail.[46] Anatomically, these lesions vary in size and gross appearance. Some are well-circumscribed, ovoid masses; others infiltrate surrounding pancreatic parenchyma so diffusely that the pancreas appears as a matted mass of tumor. Some small carcinomas that arise in the ampulla of Vater may be very difficult to detect. Tumors in the pancreatic head usually spread into the duodenum and compress the common bile duct and ampulla of Vater. Mechanical obstruction of the biliary tract causes dilatation of the ducts and frequently the gallbladder. A markedly distended and clinically palpable gallbladder, commonly referred to as a Courvoisier gallbladder, is easily demonstrated sonographically and is a reliable indicator of an otherwise unseen lesion in the pancreatic head (Fig. 6-17).[46] Other exocrine lesions—benign solid adenoma and cystadenoma, squamous cell carcinoma, and adenocanthoma—are rare.[9] Tumors of endocrine origin virtually always rise from islet cells and are, therefore, known as islet cell tumors. Depending on the hormonal effect that these neoplasms produce and on the cells of origin, they are variously known as insulinomas, gastrinomas, or glucagonomas.[63]

Solid Neoplastic Lesions. Solid pancreatic tumors usually appear as echopenic to moderately echogenic areas within the parenchyma of the organ.[73] Com-

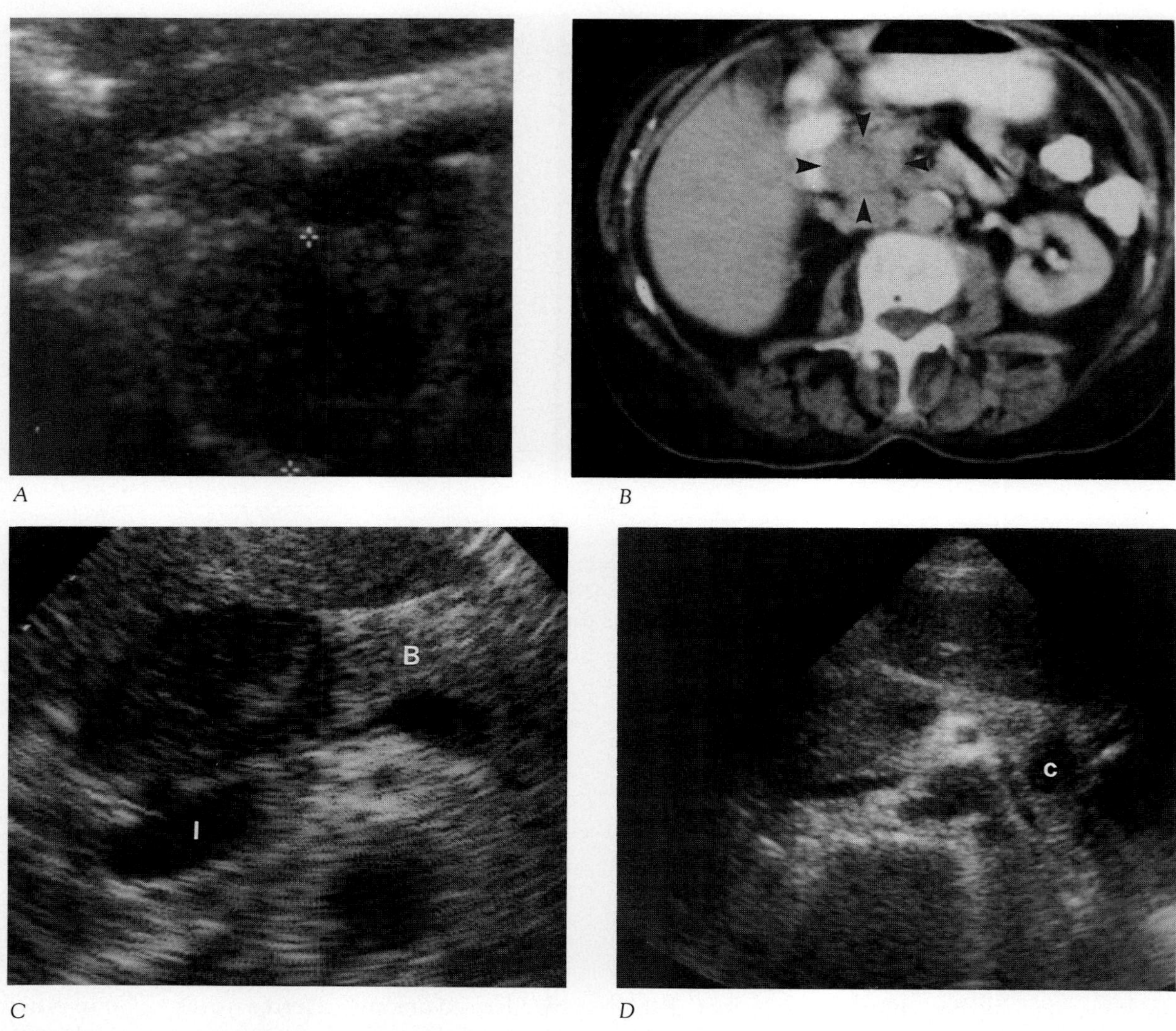

FIGURE 6-18. (*A*) A magnified view over the head of the pancreas demonstrating a well-circumscribed carcinoma (calipers). (*B*) CT of same patient (*arrowheads,* mass) (C) Hypoechoic, well-circumscribed pancreatic carcinoma (B, body of pancreas; I, inferior vena cava). (*D*) Sonogram demonstrates carcinoma of the pancreatic tail (c, mass).

pared to the surrounding pancreatic tissue, these masses appear hypoechoic (Fig. 6-18). The borders may be well-defined, but more often they appear as poorly marginated, complex masses diffusely involving the pancreatic head (Fig. 6-19).[39,65,66] Since pancreatic carcinoma is rarely detected early in the disease process, by the time the patient is referred for diagnostic imaging procedures, the neoplasm has usually spread. Enlarged lymph nodes in the porta hepatis and in the paraaortic region indicate nodal metastasis (Fig. 6-20). Inflammation of the pancreas is a common sequela in carcinomatosis, and the remainder of the organ may appear enlarged and hypoechoic.[56] Additionally, tumors in

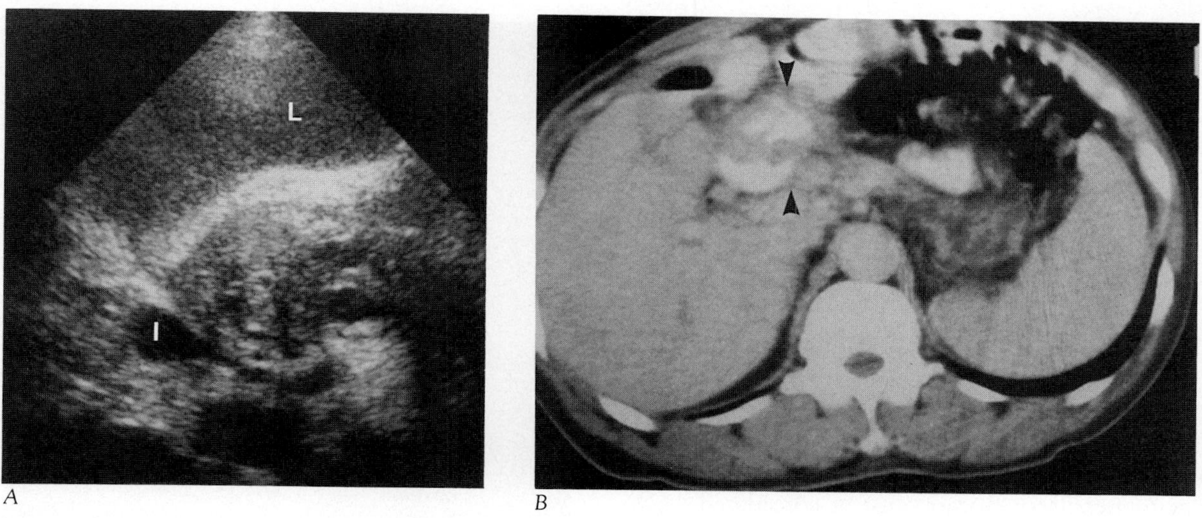

FIGURE 6-19 (*A*) Diffuse involvement of the head of the pancreas with adenocarcinoma (I, inferior vena cava; L, left lobe of liver). (*B*) CT of same patient (*arrowheads*, involved pancreatic head).

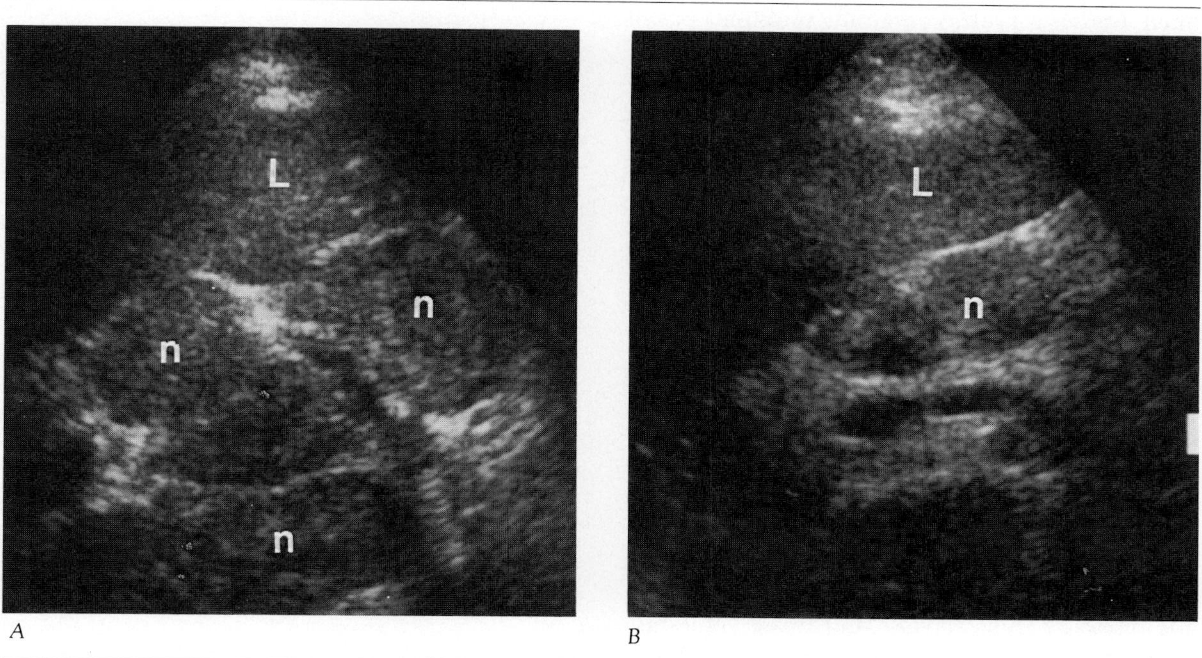

FIGURE 6-20. (*A*) Transverse sonogram demonstrates periportal lymphadenopathy in a patient with primary carcinoma of the pancreas (L, liver; n, nodal masses). (*B*) Sagittal sonogram of the same patient (L, liver; n, nodal masses).

the head of the pancreas may cause obstructive jaundice, in which case the common bile and intrahepatic ducts may appear dilated. If the neoplasm is very small, the only sonographic indicator of an intrapancreatic abnormality may be the blunt termination of a dilated common bile duct in the head of the pancreas (Fig. 6-21).

Cystic Neoplastic Lesions. The majority of pancreatic tumors are solid, but cystic neoplasms do occur. When a fluid-filled structure is seen in or around the pancreas, the most likely diagnosis is pseudocyst. Differentiation can be easily made by analyzing laboratory results, which will most likely demonstrate inflammatory disease. In the absence of clinical suspicion of acute or chronic pancreatitis, cystic neoplastic disease must be considered.[24] Cystic neoplastic lesions are divided into two groups: benign microcystic adenomas and malignant mucinous cystic adenomas.[32,35,37] Microcystic adenomas are benign lesions composed of many cysts smaller than 2 cm. They occur more frequently in the head of the pancreas and may contain calcifications.[50] Morphologically these tumors have thin, well-defined, fibrous capsules containing multiple cysts of varying size.[46] Mucinous cystic adenomas—also referred to as cystadenocarcinomas—are predominantly malignant lesions composed of larger cystic areas (more than 2 cm) and may contain peripheral rim calcifications. They are usually large, unilocular, encapsulated masses, although some rare multilocular lesions have been reported.[14] About 60% in the tail of the pancreas, and those appear to be among the few pancreatic malignancies that have excellent potential for cure.[15]

The patient with pancreatic carcinoma presents with vague, diffuse pain located in the epigastrium that radiates to the back. As with acute pancreatitis, leaning forward or sitting upright may alleviate the pain. Jaundice occurs if the lesion produces biliary obstruction, and weight loss is common. Both of these symptoms occur late in the disease. Laboratory results are generally nonspecific for pancreatic disease. Serum amylase and lipase values are occasionally elevated; steatorrhea does not occur in the absence of jaundice; occult blood may be detected in stool when the tumor is in the ampulla of Vater.

Primary cystic neoplasms have a variable sonographic appearance. Again, 85% to 90% of cystic masses in the pancreatic bed are related to inflammatory disease.[72] Microcystic adenomas appear sonographically as poorly marginated, mixed echogenic lesions. The cystic components are usually too small to be seen individually (Fig. 6-22). Mucinous cystic neoplasms contain larger (greater than 5 cm) uni- or multilocular areas, which may be seen sonographically. Mural excrescences may be seen projecting into the cystic area.[12,25,48,49] Other noninflammatory cystic lesions of the pancreas include polycystic disease and cystic fibrosis.

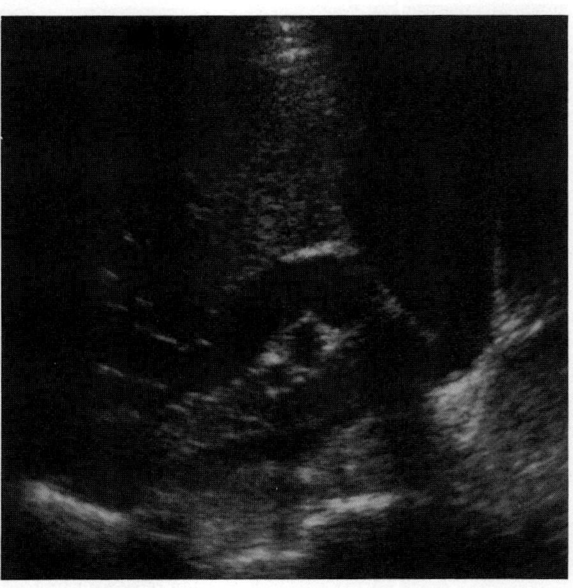

Figure 6-21. Dilated common bile duct in a patient with carcinoma in the head of the pancreas.

Nonneoplastic Cystic Lesions

Cystic fibrosis is discussed in Chapter 15. Ultrasonography is a useful tool for evaluating the degree of pancreatic involvement in children.[58,71]

Polycystic Disease. Polycystic disease is an inherited disease characterized by the presence of multiple small cysts in the kidney, liver, and pancreas.[52] Usually the patient presents with a family history of polycystic disease or is being worked up for hy-

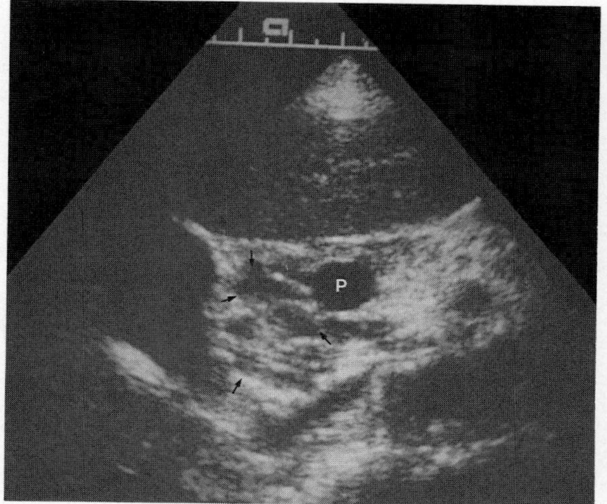

A

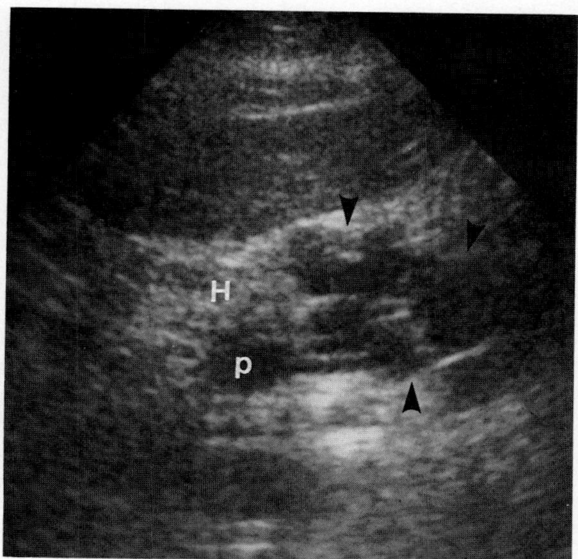

B

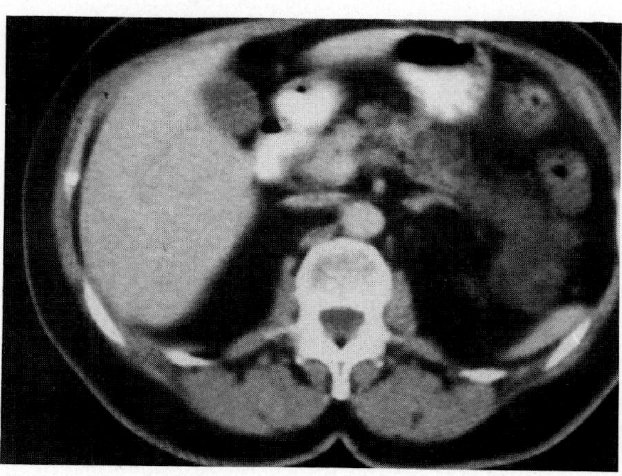

C

Figure 6-22. (*A*) Sonogram demonstrates macrocystic adenocarcinoma with cystic lesions (*arrows*) in the body and tail (P, portal venous confluence). (*B*) Macrocystic adenocarcinoma on this sonogram demonstrates the presence of cystic lesions (*arrowheads*) in the body and tail (P, portal venous confluence; H, head of pancreas). (C) Macrocystic adenocarcinoma is demonstrated on this CT.

pertension, renal insufficiency, or pyelonephritis. The pancreas is rarely the primary organ of interest in these patients. The slowly multiplying and enlarging cystic masses eventually destroy the normal pancreatic tissue. The vast majority of patients with polycystic disease, however, succumb to renal failure well before the pancreas is physiologically affected. The finding of well-defined cystic lesions in the pancreas should alert the sonographer to the possibility of polycystic disease. In such cases, the liver and kidneys should be surveyed for the classic appearance of polycystic disease. In the absence of renal or hepatic cysts, the diagnosis of polycystic disease cannot be made; instead, one of the abovementioned inflammatory or neoplastic lesions should be considered.

References

1. Alpern MB, Sandler MA, Kellman GM, et al: Chronic pancreatitis: Ultrasonic features. Radiology 1985, 155:215–219.

2. American Cancer Society: Cancer Facts and Figures. New York, American Cancer Society, 1988.
3. Ammann RW, Akobintz A, Largiader F, et al: Course and outcome of chronic pancreatitis: A longitudinal study of a mixed medical-surgical series of 245 patients. Gastroenterology 1984, 86:820.
4. Anderhub B: Manual of Abdominal Sonography. Baltimore, University Park Press, 1983.
5. Arger PH, Mulhern CB, Bonavita JA, et al: An analysis of pancreatic sonography in suspected pancreatic disease. J Clin Ultrasound 1979, 7:91–97.
6. Balthazar EJ, Subramanyam BR, Lefleur RS, et al: Solid and papillary epithethial neoplasms of the pancreas. Radiology 1984, 150:39–40.
7. Bank S: Chronic pancreatitis: Clinical features and medical management. Am J Gastroenterol 1986, 81:153–167.
8. Barkin J, Vining D, Miale A, et al: Computerized tomography, diagnostic ultrasound, and radionuclide scanning. JAMA 1977, 238:2040–2042.
9. Becker WF, Welsh RA, Pratt HS: Cystadenoma and cystadenocarcinoma of the pancreas. Ann Surg 1965, 161:845–859.
10. Bryan PJ: Appearance of the normal pancreatic duct: A study using real-time ultrasound. J Clin Ultrasound 1982, 10:63–68.
11. Bullock BL, Rosendahl PP. Pathophysiology, 2nd ed. Glenview, IL, Scott, Foresman, 1988.
12. Carroll B, Sample WF: Pancreatic cystadenocarcinoma: CT body scan and gray-scale ultrasound appearance. AJR 1978, 131:339–341.
13. Clark LR, Jaffe MH, Choyke PL, et al: Pancreatic imaging. Radiol Clin North Am 1985, 23(3):489–499.
13. Coleman BG, Arger PH, Rosenberg HK, et al: Gray-scale sonographic assessment of pancreatitis in children. Radiology 1983, 146:145–150.
14. Compagno J, Oertel JE: Microcystic adenoma of the pancreas: A clinicopathologic study of 34 cases. Am J Clin Pathol 1978, 69:289–298.
15. Compagno J, Oertal JE: Mucinous cystic neoplasms of the pancreas with overt and latent malignancy. A clinicopathologic study of 41 cases. Am J Clin Pathol 1978, 69:573–580.
16. Cubilla AL, Fitzgerald PJ: Classification of pancreatic cancer (nonendocrine). Mayo Clin Proc 1979, 54:449–458.
17. de Graaf CS, Taylor KJ, Simonds BD, et al: Gray-scale echography of the pancreas: Reevaluation of normal size. Radiology 1978, 129:157–165.
18. Didier D, Deschamps JP, Rohmer P, et al: Evaluation of the pancreatic duct: A reappraisal based on a retrospective correlative study by sonographic and pancreatography in 117 normal and pathologic subjects. Ultrasound Med Biol 1983, 9:509–518.
19. Donovan PJ, Sanders RC, Siegelman SS: Collections of fluid after pancreatitis: Evaluation by computed tomography and ultrasonography. Radiol Clin North Am 1982, 20:653–665.
20. Doust B, Pearce JD: Grey-scale ultrasonic properties of the normal and inflamed pancreas. Radiology 1976, 120:653–657.
21. Filly RA, London SS: The normal pancreas: Acoustic characteristics and frequency imaging. J Clin Ultrasound 1979, 7:121–124.
22. Fishback F: A Manual of Laboratory Diagnostic Tests. Philadelphia, JB Lippincott, 1980.
23. Fleischer AC, Parker P, Kirchner SG, et al: Sonographic findings of pancreatitis in children. Radiology 1983, 146:151–155.
24. Freeny PC, Weinstein CJ, Taft DA, et al: Cystic neoplasms of the pancreas: New angiographic and sonographic findings. AJR 1978, 131:795–802.
25. Friedman AC, Lichtenstein JE, Dachman AH: Cystic neoplasms of the pancreas: Radiological-pathological correlation. Radiology 1983, 149:45–50.
26. Goekas MC: Acute pancreatitis. Ann Intern Med 1985, 103:86–91.
27. Goldstein HM, Katragadda CS: Prone view ultrasonography for neoplasms of the pancreatic tail. AJR 1978, 131:231–236.
28. Gonzales AC, Bradley EL, Clements JL: Pseudocyst formation in acute pancreatitis—ultrasonographic evaluation of 99 cases. AJR 1976, 127:315–317.
29. Guillan RA, McMahon J: Pleomorphic adenocarcinoma of the pancreas. Am J Gastroenterol 1973, 60:379–386.
30. Guyton AC: Textbook of Medical Physiology, 7th ed. Philadelphia, WB Saunders, 1986.
31. Haaga JR, Alfidi RJ, Havrilla TR, et al: Definitive role of CT scanning of the pancreas. Radiology 1977, 124:723–730.
32. Herrera L, Glassman CI, Komins JI: Mucinous cystic neoplasm of the pancreas demonstrated by ultrasound and endoscopic retrograde pancreatography. Am J Gastroenterol 1980, 73:512–515.
33. Hessel SJ, Siegelman SS, McNeil BJ, et al: A prospective evaluation of computed tomography and ultrasound of the pancreas. Radiology 1982, 143:129–133.
34. Hill MC: Pancreatic sonography: An update. *In* Sanders RC (ed): Ultrasound Annual 1982. New York, Raven Press, 1982.
35. Hodgkinson DJ, Remine WH, Weiland LH: Pancreatic cystadenoma: A clincopathologic study of 45 Cases. Arch Surg 1978, 113:512–519.
36. Husband JE, Meire HB, Kreel L: Comparison of ultrasound and computer-assisted tomography in pancreatic diagnosis. Br J Radiol 1977, 50:855–862.
37. Itai Y, Ohhashi K, Nagai H, et al: "Ductectatic" mucinous cystadenoma and cystadenocarcinoma of the pancreas. Radiology 1986, 161:697–700.

38. Jeffrey RB, Laing FC, Wing VW: Extrapancreatic spread of acute pancreatitis: New observations with real-time US. Radiology 1986, 159:707–714.
39. Koenigsberg P: Focal lesions of the pancreas. Semin Roentgenol 1985, 20:3–21.
40. Lack EE, Lavey R: Tumors of the exocrine pancreas in children and adolescents. A clinical and pathologic study of eight cases. Am J Surg Pathol 1983, 7:319–327.
41. Laing FC, Gooding GA, Brown T, et al: Atypical pseudocysts of the pancreas: An ultrasonographic evaluation. J Clin Ultrasound 1979, 7:27–32.
42. Larsson L: Endocrine pancreatic tumors. Human Pathol 1978, 9:401–416.
43. Lawson TL: Sensitivity of pancreatic ultrasonography in the detection of pancreatic disease. Radiology 1978, 128:733–736.
44. Lawson TL: Acute pancreatitis and its complications. Computed tomography and sonography. Radiol Clin North Am 1983, 21:495–513.
45. Lawson TL, Berland LL, Foley WD: Coronal upper abdominal anatomy: Technique and gastrointestinal applications. Gastrointest Radiol 1981, 6:115–121.
46. Lawson TL, Berland LL, Foley WD: Malignant neoplasms of the pancreas, liver and biliary tract. *In* Bragg DG, Rubin P, Youker JE (eds): Oncologic Imaging. New York, Pergamon Press, 1985.
47. Lee SH, Bodensteiner D, Eisman S, et al: Chronic relapsing pancreatitis with pseudocyst erosion into the portal vein and disseminated fat necrosis. Am J Gastroenterol 1985, 80(6):452–458.
48. Lloyd TV, Antonmattei S, Freimanis AK. Gray-scale sonography of cystadenoma of the pancreas: Report of two cases. J Clin Ultrasound 1979, 7:149–151.
49. Lo JW, Fung CH, Yonan TN, et al: Cystadenoma of the pancreas. An ultrastructural study. Cancer 1977, 39:2470–2474.
50. Logan SE, Voet RL, Tompkins RK: The malignant potential of mucinous cysts of the pancreas. West J Med 1982, 136:157–162.
51. Lygidakis NJ: Biliary stricture as a complication of chronic relapsing pancreatitis. Am J Surg 1983, 145:804–806.
52. Mcgeoch JE, Darmady EM: Polycystic disease of kidney, liver and pancreas: A possible pathogenesis. J Pathol 1976, 119:221–228.
53. Marks WM, Filly RA, Callen PW: Ultrasonic evaluation of normal pancreatic echogenicity and its relationship to fat deposition. Radiology 1980, 137:475–479.
54. Miller MA, Leavell LC: Anatomy and Physiology, 16th ed. New York, Macmillan, 1970.
55. Mittlestaedt CA: Abdominal Ultrasound. New York, Churchill Livingstone, 1987.
56. Niccoloni DG, Graham JH, Banks PA: Tumor-induced acute pancreatitis. Gastroenterology 1976, 71:142–145.
57. Ohto M, Saotome N, Saisho HH, et al: Real-time sonography of the pancreatic duct: Application to percutaneous pancreatic ductography. AJR 1980, 134:647–650.
58. Phillips HE, Cox KL, Reid MH, et al: Pancreatic sonography in cystic fibrosis. AJR 1981, 137:69–72.
59. Pochammer KF, Szekessy T, Frentzel-Beyme B, et al: Cranio-caudad dimension of the pancreatic head. Radiology 1985, 155:861–868.
60. Rankin RA, Welsh JD: Gastroenterology. *In* Kaufamn CE, Papper (eds): Review of Pathophysiology. Boston, Little, Brown, 1983.
61. Raptopoulos V, Kleinman PK, Marks S: Renal fascial pathway: Posterior extension of pancreatic effusions within the anterior pararenal space. Radiology 1986, 158:367–374.
62. Robbins SL, Cotran RS: Pathologic Basis of Disease. Philadelphia, WB Saunders, 1979.
63. Schroder SA, Krupp MA, Tierney LM (eds): Current Medical Diagnosis and Treatment 1988. East Norwalk, CT, Appleton and Lange, 1988.
64. Schwartz S, Shires GT: Principles of Surgery. New York, McGraw-Hill, 1979.
65. Shawker TH, Garra BS, Hill MC, et al: Spectrum of sonographic findings in pancreatic carcinoma. J Ultrasound Med 1986, 5:169–175.
66. Shawker TH, Linzer M, Hubbard VS: Chronic pancreatitis: The diagnostic significance of pancreatic size and echo amplitude. Radiology 1985, 154:568–574.
67. Siegel MJ, Martin KW, Worthington JL: Normal and abnormal pancreas in children: US studies. Radiology 1987, 165:15–18.
68. Silverstein W, Isikokk MB, Hill MC, et al: Diagnostic imaging of acute pancreatitis: Prospective study using CT and sonography. AJR 1981, 137:497–502.
69. Sommers SC, Meissner WA: Unusual carcinomas of the pancreas. AMA Arch Pathol 1954, 58:101–111.
70. Weinstein DP, Weinstein BJ: Ultrasonic demonstration of the pancreatic duct: An analysis of 41 cases. Radiology 1979, 130:729–732.
71. Willi UV, Reddich JM, Teele RL: Cystic fibrosis: Its characteristic appearance on abdominal sonography. AJR 1980, 134:1005–1010.
72. Wolfman NT, Ramquist NA, Karstaedt N, et al: Cystic neoplasms of the pancreas: Ct and sonography. AJR 1982, 138:37–40.
73. Wolson AH, Walls WJ: Ultrasonic characteristics of cystadenoma of the pancreas. Radiology 1976, 119:203–205.
74. Zaleman M, Van Gansbeke D, Matos C, et al: Sonographic demonstration of portal venous system thrombosis secondary to inflammatory disease of the pancreas. Gastrointest Radiol 1987, 12:114–121.

CHAPTER 7

Spleen

Mimi C. Berman, Sherman S. Lipschitz,
Barbara Wajsbrot-Kandel

Every thorough sonographic examination of the upper abdomen or kidneys includes views of the spleen (Figs. 7-1, 7-2). While requests for ultrasound examinations of the spleen are relatively uncommon, the sonographer must be familiar with its normal appearance as well as the abnormal morphologic changes associated with disease. If clinical signs suggest disease of the spleen, the modality of choice is radionuclide imaging, but such scans may be unable to differentiate between a cyst and an abscess, in which case computed tomography (CT), magnetic resonance imaging (MRI), or ultrasonography will be necessary to gather additional information. Used to best advantage, ultrasound can demonstrate the existence and composition of a mass, disruption of splenic texture or outline, progressive changes in masses, and the size of the spleen.

Normal Anatomy

As always in ultrasonography, the practitioner who appreciates the normal appearance and normal variations of the organ can more readily recognize abnormalities.

The normal spleen presents several challenges to the sonographer. Its location in the nook of the left upper quadrant covered by the ninth to eleventh ribs (Figs. 7-3, 7-4) makes it difficult to scan. Its variable and rather asymmetric shape makes it a challenge to orient the transducer to find its longest axis. Variations in the body's blood needs can affect its size; its volume can decrease from 350 to 200 ml in less than 1 minute.[4] Normal irregularities in shape can simulate masses of adjoining organs such as the pancreas, kidneys, adrenals, and bowel, so knowledge of normal variants is essential to prevent misdiagnosis.

Ham compared the spleen to the size and shape of a clenched fist.[15] It is an intraperitoneal organ located in the left hypochondrium between the fundus of the stomach and the left hemidiaphragm, its long axis lying parallel to the ninth to eleventh ribs. Its medial border lies approximately 4 cm from the spine, and its lateral border at the midaxillary line in the ninth intercostal space. The hilus is the only portion that is not covered by peritoneum, but here peritoneal reflections or ligaments anchor the spleen and carry the main splenic vessels, the splenic arteries and veins (see Fig. 7-3). Average measurements of the spleen in autopsy specimens are 4 cm thick, 8 cm wide, and 12 cm long.[13,14,53]

At the hilus the splenic arteries and veins are covered by the mesentery of the lienorenal ligament. The tail of the pancreas usually abuts the hilus, since it is also within this ligament (see Fig. 7-4).[18]

While the spleen is not firmly anchored in the body, it is attached to the stomach by the gastro-

(text continues on page 225)

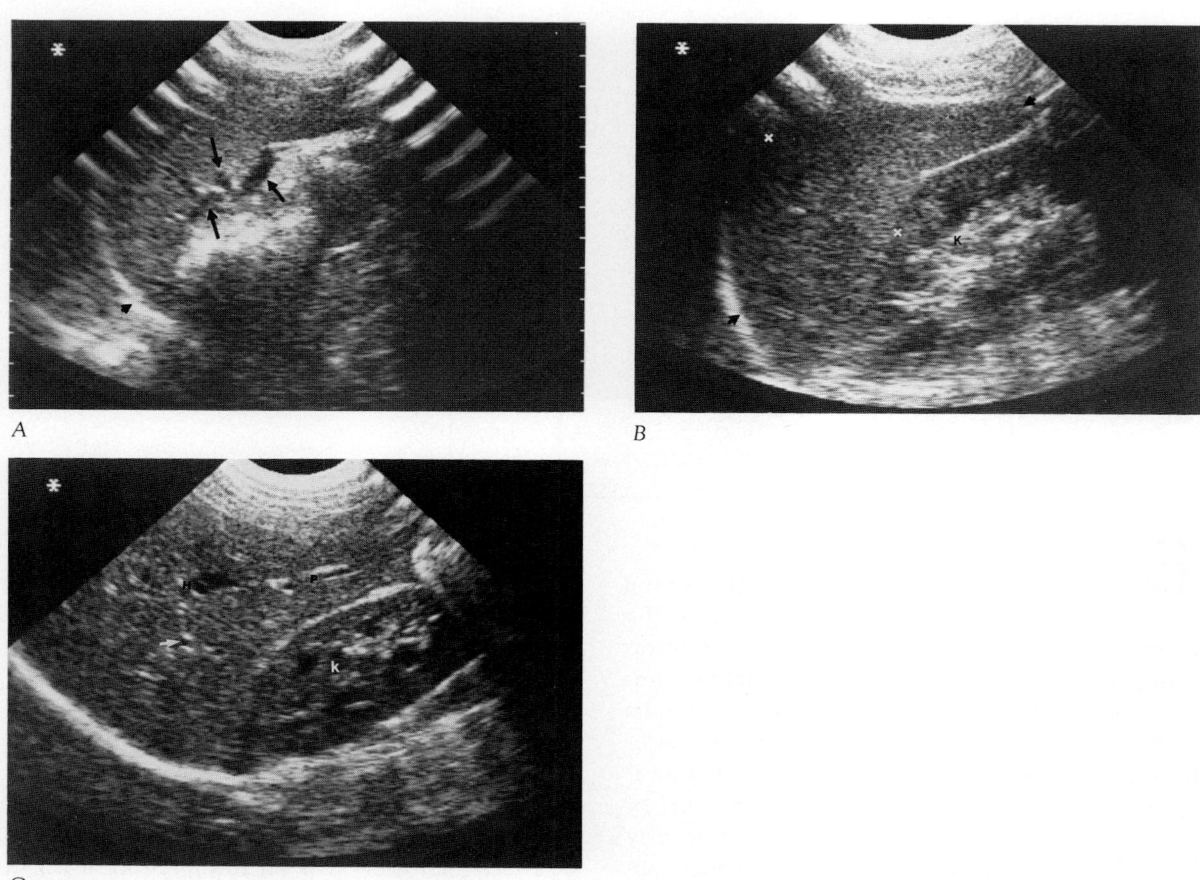

FIGURE 7-1. (A) Longitudinal scan of a normal spleen. Visible at the hilus are the splenic vessels *(arrows)* and the diffuse echoes created by the ligaments (diaphragm, *black arrowhead*). (B) A longitudinal section lateral to the hilus outlines the contour of the spleen and shows its relationship to the left kidney (K). Measurement of the long axis *(arrowheads)* and height *(between cursors)* of the spleen indicate that it is 9.5 cm long by 4.5 cm high. (C) A longitudinal scan of the liver and right kidney (K) of the same patient. The liver is isoechoic with the spleen exception for the hepatic veins (H), portal veins (P), and biliary radicles *(arrow)*, which disrupt the homogeneity of the echoes. (Courtesy Geraldine Sciabarra, Brooklyn, NY.)

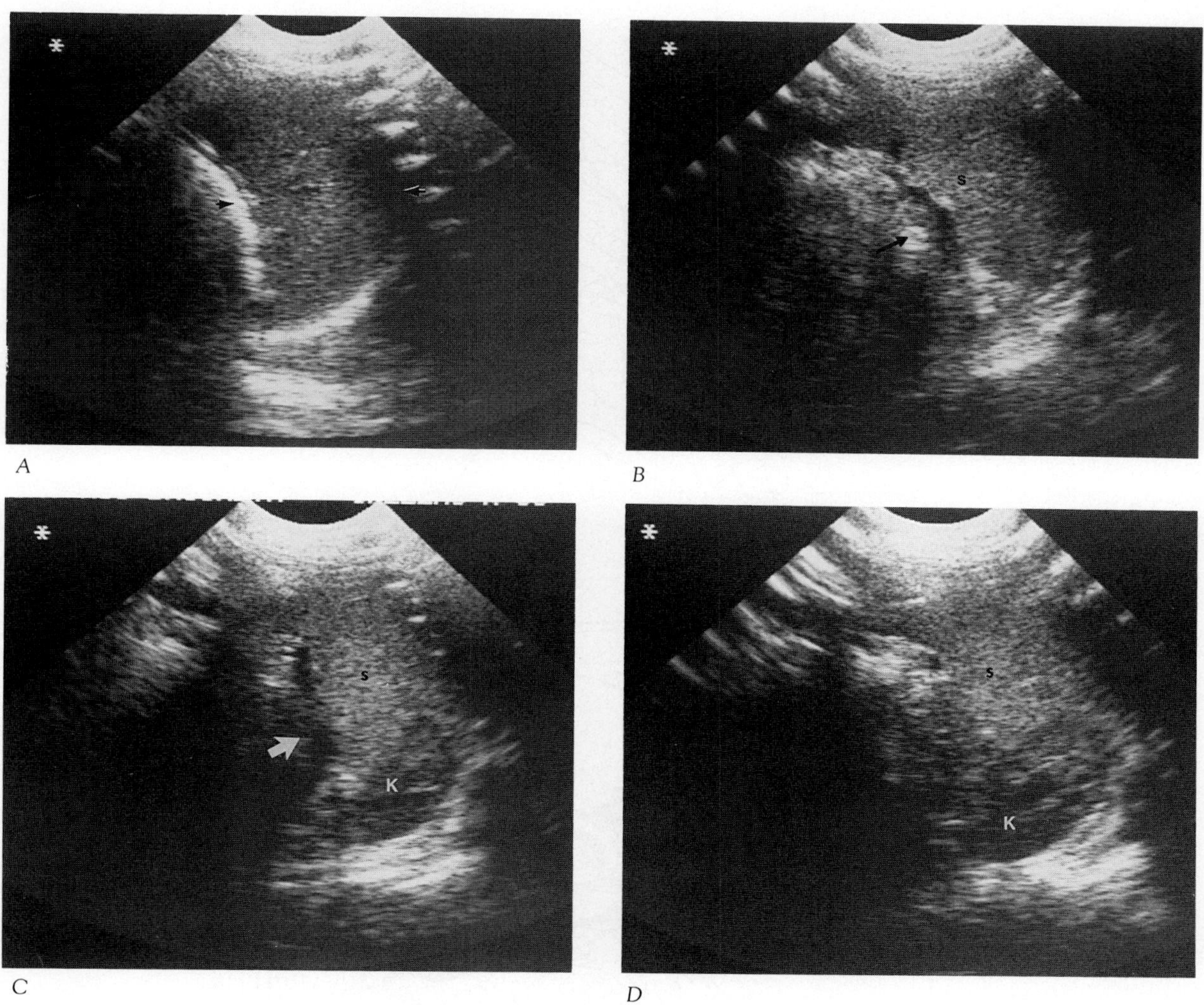

FIGURE 7-2. (*A*) A transverse section of the same normal spleen taken superior to the hilus. The width *(arrows)* should be measured here, apparently the greatest transverse diameter (5.2 cm). (*B–D*) Transverse sections of the spleen (S) moving caudad through the hilus *(arrow)* to the caudal tip. The left kidney (K) appears in sections C and *D*. (Courtesy Geraldine Sciabarra, Brooklyn, NY.)

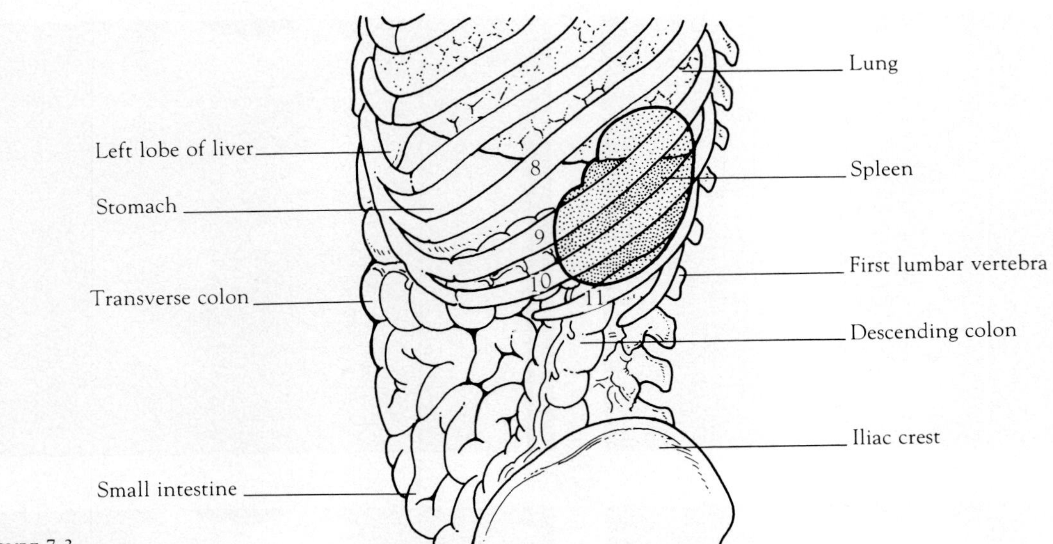

Figure 7-3.

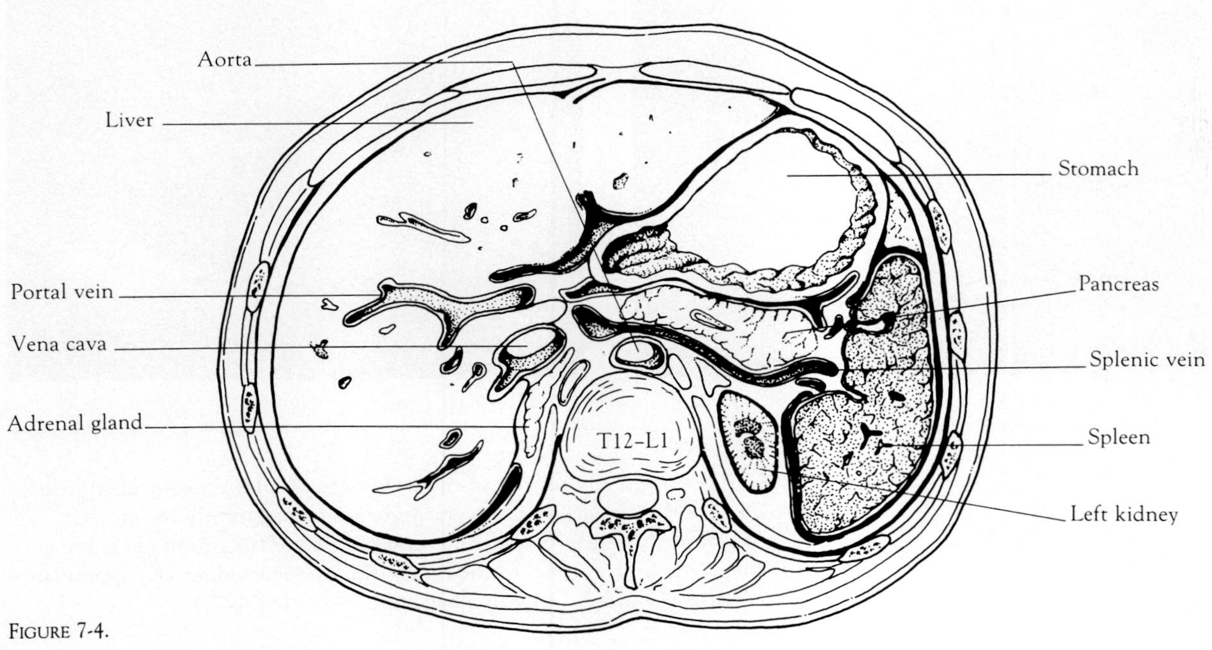

Figure 7-4.

Figure 7-3. The spleen in relationship to surrounding organs and structures.

Figure 7-4. Cross-section of the abdomen at the level of the hilus of the spleen.

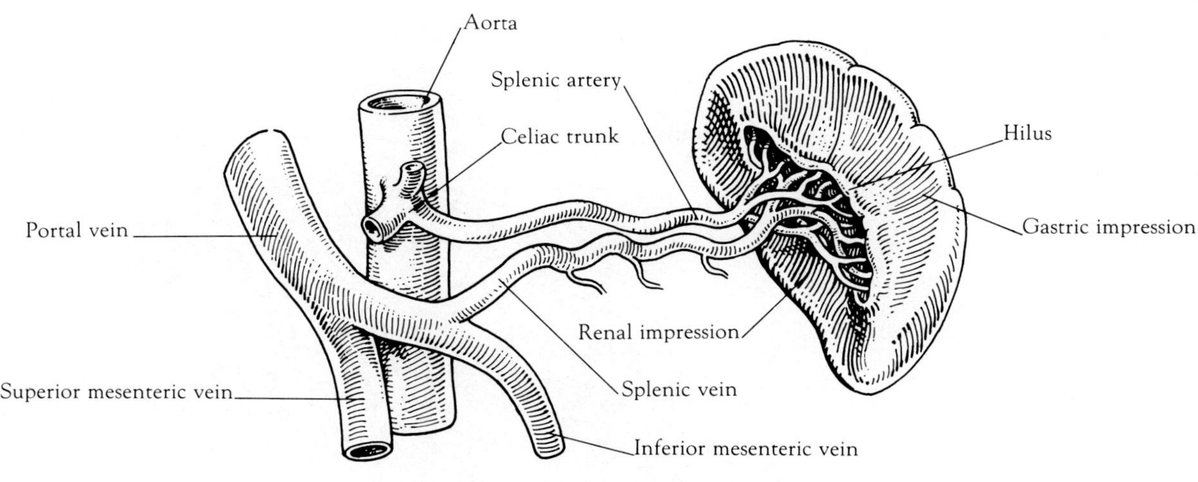

FIGURE 7-5. The circulation to the spleen, including the splenic vein and splenic artery.

lienal ligament and to the dorsal body wall by the lienorenal ligament. The phrenicocolic ligament, which is not attached directly to the spleen, supports its inferior end. These attachments allow the spleen to enlarge as much as 10 times[18] and to shift to ectopic locations.

A connective tissue capsule covers the spleen and projects fibers (trabeculae) into its pulp. The peritoneum covers the capsule. At the hilus, the splenic artery, which has divided first into two major branches and then into some six to 36 minor ones,[3] enters the spleen. The splenic veins leave the spleen in close association with the arteries (Fig. 7-5).

On entering the spleen, the splenic arteries branch into increasingly smaller arterioles, which may be visible as small echogenic lines traversing the splenic parenchyma. It is important for sonographers to remember that because there are no adequate anastomoses between arteries in the spleen, it is susceptible to infarction. The trabeculae divide the spleen into communicating compartments filled with the white and the red pulp, which filter the peripheral blood (Fig. 7-6).

The white and red pulp make the spleen a soft, friable organ, similar to a sponge. The white pulp, which makes up approximately 15% of its structure,[41] is composed of lymphatic tissue and lymphatic follicles. Lymphatic follicles are spherical thickenings of the lymphatic tissue that surrounds the arterioles as para arteriole lymphatic sheaths. The lymphatic follicles are responsible for the production of antibodies and therefore grow in number and size in response to antigens. The red pulp, composed of a framework of reticular cells and reticular fibers together termed the cords of Billroth, surrounds specialized veins, the venous sinusoids. Blood from the arterioles flows from the reticular meshwork into the venous sinusoids and then into branches of the splenic vein.[57] The branches leave the spleen, passing through the trabeculae, and converge to form the splenic vein.

Normal Variations

The spleen undergoes the same maturational changes as most body organs. It is visible as early as 5 weeks' gestation, at which time it measures 8 to 10 mm. After the sixth decade it involutes.[27]

Aplasia (congenital absence of the spleen), a failure of normal embryogenesis, is very rare and usually is associated with other lethal malformations. Partial development may also occur and may be associated with situs inversus and cardiovascular anomalies. If no splenic tissue is visualized on ul-

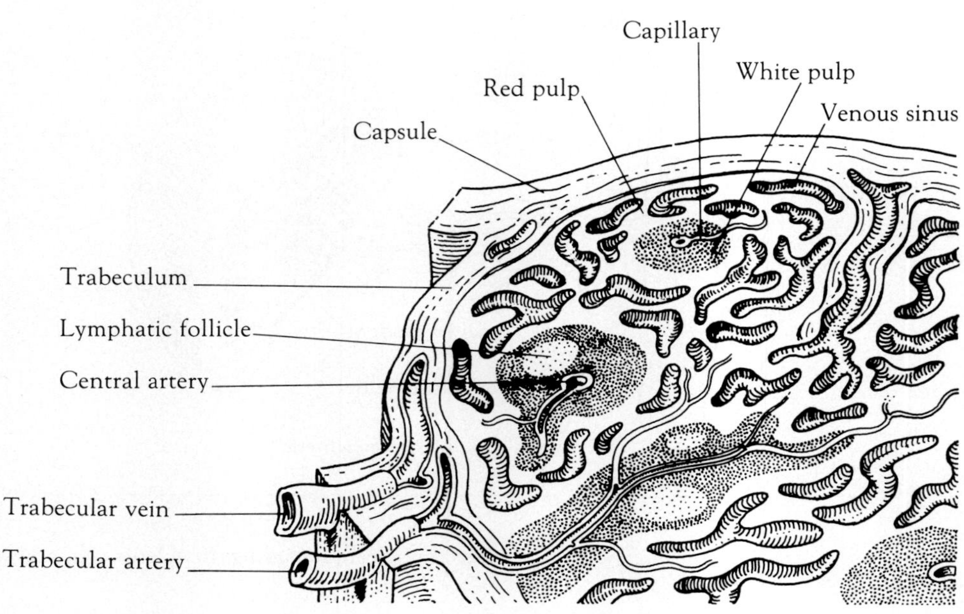

FIGURE 7-6. Schematic of the cellular structure of the spleen.

trasonography and there is no history of splenectomy, the entire left side should be examined from thorax to pelvis for an ectopic spleen. Splenic ptosis can occur if the supporting ligaments are dysfunctional or lax. The condition may be associated with a generalized visceral ptosis or absence of the abdominal musculature, as in prune belly syndrome.[48] The other causes of displaced or wandering spleen are extreme weight loss, weak abdominal muscles, splenomegaly,[2,23,27] and stretching of the supporting ligaments, which seems to occur predominantly in multiparous females between 20 and 40 years of age. The prevalence of ectopic spleen is less than 0.5%,[23] and 90% of the time females are affected.[40] The diagnosis may be made sonographically or by radionuclide studies (Fig. 7-7). Typically, when the spleen is ectopic, it is also malrotated, resulting in a high incidence of torsion and infarction. Consequently, prophylactic splenectomy may be recommended.[48]

A spleen can have prominent lobulations that should not be confused with rupture or infarction.[15] About 25% of persons have an accessory spleen (Fig. 7-8).[15,41] Approximately 80% lie in the hilus or on the gastrosplenic ligament omentum.[41] The other 20% are found in the area of the pancreatic tail and in the mesentery of the small and large intestines. Differentiating accessory spleens from pancreatic masses or from hilar lymph nodes may be difficult, unless it is possible to trace their blood supply to the splenic artery. Following splenectomy, it is not unusual for small accessory spleens to enlarge and assume the normal functions and size of the organ. This has been termed the born again spleen (Fig. 7-9).[35] Radionuclide scan may confirm the findings.

Physiology

The spleen continues to hold mysteries for physiologists. The ancients thought it was the source of melancholy and anger, probably because of its purple color.[45] Although it is rarely the primary site of disease, as the largest unit in the reticuloendothelial system it is often involved in inflammatory, hematopoietic, and metabolic disorders.[40] As a result

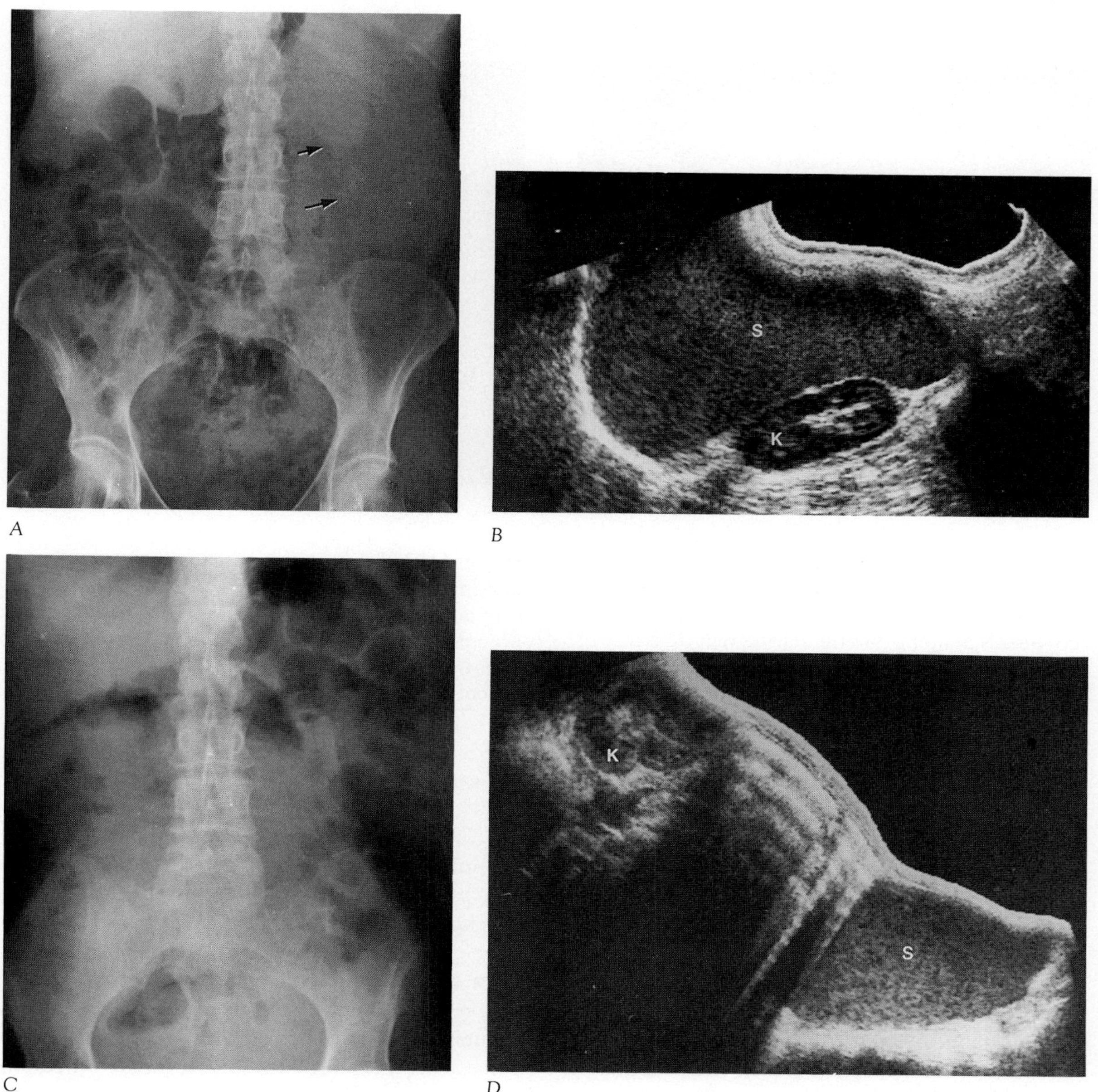

FIGURE 7-7. This case documented the movement of the spleen from its normal left side upper quadrant location into the pelvis. The initial examination demonstrated an enlarged spleen on a radiograph (*A*) and sonogram (*B*). The patient, a 58-year-old woman, continued to complain of abdominal discomfort. Eight months later, a radiograph (C) did not show the spleen in the left upper quadrant, and ultrasonography demonstrated it in the pelvis. At surgery, an enlarged spleen that was diffusely infiltrated by mixed-cell lymphoma was removed from the pelvis. (*A*) Plain radiograph of the abdomen reveals increased soft tissue density in the left upper quadrant *(arrows)*. (*B*) Sagittal sonographic image of the left upper quadrant shows an enlarged spleen (S) corresponding to the area of increased density on the plain abdominal radiograph (K, kidney). (C) Plain abdominal radiograph shows multiple loops of air-filled bowel in the left upper quadrant and absence of the previously noted splenic density. (*D*) Sagittal ultrasound image of the left side shows the left kidney (K) and the ectopic spleen (S) in pelvis separated by air-filled loops of bowel *(arrows)*. (Reprinted with permission from Kinori I, Rifkin MD: A truly wandering spleen. J Ultrasound Med 1988, 7:101–105.)

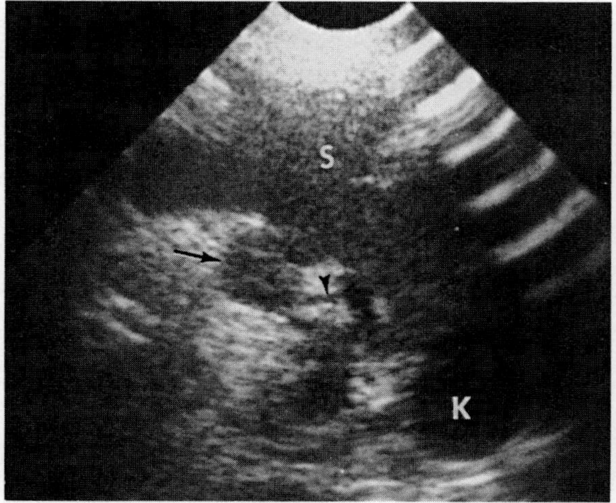

Figure 7-8. Sonogram of an accessory spleen (*arrow*). Coronal scan from the left upper flank demonstrated an isoechoic mass medial to the spleen (S) with a vein (*arrowhead*) draining into the splenic vein (K, left kidney). (Courtesy Dr. Hsu-Chong Yeh, Mt. Sinai School of Medicine, New York.)

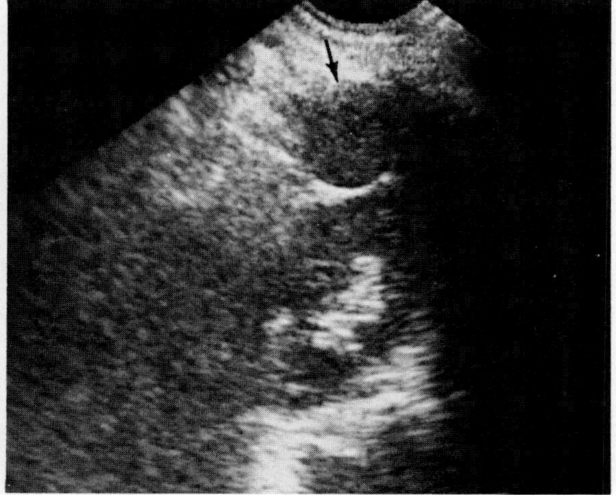

Figure 7-9. This born again spleen (*arrow*) was demonstrated lateral to the left kidney on a transverse scan taken from the left upper flank. Radionuclide scan proved this to be a spleen. The patient had undergone splenectomy. (Courtesy Dr. Hsu-Chong Yeh, Mt. Sinai School of Medicine, New York.)

of increased appreciation of the spleen's function in the body's defense against disease, splenectomy is no longer performed as hastily as in the past. It has been said that the spleen is to circulating blood what the lymph nodes are to lymph. It's major function is to filter the peripheral blood.[52,57]

Functions of the Spleen

Defense Against Disease. In the white pulp lymphocytes develop.[52] Although some of its protection against infection appears to wane in adulthood, the spleen does defend children against infection. Splenectomy is contraindicated in children younger than 3 years. The spleen's role in immune reactions is still being studied, but it is now thought that it has some unique immune functions that cannot be performed by other organs. Not merely a source of lymphocytes, macrophages, plasma cells, and antibodies, it can phagocytose bacteria that have bypassed the lymph nodes.

Erythropoiesis. We know that from about the fifth to the sixth months of fetal life the spleen is responsible for erythropoiesis. Later, the bone marrow assumes this function, but the spleen retains the capacity to produce red blood cells throughout adult life. The spleen's hematopoietic functions can be regained (so-called extramedullary hematopoiesis[41]) if chronic anemia develops or bone marrow parenchyma is lost.

Destruction and Removal of Defective Red Blood Cells. The removal of senescent, defective red blood cells occurs mainly in the cords of Billroth. Phagocytes come in contact with the blood in the reticulum cells. The blood is further exposed to phagocytes when it passes through the walls of the sinusoids on its way to the veins. The walls of the sinusoids also trap defective cells, which are then phagocytosed. As the spleen destroys aged red cells, it metabolizes their iron for reuse in hemoglobin.[15,41]

The spleen also removes defective cells such as spherocytes, sickle cells, and thalassemic cells from circulation as they pass through the walls of the sinuses because they do not possess the biconcave shape of normal red blood cells. This is referred to as the spleen's culling function.

Red blood cells that are abnormal because they

contain a granule, or even a parasite are not culled; the spleen removes only the extraneous material. Once cleaned, the erythrocyte is returned to circulation. This is the spleen's pitting function.

Normal Sonographic Appearance and Technique

The echogenicity of the spleen is comparable to that of the liver when the tissues are evaluated at the same distance from the transducer (see Fig. 7-1). It has homogenous, low- to mid-level echoes, which usually are disrupted only by the arteries and veins, in the area of the hilus. Although on cut sections the white pulp appears as gray circular or cylindrical areas, it cannot be defined on sonograms. Unlike the liver, in which the portal and hepatic veins and biliary radicles can be resolved sonographically, the splenic parenchyma appears more homogenously echogenic, except for the region of hilus, where the splenic artery and its bifurcations and the convergence of the splenic veins can be seen. It may be difficult to differentiate between these vessels without studying the Doppler signals (Fig. 7-10). Examining the spleen requires creative manipulation of the transducer and patient, but it is often performed most successfully by scanning along the axis of the ribs. This is usually best done with the patient lying with the right side down and the left arm raised over the head to separate the ribs and allow better transducer access. Newer, larger transducer heads may make intercostal scanning unfeasible. If so, the subcostal approach might be successful. In general, a sector scanner provides more maneuverability than a linear-array transducer.

Long-axis views of the spleen should be recorded, including one of the hilus with its blood vessels and several through the parenchyma. The left hemidiaphragm and the interface with the left kidney should be demonstrated. The longest axis of the spleen can be measured, as can the largest anteroposterior dimension. Once sagittal scans are complete, the transducer should be rotated 90 degrees and the transverse images recorded, measuring the organ at its widest points if the splenic volumetric index (SVI) is to be calculated, as described below.

Because of the normal variations in splenic shape and size, in ultrasound practice, length is the dimension principally monitored for enlargement. The anteroposterior diameter and width are measured if the volume is being calculated or if repeated examinations will be performed to observe for changes in size. A long axis greater than 12 cm is generally taken to indicate enlargement. Others have employed surface area[25,31] and volumetric measurements to assess splenic size. Pietri and Boscaini,[36] pointing to the close correlation between splenic size at autopsy and ultrasonographic volume measurements, developed an SVI as a reference standard. The formula is as follows:

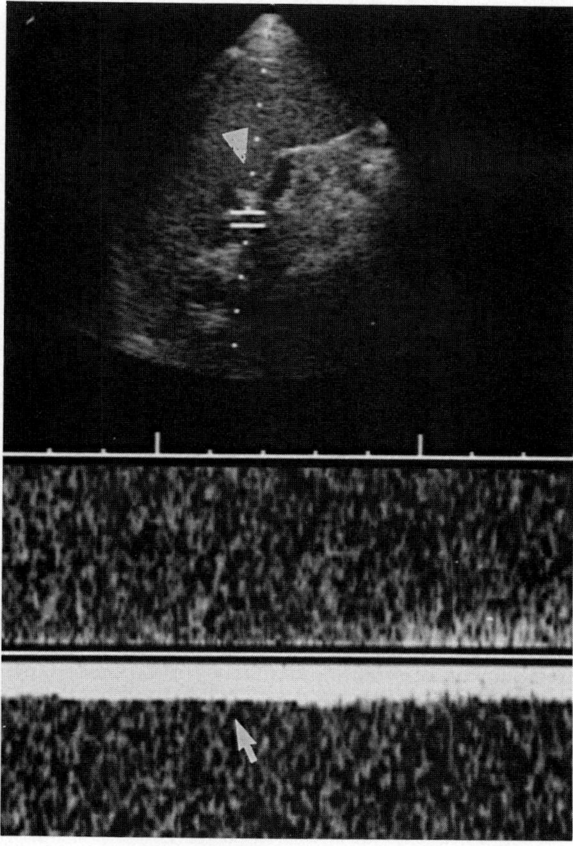

FIGURE 7-10. The splenic vein *(arrowhead)* can be differentiated from the artery by studying the Doppler signals. In this scan the vein is identified by the spectral tracing *(arrow)* of flow away from the transducer. Splenic vein thrombosis would be demonstrated as absence of venous flow.

$$SVI = \frac{\text{length} \times \text{height} \times \text{width}}{27}$$

These authors reported that for 95% of normal subjects the index was between 8 and 34.

Diseases of the Spleen

While attempts have been made to correlate alterations of splenic echogenicity with disease states, the most reliable sonographic criteria seem to be those that affect the morphology of the organ.[29,43,46,47]

SPLENOMEGALY

Although many diseases involve the spleen, they produce few sonographically demonstrable changes. The most frequent sonographically observed splenic abnormality is enlargement, which can itself cause symptoms, such as left upper quadrant fullness or pain from stretching of the capsule, stretching of the suspensory ligaments, or pressure on adjacent organs, particularly the stomach and intestines. In addition, the patient often suffers symptoms related to the underlying disease, such as jaundice, lymphadenopathy, fever, or hemorrhage.

Since many diseases affecting the spleen involve the blood, the erythrocyte and differential leukocyte counts can provide clues to the primary disease. For evaluation of spleen size, radionuclide scanning, or scintigraphy, remains the most accurate modality. Ultrasonography can be used to estimate splenic volume, but this is a cumbersome process and results are not always reproducible. While historically many criteria for splenomegaly have been developed including splenic length greater than 12 cm,[50] volume index greater than 34,[36] and surface area measurements,[33] currently only a length measurement of greater than 12 cm is commonly used. These criteria are necessary only when minimal to moderate splenomegaly exists. Visual inspection suffices when an enlarged spleen fills the abdominal cavity, extending into the pelvis (see Figs. 7-7B, 7-12, 7-16).

A wide range of pathologic processes may produce splenomegaly. These may be broadly categorized as congestive, hematologic, infiltrative, and metabolic (Table 7-1).[10] The single most common cause of splenomegaly is congestion secondary to portal hypertension, most often due to liver cirrhosis (Fig. 7-11).[50] In cirrhosis, nodular parenchymal regeneration and fibrosis cause a reduction in blood flow and an elevation in portal venous pressure (portal hypertension). Secondarily, there is a reversal of the normal flow through the portal and splenic veins toward the liver. The reversal of blood flow and damping of the normal respiratory variation in venous Doppler signal are characteristic of elevated portal pressure.[49] As pressure within the portal vein increases, it becomes enlarged and tortuous. Collateral venous pathways (varices) then appear within the splenic hilus, retroperitoneum, and gastrohepatic ligament. A recanalized umbilical vein in the ligamentum teres within the liver is also common and is pathognomonic for portal hypertension.

TABLE 7-1. Disease category or pathologic process causing splenomegaly

DISEASE CATEGORY	PATHOLOGIC PROCESS
Congestive	Portal hypertension
Hematologic	Thalassemia, hereditary spherocytosis, autoimmune hemolytic anemia, sickle-cell disease (in early stage)
Infiltrative	Leukemia, Hodgkin's lymphoma, non-Hodgkin's lymphoma
Metabolic	Gaucher's disease, Niemann-Pick disease
Chronic inflammatory conditions	Sarcoid, tuberculosis, malaria
Hematopoietic malignancies	Acute lymphocytic leukemia, chronic myelogenous leukemia, chronic lymphocytic leukemia, agnogenic myeloid metaplasia
Trauma	Parenchymal hematoma, subcapsular hematoma

In abnormalities of red cell morphology including hereditary spherocytosis, as well as in hemoglobin defects such as thalassemia, there is congestion of red cells with associated reticuloendothelial hyperplasia. These changes are associated with splenomegaly.[10]

In leukemic states and lymphoma, there may be diffuse infiltration of the spleen by malignant cell

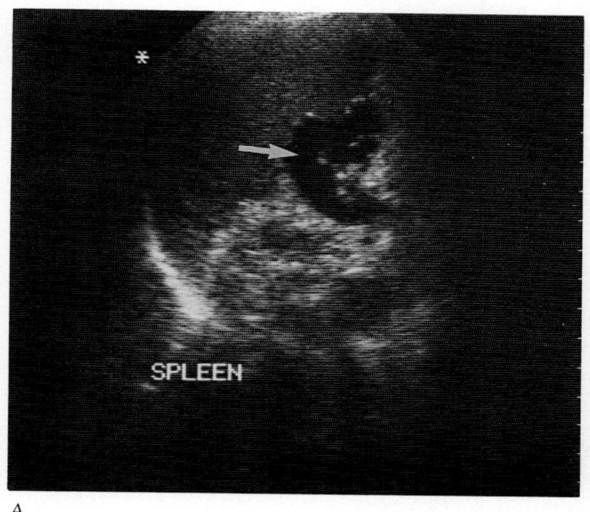

A

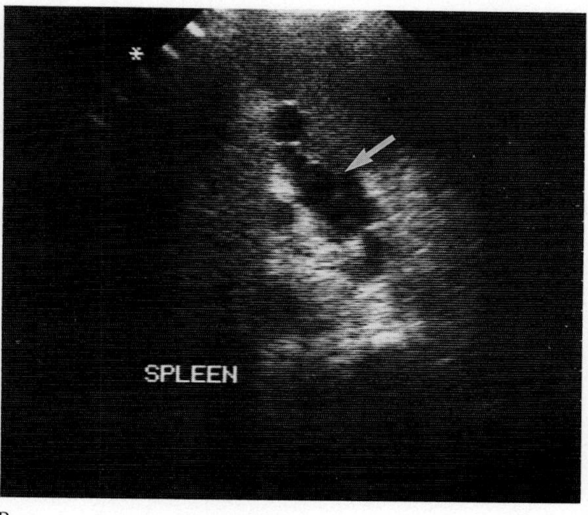

B

FIGURE 7-11. (*A*) Sagittal image of spleen with dilated splenic vein *(arrow)* secondary to portal hypertension. (*B*) A transverse section through the tortuous dilated splenic vein *(arrow)*.

lines with associated enlargement (see Figs. 7-7B, 7-12). Diffuse infiltration of the bone marrow by these malignant cells may compromise its hematopoietic capability. As a consequence the spleen may become the site of blood production, so-called extramedullary hematopoiesis. This too may enlarge the spleen.

In metabolic diseases such as Gaucher's and Niemann-Pick disease, the spleen is enlarged with macrophages distended with metabolic elements characteristic of each disease.[6,10,16]

Efforts to correlate changes in splenic echogenicity with specific disease states have been inconsistent and sometimes contradictory, making echogenicity an unreliable sonographic diagnostic criterion. Splenomegaly may produce (1) no significant change in echogenicity or (2) a diffuse decrease in echogenicity, or less commonly, (3) a diffuse increase (Table 7-2). Spinetta and coworkers[47] examined 175 cases of splenomegaly in which there was no significant alteration in parenchymal echogenicity. They noted that in these cases the primary anatomic alterations were in the red pulp, the sinusoids, and reticuloendothelium. The diseases that did not affect splenic echogenicity included

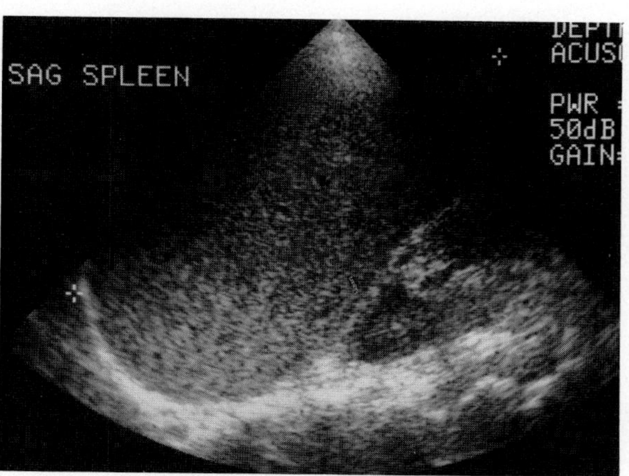

FIGURE 7-12. The enlarged spleen of a patient with acute lymphoblastic leukemia. The spleen was too large to image on one sector scan, but an estimated measurement was made of 16.7 cm.

TABLE 7-2. Sonographic characteristics of disease category or process that produces focal or diffuse lesions

SONOGRAPHIC APPEARANCE	DISEASE CATEGORY OR PROCESS
FOCAL LESIONS	
Splenic cysts	
Anechoic, well-defined walls, enhanced sound transmission	Congenital
Sharply demarcated wall, multilocular internal structure representing daughter cyst, mural calcifications	Acquired echinococcal (hydatid)
Large cysts, dense, clearly defined walls	Epidermoid or epithelial
May not have well-defined wall, mural calcifications	Posttraumatic, or post-inflammatory pseudocysts
Single or multiple simple cysts	Polycystic kidney disease lymphangioma, extension of pancreatic pseudocyst
Abscesses	
Usually multiple, range from anechoic with well-defined borders to echo-filled and septate, gas creates dirty shadowing, air-fluid or fluid-fluid level might be visible	Bacterial endocarditis, diverticulitis, osteomyelitis, pelvic or other infection
Infarcts	
Well-demarcated, wedge-shaped or round, hypoechoic in acute phase; more echogenic in later stage; measure 1–2 cm and usually located in periphery with apex pointing medially	Bacterial endocarditis, tumor embolization, hemoglobinopathy, myeloproliferative disorders, leukemia, lymphoma, vasculitis (SLE, polyarteritis nodosa)
Hematoma	
Isoechoic to echogenic mass within parenchyma, which may become hypoechoic as hematoma resolves, may demonstrate fluid-fluid level, may produce splenomegaly	Trauma, coagulation disorder
Fractured spleen may appear only as enlarging spleen with normal echogenicity; blood might be found in pelvis, flanks, Morison's pouch, lesser and greater sacs; subcapsular hematoma may appear as normal spleen, or hypoechoic, or echogenic mass adjacent to clearly defined capsule; pericapsular hematoma may efface smooth contour of splenic capsule	Ruptured spleen secondary to trauma or enlargement
Echogenic lesions	
Sometimes with hypoechoic areas and accompanying splenomegaly	Primary benign and malignant neoplasms and metastases, abscesses, hematomas
DIFFUSE CHANGES	
Calcifications	
Echogenic foci with varying degrees of acoustic shadowing	Sequelae of granulomatous disease such as histoplasmosis or tuberculosis, from previous hematoma or infarction, cysts
Hypoechoic nodules	
Irregular, multiple hypoechoic parenchymal masses; occasionally hyperechoic lesions	Hodgkin's and non-Hodgkin's lymphoma, benign (i.e., hemangioma, hematoma, isolated lymphangioma) and malignant neoplasms (metastases)

hereditary spherocytosis, hemolytic anemia, polycythemia rubra vera, agnogenic myeloid metaplasia, idiopathic thrombocytopenic purpura, erythroleukemia, and storage diseases, including amyloidosis, hemochromatosis, and lipoidosis.[31,46]

In 135 cases in which a diffuse decrease in echogenicity was observed, the disease process involved the white pulp. Diseases in this category included acute viral infections (viral hepatitis, infectious mononucleosis), and neoplasms including Hodgkin's and non-Hodgkin's lymphoma, leukemia, and multiple myeloma.

Other authors[43] suggest that an increase in parenchymal echogenicity may be observed in chronic inflammatory states that produce splenomegaly, including sarcoid, tuberculosis, malaria, and congestion. Taylor and Milan[51] observed an increase in parenchymal echogenicity in leukemic patients treated with radiation or chemotherapy. The cause of the increased parenchymal echogenicity is unknown, but it may be attributable to splenic fibrosis or to the anatomic alterations associated with the parenchymal infiltration.

Focal Lesions

In addition to the diffuse involvement described previously, a variety of processes involve the spleen focally, including true or primary cysts, secondary or pseudocysts, infarctions, granulomas, abscesses, primary benign and malignant neoplasms, and metastases (see Table 7-2).

Cysts. Cysts in the spleen may be congenital or acquired (Fig. 7-13). Within the acquired group they may be post-inflammatory, traumatic, or parasitic. Worldwide, parasitic cysts are the most common

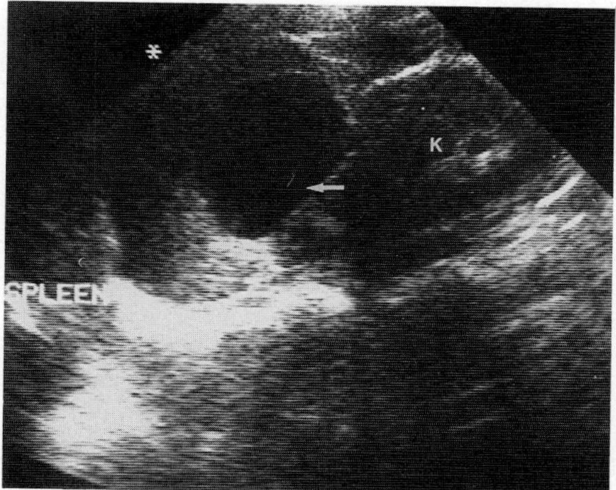

A

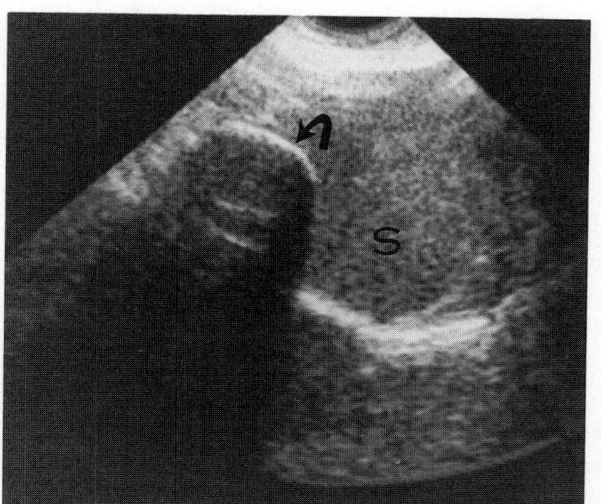

B

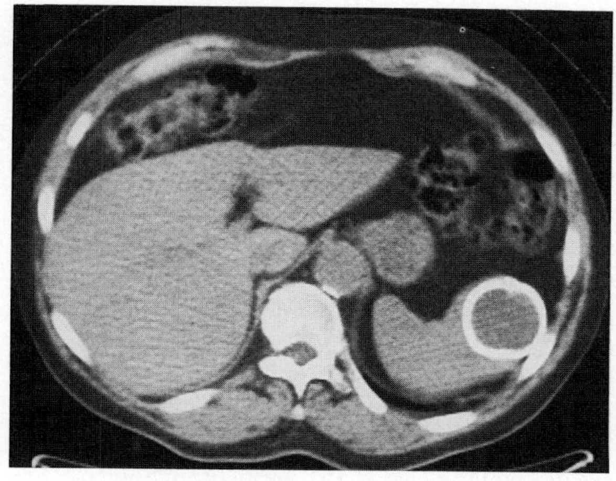

C

FIGURE 7-13. (*A*) A sagittal scan of a splenic cyst (*arrow*) discovered as an incidental finding on an abdominal sonographic examination (K, kidney). (*B*) Coronal real-time sonogram of an intrasplenic arcuate calcification (*arrow*) with posterior shadowing, obscuring the internal structure of the cyst (S, spleen). (*C*) CT of same patient revealed an intrasplenic cyst with a thick, calcified rim. (*B*, *C* reprinted with permission from Adler DD, et al: Sonographic spectrum of focal splenic lesions. J Diagn Med Sonogr 1986, 2:315–320.)

benign cysts. These are overwhelmingly echinococcal (hydatid) in origin, attributable to *Echinococcus multilocularis* or *Echinococcus granulosus*.[26] Sonographically, the appearance of hydatid cysts varies from simple and centrally anechoic to complex secondary to infolding membranes, scoleces, and hydatid sand.[11] All of these cysts should demonstrate the characteristic sonographic features of a cyst, including a well-defined posterior wall and acoustic enhancement. Mural calcification may be seen.

While parasitic cysts are the most common benign splenic cysts worldwide,[17] pseudocysts are the most common in the United States, outnumbering all other sources four to one.[1,42] Typically, these pseudocysts are post-traumatic and are the sequela of hematomas. They may also represent the final stage of organization of an abscess or infarct. They lack a true epithelial lining and are lined by debris and granulation tissue.[3,5,8,17] Calcification within the wall of a cyst occurs in approximately 50% of cases, more commonly than observed in primary cysts[9] (Fig. 7-13B).

Epidermoid or epithelial cysts constitute 10% of nonparasitic cysts (Fig. 7-14).[57] They have been described in patients 6 months to 50 years of age, but 80% occur before age 20 years. These cysts originate from the splenic capsular mesothelium, which undergoes cystic dilatation, and in some cases vascular metaplasia.[9,26,34] Such vessels are easily ruptured, often by minor trauma, accounting for the frequent presence of hemosiderin in the cyst aspirate.[26] Most often these large cysts are unifocal, with dense fibrous walls, and usually they cause no symptoms unless they are very large, up to 13 cm,[9,42] in which case symptoms may relate to compression of adjoining structures.

A rare cystic mass which can involve the spleen focally or diffusely is the lymphangioma. These are cystic, endothelial lined spaces filled with proteinaceous material. Involvement of the spleen by this entity may be localized or may be part of a generalized lymphangiomatosis of the skin, lung, bone, and viscera. Sonographically, they appear as multiseptated cystic masses.[38]

Abscesses. Single focal abscesses within the spleen are uncommon (Fig. 7-15). More often abscesses are multiple, the result of hematogenously disseminated infections, including bacterial endocarditis, diverticulitis, osteomyelitis, and pelvic infections (Fig. 7-16).[7,42,49] Typically, these lesions are complex in appearance, with mixed echogenic properties, and often they are indistinguishable from metastatic lesions or hematomas. When gas is present in the lesion, the characteristic high-level echoes and ring-down shadowing (dirty shadowing) will be observed. Similarly, the demonstration of an air-fluid level when the transducer is held in a posterior or posterolateral position is helpful.[8] Infected hematomas may present with identical sonographic properties.

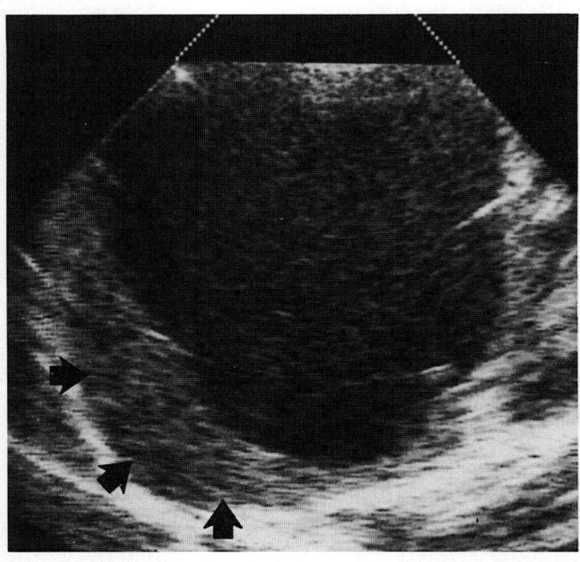

FIGURE 7-14. This large, irregularly marginated cystic mass with low-level internal echoes was proven on histologic examination to be a congenital epidermoid cyst with internal hemorrhage. Arrows point to the rind of normal splenic parenchyma. (Reprinted with permission from Adler DD, et al: Sonographic spectrum of focal splenic lesions. J Diagn Med Sonogr 1986, 2:315–320.)

Infarcts. Infarcts in the spleen are secondary to a wide range of pathologic causes, including bacterial endocarditis, tumor embolization, hemoglobinopathy, myeloproliferative disorders, leukemia, lymphoma, and vasculitis (systemic lupus erythematosus, polyarteritis nodosa). Clinically, infarcts

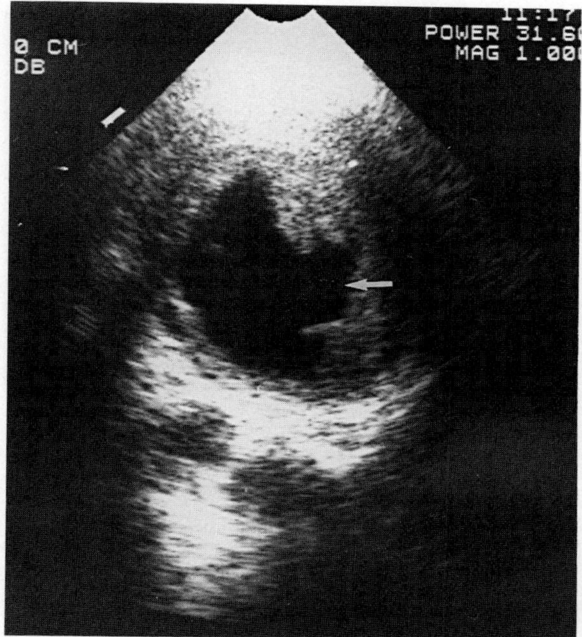

A

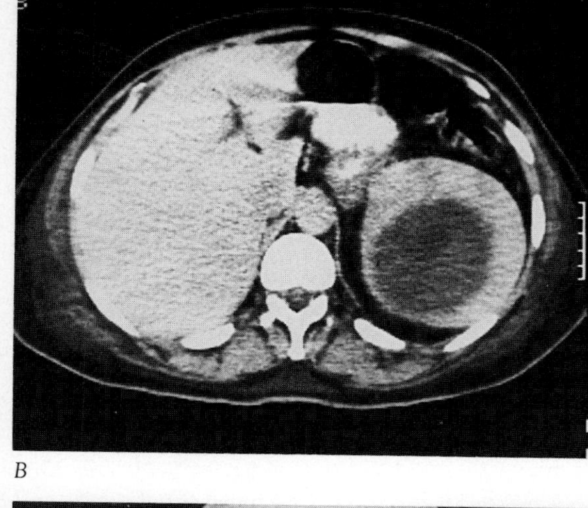

B

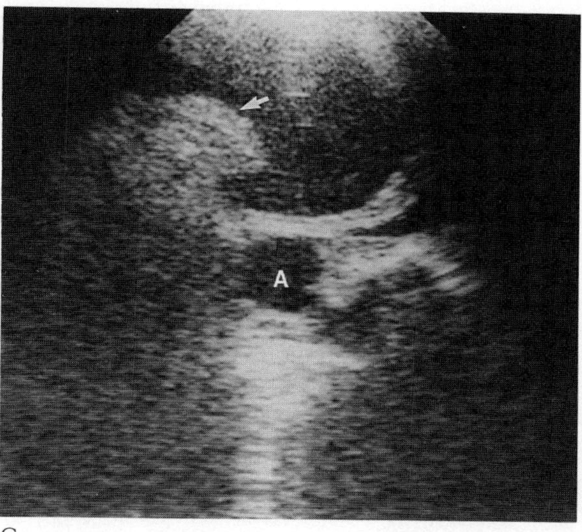

C

FIGURE 7-15. This diabetic patient presented with right upper quadrant pain, fever, and elevated white cell count. Cholelithiasis was suspected. (*A*) Transverse scan: Ultrasonography revealed an irregularly shaped and poorly marginated anechoic mass (arrow) in the spleen, which represented an abscess. (*B*) CT of the abscess. (C) Transverse sonogram through the spleen (S) of a 76-year-old woman. The echogenic area *(arrow)* was found at surgery to be an abscess. CT demonstrated the abscesses and a 4-cm accessory spleen (A) adjacent to the upper pole of the kidney. (Courtesy of KayLynn Schmitt, Rock Springs, WY.)

present with the onset of sudden left upper quadrant pain. Sonographically, these often appear as well-demarcated hypoechoic wedge-shaped or round areas located at the periphery (Fig. 7-17). In their study, Maresca and associates described two distinct patterns of echogenicity. The first, the acute inflammatory phase, presents sonographically with hypoechoic features. These changes correspond to edema, inflammation, and necrosis. Later, as organization takes place, fibrosis and shrinkage supervene, giving rise to increased parenchymal echogenicity.[24,29] Few if any features distinguish infarction from other sources of focal splenic disease, including small abscesses, metastatic disease, and lymphoma, each of which lesions ranges in size from 1 to 2 cm. It can be said that, in the absence of its classic wedge shape and peripheral location, infarction may be distinguished by its in-

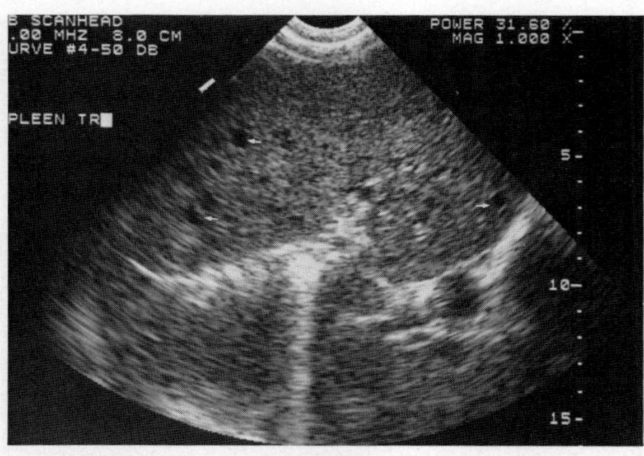

A

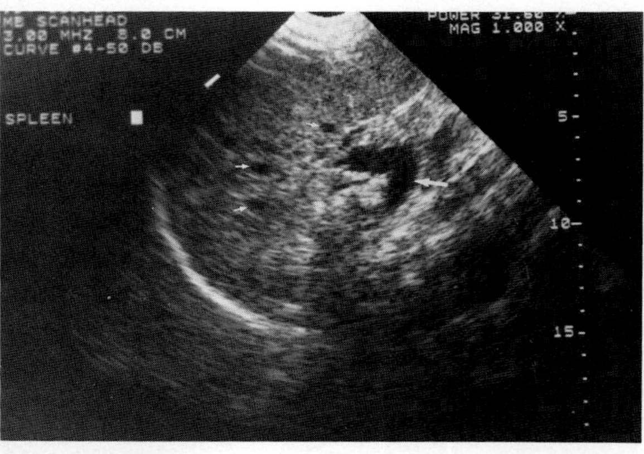

B

FIGURE 7-16. This 33-year-old female intravenous drug abuser, presented with fever, renal insufficiency, and endocarditis. The ultrasonographic examinations demonstrated multiple anechoic lesions *(arrows)* in the spleen, representing abscesses. The spleen was enlarged, probably secondary to portal hypertension. (*A*) Sagittal view; (*B*) transverse view of dilated portal vein *(large arrow)*.

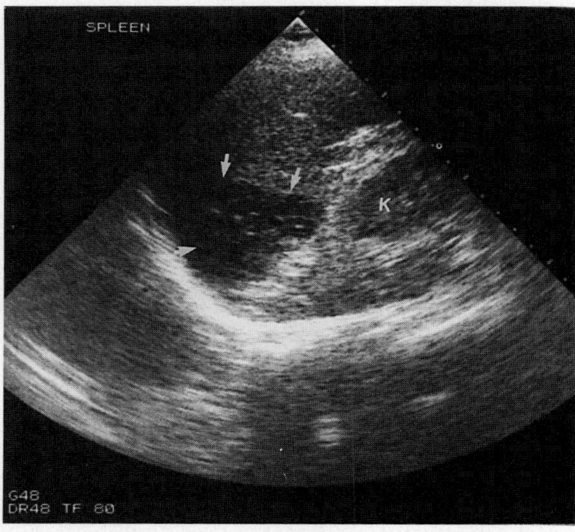

FIGURE 7-17. A hypoechoic, triangular lesion *(arrow)* in the posterior lateral aspect of the spleen represents an infarct. The gallium scan was negative, excluding the possibility of an abscess (K, kidney).

creasing echogenicity over time, although such changes may also be seen in the healing phase of leukemia or lymphoma.[21,43,51]

Trauma, Rupture and Hematoma. The spleen is the organ most frequently damaged in blunt abdominal trauma.[1,20] A range of splenic abnormalities are seen in this setting, including fracture of the capsule, parenchymal lacerations, and focal parenchymal or subcapsular hematoma (Fig. 7-18). In cases of blunt abdominal trauma when splenic involvement is suspected, CT is often the modality of choice because it can image the entire body. When ultrasonography is used, the spleen may appear normal if there is a small, fresh hematoma or it may present as a heterogeneous mass if there are extensive parenchymal injuries. A hematoma is often isoechoic and therefore difficult to identify in acute trauma, but it may become apparent on follow-up scans, as it evolves and becomes echogenic and then anechoic (possibly leading to pseudocyst formation) (Fig. 7-19).

Subcapsular hematomas may also be isoechoic to the spleen. A double contour may be seen, produced by the collection between the capsule and splenic parenchyma. With time, the hematoma

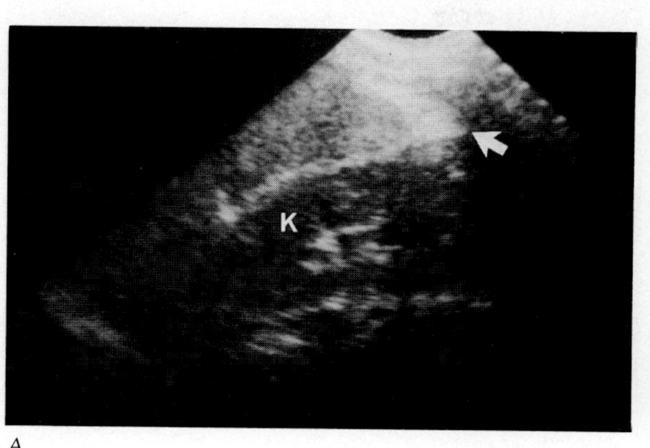

A

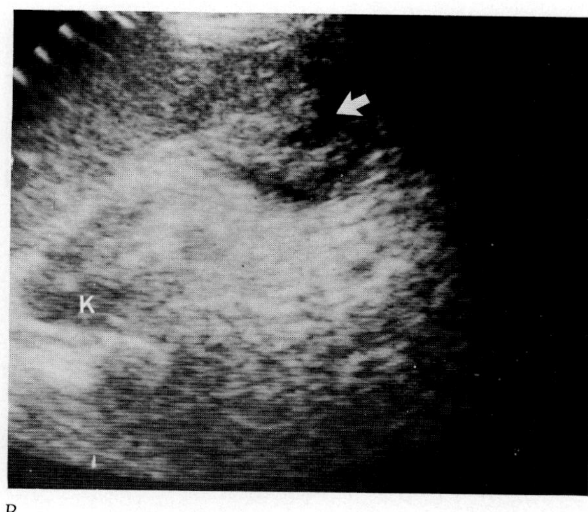

B

FIGURE 7-18. (*A*) The echogenic crescent-shaped mass (*arrow*) at the splenic tip represents a subcapsular hematoma (K, kidney). (*B*) A rupture of the spleen appears as a complex mass (*arrow*) at the area of the splenic tip (*arrow*); (K, kidney). (Courtesy of Dr. Richard Schaeffer, New York, NY).

may become echogenic, complex, and then anechoic (Fig. 7-20).[8]

An enlarging and sonographically heterogeneous spleen in the setting of acute trauma suggests the diagnosis of ruptured spleen. The sonographer must examine the pelvis, Morison's pouch, and the flanks for free blood suggesting splenic rupture. Hemoperitoneum may be suggested by the sonographic demonstration of fluid in the lesser and greater sac on both sides of the gastrosplenic ligament. Weill[55] describes this finding as the butterfly sign. Currently, patients with splenic trauma are treated conservatively so as to reduce the risk of infection arising from splenectomy. However, early identification and regular follow-up of patients with splenic trauma is important, since delayed recognition may result in catastrophic splenic rupture days or weeks following the traumatic episode.[1,8,55,58]

An enlarged spleen may rupture spontaneously, whatever the cause of the enlargement. Abnormalities that have been associated with rupture include Hodgkin's disease, infectious mononucleosis, pneumonia, chickenpox, polycythemia rubra vera, and agnogenic myeloid metaplasia. Ultrasonography may show pericapsular, subcapsular, or peritoneal blood collections.[42]

Splenic Calcifications. Calcifications in the spleen appear echogenic and may demonstrate varying degrees of acoustic shadowing (Fig. 7-20). They are usually the sequelae of granulomatous disease, most commonly histoplasmosis or tuberculosis. Calcifications may also result from previous infarction or hematoma.

Malignant Neoplasms. Although Hodgkin's disease usually begins in lymph nodes, the spleen may be the primary site.[40] In either case, eventually the spleen becomes involved. Irregular tumorlike nodules appear in the spleen. In both Hodgkin's and non-Hodgkin's lymphoma, involvement of the spleen may appear as focal hypoechoic or hyperechoic masses, diffuse splenomegaly, or normal splenic contour and size.[56] It should be noted that in this setting diffuse enlargement may or may not represent histologically demonstrable infiltration. In a study by King and coworkers, splenic ultrasonography was found to be a useful adjunct to con-

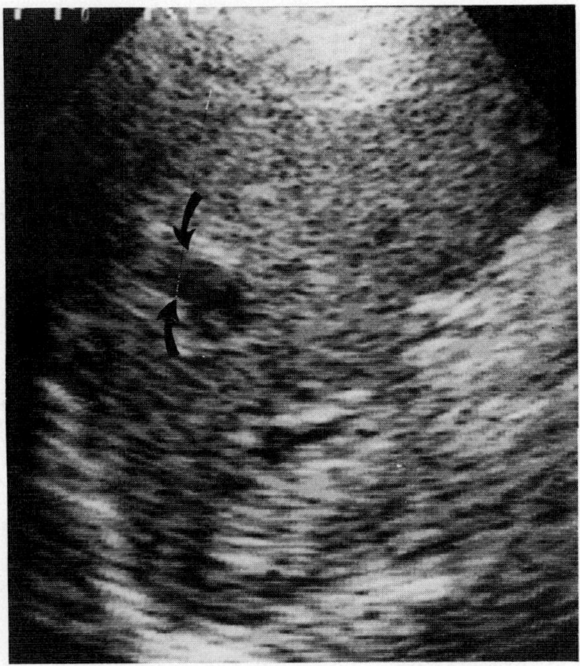

A

B

Figure 7-19. (*A*) Coronal real-time sonogram in a 30-year-old woman, 7 days after trauma and decreasing hematocrit values. Irregular echogenic and echo-free (*arrows*) intrasplenic foci were seen at surgery to represent hematomas. (Reprinted with permission from Adler DD et al: Sonographic spectrum of focal splenic lesions. J Diagn Med Sonogr 1986, 2:315–320). (*B*) Well-defined echogenic, intrasplenic mass (*arrow*) represents a hematoma. (Courtesy Richard Schaeffer, New York, NY.)

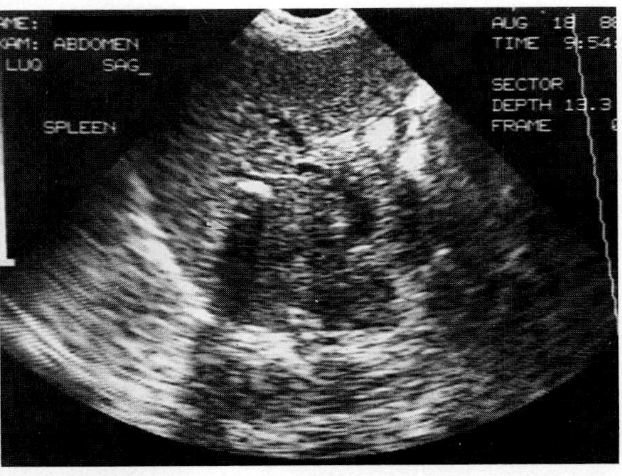

Figure 7-20. Echogenic foci with acoustic shadowing (*arrow*) were an incidental finding on sonography of the spleen. This appearance is characteristic of calcified granulomas.

firm splenomegaly and diffuse involvement by lymphoma, but it could not supplant staging laparotomy.[22] Normal spleen size did not exclude lymphomatous infiltration, nor was splenomegaly always associated with lymphomatous infiltration. As Murphy observed, 33% of patients with Hodgkin's disease may have splenomegaly with no demonstrable histologic involvement.[31] The vast majority of the splenic lymphomatous nodules have a hypoechoic appearance with ill-defined margins (Fig. 7-21). Most often they are multiple.

Primary malignant lesions of the spleen are rare. Angiosarcomas are rare primary tumors, often presenting as a large left upper quadrant mass. They are equally distributed among men and women, and clinically 70% of patients present with anemia. The prognosis is very poor: only 20% survive 6 months. Sonographically, angiosarcomas appear solid with nodular areas of mixed echogenicity. The echopenic areas within the tumor correspond to the vascular areas identified on microscopic examination.[5,33,54]

Metastatic Lesions. Despite its rich blood supply, metastases to the spleen are relatively uncommon, but they do spread from a variety of neoplasms, includ-

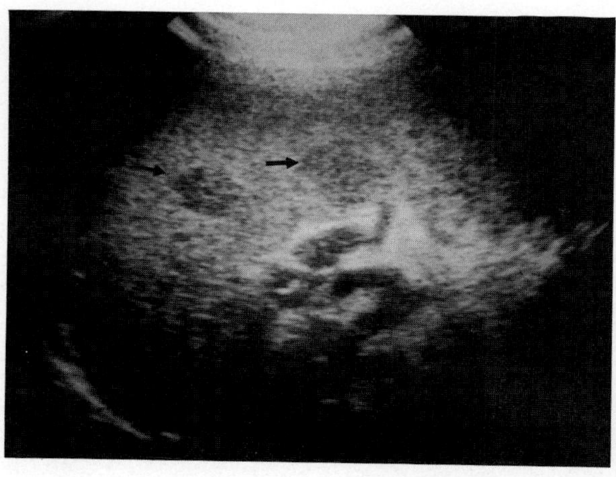

Figure 7-21. Hypoechoic masses *(arrows)* represent lymphocytic leukemic metastases to the spleen. (Courtesy Richard Schaeffer, New York, NY.)

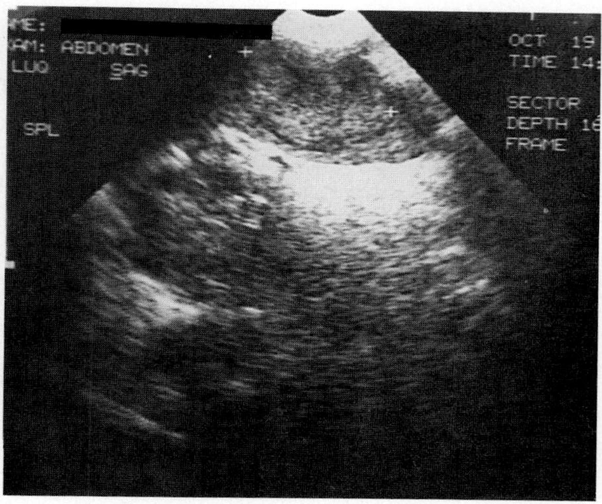

A

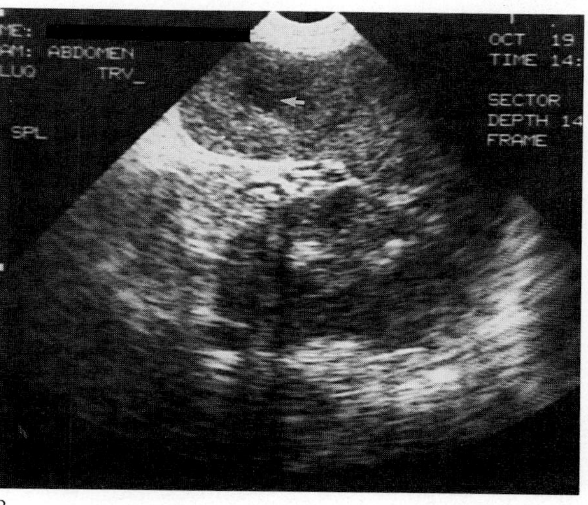

B

Figure 7-22. (*A*) Sagittal scan. A large echogenic mass in the anterior segment of the spleen *(between cursors)*. (*B*) Transverse scan demonstrates a central anechoic area *(arrowhead)* suggestive of necrosis. Echogenic masses found in the liver and the splenic mass were compatible with metastases from a primary gastrointestinal lesion.

ing those of the lung, breast, pancreas, and ovary. Overall, melanoma is the most frequent metastatic lesion of the spleen (Fig. 7-22). In one study, only 3.7% of 1140 cases of documented metastatic disease demonstrated metastatic desposits in the spleen.[56] Siniluoto reported that 52% of the patients with metastatic disease to the spleen demonstrated multifocal masses, 38% demonstrated a unifocal mass, and 10% an infiltrative pattern. Among the focal lesions, 46% were hypoechoic, 29% were mixed, and 11% were target lesions. There was no consistent correlation between the sonographic appearance of the lesions and the histologic type of primary tumor. Following therapy, some hypoechoic lesions may become hyperechoic.[31,43,44]

Acquired Aplasia and Hypoplasia. A small nonfunctional spleen is associated with repeated infarction, as occurs with sickle cell anemia (Fig. 7-23). In such cases the spleen is small, fibrotic, and often calcified. A small spleen may also be associated with celiac disease, dermatitis herpetiformis, thyrotoxicosis, and irradiation associated with Thorotrast use.[42] In all such cases, the patient has functional asplenia and no uptake of technetium-sulfur colloid is noted on scintigraphy.

Benign Hemangioma. Hemangiomas, the most common benign neoplasm of the spleen, may be broadly described as congenital hamartomas. Autopsy studies indicate that hemangiomas occur with a frequency of 1 in 600.[28] They may be divided

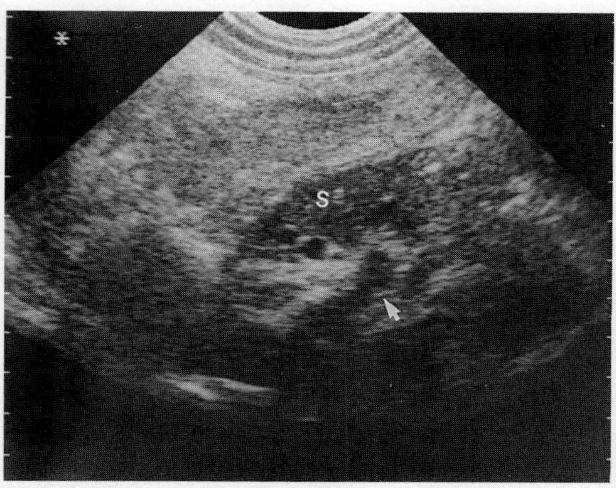

Figure 7-23. Sagittal section of a small, infarcted spleen (S) in a young man with sickle cell disease. The splenic vein *(arrow)* appears dilated. Initially the spleen is enlarged, but following repeated bouts of infarction it becomes progressively smaller until it is often not visible sonographically because of overlying bowel gas.

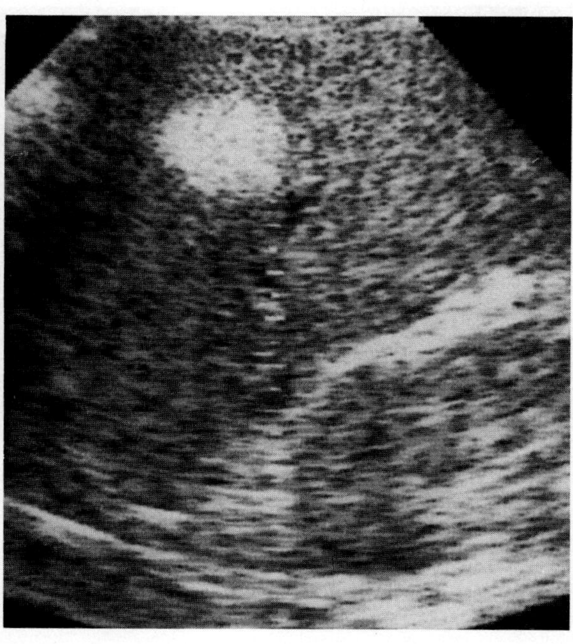

Figure 7-24. Sagittal real-time sector scan in a 43-year-old woman demonstrates a focal echogenic lesion that proved at autopsy to be a lipomatous hamartoma. (Reprinted with permission from Adler DD, et al: Sonographic spectrum of focal splenic lesions. J Diagn Med Sonogr 1986, 2:315–320.)

into capillary and cavernous types. The sonographic appearance is variable, including well-defined, echopenic foci with enhanced through-transmission, echogenic masses, and mixed complex masses.[12] Differential considerations for the complex appearance include hydatid cyst, abscess, and metastases. Symptoms are usually secondary to rupture or compression of adjoining structures. A pathologically involved spleen demonstrates enlargement, with nodular areas corresponding to cystic spaces containing serous fluid and coagulated blood. Considered to be congenital malformations, these lesions may be complicated by splenic rupture with peritoneal symptoms in as many as 25% of cases.[19] Other common benign lesions include lipomatous hamartomas and lymphangiomas (Fig. 7-24). These lesions cannot be differentiated sonographically.[28,37,46]

Acquired Immunodeficiency Syndrome (AIDS). Human immunodeficiency virus (HIV) is frequently accompanied by opportunistic infections and lymphoma, which affect the spleen as well as other abdominal viscera and the retroperitoneum. Most commonly, an enlarged spleen, with or without associated adenopathy in the splenic hilus, is identified in our HIV seropositive patients. From our experience, the most frequent opportunistic infection that affects the spleen is tuberculosis. Hodgkin's and non-Hodgkin's lymphoma, also common complications of HIV infection and AIDS, involve the spleen. Tuberculosis and lymphoma may appear as hypodense nodular implants within the splenic parenchyma (Fig. 7-25). If diffuse involvement occurs, the spleen may be enlarged. Kaposi's sarcoma, a frequent complication of the AIDS syndrome, may have the same sonographic characteristics.

In patients with extrapulmonary pneumocystis-carinii, the spleen, liver, kidneys, and adrenal glands may all demonstrate numerous punctate non-shadowing echogenic foci (Fig. 7-26), representing calcifications typical of the granulomata of pneumocystis carinii infection.[39]

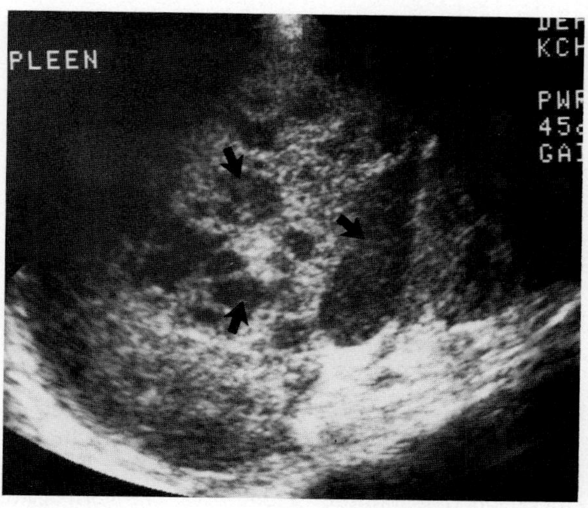

FIGURE 7-25. An intravenous drug abuser who tested HIV positive presented with splenomegaly and fever. Ultrasonography demonstrated multiple hypoechoic masses (*arrows*). At splenectomy, multiple tuberculous abscesses were found.

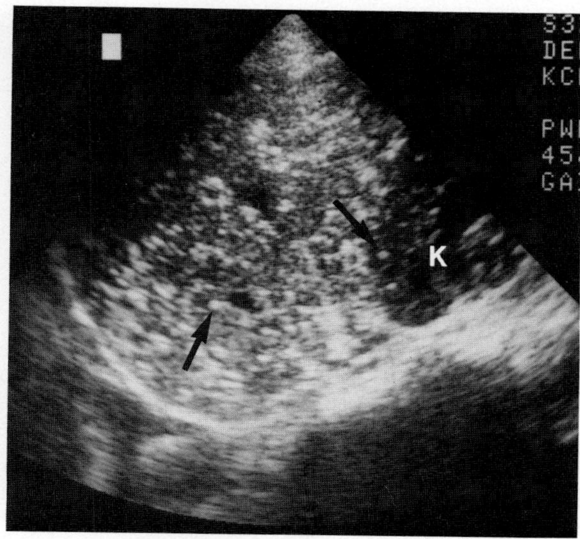

FIGURE 7-26. A sagittal scan of the spleen of an intravenous drug abuser with a history of ovarian carcinoma and HIV positive test showed multiple echogenic nonshadowing foci in the spleen and left kidney (*arrows*). The foci were also seen in the liver. These were characteristic of extrapulmonary pneumocystis carinii granuloma (K, kidney).

Conclusion

Meticulous sonographic examination of the spleen can reveal changes in its morphology and echogenicity. The latter feature may provide more definitive diagnostic information as improved resolution, computer analysis of sound waves, and Doppler investigation are conducted on splenic tissue. While radionuclide imaging and CT are often the first studies conducted of the spleen, ultrasonography is effective in characterizing masses, in identifying the nature of palpated left-side upper quadrant masses, in monitoring the course of trauma to the spleen, and in locating intraperitoneal blood collections.

Acknowledgment

Illustrations produced by the Department of Biomedical Communications, State University of New York, Health Science Center at Brooklyn.

References

1. Adler D, Blane CE, Coran AG, et al: Splenic trauma in the pediatric patient, integrated roles of ultrasound and computed tomography. Pediatrics 1986, 78:576–580.
2. Agee JH, Crepps L, Layton M: Wandering pelvic spleen. J Clin Ultrasound 1985, 13:145–146.
3. Anson BJ (ed): Morris' Human Anatomy, 12th ed. New York, McGraw-Hill, 1966.
4. Anthony AP, Kolthoff NJ: Textbook of Anatomy and Physiology, 9th ed. St. Louis, CV Mosby, 1975.
5. Aranha GV, Gold S, Grace TB: Hemangiosarcoma of the spleen. J Surg Oncol 1976, 8:481–487.
6. Beeson P, McDermott W, Wyngaarden J: Cecil Textbook of Medicine, 15th ed. Philadelpia, WB Saunders, 1979.
7. Chulay JD, Lankerani MR: Splenic abscess—report of 10 cases and review of the literature. Am J Med 1976, 61:513.
8. Cooperberg P: Diagnostic ultrasound test and syllabus. Am Coll Radiol 1988, 23:237–242.

9. Dachman AH, Ros PR, Murari PJ, et al: Nonparasitic splenic cysts. Report of 52 cases with radiologic-pathologic correlation. AJR 1986, 147:537–542.
10. Feffer A: Enlargement of Lymph Nodes and Spleen in Harrison's Principles of Internal Medicine, 9th ed. New York, McGraw Hill, 1980.
11. Franquet T, Montes M, Lecumberri FJ, et al: Hydatid disease of the spleen: Imaging findings in nine patients. AJR 1990, 154:524–528.
12. Freeny PC, Vermont TR, Barnett DC: Cavernous hemangioma of the liver ultrasonography and computed tomography. Radiology 1979, 132:143–148.
13. Goss CM (ed): Henry Gray Anatomy of the Human Body, 29 ed. Philadelphia, Lea & Febiger, 1973.
14. Gray H: Anatomy, Descriptive and Surgical, revised from the 15th English ed. New York, Bounty Books, 1977.
15. Ham AW: The structure of the spleen. *In* Blaustein A (ed): The Spleen. New York, McGraw-Hill, 1963.
16. Hill SC, Reinig JW, Baranger JA, et al: Gaucher's disease: Sonographic appearance of the spleen. Radiology 1986, 160:631–634.
17. Himji SD, Cooperberg PC: Ultrasound diagnosis of splenic cysts. Radiology 1977, 122:787–789.
18. Hollinshead WH: Textbook of Anatomy, 3rd ed. Hagerstown, MD, Harper and Row, 1974.
19. Husni EA: The clinical course of splenic hemangioma. Arch Surg 1961, 83:681–687.
20. Jordan GL, Beall AC Jr: Diagnosis and management of abdominal trauma. Curr Probl Surg 1971, 11:40–42.
21. Kauzlaric D, Passega E: Atypical sonographic findings in splenic infarction. J Clin Ultrasound 1986, 14:461–462.
22. King DJ, Dawson AA, Bayliss AP: The value of ultrasonic scanning of the spleen in lymphoma. Clin Radiol 1985, 36:473–474.
23. Kinori I, Rifkin MD: A truly wandering spleen. J Ultrasound Med 1988, 7:101–105.
24. Koehler RE: Spleen. *In* Lee JKT, Sagel SS, Stanley RJ: Computed Body Tomography. New York, Raven Press, 1983.
25. Koga T, Monkrawa Y: Ultrasonic determination of the splenic size and its clinical usefulness in various liver diseases. Radiology 1975, 115:157–161.
26. Lam AH, Parslow B: Ultrasound of splenic epidermoid cyst in children. Austral Radiol 1985, 29:(6)147–149.
27. Macpherson AIS, Richmond J, Stuart AE: The Spleen. Springfield, IL, Charles C Thomas, 1973.
28. Manor A, Starinsky R, Garfinkel D: Ultrasound features of a symptomatic splenic hemangioma. J Clin Ultrasound 1984, 12:95–97.
29. Maresca G, Mirk P, DeGaetano AM, et al: Sonographic patterns in splenic infarct. J Clin Ultrasound 1986, 14:23–28.
30. Mittelstaedt CA, Partain CL: Ultrasonic-pathologic classification of splenic abnormalities: Gray-scale patterns. Radiology 1980, 134:697–705.
31. Murphy JF, Bernardino ME: The sonographic findings of splenic metastases. J Clin Ultrasound 1979, 7:195–197.
32. Nahman B, Cunningham J: Sonography of splenic angiosarcoma. J Clin Ultrasound 1985, 13:354–356.
33. Niederay C, Sonnenberg A, Muller J: Sonographic measurements of the normal liver, spleen, pancreas and portal vein. Radiology 1983, 149:537–540.
34. Ough YD, Nash HR, Wood DA: Mesothelial cysts of the spleen and squamous metaplasia. Am J Clin Radiology 1981, 76:666–669.
35. Pearson HA, Johnson D, Smith K: The born-again spleen: Return of splenic function after splenectomy for trauma. N Engl J Med 1978, 298:1389–1392.
36. Pietri H, Boscaini M: Determination of a splenic volumetric index by ultrasonic scanning. J Ultrasound Med 1984, 3:19–23.
37. Pines B, Rabinovich J: Hemangioma of the spleen. Arch Pathol 1942, 33:487–503.
38. Pistoia F, Markowitz SK: Splenic lymphangiomatosis: CT diagnosis. AJR 1988, 150:121–122.
39. Radin DR, Baker EL, Klatt EC, et al: Visceral and nodal calcification in patients with AIDS-related pneumocystis carinii infection. AJR 1990, 154:27–31.
40. Robbins SL, Cotran RS, Kumar V: Pathologic Basis of Disease, 3rd ed. Philadelphia, WB Saunders, 1984.
41. Seufert RM, Mitrou PS: Surgery of the Spleen, rev English ed. New York, Thieme, 1986.
42. Sieler LA: Sonography of the spleen, a review. J Diagn Med Sonogr 1987, 3:69–77.
43. Siler J, Hunter TB, Weiss J, et al: Increased echogenicity of the spleen in benign and malignant disease. Am J Radiol 1980, 134:1011–1014.
44. Siniluoto T, Privansalo M, Lahde S: Ultrasonography of splenic metastases. Acta Radiologica 1989, 30:463–466.
45. Skeat WW: Etymological Dictionary of the English Language. Oxford, Oxford University Press, 1956.
46. Smith R, Gowing PC: Hemangioma of the spleen, relation to other cystic tumors. Case reports of giant cavernous hemangioma. Br J Surg 1953, 40:566–568.
47. Spinetta G, Ferrizi F, Miselli A: Sonographic patterns in diffuse splenic lesions. Rays 1986, 11:81–85.
48. Tait NP, Young JR: The wandering spleen, an ultrasonic diagnosis. J Clin Ultrasound 1985, 13:141–144.
49. Taylor KJW: Reticuloendothelial system. *In* Goldberg BB, (ed): Abdominal Sonography, 2nd ed. New York, John Wiley & Sons, 1984.

50. Taylor KJW, Burns P, Wells PNT: Clinical Applications of Doppler Ultrasound. New York, Raven Press, 1988.
51. Taylor KJW, Milan J: Differential diagnosis of chronic splenomegaly by gray-scale ultrasonography. Clinical observation and digital a scan analysis. Br J Radiol 1976, 49:519–525.
52. Vander AJ, Sherman JH, Luciano DS: Human Physiology. New York, McGraw-Hill, 1985.
53. Videbaek A, Christensen BE, Jonsson V: The Spleen in Health and Disease. Chicago, Year Book Medical Publishers, 1982.
54. Wafula SMC: Ultrasound and CT demonstration of primary angiosarcoma of the spleen. Br J Radiol 1985, 58:903–907.
55. Weill F, Romer P: Ultrasound of the traumatized spleen. Left butterfly sign in lesions masked by echogenic blood clots. Gastrointest Radiol 1988, 13:169–172.
56. Wernecke K, Peters P, Kruger KG: Ultrasonographic patterns of focal hepatic and splenic lesions in Hodgkins and non-Hodgkins lymphoma. Br J Radiol 1987, 60:655–660.
57. Wolf BC, Neiman RS: Disorders of the Spleen. Philadelphia, WB Saunders, 1989.
58. Zucker K, Brown SK, Rossman D: Nonoperative management of splenic trauma, conservative or radical treatment. Am Surg 1984, 119:400–409.

CHAPTER 8

Gastrointestinal Tract

GLENN A. ROUSE, MARIE DELANGE

The gastrointestinal (GI) tract has generally been considered more of a problem than an opportunity for sonographers. Gas in the GI tract can obscure details of the bowel wall and lumen as well as structures deep to the bowel such as the pancreas and the periaortic area of the retroperitoneum. Fluid or feces in the bowel lumen can be misinterpreted as non-GI disease. But the development of higher-resolution real-time transducers and of specialized transrectal and endoscopic sonographic instruments bodes well for the future of sonography of the GI tract, sometimes described as the last frontier of ultrasound.[32]

Methods

Real-time transducers provide the sonographic equivalent of fluoroscopy. The peristaltic activity visible on real-time examinations is nearly impossible to capture on still images, but it is invaluable to the sonographer who is identifying the GI tract and evaluating its function.

Two broad classes of ultrasonographic examinations are performed on the GI tract: transabdominal and endoluminal. Transabdominal sonography is the traditional method, often used as a screening procedure to evaluate abdominal or pelvic pain or mass. Although the GI tract is not usually the primary focus of an abdominal sonogram, the clinician will find the examination more informative if the sonographer can identify GI lesions that may cause nonspecific abdominal symptoms.

Endoluminal sonographic examinations, on the other hand, are directed specifically at the bowel or the surrounding structures. With the renewed interest in prostatic ultrasound, a variety of transrectal transducers have been developed, many of which are also suitable for evaluating the rectal wall and perirectal area, and can be used to stage rectal tumors. The advantage of the endoluminal approach is that higher-frequency transducers can be used and the layers of the bowel wall can be imaged.[6]

Endosonography is not widely employed by general sonographers. Performed by gastroenterologists using specialized endoscopes, endosonography has been a cooperative development of Japanese and European gastroenterologists and Japanese endoscope manufacturers. Its chief advantage over optical endoscopy is its ability to "see" the layers of the bowel wall, making it useful for staging bowel malignancies and evaluating lesions of the deep layers of the wall that do not involve the superficial part of the mucosa.[2,3,50] Sonographically guided biopsy of such lesions may be possible in the future. Endosonography has been performed primarily on the upper GI tract—the esophagus, stomach, and duodenum.[2,3,17,43,47–50,57] The method of examination is similar to conventional upper GI endoscopy. Following the usual premedication, the sonoendoscope is introduced into the esophagus with the patient in the left lateral decubitus position. When the lesion is identified visually, it can be examined with the attached sonographic transducer.[57]

Preparation

Preparation of the patient for transabdominal sonography of the GI tract depends on the part of the tract that is of interest. Because examination of the upper abdomen looks at the gallbladder, pancreas, bile ducts, and upper GI tract, the patient should be advised to fast for about 4 hours before the examination, to ensure distension of the gallbladder and to minimize stomach gas. If the stomach and duodenum are to be further evaluated, the patient can drink 10 to 40 ounces of water through a straw to improve visualization.[32] We have noticed that having the patient drink fluid also helps in evaluating the mucosa and peristalsis of the jejunum and ileum. Oral fluid is, of course, contraindicated if the patient has GI obstruction or ileus or is scheduled for upper GI barium studies. For transabdominal examination of the colon, no special preparation is necessary, except for the rare occasion during pelvic sonography when a water enema is required to establish the position of the rectosigmoid colon.[39] Before transrectal sonography, a cleansing enema may be helpful so that fecal material is not confused with mucosal lesions.[6]

Anatomy of the Bowel Wall

The GI tract is, essentially, a very long muscular tube, originating at the mouth and terminating at the anus (Fig. 8-1). The layers of the bowel wall are the same throughout the GI tract. Described anatomically, the innermost layer is the epithelium, which in the esophagus is squamous and elsewhere a layer of cuboidal cells atop villi and glands. Deep to the epithelium lies the lamina propria, which in the esophagus is loose areolar tissue and elsewhere is glandular tissue. Immediately below the lamina propria is a very thin, smooth muscle layer called the muscularis mucosa. Just above and below the muscularis mucosa are scattered patches of lymphoid tissue. Below the muscularis mucosa is more loose areolar tissue, called the submucosa. Deeper yet lies the muscularis propria, also known as the muscularis externa. This structure consists of an inner circumferential layer and an outer longitudinal layer of smooth muscle. The final layer of the wall is the serosa, a thin epithelial layer on the periphery of the bowel (Fig. 8-2).

The structure of the bowel wall is sonographically visible using endoluminal transducers and is sometimes visible transabdominally, particularly in the stomach (Fig. 8-2B). The innermost sonographic layer is an echogenic line that represents the fluid-mucosa interface. Deep to that is a hypoechoic layer—the mucosa, lamina propria, and muscularis mucosa. Deeper yet is the echogenic submucosa, followed by a hypoechoic layer, the muscularis propria, which in turn is followed by a thin echogenic layer, the serosa. Thus the sonographic structure of the bowel is usually described as five layers: three echogenic layers separated by two hypoechoic ones. In one study in vitro using a 10-MHz transducer, the muscularis mucosa and the two layers of the muscularis propria were resolved as well.[2] Visualizing the layers of the bowel wall is useful in detecting certain pathologic conditions that will be discussed later.

Esophagus and Esophagogastric Junction

SONOGRAPHIC TECHNIQUE

Sonographic imaging of the esophagus is accomplished only via the sonoendoscope. With proper technique and newer equipment, the examiner can visualize fairly well the layers of the esophageal wall[3] and surrounding mediastinal structures. European and Japanese esophageal sonoendoscopists are interested mainly in staging esophageal tumors.[43,49,57] At this writing, sonoendoscopy of the esophagus has not been compared with computed tomography (CT) and magnetic resonance imaging (MRI), but surgical findings indicate that sonoendoscopy is quite accurate.[49,57]

Although esophageal varices are visible with sonoendoscopy,[8,43] they can be assessed adequately with optical endoscopy. The esophagogastric junction can sometimes be viewed transabdominally (Fig. 8-3).

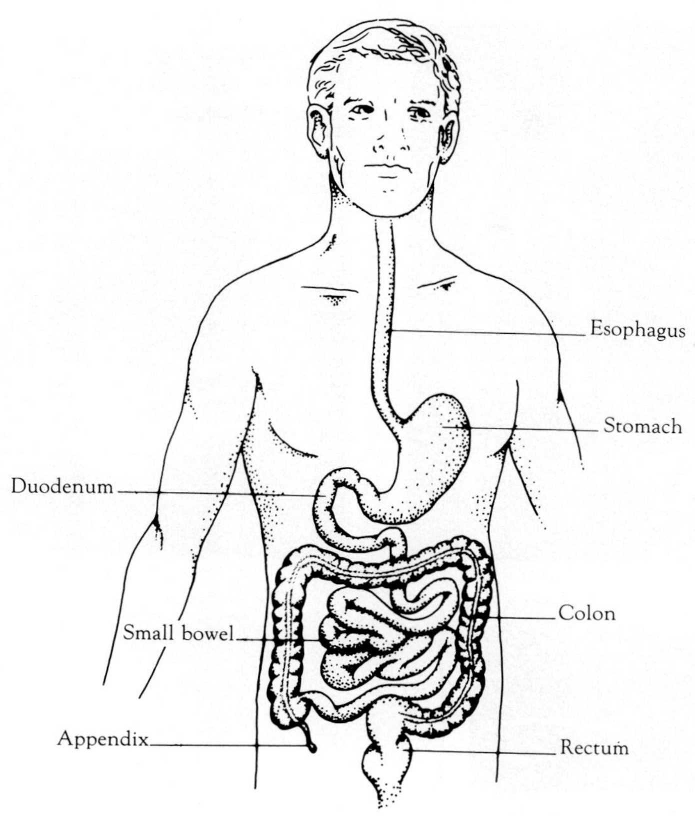

FIGURE 8-1. Anatomic drawing of the gastrointestinal tract.

DISORDERS

Carcinoma. Most carcinomas of the esophagus are squamous cell carcinomas. These occur least commonly in the upper esophagus, and with about equal frequency in the middle and lower thirds. Squamous cell carcinoma of the esophagus affects older persons and more men than women. The lesions begin as longitudinal plaquelike areas, which quickly enlarge circumferentially; subsequently strictures form and dysphagia develops. Since the esophagus lacks a serosa, extension into the surrounding mediastinum is unimpeded and few patients survive 5 years after diagnosis.[20,27]

Other Tumors of the Esophagus. Primary adenocarcinoma of the esophagus is rare; most arise from the stomach and involve the esophagus by direct extension. Other rare malignant tumors of the esophagus include carcinosarcoma, lymphoma, mucoepidermoid carcinoma, and adenoid cystic carcinoma. The most common benign tumor of the esophagus is leiomyoma.[27]

Esophagogastric Junction. The esophagogastric junction can be evaluated with endosonography or, if the left lobe of the liver is large enough, with transabdominal sonography. One can demonstrate a variety of abnormalities, including hiatus hernia, esophageal varices, and tumors.

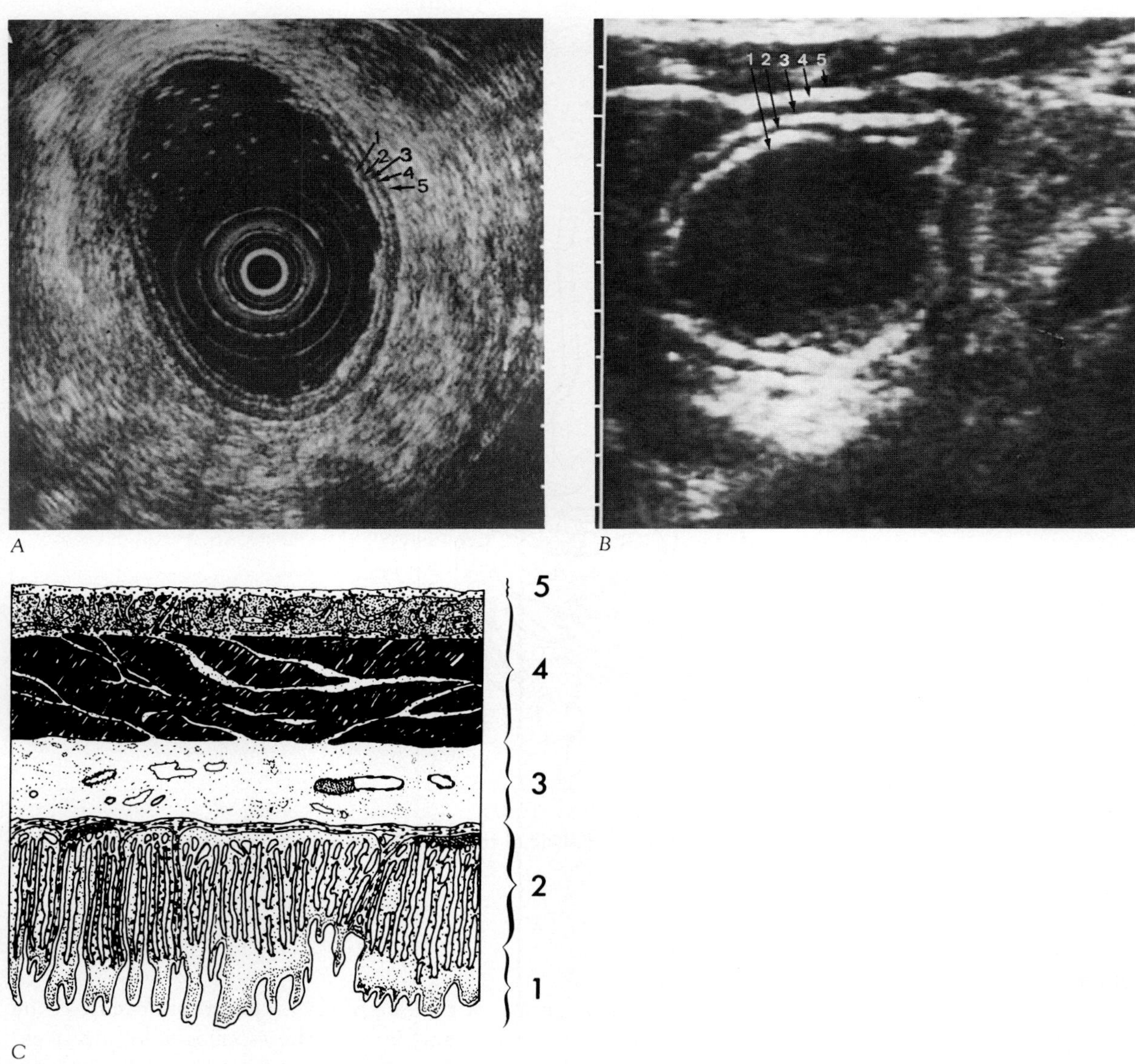

Figure 8-2. (*A*) Endoscopic ultrasonographic appearance of the normal gastric wall at the level of the body of the stomach. Five distinct layers of different echogenicity can be identified. (From Bolondi L, Casanova P, Caletti GC, et al: Primary gastric lymphoma versus gastric carcinoma: Endoscopic US evaluation. Radiology 1987, 165:821–826.) (*B*) Longitudinal transabdominal image of the gastric wall layers. (C) Drawing of the gastric wall layers. The corresponding sonographic layers are numbered: mucosal surface (1), the deeper part of the mucosa and the muscularis mucosa (2), the submucosa (3), the muscularis propria, which anatomically has a longitudinal muscle layer and a circular muscle layer (4), and the serosa (5). (From Williams D, Rouse GA, Tan-Sinn P: The gastrointestinal wall layers: An aid in sonographic detection of gastric wall lesions and rectal wall cancer staging. J Diagn Med Sonog 1990, 6:3–17.)

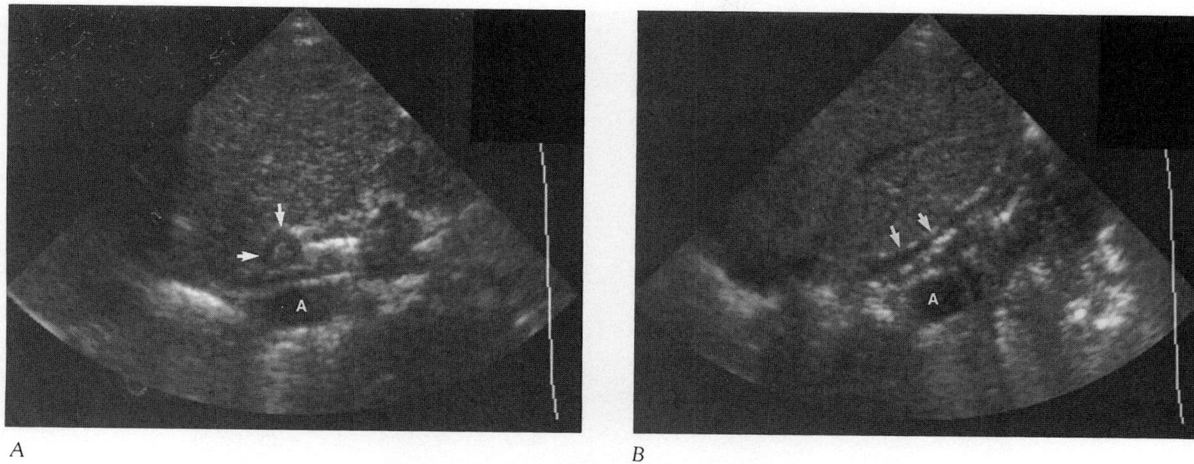

FIGURE 8-3. Longitudinal (*A*) and transverse (*B*) views of the normal esophagogastric junction *(arrows)* traversing between the aorta (*A*) and liver. Note the typical target appearance on the longitudinal view.

Stomach

SONOGRAPHIC TECHNIQUE

Of the entire GI tract, the stomach has the most potential for better sonographic diagnosis. The layers of the GI tract wall are thicker here than anywhere else and nearly always can be visualized transabdominally in the normal patient. A few special techniques are occasionally helpful. If the sonographer is uncertain whether a cystic structure in the left upper quadrant represents the stomach, giving the patient a few sips of water through a straw produces a sparkling or swirling pattern in the stomach as the water flows. Usually, the stomach contains some air when the patient is supine. Turning the patient into the right lateral decubitus position moves fluid into the antrum, providing better visualization of that part of the stomach and confirming the identity of the stomach. Similarly, turning the patient into the left lateral decubitus position often improves visualization of the fundus.[32]

When a solid-looking mass is suspected to be the stomach, or when detailed evaluation of the gastric mucosa is required, the patient should sit up and slowly drink 40 to 50 ounces of water and then be scanned in the upright, left lateral decubitus, supine, and right lateral decubitus positions, thus demonstrating most of the gastric mucosa.[32] Some investigators recommend giving 1 mg of glucagon intravenously before the patient drinks the water, to ensure retention of the fluid in the stomach; this should produce 30 to 60 minutes of gastric distention.[55]

NORMAL ANATOMY

The stomach normally lies in the left upper quadrant of the abdomen. The fundus is medial to the spleen and anterior to the left kidney. The body and antrum of the stomach lie posterior or inferior to the left lobe of the liver, anterior to the pancreas, and medial to the gallbladder and porta hepatis (Fig. 8-4). The antrum and body of the stomach often appear as a targetlike structure inferior to the left lobe on longitudinal sonograms. If the left hepatic lobe is large enough, the esophagogastric junction can also be visualized as a targetlike structure just below the diaphragm and just to the left of the spine (see Fig. 8-3A). Gas, mucus, or fluid may fill the center of the stomach. If the stomach is not distended, the bowel wall should measure 2 to 6 mm thick. When the stomach is distended to a diameter of 8 cm or more, the wall should mea-

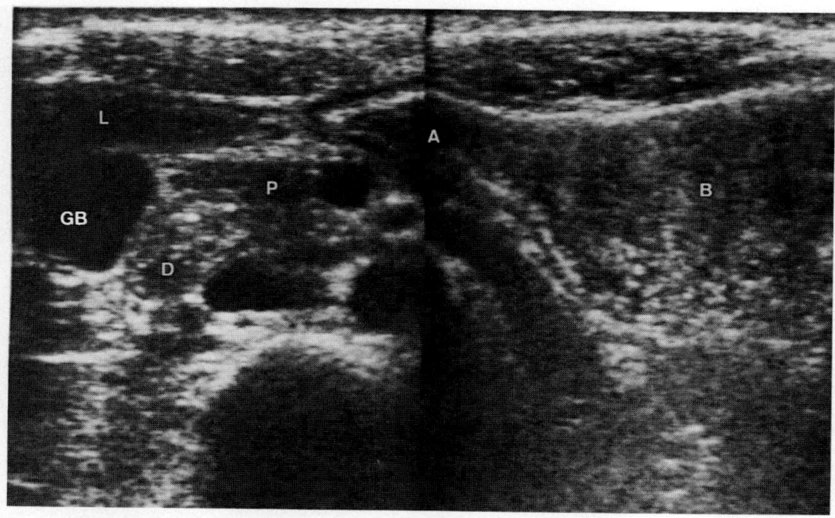

FIGURE 8-4. Normal relational anatomy of the stomach: Transverse view of the body (B) and antrum (A) of the stomach. Note the relationship to the liver (L), gallbladder (GB), second portion of the duodenum (D), and uncinate process of pancreas (P). (From Williams DM, Rouse GA, Tan-Sinn P: The gastrointestinal wall layers: An aid in sonographic detection of gastric wall layers. J Diagn Med Sonogr 1990, 6:3–17.)

sure 2 to 4 mm.[16] Often when fluid is present in the stomach, the rugal folds and posterior wall structure can be seen.

DISORDERS

Gastric Dilatation. Many disorders can cause the stomach to dilate (Fig. 8-5A). Acute dilatation can occur after surgery or after placement of a body cast. It is not clear whether this dilatation is caused by reflex paralysis of gastric motility or obstruction of the duodenum by the superior mesenteric artery impinging on it. Tumor or ulcer disease may obstruct the gastric outlet. Pyloric muscle hypertrophy is rare in adults, but when it does occur, it is usually associated with gastritis or ulcer disease. Diabetes mellitus, scleroderma, or surgical vagotomy may bring about gastric dilatation as a complication of neuropathy. The sonographer can observe gastric peristalsis to differentiate atonic from obstructive dilatation, but the distinction may be impossible in many cases because of rigidity of the stomach wall, often seen in tumor infiltration and gastric ulcer disease, and the uncoordinated peristaltic waves seen in neuropathic conditions. Volvulus is another rare cause of gastric dilatation.[9]

Gastritis and Ulcer Disease. Chronic gastritis may present as enlarged rugal folds with generalized thickening of the mucosal layer of the wall (Fig. 8-5B,C). This thickening may accompany either increased acid production, as in Zollinger-Ellison syndrome, or decreased acid production, as in Menetrier's disease. Chronic gastritis may also demonstrate hyperplastic and inflammatory polyps. Another variation is atrophic gastritis, in which the mucosa is thinned. This is difficult to see sonographically, but it is considered a precursor of gastric carcinoma.[42]

Gastric peptic ulcers are one third as common in the United States as duodenal ulcers. Benign peptic gastric ulcers can occur anywhere in the stomach, but most often appear along the antral portion of the lesser curvature. Sonographically, there may be major wall thickening, usually caused by marked

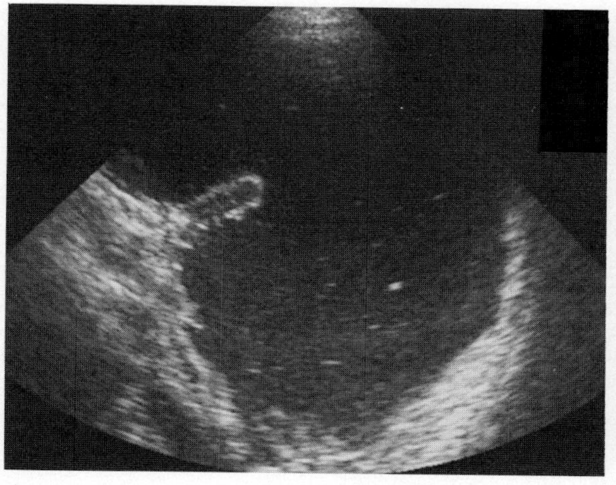

A

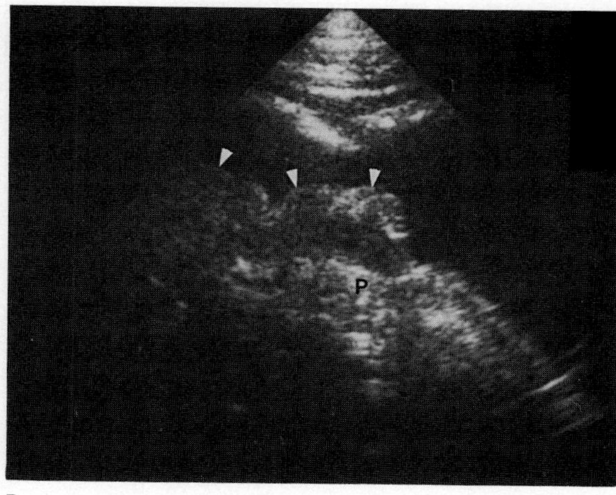

B

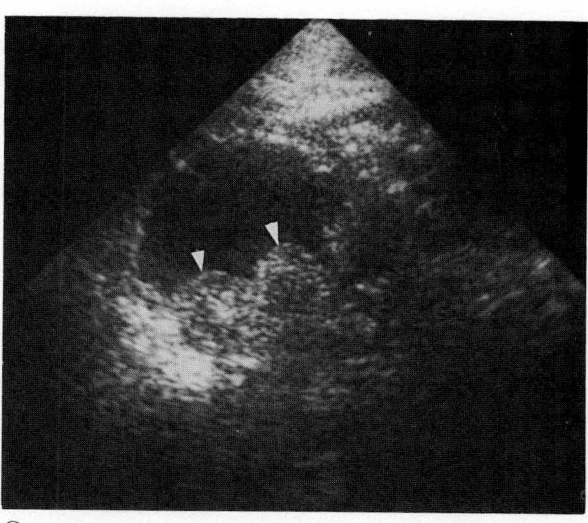

C

FIGURE 8-5. (*A*) Transverse view of the gastric fundus demonstrates marked gastric distention because of gastric outlet obstruction. (*B*) Longitudinal and (*C*) transverse views of the antrum also demonstrate distention, as well as hypertrophic gastric rugae (*arrowheads*). This patient with acute and chronic pancreatitis has focal hypertrophic gastritis adjacent to the head and body of the pancreas (P).

edema of the submucosa, with milder thickening of the gastric mucosa. Typically, the mucosa is undercut at the edge of the ulcer (Fig. 8-6). A malignant ulcer, by contrast, should show more "heaping up" of the margin of the ulcer.[42] The bowel layers adjacent to the ulcer may be obliterated in either benign or malignant ulcers.[43,50] Ulcers can be detected sonographically,[51] particularly if they are large, but often they are only suggested by focal or generalized edema of the wall. Peptic duodenal ulcers are even more difficult to identify, but mucosal edema can sometimes suggest their presence (Fig. 8-7).

Complications of peptic ulcer disease, gastric or duodenal, include anterior or posterior perforation. Usually, anterior perforation results in free intraperitoneal air, and often, subsequent peritonitis, which may appear sonographically as ascites, loculated ascites, or dense debris in the peritoneal space (Fig. 8-8). Thickening of the bowel serosa may be observed due to peritoneal irritation and

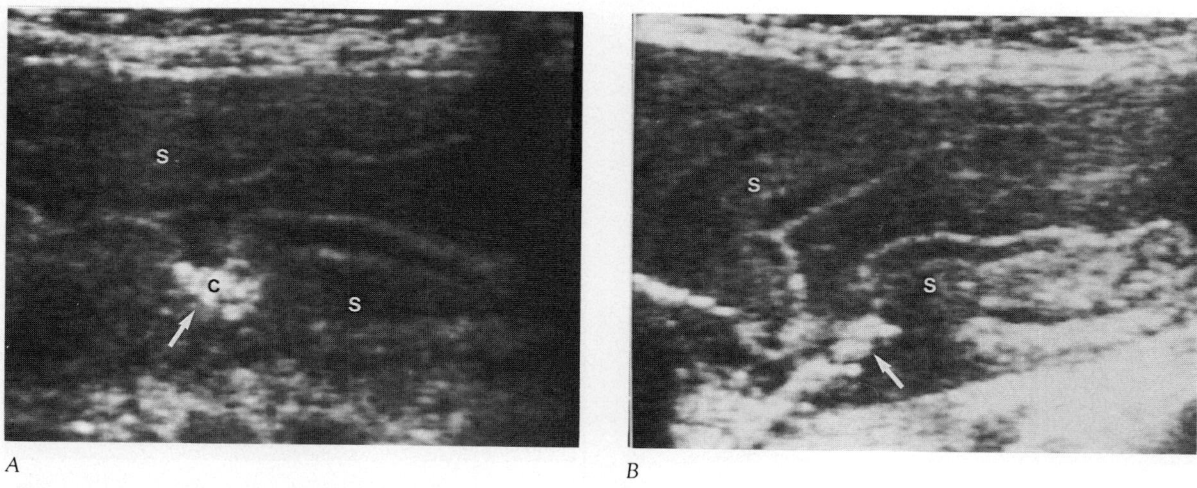

Figure 8-6. (*A*) Longitudinal and (*B*) transverse views of the gastric antrum in a patient with a benign gastric ulcer *(arrows)*. Note the markedly thickened submucosal layers (S) and the blood clot (C) in the base of the ulcer. (From Williams D, Rouse GA, Tan-Sinn P: The gastrointestinal wall layers: An aid in sonographic detection of gastric wall lesions and rectal wall cancer staging. J Diagn Med Sonogr 1990, 6:3–17).

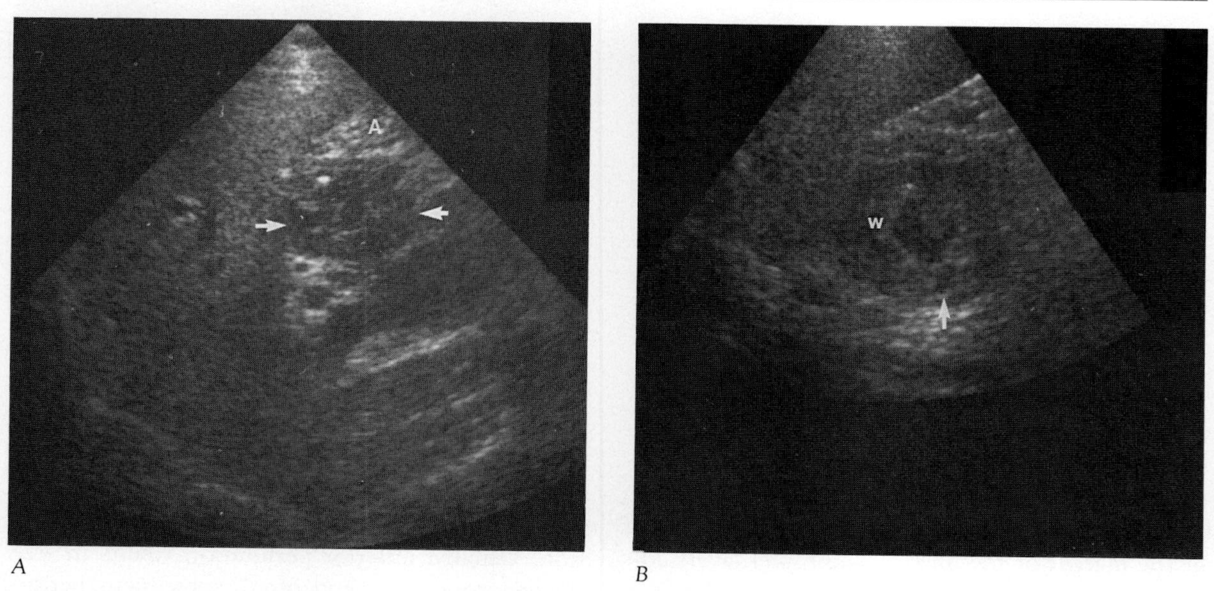

Figure 8-7. (*A*) Longitudinal view demonstrates edema of the duodenum *(arrows)* adjacent to the gastric antrum (A). (*B*) Magnified view demonstrates thickening of the duodenal wall (W) and peptic ulcer crater *(arrow)*.

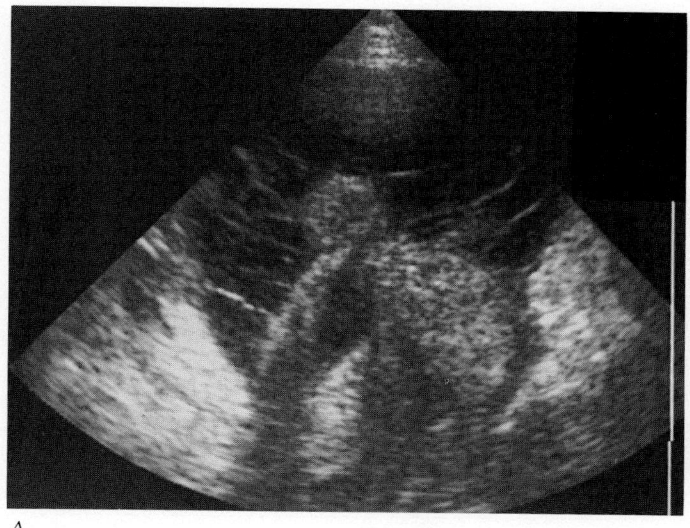

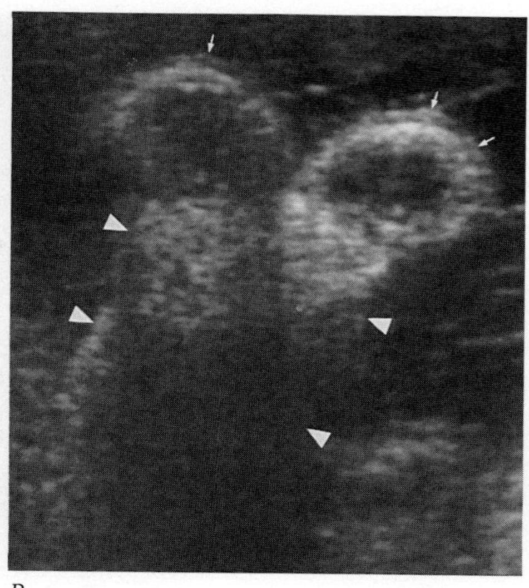

FIGURE 8-8. Ascites due to peptic ulcer perforation: (*A*) Transverse view demonstrates ascites with multiple loculations. (*B*) Magnified view of the small bowel loops again shows septations in the fluid as well as serosal edema *(small arrows)* of the bowel loops and shortening of the mesentery *(arrowheads)*. These findings result from leakage of bowel contents, such as amylase, into the peritoneal space.

reactive edema. Generalized peritoneal infection or localized abscess may also result (Fig. 8-8B).[29,32] The chief complication of posterior duodenal perforation is bleeding, but posterior perforation of the stomach may result in pancreatitis.

Gastroduodenal Crohn's Disease. Crohn's disease is an idiopathic inflammation that starts in the submucosa and spreads to all layers of the bowel wall. This disease usually occurs in young adults and affects the ileum primarily, and to a lesser extent the colon. Two to eight percent of patients have stomach or duodenal involvement.[40] Since the entire wall is involved at diagnosis, the sonographic appearance is that of a nonspecific hypoechoic target lesion if the lumen is viewed transversely. Advanced carcinoma, lymphoma, hematoma, and tuberculosis can appear similar.

Other Inflammatory Conditions. Infection of the stomach can display marked thickening of the stomach wall and swelling of the gastric rugae, a condition called phlegmonomous gastritis.[40,53] Most cases are caused by α-hemolytic streptococci, but *Staphylococcus, Escherichia coli, Clostridium welchii,* and *Proteus* species have also been found. Peritonitis occurs in 70% of cases. When gas-forming organisms such as *E. coli* or *C. welchii* are the cause, small gas bubbles may form in the gastric wall; this is a type of emphysematous gastritis.[40,53] Swallowing a corrosive substance is a more common cause of emphysematous gastritis.[40]

Benign Gastric Tumors. In order of decreasing frequency, benign tumors include hyperplastic polyp (38%), leiomyoma (24%), gastric adenoma (10%), heterotopic pancreas (7%), fibroma (4%), neurinoma (4%), leiomyoblastoma (3%), lipoma (3%), gastric cyst (2%), vascular tumors (2%), and others (2%) (Fig. 8-9).[34] Hyperplastic polyps and gastric adenomas are polypoid masses arising from the gastric mucosa, and adenomas seem to have some malignant potential. Gastric cysts develop by cystic dilatation of gastric glandular tissue and enlarge into

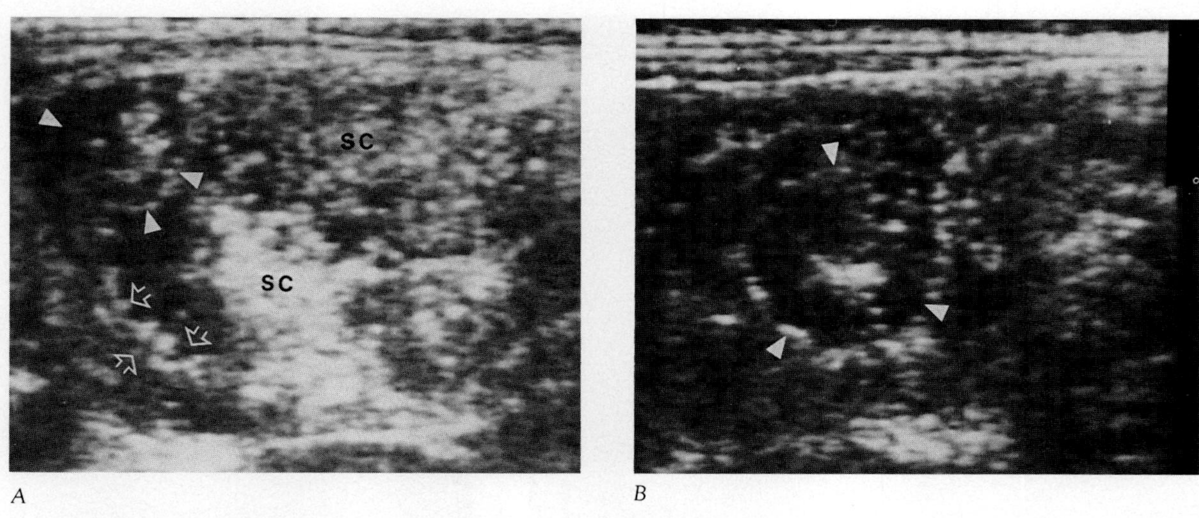

FIGURE 8-9. (*A*) Transmural and (*B*) en face views of a submucosal heterotopic pancreas *(arrowheads)*. The normal gastric wall is shown adjacent to the mass for comparison *(open arrows)*. The echogenic material on the transmural view is stomach contents (SC).

the submucosal space. Other types of tumors arise from the submucosal or muscle layer and spare the mucosa unless surface ulceration develops. Lipomas are generally echogenic.[57] Smooth muscle tumors may show a typical swirled texture if they are large enough.[57]

Carcinoma. Gastric carcinoma is the third most common GI malignancy following colon carcinoma and pancreatic carcinoma, but its incidence has been declining in the United States since the turn of the century. The relationship of diet to gastric cancer has long been debated; smoked food, nitrosamines, and high-starch diets have been implicated. Japan, Chile, Iceland, and Finland currently have gastric cancer rates up to seven times higher than the United States. A familial tendency to develop this condition has also been noted.[25]

Gastric carcinoma arises from the mucosa of the stomach,[23] invading the submucosa and muscularis propria. Various systems for classifying it have been proposed; one of the most commonly used is that of Borrman.[5] In this system, a type 1 lesion is a focal polypoid mass. A type 2 lesion is a focal ulcerating tumor; and a type 3 lesion is also a tumor ulcer but has more extensive surrounding infiltration. A type 4 lesion demonstrates extensive infiltration of the stomach wall and may involve the entire stomach (Fig. 8-10). Most gastric carcinomas spread primarily toward the serosa of the gastric wall.[23] Some gastric tumors arise in the margin of a long-standing benign peptic ulcer.[42]

Lymphoma. Primary lymphoma of the stomach accounts for 3% to 8% of gastric malignancies (Fig. 8-11).[34] It is usually a reticulum cell sarcoma or lymphosarcoma but rarely may be Hodgkin's lymphoma.[34] The stomach is the most common site of primary lymphoma of the GI tract. The cells of origin are lymphocytes located just above and below the muscularis mucosa. Typically, lymphoma initially involves the outer part of the lamina propria and the inner part of the submucosa. Endosonography characteristically reveals this involvement as well as a tendency for the tumor to spread laterally following the muscularis mucosa rather than vertically through the layers of the wall as in gastric carcinoma (Fig. 8-12).[4] The fact that the surface of the mucosa is not involved until quite late in the disease seems to be one of the primary reasons for

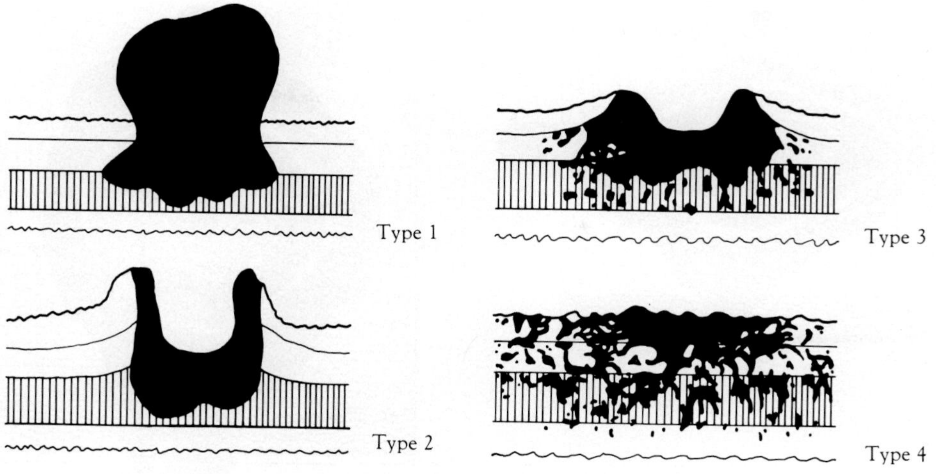

FIGURE 8-10. Borrman's classification of gastric carcinoma.[5]

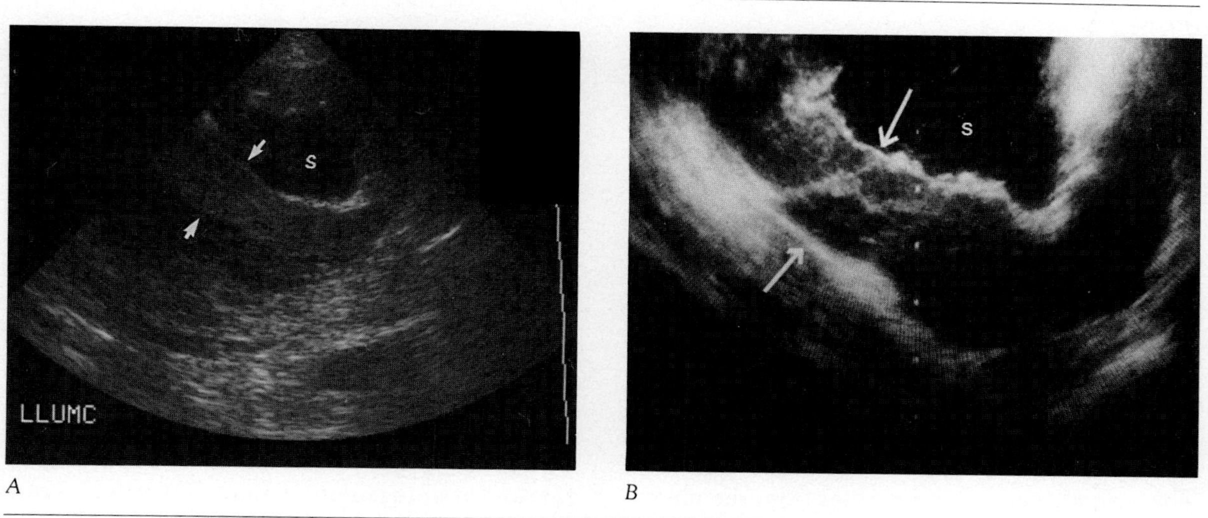

FIGURE 8-11. Gastric lymphoma. (*A*) Case 1: Transabdominal transverse view of the stomach (S) demonstrates thickened wall *(arrows)*. (From Williams D, Rouse GA, Tan-Sinn P: The gastrointestinal wall layers: An aid in sonographic detection of gastric wall lesions and rectal wall cancer staging. J Diagn Med Sonogr 1990, 6:3–17.) (*B*) Case 2: Endosonographic view of the stomach (S) also showing thickened wall *(arrows)*. (From Bolondi L, Casanova P, Caletti GC, et al: Primary gastric lymphoma versus gastric carcinoma: endoscopic US evaluation. Radiology 1987, 165:821–826.)

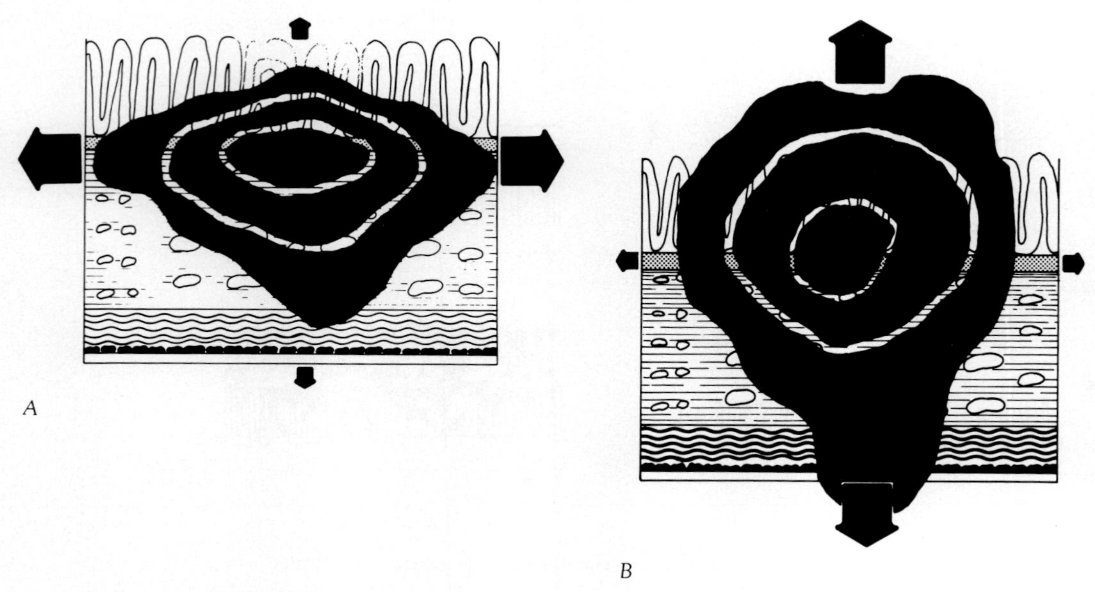

FIGURE 8-12. Growth pattern of (*A*) lymphoma and (*B*) carcinoma of the stomach.

interest in endosonography. Some lymphomatous lesions, however, do appear polypoid by endosonography and are difficult to differentiate from gastric carcinoma.[4] By transabdominal sonography, the thickened, hypoechoic gastric wall and the marked rugal thickening may be revealed.[11] Sonographically, gastric carcinoma is sometimes more echogenic than lymphoma, and in infiltrative lesions all layers are more equally involved than in lymphoma.[4,28,49]

Leiomyosarcoma. Leiomyosarcoma accounts for 1% to 3% of all malignant tumors of the stomach.[34] This smooth muscle tumor arises from the muscularis propria and is, therefore, primarily exophytic. The appearance is very similar to the sonographically familiar uterine fibroid.[57] It is difficult to differentiate sonographically or histologically from its benign counterpart, the leiomyoma.[34,57] Tumors smaller than 4 or 5 cm are considered unlikely to undergo malignant transformation; however, hemorrhage and cystic degeneration can occur.[34]

Other Malignant Gastric Lesions. Other gastric malignancies include carcinoid, hemangioendothelioma, hemangiopericytoma, Kaposi's sarcoma, liposarcoma, myxosarcoma, fibrosarcoma, and secondary tumors.[34] The epidemic of acquired immunodeficiency syndrome (AIDS) may result in many more cases of Kaposi's sarcoma than occurred in the past. The most common primary sources for metastasis to the stomach are malignant melanoma, breast carcinoma, and bronchogenic carcinoma.[34]

Duodenum

SONOGRAPHIC TECHNIQUE

The duodenum is best visualized by examining before and after ingestion of water. The valvulae conniventes—the folds in the inside bowel wall from which the microscopic villi protrude—can sometimes be demonstrated (Fig. 8-13).

NORMAL ANATOMY

The duodenal bulb, the first portion of the duodenum, normally lies to the right of the gastric antrum, anterosuperior to the pancreatic head and medial to the gallbladder (Fig. 8-14). Then the duodenum bends inferiorly to the right of the pancreatic head; this is the second portion. Next, it

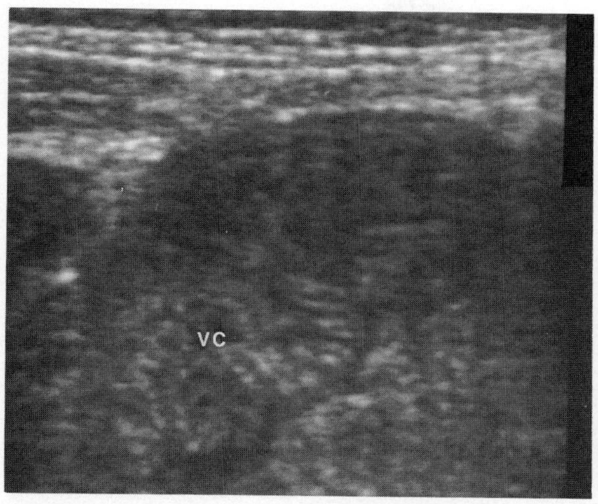

Figure 8-13. Longitudinal view of the duodenum shows multiple valvulae conniventes (VC).

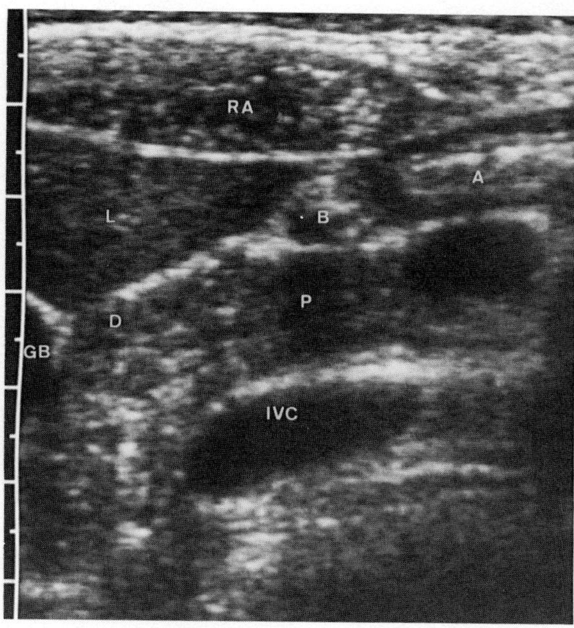

Figure 8-14. Normal relational anatomy of the duodenum. Transverse view demonstrates the gastric antrum (A), duodenal bulb (B), the second portion of the duodenum (D), the uncinate process of the pancreas (P), the liver (L), the gallbladder (GB), the inferior vena cava (IVC), and the rectus abdominis (RA).

bends to the left, extending inferior to the pancreas and passing between the superior mesenteric artery anteriorly and the aorta posteriorly, forming the third portion. The fourth extends superiorly and to the left, posterior to the stomach, becoming the jejunum at the ligament of Treitz.

Small Bowel

Sonographic Technique

Drinking fluid may enhance visualization of the mucosa of the jejunum and ileum and demonstrate peristalsis. The best time to view the small bowel depends on the transit time of the bowel. If ileus or obstruction is present, however, taking additional fluid by mouth is not helpful. If the small bowel is distended with fluid, the valvulae conniventes of the mucosa and other layers of the bowel wall are usually visible transabdominally.

Normal Anatomy

The jejunum and ileum lie in the central portion of the abdomen, inferior to the liver and stomach and superior to the urinary bladder. With modern high-resolution transabdominal transducers, loops in the small bowel can often be visualized even without distension by fluid or gas (Fig. 8-15). These sections of bowel should be smaller than 3 cm in diameter and pliable on palpation and should demonstrate peristalsis. If fluid is present in the loops, the valvulae conniventes should be visible (Fig. 8-16A,B). Sonographic visualization of the valvulae conniventes is known as the keyboard sign (Fig. 8-16C).[55]

Disorders

Ileus. Ileus, also called acute intestinal pseudo-obstruction, is characterized by failure of the intestine to propel its contents owing to diminished motility. The causes of ileus are many fold – peritonitis, spinal fracture, renal colic, acute pancreatitis, bowel ischemia, myocardial infarction, surgery, medications, hypokalemia, and infection, to name

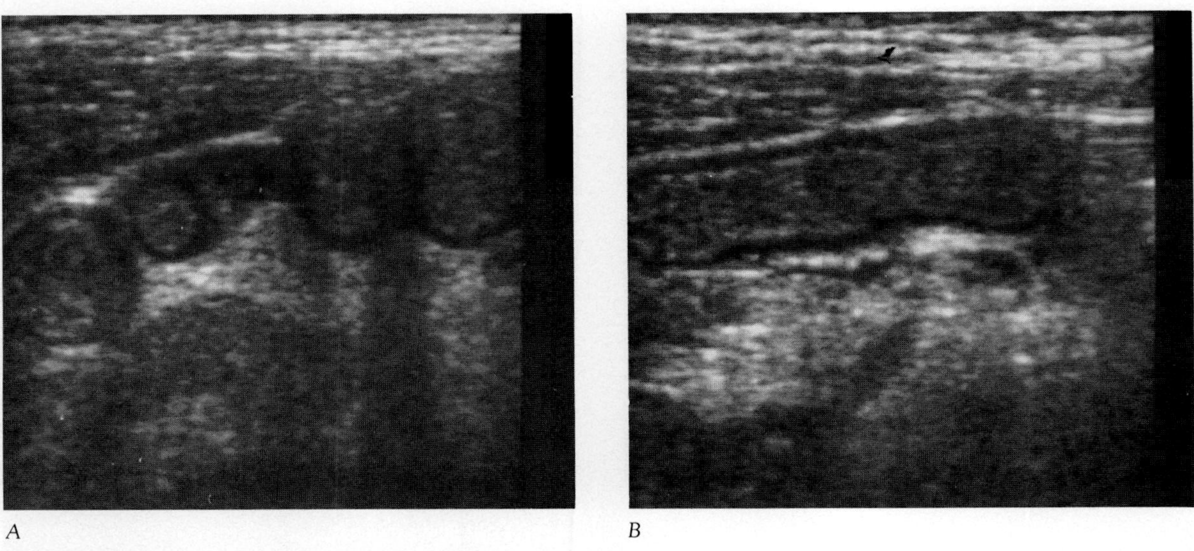

FIGURE 8-15. (*A*) Transverse and (*B*) longitudinal views of normal, nondistended small bowel loops.

just a few.[30] Sonographically, one sees small bowel distended with either air or fluid. Peristalsis is normal to somewhat increased. The bowel is less distended than when obstructed.[31]

Obstruction. Small bowel obstruction also has many causes, such as adhesions, inflammatory masses, neoplastic lesions, volvulus, intussusception, and luminal obstruction (such as fecal impaction).[10] Typically the bowel loops are perfectly round in cross section, and peristalsis can vary from none to markedly increased (Fig. 8-16).[31] The valvulae conniventes are often visible.

In volvulus, the twisted, dilated loop appears C shaped when viewed longitudinally, and often contains only fluid, no air. Intussusception, telescoping of the bowel into itself, is much rarer in adults than in children, and an identifiable bowel lesion is present in 75% to 80% of adults with this condition.[10] The sonographic appearance of intussusception can be a nonspecific target lesion,[7,52] but if one observes multiple concentric rings in the transverse view and longitudinal infolding[33] the diagnosis can be quite certain (Figs. 8-17, 8-18).

Hematoma. Hematoma of the bowel may result from trauma, ischemia, medication, or a hematologic abnormality, such as hemophilia, Henoch-Schönlein purpura, anaphylactoid purpura, or thrombocytopenic purpura.[26] Traumatic hematoma occurs most commonly in the duodenum, because it is fixed in position and less able to move out of harm's way (Fig. 8-19).[13] In adults, a common cause of bowel hematoma is anticoagulant therapy.[13] The most frequent cause of bowel ischemia is arterial obstruction.[13] Sonographically, bowel hematoma is seen as nonspecific wall thickening of variable echogenicity. The thickening may be eccentric, and the mesentery may be involved. Often there is thickening of the mucosal folds.[26]

FIGURE 8-17. Intussusception (target pattern). (*A*) Longitudinal and (*B*) transverse views of an intussusception appearing as a nonspecific target lesion (*arrows*).

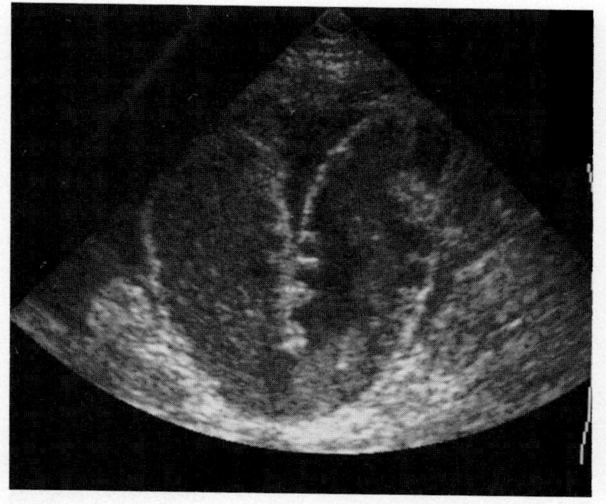
A

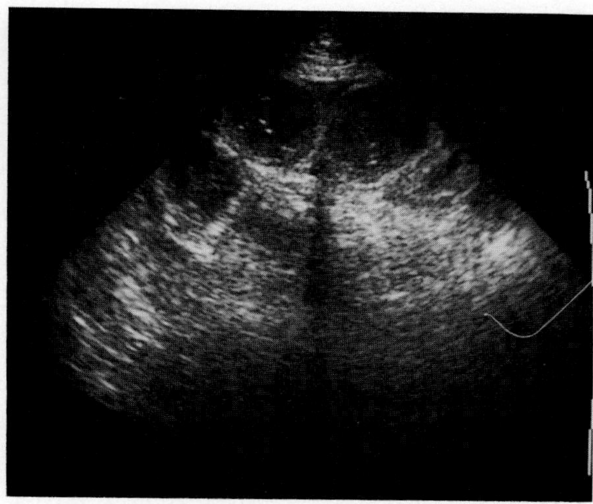
B

FIGURE 8-16. (*A*) Longitudinal and (*B*) transverse views of obstructed small bowel loops. Note that the loops are fluid filled and perfectly round. (C) The valvulae conniventes are well seen on this longitudinal view, creating the typical keyboard sign.

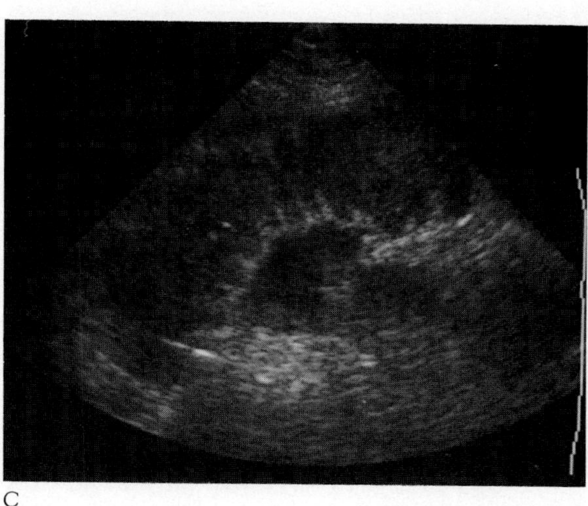
C

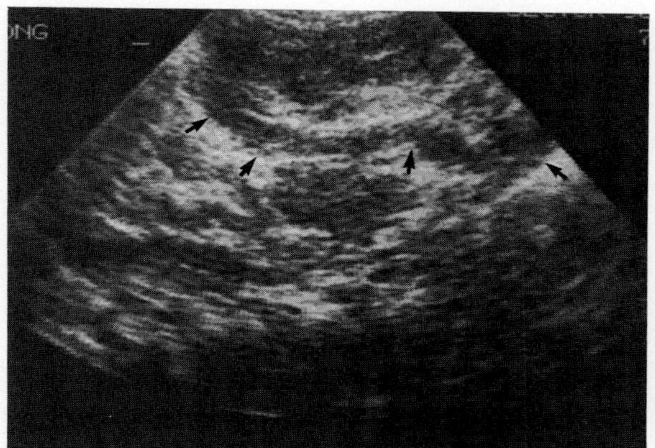

FIGURE 8-17A

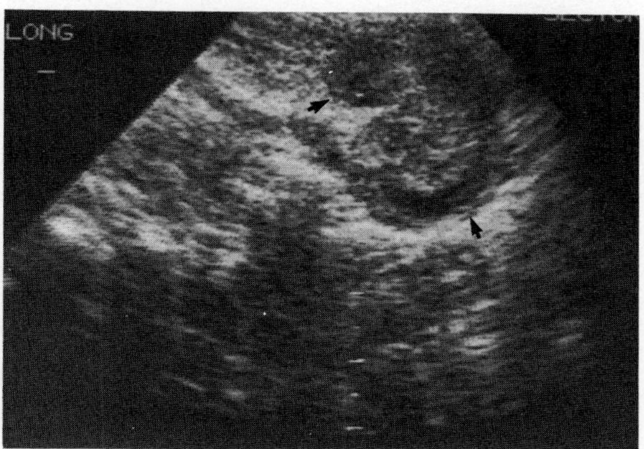

B

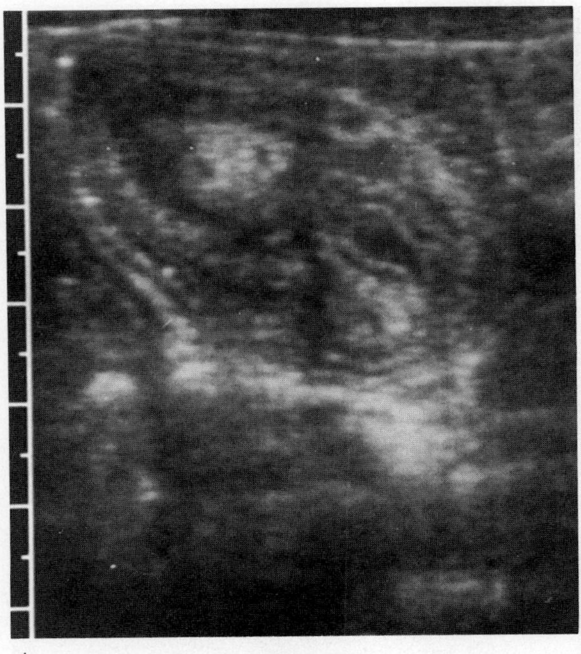

A

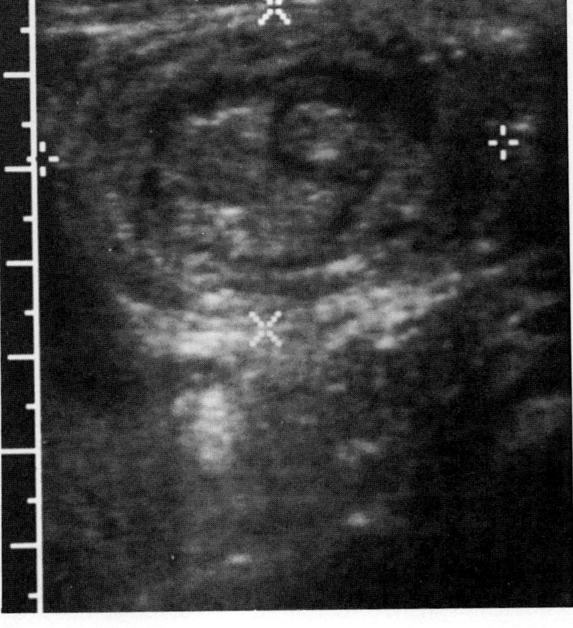

B

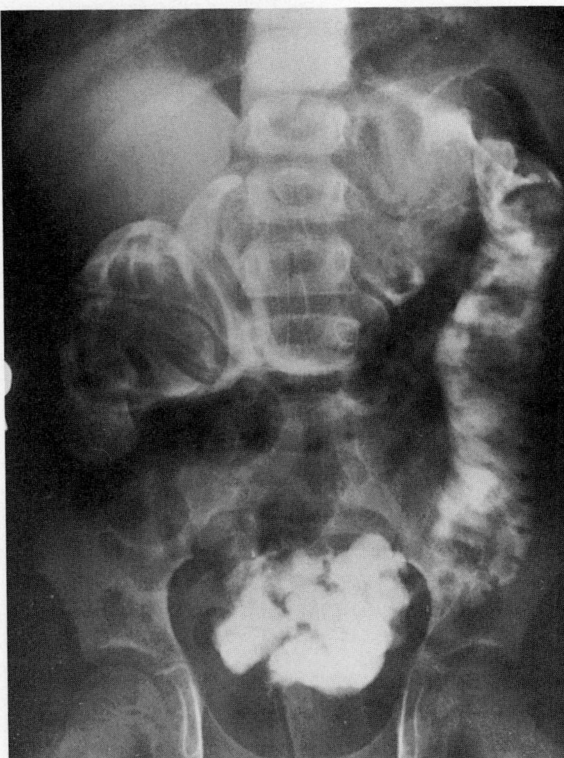

C

FIGURE 8-18. Intussusception (concentric rings). (*A,B*) Longitudinal scans show multiple concentric layers of small bowel telescoped into the large bowel. (C) Barium enema demonstrates intussusception in the transverse colon. (From Mulvihill D: Ultrasound findings of chronic intussusception in a patient with cystic fibrosis. J Ultrasound Med 1988, 7:353–355.)

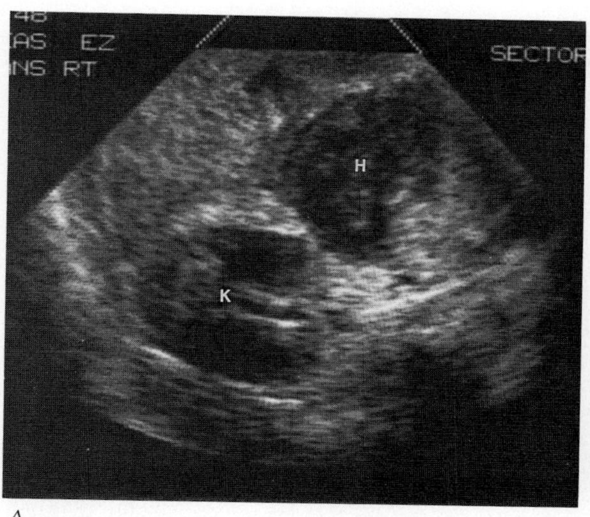

A

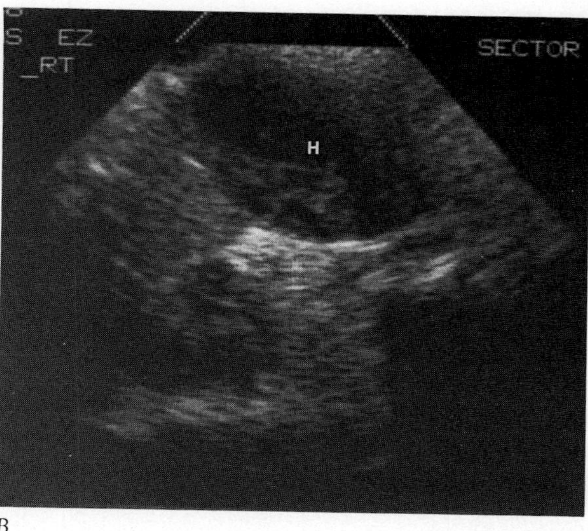

B

FIGURE 8-19. (*A*) Transverse view of the right side upper quadrant shows the duodenal hematoma (H) medial and anterior to the right kidney (K). (*B*) Longitudinal view of the duodenal hematoma (H) shows internal septations.

Edema. Swelling of the valvulae conniventes can be caused by hypoproteinemia,[13] which may be due to cirrhosis, kidney disease, or protein loss from the GI tract, as may occur in Menetrier's disease, Whipple's disease, intestinal lymphangiomatosis, inflammatory bowel disease, and GI tumors.[13] Blockage of mesenteric lymph channels, angioneurotic edema, and abetalipoproteinemia can also cause thickening of small bowel mucosal folds (Fig. 8-20).[13]

Granulomatous Enteritis (Crohn's Disease). Crohn's disease is the most common nonspecific inflammation of the small bowel. Its cause is unknown; the inflammation starts in the submucosa and becomes transmural, often with granulomatous features. The disease involves the ileum most often but may also affect the colon, jejunum, and stomach. Ulcers, fistulae, and mucosal nodularity are frequently present.[35] Sonographically, the most obvious finding is hypoechoic thickening of the bowel wall and mesentery (Fig. 8-21). The resultant bull's-eye appearance is nonspecific and is often indistinguishable from tumor, hematoma, ulcerative colitis, pericecal abscess, or ruptured small bowel diverticulum (Fig. 8-22).[12,14,41,56]

Tumors. The most common primary neoplastic lesions of the small bowel, in order of occurrence, are smooth muscle tumors, carcinoid tumors, adenocarcinomas, and lymphoma.[45] The bowel may also be involved as a part of multisystem lymphoma. When primary and multisystem lymphomatous involvements of the GI tract are combined, lymphoma is the most common neoplasia of the small bowel.[32]

Lymphoma of the small bowel is usually part of a systemic involvement, most frequently by non-Hodgkin's lymphoma (including Burkitt's, undifferentiated, and histiocytic lymphoma). Fifty percent of patients with Hodgkin's disease, however, also have involvement of the GI tract eventually.[32] The sonographer may see the bowel wall involvement as a target lesion. The mesenteric nodes may also be affected without involvement of the bowel wall.

Primary adenocarcinoma of the small bowel may present as either a constricting circumferential le-

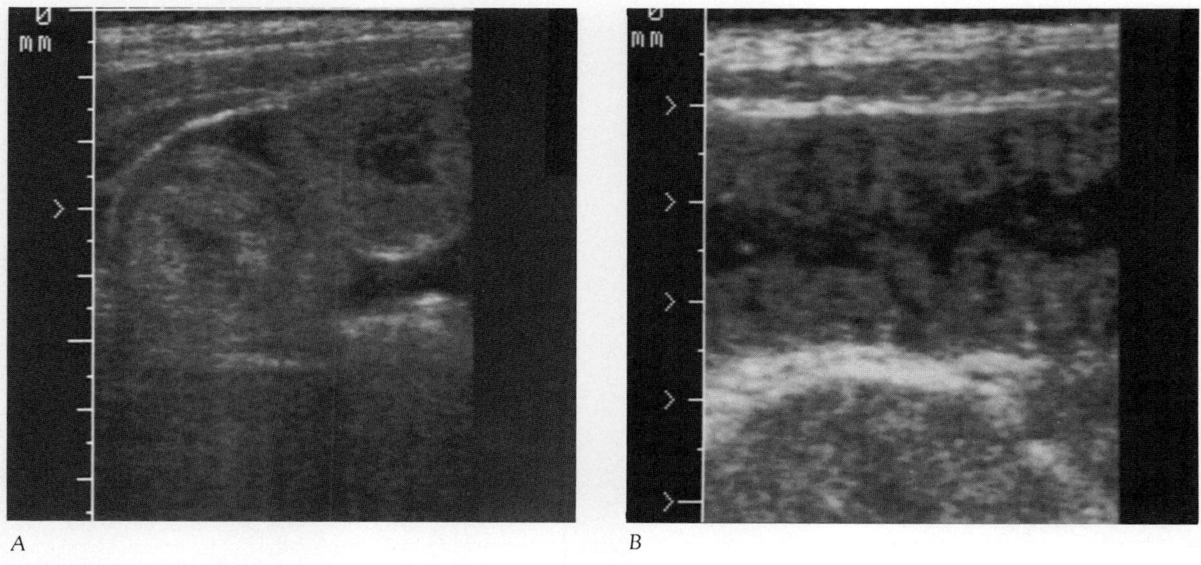

A B

Figure 8-20. (*A*) Transverse and (*B*) longitudinal views of small bowel loops with marked thickening of the valvulae conniventes and associated ascites in a patient with cirrhosis.

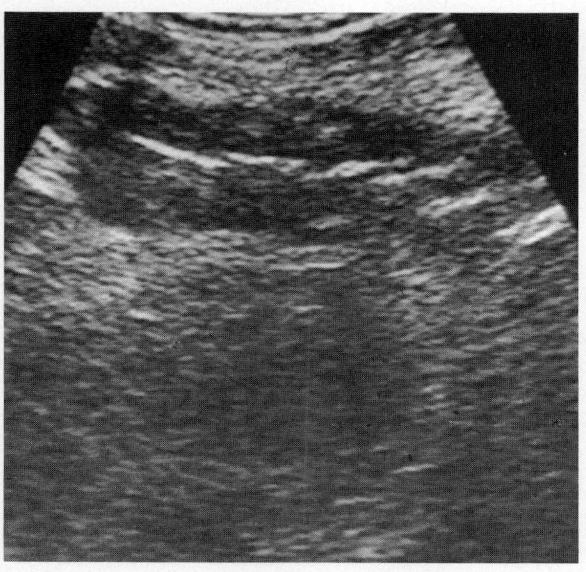

Figure 8-21. Longitudinal sonogram of granulomatous enteritis (Crohn's disease) of the ileum. Note the thickened hypoechoic wall. (From Worlicek H, Lutz H, Heyder N, Matek N: Ultrasound findings in Crohn's disease and ulcerative colitis: A prospective study. J Clin Ultrasound 1987, 15:153–163.)

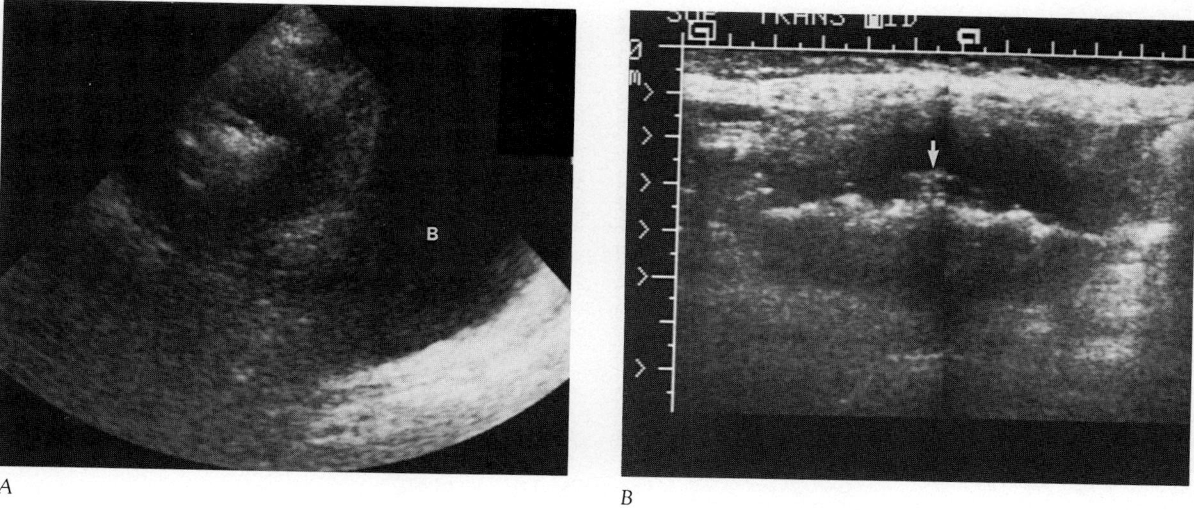

A B

Figure 8-22. (*A*) Transverse and (*B*) longitudinal views of the lower abdomen show a small bowel mass superior to the bladder (B). The inflammation resulted from rupture of an ileal diverticulum *(arrow)*.

sion or as a polypoid lesion. The lesions may range from 1 to 10 cm in diameter.[45]

Leiomyoma is the most common benign tumor of the small bowel; it looks like leiomyomas elsewhere, including in the uterus. The tumor arises from the muscularis propria and is usually eccentrically located in the wall. Leiomyosarcomas can appear identical to larger leiomyomas, but larger tumors and tumors with central necrosis are more likely to be malignant.[45]

Adenomas, lipomas, hemangiomas, and neurofibromas are other benign tumors that can arise in the small bowel.[45] Metastatic malignancies, especially from melanoma and carcinomas of the lung, kidney, and breast, occur as either single or multiple intramural or intraluminal masses. These metastases may appear similar to smooth muscle tumors or lymphoma.[13] Carcinoid tumors are discussed in the next section.

Vermiform Appendix

Sonographic Technique

The sonographic examination of the right side lower quadrant, as first described by Puylaert,[36] begins with identifying the right colon, which is then followed downward to the cecum. By placing steady pressure on the transducer, one can displace gas-filled bowel loops to search for the appendix. The cecum and terminal ileum can often be seen. One can identify the normal appendix in some persons, but only inflamed, distended appendices can be visualized consistently.

Normal Anatomy

The normal appendix is not routinely visible transabdominally but can sometimes be visualized, especially when ascites is present (Fig. 8-23). The normal appendix should measure no more than 6 mm in diameter, and the hypoechoic part of the wall should measure no more than 2 mm thick.[22]

Disorders

Appendicitis. Appendicitis is almost always associated with obstruction of the appendiceal lumen. While it may occur in any age group, young adults are most often affected. Appendicitis has generally been considered a clinical diagnosis, characterized initially by general periumbilical pain associated with leukocytosis, fever, and sometimes nausea.

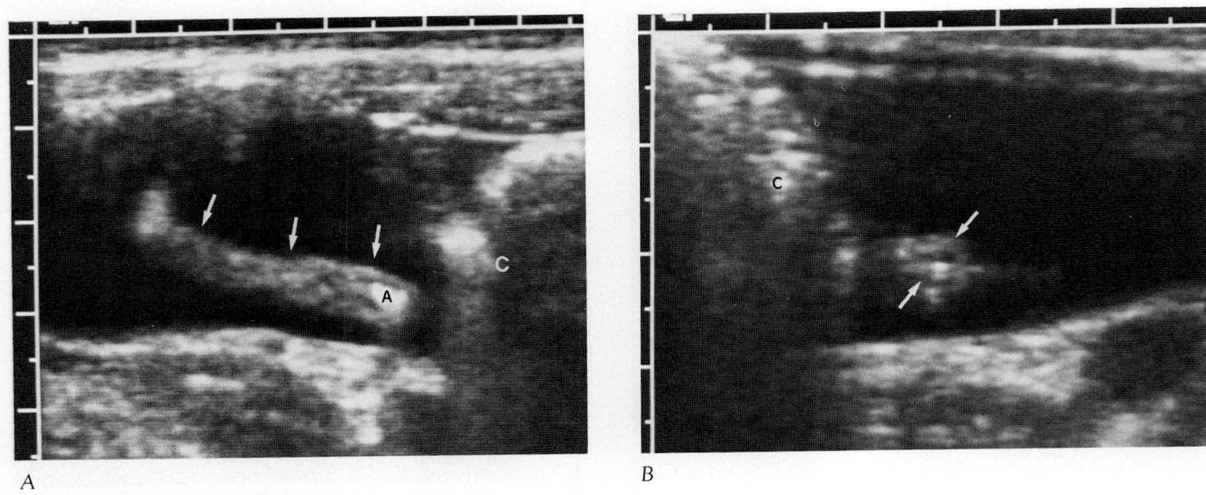

FIGURE 8-23. (*A*) Longitudinal and (*B*) transverse views of the normal appendix in a patient with ascites. Note that the appendix *(arrows)* is smaller than 5 mm in diameter and is adjacent to the cecum (C). A small amount of air (A) is noted in the base of the appendix. (From Gisler M, Rouse G, Delange M: Sonography of appendicitis. J Diagn Med Sonogr 1989, 5:57–60.)

After a few hours the pain localizes in the right lower quadrant, and there is point tenderness over the appendix and signs of peritoneal irritation such as rebound tenderness. Diagnostic studies have rarely been considered necessary traditionally; however, at appendectomy the appendix has been found to be normal in up to 40% of suspected appendicitis cases in young women, apparently because there are numerous gynecologic causes of right lower quadrant pain in this population.[21] Also, there is much variation in the clinical presentation of appendicitis; many cases do not exhibit the classical symptoms. Four sonographic series have found that ultrasonography is 80% to 90% sensitive and 95% to 100% specific in diagnosing acute unruptured appendicitis.[1,21,22,36] Visualization of an appendix larger than 6 mm in diameter with mucus in the appendiceal lumen and with associated focal pain over the appendix is sufficient to establish the diagnosis of unruptured appendicitis (Fig. 8-24).[22] Although it was initially believed that any appendix visualized sonographically was abnormal,[36] it is now clear that the normal appendix can sometimes be identified,[21,22] especially in patients with ascites (Fig. 8-23). It is also becoming clear that some cases of appendicitis can resolve without surgery, perhaps to recur later. Retrocecal appendices, however, are particularly difficult to visualize sonographically.[22] If a calcified appendicolith is identified in the appendix, it is a strong suggestion that appendicitis is present, even if a dilated appendiceal lumen is not seen (Fig. 8-25).[22]

The chief complication of appendicitis is, of course, abscess formation or generalized peritonitis. Appendiceal rupture is not required for these complications to arise, as pathogens may travel through the intact wall.[32] When the appendix has ruptured, it is much more difficult to visualize because the lumen is no longer distended and the anatomy is distorted by surrounding inflammation and adjacent abscess. Appendiceal abscesses usually are echogenic, because colon organisms form gas within them (Fig. 8-26). Gas in a tubo-ovarian abscess is less common. Characteristically, appendiceal abscesses are at the cecal tip or in the pericolic gutter, but sometimes they occur between small bowel loops medially, where they are much more difficult to find sonographically.

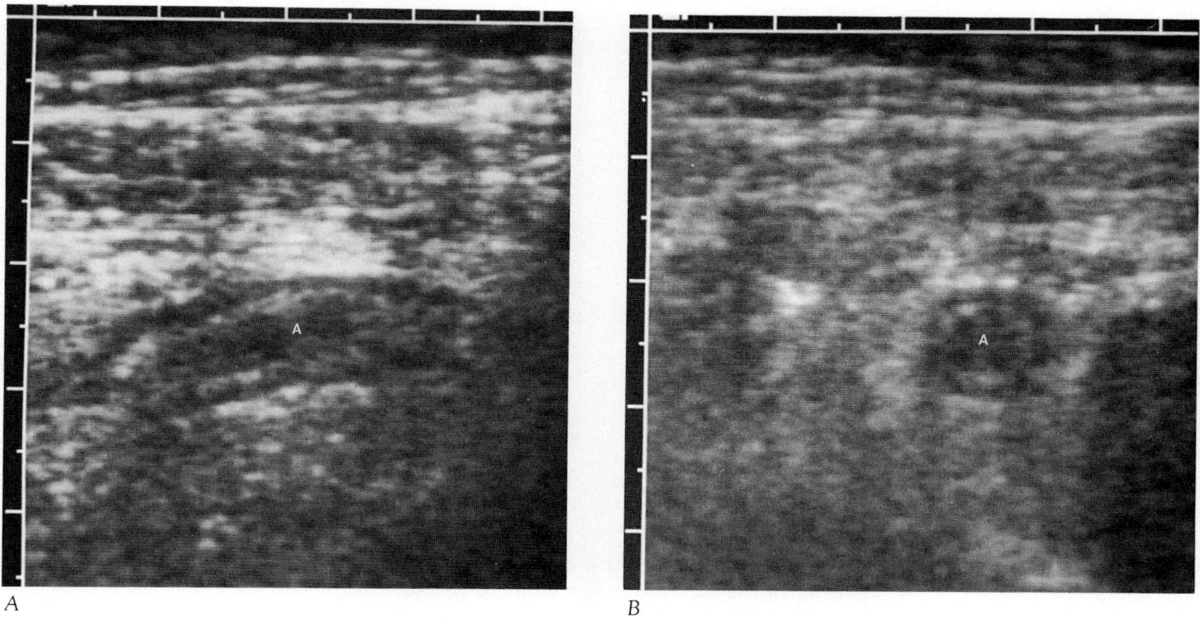

A B

FIGURE 8-24. (*A*) Longitudinal and (*B*) transverse views of a dilated, inflamed appendix (A). Note that the appendiceal diameter is greater than 6 mm and the wall is approximately 2 mm thick. (From Gisler M, Rouse G, Delange M: Sonography of appendicitis. J Diagn Med Sonogr 1989, 5:57–60.)

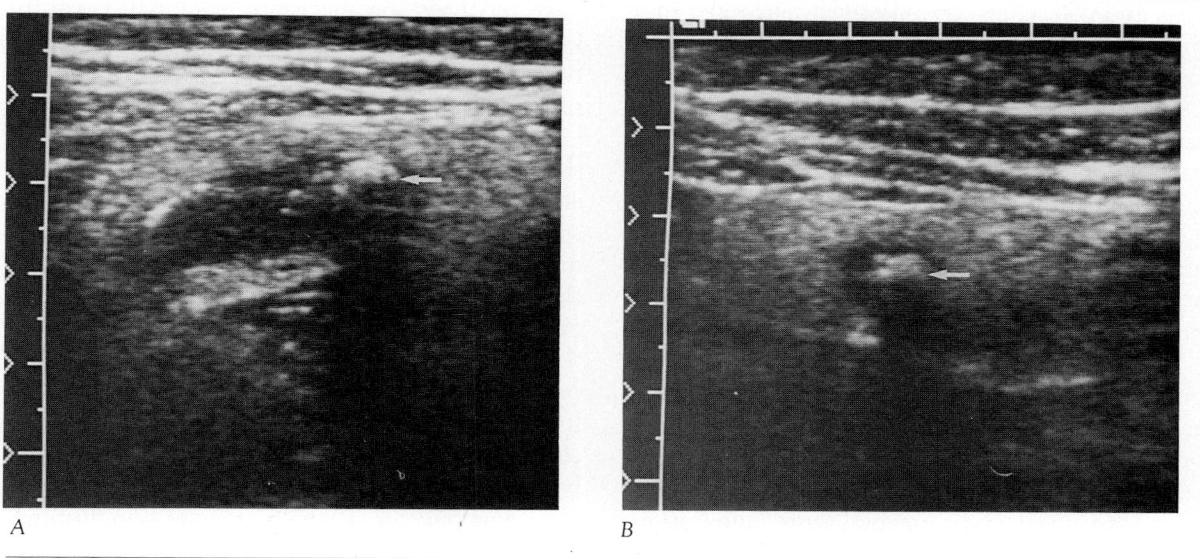

A B

FIGURE 8-25. (*A*) Longitudinal and (*B*) transverse views of a distended appendix containing an appendicolith (*arrow*).

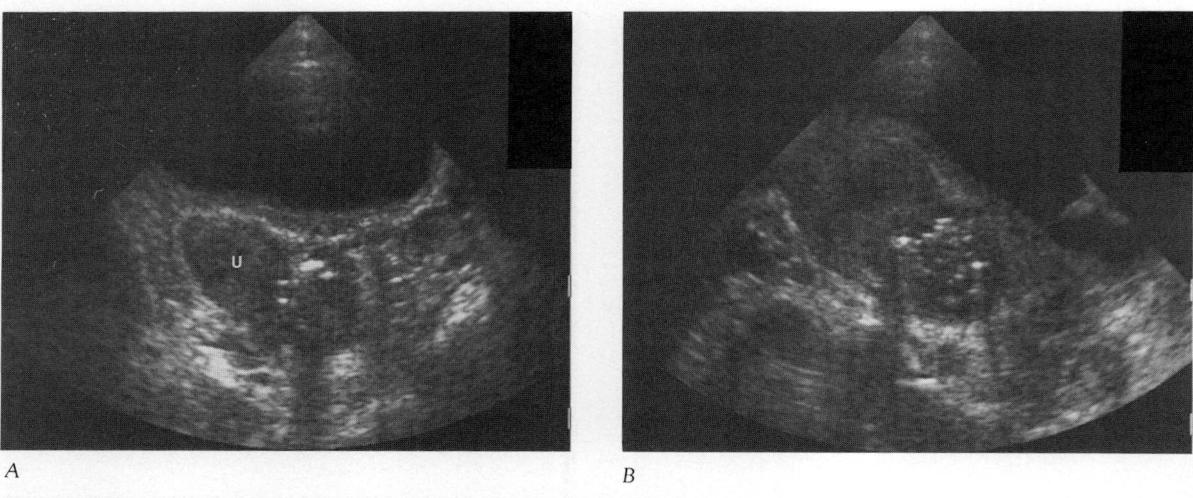

FIGURE 8-26. (*A*) Transverse and (*B*) longitudinal views of an appendiceal abscess to the left of the uterus (U). Note the air within.

Mucocele. Mucocele, distension of the appendix by mucus, is an uncommon lesion, found in 0.25% of appendectomies.[19,32] It is four times more common in women than in men and mean age at diagnosis is 55 years. Right lower quadrant pain is present in 64% of cases; 23% of patients are asymptomatic.[19] Higa and colleagues have classified mucoceles into three groups: focal or diffuse hyperplasia, mucinous cystadenoma, and mucinous cystadenocarcinoma.[18] Only the last is considered to have malignant potential.[18,19] Mucocele rupture can cause massive accumulation of gelatinous ascites, called pseudomyxoma peritonei. If the mucocele is the mucinous cystadenocarcinoma variety, ascites is malignant and the patient has a poorer prognosis. An association has been noted between mucoceles and the presence of one or more other colon tumors.[19]

Sonographically, the mucocele appears as a purely cystic or complex mass up to 7 cm in diameter, demonstrating through-transmission posteriorly and located in the right lower quadrant.[19] This lesion may be difficult to differentiate from ovarian cysts, mesenteric cysts, omental cysts, duplication cysts, renal cysts, or even abdominal abscess.

Carcinoid Tumors. Carcinoids (argentaffinomas) arise from the argentaffin cells of the mucosa. In order of decreasing frequency, they arise in the appendix, small bowel, rectosigmoid colon, lung and bronchi, esophagus and stomach, pancreas, gallbladder, biliary tract, ovary and testis, and right colon. Carcinoids have histologic features of malignancy, such as anaplasia and increased mitoses, but have relatively low metastatic potential. Local invasiveness is the best indicator of degree of malignancy. Appendiceal carcinoids rarely metastasize; small bowel lesions are the most likely to do so.[54]

Sonographically, carcinoid tumors appear as sharply marginated hypoechoic masses without acoustic enhancement.[32] The lesions are small: 73% smaller than 1.5 cm. The larger the lesion, the more likely it is to metastasize: 2% of lesions smaller than 1 cm, 50% of 1- to 2-cm lesions, and 80 to 90% of larger lesions.[54]

The tumors often produce hormones, principally serotonin and prostaglandin E, but since the liver inactivates serotonin received via the portal circulation, liver metastases are virtually always present if the patient experiences the carcinoid syndrome (Fig. 8-27), which includes skin flushing, diarrhea, cyanosis, asthmatic attacks, and cardiac valve lesions. If the primary site of the carcinoid is outside the GI tract (i.e., ovary, bronchus), metastasis is not required for the carcinoid syndrome.[54]

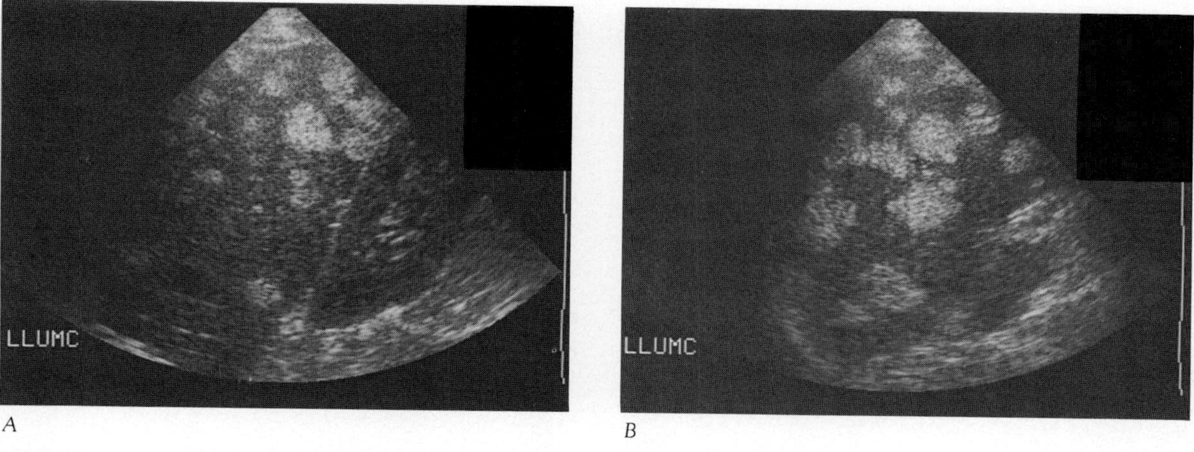

Figure 8-27. (*A*) Transverse and (*B*) longitudinal sonograms of the liver show multiple hyperechoic metastases from small bowel carcinoid tumors.

Other Disorders. Sonographic detection of adenocarcinoma of the appendix has been reported.[46] The clinical presentation may be similar to that of acute appendicitis. Crohn's disease of the appendix can occur as an isolated condition, or more commonly with Crohn's disease of the colon or ileum.[13,35] The sonographic appearance of these conditions is nonspecific.

Colon and Rectum

Sonographic Technique

No special techniques are available for evaluating the colon. A normal person usually has more air in the colon than in the small bowel, and the colon's larger diameter and prominent haustral indentations are often identifiable. A fluid-filled colon is unusual, generally indicating diarrhea or obstruction. The examiner may sometimes have difficulty differentiating a solid mass in the colon from a small bowel lesion. It is helpful to know where the colon is usually located and to note the greater amount of air in the colon.

Endoluminal examination of the rectum should be performed in both the axial and longitudinal directions if possible as this allows better evaluation of the layers of the bowel wall involved, the extent of invasion of any tumor that may be present, and evidence of local lymphadenopathy.

Normal Anatomy

The colon usually lies in the periphery of the abdomen, laterally on the right and left, and superiorly along the liver margin in the upper abdomen. Since the colon hosts gas-producing bacteria, it is more often distended with gas than the rest of the bowel. The colon can frequently be identified by its customary position, its larger diameter, and its characteristic haustral folds, which are up to 3 to 5 cm apart (Fig. 8-28). The colon wall should measure 4 to 9 mm thick when not distended, and 2 to 4 mm when the colon is distended to a diameter of 5 cm or more.[16]

Disorders of the Colon

Obstruction. The colon usually is at least partially filled with gas, and when colonic obstruction occurs, the obstructed loop is likely to be gas filled. This makes colon obstruction easy to diagnose radiographically and rather more difficult sonographically. Nevertheless, ultrasonography can visualize dilated bowel loops, particularly if linear arrays are used. While a specific diagnosis is not always possible, the location of the dilated loop may give

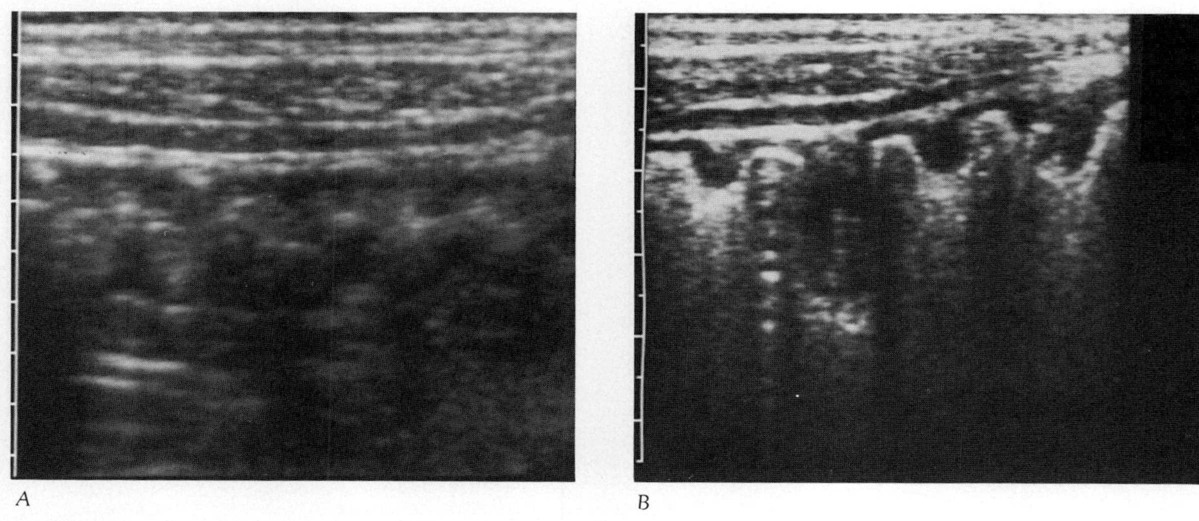

A B

Figure 8-28. Longitudinal transabdominal views of the normal colon (*A*) without distention and (*B*) with mild gaseous distention.

some clues. Cecal volvulus is manifested by dilation of the right colon only. Sigmoid volvulus shows maximum dilatation in the central abdomen. Diverticulitis with obstruction usually causes dilatation of the left, and perhaps the entire colon, and an obstructing rectal carcinoma appears similar.

Crohn's Colitis (Granulomatous Colitis). Crohn's disease of the colon produces signs identical to Crohn's disease of the small bowel (Fig. 8-29). It tends to be a transmural inflammation, potentially developing fistulae and pericolonic abscesses. Multiple separate areas of the colon may be involved; the right colon is a frequent site, and associated ileal involvement is common. In one study, 64% of patients with Crohn's disease had sonographically demonstrable lesions with hypoechoic bowel walls thickened from 4 to 22 mm.[56] The sonographers also noted lumenal narrowing, bowel wall rigidity, and absence of haustral folds.[56]

Ulcerative Colitis. Ulcerative colitis is an inflammatory disease confined to the colonic mucosa and submucosa. The cause is not known, but a hypersensitivity or autoimmune mechanism is suspected.[20] The inflammation starts in the rectal region and as the disease progresses, extends up the left colon and may eventually involve the entire colon.[20] Unlike Crohn's colitis, ulcerative colitis does not skip some areas, leaving them unaffected, but spreads in a continuous pattern. Patients with ulcerative colitis are at high risk of developing a particularly virulent form of colon carcinoma.[20]

In one series, 53% of patients with ulcerative colitis had sonographically detectable lesions, varying in length from 3 cm to the entire colon.[56] The bowel wall was thickened from 4 to 10 mm and was usually hypoechoic, although occasionally the layers of the bowel wall were visible sonographically (Fig. 8-30). Seventy-six percent of the lesions occurred in the left colon only.[56]

Figure 8-30. (*A*) Longitudinal and (*B*) transverse views of the colon in ulcerative colitis. Note the preservation of the bowel layers (b). (From Worlicek H, Lutz H, Heyder N, Matek N: Ultrasound findings in Crohn's disease and ulcerative colitis: A prospective study. J Clin Ultrasound 1987, 15:153–163.)

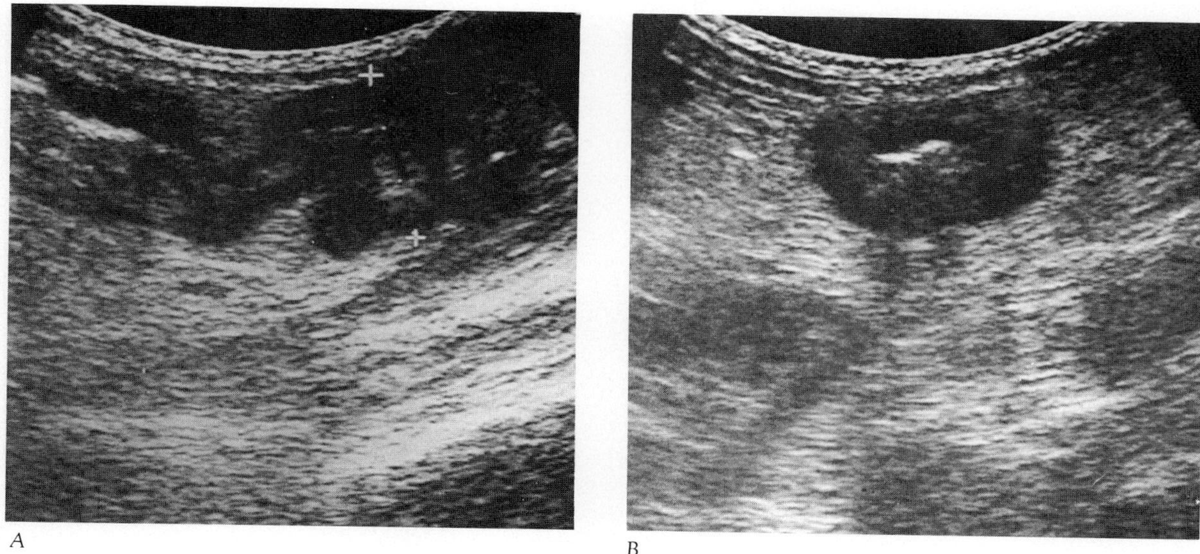

A B

FIGURE 8-29. (*A*) Longitudinal view of thickened terminal ileum (31 mm between cursors) and cecum. (*B*) Transverse view of the colon in Crohn's disease. Note the markedly thickened, uniformly hypoechoic wall. (From Worlicek H, Lutz H, Heyder N, Matek N: Ultrasound findings in Crohn's disease and ulcerative colitis: A prospective study. J Clin Ultrasound 1987, 15:153–163.)

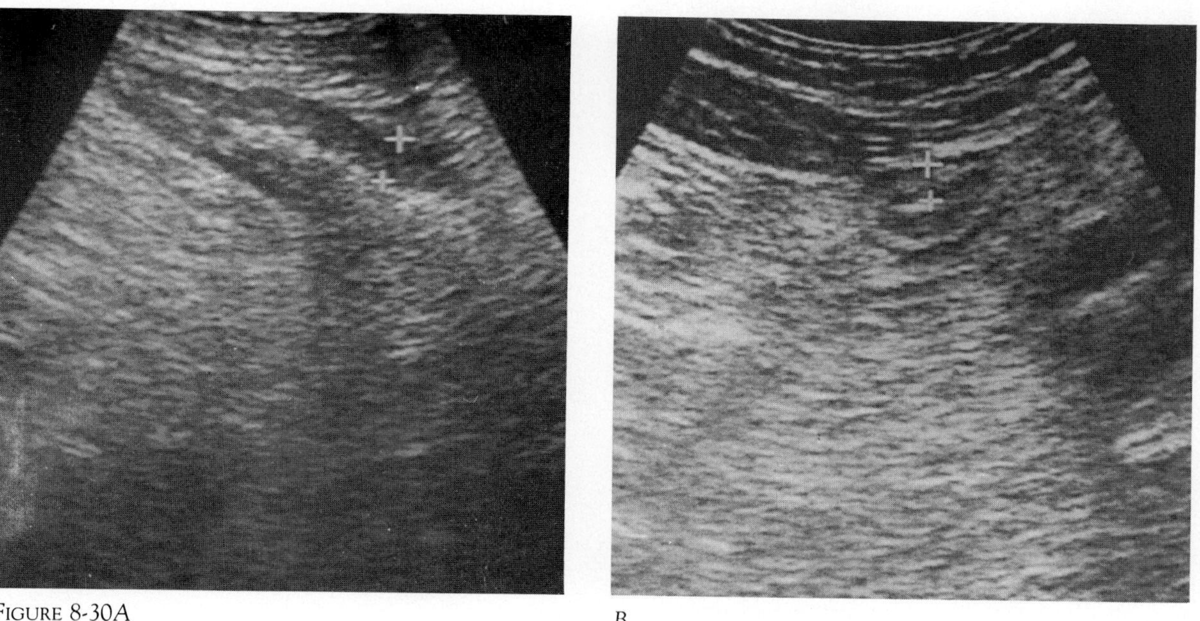

FIGURE 8-30*A* *B*

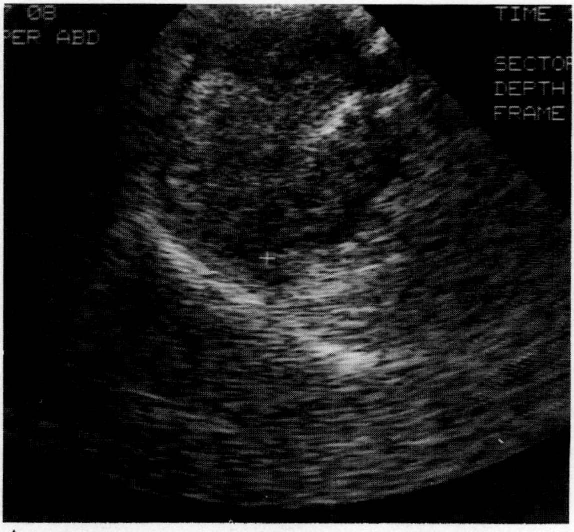

A

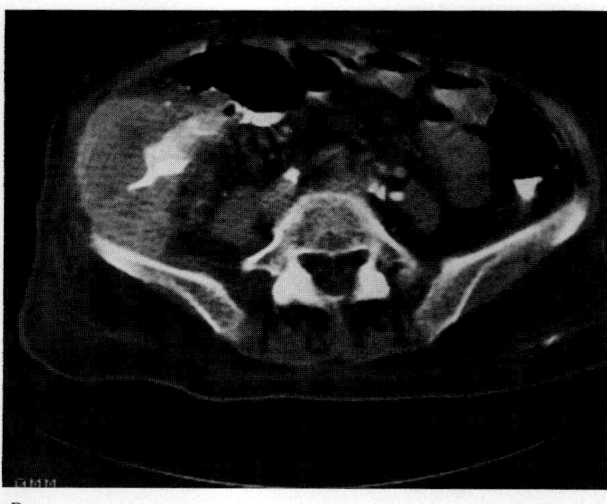

B

C

FIGURE 8-31. (*A*) Transverse sonogram of a right colon carcinoma *(between cursors)*. (*B*) Transverse CT of the same tumor. (C) Barium enema study shows eccentric right colon lesion *(arrow)*.

Diverticular Disease. Diverticulosis is an acquired condition in which small hernias of the mucosa (diverticula) form through the muscular layer of the colon. The rectosigmoid colon is most often affected. This condition, which is associated with a low-bulk diet, affects more than 50% of people older than 50 years in western countries.[15] Diverticulosis is usually asymptomatic and is not sonographically detectable unless air or barium is present in the diverticula.

If one or more diverticula become filled with inspissated fecal material and then become inflamed, diverticulitis results. Often there is also inflammatory thickening of the bowel wall. Pericolic abscesses may form, because of diverticular rupture or transmural spread of infection.[15] Sonographically, these abscesses appear as masses adjacent to the colon. They may be hypoechoic or may contain gas.

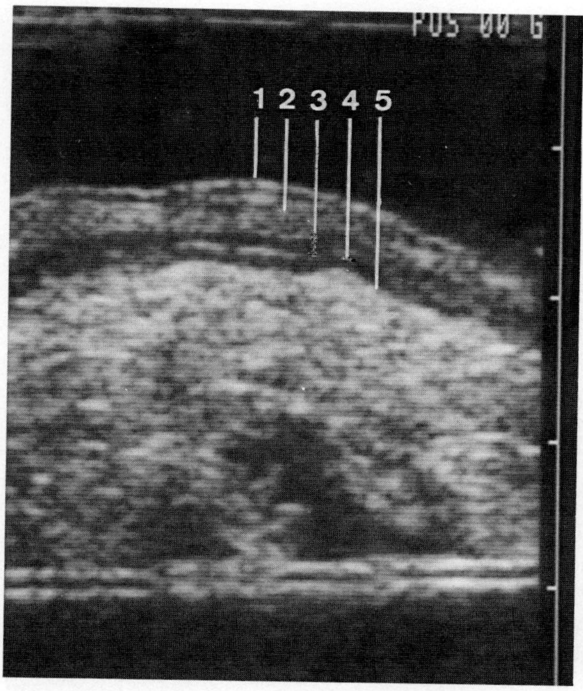

Figure 8-32. Longitudinal sonogram of normal surgical specimen of the rectal wall. Note the excellent delineation of the five sonographic layers of the bowel wall. In this case, the interface between the longitudinal and transverse parts of the muscle layer (layer 4) can be identified. (From Williams D, Rouse GA, Tan-Sinn P: The gastrointestinal wall layers: An aid in sonographic detection of gastric wall lesions and rectal wall cancer staging. J Diagn Med Sonogr 1990, 6:3–17).

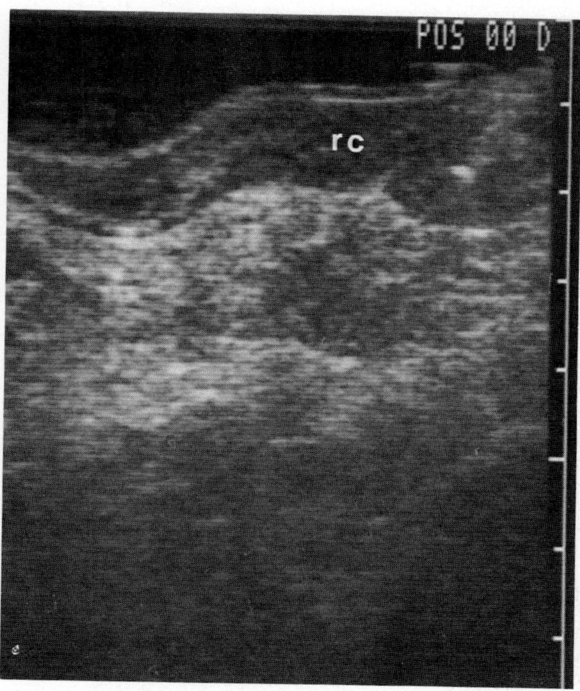

Figure 8-33. Longitudinal transrectal sonogram of a rectal carcinoma (rc). The tumor has not broken through the muscularis propria. (From Williams D, Rouse GA, Tan-Sinn P: The gastrointestinal wall layers: An aid in sonographic detection of gastric wall lesions and rectal wall cancer staging. J Diagn Med Sonogr 1990, 6:3–17.)

Other Inflammatory Disorders. Other inflammatory colon conditions that may result in colon wall thickening include ischemia, amebiasis, shigellosis, tuberculosis, pseudomembranous colitis, radiation colitis, endometriosis, and pancreatitis.[13]

Carcinoma. In western countries, colon carcinoma is the third leading cause of death from cancer, after carcinoma of the lung and breast. Fifty percent of colon carcinomas arise in the rectum and rectosigmoid colon, 25% in the sigmoid, and 25% in the rest of the colon.[44] Transabdominal sonography demonstrates a large colon cancer as a nonspecific hypoechoic target lesion (Fig. 8-31).[24] Smaller polypoid lesions are much more difficult to identify because of gas or fecal material in the colon.

With high-frequency transrectal probes, the rectum can be imaged in transverse and longitudinal planes and can demonstrate the layers of the rectal wall (Fig. 8-32).[6] When rectal carcinoma is present, transrectal sonography can determine the degree of infiltration of the rectal wall and the perirectal area (Fig. 8-33).[37,38] In one study, transrectal sonography correctly identified perirectal fat infiltration in 89% of cases, compared to 55% with CT.[38] Local lymph node involvement was correctly identified by transrectal sonography in 72% of cases but by CT in only 20%. Accurate presurgical staging of rectal

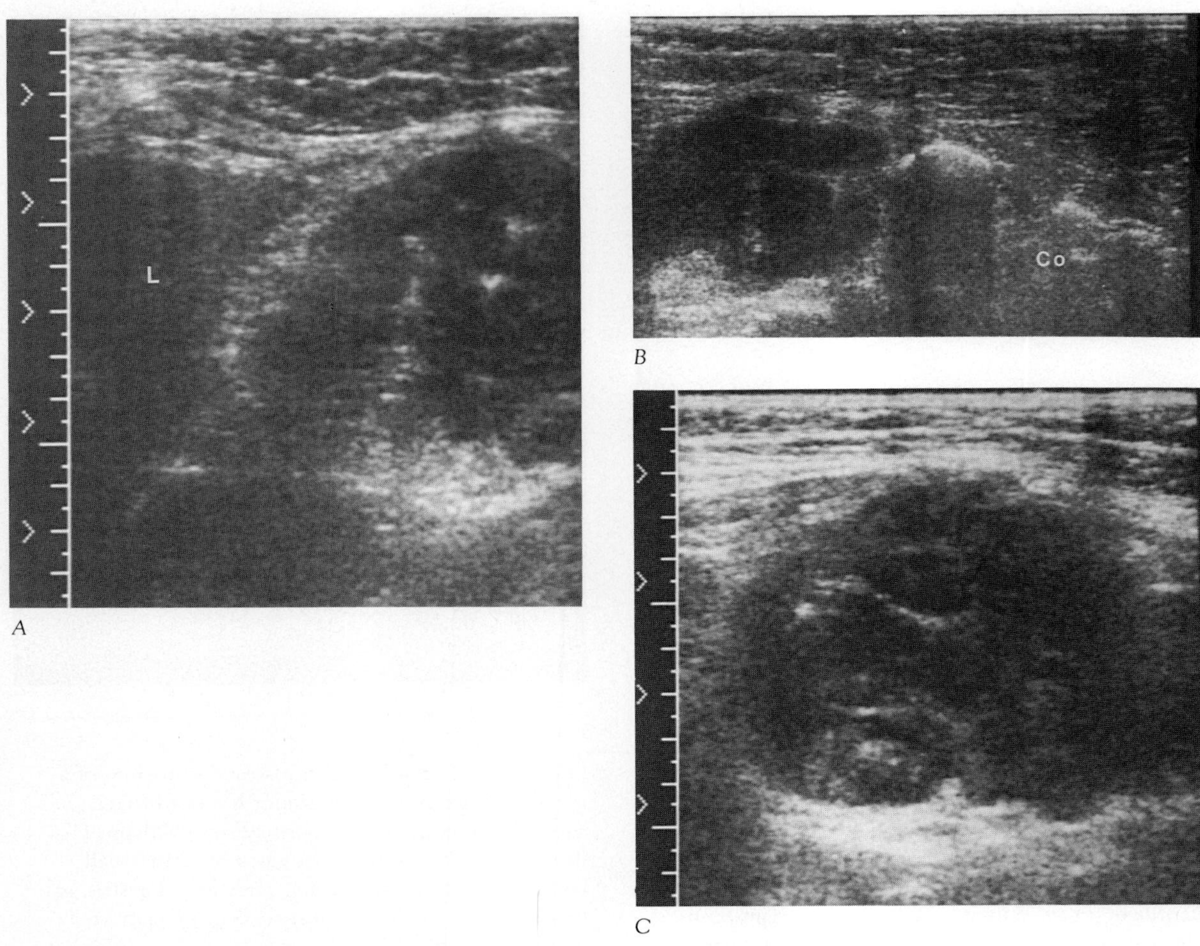

FIGURE 8-34. Immunoblastic lymphoma. (*A*,*B*) Longitudinal views of the upper and middle right abdomen show a nodular constricting hypoechoic mass adjacent to the liver (L) and constricting the colon (CO). (C) Transverse view of the lymphoma, shows marked nodularity of the mass.

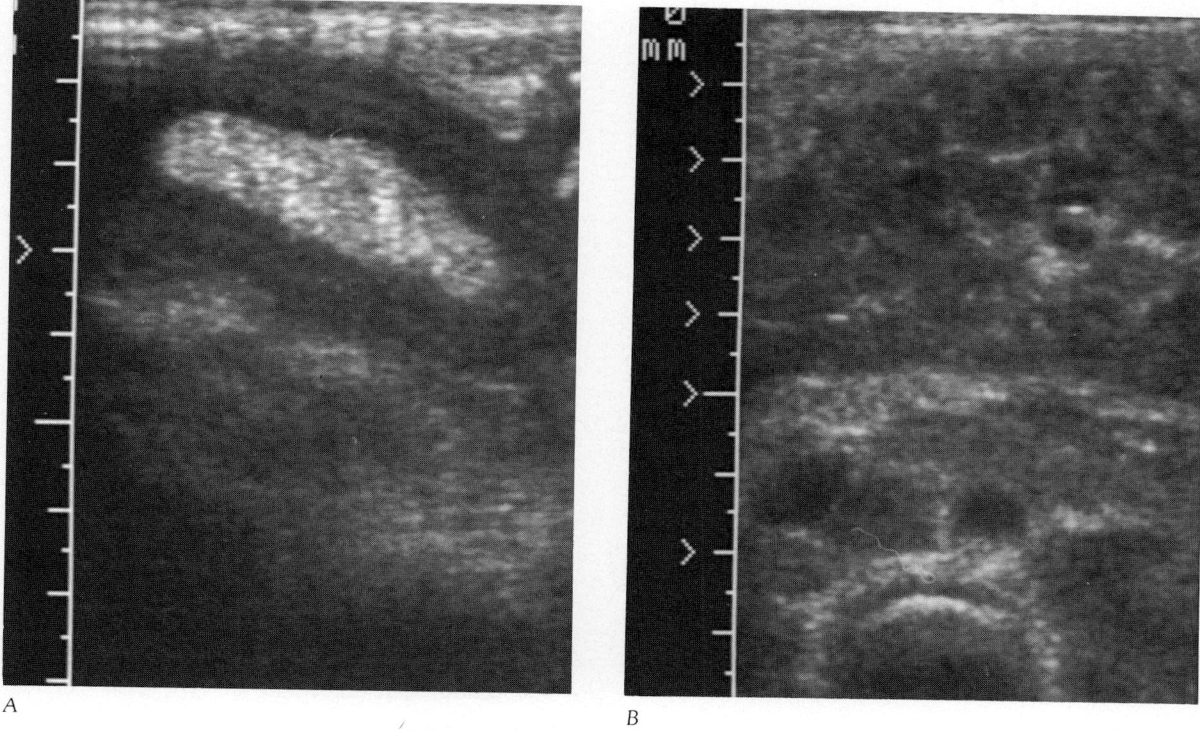

FIGURE 8-35. (*A*) Longitudinal sonogram of colon involved by Burkitt's lymphoma. Note the uniformly thickened hypoechoic wall. (*B*) Transverse view of the mesentery shows severe lymphadenopathy.

tumors is vital for optimal planning of surgery and radiation therapy.

Lymphoma. Lymphoma of the colon appears similar to lymphoma of the small bowel. A hypoechoic lesion, annular, eccentric, or diffusely involving the bowel wall, may be observed (Figs. 8-34, 8-35).

Benign Tumors. The same lesions seen elsewhere in the bowel can also involve the colon—leiomyomas, lipomas, fibromas, and hemangiomas.

Summary

Sonography will not replace barium studies of the GI tract as the principal method of visualizing GI anatomy and function, nor will it replace CT in the overall staging of GI malignancies. But in the evaluation of abdominal discomfort, transabdominal sonography can play a valuable screening role, sometimes implicating the GI tract as the cause of the symptoms. The sonographic signs of GI lesions are summarized in Table 8-1. Sonography also has the unique ability to visualize the layers of the bowel wall, either transabdominally or endoscopically, which can sometimes provide information invaluable in the diagnosis or staging of GI lesions. For most conditions, the sensitivity and specificity of ultrasound in the evaluation of GI abnormalities is not well-established, and the clinical indications for its use are still evolving, but wider use of gastrointestinal sonography in the future seems assured.

TABLE 8-1. Sonographic appearance of gastrointestinal lesions

APPEARANCE	LESION
Target or pseudokidney sign (circumferential hypoechoic thickening of the bowel wall)	Lymphoma, intussusception, nonspecific inflammation, chronic ulcerative colitis, regional enteritis, hematoma, metastatic tumor
Focal hypoechoic lesions in the submucosa of the stomach	Neuroma, fibroma, gastric cysts, varices, ectopic pancreas
Focal hyperechoic lesions in the submucosa of the stomach	Ectopic pancreas, lipoma
Focal defect in the gastric mucosa with the mucosal layer preserved to the edge of the ulcer	Benign gastric ulcer
Defect in the gastric mucosa with indistinct mucosal layer at the ulcer edge	Benign or malignant ulcer
Focal hypoechoic lesions of the muscularis propria (exophytic)	Leiomyoma, leiomyosarcoma, metastatic tumor
Large cystic lesions	Obstruction, ileus, volvulus, mucocele,
Thickening of the valvulae in the small bowel	Cirrhosis, renal disease, Menetrier's disease, Whipple's disease, lymphangiomatosis, abetalipoproteinemia, inflammatory diseases
Mild thickening of the colon wall (<1 cm)	Chronic ulcerative colitis, regional enteritis, diverticulitis, pseudomembranous colitis, amebiasis, shigellosis, radiation colitis
Multiple concentric rings of bowel wall on transverse view, folded layers on longitudinal view	Intussusception

References

1. Abu-Yousef MM, Bleicher JJ, Majer JW, et al: High-resolution sonography of acute appendicitis. AJR 1987, 149:53–58.
2. Aibe T, Fuji T, Okita A, Takemoto T: A fundamental study of normal layer structure of the gastrointestinal wall visualized by endoscopic ultrasound. Scand J Gastroenterol 1986, 21(suppl 123):6–15.
3. Bolondi L, Caletti G, Casanova P, et al: Problems and variations in the interpretation of the ultrasound features of the normal upper and lower GI tract wall. Scand J Gastroenterol 1986, 21(suppl 123):16–26.
4. Bolondi L, Casanova P, Caletti GC, et al: Primary gastric lymphoma versus gastric carcinoma: Endoscopic US evaluation. Radiology 1987, 165:821–826.
5. Borrman R, Henke F, Lubarsch O: Handbuch der Speziellen Pathologischen Anatomie und Histologie, vol 4. Berlin, Springer-Verlag 1926.
6. Boscaini M, Montori A: Transrectal ultrasonography: Interpretation of normal intestinal wall structure for the preoperative staging of rectal cancer. Scand J Gastroenterol 1986, 21(suppl 123):87–98.
7. Bowerman RA, Silver TM, Jaffe MH: Real-time ultrasound diagnosis of intussusception in children. Radiology 1982, 143:527–529.
8. Caletti GC, Bolondi L, Zani L, Labo G: Technique of endoscopic ultrasonography investigation: Esophagus, stomach and duodenum. Scand J Gastroenterol 1986, 21(suppl 123):1–5.
9. Clearfield HR, Stahlgren LH: Acute dilatation, volvulus, and torsion of the stomach. *In* Berk JE, Haubrick WS, Kalser MH, et al (eds): Bockus Gastroenterology, 4th edition, vol 2. Philadelphia, WB Saunders, 1985.
10. Cohn I Jr: Intestinal obstruction. *In* Berk JE, Haubrick WS, Kalser MH, et al (eds): Bockus Gastroenterology, 4th ed, vol 3. Philadelphia, WB Saunders, 1985.
11. Derchi LE, Banderali A, Bossi MC, et al: Sonographic appearance of gastric lymphoma. J Ultrasound Med 1984, 3:251–256.
12. Dubbins PA: Ultrasound demonstration of bowel wall thickness in inflammatory bowel disease. Clin Radiol 1984, 35:227–231.

13. Eisenberg RL: Gastrointestinal Radiology. Philadelphia, JB Lippincott, 1983.
14. Fahkry JR, Berk RN: The "target" pattern: Characteristic sonographic feature of stomach and bowel abnormalities. AJR 1981, 137:969–972.
15. Fleischer AC, Dowling AD, Weinstein ML, James AE Jr: Sonographic patterns of distended, fluid-filled bowel. Radiology 1979, 133:681–685.
16. Fleischer AC, Muhletaler CA, James AE: Sonographic assessment of the bowel wall. AJR 1981, 136:887–891.
17. Heyder N, Lux G: Malignant lesions of the upper gastrointestinal tract. Scand J Gastroenterol 1986, 21(suppl 123):47–51.
18. Higa E, Rosai J, Pizzimbono CA, et al: Mucosal hyperplasia, mucinous cystadenoma, and mucinous cystadenocarcinoma of the appendix: A reevaluation of appendiceal "mucocele." Cancer 1973, 32:1525–1541.
19. Horgan JG, Chow PP, Richter JO, et al: CT and sonography in the recognition of mucocele of the appendix. AJR 1984, 143:959–962.
20. Horn RC Jr: Alimentary tract. *In* Anderson WAD (ed): Pathology, 6th ed, vol 2. St. Louis, CV Mosby, 1971.
21. Jeffrey RB Jr, Laing FC, Lewis FR: Acute appendicitis: High-resolution real-time US findings. Radiology 1987, 163:11–14.
22. Jeffrey RB Jr, Laing FC, Townsend RR: Acute appendicitis: Sonographic criteria based on 250 cases. Radiology 1988, 167:327–329.
23. Johnson BA: A proposed new sonographic sign to aid in further differentiation of gastric neoplasms. J Diagn Med Sonogr 1987, 3:21–26.
24. Kremer H, Lohmoeller G, Zollner N: Primary ultrasonic detection of a double carcinoma of the colon. Radiology 1977, 124:481–482.
25. Kurtz RC, Sherlock P: Carcinoma of the stomach. *In* Berk JE, Haubrick WS, Kalser MH, et al (eds): Bockus Gastroenterology, 4th ed, vol 2. Philadelphia, WB Saunders, 1985.
26. Lee TG, Brickman FE, Avecilla LS: Ultrasound diagnosis of intramural intestinal hematoma. J Clin Ultrasound 1977, 5:423.
27. Livstone EM: Tumors of the esophagus. *In* Berk JE, Haubrick WS, Kalser MH, et al (eds): Bockus Gastroenterology, 4th ed, vol 2. Philadelphia, WB Saunders, 1985.
28. Machi J, Takeda J, Sigel B, Kakegawa T: Normal stomach wall and gastric cancer: Evaluation with high-resolution operative US. Radiology 1986, 159:85–87.
29. Madrazo BL, Hricak H, Sandler MA, Eyler WR: Sonographic findings in complicated peptic ulcer disease. Radiology 1981, 140:457–461.
30. Manten HD, Harary AM: Chronic ideopathic intestinal pseudoobstruction. *In* Berk JE, Haubrick WS, Kalser MH, et al (eds): Bockus Gastroenterology, 4th ed, vol 3. Philadelphia, WB Saunders, 1985.
31. Miller JH, Kemberling CR: Ultrasound scanning of the gastrointestinal tract in children: Subject review. Radiology 1984, 152:671–677.
32. Mittelstaedt CA: Abdominal Ultrasound. New York, Churchill Livingstone, 1987, pp 605–656.
33. Montali BG, Croce F, De Pra L, Solbiati L: Intussusception of the bowel: A new sonographic pattern. Br J Radiol 1983, 56:621–623.
34. Nelson RS, Lanza FL: Benign and malignant tumors of the stomach (other than carcinoma.) *In* Berk JE, Haubrick WS, Kalser MH, et al (eds): Bockus Gastroenterology, 4th ed, vol 2. Philadelphia, WB Saunders, 1985.
35. Pringot J, Bodart P: Inflammatory diseases of the small bowel. *In* Margulis AR, Burhenne JH (eds): Alimentary Tract Radiology, 3rd ed, vol 1. St Louis, CV Mosby, 1983.
36. Puylaert J: Acute appendicitis: US evaluation using graded compression. Radiology 1986, 158:355–360.
37. Rifkin MD, McGlynn ET, Marks G: Endorectal sonographic prospective staging of rectal cancer. Scand J Gastroenterol 1986, 21(suppl 123):99–103.
38. Rifkin MD, Marks GJ: Transrectal US as an adjunct in the diagnosis of rectal and extrarectal tumors. Radiology 1985, 157:499–502.
39. Rubin C, Kurtz AB, Goldberg BB: Water enema: A new ultrasound technique in defining pelvic anatomy. J Clin Ultrasound 1978, 6:28.
40. Seaman WB: Nonneoplastic lesions of the stomach and duodenum. *In* Margulis AR, Burhenne JH (eds): Alimentary Tract Radiology, 3rd ed, vol 1. St Louis, CV Mosby, 1983.
41. Sonnenberg A, Eckenbrecht J, Peter P, Niederau C: Detection of Crohn's disease by ultrasound. Gastroenterology 1982, 83:430–434.
42. Spjut HJ: Pathology of the stomach and duodenum. *In* Margulis AR, Burhenne JH (eds): Alimentary Tract Radiology, 3rd ed, vol 1. St Louis, CV Mosby, 1983.
43. Strohm WD, Classen M: Benign lesions of the upper GI tract by means of endoscopic ultrasound. Scand J Gastroenterol 1986, 21(suppl 123):41–46.
44. Talbot IC, Morson BC: Colon pathology. *In* Margulis AR, Burhenne JH (eds): Alimentary Tract Radiology, 3rd ed, vol 1. St Louis, CV Mosby, 1983.
45. Talbot IC, Morson BC: Small bowel pathology. *In* Margulis AR, Burhenne JH (eds): Alimentary Tract Radiology, 3rd ed, vol 1. St Louis, CV Mosby, 1983.
46. Tan A, Lau PH: Sonography of primary adenocarci-

noma of the appendix with pathological correlation. Am J Gastroenterol 1983, 78:488–492.

47. Tio TL, Den Hartog Jager FCA, Tytgat GNJ: Endoscopic ultrasonography in the detection and staging of gastric non-Hodgkin lymphoma: Comparison with gastroscopy, barium meal, and computed tomography scan. Scand J Gastroenterol 1986, 21(suppl 123):52–58.
48. Tio TL, Den Hartog Jager FCA, Tytgat GNJ: Endoscopic ultrasonography of non-Hodgkin lymphoma of the stomach. Gastroenterology 1986, 91:401–408.
49. Tio TL, Den Hartog Jager FCA, Tytgat GNJ: The role of ultrasonography in assessing local resectability of esophagogastric malignancies: Accuracy, pitfalls, and predictability. Scand J Gastroenterol 1986, 21(suppl 123):78–86.
50. Tio TL, Tytgat GNJ: Endoscopic ultrasonography of the normal and pathologic gastrointestinal wall structure. Scand J Gastroenterol 1986, 21(suppl 123):27–33.
51. Tomooka Y, Koga T, Shimoda Y, et al: The ultrasonic demonstration of acute multiple gastric ulcers in a child. Br J Radiol 1987, 60:290–292.
52. Verbanck JJ, Rutgeers LJ, Douterlungne PH, et al: Sonographic and pathologic correlation in intussusception of the bowel. J Clin Ultrasound 1986, 14:393–397.
53. Vilardell F: Gastritis. *In* Berk JE, Haubrick WS, Kalser MH, et al (eds): Bockus Gastroenterology, 4th ed, vol 2. Philadelphia, WB Saunders, 1985.
54. Warner RRP: Carcinoid tumor. *In* Berk JE, Haubrick WS, Kalser MH, et al (eds): Bockus Gastroenterology, 4th ed, vol 3. Philadelpia, WB Saunders, 1985.
55. Weigall SL, Wolfman NT, Watson H: The fluid-filled stomach: A sonic window. J Clin Ultrasound 1979, 7:353–356.
56. Worlicek H, Lutz H, Heyder N, Matek N: Ultrasound findings in Crohn's disease and ulcerative colitis: A prospective study. J Clin Ultrasound 1987, 15:153–163.
57. Yasuda K, Nakajima M, Kawai K: Endoscopic ultrasonography in the diagnosis of submucosal tumor of the upper digestive tract. Scand J Gastroenterol 1986, 21(suppl 123):59–67.

CHAPTER 9

Kidney

DIANE M. KAWAMURA, KATHY GILL

Anatomy

EMBRYOLOGY

As early as the third week of embryonic development, the kidneys begin to form from the columns of mesoderm (intermediate mesoderm).[167] In successive intervals, three pairs of kidneys differentiate: the pronephros, the mesonephros, and the metanephros and paramesonephric ducts.[33,101,158]

The pronephros (forekidney) is a transitory, nonfunctional structure that appears early in the fourth week of gestation. It degenerates rapidly, leaving nothing more than a duct to be utilized by the next kidney. Late in the fourth week, the mesonephros (midkidney) forms just caudad to the pronephros. This structure provides partial function while the permanent kidney continues to develop.[14,101,158,167] By the end of the embryonic period and prior to degeneration, the mesonephros claims the pronephric duct and becomes known as the mesonephric duct.[101] In the male, the mesonephric duct (wolffian) persists and develops into the male epididymis, the ductus deferens, and the ejaculatory duct.[32,50,109] In the female, the mesonephric duct develops into the paramesonephric duct (müllerian), and eventually into the uterus and vagina.[14,109]

During the fifth week of gestation, the metanephros (permanent kidney) appears as hollow ureteric buds that push upward from the mesonephric duct.[32,101] The expanded distal ends form the renal pelvis, associated calyces, and collecting tubules; the mesonephric duct, the unexpanded proximal portion, forms the ureters.[167] The nephrons, the functional units of the kidney, arise from the intermediate mesoderm around each ureteric bud. Nephron function begins at approximately 8 weeks.[158]

With fetal growth, the kidneys appear to migrate from their pelvic location to the abdomen. This results from the rapid growth of the caudad part of the kidneys.[62] As this so-called migration is not complete until 5 or 6 years of life, the kidneys in infants and young children are located more caudad.

EXTERNAL ANATOMY

The kidneys are about the size of a tightly clenched fist. Each is approximately 10 to 12 cm long, 5 to 7.5 cm wide, 2 to 3 cm thick, and weighs approximately 130 to 150 g.[14,15,101,158,167] They are paired, reddish brown organs with convex lateral borders and concave medial borders.[101,158] On the medial border is an indentation or cleft, the renal hilus, which leads into a space called the renal sinus.[5,158] Renal blood vessels, lymphatics, nerves, and the ureter enter or exit the kidney at the hilus and occupy the sinus (Fig. 9-1).[101]

Both kidneys are located retroperitoneally lying along the posterior abdominal wall. Each kidney is surrounded by three layers of supportive tissues. The innermost layer is the fibrous renal capsule,

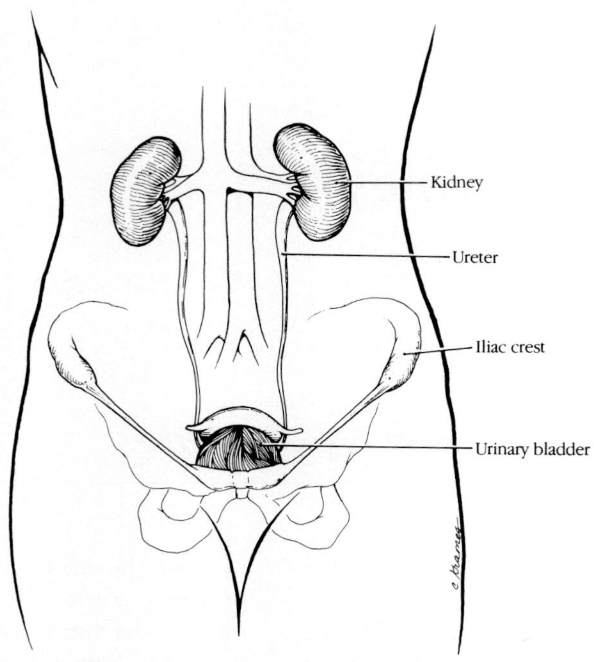

FIGURE 9-1. Anterior view of female urinary tract.

which covers the surface, is continuous with the outer layer of the ureter at the hilus, and gives a fresh kidney a glistening appearance.[101] The renal capsule serves as a barrier against physical trauma and infection.[43,78] The second, or middle, layer is a mass of perirenal fat, the adipose capsule, which helps to hold the kidney in place against the posterior trunk muscles and cushions it against blows.[167] The third, outermost layer, the renal fascia, is also referred to as Gerota's fascia. The renal fascia is a dense, fibroareolar connective tissue surrounding the kidney, the adipose capsule, and the adrenal gland, completely enclosing them and anchoring these organs to surrounding structures (Fig. 9-2).[101,112,167]

Renal vasculature and the fatty encasement are extremely important in holding the kidneys in their normal position, but it is normal for both kidneys to demonstrate 3 to 4 cm of excursion when a patient changes from a supine to an erect position. Ptosis, an abnormal displacement to a lower position,[164] occurs when the amount of fatty tissue dwindles (owing to rapid weight loss) and may precipitate a kinked ureter, resulting in hydronephrosis.[101]

INTERNAL ANATOMY

A coronal section of a kidney reveals three distinct regions: the cortex, the medulla, and the pelvis.[101,158,167] The granular-looking outer region, the renal cortex, extends from the renal capsule to the bases of the pyramids and into the spaces between them.[167] The cortical extensions passing between the renal pyramids are called renal columns or columns of Bertin.[54,150,158] Deep to the cortex, the renal medulla exhibits triangular or cone-shaped tissue masses called medullary (or renal) pyramids.[101,158,167] The broader base of each pyramid faces the cortical area; its apex or papilla points are directed toward the center of the kidney.[99] The striated (striped) appearance of the pyramids is due to the presence of straight tubules and blood vessels (Fig. 9-3).[167]

The renal pelvis is a large cavity medial to the hilus.[167] Flat and funnel-shaped, it is continuous

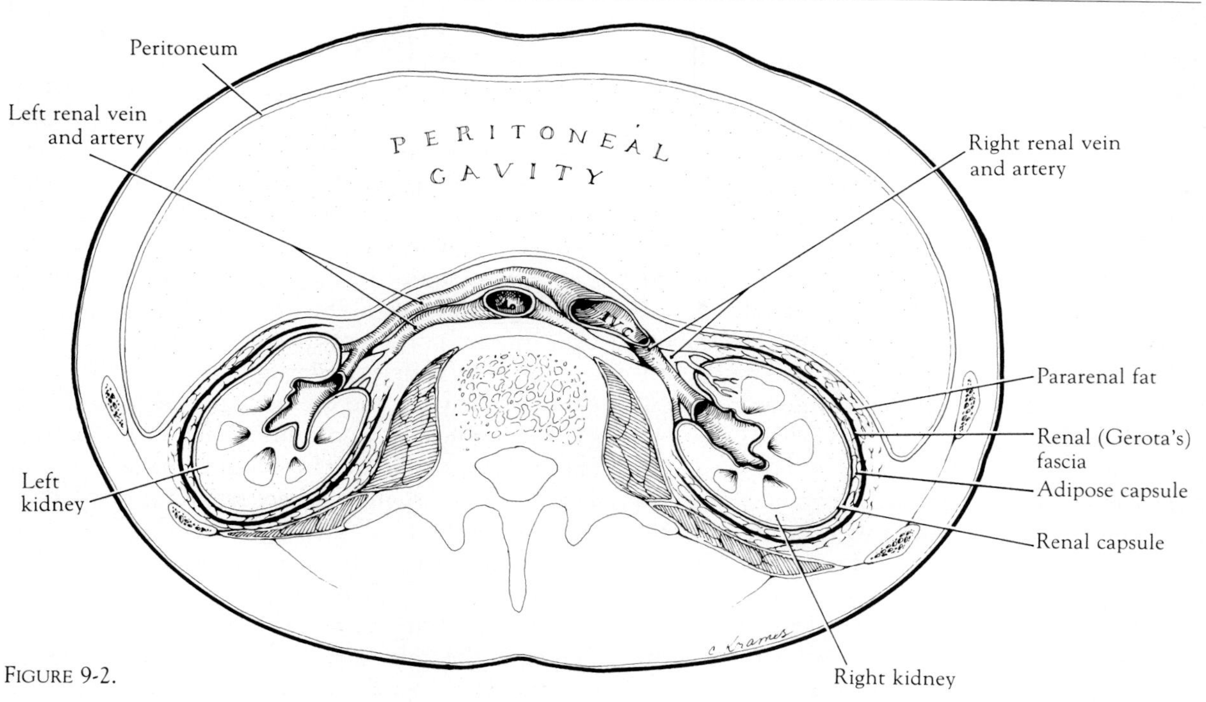

FIGURE 9-2.

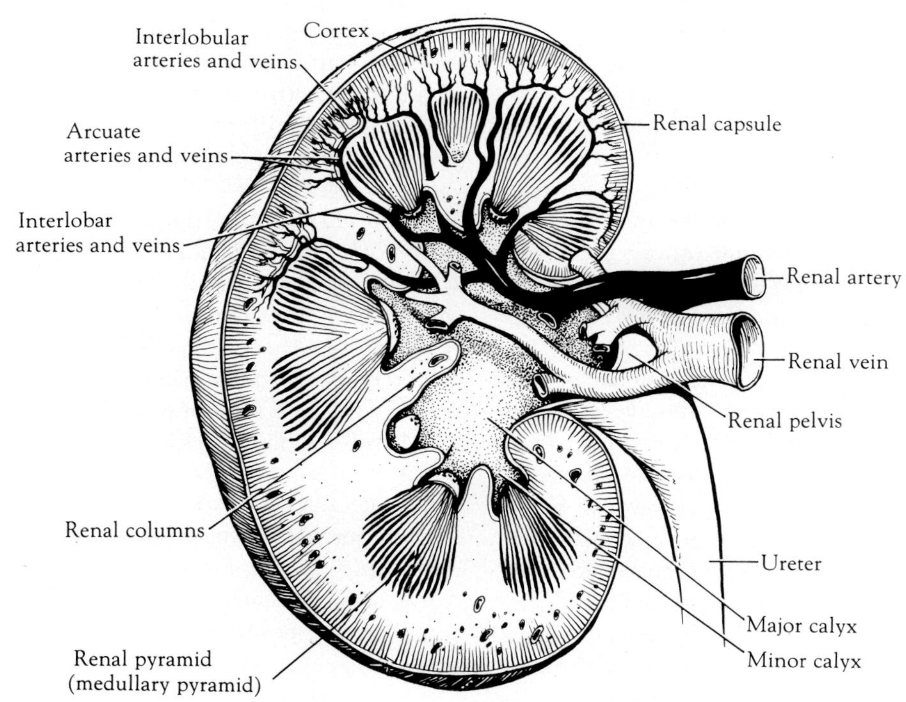

FIGURE 9-3.

FIGURE 9-2. Transverse section shows the retroperitoneal location of the kidneys surrounded by the renal capsule, the adipose capsule, and the renal (Gerota's) fascia (Ao, aorta; IVC, inferior vena cava).

FIGURE 9-3. Coronal section shows the internal renal anatomy.

with the ureter, leaving the hilus. The papillae of the renal pyramid projects into a cup-like chamber at the edge of the pelvis called the minor calyces.[101] The eight to 18 minor calyces join together to form two or three major calyces.[158] The calyces collect urine, which drains continuously from the papillae and empties into the renal pelvis. From the renal pelvis, urine flows into the epithelium-lined, fibromuscular ureters, which are approximately 25 to 30 cm long and 6 mm in diameter.[101,158,167] The smooth muscle wall of the calyces, pelvis, and ureters contracts rythmically and propels urine by peristalsis to the bladder to be stored.[150,167]

Nephron. The cortex and renal pyramids together constitute the renal parenchyma containing the kidney's basic histologic and functional unit, the nephron.[150,158] Each kidney contains more than 1,000,000 nephrons.[50,150] Each nephron consists of (1) a renal corpuscle, an enlarged terminal end comprised of the glomerular capsule and its enclosed glomerulus; (2) a renal tubule divided into a proximal convoluted tubule, a peri-nephric loop (the loop of Henle), and a distal convoluted tubule; and (3) a vascular component.[101,158] Table 9-1 describes the nephron's anatomy. Nephrons are frequently classified into two types. A cortical nephron's glomerulus is located in the outer cortical zone and the remainder of the nephron rarely penetrates the medulla. A juxtamedullary nephron's glomerulus is usually closer to the corticomedullary junction, with longer loops of Henle extending farther into the medulla (Fig. 9-4).[150,167]

Juxtaglomerular apparatus. The nuclei of the smooth muscle cells adjacent to the afferent (and sometimes efferent) arteriole is rounded instead of elongated. These modified cells are called juxtaglomerular cells, and in response to lowered blood pressure are thought to secrete an enzyme called renin.[158,167] Adjacent to the afferent and efferent arteriole, the cells of the distal convoluted tubule become narrower and taller.[167] Collectively, these cells are called the macula densa and are thought to be chemoreceptors or osmoreceptors that respond to changes in the solute concentration of the filtrate.[101] Each nephron's juxtaglomerular apparatus (JGA) is formed from these juxtaglomerular cells and the macula densa.[101]

VASCULAR ANATOMY

Just inferior to the superior mesenteric artery (SMA), the renal arteries arise from the lateral and medial aspects of the abdominal aorta.[50,109] Because the aorta lies to the left of the midline, the right renal artery is typically longer than the left.[5,101] It courses transversely across the crus of the diaphragm posterior to the inferior vena cava (IVC), the right renal vein, the head of the pancreas, and the inferior portion of the duodenum.[3,5,109] The left renal artery courses posterior to the left renal vein, the splenic vein, and the body of the pancreas.[3,109]

The right renal vein courses anterior to the right renal artery and enters the right lateral aspect of the IVC at a slightly lower transverse plane than the left renal vein.[3,50] Because the IVC is situated to the right of the midline, it is shorter than the left renal vein.[109] The left renal vein courses from the left kidney hilus, anterior to the left renal artery, crossing the aorta anteriorly, and passes posterior to the SMA before entering the medial aspect of the IVC (Fig. 9-5).[3,50,109]

To carry out the normal kidney functions of removing wastes from the blood and regulating its fluid and electrolyte content, approximately 1100 to 1200 ml of blood passes through the kidneys every minute (Table 9-2, Figs. 9-3, 9-6). This represents 20% to 25% of the total cardiac output transported by the right and left renal arteries.[150,158,167] The enormous blood flow is related to the fact that, for the kidneys to maintain blood homeostasis a considerable amount of blood must pass through the kidneys.[158] More than 90% of the blood entering the kidney perfuses the cortex, containing the nephron, and only a small amount of the blood supplies the kidney's nutritive needs.[101]

RELATIONAL ANATOMY

It is important to understand the location and relationship of the kidneys to surrounding structures, as displacement of those structures or an unusual renal position may suggest disease. The

(text continues on page 284)

FIGURE 9-4. (*A*) Location and (*B*) structure of the cortical and juxtamedullary nephrons.

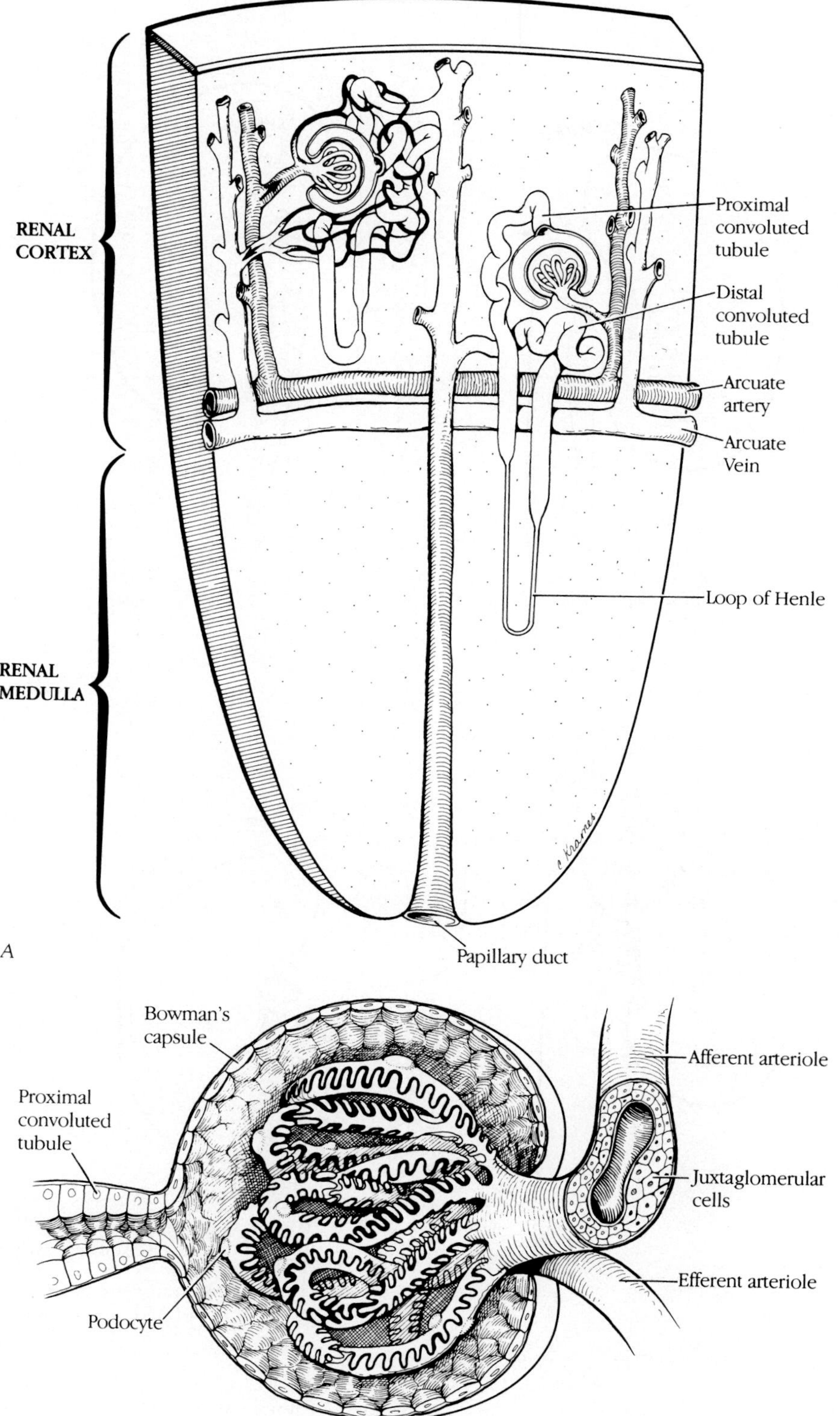
RENAL CORTEX
RENAL MEDULLA
Proximal convoluted tubule
Distal convoluted tubule
Arcuate artery
Arcuate Vein
Loop of Henle
Papillary duct
A
Bowman's capsule
Afferent arteriole
Proximal convoluted tubule
Juxtaglomerular cells
Efferent arteriole
Podocyte
B

Anterior surface

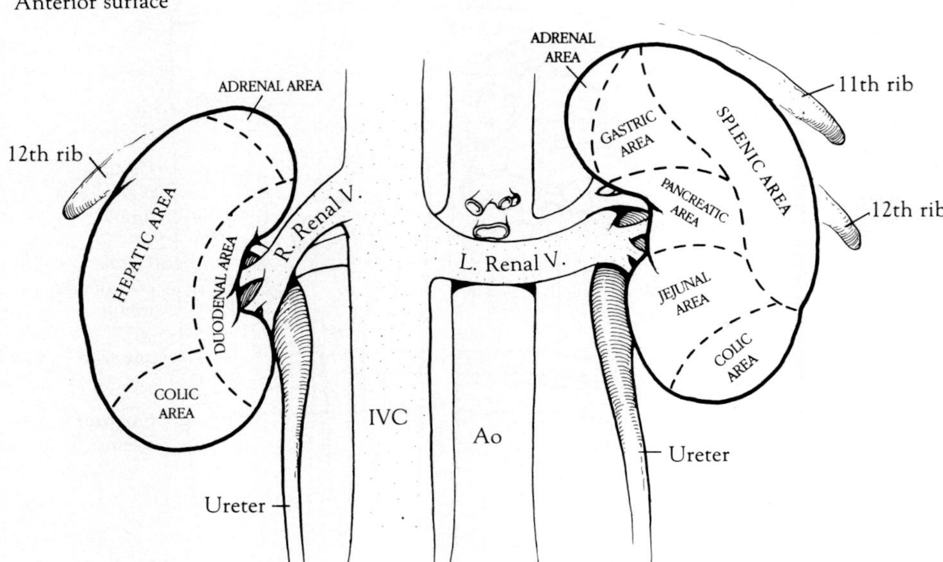

Posterior surface

11th rib
DIAPHRAGMATIC AREA
TRANSVERSE TENDON AREA
QUADRATUS LUMBORUM AREA
PSOAS AREA
Ao
R. Renal A.
IVC
DIAPHRAGMATIC AREA
12th rib
QUADRATUS LUMBORUM AREA
TRANSVERSE TENDON AREA
PSOAS AREA

✻ Transverse process of 1st lumbar vertebra

✸ Transverse process of 2nd lumbar vertebra

Figure 9-5. Topographic anatomy of renal vasculature and the anterior, posterior, lateral, and medial surfaces.

Table 9-1. Anatomy of the nephron[5,14,101,109,150,158,167]

Renal Corpuscle	
Glomerular capsule	Double-walled cup beginning in the cortex, composed of parietal and visceral layer separated by capsular space (often referred to as Bowman's capsule)
Parietal layer	Outer wall composed of simple squamous epithelium
Visceral layer	Inner wall surrounding a capillary network called the glomerulus; consists of epithelial cells called podocytes (octopus-like branches terminating in foot processes or pedicles which intertwine with one another and cling to the basement membrane of glomerulus, forming part of filtration membrane.)
Glomerulus	Tuft of capillaries associated with renal tubule. Endothelium is fenestrated so capillaries are exceptionally porous, allowing all substances, except blood cells and most plasma proteins, to pass from blood into glomerular capsule.
Renal Tubule	
Proximal convoluted tubule	(Convoluted means coiled and proximal signifies the glomerular capsule is the origin.) Wall consists of cuboidal epithelium with microvilli, cytoplasmic extensions, increasing surface area for reabsorption and secretion.
Descending limb	Renal tubule straightens, becomes thinner, dips into medulla; consists of squamous epithelium.
Loop of Henle	Diameter increases, bends into a **U** shape
Ascending Limb	Ascends toward cortex and consists primarily of cuboidal epithelium
Distal convoluted tubule	Cuboidal epithelium with few microvilli (unlike proximal convoluted tubule). Distal convoluted tubule of several nephrons empties into a common collecting tubule which transports urine back into renal pyramids in medulla.

Table 9-2. Renal vasculature[5,14,101,109,150,158,167]

Renal artery	Before or immediately after entering hilus, divides into five segmental or lobar branches
Lobar (segmental) arteries	Within renal sinus, each segmental or lobar artery branches to form interlobar arteries
Interlobar arteries	Pass between pyramids and branch into arcuate arteries at bases of pyramid
Arcuate arteries	Arching branches coursing between medulla and cortex, parallel to kidneys' surface
Interlobar arteries	Divisions of arcuate arteries produce a series of interlobar arteries, which travel through cortex toward kidney surface
Afferent arterioles	Interlobar arteries divide into several afferent arterioles, each of which supplies a renal corpuscle and forms a glomerulus, a tangled capillary network.
Glomerulus	Blood comes in close contact with cells of glomerular capsule.
Efferent arteriole	Reunited glomerular capillaries lead away from glomerular capsule, are smaller in diameter than afferent arterioles, and are unique as blood usually flows out of capillaries into venules and not into other arterioles.
Peritubular capillaries	Each efferent arteriole of a cortical nephron divides to form a network of capillaries around convoluted tubules called peritubular capillaries.
Vasa recta	Efferent arterioles of a juxtamedullary nephron form straight specialized portions from peritubular capillaries, called vasa recta and course with loops of Henle into medulla.
Interlobar veins	Peritubular capillaries unite to form interlobar veins, which unite to form arcuate veins.
Arcuate veins	Follow same course as arcuate arteries and drain into interlobar veins
Interlobar veins	Course between pyramids and unite to form single renal vein
Renal vein	Exits kidney hilus

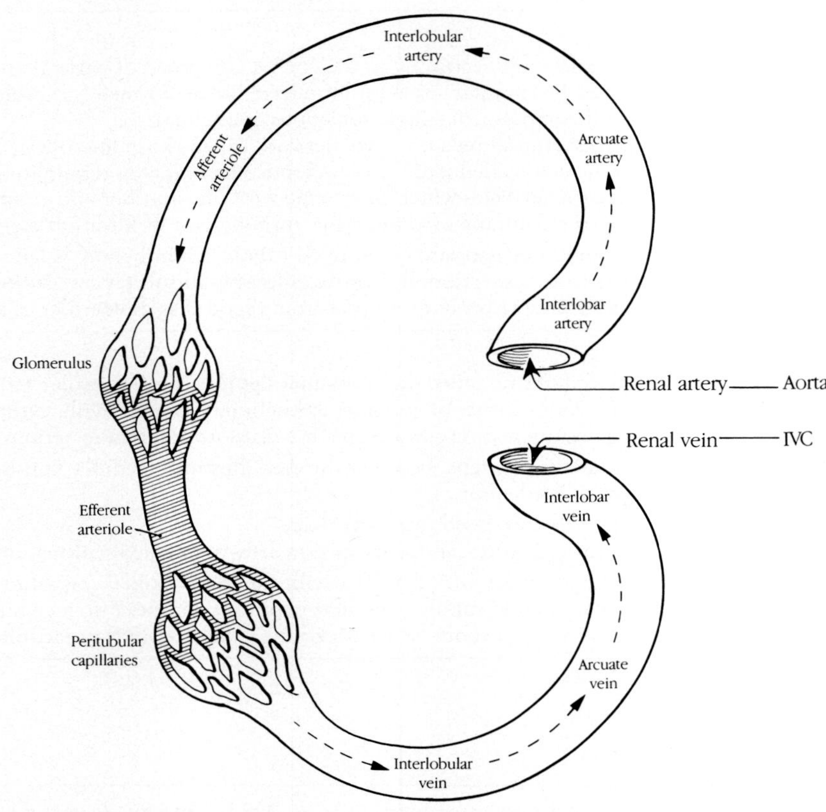

FIGURE 9-6. A schematic depiction of the sequence of renal blood flow.

relational anatomy may be easier to understand when the kidney is viewed as having anterior and posterior surfaces, lateral and medial borders, and a superior and an inferior extremity.

Anterior Surface. In most patients, the right kidney is 2 to 8 cm lower than the left owing to the presence of the liver.[109] A narrow portion of the right anterior superior surface is in relation with the right adrenal gland.[50] Inferior to this, approximately 75% of the anterior surface comes in contact with the renal impression on the visceral surface of the liver.[50] The remaining right anterior surface is in contact with the descending portion of the duodenum.[50] Laterally, the right superior anterior surface is in contact with the hepatic flexure and medially with the small intestine.[50] The areas in contact with the liver and small intestine are covered by peritoneum; the adrenal, duodenal, and colic areas are devoid of peritoneum (see Fig. 9-5).[50,109]

The left anterior superior surface of the medial border is in close proximity to the left adrenal gland.[50] Close to the left anterior lateral border, a long strip is in contact with the renal impression on the spleen.[50] At approximately the middle of the anterior surface lies a somewhat quadrilateral field marking the site of contact with the body of the pancreas.[50] Superior to this small triangular portion, between the adrenal and splenic areas, the left kidney is in contact with the posterior surface of the stomach.[50] Inferior to the pancreatic area, its lateral part is in relation with the colon's splenic flexure and its medial part lies in relation to the small intestine.[50] The areas in contact with the stomach and spleen are covered by the omental bursa type of peritoneum, whereas that in relation to the small intestine is covered by the peritoneum of the greater sac.[50] The adrenal, pancreatic, and colic areas are devoid of peritoneum (see Fig. 9-5).[50] Kidney surfaces in direct contact with other organs devoid of peritoneum are frequently referred to as bare areas.[109]

Posterior Surface. The posterior surface of both kidneys lies on the diaphragm, the medial and lateral lumbocostal arches, and the anterior surfaces of the psoas major, the quadratus lumborum, and the tendon of the transversus abdominis muscles (see Fig. 9-5).[50,109]

Lateral and Medial Border. The lateral convex border is directed toward the posterolateral wall of the abdomen.[50] On the left side, it is in contact superiorly with the spleen.[50] The median border is directed somewhat anteriorly and inferiorly.[50] The superior and inferior extremities of the medial border are convex.[50] The middle medial border is concave, presenting a deep longitudinal fissure, the renal hilus.[50] Above the hilus, the medial border is in relation with the adrenal gland, below the hilus, with the ureter.[50] The relative position of the main structures in the hilus is as follows: the renal vein is anterior, the artery is in the middle, and the ureter is posterior and directed inferiorly (see Fig. 9-5).[5,158,167]

Superior and Inferior Extremity. The superior extremity of the kidney is thick and rounded, closer to the midline than the inferior extremity, and is topped by the adrenal gland, which also covers a small portion of the anterior surface.[50] The inferior extremity is smaller and thinner and lies farther lateral and extends to within 5 cm of the iliac crest.[50]

Physiology

The kidneys, which process about 180 L (45 gallons) of blood-derived fluid daily, are involved with both excretory and regulatory activities.[101] Of the total amount of blood-derived fluid circulated through the kidneys, 99% is filtered and returned for circulation while only about 1% is eliminated from the body as urine.[101] The body depends on the efficient functioning of the glomeruli and the renal tubules (nephrons and collecting tubes) to filter the entire plasma volume approximately 60 times a day.[101,167] As the smallest structural unit capable of producing urine, the nephron is so important that one third must function simply to ensure survival.[150] Three important nephron functions are (1) controlling blood concentration and volume by removing selected amounts of water and solutes, (2) helping to regulate blood pH, and (3) removing toxic wastes from the blood.[167] The three processes involved in urine formation and the simultaneous adjustment of blood composition are described in Table 9-3.

TABLE 9-3. Urine Formation[5,101,150,158,167]

PROCESS	FUNCTION
Glomerular filtration	Nonselective process by which fluids and solutes are forced through membrane by pressure gradient; occurs in renal corpuscle across endothelial capsular membrane. Portion of fluid entering nephron is called filtrate. Filtrate consists of all raw materials in blood processed by renal tubules except formed elements and proteins too large to pass through the endothelial barrier.
Tubular resorption	A discriminating process occurring as filtrate passes through renal tubules. Depending on body needs, epithelial cells reabsorb water, glucose, amino acids, and electrolyte ions. The process allows the body to retain most of its nutrients. Wastes, such as urea, are only partially reabsorbed.
Tubular secretion	Active process that transports substances into nephron and adds materials to filtrate from blood. Secretion is for (1) disposing of substances not already in filtrate (penicillin and phenobarbital); (2) eliminating undesirable compounds reabsorbed by passive processes (urea and uric acid); (3) removing excessive potassium ions; and (4) regulating blood pH.

Antidiuretic hormone (ADH), secreted by the posterior pituitary, increases the water permeability of the collecting tubule segments (facultative reabsorption) by enlarging the pores so that water passes easily into the interstitial spaces.[16,101,150] Responsible for maintaining the body's fluid balance, ADH secretion increases in event of increased water loss (sweating or diarrhea) or reduced blood volume or blood pressure (hemorrhage).[101,167]

Aldosterone, secreted by the adrenal cortex, increases the rate of tubular resorption of sodium and effects a concurrent loss of potassium.[166] Extracellular excess of potassium promotes aldosterone secretion, which in turn produces an increase in potassium excretion and sodium retention by the kidneys.[166] Aldosterone secretion is also controlled by the renin-angiotensin system. Renin, secreted by the juxtaglomerular apparatus, increases in response to decreased blood pressure in the afferent arteriole secondary to sodium depletion or to a change from the supine to the upright position.[150,166] Renin acts as a catalyst on certain plasma proteins to produce angiotensin I, which is converted to angiotensin II by proteolytic enzymes.[150] Angiotensin II increases the systemic blood pressure: by acting as a potent vasoconstrictor, it increases the peripheral resistance and causes increased blood pressure, and by increasing the rate of aldosterone secretion and tubular reabsorption of sodium, it increases the kidney's ability to retain water and to produce a small volume of concentrated urine.[16,18,150] In response to the increased volume of filtrate and increased sodium chloride passing through the juxtaglomerular apparatus, renin secretion decreases.[150]

Kidney Function Tests

Several serum and urine laboratory tests (for urea nitrogen, creatinine, and uric acid) are used to evaluate renal function (Table 9-4). Laboratory examination of urine specimens can detect the presence of red blood cells, white blood cells, and bacteria, which could indicate infection or tumor (Table 9-4). Because normal values vary for sex, age, and geographic region, they are not presented here.

Sonographic Technique

Preparation

No patient preparation is required for ultrasonographic examination of the kidneys,[24,104] but if surrounding structures are of interest, such as the adrenal glands or the pancreas, it is recommended that the patient fast approximately 6 to 8 hours before the examination. If the examination's purpose includes associated ureteral or bladder pathology, the patient should drink 20 to 24 ounces of liquid 30 to 45 minutes before the examination to ensure a urine-filled bladder.[24]

Patient Positions

A prone position and posterior scannning site were the traditional methods of obtaining longitudinal and transverse kidney images with a static scanner,[65] but thick paraspinous muscles and rib artifacts frequently prevent optimal visualization of the renal architecture, especially the upper pole.[65,104] For patients who can be scanned only in a prone position, a pillow or rolled sheet placed under the abdomen at the kidney level compresses anterior soft tissue and stretches the posterior muscles. This results in reducing scattering and absorption of the sound beam[104] and enlarges the acoustic window between the iliac crest and the ribs.[54]

Utilizing real-time instrumentation, the kidneys can usually be accessed with the patient in a supine or decubitus position and images can be obtained from anterior or lateral approaches.[37] It is often advantageous to scan from more than one patient position and anatomic site.

Using the liver as an acoustic window, the right kidney is best imaged with the patient in either a supine or left lateral decubitus position, scanning through the anterior axillary line, intercostally or subcostally.[37,54,65,104] The left kidney is best imaged in the right lateral decubitus position requiring transducer placement in an intercostal space along the posterior axillary line and using the spleen as an acoustic window.[37,104] When the left upper pole cannot be identified owing to rib or bowel gas interference, the fluid-filled stomach can be used as an acoustic window.[130] The patient is given 500 to 1000 ml of degassed water and sits in an erect to semierect position to allow superior displacement of residual stomach gas. Starting from a supine position, it is usually necessary to try different degrees

TABLE 9-4. Renal function tests[23,71,92,120,161,166]

TEST—SPECIMEN	EXPLANATION	PATHOLOGIC VARIATION	CLINICAL INDICATIONS
Blood urea nitrogen (BUN)—serum	Measures amounr of urea nitrogen in blood. Urea, an end-product of protein metabolism, is formed in liver and carried to kidney for excretion. BUN can be used to measure renal function.	Increase	Acute or chronic disease or damaged kidneys: renal failure, congestive heart failure with decreased renal blood supply, obstructive uropathy, stress, dehydration, starvation, decreased blood volume (hemorrhage)
		Decrease	Overhydration, liver failure, pregnancy, decreased protein intake, smoking
Creatinine clearance rate (Cr,CrCl)—serum or urine	Creatinine is a nonprotein, end-product of breakdown of creatinine phosphate found in skeletal muscles. Blood concentration is proportional to amount of active body muscle tissue and is normally maintained at a constant rate. Creatinine is removed by glomerular filtration the rate of which is close to that of serum creatinine production. It is a very accurate test, since creatinine production is not affected by protein intake, urine volume, hydration, or protein metabolism.	Increase	If the creatinine level is double the normal value for a patient, it is indicative that 50% of the nephrons are not functioning
		Decrease	Muscle weakness or dystrophy, myasthenia, starvation, hyperthyroidism
Uric acid (UA)—serum or urine	Uric acid is an end-product of purine metabolism. Purines come from dietary sources and from breakdown of proteins.	Increase	Gout, leukemia, renal hypertension, septicemia
		Decrease	Renal tubular degeneration, Fanconi's syndrome, liver disease
Red blood cell count (RBC)—serum	Kidneys secrete erythropoietin, which stimulates production of RBCs in bone marrow; counted per milliliter of blood.	Increase	Hypernephromas and renal cysts increase erythropoietin, causing erythrocytosis
Total white blood cell count (WBC)—serum	Counted per milliliter of blood.	Increase	Infection or inflammation causes leukocytosis
		Decrease	Toxic reactions, chemotherapy, or radiation therapy

Table 9-4. Renal function tests[23,71,92,120,161,166] *(continued)*

Test—Specimen	Explanation	Pathologic Variation	Clinical Indications
Differential white cell count (Diff)—serum	Reports percentages of white cells: granulocytes (neutrophils, eosinophils, basophils) and nongranulocytes (lymphocytes and monocytes) in blood. With elevation of WBC, one or more cell type increases in number. The percentage increases per sample of 100 while the other cell percentages decrease, even though the absolute count does not. Diff provides specific information on stage and severity of disease or infection and host's ability to resist.	Increase neutrophils (segs, or mature cells; band or stabs, young cells)	Bacterial infection, inflammatory process, physical stress, tissue necrosis
Hematocrit (Hct)—serum	Percentage of red blood cells in plasma.	Decrease	Acute hemorrhagic processes secondary to disease or trauma
Lactic acid dehydrogenase (LDH)—serum	Enzyme found in cytoplasm of nearly all tissues.	Increase	Acute renal infarction, chronic renal disorders
Urine pH—urine	Measures relative acidity (<7) or alkalinity (>7). Normally, urine tends to be acidic due to diet (meat, eggs), whereas fruits and vegetables render it alkaline. Alkaline urine promotes growth of certain organisms and calcium phosphate calculi in susceptible persons.	Alkalinity	Renal tubular acidosis, diet, infection, respiratory alkalosis, metabolic alkalosis, drugs, bed rest
Specific gravity of urine—urine	Measures kidney's ability to concentrate urine. Density of urine is compared to density of water (1.000). The higher the number, the more concentrated the urine unless it contains abnormal constituents.	Increased	Dehydration, high number of solutes (iodinated contrast medium, glucose, IV albumin, protein), and increased secretion of ADH (trauma, stress, surgery)
		Decrease	Hydration, presence of diuretic medication

TABLE 9-4 (*continued*).

TEST—SPECIMEN	EXPLANATION	PATHOLOGIC VARIATION	CLINICAL INDICATIONS
Urine protein—urine	With proteinuria or albuminuria (excess of plasma proteins, principally albumin, in urine) blood concentration is lower.	Increase	Acute or chronic glomerulonephritis, nephrotic syndrome, lupus nephritis, amyloidosis, severe renal venous congestion, nephrotoxic effect
Casts, and cells—urine	Casts are formed in kidney as a result of agglutination of cells or cellular debris. Casts in urine imply tubular or glomerular disorders. It is associated with proteinuria or albuminuria, since protein is necessary for cast formation.	WBC casts	Pyelonephritis
		RBC casts	Glomerulonephritis
		Hyaline casts	Acute renal inflammatory disease, renal hypertension, heart failure, diabetic renal disease
		Epithelial casts or cells	Renal tubular degeneration if seen in large quantities
		Granular casts	Nephritis, acute tubular necrosis, advanced glomerulonephritis, pyelonephritis
		Waxy casts	End-stage renal disease
		Hematuria (blood cells)	Hemorrhagic cystitis or calculi in renal pelvis, tuberculosis, or tumors of renal collecting and tubule system
Urinary glucose—urine	If blood glucose level is normal (no diabetes mellitus), the presence of sugar in urine indicates a low renal threshold for resorption.	Glycosuria	Without diabetes mellitus, indicates renal tubule dysfunction (pregnancy, drugs, congenital metabolic disorders, Fanconi's syndrome)

of head elevation and of left or right posterior obliquity to optimally position the stomach over the kidney.[130]

The renal arteries and veins are best visualized on a transverse plane because of their perpendicular relationship to the ultrasound beam. The right renal vessels are best imaged with the transducer placed transversely over the right kidney and angled medially. To visualize the left renal vessels, the transducer should be placed in a transverse orientation in the midline of the abdomen, just inferior to the origination of the SMA.

A decubitus patient position provides a coronal view with better visualization of the renal parenchyma and medial and lateral borders and demonstrates the kidney's frontal plane so that lesions in the kidney and perirenal and pararenal spaces can easily be located.[104] A prone or supine position is better at demonstrating the posterior and anterior borders of the kidneys.[104]

Regardless of the approach selected, two projections at right angles to each other and views of the entire kidney should be obtained.[65] With the upper pole more medial and posterior than the lower

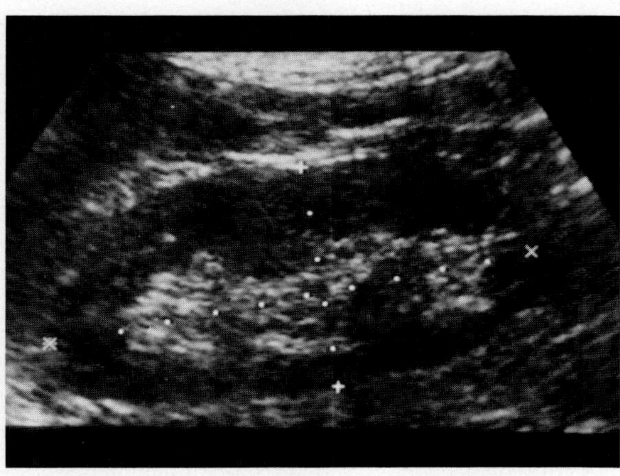

FIGURE 9-7. The left kidney's true longitudinal axis, measuring 10.5 cm by 4.8 cm is demonstrated in this coronal section.

pole,[37] the longitudinal renal axis is normally oriented in an oblique plane. Establishing the long axis can be accomplished by scanning the upper, middle, and lower poles of the kidney transversely, localizing the calyceal echoes on each section, and placing a mark on the patient's skin. After all three levels are marked, the transducer is returned to the longitudinal plane to scan along the marks, connecting them to produce a true longitudinal axis view of the kidney (Fig. 9-7).[3] If the imaging plane is skewed, the apparent renal length will be shorter.[37] A view obtained by excretory urography (intravenous pyelography or IVP) can also help identify the location and angle of the kidneys' longitudinal lie.

TECHNICAL CONSIDERATIONS

For better kidney visualization, deep inspiration helps push the liver, spleen, and kidneys down below the ribs as much as 2.5 cm.[56] It is important to visualize some portion of liver with the right kidney and the spleen with the left kidney, as their echo amplitude can be compared to that of the renal parenchyma.[65]

For adults, a 3.5- to 5-MHz transducer is generally the highest-frequency that affords adequate visualization of parenchymal detail in each projection. Since acoustic energy attenuates exponentially as it penetrates tissue and attenuation increases with frequency,[37] optimal visualization of renal parenchyma requires varied gain settings.[135,136] To minimize the effect of inappropriate time gain compensation (TGC), TGC is adjusted to achieve even-sized, uniform echo intensity throughout the depth of the homogeneous hepatic or splenic tissue and should be compared to renal cortical echo amplitude at the same depth.[37,104] The gain setting should be high enough to fill the cortex but low enough so as not to obliterate the medulla.[104,136]

PITFALLS

Although the kidneys are relatively easy to identify sonographically, there are pitfalls. Rib artifacts, especially at the upper poles of the kidneys, can cause shadowing and obscure pathologic processes. Other anatomic structures—adrenal glands, liver, spleen, pancreatic head, and pancreatic tail—lie close to the kidneys' upper pole and can simulate masses arising from this region. Congenital or developmental anomalies can make kidneys appear diseased or difficult to identify. Atrophic kidneys pose a significant challenge as they are quite small and difficult to outline. Athletic patients and young men frequently have prominent hypertrophic psoas muscles that can simulate a renal or adrenal tumor and should not be mistaken for retroperitoneal fibrosis. Large or multiple cysts can be mistaken for hydronephrosis, and pseudohydronephrosis can appear secondary to overfilling of the bladder[24] or rapid hydration. An ectopic or transplanted kidney can be confused with a pelvic mass. Inappropriate TGC settings do not allow the determination of solid versus cystic masses. Respiratory motion or failure to visualize the true long axis of the kidney can lead to under- or overestimation of renal size.[3,24]

A repertoire of scanning skills must be developed to help overcome these pitfalls. With careful scanning technique, the origin of any mass can be determined. In scanning pelvic masses, visualizing the kidneys in their normal position rules out a pelvic kidney. Likewise, if one of the kidneys is not found in its proper location, it is important to check the pelvic region. Postvoiding studies should be performed whenever any degree of hydronephrosis is encountered or when scanning a transplanted kidney.[24] A technique helpful in differentiating muscle from mass is to instruct the patient (lying in a supine position) to flex or pull up the legs while observing muscle contraction with real-time sonography. Obtaining the patient's clinical history and correlating it with the images is the most useful measure for avoiding scanning pitfalls.

Normal Sonographic Anatomy

Ultrasonography is excellent for imaging all renal and juxtarenal tissue. Current sonographic equipment permits identification and assessment of renal length, width, and thickness; appearance, size, and echogenicity of the renal sinus, and parenchymal cortex and medulla; and the distinctness of the corticomedullary junction produced by the interfaces of the arcuate vessels and the inward extensions of the column of Bertin.[67,104,134]

Although the kidney's position varies from patient to patient, they are normally located between the lower ribs and the iliac crest. For proper localization, surrounding structures should be identified. In relative scanning planes, the liver, gallbladder, second portion of the duodenum, right adrenal gland, and IVC can be identified on the right.[65] On the left, potentially identifiable structures include the spleen, pancreas, fourth portion of the duodenum, left adrenal gland, and aorta.[65] The crus of the diaphragm, psoas muscle, and quadratus lumborum can be identified bilaterally.

Once normal position and location of the kidneys have been established, the contour and internal architecture are observed. The shape and contour of a normal kidney appears smooth. Renal architecture presents specific echo amplitudes.[65] Table 9-5 shows this normal echo amplitude and should assist in defining disease when alterations are encountered (Fig. 9-8).

The renal capsule is closely applied but not adherent to the renal parenchyma and appears sonographically as a strong continuous, linear, specular reflector surrounding the cortex.[112] Sparse perinephric fat, such as in infants, makes this line difficult to visualize.[54]

Renal Sinus

The renal sinus is imaged as an intense compact zone, of homogeneous central echoes within the kidney sinus (see Table 9-5).[25,37,65,104,137] The echo intensity is caused primarily by hilar adipose tissue and secondarily by blood vessels and the collecting system.[25,65] The echo amplitude results from the inherent scattering properties of fat cells and is not attributable to coexisting fibrous tissue septa.[10,65,70] If renal sinus fat is minimal, as it is in infants, the central renal complex is less echogenic.[25] In obese patients or patients with renal sinus lipomatosis, the central renal complex appears as an enlarged central echogenic complex,[104,140] an anechoic to hy-

Table 9-5. Normal sonographic anatomy of kidney and related structures[37,65,67,104,137]

Echo amplitude of stuctures in ascending order	Renal medulla, renal cortex, spleen, liver, pancreas, diaphragm, renal sinus & capsule (isoechoic)
Renal capsule	Strong continuous, linear, specular reflector surrounding the cortex
Renal sinus	Intense compact zone of central homogeneous echoes within the kidney sinus having an echo amplitude equal to that of the renal capsule
Renal parenchyma	Resolves into more echogenic outer cortex and column of Bertin from the hypoechoic inner
Renal cortex	Homogeneously echogenic with closely spaced, relatively low-level intensity echoes less than normal liver and spleen
Renal medulla	Rounded or blunted geometric hypoechoic zones are best demonstrated on coronal sections, becoming more prominent with increased diuresis
Corticomedullary junction	Recognized by columns of Bertin extending inward and arcuate vessels
Arcuate vessels	Discrete, high-level, commalike, specular echoes arching over the tops of the pyramids
Vasculature	Linear anechoic tubular structures entering and exiting the renal hilus
Renal volume	$V = 0.49 \times$ length $\times$ width $\times$ thickness

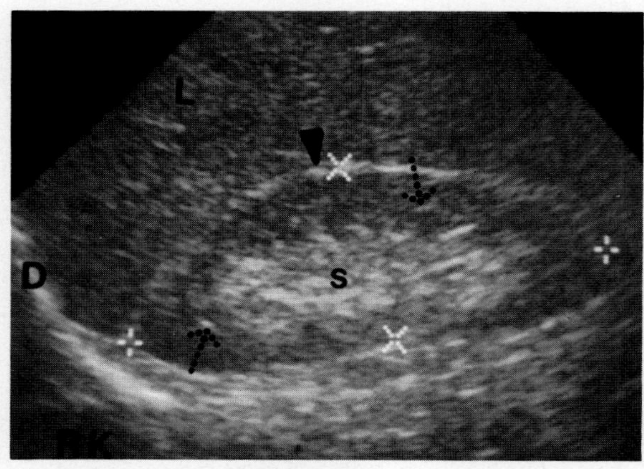

A

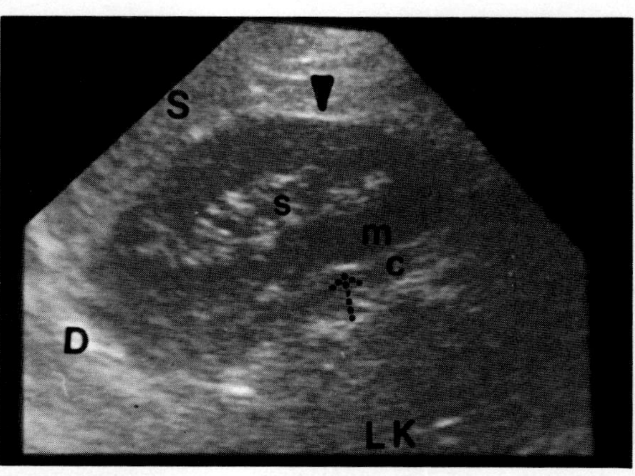

B

Figure 9-8. (*A*) With the patient in the supine position, a sagittal section of the normal right kidney (RK) is identified distal to the liver (L) and anterior to the diaphragm (D). The right kidney *(cursors)* measures 4.59 cm thick and 12.3 cm long (*Dotted arrows,* arcuate vessels; *arrowhead,* renal cortex). (*B*) With the patient in a decubitus position, a coronal section of the normal left kidney (LK) is identified anterior to the diaphragm (D) and medial to the spleen (S). On both images the renal sinus (s) contains intense specular echoes, the cortex (c) contains homogeneous low-level echoes, and the medulla (m) is mostly anechoic. Arcuate vessels are seen as punctate echoes *(dotted arrows)* and may be used to identify the corticomedullary junction. The renal capsule is seen as a strong, continuous, linear, specular reflector surrounding the cortex *(arrowheads)*.

poechoic mass lesion,[24,140] or densely echogenic[10,140] with splaying of infundibular structures secondary to the increase in surrounding fat.[2,25] When two lobulations of renal sinus fat are identified, a bifid renal pelvis or a double intrarenal collecting system should be suspected.[37,104,143] The earliest renal sinus architectural change resulting from any infiltrative disease process, regardless of cause, is uneven widening of the interlobar septum.[65,70]

Renal Parenchyma

Surrounding the renal sinus, the two distinct areas of the kidney parenchyma can be sonographically resolved (see Table 9-5). Differentiation between cortex and medulla is clearest in thin patients and in children.[37] The echogenicity of normal adult renal cortex is comparable to that of spleen and liver at the same depth and is valid only in the absence of hepatic or splenic disease.[37,104,112] Scanning through a bile-filled gallbladder lying anterior to the kidney should be avoided as it enhances the echoes.[65] A hyperechoic cortex is abnormal and should make the sonographer suspicious of infiltrative disease. The medullary region is larger in children.[65] In infants and young children, compound calyces are frequently associated with compound pyramids and are commonly present in the upper and lower renal poles. This normal hypoechoic complex can mimic obstruction of the upper pole of a duplex system, focal calicectasis, simple cyst, hydrocalyx due to infundibular stenosis from a crossing vessel, or a hypoechoic mass.[79] The diuretic status of the kidney affects the detectability and sonographic characteristics of the medulla.[65] With increased diuresis, the medullary pyramids become more prominent, anechoic, and more readily visible.[65]

In addition to the columns of Bertin extending inward, the corticomedullary junction is recognized by discrete, high-level, comma-shaped, specular echoes from the arcuate vessels.[37,104] The arcuate arteries are identified arching over the tops of the pyramids and serve as a marker for evaluation of cortical thickness (Fig. 9-9).[104,135,136]

Vasculature

The renal arteries are identified entering the hilus, posterior to the renal veins. They are not visualized as frequently as the veins, and care must be taken not to confuse them with the crus of the diaphragm. Longer than the left, the right renal artery is retrocaval.

The renal veins are visualized at about the same level as the renal arteries. The right renal vein's size is altered by respiration and transmitted pulses from the IVC (Fig. 9-10).[65] The left renal vein can be seen coursing between the SMA and the aorta to enter the lateral aspect of the inferior vena cava. The narrowing of the left renal vein between the aorta and the SMA is termed the nutcracker phenomenon and should not be mistaken for pathologic change.[65] The prominence of the left renal vein and the incompletely imaged normal aortic wall adjacent to it may give the false impression of a left renal artery aneurysm.[90] In a patient with renal cell carcinoma, determining the patency of the renal veins is an important aspect of staging the disease.[56,65,82,95,149] Venous tumor thrombus is diagnosed by the sonographic appearance of diffuse, low-intensity, intraluminal echoes or focal nodules with or without luminal distension.[95,165] Chapter 3 covers the vasculature in detail.

Measurements

Changes in renal mass accompanied by changes in renal architecture are easily detected by qualitative visual inspection of sonographic images. Alterations of renal mass without significant alterations in architecture require a quantitative method of detection.[80] Accurate bilateral kidney length, width, and thickness measurements are normally obtained in the routine procedure. From a physiologic standpoint,[15] renal volume is more sensitive than any single linear kidney measurement and is the most useful and important variable in detecting disease and in evaluating renal allografts, mon-

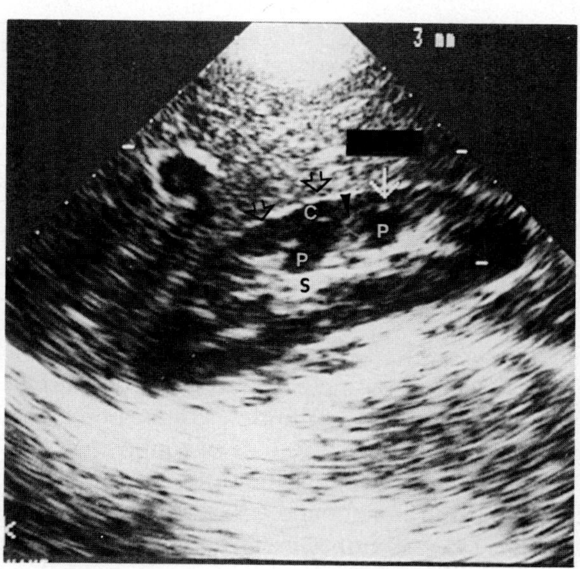

FIGURE 9-9. The medullary pyramids (P), cortex (C), an arcuate vessel *(open arrow)*, and column of Bertin *(arrowhead)* are visualized on this sagittal section through the right kidney. The renal sinus (s) and renal capsule produces the most intense echoes in comparison to the hypoechoic parenchymal pattern.

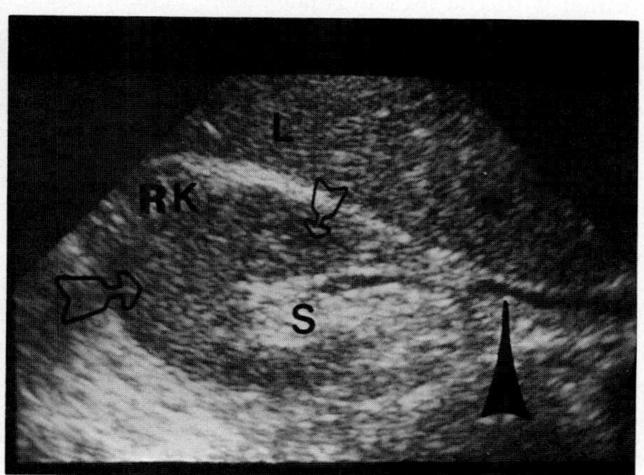

FIGURE 9-10. On a transverse section of a normal right kidney (RK), the renal vein *(large arrowhead)* is identified entering the inferior vena cava *(small arrowhead)*. The renal sinus (S) has intense specular echoes, and the medullary pyramids *(open arrows)* can be identified in the renal parenchyma (L, liver).

itoring children with urinary tract disease, or assessing patients after unilateral nephrectomy.[69,80,104] Renal length is only indirectly useful, since the kidney's size depends on a number of variables, including age, sex, body habitus, and hydration.[15] The adjusted three-dimensional ellipsoid method of determining volume is considered more accurate than the traditional stepped-section method for predicting renal mass.[80] Renal volume can be calculated using the formula in Table 9-5 after obtaining the greatest measurements of length, width, and thickness.[69,80,104]

Congenital Anomalies

It has been estimated that 10% of infants have some form of urinary tract abnormality.[65] Congenital kidney anomalies can be classified according to (1) amount of renal tissue; (2) number; (3) position, form, and orientation; or (4) differentiation leading to various cystic disease.

Amount of Renal Tissue

Agenesis and Hypoplasia. Renal agenesis is presumed to be due to unilateral absence of the nephrogenic primordium or failure of the wolffian duct to make contact with the mesodermal mass.[104] The absence of function resulting from unilateral renal agenesis (absence of one kidney and ureter) or the diminished function caused by unilateral hypoplasia (reduced number of renal lobules and calyces[129]) often produces hypertrophy of the opposite kidney. Unilateral renal agenesis and hypoplasia are not considered life threatening, as the body can sustain life with one kidney. Sonographically, the two entities are difficult to visualize. If no kidney or a small kidney is identifiable in the renal fossa along with hypertrophy of the contralateral kidney, agenesis or hypoplasia may be suspected, but an ectopic kidney cannot be excluded.[104]

Bilateral renal agenesis, complete absence of both kidneys is not compatible with life. Bilateral renal agenesis can be detected in utero and is associated with oligohydramnios and absence of fetal urinary bladder filling.[29,73]

Anomalies of Number

Collecting System Duplications. Complete duplication of the ureter is a common congenital anomaly of the genitourinary tract found at autopsy in one in 157 adult patients and in one in 270 pediatric patients.[93,103] More frequent in women than in men, it is associated with early development of renal diseases.[93] Two ureteral buds arise in the fourth gestational week from the wolffian duct, and initially the caudal ureter drains the lower pole while the cephalic ureter drains the upper one. As the fetus develops, the cephalad ureter continues to migrate with the wolffian duct and enters the bladder at the trigone; however, it is usually associated with a short or absent submucosal tunnel and may become dilated due to vesicoureteral reflux or from an upper pole system obstruction.[65,93] The upper pole ureter is malpositioned, enters the bladder below the trigone, and may be obstructed, leading to ectopic ureterocele.[65,104]

Sonographically, identifying separation in the normal renal sinus echodensities contributes to the diagnosis (Fig. 9-11). If dilatation is present, the sonographic characteristics are those of hydronephrosis.[104] If an associated dilated ureter is present, its course should be followed in search of a ureterocele.[93,104] If the obstructed upper pole system does not function and if the kidney is small, identification by IVP may be difficult.[75] When there is a question of possible collecting system duplication, sonography, which is independent of renal function, can be substituted for urography to (1) determine the presence of kidneys, (2) exclude hydronephrosis, (3) exclude a duplication anomaly,[147] (4) identify a ureterocele in the bladder, and (5) guide percutaneous puncture, if indicated.[65]

Supernumerary Kidneys. Complete duplication of the kidney, pelvis, and ureter is a rare condition believed to be due to splitting of the nephrogenic blastema before or at the time of union with the ureteric bud. This duplication occurs with equal frequency on the right and left side and can be bilateral. The extra kidney usually is ectopic, and the ureter usually joins the upper kidney ureter, so that there is a common ureteral opening into the bladder trigone on the affected side.[109]

If the condition is suspected, ultrasonography can outline two separate kidneys, but if an extra kidney is not suspected and is ectopic it may be overlooked during a routine examination.[56] With normal functioning, an IVP demonstrates an accessory kidney.

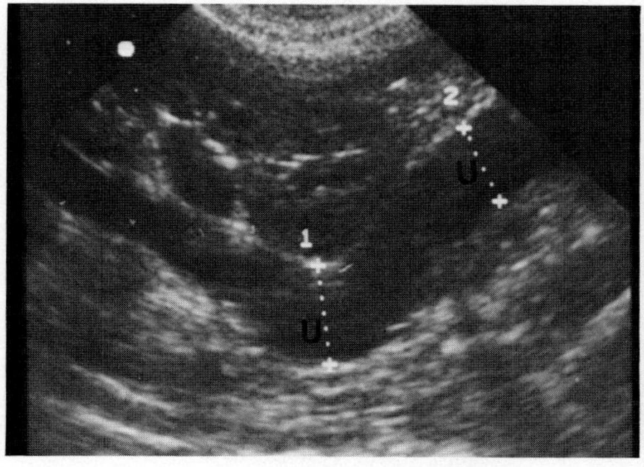

A

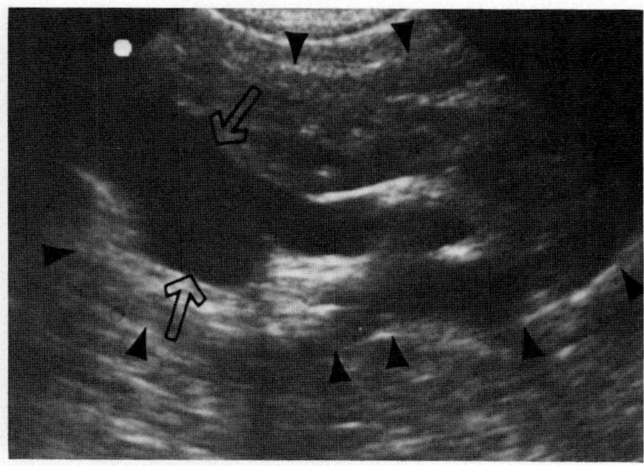

B

FIGURE 9-11. In a 14-year-old girl, a left renal collecting duplication is recognized. (*A*) An upper ureter (U 1) measuring 1.74 and a lower ureter (U 2) measuring 1.42 cm are identified. (*B*) The left kidney is identified with arrowheads and the lower pole collecting system was normal. The upper pole collecting system is dilated *(open arrows)* and demonstrates the sonographic characteristics of hydronephrosis. The patient underwent surgery for partial left nephrectomy. (Courtesy Steven Trawick, Phoenix AZ.)

ANOMALIES OF POSITION, FORM, AND ORIENTATION

Ectopic Kidneys. If early fetal vascular connections persist[109] or if the metanephros develops in an abnormally low position, normal ascension of the kidney may not always occur.[129] These kidneys are normal or slightly smaller in size and lie just above the pelvic brim, or sometimes even within the pelvis (Fig. 9-12).

An intrathoracic kidney is a rare developmental anomaly that results when the kidney continues its craniad ascent. It is thought to be associated with delayed closure of the thoracic cavity. The pleuroperitoneal canal normally closes between the seventh and eighth week of fetal life.[105] With an intrathoracic ectopic kidney, the diaphragm closes below or around the kidney.[109] If kidney infection or obstruction develops, thoracic symptoms may be produced.[109]

In the third type of renal ectopy, both kidneys are located on one side of the body. It is relatively uncommon, and fusion to the contralateral kidney is more common than the unfused type.[99,131] The upper pole of the crossed ectopic kidney is usually fused to the lower pole of the normally rotated ipsilateral kidney, and the ureter of the ectopic kidney crosses the midline to enter the bladder on the opposite side (Fig. 9-13).

With all three types of ectopy, an associated rotational anomaly is common in which the kidney pelvis faces anteriorly.[105,109] Vascular insertion into the aorta and IVC may be displaced, and the longer renal vessels have a more tortuous path, making kidney obstruction and infection more likely.[109] Ipsilateral crossed ectopia and pelvic kidneys are associated with a higher incidence of bacterial infection and calculi because the ureter is kinked or tortuous,[11,109,129] although it enters the bladder trigone in its normal position.[109] Pelvic kidney can be confused with a palpable pelvic mass.[109]

Sonography should be used to seek ectopic kidney or renal vasculature.[65] Bowel gas may make a pelvic kidney more difficult to locate. Associated malrotation of the kidneys may require oblique scanning planes to image renal structures. The crossed fused kidney may mimic a single kidney with a duplicated system or a kidney with a renal mass.[101,104] Two separate sinuses should be demonstrated as well as the absence of the contralateral

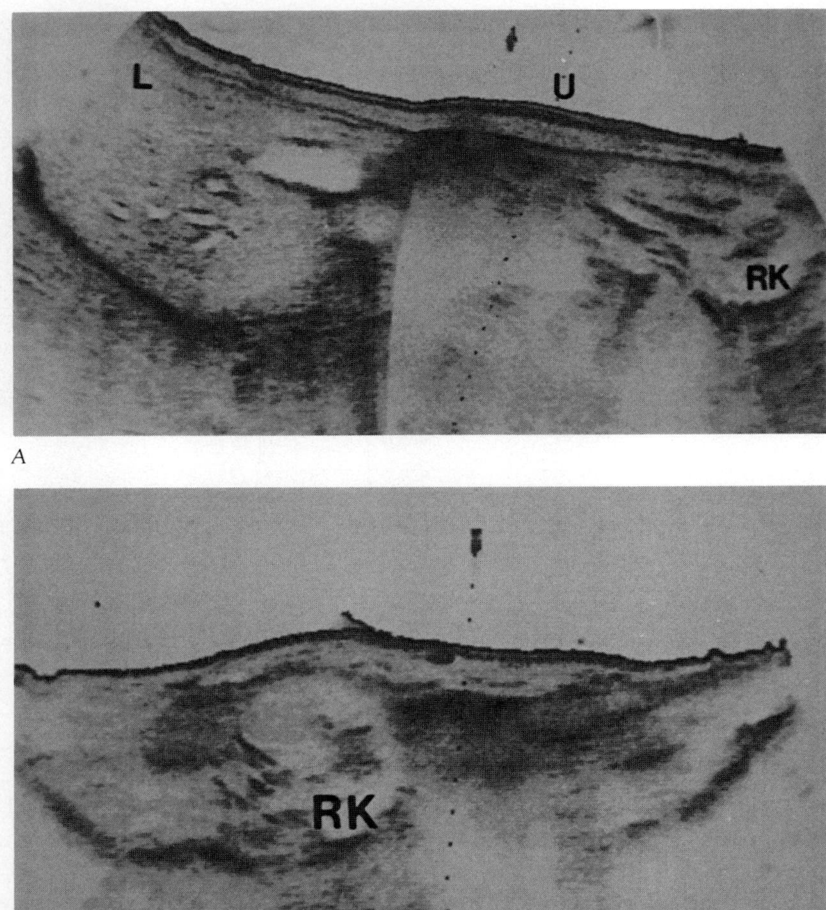

Figure 9-12. On (*A*) sagittal and (*B*) transverse static images, an ectopic right kidney (RK) is identified in the pelvis (L, liver; U, umbilicus). (Courtesy Cathy Carr-Hoefer, Corvallis, OR.)

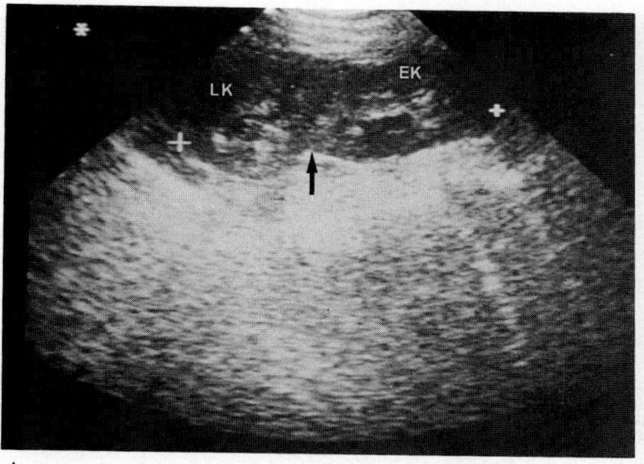

A

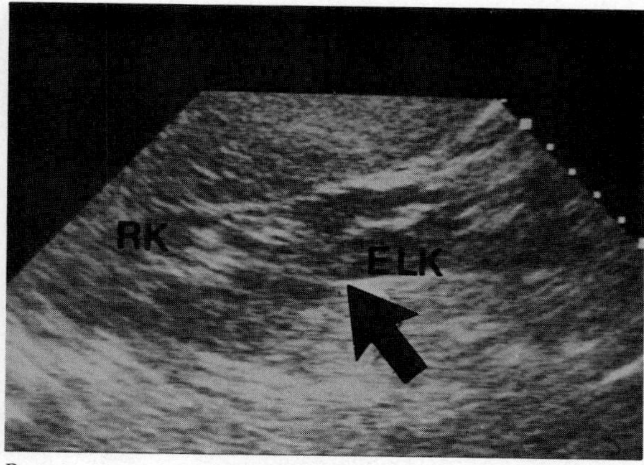

B

FIGURE 9-13. (*A*) The left kidney's (LK) lower pole fusing with the upper pole (*arrow*) of the ectopic right kidney (EK) can be identified on this sagittal section. The crossed-fused renal ectopia measured 23 cm, and two collecting systems are identified. Demonstrating the area of fusion is important to avoid misinterpretation of double collecting system. Scans of the right side failed to demonstrate a normally positioned right kidney. (*B*) The right kidney's (RK) lower pole fuses with the upper pole (*arrow*) of the ectopic left kidney (ELK). Two collecting systems are identified on this sagittal section made on the right side. Scans made on the left side failed to demonstrate a normally positioned left kidney. (Courtesy James Hansen, Ogden, UT.)

kidney.[11] Feces-filled colon or small bowel may occupy the normal renal fossa and mimic a renal mass or a hydronephrotic kidney.[11,99,104,131] Real-time sonography should be able to discern colon peristalsis or a change in configuration over time.[11]

Horseshoe Kidney. Fusion of the upper or lower kidney poles during fetal development produces a horseshoe-shaped structure continuous across the midline and anterior to the great vessels.[109,129] This is a common anomaly (one in 500 to 1000 autopsies).[129] The majority are fused, with an isthmus composed of a simple cord or a fibrous band at the lower pole,[146] although approximately 10% are fused at the upper pole.[109] With lower pole fusion the ureters usually pass anterior to the renal parenchyma. Generally asymptomatic and capable of normal function, horseshoe kidneys can be associated with hydronephrosis, infection, or calculus formation.[65]

Patients with horseshoe kidney are often referred for evaluation of a pulsatile abdominal mass.[104,146] Sonographically, when a mass is identified anterior to the abdominal aorta a horseshoe kidney should be considered, along with an abdominal aortic aneurysm,[65] lymphadenopathy,[56] and pancreatic enlargement.[104] Bowel gas may obstruct visualization.[102] After locating the long axis of the kidneys, follow the lower pole by angling and obliquing the scanning plane to determine if they fuse into the mass.[104] Lower fused poles are usually identified as a solid renal mass at the level of the iliac crest crossing the fourth or fifth lumbar vertebra (Fig. 9-14).[102] Occasionally, a patient has very superficial renal tissue due to an exaggerated anteroposterior kidney axis.[104]

Lobulations. Fetal lobulation can persist into adulthood and give the kidney contour a scalloped appearance that should not be confused with scarring or cystic disease.[109] A common renal variation is a local bulge of the lateral border, called dromedary

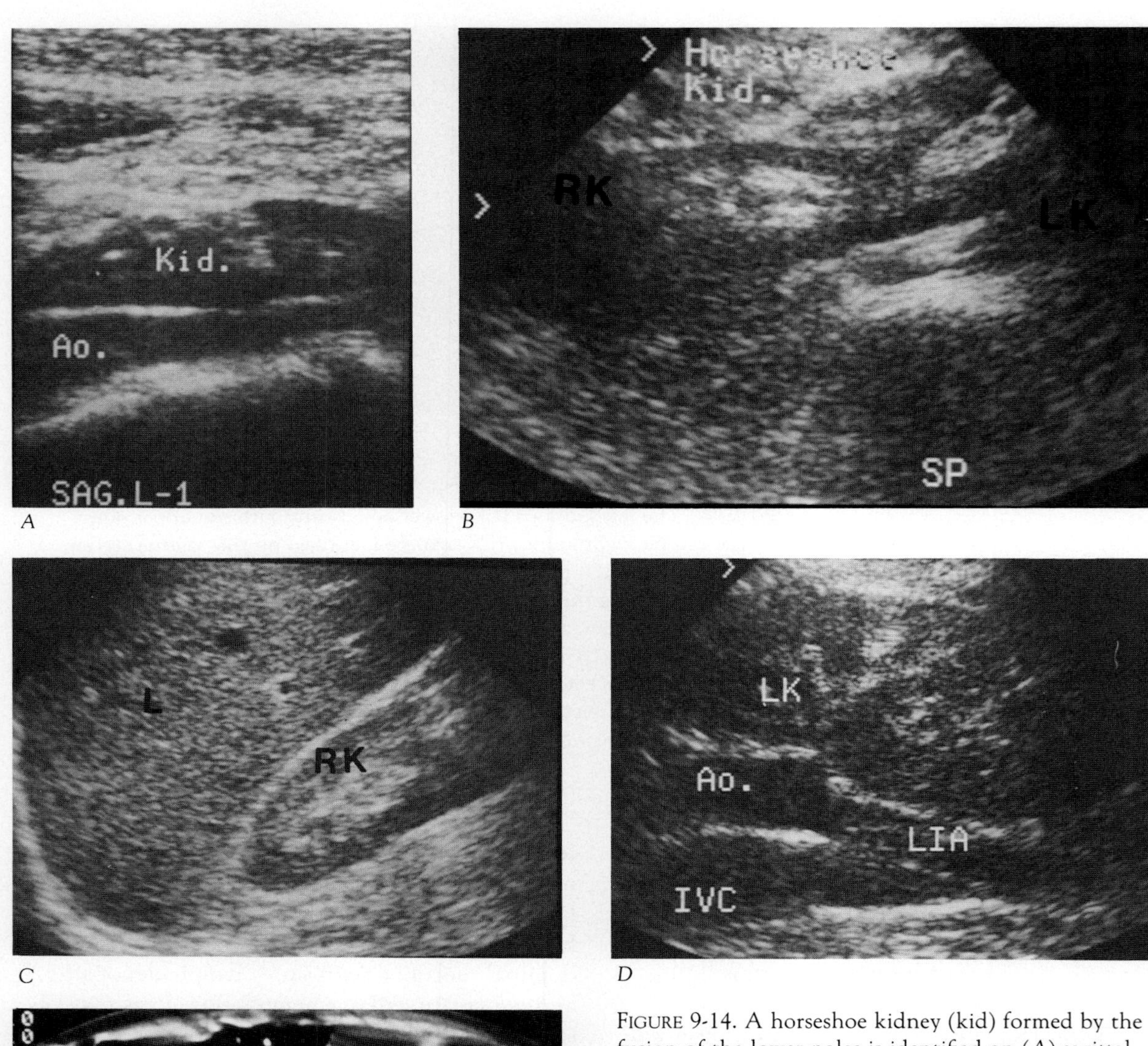

FIGURE 9-14. A horseshoe kidney (kid) formed by the fusion of the lower poles is identified on (*A*) sagittal and (*B*) transverse sections. The fusion of the renal structures is continuous across the midline and lies anterior to the aorta (Ao), inferior vena cava (IVC), and spine (SP). (*C*) Posterior to the liver (L), the right kidney's (RK) inferior pole is visualized angling upward. (*D*) The left kidney (LK) is located closer to the midline (LIA, left iliac artery) (Courtesy Cathy Carr-Hoefer, Corvallis, OR.) (*E*) A transverse CT section demonstrates the appearance of a horseshoe kidney. The fused lower poles (*arrow*) of the right kidney (RK) and left kidney (LK) drape over the prevertebral vessels (A, aorta; IVC, inferior vena cava.)

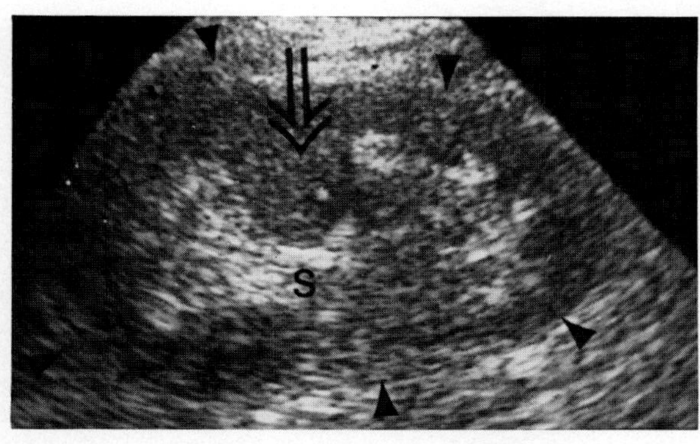

FIGURE 9-15. Sagittal section of the left kidney (arrowheads) demonstrates a small masslike solid tissue area *(open arrow)* projecting into the lateral aspect of the left renal sinus (S). This was thought to be a hypertrophied column of Bertin rather than a pathologic mass, but because of its somewhat bulbous appearance a radionuclide renal scan was recommended. It confirmed that this was functioning renal tissue rather than a neoplasm. (Courtesy Steven Trawick, Phoenix, AZ.)

hump.[34] This can be distinguished from an abnormal mass because it has the same echo texture as the adjacent parenchyma with no identifiable margin. Usually a projection from the renal sinus can be identified pointing toward the dromedary hump.[37]

Renal Column of Bertin. A mass effect may be produced by hypertrophy of the renal column of Bertin. If this is suspected, a coronal sonographic image should be obtained of the renal column. The image should have the following characteristics: (1) it indents the renal sinus laterally; (2) it is clearly defined from the renal sinus; (3) its largest dimension is less than 3 cm; (4) it is continuous or contiguous with the renal cortex; and (5) its echogenicity is close to that of the cortex (Fig. 9-15).[104]

Cystic Diseases

Cystic diseases of the kidney may be hereditary alterations in differentiation, nonhereditary but developmental, or acquired disorders.[129] For convenience and simplicity, they are discussed collectively here. Cystic dysplastic kidneys, multicystic kidneys, and infantile polycystic kidneys (found in newborns and children) are discussed in Chapter 17. As a group, renal cysts are important because they are reasonably common and often present diagnostic problems, some forms are major causes of renal failure, and occasionally they can be confused with malignant tumors.[129]

Renal cysts are nonfunctioning and so are not visualized directly on IVP. Ultrasound is an excellent modality for defining the type of cystic disease because it is an anatomic examination, it is capable of distinguishing cystic from solid lesions, it is particularly suitable for renal imaging and it is portable.[104]

ADULT POLYCYSTIC KIDNEY DISEASE

Adult polycystic kidney disease (APKD) is a relatively common disease (1 in 500) and accounts for 5% to 8% of the patients who require chronic dialysis or renal transplantation.[129] The cause of this form of polycystic disease is unknown, and it is inherited as an autosomal dominant trait.[119,124] The gene penetrance is such that morphologic evidence is seen in almost 100% of patients who survive to 70 and 80 years of age (1 in 1000 population).[109,133,170] Even though victims may remain asymptomatic throughout life,[124] APKD usually becomes clinically manifest in the fourth decade[53] and tends to cause kidney failure at the same age in members of an affected family.[119] With this type of cystic disease, cystic dilatations form in the proximal convoluted tubules, Bowman's capsule, and the collecting tubules. With age, the cysts enlarge and renal function begins to decrease. The most frequent complication is infection and renal calculi,[124] but cyst rupture, hemorrhage, and ureteric obstruction may also occur.[104] The patient presents with abdominal and lumbar pain, hematuria, and hypertension.[124] If calcification is present and is associated with the cysts, it appears thin, ringlike, curvilinear, or as small flecks and amorphous concretions.[104] Death usually occurs about 10 years after onset of symptoms.[124] The most common causes of death are uremia (59%), cerebral hemorrhage (13%), and cardiac disease, usually associated with hypertension.[124] Concurrent with the disease, patients can also have cysts in the liver (25% to 50%), pancreas (9%), lungs, spleen, ovaries, testes,

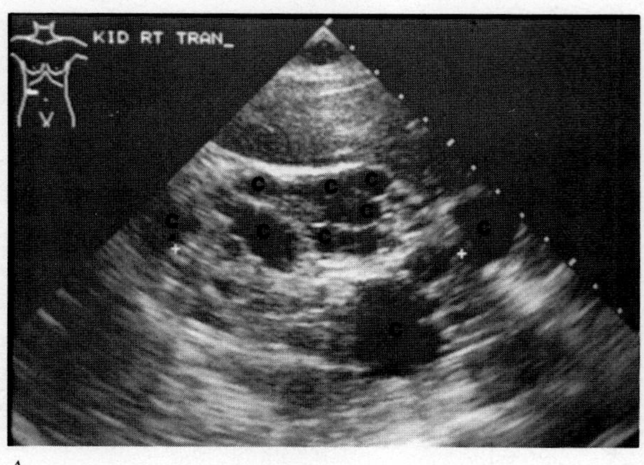

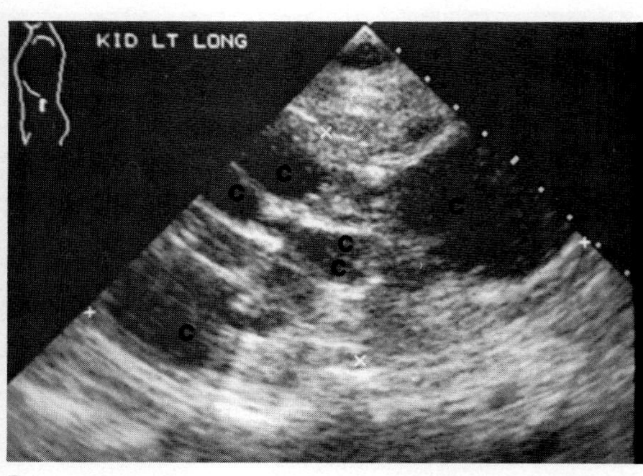

A B

FIGURE 9-16. Adult polycystic kidney disease is identified in both the (*A*) right and (*B*) left kidney. Numerous discrete cysts (c) in the cortical regions, distortion of the central echo complex, and poorly demarcated renal contour are seen.

epididymis, thyroid, uterus, and bladder.[104] Berry aneurysms in the circle of Willis occur in 11% to 20% of patients.[124]

Ultrasonography can safely be used to screen family members to diagnose polycystic disease that is not clinically manifest,[144] to provide genetic counseling prior to procreation, and to learn more about the natural history of the disease.[104] The examintion protocol should include scanning both kidneys and making the routine kidney measurements and measurements of major cysts. Since the disease may manifest cyst formation in other organs, the liver, pancreas, spleen, and ovaries should be imaged.

Sonographically, both kidneys are usually enlarged, with numerous discrete cysts in the cortical regions.[53,104,117] If the many cysts are too small to be resolved individually, innumerable abnormal, small echo complexes representing distorted renal cortex and medulla may be seen dotting the parenchyma.[117] There may be distortion of the central echo complex.[117] A poorly demarcated renal contour is secondary to multiple peripheral cysts causing distortion and a decrease in specular reflections from the renal capsule (Fig. 9-16).[104] Once APKD is identified, the liver, pancreas, and spleen should carefully be scanned for evidence of cystic involvement (Table 9-6).

APKD is usually diagnosed quickly and accurately with ultrasound because the differential diagnosis of bilateral renal masses is limited (Fig. 9-17). On IVP, multiple metastases, multiple hamartoma, and renal lymphoma may resemble polycystic disease; but all of these appear sonographically as solid lesions.[117]

MEDULLARY CYSTIC DISEASE

Medullary Sponge Kidney. The pathogenesis of medullary sponge kidney is unknown. It is a relatively common and usually innocuous structural change restricted to lesions of multiple cystic dilatation of the collecting ducts in the medulla.[124,129] The condition occurs in adults, usually bilaterally,[124] and is normally discovered as an incidental finding or sometimes in relation to secondary complications (calcifications in the dilated cysts, infection, urinary calculi). Renal function is usually normal.

Sonography does not have a defined role in documenting medullary sponge kidney, as the cysts tend to be very small.[35,124]

Uremic Medullary Cystic Disease. Nephronophthisis, or uremic medullary cystic disease, is a progressive familial hereditary disorder that usually has its onset in childhood; there are dominant and recessive modes of transmission.[104] It is characterized by

TABLE 9-6. Congenital cystic diseases of the kidney[35,53,104,109,119,124,125,133,170]

ENTITY	CAUSE	CLINICAL FEATURES	LABORATORY VALUES	SONOGRAPHIC FEATURES
Adult polycystic kidney disease	Autosomal dominant inheritance; multiple cyst formation on both kidneys leads to decreased function	Affects both sexes; onset usually in forth decade; hypertension; abdominal, back and flank pain	Proteinuria (50% of patients), azotemia, hematuria, uremia	Bilateral enlarged kideys contain numerous cysts of various sizes; poorly demarcated renal capsule contour; may distort central echo complex; associated cysts in liver, pancreas, or spleen may be seen
Uremic medullary cystic disease	Dominant and recessive hereditary disorder; multiple medullary and corticomedullary cysts 1 to 5 cm	Onset 3–5 years to early adulthood; renal failure, polyuria, thirst, renal salt wasting	Hyposthenuria, severe anemia, elevated serum alkaline phosphatase	Small cysts confined to the medullary portions of both kidneys; may have widening of central echoes with small cysts; normal-sized or moderately small kidneys; loss of corticomedullary differentiation and increased parenchymal echogenicity

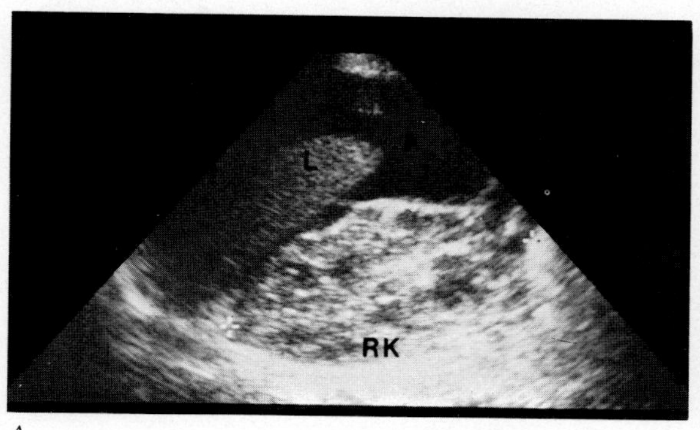

A

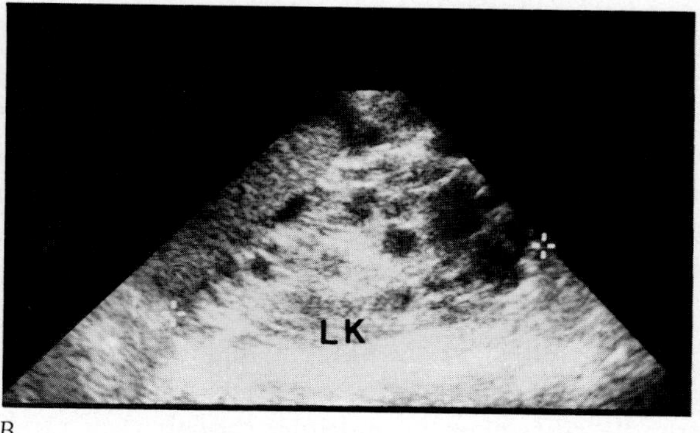

B

FIGURE 9-17. This patient was admitted with known esophageal cancer and was evaluated with ultrasonography for abdominal distension. Ascites (A) was found throughout the abdomen, and numerous discrete cysts were demonstrated in the cortical regions with distortion of the central echo complex consistent with adult polycystic kidney disease. (*A*) The right kidney (RK) measured 12.3 cm long, and (*B*) the left kidney (LK) measured 12.8 cm. (Courtesy Marsha McIntosh, Salt Lake City, UT.)

the presence of variable numbers of cysts in the medulla associated with significant cortical tubular atrophy and interstitial fibrosis. The cortical tubulointerstitial damage is the cause of eventual renal insufficiency and progresses to terminal renal failure over a period of 5 to 10 years.[129]

The most characteristic sonographic findings are multiple small cysts confined to the kidney's medullary portion.[35,104,125] The presence of these cysts, associated loss of corticomedullary differentiation and increased parenchymal echogenicity,[104] with anemia, salt wasting, progressive azotemia, and often polyuria,[53] suggests the diagnosis of juvenile nephronophthisis (see Table 9-6). The diagnosis is assisted by visualizing small kidneys, with a sharply defined cortical surface; polycystic disease presents with cysts of variable size and location and enlarged kidneys with irregular cortical outlines.[35,104,125] Furthermore, the capacity of ultrasound to identify cysts in the medullary region is limited. IVP visualizes cysts that communicate with the pelvicalyceal systems and includes pyogenic cysts, abscesses, diverticula, papillary necrosis, and medullary sponge kidney.[104] Simple cyst, parapelvic cyst (usually only one), and medullary cystic disease do not communicate with the pelvicalyceal systems.[104]

SIMPLE CYST

Of unknown origin, the most often encountered type of renal cyst is a simple serous fluid collection originating in the renal cortex.[124] Uncommon before age 40 years, the prevalence of cysts increases markedly thereafter and is approximately 50% for persons older than 55 years.[31,104,124] Presumably, so as not to confuse these with polycystic disease, they are referred to in the singular (simple or solitary renal cyst). Single cysts are more common,[53] but simple cysts may be multiple, though they rarely number more than four per kidney.[117] They have an epithelial lining and vary in size from 1 mm to giant cysts containing 5000 ml of clear amber fluid.[31,117] Simple cysts are usually unilocular but many contain some septation or loculation.[117] These cysts can be located anywhere in the kidney, including the adjacent tissues of the renal pelvis (peripelvic cyst) and the small collecting system subdivisions (Fig. 9-18).[31] Unless they obstruct portions of the collecting system, they remain asymptomatic and are most often discovered as an incidental finding.[31] Simple cysts rarely cause other symptoms, although hypertension has been attributed to these lesion.[31]

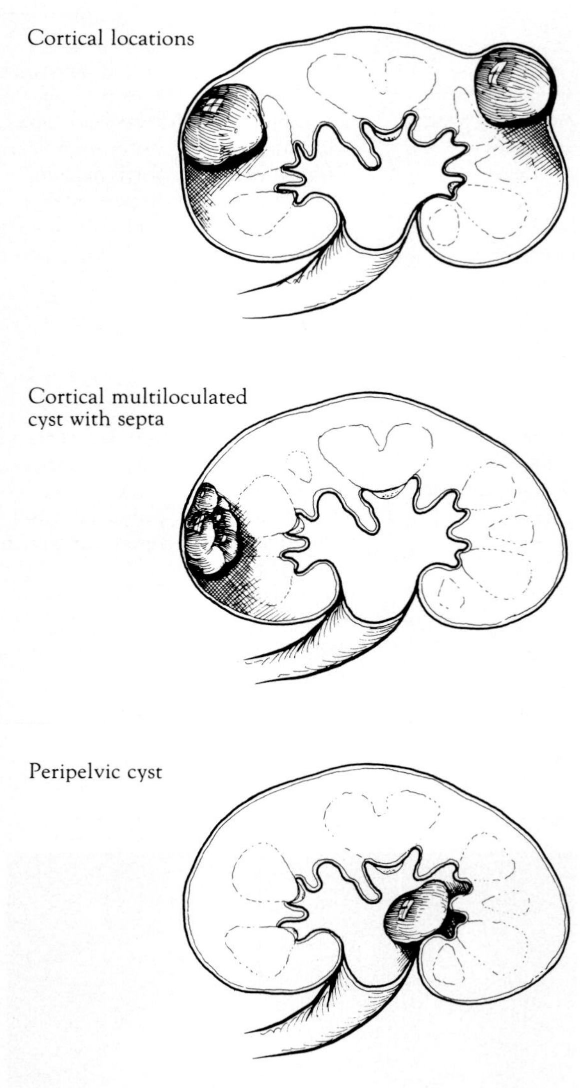

FIGURE 9-18. Common locations of renal simple cysts.

For sonographic differential diagnosis, these lesions must meet classic cyst criteria: (1) clear, smooth wall demarcation, especially a sharply defined far wall; (2) spheric or slightly ovoid shape; (3) absence of internal echoes; and (4) acoustic en-

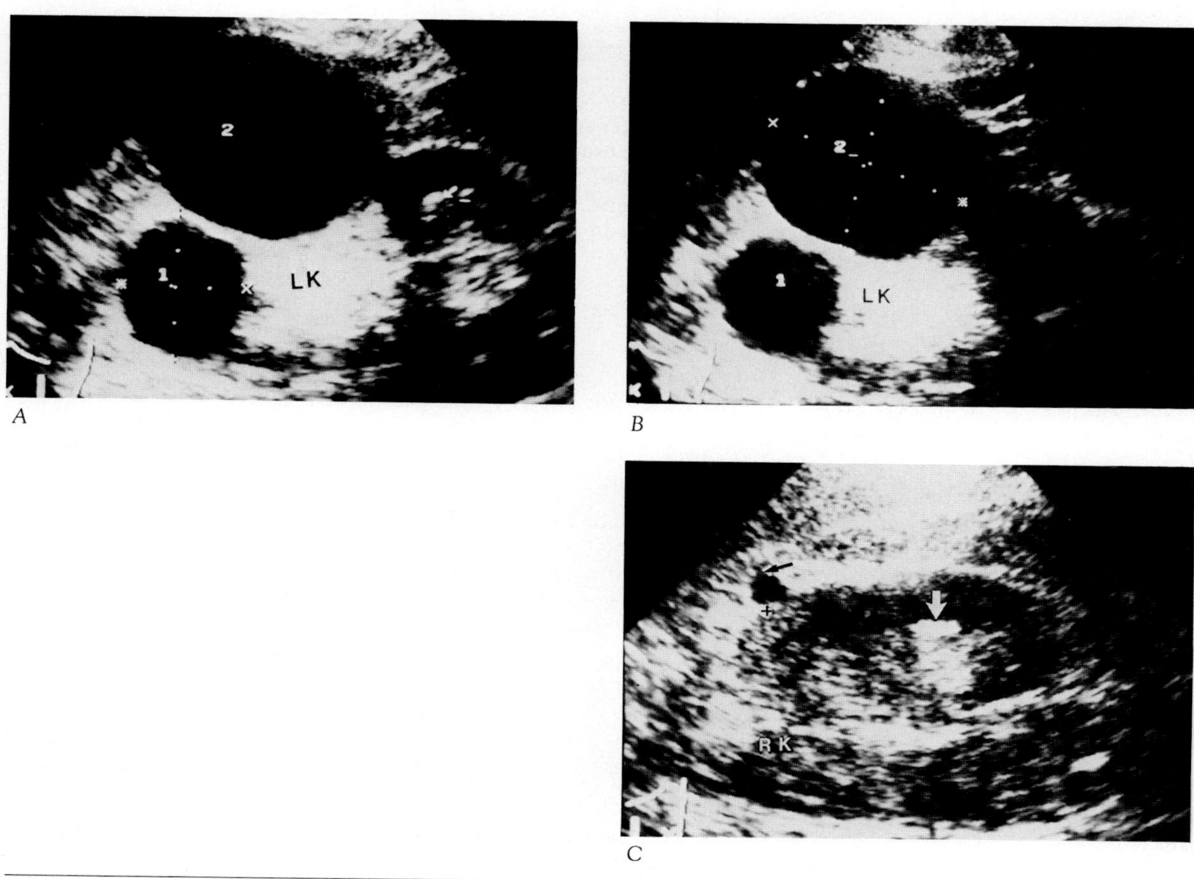

FIGURE 9-19. Incidental to a gallbladder examination, two large simple cysts were found involving the upper pole of the left kidney (LK) and one simple cortical cyst was found in the right kidney (RK). Renal calculi were also identified *(arrows)*. In the sagittal plane of the left kidney, the first cyst (1) measured 3.3 × 4 cm and the second cyst (2) measured 5.7 × 5.8 cm. In the sagittal plane of the right kidney, the cortical cyst measured 1.0 cm. (Courtesy Tally Call, Logan, UT.)

hancement beyond the cyst compared to the intensity of echoes of normal adjacent renal parenchyma (Fig. 9-19).[19,56,104,117] An additional finding just beyond the outer margin of the cyst at the acoustic enhancement borders is a narrow band of acoustic edge shadowing secondary to refraction and deflection of the echoes around the curved surface of a cystic mass (Table 9-7, Fig. 9-20).[31,36,157]

If all cyst criteria are followed, a firm and accurate diagnosis of a simple renal cyst is 95% to 98% accurate; another 2% are due to hematomas, localized hydronephrosis, or septa in cysts.[104,117,124] The causes of incorrect diagnosis include lesions smaller than 2 cm, other left upper pole masses, diffusely infiltrating urothelial tumors, echogenic fatty lesions or acute abscesses, and hematomas.[104] Sonography cannot determine whether the cyst is benign or malignant. Most are benign, but if mural growth is seen on follow-up examination, the cyst could be malignant. Accuracy approaches 100% when the ultrasound examination is combined with cyst aspiration for cytologic and biochemical studies of

TABLE 9-7. Developmental and acquired renal cystic masses[19,31,36,53,56,104,157]

Mass	Cause	Clinical Signs	Laboratory Values	Sonographic Features
Simple cyst	Unknown	Discovered in 50% of patients after age 55 years; usually asymptomatic and discovered incidentally; rarely produces hypertension	Negative	Anechoic, clear, smooth wall demarcation, spheric or slightly ovoid, through-transmission; may be narrow band of acoustic shadowing edge artifact; single or multiple, but usually not more than four per kidney; usually 1–5 cm unilocular, but may contain septation or loculation
Hemorrhagic cyst	Benign cysts can be transformed	Asymptomatic to abdomen, back, and flank pain	Hematuria	Anechoic to complex masses, with or without acoustic enhancement, with smooth to irregular walls
Septate or multiloculated cyst	Unknown, septation has no pathologic significance	Asymptomatic to abdomen, back, and flank pain	Negative	Anechoic with one or more groups of linear, internal, thin echoes; wall infolding or sacculations can also produce irregularity
Infected or inflammatory cyst	Unknown	If symptomatic, pain and fever	Leukocytosis	Anechoic mass meeting cyst criteria to complex mass, with or without particulate debris, smooth, thin to thick, irregular, ill-defined margins
Calcified cyst	Can be acquired in benign cysts; many were hemorrhagic or infected previously	Asymptomatic to abdomen, back, and flank pain	Negative	Hyperechoic cyst wall with decreased sound transmission due to mural calcification; calcification may reflect enough sound, suggesting the mass is solid; second scanning plane a calcium-free, anechoic portion
Milk of calcium cyst	Formation is believed to be associated with low-grade inflammation and partial or complete obstruction in a calyceal diverticulum	Asymptomatic, incidental finding	Negative	Within calyx, an anechoic area with hyperechoic foci with acoustic shadowing; foci may show movement with changing patient position
Parapelvic cyst	Unknown, follows extravasation into renal sinus	Asymptomatic, may be associated with hypertension or hydronephrosis	Hematuria, leukocytosis	Anechoic, well-defined, sharp borders with through-transmission; solitary, multiple, or multilocular interconnecting network of cysts along the calyceal infundibulum or around the renal pelvis

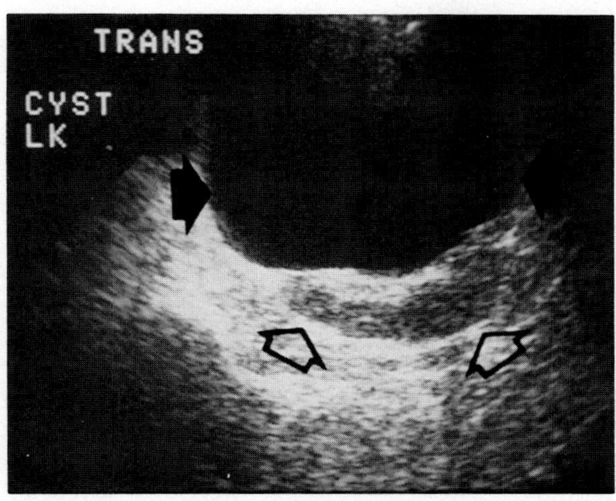

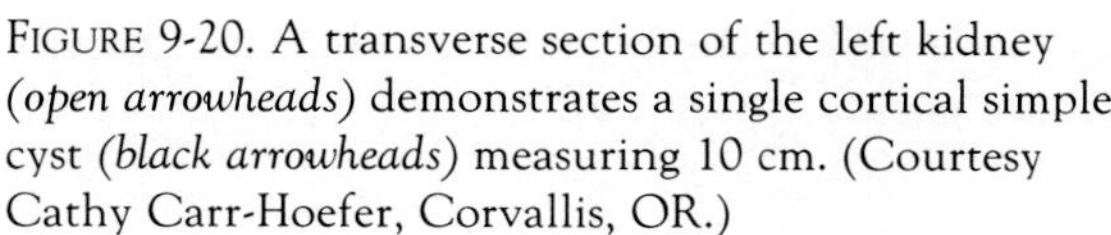

FIGURE 9-20. A transverse section of the left kidney *(open arrowheads)* demonstrates a single cortical simple cyst *(black arrowheads)* measuring 10 cm. (Courtesy Cathy Carr-Hoefer, Corvallis, OR.)

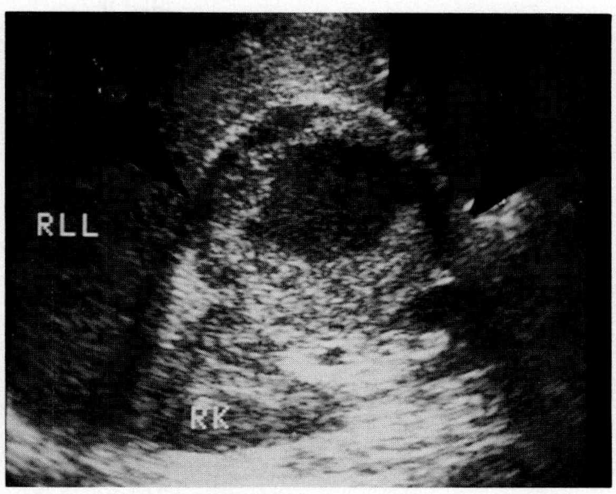

FIGURE 9-21. A complex mass representing a hemorrhagic cortical cyst *(arrowheads)* is identified on this sagittal section of the right kidney (RK). The patient presented with right upper quadrant pain and hematuria but without hypertension (RLL, right liver lobe). (Courtesy Cathy Carr-Hoefer, Corvallis, OR.)

the aspirate; double-contrast cystography is recommended.[117]

HEMORRHAGIC CYST

Approximately 6% of simple renal cysts hemorrhage,[31,56,117] and the prevalence increases in polycystic kidney disease.[104] The reported incidence of neoplasm in these lesions approaches 31%.[49] Depending on the age of the bleed, clot, and resorption, hemorrhagic cysts sonographically vary from anechoic to complex masses with or without acoustic enhancement (Table 9-7, Fig. 9-21).[31,49,104,117] Not always meeting classical criteria for a cyst on ultrasound, these lesions should be investigated by aspiration or computed tomography (CT).[104] On CT, the presence of blood in any form increases attenuation and hemorrhagic cysts appear hyperdense.[104,117]

SEPTATE OR MULTILOCULATED CYST

The interior of a renal cyst is usually a single smooth cavity, although some cysts are trabeculated or divided by fibrous septa into two or more compartments.[31,117] Usually there is free communication between loculi, as the septa are usually incomplete.[31,117] Septation has no pathologic significance[117] unless papillary projections are demonstrated.

Sonographically, septa appear as groups of linear, internal echoes and should be evaluated to make sure they are thin.[31,104] If the transducer is not perpendicular to the septum, the septal echoes may not appear linear and may suggest a solid mass within the cyst wall.[31] Minimal cyst wall infoldings or small sacculations can also produce irregularity of the wall image.[31] In such cases, cyst puncture becomes a vital diagnostic tool (see Table 9-7, Fig. 9-22).[31,117]

INFECTED OR INFLAMMATORY CYST

Like hemorrhagic cysts, simple renal cysts can become infected. Their walls become thicker and they usually contain cloudy fluid rather than the purulent contents of abscesses.[117]

If the cyst content is sonographically clear and free of debris, it meets the classic ultrasound criteria for a cyst,[117] but a complex echo pattern is seen

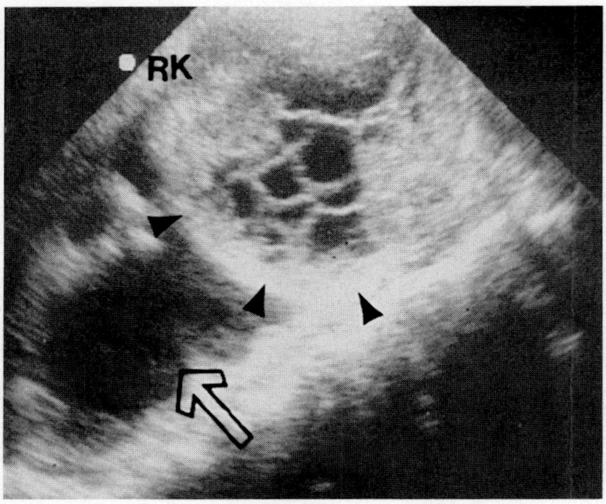

Figure 9-22. A 64-year-old man presented with acute abdomen and back pain. A complex, multiloculated mass *(arrowheads)* containing septa measuring 9.7 × 9.8 cm is identified in the lower pole of the right kidney (RK). Hydronephrosis *(open arrow)* is also seen. Septation may be seen within a simple cyst as a linear echo density and should be evaluated to make sure it is thin. The differential diagnosis for this mass included an infected cyst and a neoplasm such as renal cell carcinoma. (Courtesy Lisa Schneiter, Ogden, UT.)

when particulate material floats in the fluid.[117] This debris often shifts when the patient changes position.[117] Necrotic exudate adherent to the cyst wall can sometimes be identified as discrete, hyperechoic, thickened mural masses[31,117] with ill-defined borders (see Table 9-7, Fig. 9-23).[56]

Calcified Cyst

Mural calcification occurs in approximately 1 to 2% of all simple renal cysts,[117] many of which were hemorrhagic or infected at one time. Sonographically, the layered, eggshell-thin cyst wall is hyperechoic, decreasing sound transmission and making an accurate diagnosis difficult.[31] In certain areas, a densely calcified cyst can reflect enough sound to suggest, falsely, that it is solid. In these cases, it is important to obtain images from two scanning planes, as the cyst pattern can be identified in the calcium-free portions.[117] Since mural calcifications are also associated with malignancy, correlation with other imaging procedures and chemical analysis of the aspirate may be necessary to make a diagnosis (see Table 9-7).

Milk of Calcium Cyst

Milk of calcium cysts are actually calyceal diverticula, which may or may not have lost their communications with the calyceal system.[31] In most cases, the formation of milk of calcium occurs in a calyceal diverticulum with low-grade inflammation and partial or complete obstruction to urine flow with stasis.[104] The milk of calcium represents primarily small calcium carbonate crystals, which normally are asymptomatic and are found only incidentally.[31,56] Sonographically, there is a layering, linear band of hyperechoic echoes associated with an acoustic shadow representing the crystals that may move within the cystic mass when the patient changes positions (see Table 9-7).[31,56]

Parapelvic Cyst

Parapelvic cysts are located in the renal hilus and have no communication with the collecting system.[104] Their cause is not known, but they have been known to develop following urine extravasation into the renal sinus.[117] Strictly speaking, parapelvic cysts develop from lymphatic or other non-

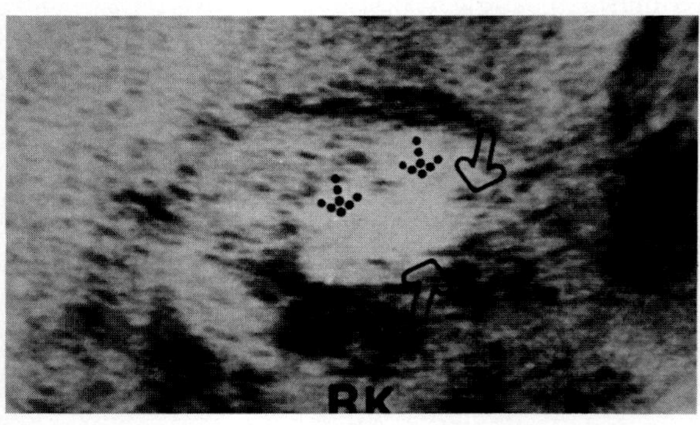

Figure 9-23. Both septa *(open arrows)* and a multiloculated *(dotted arrows)* complex mass are seen on this sagittal section of the right kidney (RK). The differential diagnosis favored an infected cyst, since the contents shifted with changes in the patient's position.

parenchymal tissues.[60,117] In practice, however, the term is frequently applied incorrectly to describe renal cysts that originate near the hilus and extend anterior or posterior to the renal pelvis.[117] Patients are usually asymptomatic but may have hypertension, hematuria, or hydronephrosis.[60,104] The cysts may become secondarily infected.[60,104]

Sonographically, its hilar location should differentiate a pararenal cyst from a perirenal cyst. They can be solitary, multiple, or a multilocular interconnecting network of small cysts appearing in the characteristic location in the normally compact central echo complex.[117] Distributed along the calyceal infundibula or around the renal pelvis, they usually are not mistaken for the sonographic manifestations of hydronephrosis but are more often confused with sinus lipomatosis.[60,117] Parapelvic cysts are anechoic, well-defined masses with sharp borders compared to the hypoechoic, ill-defined sinus fat deposits seen with lipomatosis (see Table 9-7, Fig. 9-24).[117]

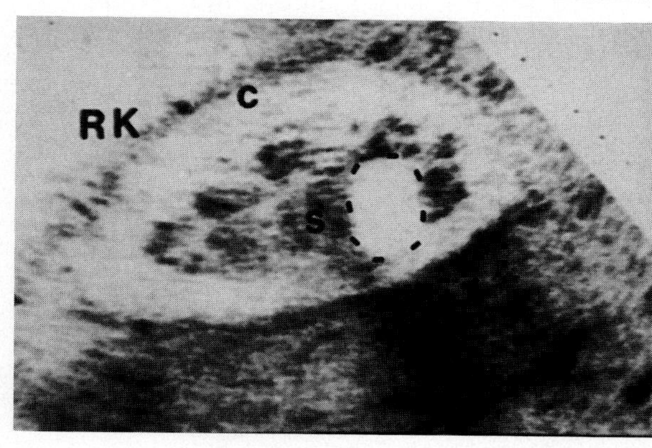

FIGURE 9-24. A sagittal section of the right kidney (RK) demonstrates a pararenal cyst *(dotted line)*. This should not be confused with early dilatation of the renal pelvis (c, renal cortex; s, renal sinus).

ACQUIRED CYSTS

Most acquired cysts of the kidney occur when some process destroys renal tissue, leaving a lesion in the parenchyma that may or may not communicate with the collecting system.[124] This category includes cavitating hematomas, inflammatory cysts (pyogenic and tuberculous abscess, parasitic cysts), necrotic neoplasm, calyceal diverticula, other unusual lesions,[124] and uremic renal cystic diseases in patients receiving dialysis.[52] There is no specific sonographic presentation of these acquired cysts, although location within the kidney, configuration of the lesion, and clinical history allow for more limited differential diagnosis.[124]

Cystic lesions arising outside renal tissue, such as pancreatic pseudocysts, necrotic metastatic neoplasm, posttraumatic urinomas, renal artery aneurysms, and other less common lesions may occasionally be noted within the kidney on ultrasound examination.[124]

Obstructive Uropathy

Obstructive disorders can occur at any age and cause impairment of urine flow by involving any urinary tract structure from the renal tubules to the urinary meatus. In 90% of cases, the obstruction is located below the level of the glomeruli.[119] As the severity and duration of obstruction increases, the kidneys become more susceptible to infection, calculus development, and permanent damage. When urine flow is obstructed, urine filtration continues, the calyces become distended, the renal pelvis dilates, and its pressure is elevated. Transmitted back to the collecting ducts, the elevated pressure causes blood vessel compression.[129] If the obstruction is complete, serious and irreversible kidney damage occurs after about 3 weeks, and if incomplete, after about 3 months.[119]

HYDRONEPHROSIS

Hydronephrosis represents urine dilatation of the renal pelvis, calyceal structures, and infundibula.[112] Table 9-8 presents the intrinsic and extrinsic causes of obstruction leading to dilatation.[119,124] Depending on the cause, symptoms and laboratory values vary.

Ultrasonography is extremely sensitive to the presence of hydronephrotic changes and can be recommended as the initial procedure when obstructive uropathy is a clinical consideration.[35] The sonographic hallmark of hydronephrosis is splaying, spreading, or ballooning of the central echo complex.[117,124] Since this is not ordinarily character-

TABLE 9-8. Sonographic features of hydronephrosis[117,119,124,143]

CAUSE	CLINICAL SIGNS	SONOGRAPHIC FEATURES
Intrinsic: Calculi, hematoma, neoplasm, stricture, ureterocele, sloughed papilla, pyelonephrosis, congenital (aberrant vessels, posterior urethral valves, ureteropelvic junction obstruction, ectopic ureterocele collecting system duplication) Extrinsic: Neoplasm, trauma, neurogenic bladder, surgery (ligation, transection, edema, etc.), bladder outlet obstruction (neoplasm, prostatic hypertrophy, urethral problems), retroperitoneal fibrosis, gynecologic (tuboovarian abscess, endometriosis, etc.), pregnancy, inflammatory lesions (pelvic, GI, retroperitoneal)	Asymptomatic if unilateral, mild or moderate, or associated with other entities (pregnancy); abdomen, back, and flank pain	Distortion of pelvocalyceal structure with dilated fluid-filled calyces, infundibula, and pelvis, causing splaying of central echo complex; depending on point of obstruction, may be unilateral or bilateral. With moderate hydronephrosis: (1) continuous broad anechoic band with distension of intrarenal pelvis; (2) oval anechoic collections along the periphery of central echo complex when calyceal enlargement is greater than renal pelvis enlargement; or (3) mixed pattern with pelvis and calyces enlarged. With chronic hydronephrosis: (1) single, blown-out, ellipsoid, anechoic collection spreading central echo complex with loss of individual calyceal structures into markedly distended pelvis; (2) lobulated or large septate anechoic pattern representing markedly distended individual calyces; or (3) anechoic dumbbell configuration due to a ureteropelvic obstruction with marked extrarenal pelvis and intrarenal infundibulum enlargement.

istic of parenchymal renal masses, it is highly suggestive of obstruction in the collecting system (Table 9-8, Figs. 9-25, 9-26).[117]

Hydronephrosis is often found incidentally in asymptomatic patients during routine obstetric ultrasonography. The incidence is greater in the right kidney (90%) than in the left (67%).[42,44,115] The cause of hydronephrosis and reason for the right-sided preponderance remain controversial.[44,104] There is a wide variation in the extent of dilatation with an increasing calyceal diameter as the pregnancy progresses.[44] Bladder filling, parity, and history of urinary tract problems are not related to the degree of dilatation (Fig. 9-27).[104] These findings are most often not considered pathologic.[44]

It is difficult to distinguish mild hydronephrosis from conditions that simulate it:[124] (1) normal variants (distensible collecting system, extrarenal renal pelvis,[144] full bladder, congenital megacalyces, calyceal diverticulum); (2) increased urine flow (overhydration, medications, osmotic diuresis during or immediately after urography, diabetes insipidus, diuresis in nonoliguric azotemia); (3) inflammatory disease (acute pyelonephritis, chronic pyelonephritis);[35] (4) renal cystic disease (single cyst, parapelvic cysts, adult polycystic kidney disease, medullary cystic disease, multicystic-dysplastic kidney);[35] and (5) other causes such as postobstructive or postsurgical dilatation, vesicoureteral reflux, papillary necrosis, and renal sinus lipomatosis.[104,124] It is important to remember that hydronephrosis causes spreading of the calyceal echoes and that some entities that simulate hydronephrosis (cystic disease) compress the central sinus echoes.[35] With hydronephrosis, evaluating the remaining kidney cortex is important, as it indicates how much functioning tissue remains. Identifying a dilated ureter in continuity with an upper pole cystic mass is extremely helpful in diagnosis.[35,117]

UROLITHIASIS

Calculi can develop anywhere in the urinary system, but most develop in the kidney. Urolithiasis

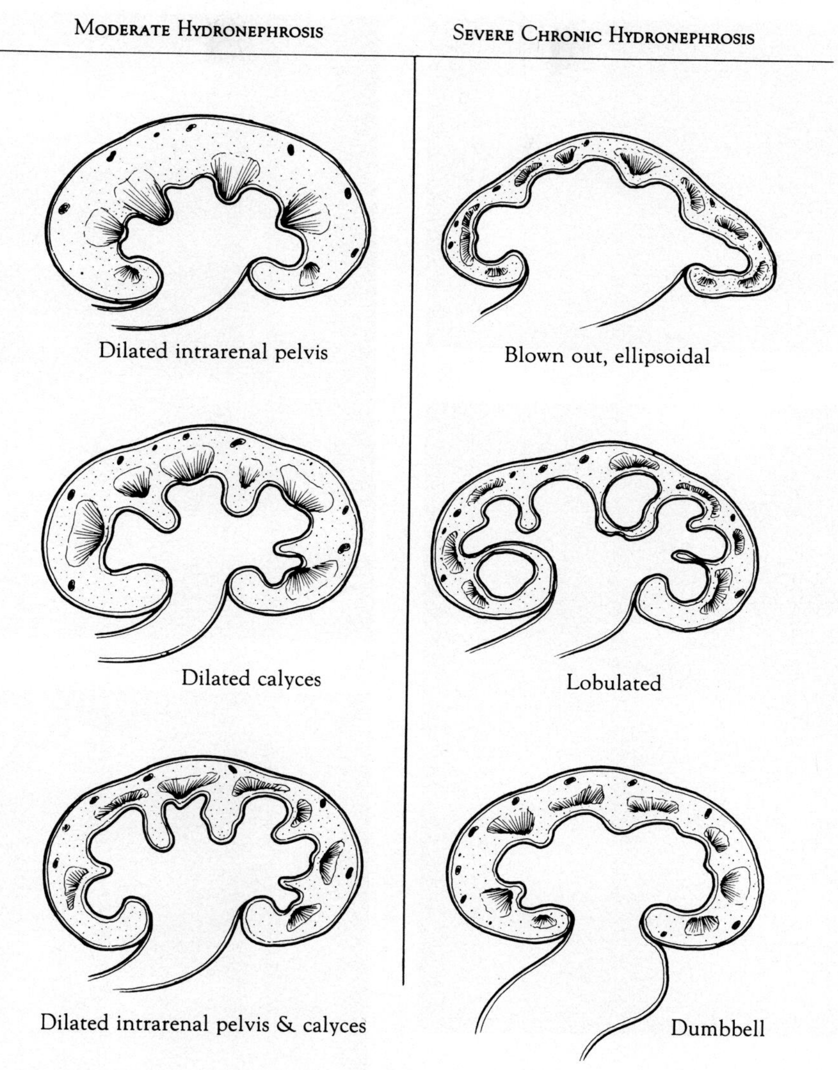

FIGURE 9-25. Schematic illustration of the sonographic patterns of moderate hydronephrosis and severe chronic hydronephrosis.

is calculi in the urinary tract and nephrolithiasis is calculi in the kidney. The prevalence of nephrolithiasis is 0.1% to 6%. It is more common in males than females, and in patients between 30 and 55 years of age, and is the third most common urinary disorder in hospitalized patients.[104,109,119] Because of the increased incidence of urolithiasis, the southeastern part of the United States is referred to as a geographic "stone belt." Hot climates favor stone formation. The prevalence is higher among people new to these areas, owing to unsuspected water loss leading to concentrated urine and increased precipitation of dissolved salts.[109]

A clearly defined cause for urinary calculi has not yet been established. What is known is that their development requires the presence of a nidus

(text continues on page 312)

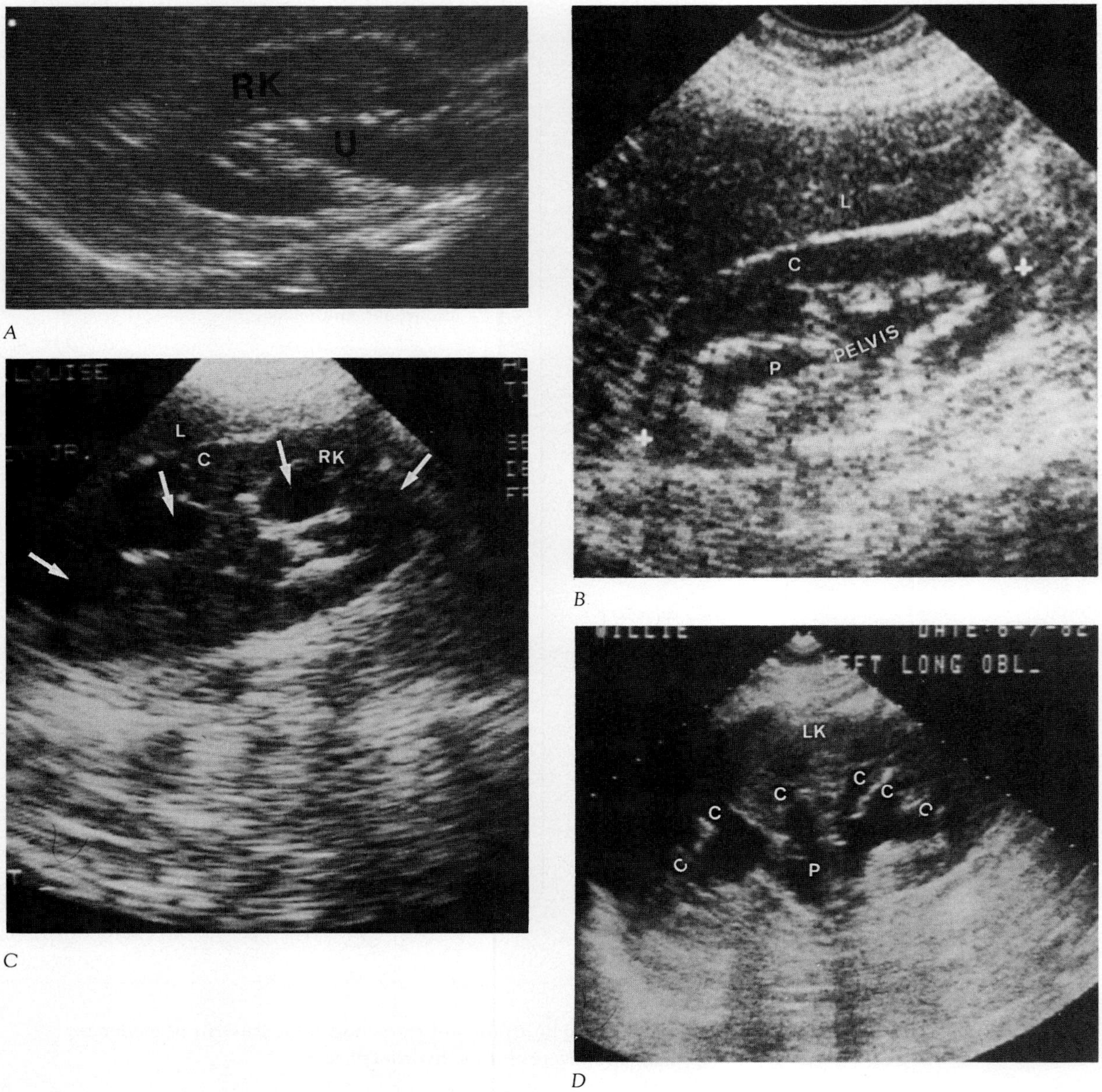

A

B

C

D

FIGURE 9-26. (*A*) Transverse section of the right kidney (RK) with moderate hydronephrosis. The intrarenal pelvis is dilated and the ureter (U) exiting the renal pelvis can be identified. (Courtesy Jullee Ballingham, Ogden, UT.) (*B*) Moderate hydronephrosis presents with a continuous broad anechoic band and a dilated intrarenal pelvis. It is diagnosed by observing the spreading of the central echo complex, as seen in this right renal sonogram (C, cortex; P, medullary pyramid; L, liver). (C) On a sagittal image of the right kidney (RK), moderate hydronephrosis presents an oval anechoic pattern along the periphery of the central echo complex.

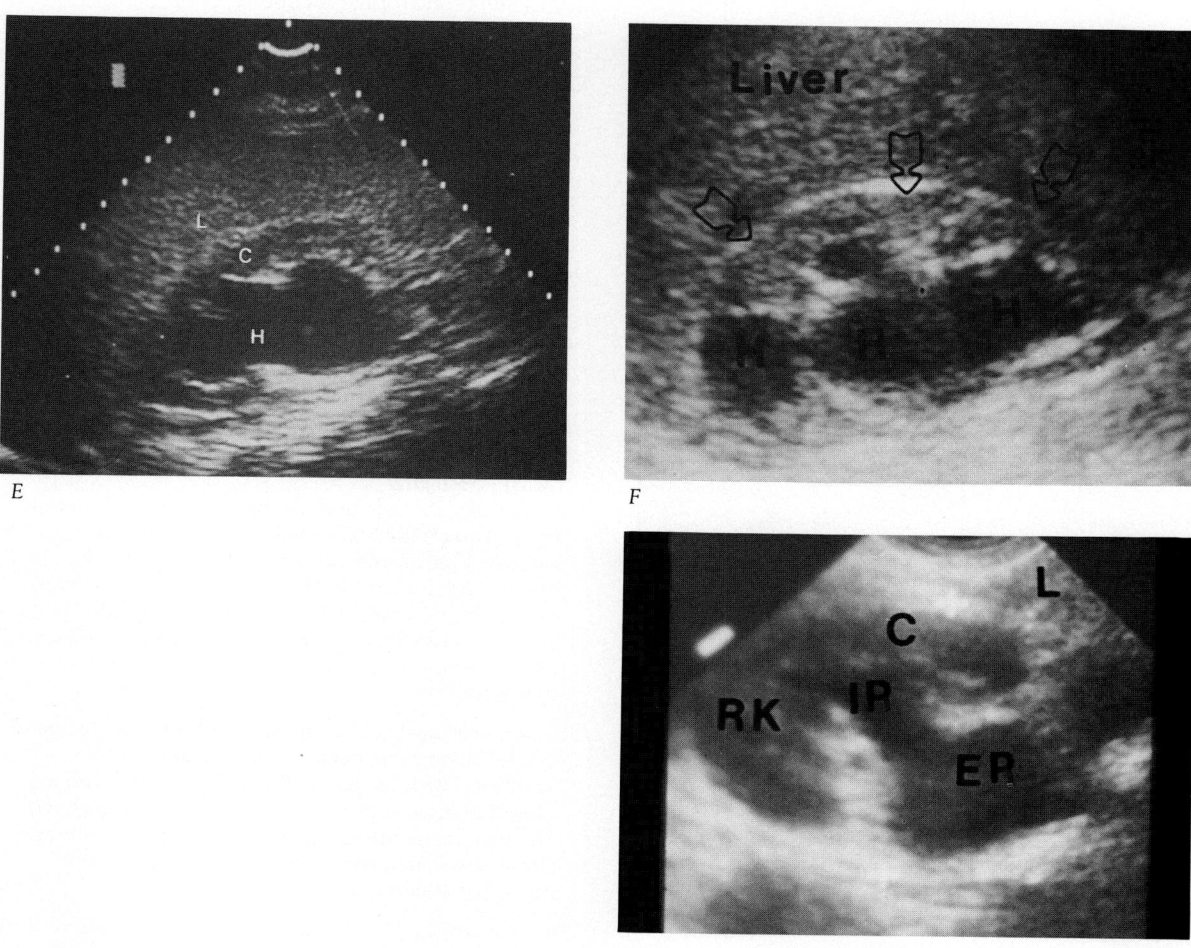

FIGURE 9-26 *(continued)*. Calyceal enlargement *(arrows)* is greater than renal pelvis enlargement. Dilated calyces can simulate cystic lesions (C, cortex; L, liver). *(D)* A sagittal section of the left kidney (LK) demonstrates moderate hydronephrosis presenting as a mixed pattern with dilated intrarenal pelvis (P) and calyces (C). *(E)* Chronic hydronephrosis (H) is demonstrated by severe dilatation of the renal pelvis in a single, blown-out ellipsoidal pattern with spreading of the central echo complex and a loss of individual calyceal structures due to blunting. There is thinning of the right renal cortex (C; L, liver). *(F)* Severe chronic hydronephrosis of the right kidney *(open arrows)* was diagnosed in a 63-year-old woman who had urinary incontinence and a history of colon cancer metastasizing to the liver. A lobulated and large septate anechoic pattern representing markedly distended individual calyces (H) can be identified. (G) In a patient with severe, chronic hydronephrosis, an anechoic dumbbell configuration due to an ureteropelvic obstruction causing marked extrarenal (EP) and intrarenal (IP) infundibulum enlargement is visualized on a coronal transverse section of the right kidney (RK; L, liver; C, renal cortex).

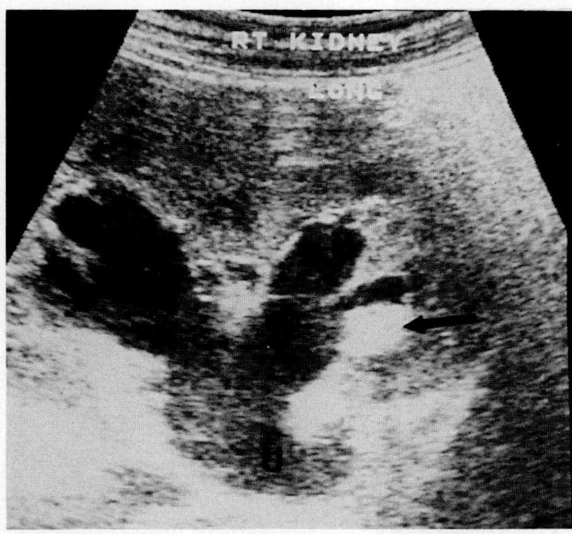

FIGURE 9-27. Moderately severe maternal hydronephrosis and proximal ureteral dilatation is identified in a sagittal section of the right kidney of a 23-year-old, multiparous woman with a 23-week gestation. Another incidental finding during the obstetric ultrasound examination is a bright echo at the junction of the pelvis and ureter *(arrow)* that is not obstructing the ureteropelvic junction. This was diagnosed as renal sinus fat. The left kidney is normal.

for stone formation and an environment that supports the continued precipitation of stone components.[109,119] Calculus formation is influenced by hereditary and familial predisposition, high concentration of stone constituents, changes in urinary pH, or the presence of bacteria, but many calculi form in the absence of these factors.[129] The three major theories of stone formation and the four types of urolithiasis are presented in Table 9-9. Urine cultures, urine analysis, and serum protein, bicarbonate, and uric acid levels help determine the cause of stone formation.

Depending on size and location of the urolithiasis, clinical symptoms can be hematuria (resulting from tissue damage), oliguria (resulting from obstruction), or renal colic (as calculi are passed).[18] Renal colic is painful spasms radiating from the costovertebral angle to the flank and the suprapubic region to the external genitalia. When nephrolithiasis is confined to the renal pelvis and calyces, the pain is more constant and dull. Nausea, vomiting, fever, chills, abdominal distension, and pyuria can also be included in the list of symptoms. Anuria is present only with bilateral obstruction (or unilateral obstruction in a patient with only one kidney).

Within the resolving capabilities of the equipment, and regardless of their chemical composition, ultrasonography images calculi as echogenic structures.[72,104] Unlike cholelithiasis situated in a bile-filled gallbladder, highly reflective nephroli-

TABLE 9-9. Stone formation and types of urolithiasis[6,18,104,109,119]

Theories of Stone Formation

1. Saturation theory: Urine saturated with calcium salts, uric acid, magnesium ammonium phosphate, or cystine
2. Deficiency of stone formation inhibitors theory: Kidney lacks a normal product that inhibits stone formation
3. Matrix theory: Organic materials derived from tubule cells act as a nidus for stone formation (based on observation that organic matrix materials are found in all layers of kidney stones, although it is not known whether matrix material contributes to initiation of formation or material is entrapped in stone as it forms)

Types of Urolithiasis

Calcium oxalate, calcium phosphate, or a combination of the two (80%–90%) usually associated with increased blood and urinary concentrations of calcium predisposed by excessive bone reabsorption caused by immobility, bone disease, renal tubular acidosis, milk-alkali syndrome, hyperparathyoidism, hypervitaminosis D, medullary sponge kidney, hyperoxaluria

Struvite or magnesium ammonium phosphate (recurs in 27% of susceptible persons), most commonly associated with bacterial *(Proteus)* infections and are caused by urea-splitting action of bacteria; staghorn calculus (stone filling the entire renal pelvis) almost always associated with urinary tract infections or persistent alkaline urine

Uric acid stones (8%) caused by high concentration of uric acid (urine pH about 5.5) associated with gout and dehydration

Cysteine formed in acid urine due to an inherited renal tubule defect affecting the absorption of urine amino acids

thiasis situated within the highly reflective central echoes of the collecting system are difficult to discern unless they are large and cast an acoustic shadow.[144] For optimal visualization of an acoustic shadow, varying gain settings must be used, usually lower, and the narrow portion of the focal zone is positioned in the region of the suspected calculus.[104] When a renal calculus is identified by its characteristic dense echo pattern and associated sound attenuation and strong acoustic shadow,[72] observation of associated hydronephrosis can enable the examiner to localize the area of obstruction (Fig. 9-28). Ureteral stones are more difficult to visualize sonographically and will be detected only if the ureter is dilated significantly. Most urolithiasis can be detected on a kidney-ureter-bladder (KUB) radiograph; follow-up with an IVP determines its size and location. Radiography does not demonstrate early calculus formation or uric acid stones.[104]

Since most urolithiases are smaller that 5 mm, the treatment of choice is to facilitate natural passage of the stones. Vigorous hydration and administration of diuretics flushes the kidneys and ureters. Calculi too large to be passed require a more invasive procedure. Cystoscopy, with retrieval instruments, can aid in the removal of stones. Removal of calculi confined to the renal pelvis, parenchyma, or calyces may require a flank or lower abdominal incision. Extracorporeal shock-wave lithotripsy (ESWL) focuses shock waves on localized renal calculi to disintegrate them so they can be passed naturally.[84] Prophylaxis to prevent recurrent calculus formation in predisposed patients includes a low-calcium diet to prevent hypercalciuria, parathyroidectomy for hyperthyroidism, allopurinol for uric acid calculi, and daily doses of ascorbic acid to acidify the urine.

Inflammatory Diseases

Urinary tract inflammatory diseases cover a wide spectrum. Urinary tract infections (UTI) cause significant morbidity; they are second only to respiratory infections in prevalence.[119,129] Bacterial infections may remain asymptomatic or localized to the bladder but carry the potential for spread to the kidneys.[129] The incidence is higher for women: approximately 20% develop at least one UTI during their lifetime.[119] Among all patients receiving dialysis to sustain life, infections are responsible for 13% to 22% of disease.[119]

Escherichia coli and *Enterobacter, Klebsiella, Pseudomonas,* and *Proteus* species are the gram-negative bacilli responsible for 85% of UTI. Any interference with normal voiding, incomplete emptying, stasis, or instrumentation leaves residual urine in the bladder and enhances bacterial multiplication.[87,119,129] The bacteria ascend the urinary tract through the urethra (urogenous ascending route) or along the lymphatics (lymphogenous).[106,109,171] It is believed that lymphogenous spread is facilitated by lymphatic connections between the upper and lower urinary tract along the adjacent mucosa of the collecting system and there may be lymphatic channels between the colon and the right kidney.[87,171]

The incidence of these infections is greatest in women 15 to 24 years of age, suggesting that the shorter female urethra located close to the vagina and rectum and associated hormonal and anatomic changes contribute to the higher incidence. Sexual activity may contribute in predisposed women, but the association with the development of urethritis and cystitis is controversial.[119] The higher incidence during pregnancy is believed to be related to anatomic and physiologic changes and to the fact that estrogen and progesterone play a part in smooth muscle relaxation affecting the normal peristalsis in the ureters.[44] In men, the length of the urethra and the antibacterial properties of prostatic fluid provide some protection from urogenous spread until age 50 years. After this age, prostatic hypertrophy becomes more common, and with it may come obstruction and urinary tract infections.

The second pathway for UTI is hematogenous dissemination. *Staphylococcus aureus* organisms from skin furuncles, skin infections, osteomyelitis, or endocarditis can reach the renal and perirenal tissues from remote sites months after initial exposure by hematogenous dissemination.[109,129] Lymphogenous seeding of *S. aureus* is believed to be responsible for some UTIs.[109]

Once bacteria have gained access to the kidney, the virulence of the infecting organism, host immunity, and other factors determine the extent of UTI involvement.[87] Persons with diabetes and

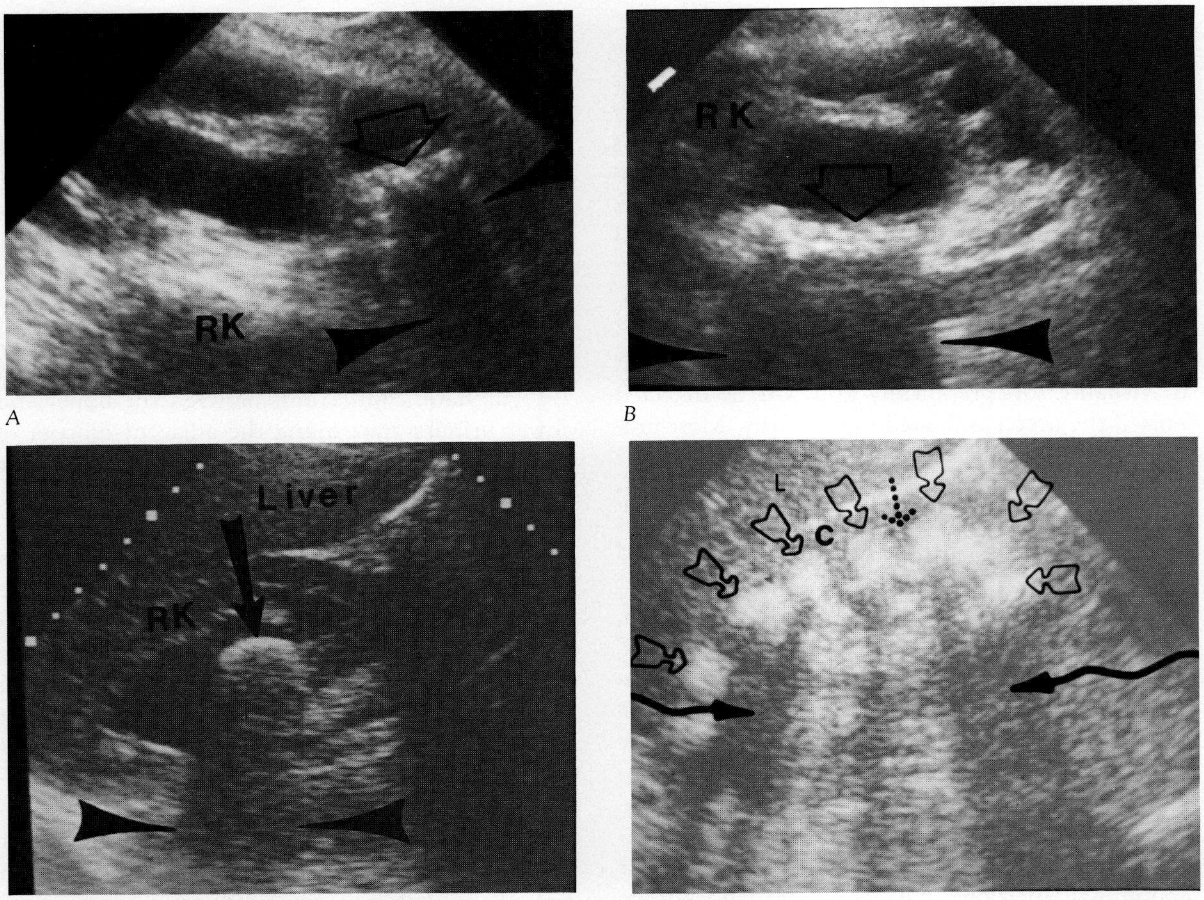

A

B

C

D

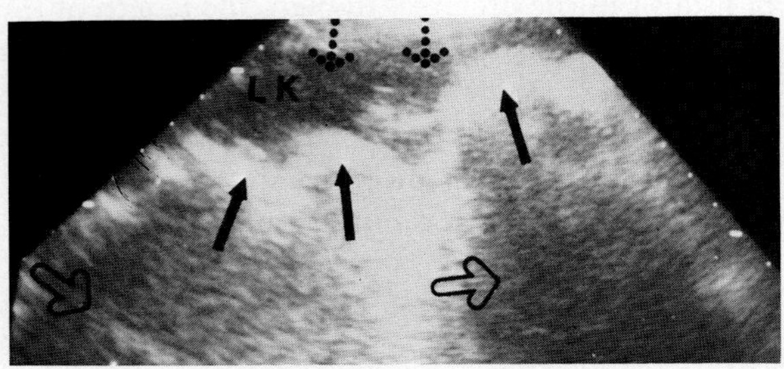

E

Figure 9-28. Dilated infundibulum, calyceal structures, and renal pelvis are visualized on (*A*) sagittal and (*B*) transverse right kidney (RK) sections. Calculi clusters (*open arrows*) are visible in the inferior pole and over the pelvis, collectively casting an acoustic shadow (*arrowheads*). (C) A large calculus (*arrow*) casting an acoustic shadow (*arrowheads*) is identified in the right renal pelvis (RK). (*D*) Calcium oxalate urolithiasis (*open arrows*) casting acoustic shadows (*curved arrows*) is identified in the right renal pyramids of this 33-year-old woman with renal tubular acidosis (*dotted arrow*, column of Bertin; c, renal cortex; L, liver). (Courtesy James Hansen, Ogden, UT.) (*E*) On a sagittal section of the left kidney (LK), the collecting system is calcified (*black arrows*), which confirms a radiographic finding. Normal tissue is identified (*dotted arrows*) along with acoustic shadowing (*open arrows*). (Courtesy Steven Trawick, Phoenix, AZ.)

other states of immune compromise are more likely to develop infections than patients with normal immunity.[87,119]

For 75% of patients with documented acute renal infection findings of excretory urography are normal and an enlarged, poorly functioning kidney is demonstrated only 25% of the time.[87,168,171] Ultrasonography's sectional imaging methods provide an excellent modality for assessing the internal renal architecture.[87,106] Abnormalities can be recognized early in the course of the disease, diffuse renal inflammatory disease is differentiated from focal lesions, and extension into the retroperitoneum is demonstrated.[87,106] Sonography is an important initial screening examination for patients with urosepsis resulting from pyelonephritis, pyonephrosis, or a large renal or perirenal abscess.[77] Urosepsis represents a true urologic emergency and requires urgent drainage.[77] Serial examinations are easily performed to define different phases of the disease when there is inadequate clinical response to antibiotic therapy or suspicion of an underlying lesion that predisposes to infection, such as obstruction by a urinary tract anomaly.[87] Ultrasonography does not depend on renal function or expose the patient to the risk of allergic reactions to contrast media.[19,87] For women of childbearing age, its greatest advantage is the nonionizing radiation.

ACUTE PYELONEPHRITIS (BACTERIAL NEPHRITIS)

Acute pyelonephritis (APN) is an acute suppurative bacterial inflammation of renal tubulointerstitial tissues, unilateral or bilateral, and is associated with UTI.[119,129] In its earliest stages, the histopathologic appearance is diffuse edema producing renal enlargement with intense inflammatory foci, which may lead to microabscess formation throughout the involved renal interstitium.[87,119,129]

The onset is usually abrupt. The usual presenting signs, symptoms, and laboratory values are presented in Table 9-10.[107,154,171] Bladder irritation—symptoms such as dysuria, frequency, and urgency—is usually present.[119] Without other symptoms, pyuria is not diagnostic for APN because it is also present in lower UTIs.

Acute pyelonephritis is most common in women aged 15 to 35 years.[106,107] It is postulated that the most common routes of infection are ascending infection along the lymphatics[171] and urogenous spread facilitated by reflux,[45] obstruction, or congenital renal anomaly.[107] The most common organism is *E. coli.*[129] The widespread use of antibiotics makes hematogenous seeding of *S. aureus* from a remote site a rarer cause.[106] The sonographic appearances of APN is described in terms of the phases of renal infection.

Diffuse Bacterial Nephritis. The phase of APN in diffuse bacterial nephritis demonstrates a sonographically normal-looking kidney or one that appears homogenous and enlarged owing to the inflammatory edema.[104,107] Compared to normal parenchyma and to the unaffected kidney, the increased fluid content decreases the echogenicity[106,107] and gives a stronger back wall.[104] Changes in the renal sinus central echo pattern are sensitive indicators of the severity of the inflammatory process.[87,106,107] As the infection progresses, the central echo complex blends into the homogenous edematous parenchyma and disappears completely (see Table 9-10, Fig. 9-29).[87,104]

Acute Focal Bacterial Nephritis. Also known as acute lobar nephronia, acute focal bacterial nephritis is an inflammatory mass caused by acute focal infection infiltrating into the renal parenchyma without drainable pus.[104,132,152,161] Sonographically, acute focal bacterial nephritis appears as an indistinct, hypoechoic solid mass without definable walls.[87,94,104] This focal mass disrupts normal corticomedullary differentiation and contains scattered low-level echoes.[30,47,68,88,132,152] Through-transmission cannot be demonstrated.[87] Serial examinations on patients undergoing antibiotic therapy may show anechoic areas representing liquefaction. Continued follow-up should demonstrate the resolving mass (see Table 9-10).[104]

Acute Diffuse Bacterial Nephritis. Acute diffuse bacterial nephritis is also referred to as acute suppurative nephritis.[87] Sonographically, the phase of APN involves the entire kidney.[87] The affected kidney appears homogenous and enlarged, producing a patchy disorganized parenchymal pattern.[85,87,161] In the acute stage, the central renal sinus echo blends with abnormal parenchyma.[87,107] Serial examinations on patients undergoing antibiotic therapy should show the central sinus echoes reap-

(text continues on page 318)

TABLE 9-10. Inflammatory diseases of the kidney[22,32,38,47,48,58,68,75,87,88,104,107,117,129,132]

DISEASE	CAUSE	CLINICAL SIGNS	LABORATORY VALUES	SONOGRAPHIC FEATURES
Acute bacterial nephritis	Most often gram-negative bacilli by urogenous or lymphogenous ascent; *S. aureus* by hematogenous or lymphogenous seeding	Chills, fever, headache, back pain, costovertebral tenderness, malaise, dysuria, frequent and urgent urination	Leukocytosis, hematuria Pyuria Bacteriuria	Homogeneous, enlarged kidney, hypoechoic and strong back wall compared to normal renal parenchyma; as infection progresses, central sinus echoes blend into edematous homogeneous parenchyma.
Acute focal bacterial nephritis	As for above acute bacterial nephritis	As for acute bacterial nephritis	As for acute bacterial nephritis	Indistinct, hypoechoic solid mass without definable wall; normal corticomedullary differentiation disrupted with scattered low-level echoes.
Acute diffuse bacterial nephritis (acute lobar nephronia)	As for acute bacterial nephritits	As for acute bacterial nephritis	As for acute bacterial nephritis	An enlarged, homogeneous kidney produces patchy disorganzied parenchymal pattern; central renal sinus echo blends with abnormal parenchyma.
Chronic atrophic pyelonephritis	Recurrent infections superimposed on diffuse or localized obstructive lesions or vesicoureteral reflux resulting in renal scarring and atrophy	As for acute bacterial nephritis	As for acute bacterial nephritis	Small kidney with increased echoes in the involved area of the cortex and medulla from focal fibrosis; focal or multifocal processes with loss of renal parenchyma; with one or more calyces retracted and not distended, an echogenic zone extends beyond normal area of sinus.

Table 9-10 (*continued*).

Disease	Cause	Clinical Signs	Laboratory Values	Sonographic Features
Xanthogranulomatous pyelonephritis	Chronic infection and obstruction of ureteropelvic junction, staghorn calculus, gram-negative (*Proteus*) infection, females and diabetes patients	As for acute bacterial nephritis, plus weight loss, palpable mass	As for acute bacterial nephritis	Enlarged kidney maintains its reniform shape with a smooth contour; staghorn or other central calculus will cast an acoustic shadow; anechoic to hypoechoic, smooth- to irregular-bordered masses corresponding to debris-filled dilated calyces or foci of parenchymal destruction. In diffuse pattern, parenchyma is replaced by multiple, circular masses surrounding the central echo complex; in segmental disease, one or more masses surround a single calyx containing calculus.
Renal abscess	*S. aureus* by hematogenous or lymphogenous seeding; gram-negative bacilli by urogenous or lymphogenous ascent	As for acute bacterial nephritis	Leukocytosis	Anechoic to hypoechoic complex mass with irregular borders; if present, debris provides numerous interfaces; if chronic, can contain internal septa; gas if present, may cause acoustic shadowing or highly reflective with microbubbles.
Perinephric abscess Pyonephrosis	*S. aureus* by hematogenous or lymphogenous seeding, rupture of renal abscess, renal calculi, stricture, congenital anomaly	Acute bacterial nephritis, plus weight loss, chills, fever, unilateral or bilateral impairment of kidney function, urosepsis	Acute bacterial nephritis, leukocytosis	Anechoic to hypoechoic complex mass displacing the kidney; normal size and contour separate from the mass; anechoic (hydronephrosis) to hypoechoic with very fine echoes throughout collecting system; may have a sludge-fluid level that remains in horizontal plane when patient changes position; may present with intense linear echoes, with or without shadow representing air from gas-forming organism.

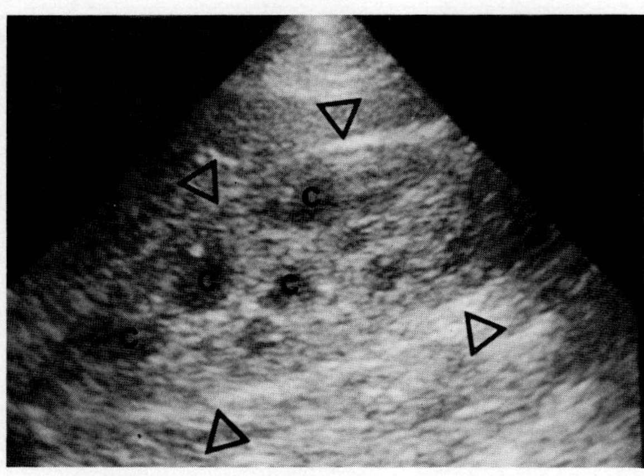

FIGURE 9-29. In a 27-year-old woman with right-sided abdominal pain and fever, a sagittal section demonstrates a homogeneous, hypoechoic right kidney *(arrowheads)* with more prominent renal calyces (c). The patient experienced extreme pain over the right flank during the examination. A normal IVP examination helped exclude the possibility of hydronephrosis. This led to the diagnosis of acute bacterial pyelonephritis. (Courtesy Jo Semon, Salt Lake City, UT.)

pearing to their normal high intensity (see Table 9-10).[87]

CHRONIC ATROPHIC NEPHRITIS

In morphologic terms, chronic pyelonephritis (CPN) is a chronic and progressive renal disorder in which renal scarring, unilateral or bilateral, is associated with pathologic involvement of the calyces and pelvis.[109,119,129] The disorder results from recurrent infections superimposed on diffuse or localized obstructive lesions or vesicoureteral reflux.[18] These recurrent renal inflammatory bouts eventually scar the kidney, and the obstructions contribute to parenchymal atrophy.[129] New evidence suggests that autoimmune mechanisms may contribute to the pathogenesis of CPN.[119] Many of the symptoms of APN are identified, but onset may be insidious. Owing to the loss of tubular function and the ability to concentrate urine, polyuria and nocturia with associated mild proteinuria is common.[18] Severe hypertension contributes to the progress of the disease. Chronic pyelonephritis is a significant cause of renal failure, being responsible for 25% of all cases of renal insufficiency and end-stage renal disease.[119] The sonographic findings of CPN are presented in Table 9-10.

Xanthogranulomatous Pyelonephritis. Xanthogranulomatous pyelonephritis is a rare type of CPN characterized by replacement of normal renal parenchyma with lipid-laden (foamy) macrophages,[48,58,131] plasma cells, and multinucleated giant cells.[87,104,129] The most common predisposing factors are chronic infection and obstruction of the ureteropelvic junction, generally from a staghorn calculus.[104,129,141] It is commonly associated with *Proteus* infections.[129] Females and diabetes patients seem more susceptible.[58,107]

The pathologic spectrum is variable and depends on the chronicity of the disease process.[58,104] The process begins in the calyces and pelvis and subsequently destroys the mucosa and extends into the adjacent medulla and cortex. Distended calyces compromise the medullary perfusion, leading to papillary necrosis.[104,169] Pus-filled, dilated calyces may predominate, or there may be replacement of the kidney with xanthogranulomatous tissue and less purulent components.[58,104]

Generally, patients present with malaise, flank pain, mass, weight loss, and UTI.[58,104] Because the disease is usually bilateral with total renal involvement, the treatment is nephrectomy.[35]

Sonographically, the varying diffuse or segmental patterns of involvement are presented in Table 9-10 (Fig. 9-30).[56,58,87,104,169] In cases of obstructive uropathy, secondary hydronephrosis may be present.[141] The presence of pelvic calculus, obstructive uropathy, marked hydronephrosis with replacement of the normal renal architecture by multiple fluid-filled masses, poor definition of the central echo complex,[48,58] or diminished renal function is instrumental in helping to differentiate xanthogranulomatous pyelonephritis from other focal complex lesions, including neoplasms, other inflammatory processes, and hematomas.[38,117]

RENAL AND PERIRENAL ABSCESS

Abscesses, either acute or chronic, are septic conditions that produce unilateral flank pain, chills, fever, and point tenderness in the costovertebral angle.[109] A renal carbuncle is an abscess in the renal cortex, usually resulting from the union of several small abscesses. Occasionally a carbuncle ruptures into the collecting system or through the capsule and causes a perirenal abscess,[109] a pus collection in the space between the kidney and renal fascia.[35]

In 20% of cases of renal or perirenal abscess it is impossible to isolate the pathogen by urinalysis or culture.[35,104,106,107] In the past, *S. aureus* was the most common agent of renal abscess.[87] Today, gram-negative bacilli are found increasingly to be the cause of renal abscess formation, spread either by the hematogenous or the ascending route,[87] resulting from a ruptured carbuncle, infected renal cysts, CPN, tuberculosis, renal trauma, or obstruction.[107,171] Abscesses most often are confined by the fascia and may extend in several directions presenting as a draining flank abscess or a subphrenic abscess.[35,107,171]

Table 9-10 presents the variable sonographic appearances of renal and perirenal abscesses.[35,87,106,117,146] With a perirenal abscess, as with any perirenal mass, displacement is the striking abnormality.[35,87] A perirenal abscess immobilizes the kidney so that deep inspiration and expiration do not produce the normal excursion of the organ.

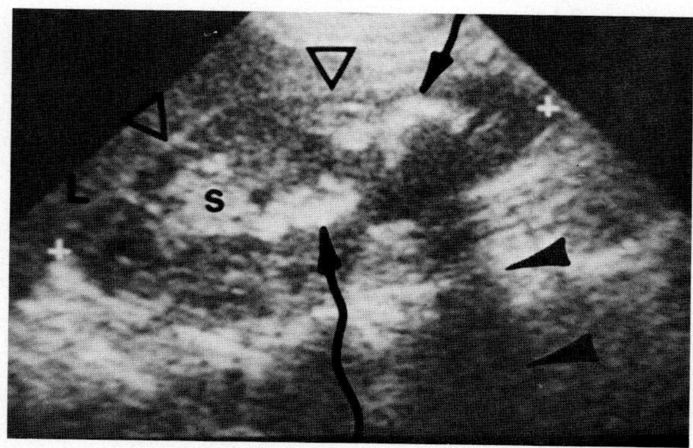

FIGURE 9-30. This 38-year-old woman has right-sided pain, elevated temperature, and may be suffering the early stages of xanthogranulomatous pyelonephritis. This sagittal section of the right kidney was imaged one month after lithotripsy on a staghorn calculus. Multiple calculi persist *(curved arrow)* and cast an acoustic shadow *(black arrowheads)* in an enlarged kidney (15.37 cm long), which maintains its normal shape (*open arrowheads;* L, liver; s, renal sinus). (Courtesy Janet Huber, Worland, WY.)

PYONEPHROSIS

Pyonephrosis (pyohydronephrosis) is the presence of purulent material in a dilated, often obstructed, renal collecting system.[22,76,77,107] The cause and clinical signs are presented in Table 9-10.[107]

When pyonephrosis is suspected, ultrasonography is the imaging procedure of choice following IVP.[22,75,107,172] Minimal to marked hydronephrosis,[106] thickness of the renal cortex, and inflammatory extension outside the kidney can be evaluated.[105] Sonographic findings are variable, owing to the stage and duration of inflammation and the extent of proteolysis of the purulent material.[87,162] The presence of tissue and cellular debris help make the diagnosis by producing low-level echoes in the dilated collecting system.[35,162,173] With tissue and debris, the most common and reliable sonographic finding of pyonephrosis is the presence of a sludge-fluid level in the collecting system that remains in the horizontal plane when the patient's position is changed.[76,106,107,162,172,173] Without the tissue and debris, pyonephrosis may present with very fine echoes throughout the dilated collecting system,[107] or it may occasionally be anechoic and simulate hydronephrosis.[35,87] With a gas-forming organism secondary to infection, air in the collecting system may be detected by the presence of intensely echogenic linear densities.[107] Although these echoes are found in the nondependent portion of the dilated system, they may cast a shadow, simulating calculi (see Table 9-10).[107]

If the pyonephrosis is chronic (several months' symptoms), diffuse xanthogranulomatous pyelonephritis may result.[48,58,107] It is important to distinguish pyonephrosis from other causes of urosepsis, so that immediate percutaneous or surgical drainage can be instituted.[77,107]

Infiltrative Diseases

When evaluating the kidney for medical disease, it is important to correlate abnormal antomic presentation with the patients' clinical history and laboratory values. Renal pathology involves interrelated nephron, vascular, or interstitial tissues as (1) nephron changes result from vascular disease; (2) vascular disease causes nephron and interstitial tissue changes; and (3) interstitial tissue changes inevitably accompany and follow vascular and nephron disease.[67] Over the long term, a seriously injured kidney shows atrophy and scarring and loses the distinguishing features of the specific original disease, regardless of whether it was glomerular, tubular, interstitial, or vascular.[67] In end-stage kidney disease, the primary renal disease often is not identifiable sonographically.

RENAL CORTICAL DISEASE

Based on cortical echo pattern criteria Rosenfield and coworkers divide diseases of the renal parenchyma into two types (Table 9-11).[134–136] The increased cortical echoes in type I are found in disease processes in which there is deposition of collagen or calcium and in some acute processes.[136] With chronic disease, the kidney becomes smaller, the cortex has increased echogenicity, and the medulla eventually becomes equally echogenic (Fig. 9-31).[104]

The following conclusions are drawn from two separate correlation studies of histopathologic and sonographic findings: (1) There is no correlation between the clarity of the corticomedullary junction and any histopathologic finding, type of disease, or laboratory finding.[67] (2) There is no correlation between the nature and severity of the glomerular lesion on renal biopsy and the sonographic findings.[134] (3) There is a correlation between cortical echogenicity and the value of BUN and serum creatinine levels.[67] (4) There is a definite relation between the nature and severity of interstitial changes on biopsy and the echo intensity of the cortex.[134] Focal interstitial changes tend to produce a minimal increase in cortical echogenicity, diffuse scarring produces a greater increase in echogenicity, and active interstitial infiltration produces the highest echo level.[134] The lack of sonographic specificity and the limited responses of the kidney to various pathologic insults may continue to limit specific sonographic diagnosis, even when accurate quantitative measurements are made.[67] After the initial diagnosis has been made by biopsy, however, the good correlation between cortical echogenicity and the severity of histopathologic changes indicates sonography is a promising noninvasive method of monitoring the progression of renal disease.[67]

TABLE 9-11. Sonographic patterns of renal cortical disease[17,104,134,135,136]

PATTERN	SONOGRAPHIC FINDINGS
Type I Acute glomerulonephritis, chronic glomerulonephritis, lupus nephritis, hypertensive nephrosclerosis, diabetic nephrosclerosis, acute tubular necrosis, renal transplant rejection, renal cortical necrosis, methemoglobinuric renal failure, Alport's syndrome, amyloidosis, some chronic diseases	Cortical echo intensity equal to or greater than adjacent liver, spleen, and renal sinus; corticomedullary definition preserved or enhanced
Type II Cysts, calyceal diverticuli, renal artery aneurysms, tumors, some abscesses, hematomas	Distorted normal anatomy and obliteration of corticomedullary definition focally or diffusely

RENAL MEDULLARY DISEASE

If the height of the pyramids exceeds or is thicker than that of the overlying cortex they are considered enlarged.[104] Medullary echo intensity equal to or greater than that of renal cortex is considered pathognomonic of medullary disease. Clinical history, laboratory values, and biopsy findings all contribute to identifying the pathogenesis of any quantifiable deviation in renal contour, size, or echogenicity.

Three chemical imbalances that are associated with a hyperechoic medulla are hyperuricemia, medullary nephrocalcinosis, and hypokalemia. The disease entities found in patients with these chemical imbalances and with a diffusely hyperechoic medulla include (1) gout;[168] (2) medullary nephrocalcinosis associated with hyperparathyroidism, chronic pyelonephritis, distal renal tubular acidosis (Wilson's disease), chronic glomerulonephritis, milk-alkali syndrome, malignant tumors,

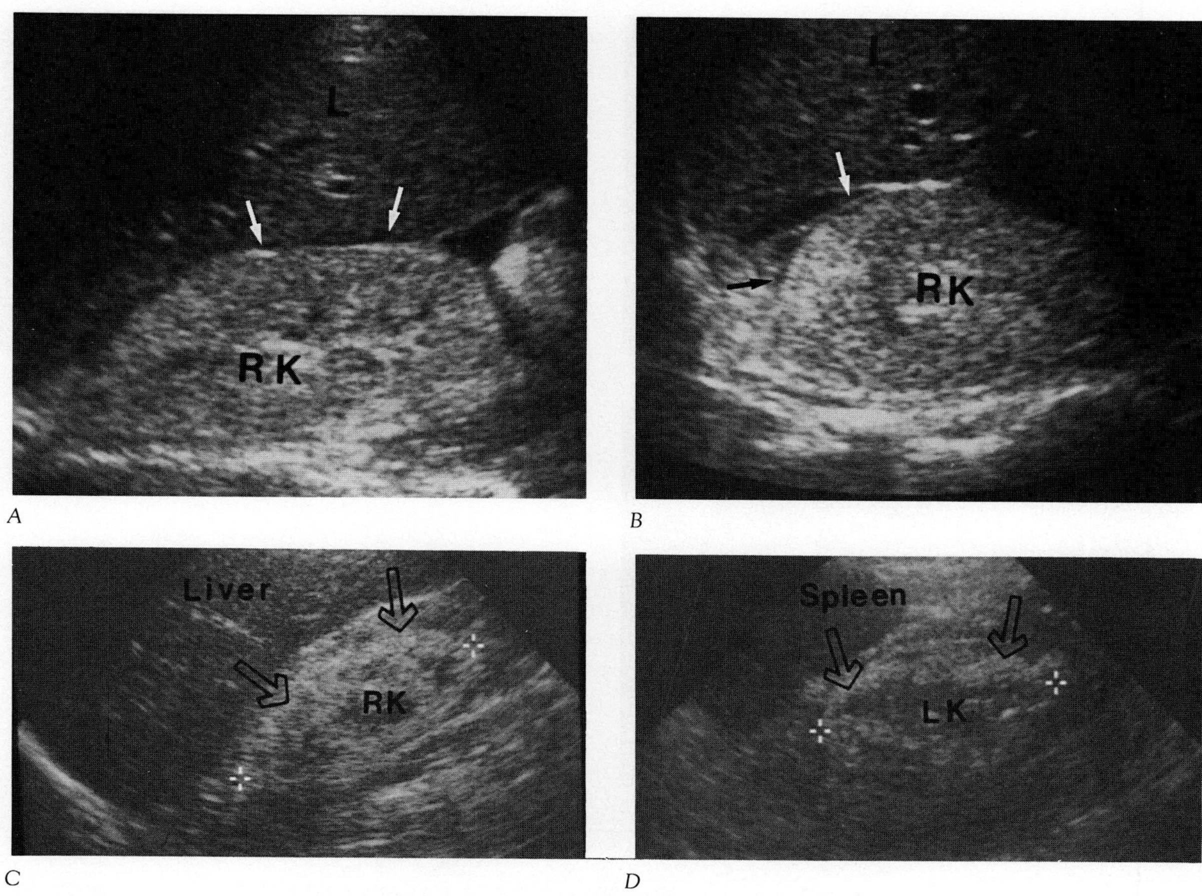

FIGURE 9-31. Both (*A*) sagittal and (*B*) transverse sections of the right kidney (RK) visualize the cortex's *(arrows)* density exceeding that of the liver (L) parenchyma. This indicates type I chronic renal cortical disease. (Courtesy Jim Baun, San Francisco, CA.) (*C*, *D*) This patient has type I chronic renal cortical disease. The kidneys become smaller as the disease progresses: right kidney (RK) is 7.2 cm long, left kidney (LK) is 6.5 cm. (Courtesy James Hansen, Ogden, UT.)

hypervitaminosis D, primary hypercalcemia, sarcoidosis, and medullary sponge kidney; and (3) renal papillary necrosis associated with pyelonephritis, diabetes, and obstructive uropathy (Fig. 9-32).[104,129] Acoustic shadowing depends on the presence, size, and composition of diffuse calcifications in the medulla.[168] With sickle cell hemoglobinopathies, a larger than normal, diffusely hyperechoic medulla is attributed to vascular dilatation, engorgement of vessels, glomerular enlargement, and interstitial edema.[43]

The patient presents with various clinical signs. Symptoms vary and are associated primarily with the type of disease process causing one of the three chemical imbalances.

RENAL SINUS DISEASE

Renal sinus lipomatosis (fibrolipomatosis), excessive fatty infiltration of the renal pelvis, is often a consequence of aging[140] and is common in the sixth to seventh decades of life.[104] It is associated with obesity, parenchymal atrophy, or destruction and

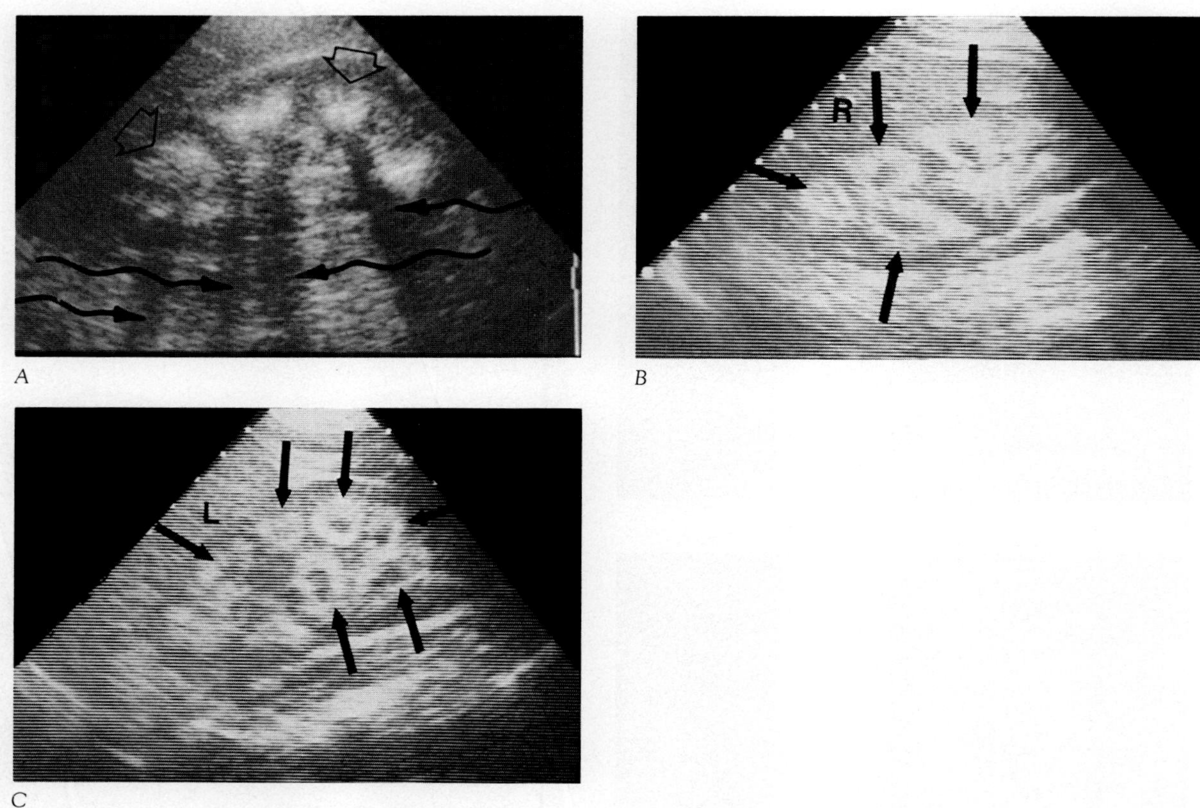

Figure 9-32. (*A*) Acoustic shadowing *(curved arrows)* is identified in this patient with medullary nephrocalcinosis associated with a history of renal tubular acidosis. The thicker than normal pyramids *(open arrows)* exceed the height of the overlying cortex. (Courtesy James Hansen, Ogden, UT.) (*B*, *C*) There is a bilateral symmetric pattern of increased echoes in the configuration of the renal medulla *(arrows)* as seen in these sagittal sections of (*B*) the right (R) and (C) left kidney (L) of a teenage girl with a history of recurrent UTI. One possible diagnoses is symmetric medullary nephrocalcinosis seen in hyperparathyroidism, Fanconi's anemia, and other unusual entities. The renal cortex appears somewhat thinned, which may be related secondarily to the medullary findings, which makes them appear thinner. There may actually be no parenchymal loss at all. The renal measurements were within normal limits. (Courtesy James Hansen, Ogden, UT.)

can be a normal variant.[3,25] Often, it begins with renal calculi, which are found in 70% of cases.[104] Nephrolithiasis is one of the predisposing factors for hydronephrosis leading to associated infection that results in renal parenchymal atrophy. The void created by ongoing parenchymal atrophy may be filled by an abundant amount of fatty tissue.[10] Thus, replacement lipomatosis can be seen as a sequela of atrophy, chronic calculous disease, and inflammation.[104]

The sonographic presentation of lipomatosis may be an enlarged, well-maintained reniform kidney that is outlined by the hypoechoic rim representing the residual parenchyma, renal capsule,

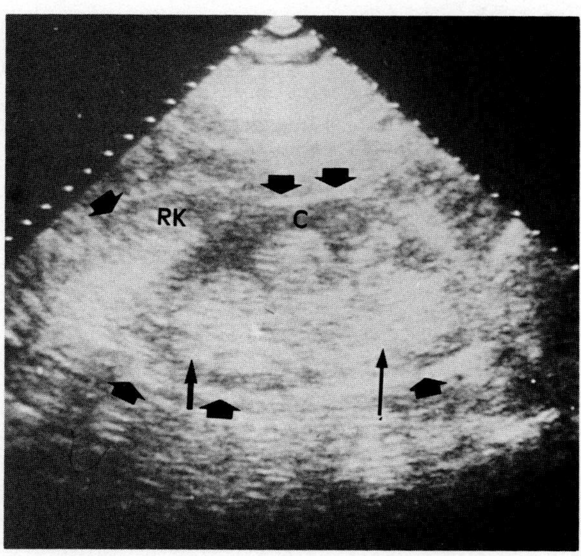

FIGURE 9-33. One of the sonographic patterns seen with renal sinus lipomatosis is increased echogenicity in the renal sinus *(arrows)*, which is demonstrated on this sagittal section of the right kidney (RK). (C, renal cortex; *arrowheads*, renal capsule).

and thick renal fascia.[25,104] The sinus echo appearances are variable: (1) an enlarged central echogenic complex;[104,140] (2) adipose tissue that may be relatively anechoic to hypoechoic, giving the impression of mass lesions;[24,140] or (3) adipose tissue that may be densely echogenic (Fig. 9-33).[10,140]

Vascular Pathology

HEMATOMAS

Renal hematomas may result from a variety of causes and are divided into spontaneous and posttraumatic types.[117] Spontaneous intrarenal hematomas usually occur as a result of a bleeding diathesis, commonly related to anticoagulant drugs such as coumadin or heparin. They are associated with renal infarcts, necrotizing arteritis, intratumoral hemorrhage,[117] and hemophilia. An intrarenal hematoma is often accompanied by a subcapsular or perinephric component, making the diagnosis somewhat more apparent.[117]

Depending on the age of the bleed, hematomas have varying echo patterns. Early in their evolution, they appear as typical cystic masses.[31,117] Gradually, as they become organized and develop a clot, the hematoma reveals a complex pattern of internal echoes.[117] Eventually, they undergo complete liquefaction and become seromas, reverting to a cystic pattern.[31,117] Chronic hematomas may become calcified, producing the characteristic acoustic shadows. (Table 9-12, Fig. 9-34).[117]

A subcapsular hematoma lies between the kidney cortex and the capsule.[142] The renal capsule's hyperechoic pattern outlines the hematoma as a well-defined linear echo. The renal cortex may appear flattened by the surrounding fluid collection.[142] Hematomas can also develop along or within any of the spaces surrounding the kidney and usually appear elongated. Whenever a fluid collection following the contour of the kidney is identified, the first impression should be a hematoma, and this finding should be considered in the context of the patient's clinical history.

INFARCTION

A renal infarction is caused by obstruction of blood supply or blood drainage by occlusion or stenosis of a vessel. Immediately after an infarction, a little parenchymal loss may not be sonographically evident,[141] or the affected area may appear echopenic.[139] In a study evaluating the sonographic pattern of a renal infarction over time, the mass appeared hypoechoic within 24 hours following an arterial occlusion.[159] Within 7 days, echoes began to appear within the mass, and by 17 days it once again appeared echogenic, with no appreciable change in cortical echogenicity.[104,159] Also reported is the appearance of a hyperechoic focal renal mass believed to be secondary to fibrosis mixed with acoustically dissimilar tissues and thinning of the involved cortex (see Table 9-12).[33,104]

Trauma

Renal injuries are divided into those resulting from blunt trauma (70%) and those resulting from penetrating trauma or secondary to operative intervention.[35,104] Athletic injuries, automobile or motorcycle accidents, and various types of crush injuries account for the majority of blunt injuries, whereas, gunshot and knife wounds account for most pen-

Table 9-12. Vascular pathology[31,33,104,117,139,141,142,159]

Lesion	Cause	Clinical Signs	Laboratory Signs	Sonographic Features
Hematoma	Trauma, anticoagulant therapy, renal infarct, necrotizing arteritis, intratumoral hemorrhage, hemophilia	Mass may be palpable, unilateral flank pain	Decreased hematocrit	Irregular, thick wall; depending on stage of the bleeding process, varying echo patterns from anechoic to complex masses with both cystic and solid components; chronic hematoma may develop calcifications with characteristic acoustic shadowing
Infarction	Obstruction of blood supply or drainage	Hypertension, lower extremity pulses absent	Elevated LDH, hematuria	Depending on the time frame following occlusion, renal parenchyma appears normal, hypoechoic, or hyperechoic

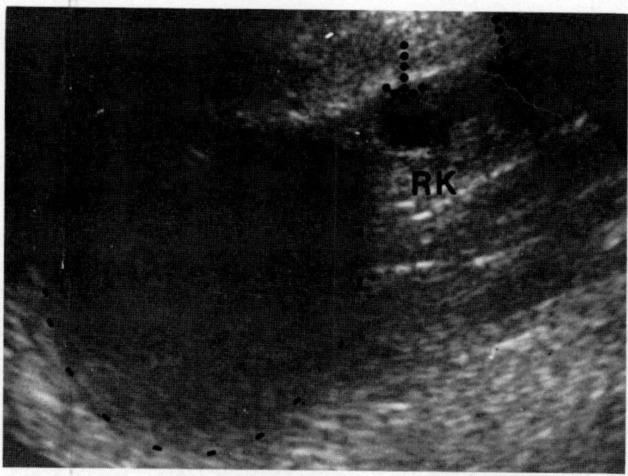

Figure 9-34. This patient presented with a history of hematuria, right side flank pain, and recent trauma to the abdomen. A sagittal section of the right kidney's (RK) upper pole demonstrates a hematoma (slashed lines), with internal echoes reflecting organization of the clot. Also identified were several cortical cysts *(dotted arrows)* on both the right and left kidney.

etrating injuries.[35] Even when the traumatic event is mild, preexisting renal abnormalities such as ectopia, anomalies, or tumor predispose to significant renal damage.[104,131]

Following an IVP examination to determine function, the role of sonography to delineate the anatomic detail in trauma to the kidney is diagnostically significant.[35] A reproducible linear absence of echoes seen in the area of a traumatized kidney suggests renal fracture.[104] Depending on the interval since the trauma, sonography demonstrates either an anechoic or a hyperechoic region in a kidney fracture with bleeding into the retroperitoneal space.[104] Focal areas of internal hemorrhage and edema are hypoechoic.[104] A blood clot in the collecting system can be identified as a low-level echo mass separating the walls of the affected system.

Neoplasms

Renal neoplasms are classified as benign or malignant and by the area of involvement. They can damage the renal parenchyma.

Benign

Ultrasound is extremely valuable in detecting some benign tumors, especially when no function is demonstrated on IVP, but it is rare that the sonographic appearance can determine the tumor type. From the literature,[18,35,104,129] Table 9-13 presents benign tumors that are less easily visualized sonographically or not visualizable at all (Fig. 9-35).

Adenoma. Often an incidental finding at surgery or autopsy, cortical adenomas are the most prevalent benign kidney tumors.[18] Usually measuring 1 cm or less and rarely larger than 3 cm in diameter, they are asymptomatic unless they enlarge.[18,117] Originating from renal tubular epithelium, these vascular benign masses are believed to be the counterpart of malignant renal cell carcinomas.[31,81,117] One theory is that adenomas smaller than 3 cm rarely metastasize, but adenomas and adenocarcinomas usually occur in the sixth or seventh decade of life and show the same male-to-female ratio, 3:1.[35,155] Adenomas may be responsible for painless hematuria.[18]

Sonographically, renal adenomas present a similar pattern to renal cell carcinoma. The highly vascular tumor has many internal echoes and associated sound attenuation (Fig. 9-36).[31,81]

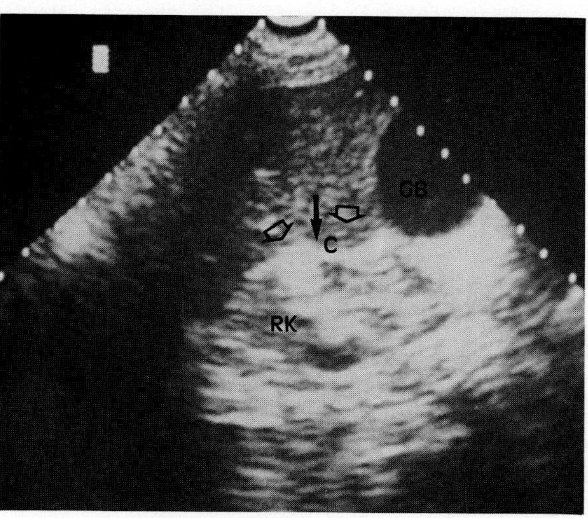

Figure 9-35. A renal fibroma (*black arrow*) confined within the renal cortex (C; *open arrows*) is seen on this transverse image of the right kidney (RK; GB, gallbladder; L, liver).

Table 9-13. Benign mesenchymal renal tumors[12,35,104,129]

Lesion	Characteristics
Leiomyoma, lipoma	Most common, female-male ratio 6:1, less than 5 mm diameter, sharply circumscribed
Hemangioma	Rare, less than 1 cm in diameter, no sex preference, occurs in 3rd and 4th decades, patients may have hematuria (capillary more common than cavernous); both types are intermixed with fibrous stroma.
Juxtaglomerular tumor	Hypovascular, solid renal mass containing large amounts of renin, mean age 31 years, normally well-circumscribed or encapsulated, arising near corticomedullary junction; associated with elevated plasma renin and secondary aldosteronism with severe diastolic hypertension.
Fibroma	Commonly occurs in medulla, rarely in cortex, 2 to 3 mm in diameter, frequently multiple, patients over 60, finding in 26%–42% of autopsies (Fig. 9-35).

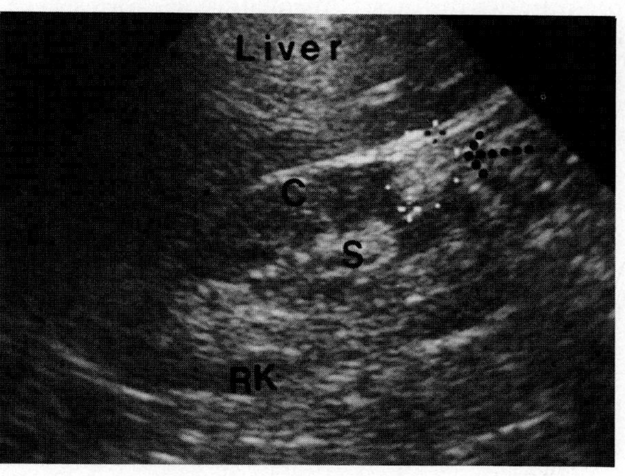

Figure 9-36. A 2× 1.5 cm echogenic lesion (*dotted arrow*) identified in the right kidney's (RK) cortex (C) could represent a benign adenoma, although angiomyolipoma and hypernephroma are also part of the differential diagnosis. Otherwise, the kidney appears normal (S, renal sinus). (Courtesy Jo Semon, Salt Lake City, UT.)

Oncocytoma. Oncocytomas, or oxyphilic adenomas, are a class of very large vascular adenomas[31,81,118] that usually occur in middle to old age with a male-to-female ratio of 1.7:1.[104,121] Patients are usually asymptomatic but may have pain or hematuria.[104] An enlarging mass may outstrip its blood supply with concurrent infarction, hemorrhage, and necrosis which produces a central stellate fibrotic scar resulting from the organization and healing of the hemorrhage.[46,104]

Sonographically, they usually cannot be distinguished from typical renal cell carcinomas,[31,81,117] which may explain why oncocytomas account for 2% to 14% of renal tumor preoperatively thought to be cancer.[46,104] Typically, they range from 0.3 to 26 cm in diameters and are well-defined, smooth, and homogeneous, similar to renal cell carcinoma.[20,46,104,121] If a central stellate scar is imaged, an oncocytoma should be suspected, as these are not present in renal cell carcinomas.[46,104,121]

Angiomyolipoma. An angiomyolipoma is an uncommon hamartomatous mesenchymal mixed benign tumor composed of fat cells intermixed with smooth muscle cells and aggregates of thick-walled blood vessels in varying proportions.[35,81,104,117] They occur in two distinct, clinicopathologic forms: (1) a unilateral solitary mass, three times more common in women and 80% on the right side, usually developing in the fourth to sixth decades, but not associated with tuberous sclerosis, and (2) multiple bilateral masses, occurring in 80% of patients with the tuberous sclerosis complex.[31,35,81,104] The diameter varies from 3 to 20 cm.[35]

Most are asymptomatic.[104] Patients with symptomatic larger lesions often present with acute onset of flank or abdominal pain or shock secondary to hemorrhage.[35,104] Focal hemorrhage with evidence of necrosis, cystic degeneration, and calcification is common within the lesion;[104,117] however, malignant transformation is thought to be extremely rare if, indeed, it ever occurs.[117]

Angiomyolipomas' striking sonographic appearance alone often leads to the diagnosis.[117] They are among the most acoustically reflective of all renal masses, hyperechoic lesions more dense than renal parenchyma.[20,59,104,122] The strong echogenicity, even at low gain settings, is due to the high fat content and the heterogeneous cellular architecture of the hamartoma as well as to its hypervascularity.[31,117] In spite of its numerous interfaces and solid nature, it still displays good sound transmission (Fig. 9-37).[117] Renal cell carcinomas have a similar pattern[31] but are usually less dense.[104]

MALIGNANT

Renal Cell Carcinoma. Renal cell carcinoma, also referred to as hypernephroma or adenocarcinoma, represents 1% to 3% of all visceral cancers.[104] They are the most common malignant tumor of the kidney, accounting for approximately 80% to 90% of all renal malignancies in adults.[21,81,104,117,129] The lesion is seen in the sixth to seventh decade and has a 3:1 male-to-female ratio.[117,129] Originating from renal tubular epithelium, the neoplasm is believed to represent the malignant counterpart of renal adenoma.[117] Classically, patients present with costovertebral angle pain, a palpable mass, and hematuria.[28,104] Only 15% of patients present with all three symptoms,[28] and hematuria is the most significant of the three.[104] Other symptoms include fever, hypertension, and possible masculinization or feminization if the tumor produces gonadotropin.[28] Tumor size varies greatly and sometimes is enormous.[117] Tumors may infiltrate throughout the kidney even though they often appear to have a capsule or pseudocapsule sharply delimiting them from adjacent normal parenchyma.[117] By local extension, renal cell carcinoma spreads into the perinephric fat and renal vein.[117] Lymphogenous and hematogenous spread often allow metastases to develop before there are any local symptoms of the primary lesion.[104] More than 50% of patients have metastases or develop them within 10 years of the diagnosis.[28] The pattern of the disease is spread to regional nodes, lungs (50%), bone (33%), opposite kidney (10% to 15%), liver, adrenal, and brain.[104,117,129] The survival rate is based on the stage of the disease. The average survival time after surgical removal for lesions at each stage is presented in Table 9-14 (Fig. 9-38).

Often highly vascular, renal cell carcinomas contain numerous areas of hemorrhage, necrosis, or cystic degeneration.[81,117] Approximately 10% are hypovascular, and many of these represent a microscopic subclassification referred to as papillary cystadenocarcinoma.[104,117] Compared to the renal parenchymal malignancy, the papillary cystadeno-

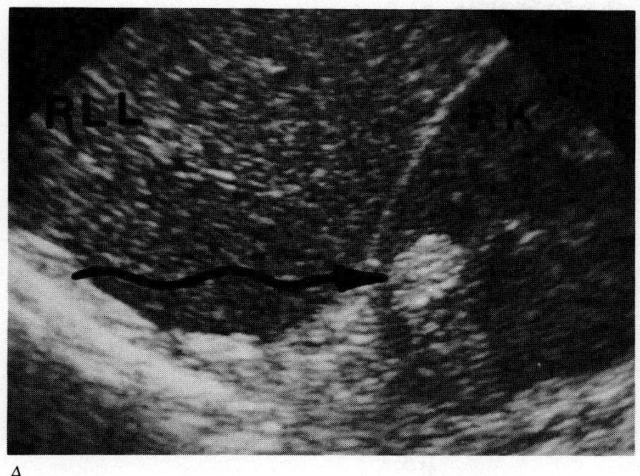

A

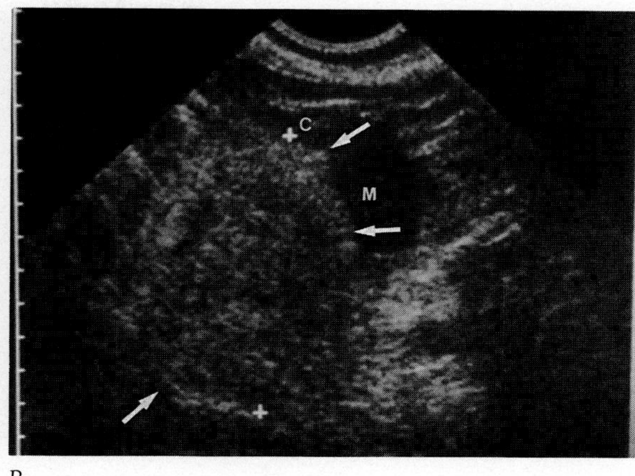

B

FIGURE 9-37. (*A*) This benign cortical angiomyolipoma (*curved arrow*) was found incidentally in the right kidney (RK) and appears hyperechoic with good sound transmission. (RLL, right liver lobe). (Courtesy Cathy Carr-Hoefer, Corvallis, OR.) (*B*) An irregular, ill-defined, hyperechoic, unilateral solitary angiomyolipoma (*arrows* and cursors) measuring 20 cm is identified on this transverse section of the right kidney. These benign tumors mixed with blood vessels, fat, and muscle tissue cannot be differentiated sonographically from a malignant process (C, renal cortex; M, renal medulla).

carcinoma is characterized by slower growth, less extensive involvement at the time of diagnosis, and a better prognosis.[104]

The IVP is reliable as a function test but is notoriously unreliable in differentiating benign and malignant renal masses. Any radiographic evidence of a renal mass requires a more definitive study such as sonography.[81,117,155] Sonographically, the echogenicity of renal cell carcinomas is less than that of normal renal parenchyma, although isoechoic and even extremely hyperechoic tumors can be seen.[21,83] Two main features characterize solid renal cell masses: the attenuation of sound by the mass (seen in almost all cases) and the presence of echoes within the mass (seen in the vast majority of cases; Fig. 9-39).[21,117]

The extent of sound attenuation is ascertained by comparing the intensity of the echoes at the far wall of the mass with those at the near wall and with those transmitted through the normal kidney,[117] liver, and spleen. Also noted are irregular wall contours.[21,56,117] The rare renal cell carcinoma

TABLE 9-14. Staging of renal carcinoma[17,18,28,35,129]

EXTENT OF DISEASE	STAGE	SURVIVAL RATE 5-YEAR
Tumor within kidney (small or large)	I	60%–70%
Tumor in perinephric fat but confined to Gerota's fascia	II	
Tumor in renal vein, regional lymph nodes, or vena cava	III	15%–20%
Adjacent organ invasion, distant metastases, tumor in juxtaregional lymph nodes	IV	5%–13%

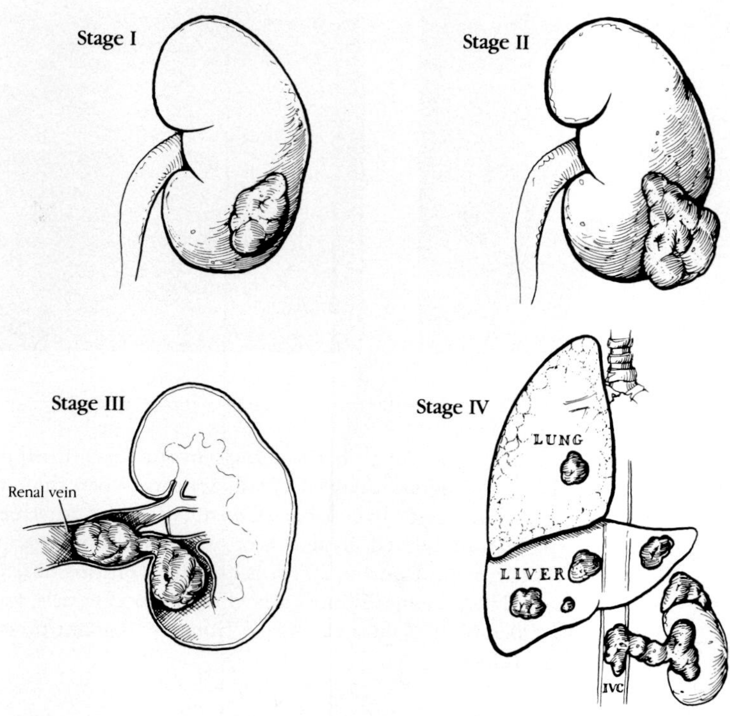

Figure 9-38. Schematic illustration of staging of renal cell carcinoma.

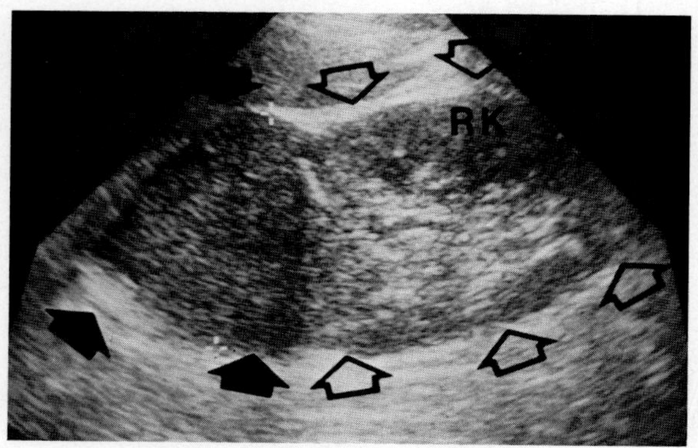

Figure 9-39. A 5.6 cm *(cursors)* stage I hypernephroma *(dark arrowheads)* located at the right kidney's (RK) upper pole can be differentiated from the normal portion *(open arrowheads)* on this sagittal section. The patient presented with hypertension and hematuria. (Courtesy Cathy Carr-Hoefer, Corvallis, OR.)

that does not attenuate sound is one that has undergone complete cystic or hemorrhagic transformation.[117] Complex patterns are encountered, with localized areas of hemorrhage, necrosis, or cystic degeneration.[117]

Solid masses are also typically characterized as containing internal echoes.[117] The size of the mass, vascularity, cholesterol,[83] and fibrous tissue content are believed to be related to the internal echo phenomenon.[31,117] With large masses, greater sound absorption decreases the possibility of weaker echoes returning to the transducer.[117] Solid, very vascular masses appear echogenic, as the multiple blood vessel wall interfaces are excellent reflectors.[117] Collagen is believed to be responsible for reflectivity of soft tissues.[117] Fibrous tissue is a principal source of collagen and is abundant in most renal tumors.[117] Calcifications and alternating areas of cystic and solid components also generate multiple sound reflections.[31,117]

Recent investigation of renal cell carcinoma with Doppler sonography indicates that hypoechoic, hypervascular, or vascular renal carcinomas exhibit high-frequency Doppler shifts of 4 kHz or more.[86] Doppler detection of vascular signals in tumors may be useful for noninvasive tissue characterization.[86] Papillary cystadenocarcinoma is usually a hypovascular tumor that returns few low-level echoes and may even appear anechoic at lower gain settings.[117]

The detection of any solid renal mass requires a concerted effort to visualize the renal vein, the IVC, the renal hilar, paraaortic lymph nodes, and the contralateral kidney to complete the examination (Fig. 9-40).[31,56,104,117,149] Invasion of the IVC is more common with hypernephromas of the right kidney than with lesions involving the left kidney.[31,51] Extension of renal cell carcinoma into the renal vein and inferior vena cava occurs in 5 to 24% of cases[149] and should be analyzed with duplex Doppler sonography to provide real-time imaging with Doppler waveform analysis for flow characteristics.[85] The normal IVC and renal vein Doppler waveform illustrates a wide spectrum of low frequencies that are phasic with respiration. In the presence of thrombus or obstruction, the Doppler signal may be damped, absent, or continuous.[85] With renal vein and IVC involvement, angiography prior to surgery affords a more complete picture of the extent of involvement, but duplex Doppler sonography provides excellent quantitative data preoperatively and for postoperative monitoring.[85]

Discrete intraluminal echoes within involved fistula formation, distention by the thrombus, compression secondary to adenopathy, and displacement of the IVC all indicate extension and are all readily imaged with real-time sonography.[117] Hilar adenopathy is imaged as solid hypoechoic masses surrounding the renal pedicle and the aorticorenal junction.[117] Paraaortic nodes obscure the outline of the great vessels or present as solid masses in the midline of the retroperitoneum.[117]

Wilms' Tumor. Wilms' tumor, a highly malignant childhood tumor also referred to as a nephroblastoma, is discussed in Chapter 17.

Urothelial Carcinoma of the Renal Pelvis. Approximately 5% to 10% of primary renal tumors occur in the renal pelvis and become clinically apparent within a relatively short time because their growth causes fragmentation, producing noticeable but painless hematuria.[129] They are small and usually not palpable but may block urinary outflow, causing palpable hydronephrosis.[129] These tumors are invasive without the bulky mass,[56] infiltrating the wall of the pelvis, calyces, and renal vein.[129] Despite the apparently small and deceptively benign mass and adequate surgical removal, the 5-year survival rate is less than 10%.[129]

Transitional Cell Carcinoma. Transitional cell carcinomas represent 7% of all renal neoplasms and 85% of primary renal pelvis tumors.[104] The patient usually presents with painless hematuria. Sonographically, it appears isoechoic with the renal parenchyma.[20] Two sonographic patterns have been described: splitting or separation of the central echo complex similar to hydronephrosis[72,104] and a bulky, hypoechoic mass lesion (Fig. 9-41).[31,56,104] The tumor is usually detected as a filling defect on IVP.[104] Sonography is helpful in determining the cause of the filling defect: calculi (keratin pearls) are hyperechoic with associated acoustic shadow;[72] tumors and blood clots appear echogenic without acoustic shadowing; and urothelial tumors are seen as low level echoes separated from the renal paren-

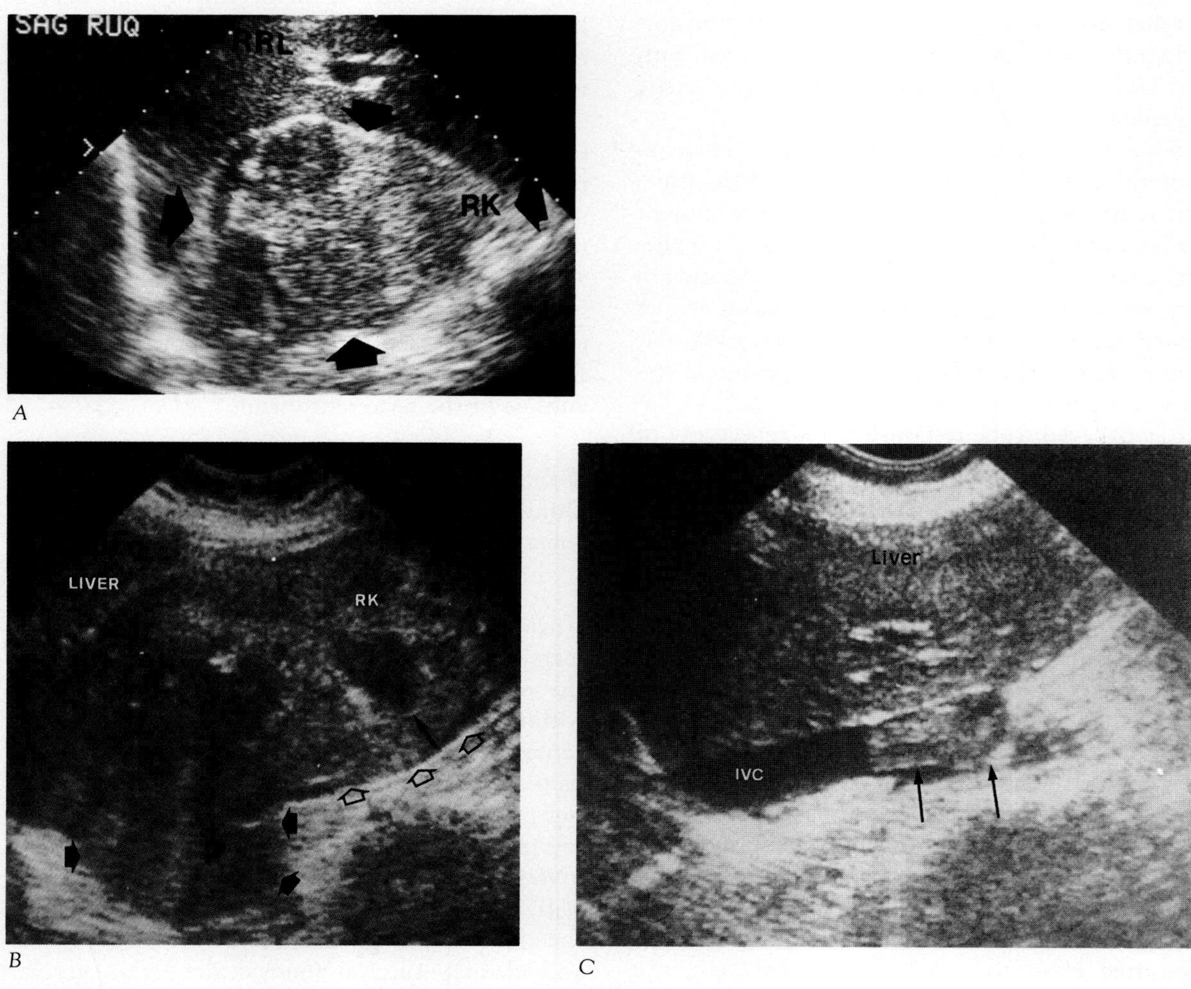

Figure 9-40. This sagittal section demonstrates a stage I hypernephroma *(dark arrowheads)* replacing the normal right kidney (RK) but still contained within the renal capsule (RRL, right liver lobe). (Courtesy Cathy Carr-Hoefer, Corvallis, OR.) (B) A coronal section of the right kidney (RK) demonstrates a large stage III hypernephroma *(closed arrowheads)* that has broken through the renal capsule *(open arrowheads)* and has caused some mild dilatation in part of the collecting system *(arrow)*. (C) A stage III hypernephroma *(arrows)* invading the inferior vena cava (IVC) is seen on this sagittal section. This demonstrates the importance of including vascular investigation with routine examination technique.

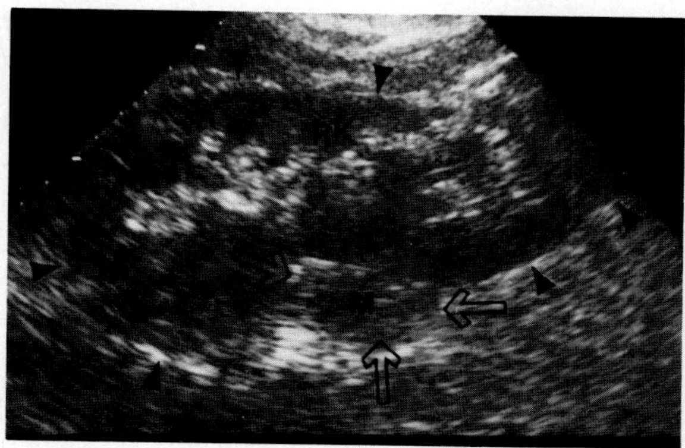

FIGURE 9-41. A filling defect in the lower pole on a male patient's cross-fused ectopic right kidney was seen on IVP and CT. On the sagittal section, the right kidney (RK, *arrowheads*) measured 15.5 cm long and 7.6 cm wide, and a hypoechoic mass *(open arrows)* producing little if any acoustic shadowing is identified. The differential diagnosis included a slowly growing neoplasm and a slowly enlarging nonopaque calculus. The mass was later diagnosed as transitional cell carcinoma. (Courtesy Steven Trawick, Phoenix, AZ.)

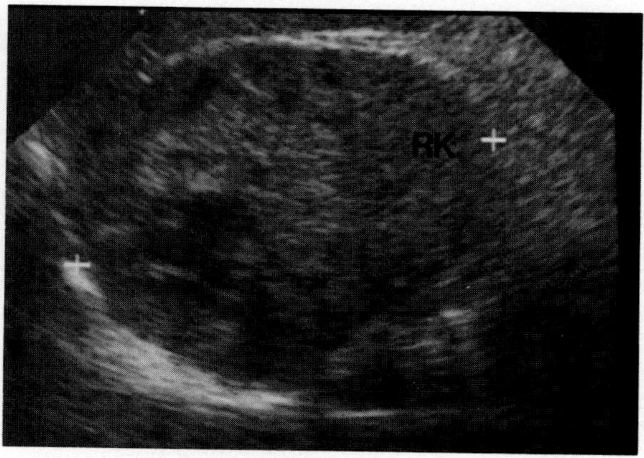

FIGURE 9-42. This patient has right lower lobe lung cancer, which metastasized to the right kidney (RK), resulting in both a cystic and a solid mass. (Courtesy Kelly Smith, Ogden, UT.)

chyma by a distinct echogenic zone of interposed renal sinus fat.[72,104]

Squamous cell carcinoma. The remaining 15% of all urothelial tumors are the highly malignant squamous cell carcinomas. This tumor has an insidious onset, metastasizes early with a poor prognosis, and is associated with renal calculi and infection.[109] Sonographically, the diagnosis is suggested by the presence of faceted calculi and marked hydronephrosis from ureteropelvic junction obstruction.[104]

METASTATIC RENAL TUMORS

Because of its profuse blood flow, the kidney is frequently the site of metastasis of carcinomas and sarcomas that arise in other organs.[129] Lung and breast tumors are the main sources.[81] Renal cell carcinoma of the kidney is the only malignancy that selectively metastasizes to the opposite kidney.[109,129] There is no specific pattern that distinguishes these lesions from other solid masses, and they may present as hypoechoic to hyperechoic (Fig. 9-42).[81,104]

Lymphoma. Secondary involvement of the kidney by lymphoma, including Hodgkin's and leukemia, occurs with significant frequency and is manifested with nonspecific enlargement of the kidney.[31,35] In Hodgkin's disease the incidence is approximately 10%, whereas in malignant lymphoma its incidence varies from 35% to 60%.[35] Sonographically, most lymphomas present as anechoic or hypoechoic, single or multiple masses.[104,117] Characteristically, lymphosarcoma is bilateral.[35]

Renal Failure

Renal failure is the inability of the kidneys to remove accumulated metabolites from the blood.[18] The situation causes alterations in electrolyte, acid-base, and water balance and accumulation of substances that normally are completely excreted.[18,109] Table 9-15 lists the three major categories. The underlying causes of renal failure are renal pathology, systemic disease, and urologic defects of nonrenal origin[129] attributed to surgery or trauma (43%), various medical conditions (26%), pregnancy (13%), and nephrotoxis (9%).[18] Acute renal failure (ARF) affects approximately 10,000 persons annually in

TABLE 9-15. Causes of acute renal failure[18,109,129]

Prerenal Conditions	Impaired renal blood flow due to hypovolemia (dehydration, hemorrhage, fluid sequestration), heart failure, septicemia
Intrarenal Conditions	Renal ischemia; glomerular membrane injury from exposure to nephrotoxic wastes (aminoglycosides, heavy metals, organic solvents, radiopaque contrast media, sulfonamides); acute tubular necrosis; intratubular obstruction (uric acid crystals, hemolytic reactions, precipitated proteins from multiple myeloma, rhabdomyolysis); acute inflammatory conditions (pyelonephritis, necrotizing papillitis)
Postrenal Conditions	Obstructive uropathy: Ureteral obstruction (calculi, tumors); bladder outlet obstruction (prostatic hypertrophy, urethral strictures)

the United States and the mortality rate is about 60%.[119] Both acute and chronic renal failure (CRF) result in azotemia, an overload of nitrogenous wastes (blood urea nitrogen, uric acid, and serum creatinine) in the blood.[119]

ACUTE RENAL FAILURE

The clinical manifestations of ARF are frequently superimposed on the signs and symptoms of the underlying disease. As ARF is potentially reversible, early signs and symptoms are important to recognize.[18] If untreated, the severe reduction in the glomerular filtration rate causes irreversible damage. The two phases of ARF are oliguric and diuretic. In the oliguric phase, urine output is greatly reduced. If there is severe oliguria and associated tissue breakdown, the patient exhibits elevated BUN, creatinine, potassium, and phosphate serum levels causing metabolic acidosis.[119] If this phase is prolonged, hypertension, neuromuscular irritability, muscle weakness, gastrointestinal bleeding, and infection are serious complications of the disease. After a few days to 6 weeks, the diuretic phase of ARF begins, which indicates that the nephrons have recovered to the extent that urine excretion is possible. The diuretic phase often occurs before renal function returns to normal, which explains why BUN, serum creatinine, potassium, and phosphate levels remain elevated or continue to rise even though urine output has increased.[119] Excessive loss of water and electrolytes occurs if the diuresis is associated with impaired nephron function.

Sonography plays an important role in the clinical evaluation and management of patients with renal failure. ARF can occur suddenly or can develop over days or weeks.[104] Once ARF has been established as the diagnosis, sonography's most important role is accurate evaluation of hydronephrosis, distinguishing postrenal or obstructive causes, and screening for parenchymal diseases.[52,65] Distinguishing the cause is important in relieving obstruction, a feature of 5% of cases of ARF, and to facilitate appropriate treatment of other renal medical disease.[52,65] Prompt intervention prevents secondary loss of renal parenchyma.[65]

The prerenal conditions related to hemorrhage and dehydration were presented earlier in this chapter, and hyperfusions due to thrombosis are presented in Chapter 3. Postrenal conditions are presented as follows: obstruction, hydronephrosis, and pregnancy, in this chapter under Obstructive Uropathy; pyonephrosis, in this chapter under Inflammatory Disease; and ureteral strictures, in Chapter 10. Prostatic hypertrophy is also a postrenal condition.

Intrarenal Conditions. The intrarenal conditions that cause renal failure from infantile polycystic disease are presented in Chapter 17. Other intrarenal conditions not repeated in this section but presented in this chapter are adult polycystic disease, medullary cystic disease, and nephronophthisis, under Cystic Diseases; bacterial interstitial nephritis (pyelonephritis) and xanthogranulomatous pyelonephritis, under Inflammatory Diseases; and nephrocalcinosis, under Renal Pathology.

Acute tubular necrosis. The most common cause of ARF is acute tubular necrosis (ATN), which is the mechanism of many forms of renal failure resulting from a variety of toxic and ischemic insults leading to widespread tubular epithelial cell destruction.[18,52] In such cases, renal insufficiency develops abruptly, although the process may be reversible.[52] Histologically there is necrosis of tubule cells and cellular casts in the collecting tubules, and grossly the kidneys are often swollen and edematous.[52]

Sonographically, most patients with ATN have normal kidneys with no changes in renal architecture, cortical echogenicity or thickness, or the appearance of medullary pyramids.[41,52] Occasionally, increased cortical echogenicity, accentuated corticomedullary definition, and a slightly enlarged kidney are observed.[52,138] When ATN is secondary to nephrotoxicity, such as myoglobinuria following renal trauma or in ethylene glycol poisoning, sonography demonstrates an increase in bilateral cortical echogenicity with preservation of the corticomedullary definition.[138]

Acute cortical necrosis. Acute cortical necrosis (ACN), a rare form of ARF, occurs most commonly in patients with shock, sepsis, hemorrhage, burns, renal vein thrombosis, hemolytic uremic syndrome, pregnancy-induced hypertension with abruptio placentae, and severe dehydration.[52,151] Although the actual mechanism of ACN is uncertain, it may be capillary damage and vasospasm secondary to intravascular thrombus or toxin production, resulting in ischemia.[52] Histologic findings are those of acute ischemic infarction limited to the cortex, necrosis of tubular cells, and cellular infiltration in the interstitium.[52] The medulla and a thin rim of subcapsular tissue remain intact.[52] Punctate or linear calcifications can be identified within 6 days after infarction, at the junction of necrotic and viable tissue or diffusely throughout the renal cortex.[104,151]

The sonographic findings are of bilateral, normal-sized kidneys.[104] Initially, the renal cortex appears hypoechoic and there is a loss of normal corticomedullary definition.[104,151] As the disease progresses to the chronic stage, follow-up studies demonstrate progressive decreases in renal size and various degrees of increased renal cortical echogenicity directly related to the degree of calcification and collagen deposition.[52]

Myoglobinuria. Myoglobinuria is the cause in 5% to 7% of patients with ARF and occurs in 33% of patients with myoglobinemia.[104,114] Normally, myoglobin is cleared by metabolism to bilirubin.[114] Increased amounts of myoglobin are released into the tissues and bloodstream following rhabdomyolysis (an acute, sometimes fatal disease characterized by destruction of skeletal muscle)[164] or as a result of other causes including alcohol and drug addiction, crush injuries, strokes, toxins, fever, or myositis.[52] Renal failure is thought to be secondary to nephrotoxicity with tubular obstruction.[114] Histologic findings include ATN, brown casts, interstitial edema, cellular infiltration, and possibly, engorgement of medullary and glomerular vessels.[52] Fibrosis and atrophy are seen in chronic cases.

The histologic changes create various sonographic appearances, from completely normal kidney in ATN to enlarged and echogenic kidneys in cases where changes reflect cellular interstitial infiltration.[52] With enlarged, distended medullary vessels, the pyramids may be prominent and hypoechoic.[52,104] In end-stage fibrosis, the kidneys may be shrunken and echogenic.[114]

Acute glomerulonephritis. Acute glomerulonephritides are renal inflammations that may be categorized as (1) renal inflammatory response caused by an autoimmune reaction resulting in glomerular damage or (2) interstitial inflammation due to infection (by gram-negative bacilli), exposure to toxins and drugs, or infiltration of inflammatory cells into the renal interstitium.[52,129] Histologically, there is proliferation of endothelial and mesangial cells in glomeruli and exudate of white blood cells.[129] The process may reverse or progress to end-stage renal disease.[52] Typically, patients present with hematuria, hypertension, azotemia, and red cell casts in the urine.[129]

The sonographic appearance varies from normal size early in the disease process to enlargement, with markedly increased echogenicity equal to that of the central echo of the renal sinus.[52,124] On follow-up examination the kidneys progressively shrink. With reversal of azotemia, renal echogenicity may become more normal.[52]

Amyloidosis. Amyloidosis, a metabolic disorder, is associated with extensive amyloid deposits in the glomeruli, arterioles, and interstitium[52,129] that eventually causes complete obliteration of the glomerulus. Patients present with excessive proteinuria or the nephrotic syndrome. As glomerular destruction progresses, the patient dies of uremia.[129] Amyloid deposits are commonly associated with abnormal serum proteins or chronic infection or inflammation such as rheumatoid arthritis.[52] At postmortem examination, 14% to 26% of patients have histologic evidence of amyloidosis.[52]

Depending on the stage of amyloidosis, the sonographic appearance of the kidneys may be large, normal, small, and eventually shrunken in end-stage.[52] Increased cortical echogenicity and accentuated corticomedullary definition are more pronounced in chronic disease. In patients with a history of collagen vascular disease or chronic illness these nonspecific findings should raise the possibility of amyloidosis.[52]

CHRONIC RENAL FAILURE

Chronic renal failure is an irreversible condition characterized by diminished function of the nephrons resulting in decreased glomerular filtration rate, renal blood flow, tubular function, and resorptive capability.[18] Progressive renal impairment leads to end-stage renal disease. The multiple causes of CRF include nephrotic syndrome, glomerulonephritis, collagen vascular disease, diabetes, hypertension, nephrosclerosis, analgesic nephropathy, and chronic pyelonephritis.[18,52,119] Having only a limited number of ways to respond to various insults, the end-stage kidney, regardless of the cause of renal failure, usually has a similar appearance pathologically and sonographically.[52,67,134] The sonographic findings are not disease specific, and there is no correlation between the type and severity of glomerular disease and the kidney's echogenicity.[67,134] Sonographically, a small, shrunken, echogenic kidney is quite definitive for end-stage renal disease, which can be the result of a variety of processes.[52]

When conservative management of end-stage renal disease is no longer effective, dialysis or renal transplantation becomes necessary. The choice is dictated by age, related health problems, donor availability, and personal preference.[119]

DIALYSIS PATIENT

During dialysis, blood from an artery moves through an artificial kidney unit designed to assume the physiologic function of the nephrons, after which it is returned to a vein. Sonography is useful for monitoring the kidneys of patients who are receiving long-term hemodialysis.[52]

Uremic Renal Cystic Disease. Many patients with CRF who receive hemodialysis develop bilateral cystic disease[4,91,145]: 43% of patients on dialysis 3 years and more than 79% of patients on dialysis longer than 5 years.[4,91] The pathogenesis of these multiple, 0.5- to 3-cm diameter acquired lesions is unknown.[52] Suggested mechanisms include obstruction secondary to fibrosis or oxalate crystals, vascular insufficiency, and direct toxicity of circulating metabolites.[100] The cysts are located throughout the kidney and involve the cortex, corticomedullary junction, and medulla.[4,52,91,145]

Sonographically, the kidneys may appear somewhat small and echogenic, and cysts are seen throughout the parenchyma. As the cysts grow, the kidney may enlarge.[52] Hemorrhage often occurs into acquired renal cysts, resulting in perirenal and retroperitoneal hematoma,[98] pain, hematuria, and echogenic collections in the cysts on sonography.[52] Hemorrhagic cysts may be indistinguishable from neoplasms.[52] Without the history of dialysis, the differential diagnosis includes hydronephrosis and polycystic disease, though with acquired cysts the kidneys usually are smaller.[52]

Carcinomas. The incidence of papillary adenomas and renal cell carcinomas in the cystic kidneys of hemodialysis patients is estimated to be between 10% and 40%.[98] The incidence is usually associated with the presence of atypical cysts.[104] Sonographically, neoplasms may be multiple and bilateral, arise adjacent to or within cysts, and appear hyperechoic to anechoic without posterior acoustic enhancement.[52]

TRANSPLANTS

Since the first successful transplant (allograft) between identical twins was performed in 1956,[96] renal transplantation has evolved into a standard treatment modality for irreversible CRF.[68,104] More than 50,000 renal transplant procedures have been performed worldwide, and the frequency is increasing.[68] The greater rate of allograft survival can be attributed to the significant progress in transplant immunology and immunosuppressive therapy, which allows more favorable selection of donor

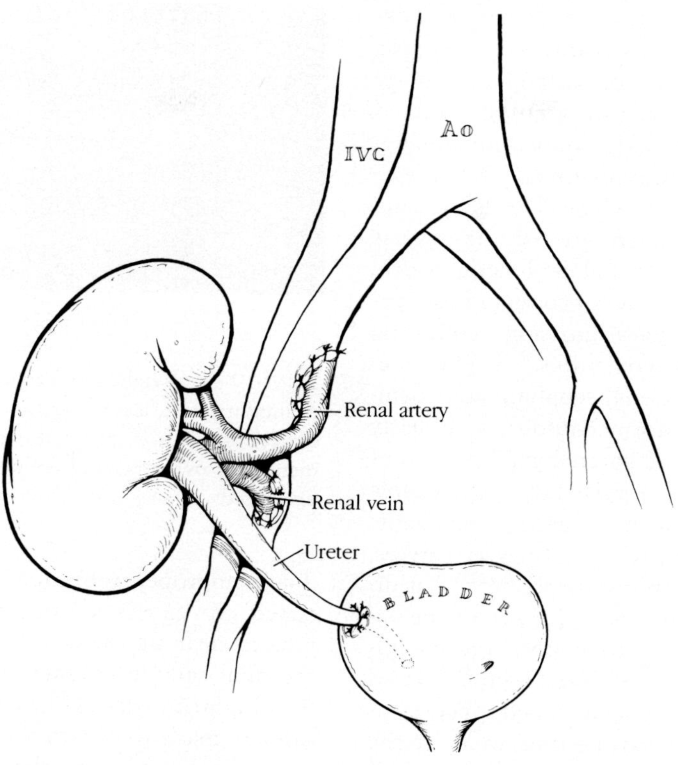

FIGURE 9-43. Schematic illustration of a renal allograft (IVC, inferior vena cava; Ao, aorta).

and recipient combinations while diminishing the incidence of severe or life-threatening infections.[68] These improvements, along with the technical aspects of organ perfusion and transplantation, have been nearly perfected: the 2-year allograft survival rate is 60% to 80%.[36,68]

Normal Scanning Technique and Appearance. Most often the renal allograft is placed retroperitoneally in an oblique orientation into the recipient's contralateral iliac fossa, anterior to the psoas muscle and iliac veins.[55,68] The surrounding bony pelvis provides a safe, well-protected location close to the bladder. The normal kidney allograft is inverted so that the dorsal aspect is oriented toward the ventral aspect of the patient.[68] The allograft renal artery and renal vein are anastomosed end-to-side to the external iliac artery and the internal vein, respectively.[68] The renal hilar structures are medial to the renal parenchyma, but the surgical placement changes the orientation so that the renal pelvis is most anterior, the renal vein is posterior, and the renal artery is between them.[68] The allograft ureter is anastomosed to the bladder (Fig. 9-43).[55,68] The patient's own kidneys (native kidneys) and ureters usually are not removed.[55]

The superficial position of the transplanted kidney allows excellent sonographic delineation of its anatomy and pathology.[65,78] Although sonography depicts gross anatomy and not function, it is affected by the tissue texture and thus gives clues to the histologic character of the allograft kidney.[68]

Following transplantation, the kidney undergoes normal renal hypertrophy.[65,66] A sonographic examination should be performed within 48 to 72 hours to determine shape and echo characteristics, to establish the baseline measurements and renal volume,[69,100] and to evaluate the renal and perirenal area to rule out hemorrhage or fluid.[63,68,78] Baseline studies increase the diagnostic accuracy of serial examinations.[63] The patient is scanned in a supine position with a full, but not distended, urinary bladder.[56] Adequate images can often be obtained by scanning alongside the surgical incision, angling toward the allograft, and obtaining the images along the anatomic coronal plane. This affords optimal quantitative assessment in both transverse and longitudinal views (to obtain length, width, and thickness) and evaluation of configuration, parenchyma, corticomedullary junction, collecting system, and the central renal sinus.[68,100] The baseline sonograms of the normal renal allograft demonstrate a smooth, reniform contour, a diffusely homogeneous, hypoechoic parenchymal pattern of uniform thickness, and a relatively hyperechoic central echo complex with a coarsely echogenic dense band representing the renal pelvis, calyces, blood vessels, and fatty fibrous tissues.[56,78,123] Within the normal homogeneous grainy pattern of the parenchyma, small anechoic to hypoechoic medullary pyramids are identified (Fig. 9-44).[56,78] Fried and coworkers have developed a medullary pyramid index (MPI), which can be used to assess the normal measurements of native and allograft kidneys and to predict renal transplant rejection:[41]

$$\text{MPI} = \frac{\frac{1}{2}\,(\text{pyramid length} \times \text{pyramid width})}{\text{cortical thickness}}$$

The median MPI was 4.17 for normal native kidneys, 6.0 for nonrejected allografts, and 7.50 for rejected allografts. There was considerable overlap between rejected and nonrejected kidneys; however, in serial examinations using the allograft as the control measurement, correlation with clinical observations and other laboratory parameters determines the MPI value.[41]

Doppler Evaluation. Immediate posttransplant duplex Doppler sonography establishes the baseline for monitoring the response to immunosuppressive therapy[128] and for later monitoring to rule out vascular occlusion and detect renal artery stenosis.[108,156,163] Before establishing the baseline, it is useful to study the aorta or inferior vena cava, to establish the proper gain settings that ensure that failure to receive signals from the allograft is not due to improper technique.[108] Once the signal is detected, the gate is reduced from the usual 5 to 10 mm, to clean up the waveform. The axial length of the final sample volume is usually 2 to 3 mm.[108] Small adjustments of the angle or position of the gate are made to obtain the best signal and are assessed by listening to the signals over the loudspeaker.[108]

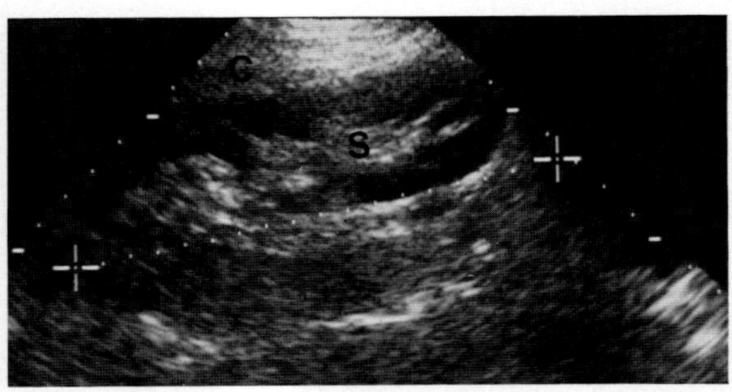

FIGURE 9-44. A right renal transplant baseline examination indicates a kidney length *(between cursors)* of 12.7 cm. A normal renal parenchyma (C, cortex, P, medullary pyramid) and renal sinus (S) are clearly visualized.

Normal renal arterial waveforms show the characteristic low-impedance pattern of antegrade flow throughout the cardiac cycle (Fig. 9-45).[108,127,128] Progressively decreasing pulsatility from the main renal artery to the arcuate arteries is normal. Sampling should be done at the arcuate arteries, the segmental arteries, and the main renal artery; and the superior, middle, and inferior aspects of the kidney should be evaluated.[108] It is normal to see a small amount of turbulence near the anastomosis of the main renal artery with the iliac artery.[108,163] Recording one or two sets of waveforms is usually adequate (Fig. 9-46).

Sampling the interlobar arteries is important when there are no signals in the more proximal or distal vessels or when there are abnormalities in the other arterial signals.[108] Renal venous waveforms may be sampled from the renal hilus, the main renal vein, and the parenchyma.[108]

Complications. The possible causes of allograft failure in the posttransplant period include (1) arterial

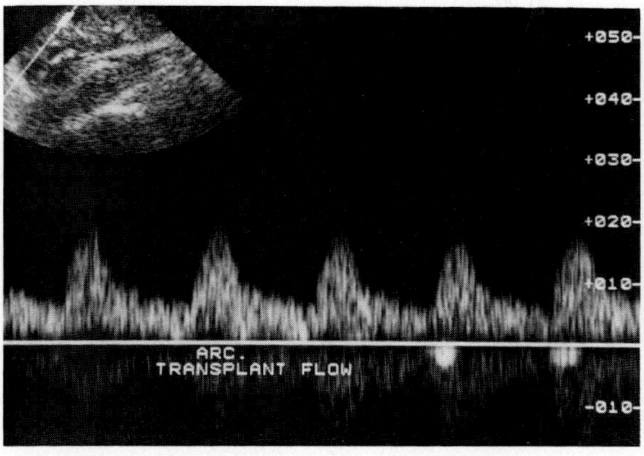

FIGURE 9-45. Doppler signals are seen from a normal, rejection-free allograft obtained from an arcuate renal artery. On the frozen real-time image, the long white line represents the path of the acoustic beam and the small white bar shows the position of the cursor in the arcuate artery. The vertical axis represents Doppler shift frequency, the horizontal axis, time. A peak in frequency shift in systole is followed by a gradual decrease throughout diastole that remains continuous and antegrade. Venous flow is seen below the horizontal axis. (Courtesy Lisa Schneiter, Ogden, UT.)

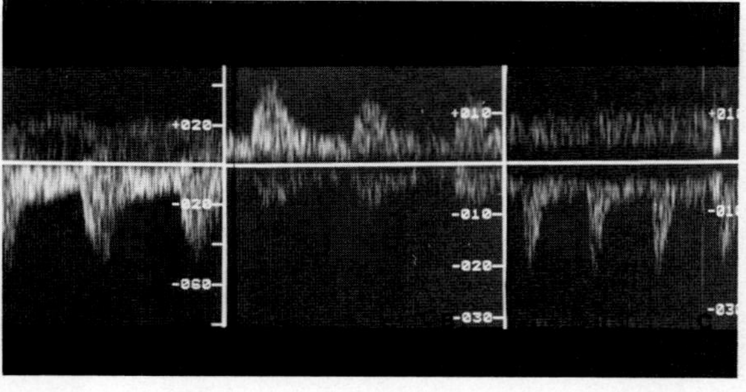

FIGURE 9-46. Doppler signals are demonstrated from a normal, rejection-free allograft obtained from (*A*) the main renal artery (*B*) segmental artery, and (C) the interlobar artery. (Courtesy Lisa Schneiter, Ogden, UT.)

or venous compromise; (2) obstruction of the collecting system; (3) viral, bacterial, or fungal infection; (4) hyperacute, accelerated acute, acute, or chronic rejection;[35] and (5) acute tubular necrosis.[68] Acute rejection may be divided into two histologic forms, interstitial and vascular. Interstitial rejection results from a cellular immune reaction, whereas acute rejection may be the result of both humoral and cellular immune mechanisms.[128]

Rejection. Reflecting the ongoing pathologic process, the sonographic parenchymal markers of renal allograft rejection include enlarged pyramids of decreased echogenicity (the edema), congestion, and hemorrhage of the interstitial tissue (Fig. 9-47).[7,40,68,123,146] The hyperechogenicity of the cortex is thought to be related to ischemia and cellular infiltration of the cortex, usually by small lymphocytes and plasma cells.[56,100,123] Necrosis and liquefaction are seen as patchy anechoic areas in the parenchyma (Fig. 9-48).[40,66,123] Reniform distortion and compression of the renal sinus echoes reflects the generalized edema, cellular infiltration, and vascular congestion of the rejecting renal allograft.[66,100,123] Thickening of the renal collecting system wall greater than 2 mm due to edema and lymphocyte infiltration is associated with rejection.[110] Thickening of the collecting system has also been noted with urinary tract infection, reflux, and chronic obstruction in both transplanted and native kidneys.[110] As focal allograft rejection is atypical, diagnostic accuracy increases with multiple sonographic findings of rejection[63] associated with markedly elevated creatinine values (Fig. 9-49).[96] A normal sonogram does not rule out rejection.[63]

In severe rejection, the renal sinus blends with the adjacent parenchyma so that the boundary between the two compartments cannot be identified.[70] In its early stages, decreased blood flow to the kidney results in cortical ischemia. The value of Doppler investigation has been reported to be limited in evaluating renal failure due to interstitial rejection,[12] useful in moderate to severe interstitial rejection in which the edema and enlargement of the interstitium may offer increased resistance to flow,[39] and very useful in demonstrating a change in the pattern of blood flow with a decrease in the diastolic flow and a sharpening (rapid rise and fall off) of the systolic flow.[108,127]

Acute tubular necrosis. ATN, a misnomer for renal failure resulting from renal tubule damage, is the most common cause of acute posttransplant renal

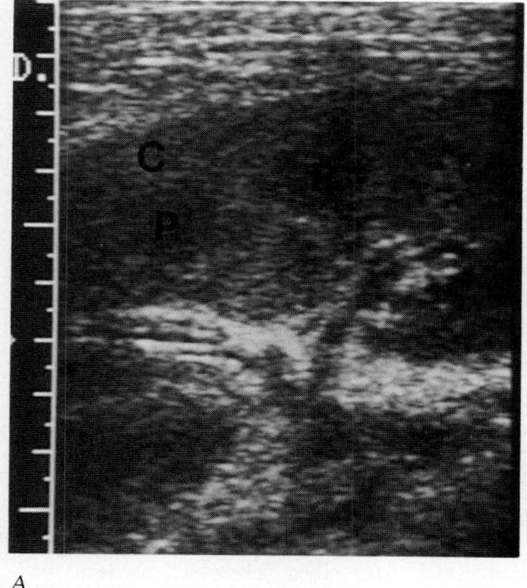

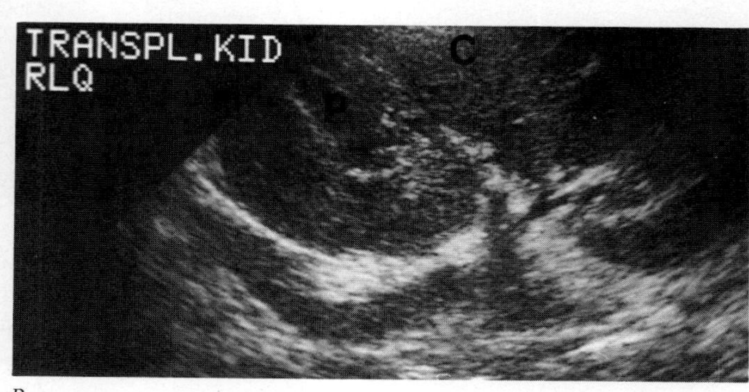

A B

FIGURE 9-47. Early signs of rejection are seen in this patient with polycystic kidney and liver disease. There is some compression of the renal sinus echoes, reflecting generalized edema, cellular infiltration, and vascular congestion of the rejecting allograft. Enlarged pyramids (P) are visualized with a hyperechoic cortex (C) having some patchy anechoic areas within the parenchyma. At the time of the examination, vascular flow was diminished but adequate. (Courtesy Cathy Carr-Hoefer, Corvallis, OR.)

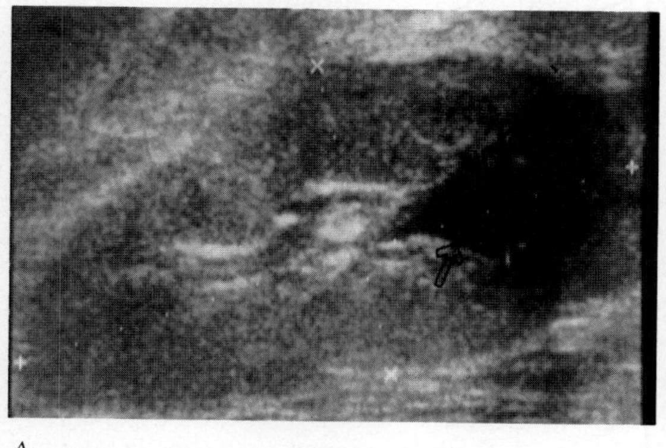

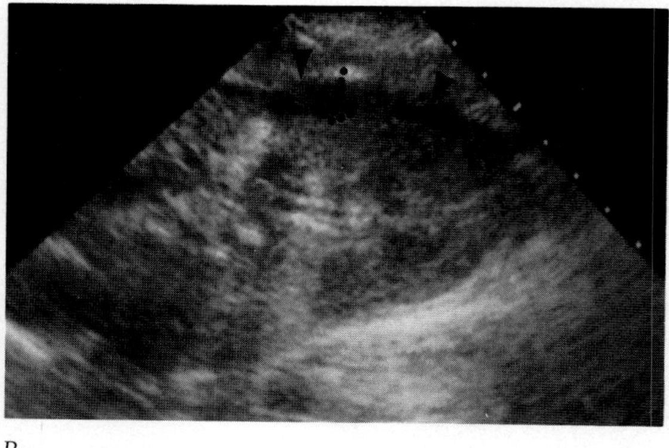

A B

FIGURE 9-48. In these transverse sections imaged after renal allograft *(cursors)* in the left iliac fossa, a thin layer of subcapsular fluid *(arrowheads)* compresses the renal parenchyma *(dotted arrows)*. The allograft measures 13.2 cm long, 6.3 cm wide, and 6.5 cm thick (AP). (*A*) The upper pole renal collecting system is dilated *(open arrows)*, whereas (*B*) the lower pole is decompressed. The unusual kidney density is characteristic of a diffuse parenchymal process. These findings correlated with this 55-year-old woman's clinical data, which indicate signs of rejection or obstruction. (Courtesy Sandra Bringhurst, Salt Lake City, UT.)

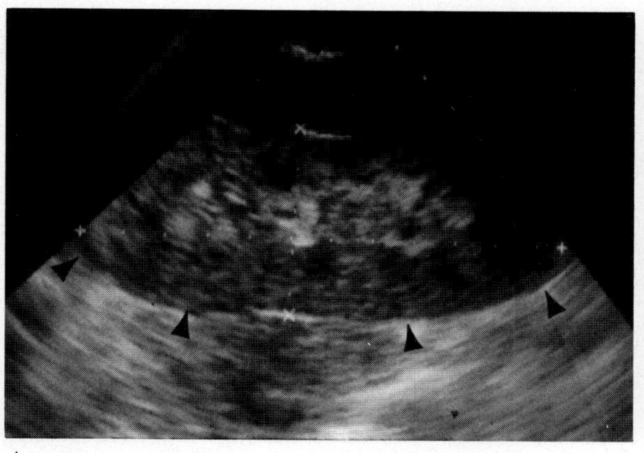

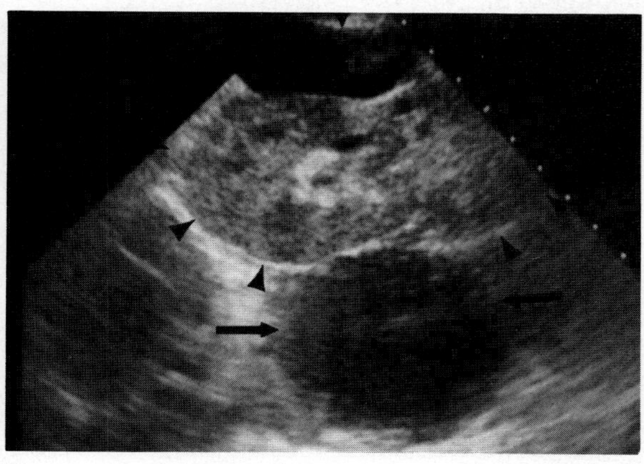

A B

FIGURE 9-49. These transverse sections of a renal allograft (cursors) in the left iliac fossa are from a follow-up examination of a 50-year-old woman. Fluid collections found on a previous examination persist anterior and posterior *(arrows)* to the allograft. Although the patient has a history of aspiration to the anterior fluid collection, it appears larger and measures 6.8 cm in the greatest length and 2.6 cm thick. The posterior fluid collection measures 7.1 cm in its greatest diameter and 5.3 cm cross-sectionally. The allograft *(arrowheads)* measures 11.6 cm long, 5.0 cm wide, and 4.5 cm thick (AP). Also, in comparison to its appearance on earlier studies, the allograft is now unusually dense, indicative of a diffuse renal parenchymal process. The renal pyramids are bright echoes, which could represent nephrocalcinosis, although no acoustic shadowing is identified. Doppler findings were normal. (Courtersy Sandra Bringhurst, Salt Lake City, UT.)

failure, appearing in as many as 50% of transplant recipients at autopsy.[56,80,104] Elevated serum creatinine levels and BUN are associated with oliguria progressing to anuria in later stages of the disease.[56,68] If uncomplicated, ATN can be reversed with an alteration in immunosuppressive therapy.[68] The diagnosis is commonly one of exclusion.[104] Associated with the sonographic appearance of no changes seen in the renal parenchyma, a clinical history and laboratory values indicative of acute renal failure strongly suggests the diagnosis of acute tubular necrosis.[55,56,68,104]

Obstructive nephropathy. Ureteral obstruction, requiring repeat surgery, occurs in 1% to 10% of transplant recipients.[7,104] Causes of obstructive uropathy include primarily ureteral necrosis,[78] followed by intrinsic blockage (blood clot, calculus, fungus ball), stricture formation, and extrinsic pressure from any pelvic mass, including a periallograft fluid collection.[7,68,104] Early in the postoperative period, the sudden onset of anuria or severe oliguria provides a clue, but the more common late obstruction usually produces nonspecific progressive azotemia, which makes clinical diagnosis difficult.[78]

Dilatation of the intrarenal collecting structures may be observed sonographically, but absence of a consistent acoustic window makes visualizing the entire ureter difficult. It should be noted that hydronephrosis and obstruction are not synonymous, and the degree of hydronephrosis does not adequately depict the severity of obstruction, or even its presence.[68] The degree of collecting system dilatation is a product of urine production, compliance of the collecting system, and the resistance to flow in the ureter and collecting system.[68] With a poorly functioning renal allograft and diminished ureteral compliance due to edema and cellular infiltration, complete obstruction can result in only modest hydronephrosis and hydroureter.[68] It is normal to see mild dilatation of the collecting structures in the immediate posttransplant period.[104] Making the diagnosis more difficult is the fact that the ureter may be dilated during episodes of acute or chronic rejection, with or without anatomic obstruction.[68,104]

If hydronephrosis is identified, it may be possible to identify an extrinsic pelvic mass, such as a lymphocele or hematoma compressing the ureter and obstructing urine flow.[7,68] Accurate diagnosis of obstruction of the urinary tract can be made in conjunction with radionuclide scanning, an IVP, or retrograde pyelography.[49,68]

Vascular compromise. Postoperatively, a renal allograft is at risk for a number of vascular lesions.[68] Since B-scan sonography alone is nonspecific, a more definitive diagnosis of both venous and arterial vascular compromise is accomplished with duplex Doppler sonography. In conjunction with clinical findings and creatinine levels, duplex Doppler findings help the clinician arrive at an accurate diagnosis.[39]

RENAL VEIN THROMBOSIS. Renal vein thrombosis is predominantly a postsurgical complication due to ischemic alteration of the vessel wall[126] or to placement of the graft into too tight a retroperitoneal pocket.[108] It is a rare cause of acute renal failure. The sonographic findings in acute renal vein thrombosis include immediate renal enlargement, increased cortical thickness, sparsely distributed cortical echoes, diminished echogenicity of the renal cortex, indistinct corticomedullary junction, and hypoechoic regions within the renal parenchyma due to hemorrhage, dilated renal vein, or renal rupture.[68] As many of these findings are similar in sonographic appearance to the morphologic changes of acute allograft rejection, interrogation of the renal vein with both real-time and Doppler sampling is recommended. No definitive signal pattern has yet been identified, but an arterial pulsed Doppler pattern of peaked antegrade systolic frequency shift, retrograde, plateaulike diastolic frequency shift,[126] and absence of the venous Doppler signal may be considered characteristic findings of acute occlusive renal vein thrombosis.[108,126] A Doppler sample with the appearance of diffuse, low-intensity intraluminal echoes or focal nodules, with or without luminal distension,[95,165] is highly suggestive of renal vein thrombosis.

VASCULAR OCCLUSION. Arterial occlusion may be due to technical difficulties at the time of surgery or to severe rejection.[108] If no arterial signals are obtained and technical factors have been excluded, arterial occlusion is present. Segmental infarction may be diagnosed by the local absence of signals within one portion of the kidney when signals are normal elsewhere in the transplant.

Diagnosing renal artery stenosis by Doppler technique depends on interrogating the main renal artery throughout its course and detecting increased velocity of blood through the stenotic segment, decreased peak frequency distal to the stenosis, and turbulence downstream from it.[108,156,163] With renal artery stenosis, the arteries of the renal hilus or parenchyma may have normal waveforms or be damped.[108] The incidence of renal artery stenosis appears to vary much, from 1.6% to 16% of allografts, but the condition is correctable.[108,156,163]

Extraperitoneal fluid collections. Peritransplant fluid collections are another frequent complication in recipients of renal allografts.[56,68,78] Common to several of these fluid complications is a decrease in renal function manifested by increased creatinine values.[56] Hematomas and abscess collections occur less frequently, and correlation to the patient's clinical presentation and laboratory values frequently aids in the diagnosis. The patient with hematoma may present with a palpable mass or enlargement of the transplant, pain and tenderness, dropping hematocrit, and hypertension.[100] The clinical signs of an abscess are leukocytosis, localized tenderness, flank pain, and fever (Fig. 9-50).[100] The sonographic features are the same as those in Table 9-12 for hematomas and Table 9-10 for abscess.

It is important to discern peritransplant fluid collections as soon as possible. Renal transplant recipients are usually in poor general health and are therapeutically immunosuppressed.[153] Following transplantation, abscesses and other infections are frequent complications, owing to the degree and duration of immune suppression.[8]

LYMPHOCELE AND LYMPH FISTULA. During renal transplant surgery, many lymphatic vessels in and around the recipient's transplant bed may be ligated.[13,56,78] If the ligated lymphatics do not rean-

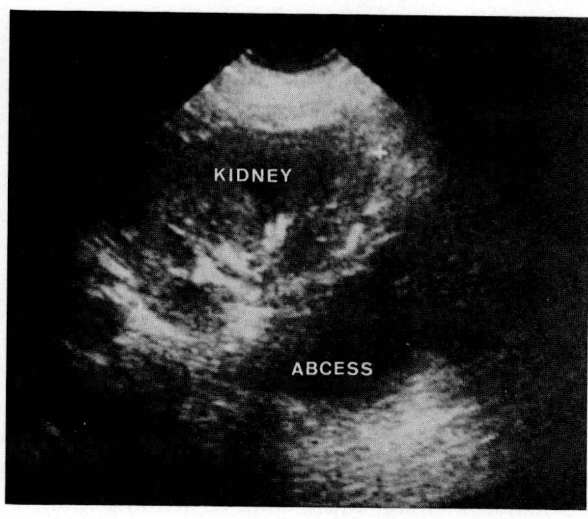

FIGURE 9-50. An abscess is visualized along the medial aspect of this right kidney allograft.

astomose spontaneously or as a reaction to the graft lymphatic,[100] a lymphocele (an accumulation of lymph) forms around the allograft.[56,78] This actually occurs in approximately 20% of transplant recipients and takes approximately 2 to 6 weeks to develop.[56,68] Clinical presentations include a palpable mass, ipsilateral leg edema, wound drainage of lymph, and variable impairment of renal function 2 weeks to 6 months after transplantation.[56,68,78]

Sonographically, lymphoceles have a variable appearance, but typically they are single, anechoic masses with well-defined borders, and occasionally they appear with numerous septations.[55,56,78] This appearance is similar to urinomas, which usually appear earlier than lymphoceles.[56] If the mass is complex with solid components, hematoma or abscess should be considered.[56,78]

URINARY FISTULA. Bladder leaks occur in approximately 10% of transplant recipients, owing to faulty surgical technique or overdistention.[56,68,78,100] Early diagnosis of a urinoma or a urinary fistula is essential, since it may lead to wound sepsis, loss of the allograft, or generalized sepsis.[68] Usually these manifest within the first 2 postoperative weeks.[56,78] Clinical presentation include local tenderness, fever, sudden decrease in urine output, or urine leakage from the wound.[56]

Sonographically, these perirenal fluid collections are anechoic with variable shapes. Typically they are walled-off urinomas adjacent to the lower pole of the allograft.[68] Septations are unusual and, unlike other peritoneal fluid collections, they have a tendency to dissect along tissue planes, necessitating careful sonographic evaluation of the flanks, scrotum, and labia.[68]

Graft rupture. Single or multiple ruptures of a graft occur in 3% to 6% of cases, within the first 2 weeks following transplantation.[56,78,113] The pathogenesis of rupture is not known[113]; however, most cases are associated with acute or hyperacute rejection.[56,78] The most common clinical presentation is pain, swelling over the graft, signs of vascular collapse, oliguria, and shock.[56,113] The sonographic finding is gross distortion of the graft contour and a perinephric or paranephric hematoma.[56,78]

Sonographically Guided Percutaneous Nephrostomy

Percutaneous nephrostomy is becoming increasingly important in the diagnosis and treatment of a wide variety of benign and malignant disorders of the genitourinary tract.[1,9,61,74,111,160] The recent advances in real-time equipment that provide high resolution, cross-sectional anatomic images has contributed to the greater safety and accurate localization and monitoring of the advancing needle or drainage catheter and identification of adjacent structures in the path.[9,61,74,111] Advances in cytologic diagnosis allow the use of small needles that permit adjacent organs and major blood vessels to be circumvented without fear of bleeding or laceration.[111]

In addition to providing tissue samples important in cytological examination of the aspirate for cysts, abscesses, and masses, percutaneous nephrostomy has been performed in patients with azotemia and urosepsis to relieve obstruction of the upper urinary tract.[77] Urine drainage, which can be a lifesaving procedure, may be accomplished by placing a catheter under sonographic guidance.[1] Renal and retroperitoneal abscesses and urine are drained extraperitoneally through the flank so as to avoid peritoneal contamination.[74] Evaluating patients following percutaneous or surgical drainage, Yoder and colleagues found that 25 of 26 patients recovered renal function even after extended periods of obstruction.[173] The low morbidity of this interventional technique is of obvious benefit to the many patients with renal infections and multisystem disorders that make them poor surgical candidates.[74]

Duplex Doppler sonography is ideal for evaluating the success of nephrostomy drainage. Platt and coworkers found a statistical significance using a threshold resistive index (RI) value of 0.70.[116] An RI value greater than 0.70 showed excellent sensitivity and specificity in distinguishing renal obstruction from unobstructed dilatation.[116] A decreased RI following percutaneous nephrostomy for relief of obstruction is highly indicative that renal obstruction is being properly relieved by a functioning tube or stent, despite persistent dilatation of the collecting system.[116]

Other Imaging Procedures

RADIOGRAPHY

Standard radiographic techniques fail to accurately outline the kidneys in many patients and provide no information about their internal structure.[26] Radiographic imaging after intravenous injection of iodinated contrast material (excretory nephrogram or IVP) provides valuable information about renal function and structural integrity,[26] but visualization of the kidneys is unlikely with elevated creatinine levels.[57] Also, the examination is contraindicated for patients with a history of severe contrast reactions and moderate renal failure.[57]

RADIONUCLIDE STUDIES

If allograft function is compromised following renal transplant, the initial imaging modality should be a radionuclide renogram using technetium^{99m}-DTPA(diethyltriamine pentaacetic acid).[89] The vascular, excretory, and drainage phases of the examination permit the evaluation of renal perfusion, renal parenchymal function, and the status of the collecting system.[89] This provides useful diagnostic distinction of rejection from acute tubular necrosis and demonstrates several less common complications, such as vascular occlusion, urinary extravasation, obstruction, and lymphocele.[14]

COMPUTED TOMOGRAPHY

CT, like sonography, is capable of imaging the kidneys in cross-sectional planes. Because of cost, availability, and ionizing radiation, CT is rarely indicated as a primary modality for assessing abnormalities of renal size.[26] CT is an excellent adjunctive procedure for the detection, characterization, and staging of renal masses.[27] Contrast-enhanced CT is excellent for distinguishing an organizing abscess from inflammatory edema and in evaluating the perinephric spaces.[57] In patients with hypertension, CT is the imaging modality of choice to determine if the underlying cause is an adrenal or extraadrenal pheochromocytoma.[148] In the diagnosis of renal and perirenal abscesses, CT may be more sensitive, in that it is capable of detecting poorly defined, smaller abscesses and of defining subtle alterations in perinephric fat.[64] CT has a limited role in evaluating failing renal transplants.[89]

MAGNETIC RESONANCE IMAGING

MRI has advantages in staging renal cell carcinoma because of its ability to clearly demonstrate any perivascular adenopathy or tumor thrombus within a vascular lumen without the need for intravenous contrast material.[27] Even though abscesses cannot be distinguished from necrotic tumors, MRI is valuable in the detection of fluid-filled processes in the retroperitoneum, and better specificity has been demonstrated in the case of hematomas.[57] MRI is rarely used to evaluate suspected secondary hypertension[148] or suspected renal transplant failure.[89]

Conclusion

This chapter details the importance of understanding how vital the kidneys are to normal body function and of recognizing the sonographic presentation of the kidneys' normal location, contour, size, and internal architecture. Identifying deviations from the norm and correlating these findings with the clinical history, laboratory values, and radiographic images narrows the differential diagnosis. The superb imaging obtained without dependence on renal function, coupled with equipment availability, the lack of ionizing radiation, and removal of the risk of exposing the patient to the parenteral administration of potentially nephrotoxic contrast material, makes ultrasonography an invaluable modality in the evaluation of the kidneys.

References

1. Alter AJ: Percutaneous nephropyelostemy. Semin Ultrasound 1981, 2:61–70.
2. Ambos MA, Bosniak MA, Gordon R, et al: Replacement lipomatosis of the kidney. AJR 1978, 130:1087–1091.
3. Anderhub B: Manual of Abdominal Sonography. Baltimore, University Park Press, 1983.
4. Anderson BL, Curry NS, Gobien RP: Sonography of evolving renal cystic transformation associated with hemodialysis. AJR 1983, 141:1003–1004.
5. Anthony CP, Thibodeau GA: Textbook of Anatomy and Physiology, 10th ed. St. Louis, CV Mosby, 1979.
6. Babcock DS: Medical disease of the urinary tract and adrenal gland. Clin Diagn Ultrasound 1981, 8:113–134.
7. Balchunas WR, Hill MC, Isikoff MB, et al: The clinical significance of dilatation of the collecting system in the transplanted kidney. J Clin Ultrasound 1982, 10:221–225.
8. Balsara VJ, Raval B, Maklad NF: Emphysematous pyelonephritis in a renal transplant: Sonographic and computed tomographic features. J Ultrasound Med 1985, 4:97–99.
9. Baron RL, Lee JKT, McClennan BL: Percutaneous nephrostomy using real-time sonographic guidance. AJR 1981, 136:1018–1019.
10. Behan M, Kazam E: The echographic characteristic of fatty tissues and tumors. Radiology 1978, 129:143–151.
11. Benitez CM, Cyr DR, Mack LA: Crossed fused renal ectopia: A sonographic diagnosis. J Diagn Med Sonogr 1985, 1:218–220.
12. Berland LL, Lawson TL, Adams MB, et al: Evaluation of renal transplants with pulsed Doppler duplex sonography. J Ultrasound Med 1982, 1:215–222.
13. Birnholz JC, Merkel FK: Submucosal edema of the collecting system: A new ultrasonic sign of severe, acute renal allograft rejection. Radiology 1985, 154:190.
14. Blumhardt R, Growcock G, Lasher JC: Cortical necrosis in a renal transplant. AJR 1983, 141:95–96.
15. Brandt TD, Neiman HL, Dragowski MJ, et al: Ultrasound assessment of normal renal dimensions. J Ultrasound Med 1982, 1:49–52.
16. Brenner B, Coe FL, Rector FC: Renal Physiology in Health and Disease. Philadelphia, WB Saunders, 1987.
17. Brown JM: The ultrasound approach to the urographically nonvisualizing kidney. Semin Ultrasound 1981, 2:44–48.
18. Bullock BL, Rosendahl PP: Pathophysiology: Adaptations and Alterations in Function, 2nd ed. Glenview, IL, Scott, Foresman, 1988.
19. Bush WH, Allen FH: Ultrasonography in the evaluation of renal masses. Appl Radiol 1979, 8(4):87–91.
20. Charboneau JW, Hattery RR, Ernest EC, et al: Spectrum of sonographic findings in 125 renal masses other than benign simple cyst. AJR 1983, 140:87–94.
21. Coleman BG, Arger PH, Mulhern CB, et al: Grayscale sonographic spectrum of hypernephromas. Radiology 1980, 137:757–765.
22. Coleman BG, Arger PH, Mulhern CB, et al: Pyonephrosis: Sonography in the diagnosis and management. AJR 1981, 137:939–943.
23. Corbet JV: Laboratory Tests and Diagnostic Procedures with Nursing Diagnosis, 2nd ed. Norwalk, CT, Appleton and Lange, 1987.
24. Craig M: Pocket Guide to Ultrasound Measurements. Philadelphia, JB Lippincott, 1988.
25. Cronan JJ, Yoder IC, Amis ES, et al: The myth of anechoic renal sinus fat. Radiology 1982, 144:149–152.
26. Davidson AJ: Abnormal renal size. *In* Eisenberg RL (ed): Diagnostic Imaging: An Algorithmic Approach. Philadelphia, JB Lippincott, 1988.
27. Demas BE, Fisher MR: Renal masses. *In* Eisenberg RL, (ed): Diagnostic Imaging: An Algorithmic Approach. Philadelphia, JB Lippincott, 1988.
28. Dierks PR, Berman MC: Renal cell carcinoma: Ultrasound, CT, and MRI correlation. J Diagn Med Sonogr 1987, 3:136–140.
29. Dubbins PA, Kurtz AB, Wapner RJ, et al: Renal agenesis: Spectrum of in utero findings. J Clin Ultrasound 1981, 9:189–193.
30. Edell SL, Bonavita JA: The sonographic appearance of acute pyelonephritis. Radiology 1979, 132:683–685.
31. Elyaderani MK, Gabriele OF: Ultrasound of renal masses. Semin Ultrasound 1981, 2:21–43.
32. England MA: Color Atlas of Life Before Birth: Normal Fetal Development. Chicago, Year Book Medical Publishers, 1983.
33. Erwin BC, Carroll BA, Walter JF, et al: Renal infarction appearing as an echogenic mass. AJR 1982, 138:759–761.
34. Felman AE, Pollack HM, Perri AJ, et al: Renal pseudotumors: An anatomic-radiologic classification. J Urol 1978, 120:133–139.
35. Ferris EJ, Seibert JJ: Urinary Tract and Adrenal Glands: Imaging and Diagnosis. New York, Grune & Stratton, 1980.
36. Filly R, Sommet R, Minton M: Characterization of

biologic fluid by ultrasound and computed tomography. Radiology 1980, 134:161–171.
37. Finberg H: Renal ultrasound: Anatomy and technique. Semin Ultrasound 1981, 2:7–20.
38. Finberg HJ, Hillman B, Smith EH: Ultrasound in the evaluation of the nonfunctioning kidney. Clin Diagn Ultrasound 1979, 2:105–123.
39. Fleischer AC, Hinton AA, Glick AD, et al: Duplex Doppler sonography of renal transplants. J Ultrasound Med 1989, 8:89–94.
40. Frick MP, Feinberg SB, Sibley R, et al: Ultrasound in acute renal transplant rejection. Radiology 1981, 138:657–660.
41. Fried AM, Woodring JH, Loh FK, et al: The medullary pyramid index: An objective assessment of prominence in renal transplant rejection. Radiology 1983, 149:787–791.
42. Fried AM, Woodring JH, Thompson DJ: Hydronephrosis of pregnancy: A prospective sequential study of the course of dilatation. J Ultrasound Med 1982, 3:255–259.
43. Gardiner KL: The renal sonographic appearance of sickle cell disease. J Diagn Med Sonogr 1987, 3:14–19.
44. Garten KJ, Pulliam RP: Hydronephrosis in pregnancy. J Diagn Med Sonogr 1985, 1:95–99.
45. Gerzof SG, Gale ME: Computed tomography and ultrasonography for diagnosis and treatment of renal and retroperitoneal abscesses. Urol Clin North Am 1982, 9:185–193.
46. Goiney RC, Goldenberg L, Cooperberg PL, et al: Renal oncocytomas: Sonographic analysis of 14 cases. AJR 1984, 143:1001–1004.
47. Gold RP, McClennan BL, Rottenberg RR: CT appearance of acute inflammatory disease of the renal interstitium. AJR 1983, 141:343–349.
48. Goldman SM, Hartman DS, Fishman EK, et al: CT of xanthogranulomatous pyelonephritis: Radiologic-pathologic correlation. AJR 1984, 142:963–969.
49. Gooding GAW: Sonography of hemorrhagic cysts with computed tomographic correlation. J Ultrasound Med 1986, 5:699–702.
50. Gray H: Gray's Anatomy: Anatomy of the Human Body, 29th ed (American Edition, edited by Charles Mayo Goss). Philadelphia, Lea & Febiger, 1973.
51. Green B, Goldstein H, Weaver R: Abdominal pansonography in evaluation of renal cancer. Radiology 1979, 132:421–424.
52. Green D, Carroll BA: Ultrasound of renal failure. Clin Diagn Ultrasound 1986, 18:55–88.
53. Grossman H, Rosenberg ER, Bowie JD, et al: Sonographic diagnosis of renal cystic diseases. AJR 1983, 140:81–85.
54. Guidi SM, Sanders RC: Renal failure. *In* Sanders RC: Clinical Sonography: A Practical Guide. Boston, Little Brown and Company, 1984.
55. Guidi SM, Sanders RC: Renal transplant. *In* Sanders RC: Clinical Sonography: A Practical Guide. Boston, Little Brown and Company, 1984.
56. Hagen-Ansert SL: Textbook of Diagnostic Ultrasonography, 3rd ed. St. Louis, CV Mosby, 1989.
57. Hahn PF, Yoder IC: Fever and flank pain: Suspected infection of the upper urinary tract in adults. *In* Eisenberg RL (ed): Diagnostic Imaging: An Algorithmic Approach. Philadelphia, JB Lippincott, 1988.
58. Hartman DS, Davis CJ, Goldman SM, et al: Xanthogranulomatous pyelonephritis: Sonographic-pathologic correlation of 16 cases. J Ultrasound Med 1984, 3:481–488.
59. Hartman DS, Goldman SM, Friedman AC, et al: Angiomyolipoma: Ultrasonic-pathologic correlation. Radiology 1981, 139:451–458.
60. Hidalgo H, Dunnick NR, Rosenberg ER, et al: Parapelvic cysts: Appearance on CT and sonography. AJR 1982, 138:667–671.
61. Hightower DR, Laing FC, Jeffrey B: A tandem guide for renal biopsy. J Ultrasound Med 1985, 4:441–443.
62. Hill LM, Peterson CS: Antenatal diagnosis of fetal pelvic kidneys. J Ultrasound Med 1987, 6:393–396.
63. Hoddick W, Filly RA, Backman U, et al: Renal allograft rejection: US evaluation. Radiology 1986, 161:469–473.
64. Hoddick W, Jeffrey RB, Goldberg HI, et al: CT and sonography of severe renal and perirenal infections. AJR 1983, 140:517–520.
65. Hricak, H: Renal ultrasound. *In* Sarti DA (ed): Diagnostic Ultrasound: Text & Cases, 2nd ed. Chicago, Year Book Medical Publishers, 1987.
66. Hricak H, Cruz C, Eyler WR, et al: Acute post-transplantation renal failure: Differential diagnosis by ultrasound. Radiology 1981, 139:441–449.
67. Hricak H, Cruz C, Romanski R, et al: Renal parenchymal disease: Sonographic-histologic correlation. Radiology 1982, 144:141–147.
68. Hricak H, Hoddick WK: Ultrasound in renal transplantation. Clin Diagn Ultrasound 1986, 18:161–179.
69. Hricak H, Lieto RP: Sonographic determination of renal volume. Radiology 1983, 148:311–312.
70. Hricak H, Romanski RN, Eyler WR: The renal sinus during allograft rejection: Sonographic and histopathologic findings. Radiology 1982, 142:693–699.
71. Jacobs D, Kasten B, Demott W, et al: Laboratory Test Handbook with DRG Index. St Louis, CV Mosby, 1984.
72. Janetschek G, Putz A, Feichtinger H: Renal transi-

tional cell carcinoma mimicking stone echoes. J Ultrasound Med 1987, 7:83–86.

73. Jeanty P, Dramaix-Wilmet M, Elkhazen N, et al: Measurement of fetal kidney growth on ultrasound. Radiology 1982, 144:159–162.
74. Jeffrey RB, Kuligowska: Interventional ultrasound. Clin Diagn Ultrasound 1986, 18:113–134.
75. Jeffrey RB, Laing FC, Wing VW, et al: Sonography of the fetal duplex kidney. Radiology 1984, 153:123–124.
76. Jeffrey RB, Laing FC, Wing VW, et al: Sensitivity of sonography in pyonephrosis: A reevaluation. AJR 1985, 144:71–73.
77. Jeffrey RB, Vernacchia FS: The role of sonography and CT in urosepsis. J Diagn Med Sonogr 1986, 2:141–144.
78. Johnson ML, Dunne MG, Watts B, et al: Ultrasonography in renal transplantation. Clin Diagn Ultrasound 1979, 2:89–104.
79. Jones BE, Hoffer FA, Teele RL, et al: The compound renal pyramid: A normal hypoechoic region on the pediatric sonogram. J Ultrasound Med 1987, 6:515–518.
80. Jones TB, Riddick LR, Harpen MD, et al: Ultrasonographic determination of renal mass and renal volume. J Ultrasound Med 1983, 2:151–154.
81. Joseph N, Neiman HL, Vogelzang RL: renal masses. Clin Diagn Ultrasound 1986, 18:135–160.
82. Karp W, Ekelund L, Olafsson G, et al: Computed tomography, angiography and ultrasound in staging of renal carcinoma. Acta Radiol 1981, 22:625–633.
83. Katz JF, Nichols L, Kane RA, et al: Renal cell carcinoma: An unusual sonographic appearance. J Ultrasound Med 1986, 5:517–519.
84. Kaude JV, Williams CM, Millner MR, et al: Renal morphology and function immediately after extracorporeal shock-wave lithotripsy. AJR 1985, 145:305–313.
85. Krebs CA, Giyanani VL, Nall LA: Duplex sonography and Doppler evaluation of renal cell carcinoma with inferior vena cava involvement. J Diagn Med Sonogr 1989, 5:126–130.
86. Kuijpers D, Jaspers R: Renal masses: Differential diagnosis with pulsed Doppler US. Radiology 1989, 170:59–60.
87. Kuligowska E: Renal infections. Clin Diagn Ultrasound 1986, 18:89–112.
88. Kuligowska E, Newman B, White SJ, et al: Interventional ultrasound detection and treatment of renal inflammatory disease. Radiology 1983, 147:521–526.
89. Kumar R: Complications of renal transplantation. *In* Eisenberg RL (ed): Diagnostic Imaging: An Algorithmic Approach. Philadelphia, JB Lippincott, 1988.
90. Kurtz AB, Dubbins PA, Zegel HG, et al: Normal left renal vein mimicking left renal artery aneurysm. J Clin Ultrasound 1981, 9:105–108.
91. Kutcher R, Amodio JB, Rosenblatt R: Uremic renal cystic disease: Value of sonographic screening. Radiology 1983, 147:833–835.
92. Lamb JA: Laboratory Tests for Clinical Nursing. Bowie, MD, RJ Brady, Prentice-Hall, 1984.
93. Lavallee G, Lafortune M, Gilchrist L, et al: Obstructed duplex kidney in an adult: Ultrasonic evaluation. J Clin Ultrasound 1985, 13:281–283.
94. Lee JKT, McClennan BL, Melson GL, et al: Acute focal bacterial nephritis: Emphasis on gray-scale sonography and computed tomography. AJR 1980, 135:87–92.
95. Levine E, Maklad NF, Rosenthal SJ, et al: Comparison of computed tomography and ultrasound in abdominal staging of renal cancer. Urology 1980, 16:317–322.
96. Linkowski GD, Warvariv V, Filly RA, et al: Sonography in the diagnosis of acute renal allograft rejection and cyclosporine nephrotoxicity. AJR 1987, 148:291–295.
97. Lubat E, Hernanz-Schulman M, Genieser NB, et al: Sonography of the simple and complicated ipsilateral fused kidney. J Ultrasound Med 1989, 8:109–114.
98. McArdle CR, Grumbach K: Sonographic and computed tomographic appearances of acquired renal cystic disease. J Ultrasound Med 1983, 2:519–520.
99. McCarthy S, Rosenfield AT: Ultrasonography in crossed renal ectopia. J Ultrasound Med 1984, 3:107–112.
100. Maklad NF: Ultrasonic evaluation of renal transplants. Semin Ultrasound 1981, 2:88–96.
101. Marieb EN: Human Anatomy and Physiology. Redwood City, CA, The Benjamin/Cummings Publishing Company, 1989.
102. Mindell HJ, Kupic EA: Horseshoe kidney: Ultrasonic demonstration. AJR 1977, 129:526–527.
103. Mines EG, Berne AS: Radiologic evaluation of ureteral duplications. Med Radiog Photog 1973, 49:30–58.
104. Mittelstaedt CA: Abdominal Ultrasound. New York, Churchill Livingstone, 1987.
105. Morcos SK: Intrathoracic kidney with a simple cyst in its upper pole diagnosed by ultrasound. J Clin Ultrasound 1985, 13:127–129.
106. Morehouse HT, Weiner SN, Hoffman JC: Imaging in inflammatory disease of the kidney. AJR 1984, 143:135–141.
107. Morehouse HT, Weiner SN, Hoffman-Tretin JC: Inflammatory disease of the kidney. Semin Ultrasound CT MR 1986, 7:246–258.

108. Needleman L, Kurtz AB: Doppler evaluation of the renal transplant. J Clin Ultrasound 1987, 15:661–673.
109. Netter FH: The CIBA Collection of Medical Illustrations, vol 6, Kidney, Ureters, and the Urinary Bladder. Rochester, NY, The Case-Hoyt Corporation, 1965.
110. Nicolet V, Carignan L, Dubuc G, et al: Thickening of the renal collecting system: A nonspecific finding at US. Radiology 1988, 168:411–413.
111. Nosher JL, Amorosa JK, Leiman S, et al: Fine needle aspiration of the kidney and adrenal gland. J Urol 1982, 128:895–899.
112. Odwin CS, Dubinsky T, Fleischer AC: Ultrasonography Examination Review and Study Guide. Norwalk, CT, Appleton and Lange, 1987.
113. Ostrovsky PD, Carr L, Goodman JD, et al: Ultrasound findings in renal transplant rupture. J Clin Ultrasound 1985, 13:132–133.
114. Pardes JG, Yong HA, Kazam E: Sonographic findings in myoglobinuric renal failure and their clinical implications. J Ultrasound Med 1983, 2:391–394.
115. Peake SL, Roxburgh HB, Langlois SL: Ultrasonic assessment of hydronephrosis of pregnancy. Radiology 1983, 146:167–170.
116. Platt JF, Rubin JM, Ellis JH, et al: Duplex Doppler US of the kidney: Differentiation of obstructive from nonobstructive dilatation. Radiology 1989, 171:515–517.
117. Pollack HM, Banner MP, Arger PH, et al: Comparison of computed tomography and ultrasound in the diagnosis of renal masses. Clin Diagn Ultrasound 1979, 2:25–72.
118. Pollack HM, Banner MP, Arger PH, et al: The accuracy of gray-scale ultrasonography in differentiating cystic neoplasms from benign cysts. Radiology 1982, 143:741–745.
119. Porth CM: Pathophysiology: Concepts of Altered Health States. Philadelphia, JB Lippincott, 1986.
120. Price SA, Wilson LM: Pathophysiology: Clinical Concepts of Disease Processes, 2nd ed. New York, McGraw-Hill, 1982.
121. Quinn MJ, Hartman DS, Friedman AC, et al: Renal oncocytoma: New observations. Radiology 1984, 153:49–53.
122. Raghavendra BN, Bosniak MA, Megibow AJ: Small angiomyolipoma of the kidney: Sonographic-CT evaluation. AJR 1983, 141:575–578.
123. Raiss GJ, Bree RL, Schwab RE, et al: Further observations in the ultrasound evaluation of renal allograft rejection. J Ultrasound Med 1986, 5:439–444.
124. Ralls PW, Halls J: Hydronephrosis, renal cystic disease, and renal parenchymal disease. Semin Ultrasound 1981, 2:49–60.
125. Rego JD, Laing FC, Jeffrey RB: Ultrasonographic diagnosis of medullary cystic disease. J Ultrasound Med 1983, 2:433–436.
126. Reuther G, Wanjura D, Bauer H: Acute renal vein thrombosis in renal allografts: Detection with duplex Doppler US. Radiology 1989, 170:557–558.
127. Rigsby CM, Burns PN, Weltin GC, et al: Doppler signal quantitation in renal allografts: Comparison in normal and rejecting transplants, with pathologic correlation. Radiology 1987, 162:39–42.
128. Rigsby CM, Taylor KJW, Weltin G, et al: Renal allografts in acute rejection: Evaluation using duplex sonography. Radiology 1986, 158:375–378.
129. Robbins SL, Cotran RS: Pathologic Basis of Diseases, 2nd ed. Philadelphia, WB Saunders, 1979.
130. Rosenberg ER, Clair MR, Bowie JD: The fluid-filled stomach as an acoustic window into the left kidney. AJR 1982, 138:175–176.
131. Rosenberg HK: Traumatic avulsion of the vascular supply of a crossed unfused ectopic kidney: Complementary roles of ultrasonography and intravenous pyelography. J Ultrasound Med 1984, 3:89–91.
132. Rosenfield AT, Glickman MG, Taylor KJW, et al: Acute focal bacterial nephritis (acute lobar nephronia). Radiology 1979, 132:553–561.
133. Rosenfield AT, Lipson MH, Wold B, et al: Ultrasonography and nephrotomography in the presymptomatic diagnosis of dominantly inherited (adult onset) polycystic kidney disease. Radiology 1980, 135:423–427.
134. Rosenfield AT, Siegel NJ: Renal parenchymal disease: Histopathologic-sonographic correlation. AJR 1981, 137:793–798.
135. Rosenfield AT, Taylor KJW, Crade M: Renal ultrasound 1979: Gray-scale, real-time, Doppler. Clin Diagn Ultrasound 1979, 2:1–24.
136. Rosenfield AT, Taylor KJW, Crade M, et al: Anatomy and pathology of the kidney by gray-scale ultrasound. Radiology 1978, 128:737–744.
137. Rosenfield AT, Taylor KJW, Jaffe CC: Clinical applications of ultrasound tissue characterization. Radiol Clin North Am 1980, 18:31–58.
138. Rosenfield AT, Zeman RK, Cicchetti DV, et al: Experimental acute tubular necrosis: US appearance. Radiology 1985, 157:771–774.
139. Sanders RC: Examination of kidneys not seen at excretion urography. *In* Resnick MI, Sanders RC (eds): Ultrasound in Urology. Baltimore, Williams & Wilkins, 1979.
140. Sanders RC: Possible renal mass. *In* Sanders RC: Clinical Sonography: A Practical Guide. Boston, Little, Brown, 1984.

141. Sanders RC: Kidneys not seen on intravenous pyelogram. *In* Sanders RC: Clinical Sonography: A Practical Guide. Boston, Little, Brown, 1984.
142. Sanders RC: Unexplained hematocrit drop: Rule out perinephric hematoma; possible perinephric mass. *In* Sanders RC: Clinical Sonography: A Practical Guide. Boston, Little, Brown, 1984.
143. Sanders RC, Conrad MR: The ultrasonic characteristics of the renal pelvicalyceal echo complex. J Clin Ultrasound 1976, 5:372–377.
144. Sarti DA: Diagnostic Ultrasound: Text & Cases, 2nd ed. Chicago, Year Book Medical Publishers, 1987.
145. Scanlon MH, Karasick SR: Acquired renal cystic disease and neoplasia: Complications of chronic hemodialysis. Radiology 1983, 147:837–838.
146. Sceusa DK, Klein PE: Ultrasonography of horseshoe kidney: A new technique. J Diagn Med Sonogr 1987, 3:38–41.
147. Schaffer RM, Shih YH, Becker JA: Sonographic identification of collecting system duplications. J Clin Ultrasound 1983, 11:309–312.
148. Schwarten, DE: Hypertension. *In* Eisenberg RL (ed): Diagnostic Imaging: An Algorithmic Approach. Philadelphia, JB Lippincott, 1988.
149. Schwerk WB, Schwerk WN, Rodeck G: Venous renal tumor extension: A prospective US evaluation. Radiology 1985, 156:491–495.
150. Seeley RR, Stephens TD, Tate P: Anatomy and Physiology. St. Louis, Times Mirror/Mosby College Publishing, 1989.
151. Sefczek RJ, Beckman I, Lupetin AR, et al: Sonography of acute renal cortical necrosis. AJR 1984, 142:553–554.
152. Siegel MJ, Glasier CM: Acute focal bacterial nephritis in children: Significance of ureteral reflux. AJR 1981, 137: 257–260.
153. Silver TM, Campbell D, Wicks JD, et al: Peritransplant fluid collections. Radiology 1981, 138:145–151.
154. Silver TM, Kass EJ, Thornbury JR, et al: The radiologic spectrum of acute pyelonephritis in adults and adolescents. Radiology 1976, 118:65–71.
155. Smith SJ, Bosniak MA, Megibow AJ, et al: Renal cell carcinoma: Earlier discovery and increased detection. Radiology 1989, 170:699–703.
156. Snider JF, Hunter DW, Moradian GP, et al: Transplant renal artery stenosis: Evaluation with duplex sonography. Radiology 1989, 172:1027–1030.
157. Sommer FG, Filly RA, Minton MJ: Acoustic shadowing due to reflective and refractive effects. AJR 1979, 132:973–977.
158. Spence AP, Mason EB: Human Anatomy and Physiology. Menlo Park, CA, Benjamin/Cummings, 1987.
159. Spies JB, Hricak H, Slemmer TM, et al: Sonographic evaluation of experimental acute renal arterial occlusion in dogs. AJR 1984, 142:341–346.
160. Stables DP, Johnson ML: Percutaneous nephrostomy: The role of ultrasound. Clin Diagn Ultrasound 1979, 2:73–88.
161. Starrett ES: Laboratory values associated with renal function and disease processes. J Diagn Med Sonogr 1986, 2:206–218.
162. Subramanyam BR, Raghavendra BN, Bosniak MA, et al: Sonography of Pyonephrosis: A prospective study. AJR 1983, 140:991–993.
163. Taylor KJW, Morse SS, Rigsby CM, et al: Vascular complication in renal allografts: Detection with duplex Doppler US. Radiology 1987, 162:31–38.
164. Thomas CL (ed): Taber's Cyclopedic Medical Dictionary, 16th ed. Philadelphia, FA Davis, 1989.
165. Thomas JL, Bernandino ME: Neoplastia-induced renal vein enlargement: Sonographic detection. AJR 1981, 136:75–79.
166. Tilkian SO, Conover MB, Tilkian AG: Clinical Implications of Laboratory Tests, 3rd ed. St. Louis, CV Mosby, 1983.
167. Tortora GJ, Anagnastakos NP: Principles of Anatomy and Physiology, 5th ed. New York, Harper and Row, 1987.
168. Toyoda K, Miyamoto Y, Masahiro I, et al: Hypoecoic medulla of the kidneys. Radiology 1989, 173:431–434.
169. Van Kirk OC, Go RT, Wedel VJ: Sonographic features of xanthogranulomatous pyelonephritis. AJR 1980, 134:1035–1039.
170. Walker FC, Loney LC, Root ER, et al: Diagnostic evaluation of adult polycystic kidney disease in childhood. AJR 1984, 142:1273–1277.
171. Wicks JD, Thornbury JR: Acute renal infections in adults. Radiol Clin North Am 1979, 17:245–260.
172. Yoder IC, Lindfors KK, Pfister RC: Diagnosis and treatment of pyonephrosis. Radiol Clin North Am 1984, 22:407–414.
173. Yoder IC, Pfister RC, Lindfors KK, et al: Pyonephrosis: Imaging and intervention. AJR 1983, 141:735–740.

CHAPTER 10

Urinary Bladder

SHARON ROBERTS, DIANE M. KAWAMURA

The urinary bladder, ureters, and urethra are important in urine transport and storage. The urine-filled bladder is one of the most accessible abdominopelvic organs for ultrasound examination. Recognizing normal position, size, and appearance helps the sonographer identify bladder anomalies and pathologies.

Anatomy and Organogenesis

The ends of the mesonephric ducts (wolffian and müllerian) and the endodermal cloaca form the urinary bladder.[13] The cloaca, the terminal, caudal, blind-ended portion of the hindgut, is the major structure that forms the lower part of the urinary and genital tract.[28,43] Its primary function is to serve as the primitive receptacle into which the reproductive and excretory tracts empty. At approximately the sixth week of gestation, the urorectal septum migrates caudad and eventually divides the cloaca into the rectum dorsally and the urogenital sinus ventrally.[24,28] This division of the cloaca is the initial step in the development of the urinary bladder.[30]

A prominent excretory structure becomes apparent in the 4- to 6-week-old embryo.[29] The distal wolffian duct and the point of origin of the ureter are incorporated into the urogenital sinus and form the area that will become the bladder trigone. The urogenital sinus then divides into a distal pars phallica, into which the wolffian duct opens, and a proximal pars pelvina, into which the ureters open. By the fourth fetal month, these two parts form the characteristic shape of the adult bladder and proceed to further develop the urethra.[2,21,28] The wolffian ducts give origin to the ureters, form the efferent tubules, duct of the epididymis, vas deferens, seminal vesicles, and ejaculatory ducts in males, and the epoophoron, paraoophoron, and Gartner's duct in females.[27]

The müllerian ducts develop in the embryo by the end of the second month.[27] These ducts terminate in the primitive urogenital sinus and fuse together. In males, most of the müllerian duct degenerates but the caudal end forms the prostatic urethra.[28] In females, the müllerian duct forms the uterus, proximal vagina, and fallopian tubes.[27,28]

The urachus, an embryonic communication between the bladder and the allantoic stock, develops into the fibrous medial umbilical ligament. It extends from the apex of the bladder to the umbilicus.[28]

URINARY BLADDER

The bladder develops into a hollow muscular viscus that serves as a reservoir for urine.[41] The urinary bladder is lined with a mucous membrane of transitional epithelium.[39,41] The mucous membrane lining of the bladder contains rugae, or folds.[45,46] When the bladder is empty, the membrane appears folded or wrinkled.[2] It is loosely attached to the underlying muscle coat, except in the trigone region where it is firmly attached to the muscular coat, appears smooth, and does not expand during bladder filling.[24,39,41]

Covering the transitional epithelium, the bladder wall is composed of three layers of smooth muscle fibers; a connective tissue submucosa, a muscle layer, and a fibrous adventitia.[24,41] The outer fibrous adventitia is continuous except on the superior surface of the bladder, which is covered by the parietal peritoneum.[24] The inner connective tissue submucosa and the outer fibrous adventitia are characterized by longitudinal layers. They enclose the detrusor muscle; the prominent circular middle muscle layer.[41]

Because of the lining's elasticity and rugae and the wall's elasticity, the bladder is capable of considerable distension, which is advantageous for an organ that continuously inflates and deflates.[3,32,46] Individual bladder capacity varies greatly, and the normal adult bladder is generally emptied before it reaches its potential capacity of 600 to 800 ml.[41,46] The bladder's size, position, and relationship to other structures vary according to its fluid content.

RELATIONSHIPS

Like the other urinary structures, the urinary bladder is located retroperitoneally on the pelvic floor.[24,41] Normally, the bladder is a round-edged tetrahedron with a superior, a posterior, and two inferior surfaces.[28] The superior surface has two regions: the fundus located posteriorly and the apex located anteriorly.[28] The two ureteral orifices are located in the body on the posteroinferior portion. The urethral orifice is located in the neck of the bladder and is the most inferior region.[28]

When empty, the anterior surfaces lies just behind and rarely superior to the symphysis in both males and females.[28,39] The fibrous medial umbilical ligament (obliterated urachus) extends from the apex upward as a blunt cone with a solid, slender continuation in the midline of the abdominal wall and attaches to the umbilicus.[27,28]

When distended with urine, the bladder can rise approximately 16 cm above the symphysis pubis. It ascends into the abdominal cavity, comes in contact with the lower anterior abdominal wall, and can be readily palpated or percussed. With overdistension, such as acute or chronic urinary retention, the lower abdomen may bulge visibly. As the bladder enlarges, it loses its ovoid or spherical configuration and becomes more globular. Coils of the small intestine lie adjacent to the upper surface of the bladder and are displaced posteriorly as the bladder enlarges.

In the female, the fundal region of the bladder lies in contact with the anterior wall of the vagina and cervix (Fig. 10-1). The uterus and vagina are interposed between bladder and rectum. When the bladder is empty the uterus rests on its superior surface.

In the male, the fundus and the body of the bladder are related to the rectum, separated above by the rectovesical pouch of peritoneum and inferolaterally on each side by a ductus deferens and seminal vesicle. The base of the prostate is applied to the caudal surface of the bladder. The greater part of this surface is directly continuous with the bladder wall (Fig. 10-2).

TRIGONE

The trigone is outlined by the three openings in the bladder—two from the ureters and one into the urethra. The ureteral orifices are situated superiorly and laterally at the extremities of the crescent-shaped interureteric ridge that forms the proximal border of the trigone.[4] The urethral opening is located at its anterior, midline, lower corner (Fig. 10-3).

URETHRA

The urethra is a small muscular tube lined with mucous membrane leading from the interior surface of the bladder to the exterior. It is the terminal portion of the urinary tract and serves as the conduit for eliminating urine.[41,46] In addition, the male urethra is the terminal portion of the reproductive tract and serves as the passage for ejaculate (semen). The female urethra serves only the urinary tract.[41]

At the bladder surface, smooth bladder muscle serves as the internal urethral sphincter. The external sphincter, or bladder neck, is not a true circular sphincter but a thickening formed by interlaced and converging fibers of the detrusor muscle as they pass distally to become the smooth musculature of the urethra.[3,6] The opening of the urethra to the exterior is referred to as the urinary meatus.

The female urethra lies directly posterior to the

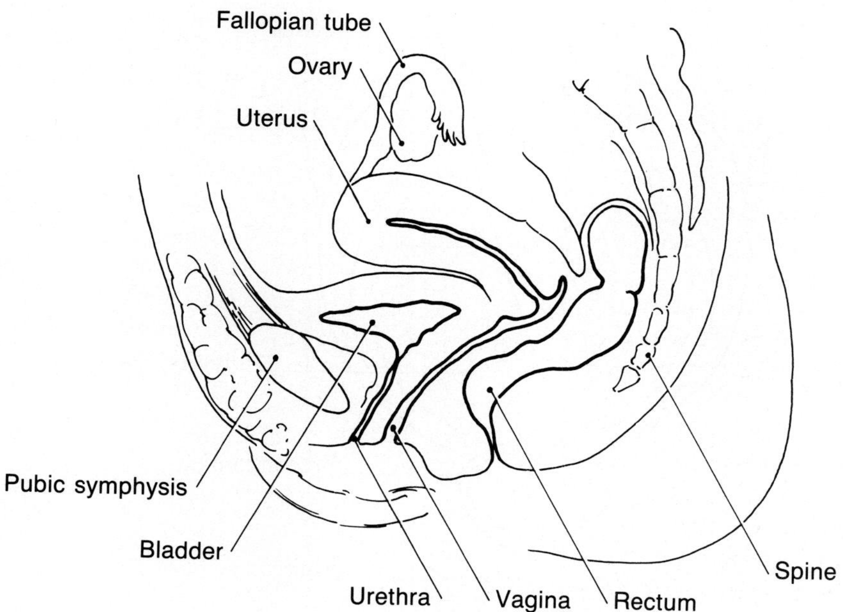

FIGURE 10-1. Sagittal view of the female pelvis.

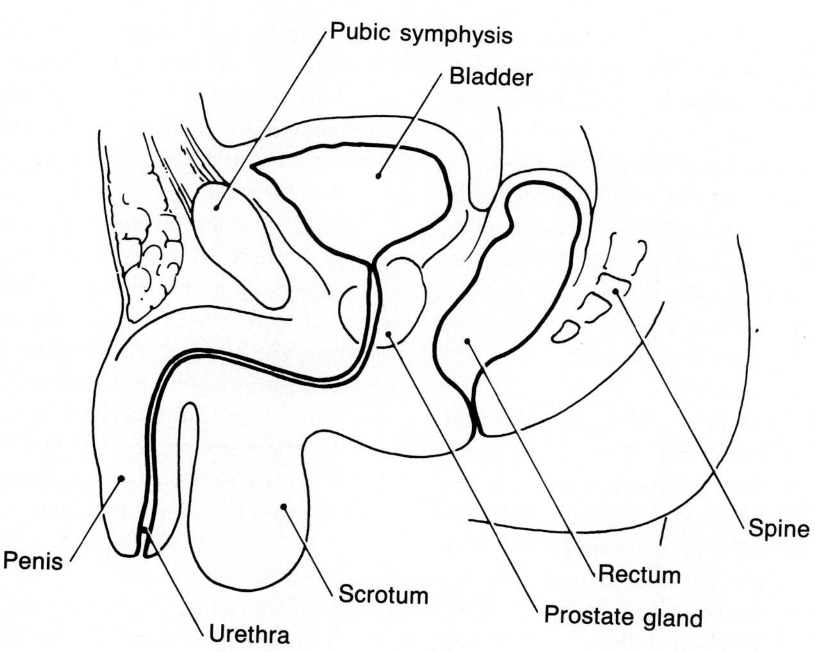

FIGURE 10-2. Sagittal view of the male pelvis.

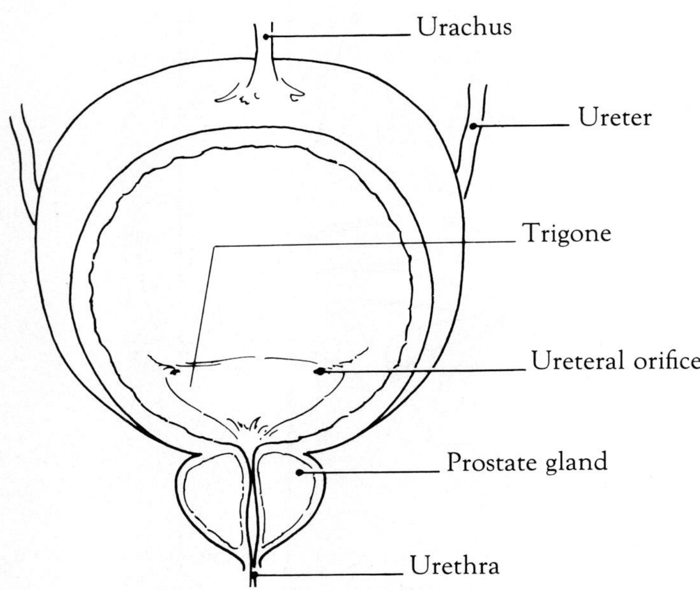

FIGURE 10-3. Inferior view of the male urinary bladder and prostatic urethra.

symphysis pubis and anterior to the vagina.[46] Its undilated diameter is 6 mm, and it is approximately 4 cm long.[41,46] It is directed obliquely downward and anteriorly.[13]

The male urethra follows a tortuous course for a distance of approximately 20 cm.[46] Immediately below the bladder, it passes through the center of the prostate gland (prostatic portion), then between two sheets of white fibrous tissue connecting the pubic bones (membranous portion), and then through the penis (cavernous portion), the external male reproductive organ.[41]

In the male, the prostate is a fibromuscular and glandular organ that lies just inferior to the bladder. The normal prostate contains the posterior urethra, which is 2.5 cm long.[24] The seminal vesicles lie just cephalad to the prostate under the base of the bladder.[41,46] They are approximately 6 cm long and quite soft. Each vesicle joins its corresponding vas deferens to form the ejaculatory duct (Fig. 10-4).[24]

URETERS

The ureters enter the bladder posteroinferiorly in an oblique manner approximately 5 cm apart (Fig. 10-5). The average length of the ureter is 30 cm and the diameter is 6 mm.[24] In three places the ureters are constricted: (1) at the ureteropelvic junction; (2) as they cross the iliac vessels; and (3) at the junction with the bladder.[7,31] The course of the ureter is retroperitoneal.

The extravesical ureter is composed of helically oriented fibers that allow peristaltic activity. As these fibers approach the vesical wall, they are reoriented into the longitudinal muscle fibers. In contrast, the intravesical ureteral segment is composed of longitudinal muscle fibers only and therefore cannot produce peristalsis. As these smooth muscle fibers approach the ureteral orifice, those that form the roof of the ureter swing to either side to join those that form the floor.[13]

CONGENITAL ANOMALIES

Bladder Duplication. Complete duplication of the urinary bladder is rare.[9,34] Although a double bladder may be an incidental finding, one must be aware that complications may arise from variations of this anomaly. Unilateral reflux, obstruction, or infection may occur secondary to stenosis or atresia of the urethra.

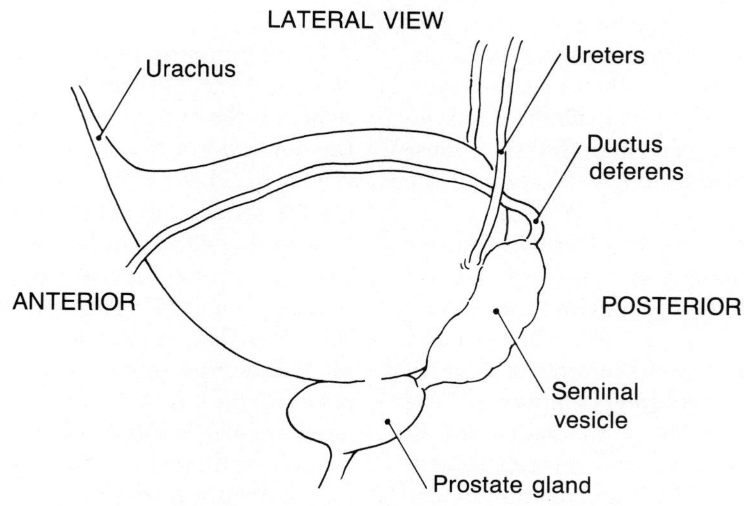

FIGURE 10-4. Lateral view of the male pelvic organs.

Ureteral Duplication. Duplication of the ureters results when the embryonic ureteric bud branches prematurely and leads to partial division and separation of the related blastema. The duplication may be complete, with two separate ureters opening into the lower urinary tract.[28] The ureter from the upper pole of the kidney inserts into the bladder caudad to the ureter from the lower pole. In females, the more caudad ureter may drain ectopically into the trigone, perineum, uterus, vagina, or urethra; in males, the distal insertion can occur in the trigone, urethra, or seminal vesicles.[25] Duplications may be unilateral or bilateral and are more common in females than in males.

Duplicate or Accessory Urethra. An accessory urethra is an uncommon malformation that occurs almost exclusively in males. True duplication is associated with duplication of the bladder, and usually of the genitalia.[2,17]

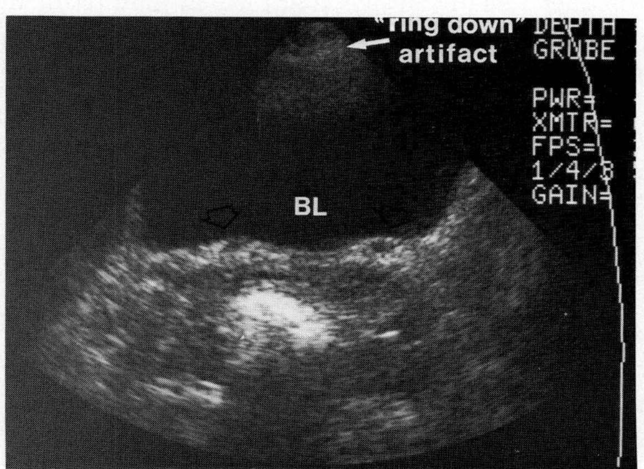

FIGURE 10-5. Transverse scan of the bladder. The ureteral orifices are seen as small mucosal elevations *(arrows)* as they enter the bladder. The anterior wall of the bladder demonstrates a ring-down artifact.

Physiology

The mechanism for voiding urine (micturition) starts with involuntary and voluntary nerve impulses.[24,46] Even though the bladder has a greater capacity, when the volume of urine exceeds 200 to 400 ml, stretch receptors trigger transmission of impulses to the lower portion of the spinal cord initiating the conscious desire to expel urine and a subconscious reflex, the micturition reflex.[3,32,41,46]

The combination of voluntary relaxation of the external sphincter muscle of the bladder, reflex contraction of linear smooth muscle fibers along the urethra, and then contraction of the detrusor muscle squeezes urine out of the bladder.[24,41] Parasympathetic fibers transmit the impulses that cause contractions of the bladder and relaxation of the internal sphincter.

Voluntary contraction of the external sphincter to prevent or terminate micturition is learned and is possible only if the nerves supplying the bladder and urethra, the projection tracts of the cord and brain, and the motor area of the cerebrum are all intact. Incontinence—involuntary emptying of the bladder—results from aging or trauma to any of these parts of the nervous system by cerebral hemorrhage or cord injury.[24,46] When neuromuscular dysfunction occurs, it can affect different parts of the lower urinary tract, including the detrusor, the bladder neck, or the proximal or distal half of the urethra.[8,33]

When there is obstruction, the pressure in the bladder remains always high, which may result in detrusor hypertrophy, the formation of diverticula, and vesicoureteral reflux. Since the urine is always infected in such patients, the result may be chronic reflux pyelonephritis or struvite stones.

There are two common causes of bladder neck obstruction in patients with neuromuscular dysfunction: detrusor–bladder neck dyssynergy and detrusor-sphincter dyssynergy.[8,33] Bladder neck obstruction can also be caused by benign prostatic hyperplasia.

Retention results from inability to void even though the bladder contains an excessive amount of urine.[24,46] Catheterization is used to relieve the discomfort accompanying retention. Thirty percent of patients who are catheterized intermittently for a long time eventually develop a "ledge" posteriorly at the bladder neck, from catheter trauma. The ledge makes voiding difficult and considerably complicates the catheterization process.

Sonographic Examination Techniques

The three basic approaches to scanning the urinary bladder are transabdominal, transrectal, and transurethral. Only the transabdominal approach is discussed here. In order to visualize the bladder sonographically, it is important that the patient prepare properly.

Bladder distension is critical to visualization and can be accomplished by three methods: (1) instructing the patient to drink water 1 hour before the test and not to void; (2) instructing the patient not to void before the examination; (3) catheterizing the patient and instilling fluid into the bladder. Having the bladder fully distended facilitates identification of many pelvic structures. In males, the bladder, seminal vesicles, prostate, and rectum should be imaged routinely; in females, the vagina, bladder, uterus, ovaries, and rectum.[19] Disease processes in one structure can involve other closely related organs. A full bladder also facilitates identification of dilated ureters. Normal ureters are not usually seen sonographically.

In preparation for scanning the bladder transabdominally, it is not necessary to restrict the diet or use catheters or enemas to reduce intestinal contents or air, but studies should be done before any anticipated radiographic examinations of the intestinal tract, as barium from contrast medium could block sound waves and interfere with imaging.[5]

The patient should lie supine when the bladder is scanned transabdominally. Sometimes it is necessary to position the patient obliquely or to roll the patient in a lateral decubitus position.

A suitable coupling agent, such as ultrasonic gel, is used on the skin surface. The highest-frequency transducer possible should be used, making sure all pelvic structures are visualized adequately.

The bladder should be scanned in both longitudinal and transverse planes. The normal bladder appears as an anechoic structure with sharply demarcated walls.[19] The bladder wall is seen as a rather smooth, thin, echogenic interface and it varies in thickness from 3 to 6 mm, depending on the degree of bladder distension.[2,10] Reverberation echoes are often seen anteriorly.[4,11]

The sonographer should identify the predictable contours of the urine-filled bladder. If the patient has never had bladder or pelvic surgery, any deviation from the normal bladder shape, especially asymmetry, should be considered abnormal and a thorough investigation should be performed of the site of the distortion to rule out a mass.[19] On transverse sections, the bladder should appear symmetric. Superiorly, the bladder appears rounded, but scanning more inferiorly, it appears square owing to the parallel walls of the acetabulum. On longitudinal sections, the bladder appears almost triangular, with the base of the triangle parallel with the anterior abdominal wall. In both longitudinal and transverse scans, the lateral walls appear straight and indented if iliopsoas muscles are prominent.[19] As the different pelvic structures are encountered, it may be necessary to angle the transducer caudad and cephalad, then medial to lateral. This also produces a sharper image of the bladder wall.

Frequently, it is possible to visualize the prostate in males using the transabdominal approach (Fig. 10-6).[11,12] By angling the transducer caudad under the symphysis, the prostate is seen posteroinferior to the bladder. A hypertrophic prostate is easy to see (Fig. 10-7). Nevertheless, the best way to visualize it is via the transrectal approach.

As mentioned earlier, the normal ureters usually are not identified by ultrasound unless they are dilated. The distal dilated ureter can be visualized as a round, anechoic structure posterior to the bladder in the transverse plane (Fig. 10-8). In the lon-

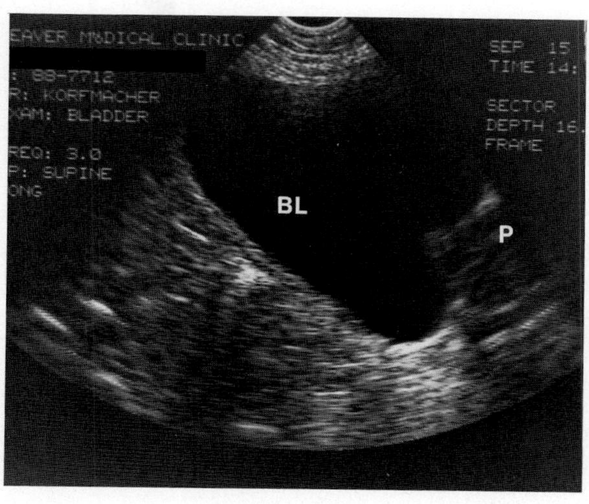

FIGURE 10-6. Longitudinal scan of the bladder (BL) and prostate (P) using a transabdominal suprapubic approach. Note the relationship between the bladder and the inferiorly located prostate gland *(arrow)*.

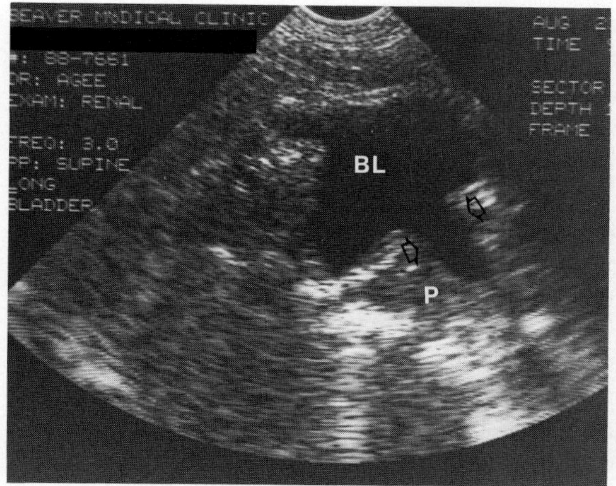

A

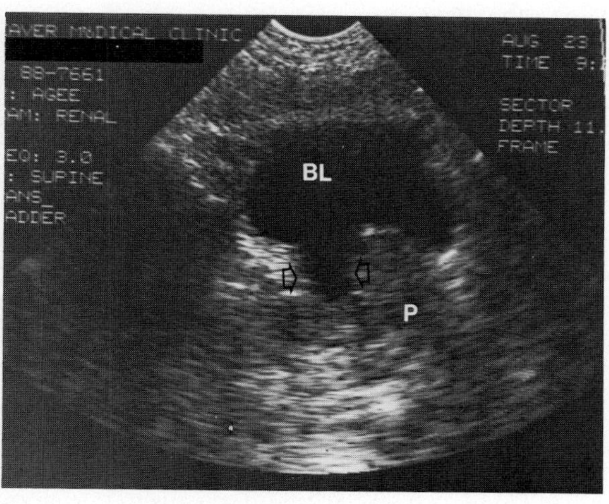

B

FIGURE 10-7. (*A*) Longitudinal scan of the bladder (BL) demonstrates enlarged prostate (P) after transurethral prostatic resection (TURP). A fluid-filled defect that developed after previous prostatectomy is visualized at the urethral orifice *(arrows)*. (*B*) Transverse scan of the bladder (BL) after TURP *(arrows)* demonstrates enlarged prostate gland (P).

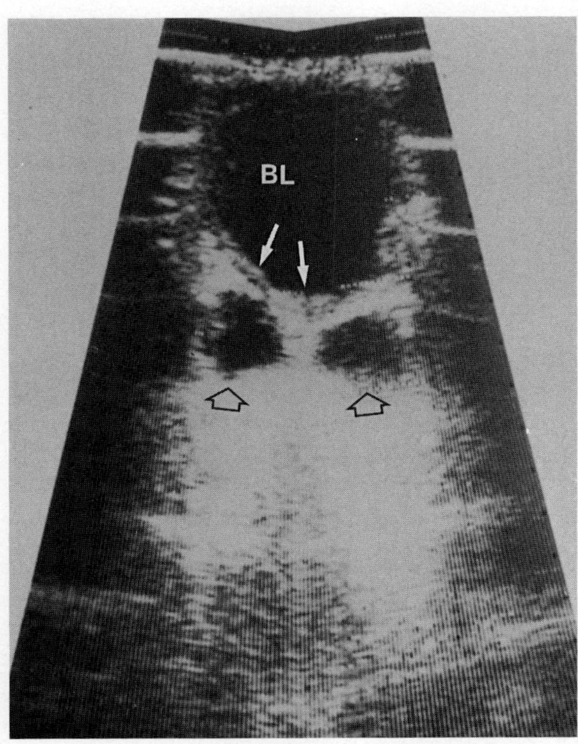

FIGURE 10-8. Transverse scan of the urinary bladder (BL). The dilated distal ureters appear as round, anechoic structures posterior to the bladder *(open arrows)*. There is a small amount of bladder wall thickening *(black arrows)*.

gitudinal plane, the dilated ureter can be visualized as a long, linear structure, usually posterior and to the right or to the left of the midline.

Bursts of echoes are seen entering the bladder from the region of the trigone.[8,11] At intervals of 5 to 20 seconds, a jet of low-intensity echoes, which lasts a few seconds, starts at the area of the ureteral orifices and flows toward the center of the bladder.[18] The jets can occur simultaneously, but more commonly are separate (Fig. 10-9). Such a jet extends up to 3 cm and broadens. After a few seconds, the low-intensity echoes become distributed in the bladder and lose intensity until they can no longer be distinguished.

In the male, the seminal vesicles are seen as two small oval, hypoechoic structures posterior to the bladder and superior to the prostate (Fig. 10-10).

The bladder volume can be calculated using the formula $V = width \times height \times depth$.[13,23] This formula is sometimes presented as $V = transverse \times AP \times length$. Bladder capacity should be noted. The capacity decreases in association with large pelvic masses, in urinary and pelvic inflammatory disease, in patients receiving radiation therapy, in advanced stages of tumor infiltration, and after recent surgery.[25]

To document the presence of residual urine and calculate its volume the patient should be asked to empty the bladder. Then the longitudinal and transverse scans should be repeated.[12,30] and another bladder volume calculated. Determining the amount of residual urine in patients with suspected bladder outlet obstruction has improved the treatment of these patients.

Anomalies

DIVERTICULA

Diverticula of the bladder are pouchlike eversions of the wall.[45] Bladder diverticula are produced by mucosal herniation through defects in the muscle wall arising as congenital defects or as acquired lesions, usually associated with diseases resulting in bladder outlet obstruction or neurogenic conditions resulting in abnormalities in bladder function.[26] One frequent form is the paraureteral (Hutch) diverticulum, which forms because the ureter is inserted at an inherently weak point in the bladder wall.[2,17]

Bladder diverticula are demonstrated sonographically as urine-filled outpouchings.[21] Careful scanning may show the narrow communication between a diverticulum and the bladder, which leads to the diagnosis (Fig. 10-11).[38] Intradiverticular tumors or stones may also be identified. Since diverticula may not empty and occasionally actually increase in size with voiding, postvoiding scans can demonstrate urine-filled diverticula.[21] Very large diverticula may be mistaken for the bladder itself, duplication of the bladder, or seminal vesicle[21] or ovarian cysts (Table 10-1).[38]

POSTERIOR URETHRAL VALVE SYNDROME

With posterior urethral valve syndrome, the prostatic urethra is markedly dilated because of an obstruction at or just below the verumontanum (an elevation on the floor of the prostatic portion of

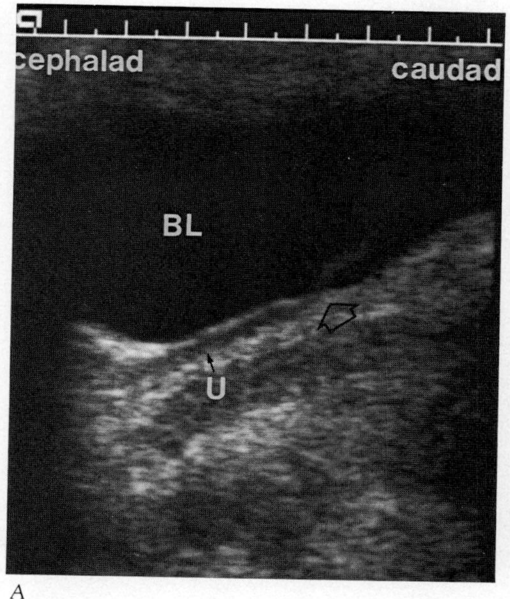

A

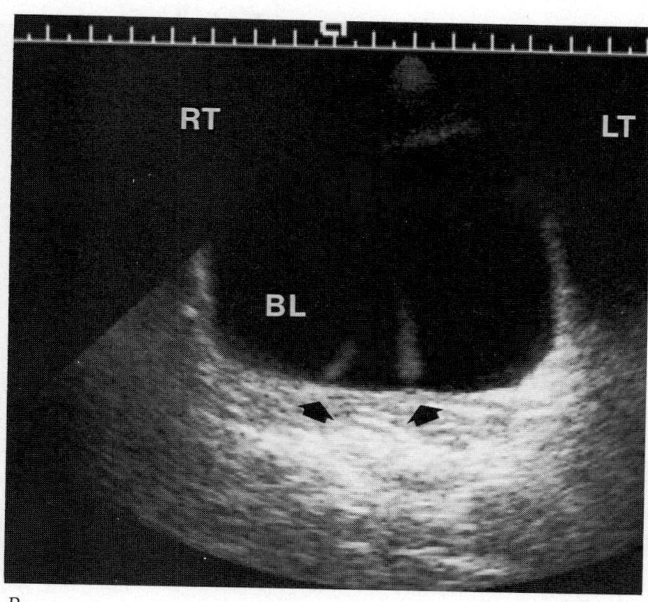

B

FIGURE 10-9. (*A*) Longitudinal scan of the right distal ureter (U). A jet of low-intensity echoes *(arrow)* is seen entering the bladder (BL). (*B*) Transverse scan of the bladder (BL). Simultaneous jets of low-intensity echoes *(arrows)* are visualized.

the urethra where the seminal ducts enter).[2,5,17] The usual form of a posterior urethral valve consists of a mucosal flap originating from the verumontanum. Posterior urethral valve syndrome is the most common cause of urinary obstruction in male infants.[11,15,22] Almost 75% are discovered during the first year of life. They may present in older children but rarely occur in adults. Approximately 40% of patients have associated vesicoureteral reflux, which is usually due to a periureteral diverticulum.[11]

The sonographic recognition of a dilated and elongated prostatic urethra helps differentiate posterior urethral valves, from neurogenic bladder dysfunction (Fig. 10-12). Also, with posterior urethral valves, the bladder wall appears thickened and hydroureters, with dilation of the upper urinary tract, may be seen (Table 10-1).

Other causes of bladder outlet obstruction include agenesis of the urethra, congenital urethral strictures, urethral tumors, and anterior urethral valves, all of which are rare. Thickening of the bladder wall can also occur with cystitis.

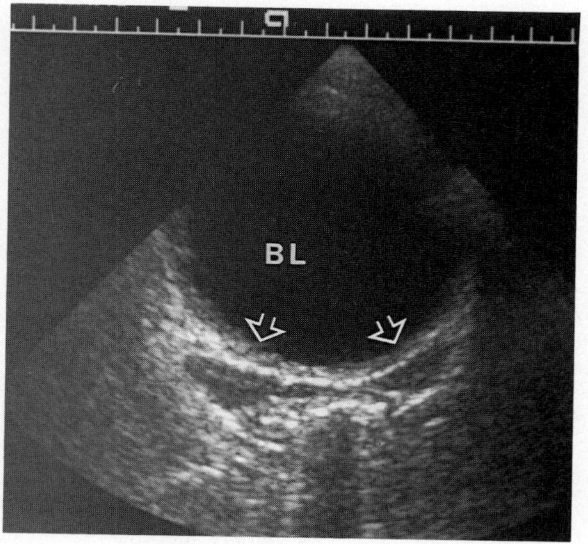

FIGURE 10-10. Transverse scan of the male urinary bladder (BL). The seminal vesicles *(arrows)* are located posterior and inferior to the bladder.

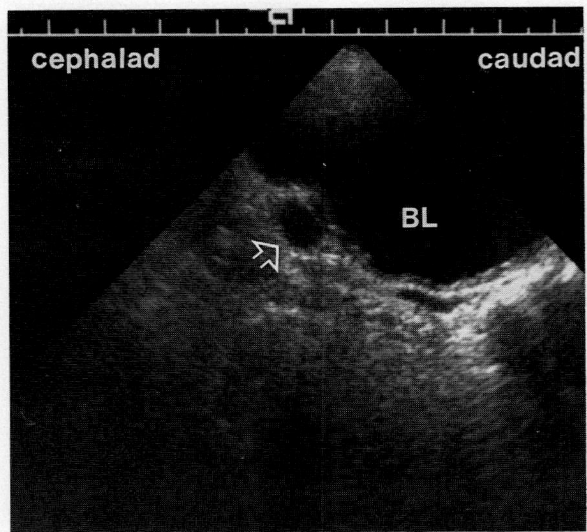

FIGURE 10-11. Longitudinal scan of the right lateral border of the bladder (BL). A bladder diverticulum is demonstrated as a round, well-defined, distinctly fluid-filled mass (*arrow*).

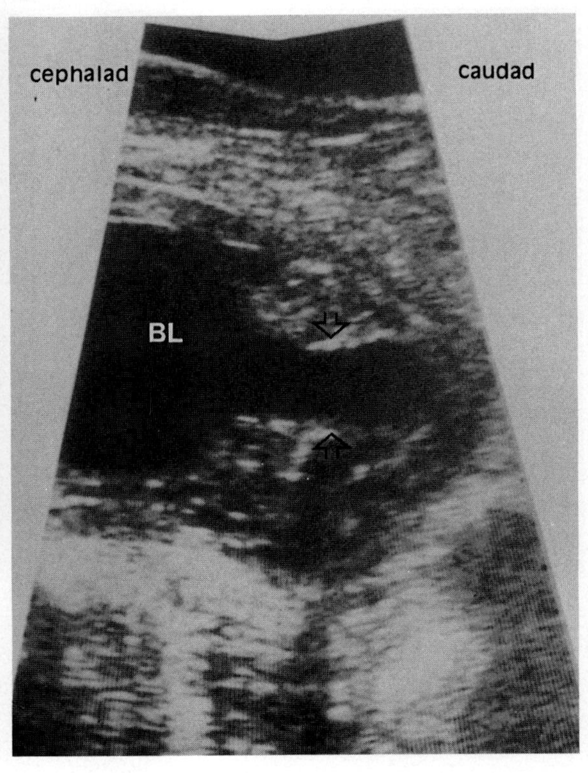

FIGURE 10-12. Longitudinal scan of the fetal bladder (BL). There is demonstration of a dilated prostatic urethra (*arrows*), also termed the keyhole sign. At birth, this boy infant had posterior urethral valves.

TABLE 10-1. Urinary bladder anomalies

ANOMALY	SONOGRAPHIC APPEARANCE
Bladder diverticula	Round, well-defined, thin-walled, fluid-filled masses with acoustic enhancement, variable in size
Posterior urethral valves	Dilated and elongated prostatic urethra (peculiar to males), subsequently, thickened bladder wall, hydroureters, or dilated upper urinary tract may develop
Bladder exstrophy	Eversion through anterior abdominal wall; other findings include hydronephrosis caused by ureterovesical obstruction
Contracture of the bladder neck	Secondary abnormalities include: vesicoureteral reflux, vesical diverticula, or large-capacity bladder
Ectopic ureter	More common for ureter to arise from the upper moiety of a duplex kidney; 10 to 20% arise from a solitary renal pelvis; may be massively dilated, may mimic multiseptate, cystic abdominal masses
Ectopic ureteroceles	Cystlike, thin-walled mass of variable size and shape, projecting into the bladder (sometimes described as a cyst within a cyst)

Anterior urethral obstruction in males is uncommon but may be secondary to strictures, diverticula, or urethral duplication. Urethral obstruction in females is rare but may be seen in cloacal or female intersex anomalies.[11]

EXSTROPHY

Exstrophy of the bladder is a complete ventral defect of the urogenital sinus and the overlying skeletal system, frequently associated with other congenital anomalies.[28,45] Classically, exstrophy of the bladder represents eversion of the viscus through a defect in the anterior abdominal wall associated with separation of the pubic symphysis.[36] The mucosal edges of the bladder and distal ends of the ureters fuse, with the skin protruding through the lower central abdominal wall, which has failed to close. Urine spurts onto the abdominal wall from the ureteral orifices.

The rami of the pubic bones are all widely separated. The pelvic ring thus lacks rigidity, the femurs are rotated externally, and the child duck-waddles. Since the rectus muscles insert on the rami, they are widely separated from each other inferiorly. A hernia, made up of exstrophic bladder and surrounding skin, is therefore present. Bladder exstrophy is almost always accompanied by epispadias, a congenital opening of the urethra on the dorsum of the penis in males or by separation of the labia minora and a fissure of the clitoris in females. Renal infection is common, and hydronephrosis caused by ureterovesical obstruction may be found.[28,36] In this disorder, abnormal persistence of the cloacal membrane acts as a mechanical barrier to mesodermal movement during the first 6 weeks of embryonic life. Since this membrane extends from the hindgut to the allantoic duct, the associated anomalies may involve portions of the urinary, genital, musculoskeletal, and gastrointestinal system (see Table 10-1).[28]

CONTRACTURE OF THE BLADDER NECK

Narrowing of the bladder neck is a common cause of vesicoureteral reflux, vesical diverticula, large bladder capacity, and the syndrome of irritable bladder associated with enuresis. This contracture has been considered a rare phenomenon. In females, the obstructive liaison is spasm of the periurethral striated muscle, which develops secondary to distal urethral stenosis.[28]

ECTOPIC URETER AND ECTOPIC URETEROCELE

An ectopic ureter does not insert near the posterolateral angle of a normal trigone.[17,29] Most ectopic ureters arise from the superior pelvis (upper moiety) of a duplex kidney, but 10 to 20% arise from a solitary renal pelvis.

An ectopic ureterocele is formed when the ectopic ureter is obstructed in the area where it enters the bladder, causing its anterior wall to balloon into the bladder (Fig. 10-13). The ureterocele is a cystlike enlargement of the lower end of the ureter (Fig. 10-14). Problems arise because (1) the ureteral opening in the wall of the sac is stenotic, and therefore hydroureter, hydronephrosis, and infection proximal to the ureterocele are common, and (2) the ureterocele sac itself may obstruct the bladder outlet or even prolapse through the urethra.

Ectopic ureters usually insert into the bladder distal to the orifice of the ureter draining the lower pole.[18,43] In males, ectopic ureters may insert in the seminal vesicle, vas deferens, or ejaculatory duct. In females, they may insert in the vestibule, vagina, or uterus.[10,22]

Sonographic diagnosis of ectopic ureters and ectopic ureteroceles must include scanning of the kidneys. The duplex kidney may demonstrate two ureters arising from within, although frequently they are difficult to distinguish. The ectopic ureter may be massively dilated and tortuous in the distal portion and mildly dilated proximally. Many variations are reported.[10,22] These extremely large ureters sometimes mimic multiseptate, cystic abdominal masses. Ectopic ureteroceles are dynamic structures that change shape and size according to intravesical pressure (Fig. 10-15). Occasionally, a dilated ectopic ureter may indent the lower vesical wall of the bladder, simulating an ectopic ureterocele on ultrasound (see Table 10-1).[10]

ANOMALIES OF THE URACHUS

In the fetus, the bladder is located at the umbilicus and communicates with the allantoic canal. The urachus is formed as the bladder begins its descent into the true pelvis. As this occurs, the vertex of the bladder elongates, forming a fibromuscular appendage approximately 5 cm long and surrounding the allantoic canal. This canal is normally obliterated by the time of birth.[2,17]

A patent urachus is the result of persistence of

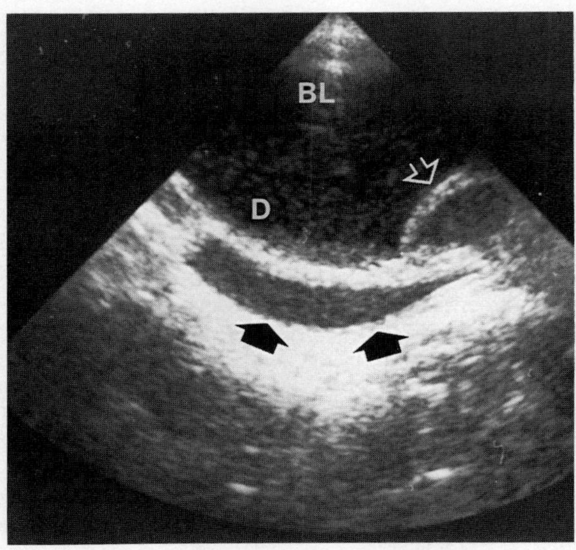

Figure 10-13. Longitudinal scan of a left dilated distal ureter *(solid arrows)*. The ureterocele *(open arrow)* is separated from the lumen of the bladder (BL) by a thin curvilinear rim of echoes. Diffuse, low-level echoes in the bladder represent debris (D).

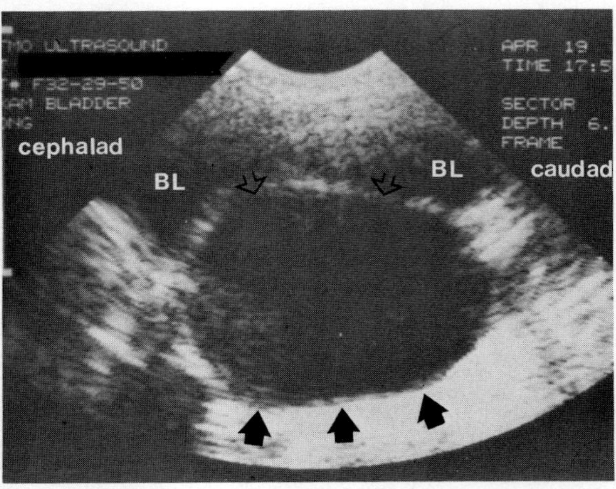

Figure 10-14. Longitudinal scan of an anechoic thin-walled mass *(black arrows)* projecting into the bladder (BL). This is a large ectopic ureterocele *(open arrows)*.

the allantoic canal between the bladder and the umbilicus. Urine may drain constantly from the umbilicus. A partially patent urachus means that the urachus communicates with either the umbilicus (urachal sinus) or the bladder but not both. If the allantoic canal is obliterated at both ends but patent in between, a urachal cyst forms.[28]

A persistent urachus is the result of the urachus communicating continuously with the bladder, and is usually asymptomatic.[28] Complications of a persistent urachus may occur: if the ends of the urachus seal off, a cyst may form; adenocarcinoma may occur in a urachal cyst; and stones may develop in such a cyst.

Pathologic Changes

Bladder Tumors

Bladder tumors are usually epithelial or uroepithelial in origin and are one of the most common tumors of the genitourinary tract.[4,20] The malignant tumors account for 3% of all cancer deaths, with a male preponderance in the fifth to sixth decade.[25] Malignant tumors are usually transitional cell carcinomas (90%), squamous cell carcinoma (5%), and rarely adenocarcinoma.[25] The most frequent symptom is painless hematuria.

Cystoscopy with biopsy is considered the most accurate method for detecting and evaluating bladder tumors, but it is invasive and requires anesthesia. For initial screening of suspected bladder tumor, ultrasound is an excellent noninvasive imaging modality. Bladder tumors located in the bladder neck or dome are difficult to detect with ultrasound.[15,25] The ability of sonography to detect the presence or absence of bladder tumors has varied from 33% for tumors smaller than 0.5 cm in diameter, 83% of tumors 1 to 2 cm, and 95% of tumors larger than 2 cm.[15] Other than the size and location of the tumor, the degree of bladder distension or obesity may affect the accuracy of tumor detection.

The normal bladder wall, usually 3 to 6 mm thick, has a uniform echo pattern, whereas an infiltrating tumor disrupts the uniformity (Fig. 10-16), (Table 10-2).[29] Blood clot, benign prostatic hypertrophy, cystitis, and bladder trabeculae can mimic bladder tumors (Figs. 10-17, 10-18).[4]

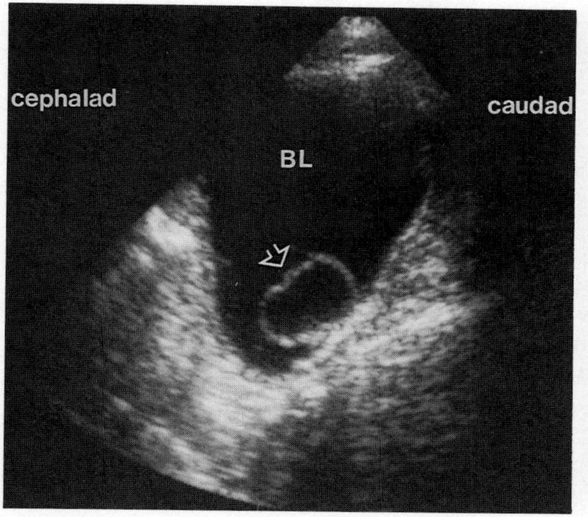

A

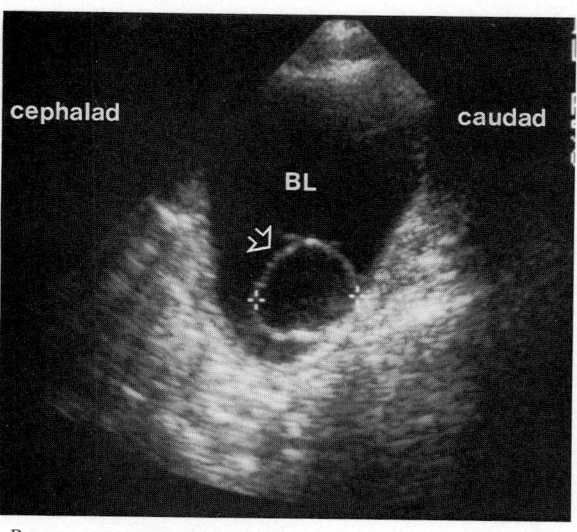

B

FIGURE 10-15. Longitudinal scans of the bladder (BL) demonstrate an ectopic ureterocele *(cursor and arrow)* changing shape from smaller (*A*) to larger (*B*) as a result of intravesical pressure.

Transvaginal longitudinal scanning has proven effective in the diagnosis of tumors located in any part of the urinary bladder. The transvaginal approach provides good image quality, allowing the tumor to be studied in detail through the anterior wall, the neck, and the apex of the urinary bladder. Bladder tumors situated on the side wall are harder to stage by transvaginal sonography.[7,31]

Following the diagnosis of carcinoma of the bladder, ultrasonography can also be helpful in staging bladder tumors. The bladder wall infiltration depth is the single most important factor; a simple and popular classification system of 0, A, B, C, and D is used.[1,2,16] The Union Internationale Contre le Cancre (UICC) proposed the tumor, node, and metastasis (TNM) classification, which is more helpful and widely accepted (Table 10-3).[1,2,33,34,42] Evidence indicates that the stage of the tumor profoundly influences curability and survival time (Fig. 10-19).[20]

Tumor response to chemotherapy is the primary determinant of whether to continue therapy. Sonography is a reliable method when scanning patients whose tumor is stable or regressing and is a

(text continues on page 364)

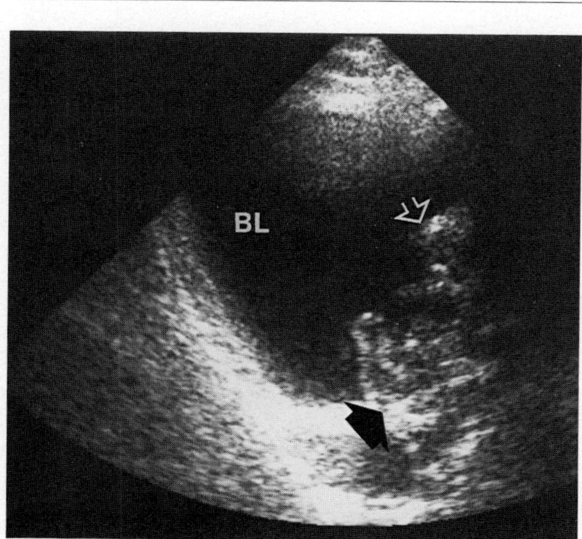

FIGURE 10-16. Longitudinal scan of the bladder (BL) reveals a bladder tumor *(open arrow)* with irregular borders and a mixed sonographic echo pattern. Note the disruption in the uniformity of the bladder wall *(solid arrow)*.

Table 10-2. Urinary bladder disorders

Lesion	Sonographic Appearance
Bladder tumor	Echogenic structures protruding into the echo-free bladder lumen; infiltrating tumors disrupt uniformity of bladder wall
Cystitis	Usually presents as thickened bladder mucosa with hypoechoic or cystic structures along the wall; can mimic bladder tumors
Bladder calculi	High-intensity echoes within the bladder associated acoustic shadowing; echogenic focus shifts to the dependent portion of the bladder with position changes
Bladder rupture	Usually difficult to visualize by ultrasound; urinoma formation may be detected as an anechoic mass with enhanced through-transmission; may have irregular borders and contain septa; may compress surrounding tissue
Distal ureteral obstruction	Sonography may demonstrate megaureter; upper urinary tract dilatation, ureterocele, ectopic ureterocele and ectopic ureter

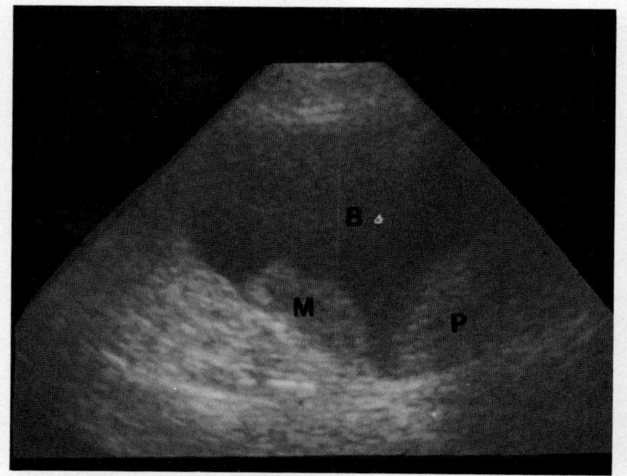

A

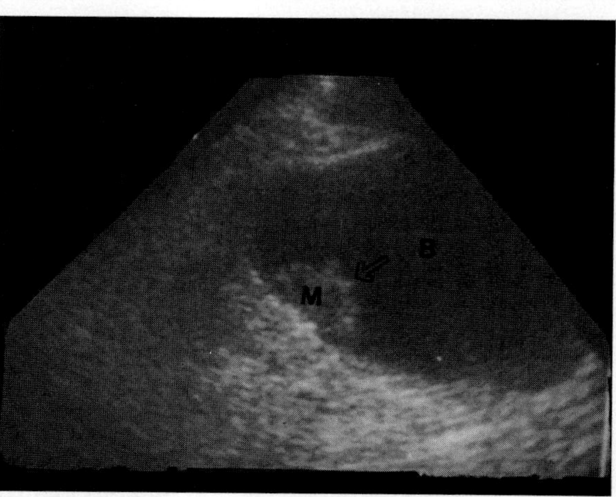

B

Figure 10-17. (*A*) Longitudinal scan of the bladder (B) demonstrates the bladder base is indented by a markedly enlarged prostate (P) on a 71-year-old man. A mass (M) emanating from the right bladder wall measures approximately 3 cm. (*B*) The transverse scan of the bladder (B) in the same patient demonstrates the mass (M) on the right bladder wall. The papillary, irregular contour *(arrow)* suggests transitional cell carcinoma. (Courtesy Brent Guernsey, Salt Lake City, UT.)

TABLE 10-3. Bladder cancer staging systems

PATHOLOGIC FINDING	SYSTEM		
	JEWETT 1952	MARSHALL 1952	UICC-TNM 1974
No tumor-definitive specimen			T0
Carcinoma in situ		0	Tis
Papillary tumor, noninvasive	A		Ta
Papillary tumor, lamina propria infiltration		A	T1
Superficial muscle invasion	B1	B1	T2
Deep muscle invasion	B2	B2	T3a
Invasion of extravesical spread (perivesical fat)	C	C	T3b
Invasion of contiguous viscera (prostate, uterus, vagina)			T4a
Invasion of pelvic or abdominal wall			T4b
No lymph node involvement			N0
Involvement of single ipsilateral node	D1	D1	N1
Involvement of multiple contralateral or bilateral regional nodes			N2
Fixed regional nodes			N3
Common iliac, aortic, inguinal nodes			N4
No metastases			M0
Distant metastases	D2	D2	M1

(Data from references 1, 2, 14, 20 and 42.)

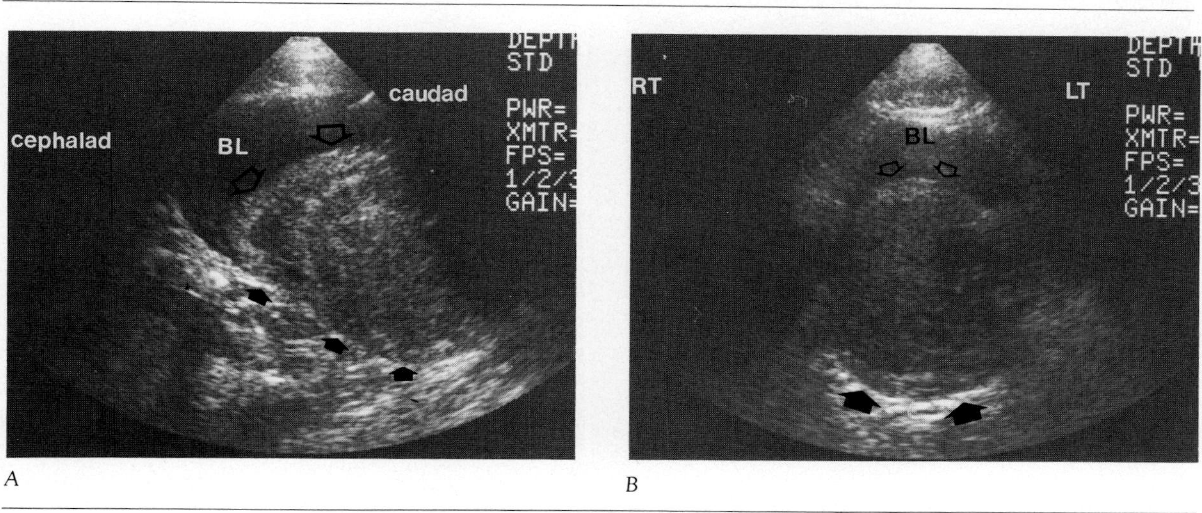

FIGURE 10-18. Longitudinal and transverse scans of the bladder (BL) reveal a large mass (*arrows*) with a complex, but predominantly solid echo pattern. The mass was confirmed to be immunoblastic sarcoma. Sarcoma of the bladder in adults accounts for fewer than 1% of adult bladder tumors.

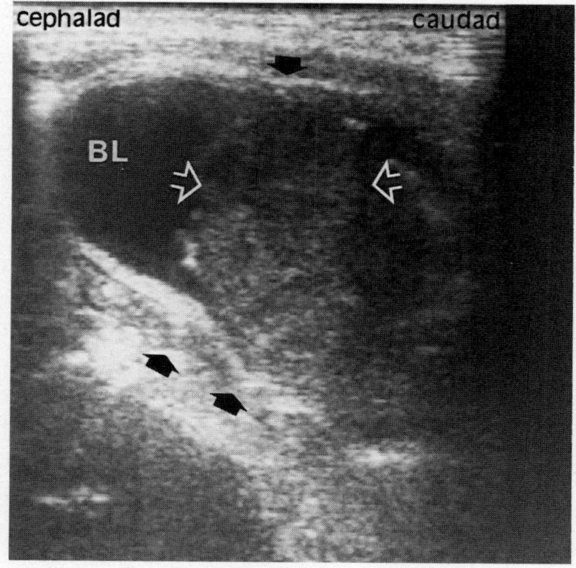

A

B

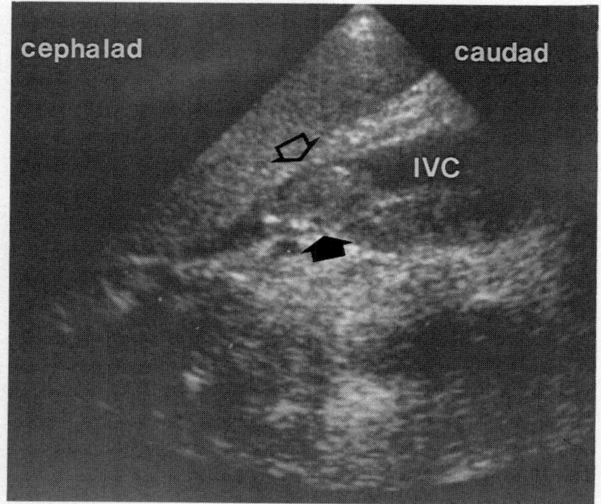

C

FIGURE 10-19. On (*A*) longitudinal and (*B*) transverse scans of the bladder (BL), a large, complex mass (*arrows*) is visualized projecting from the posterior surface. It proved to be a poorly differentiated squamous cell carcinoma. (C) Longitudinal scan of the IVC in the same patient. Low-level echoes in the IVC reveal a thrombus within (*arrows*). Pelvic malignancies predispose patients to having venous thrombosis.

useful adjunct to cystoscopy when serial scans of bladder tumors are performed. When sonography and cystoscopy are used together, the staging of bladder tumors can be more accurate than when either study is used alone.[30,47] Computed tomography (CT) is the imaging modality of choice for identifying contiguous extension of bladder neoplasms and has reduced the number of over-and understaging errors.[20]

CYSTITIS

Focal lesions in the bladder due to cystitis can mimic bladder tumors (Fig. 10-20). Bullous cystitis, a common finding, is known to urologists as catheter cystitis.[1] Patients with bullous cystitis usually need constant Foley catheter drainage, which maintains an empty bladder and results in continuous contact and irritation of the bladder mucosa with the catheter tip or balloon.[3] Changes are seen;

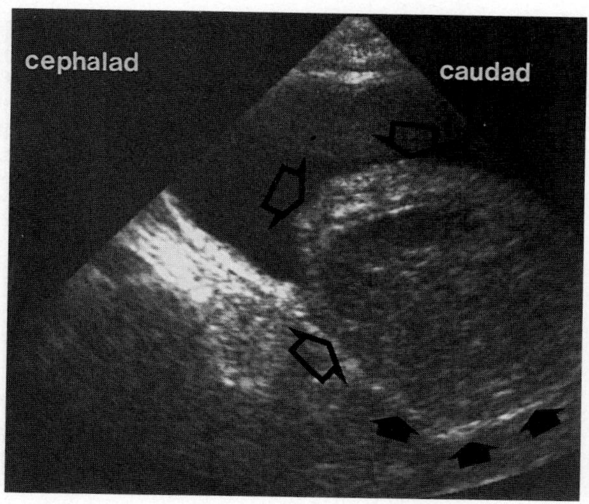

FIGURE 10-20. On a longitudinal scan of the bladder (BL) in a female with hemorrhagic cystitis, a blood clot with necrotic areas *(open arrows)* is seen adherent to the posterior bladder wall *(black arrows)*.

first thickened bladder mucosa that is smooth in early stages then becomes redundant and polypoid in the later stages. The thickened mucosa is usually hypoechoic, and the outline often smooth. The underlying muscle wall is always intact. Bladder tumors tend to have more shaggy, irregular outlines and are more echogenic. The transition between the tumor and the adjacent normal mucosa is abrupt (see Table 10-2).[3,32]

The final distinction between benign inflammatory changes and malignancy must be made by cytologic and histologic examination of biopsy material.[33,35]

CALCULI

Bladder calculi are usually single and may be asymptomatic. They may cause inflammatory changes or acute bladder neck obstruction.[23,25] They usually appear as high-intensity echoes in the bladder, have an associated acoustic shadow, and shift to the dependent portion of the bladder with position changes (Fig. 10-21).[35,37] The anterior, fluid-filled bladder provides an excellent acoustic window for the identification of bladder calculi. Stones do not have to be calcified to be identified

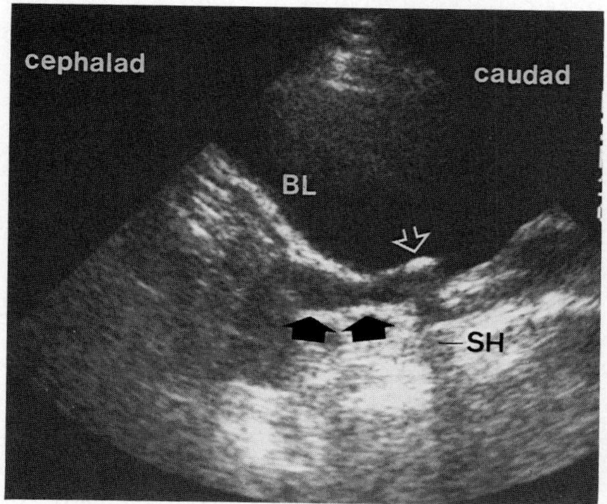

A

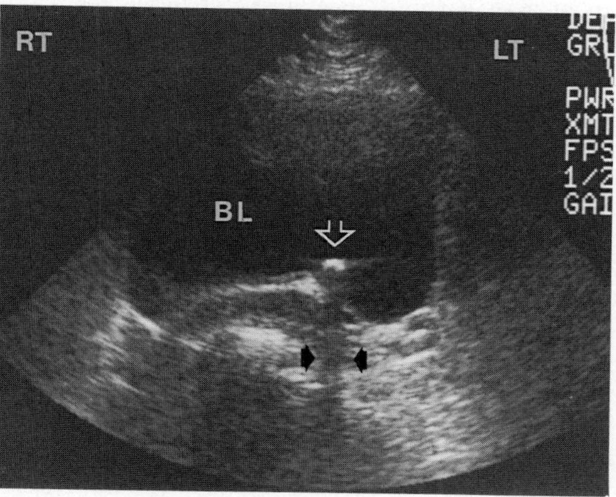

B

FIGURE 10-21. (*A*) Longitudinal scan of the bladder (BL) with a bright hyperechoic density in the area of the left ureterovesical junction *(open arrow)*. The left distal ureter is dilated (*black arrow*, SH, shadowing). (*B*) Transverse scan of the bladder (BL) in the same patient. Shadowing *(solid arrows)* is noted posterior to the well-defined bladder calculus *(open arrow)*.

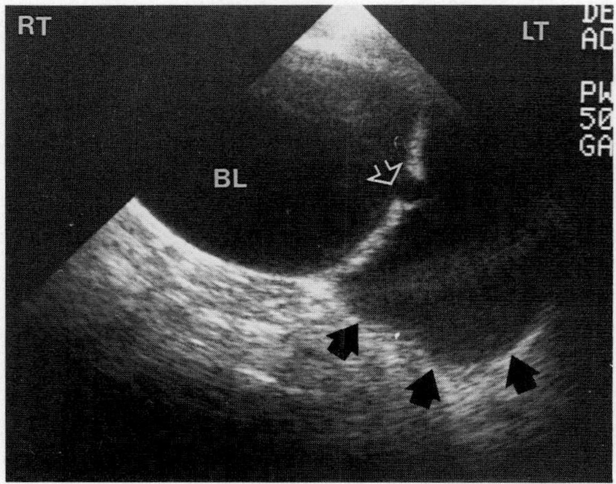

Figure 10-22. Transverse scan of the bladder (BL) of a male who experienced trauma to the pelvis. A large anechoic mass *(solid arrows)* is noted to the left of the bladder. This represents the formation of a urinoma caused by a rupture in the bladder wall *(open arrow)*.

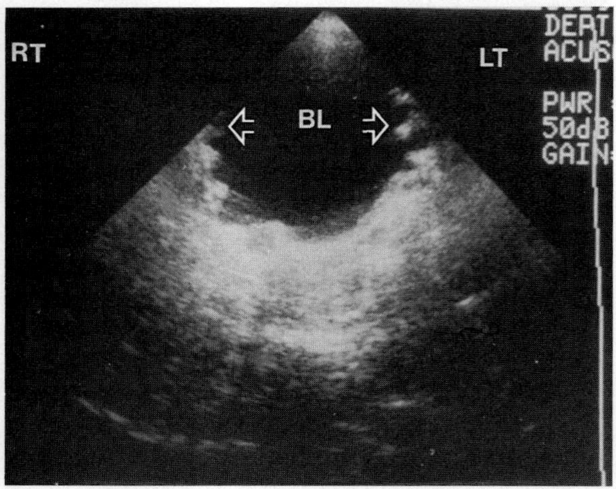

Figure 10-23. Transverse scan of the bladder (BL) demonstrates the presence of bladder saccules *(open arrows)*, a sign that bladder outlet obstruction has begun to have adverse effects on the urinary tract.

sonographically. Sonography can distinguish uric acid stones that have an acoustic shadow and shift position from a bladder tumor that appears as a fixed mass without an acoustic shadow (see Table 10-2). Intradiverticular calculi can also be identified sonographically. In a patient with diverticula, infection and stone formation are common occurrences owing to the stasis of urine.[21]

Rupture

Bladder rupture follows severe blunt, lower abdominal or pelvic trauma or penetrating abdominal or perineal injury. If the bladder was full at the time of blunt injury, rupture occurs, spilling urine into the peritoneum. Pelvic crush injuries cause bladder rupture in 1 to 15% of cases, four-fifths being extraperitoneal. A urinoma may result from temporary sealing of small tear (Table 10-2, Fig. 10-22). The best diagnostic procedure for visualizing bladder rupture is cystography.[37,44]

Bladder Wall Abnormalities

Patients with inflammatory bladder pathology may have signs and symptoms similar to those of bladder or kidney neoplasm.[7,40] Endometriosis can present as an intravesical lesion by either direct extension or implantation.[40] Regional enteritis (Crohn's disease) has been reported as a loop of small bowel with thick walls and a narrowed lumen adhering to the bladder dome.[6,43]

Neurogenic Bladder

Myelodysplasia is the most common cause of neurogenic bladder in infants and children. Most patients have a mixed upper and lower motor neuron lesion. Many patients have a trabeculated bladder and spasm of the external sphincter, causing relative obstruction and narrowing of the urethra as it courses through the urogenital diaphragm.[2,17] The patient may find it extremely difficult or impossible to void. Because of the obstruction, the pressure in the bladder remains constantly high, which may result in detrusor hypertrophy, the formation of saccules and diverticula, and vesicoureteral reflux (Fig. 10-23).[8,33] Since the urine is chronically infected in such patients, the result may be chronic reflux pyelonephritis, the formation of struvite stones, or bladder debris (Fig. 10-24).

Patients with neurogenic bladder usually un-

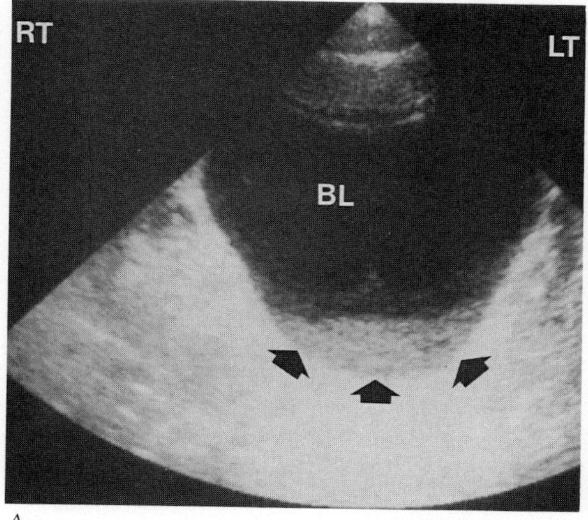

A

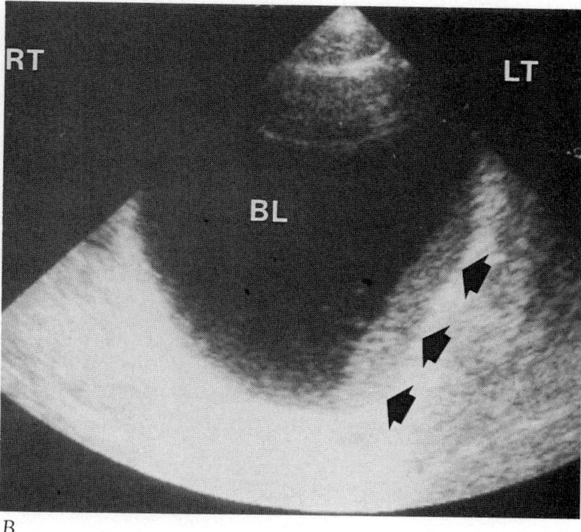

B

FIGURE 10-24. (*A*) Transverse scan of the bladder (BL). The patient lies supine while the scan is performed. A layer of debris (*arrows*) is noted along the posterior wall of the bladder. (*B*) Transverse scan of the bladder (BL) in the same patient. As the patient changes to the left lateral decubitus position, the debris (*arrows*) moves into the dependent left portion of the bladder.

dergo serial excretory urography and voiding cystourethrograms. Sonography is performed to aid in the diagnosis of trabeculated bladder, ureterectasis, vesicoureteral reflux, hydronephrosis, or bladder calculi.

Patients may need surgery for the urinary tract complications that arise. Vesicotomy or urinary diversion may be the procedure of choice.

REFLUX

Normally, the uretero vesical junction allows urine to enter the bladder but prevents it from being regurgitated into the ureter, particularly at the time of voiding. In this way, the kidney is protected from high pressure in the bladder and from contamination by infected vesical urine. When this valve is incompetent, the chance for development of urinary infection is secondary to vesicoureteral reflux.

Reflux may occur as a result of an abnormality of the trigone and secondary to anomalies such as ectopia, posterior urethral valves, paraureteric cyst, prune belly syndrome, and neurogenic bladder.[23,25]

Vesicoureteral reflux is a common urinary tract abnormality of children. High-pressure reflux (with or without associated urinary tract infection) may be a major cause of chronic renal failure with marked scarring and atrophic changes in the kidneys.[23,25]

Ultrasound examination is valuable in the management of children with reflux. In the transverse plane, the sonographer must scan meticulously in the area where the ureters enter the bladder. Many times the ureter dilates with urine as the reflux is in progress.

DISTAL URETERAL OBSTRUCTION

To differentiate a ureterovesical junction obstruction from nonobstructive causes such as reflux, a voiding cystourethrogram may be necessary. The causes of distal ureteral obstruction may be congenital or acquired. Congenital causes include primary megaureter, primary megaureter with coexisting reflux, primary megaureter with coexisting bladder saccule, simple ureterocele, and ectopic ureter and ectopic ureterocele. Acquired causes include ureteral reimplantation procedures, infection, and stricture following passage of stones.[34] The sonographic appearance is described in Table 10-2.

Conclusion

Since the urine-filled bladder is an accessible abdominopelvic organ for ultrasound imaging, the sonographer's careful and systematic scanning technique can make a substantive contribution to the diagnosis of a number of bladder anomalies and diseases. These lesions are readily identified because of the bladder's predictable shape and the neutral background of the urine.

References

1. Abu-Yousef MM:Ultrasound of bladder tumors. Semin Ultrasound CT MR 1986, 7:275–286.
2. Abu-Yousef MM, Narayana AS, Brown RC, et al: Urinary bladder tumors studied by cystosonography. Part II: Staging. Radiology 1984, 153:227–231.
3. Abu-Yousef MM, Narayana AS, Brown RC: Catheter-induced cystitis: Evaluation by cystosonography. Radiology 1984, 151:471–473.
4. Abu-Yousef MM, Narayana AS, Frankenea EA Jr, et al: Urinary bladder tumors studied by cystosonography. Part I: Detection. Radiology 1984, 153:223–226.
5. Anderhub B: Manual of Abdominal Sonograhy. Baltimore, University Park Press, 1983.
6. Boag GS, Nolan RL: Sonographic features of urinary bladder involvement in regional enteritis. J Ultrasound Med 1988, 7:125–128.
7. Bree RL, Silver TM: Sonography of bladder and perivesical abnormalities. AJR 1981, 136:1101–1104.
8. Deeshaw DD, Scher HI: Serial transabdominal sonography of bladder cancer. AJR 1988, 150:1055–1059.
9. Dubbins PA, Kurtz AB, Darby J, et al: Ureteric jet effect: The echographic appearance of urine entering the bladder. Radiology 1981, 140:513–515.
10. Friedland GW, Cunningham J: The elusive ectopic ureteroceles. AJR 1972, 116:792–811.
11. Gilsanz VG, Miller JH, Reid BS: Ultrasonic characteristics of posterior urethral valves. Radiology 1982, 145:143–145.
12. Greenberg M, Neiman HL, Brandt TD, et al: Ultrasound of the prostate. Radiology 1981, 141:757–762.
13. Gray H: Gray's Anatomy: Anatomy of the Human Body, 29th ed, (American Edition, edited by Charles Mayo Goss.) Philadelphia, Lea & Febiger, 1973.
14. Husband JE, Olliff JF, Williams MP, et al: Bladder cancer: Staging with CT and MR imaging. Radiology 1989, 173:435–440.
15. Itzchak Y, Singer D, Fischelovitch Y: Ultrasonographic assessment of bladder tumors. I. Tumor detection. J Urol 1981, 126:31–33.
16. Jewett HJ, Strong GH: Infiltrating carcinoma of the bladder: Relation of depth of penetration of the bladder wall to incidence of local extension of metastases. J Urol 1946, 55:366–372.
17. Kangarloo H, Sample WF: Ultrasound of the Pediatric Abdomen and Pelvis. Chicago, Year Book Medical Publishers, 1980.
18. Kremer H, Dobrinski W, Mikyska M, et al: Ultrasonic in vivo and in vitro studies on the nature of the ureteral jet phenomenon. Radiology 1982, 142:175–177.
19. Kurtz AB, Rifkin MD: Normal anatomy of the female pelvis: Ultrasound with computed tomography correlation. *In* Sanders RC, James AE (eds): The Principles and Practice of Ultrasonography in Obstetrics and Gynecology. Norwalk, CT, Appleton-Century-Crofts, 1985.
20. Lang EK: Carcinoma of the bladder. *In* Eisenberg RL (ed): Diagnostic Imaging: An Algorithmic Approach. Philadelphia, JB Lippincott, 1988.
21. Leopold GR: Pelvic ultrasonography. *In* Sarti DA (ed): Diagnostic Ultrasound: Text & Cases, 2nd ed. Chicago, Year Book Medical Publishers, 1987.
22. McAlister WH: Demonstration of the dilated prostatic urethra in posterior urethral valve patients. J Ultrasound Med 1984, 3:189–190.
23. McLean GK, Edell SL: Determination of bladder volumes by gray-scale ultrasonography. Radiology 1978, 128:181–182.
24. Marieb EN: Human Anatomy and Physiology. Redwood City, CA, The Benjamin/ Cummings Publishing Company, 1989.
25. Mittelstaedt CA: Abdominal Ultrasound. New York, Churchill Livingstone, 1987.
26. Morley P: The bladder. Clin Diagn Ultrasound 1986, 2:139–157.
27. Netter FH: The Ciba Collection of Medical Illustrations, vol 2, Reproductive System. Rochester, NY, The Case-Hoyt Corporation, 1965.
28. Netter FH: The Ciba Collection of Medical Illustrations, vol 6, Kidney, Ureters, and the Urinary Bladder. Rochester, NY, The Case-Hoyt Corporation, 1965.
29. Nussbaum AR, Dorst JP, Jeffs RD, et al: Ectopic ureter and ureterocele: Their varied sonographic manifestations. Radiology 1986, 159:227–235.
30. Orgaz RE, Gomez AZ, Ramirez CT, et al: Applications of bladder ultrasonography. I. Bladder content and residue. J Urol 1981, 125:174–176.

31. Pansky B, House EL: Review of Gross Anatomy, 3rd ed. New York, Macmillan Publishing, 1975.
32. Parker-Anthony C, Thibodeau GA: Textbook of Anatomy and Physiology, 11th ed. St. Louis, CV Mosby, 1983.
33. Perkash I, Friedland GW: Transrectal sonographic urodynamics. Clin Diagn Ultrasound 1986, 18:181–193.
34. Richman TS, Taylor KJW: Sonographic demonstration of bladder duplication. AJR 1982, 139:604–605.
35. Rifkin MD, Kurtz AB, Pasto ME, et al: Unusual presentations of cystitis. J Ultrasound Med 1983, 2:25–28.
36. Robbins SL, Cotran RS: Pathologic Basis of Diseases, 2nd ed. Philadelphia, WB Saunders, 1979.
37. Rosenfield AT, Taylor KJW, Weiss RM: Ultrasound evaluation of bladder calculi. J Urol 1979, 121:119–120.
38. Sarti DA: Diagnostic Ultrasound: Text & Cases, 2nd ed. Chicago, Year Book Medical Publishers, 1987.
39. Seeley RR, Stephens TD, Tate P: Anatomy and Physiology. St. Louis, Times Mirror/Mosby College Publishing, 1989.
40. Singer D, Itzchak Y, Fischelovitch Y: Ultrasonographic assessment of bladder tumors. II. Clinical staging. J Urol 1981, 126:34–36.
41. Spence AP, Mason EB: Human Anatomy and Physiology. Menlo Park, CA, Benjamin/Cummings, 1987.
42. Spiessell B, Hermanek P, Scheibe O, et al: TNM Atlas: Illustrated Guide to the Classification of Malignant Tumours. Berlin, Springer-Verlag, 1982.
43. Sumner TE, Crowe JE, Resnick MI: Diagnosis of ectopic ureterocele using ultrasound. Urology 1980, 15:82–85.
44. Talner LB: Imaging in urinary tract trauma. *In*: Radiology of the Abdomen, Syllabus. CA, 1983.
45. Thomas CL (ed): Taber's Cyclopedic Medical Dictionary, 16th ed. Philadelphia, FA Davis, 1989.
46. Tortora GJ, Anagnastakos NP: Principles of Anatomy and Physiology, 5th ed. New York, Harper and Row, 1987.
47. Tsyb AF, Slesarev VI, Komarevtsev VN: Transvaginal longitudinal ultrasonography in diagnosis of carcinoma of the urinary bladder. J Ultrasound Med 1988, 7:178–182.

CHAPTER **11**

Adrenal Glands

DIANE M. KAWAMURA, SUE ELLEN BEAVERS

The ability to sonographically study the adrenal glands has improved, although they continue to challenge the skills of the sonographer. Knowing their exact anatomic location and landmarks, acquiring scanning competency, and using the flexibility, maneuverability, and improved lateral resolution available with modern real-time scanners increases the likelihood of producing quality sonographic images of the adrenal glands.[8,12,20,29]

Anatomy

EMBRYOLOGY

The adrenal gland is comprised of two distinct parts, the cortex and the medulla. Each develops from different embryonic tissues, forms different structures, and combines within a common capsule.[11,31,40] The result is two endocrine glands in one.[27] Most glands of the body develop from epithelial tissue. The adrenal cortex, however, is derived from the mesoderm of the same region that gives rise to gonadal tissue.[39,40,43] The adrenal medulla, or center, is functionally part of the sympathetic nervous system, as it develops from the neural crest cells that also give rise to postganglionic sympathetic neurons.[11,28,39]

Cortex. At approximately gestational week 6, the fetal cortex is first recognized bilaterally as a groove between the developing dorsal mesentery and gonad.[11,17] During week 7 or 8, the cells arrange into cords with dilated blood spaces and a thin capsule of connective tissue encloses the gland.[11,17,31] At this time, the gland assumes an intimate relationship with the superior pole of the kidney.[31] The fetal adrenal gland is larger than the kidney and approximately 20 times the *relative* size of the adult adrenal gland.[11,36] During the remainder of fetal life, the cortical tissue is composed of two zones comprising approximately 80% of the entire bulk of the gland.[16,17] Undifferentiated cells are found in the outer zone, whereas the inner zone is composed of differentiated cell cords that are active in secretion.[17,40] By week 8, the cortex produces precursors to androgen, estriol, and corticosteroids.[11] After birth, the inner zone undergoes involution while the thinner outer zone continues to develop. By age three years, the cortex differentiates into three zones (1) zona glomerulosa, (2) zona fasciculata, and (3) zona reticularis. Each zone develops different cellular arrangements and becomes functionally specialized (Fig. 11-1).[17,31,39,40]

Medulla. Specific ectodermal cells ascend from the neural crest, migrate from their origin, and differentiate into sympathetic neurons of the autonomic nervous system.[17,31] Some of these primitive autonomic ganglia differentiate even further, into endocrine cells, designated as chromaffin cells, and migrate to form a mass on the medial surface of the fetal cortex.[11,17,31] Soon these chromaffin, or pheochrome, cells (from Greek *chroma*, color[41]) invade

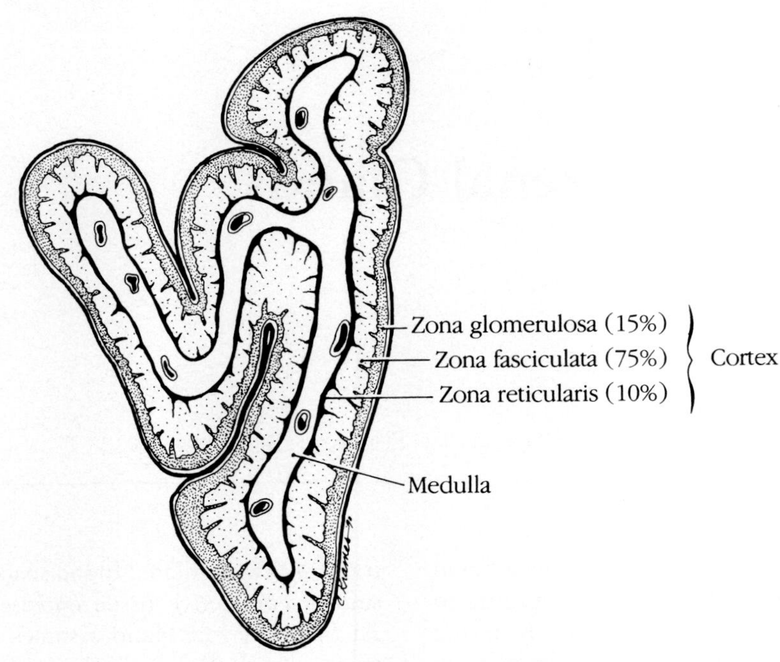

FIGURE 11-1. Cross-sectional anatomic plane of the adrenal gland demonstrates the medulla surrounded by three differentiated zones of cortex.

the developing cortex, establishing the primordium of the adrenal medulla.[11,17,31,40] The outer area of the medulla is stained a distinctive brownish color by chromic acid salts, believed to be the precursors of epinephrine.[17,31]

RELATIONAL ANATOMY

Like the kidneys, the adrenal glands are retroperitoneal.[40,43] They are generally anterior, medial, and superior to the kidneys.[17,28] The cortex and medulla are encapsulated by a thick inner layer of fatty connective tissue.[28,39,43] A thin, fibrous outer capsule attaches to the gland by many fibrous bands, providing the adrenals with their own fascial supports so they do not descend if the kidneys are displaced.[28,31] The glands are attached to the anteromedial aspect on top of Gerota's fascia, and abundant adipose tissue (perinephric fat) surrounds each gland, separating it from the kidneys (Fig. 11-2).[20,39]

Right Adrenal. The right adrenal gland is located posterior and lateral to the inferior vena cava (IVC), medial to the right lobe of the liver, and lateral to the crus of the diaphragm.[17,31]

The anterior surface of the right gland is shaped like a pyramid.[20,31] Two areas make up the anterior surface: the medial area is narrow and lies posterolateral to the inferior vena cava; the lateral, somewhat triangular portion, is in contact with the liver. The superior end of the lateral area is devoid of peritoneum as it comes in contact with the bare area of the liver, and the inferior portion is covered by reflected peritoneum from the inferior layer of the coronary ligament (Fig. 11-3A).[17]

A curved ridge separates the posterior dorsal surface into superior and inferior parts. The superior convex portion rests on the diaphragm, and the inferior concave portion is in contact with the superior, anterior surface of the right kidney (Fig. 11-3B).[17,20]

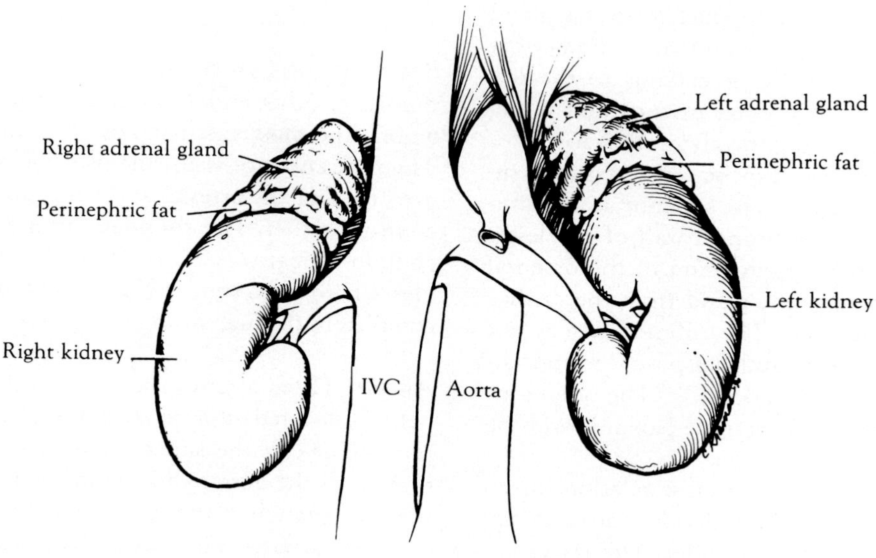

Figure 11-2. Adrenal glands are anteromedial to the kidneys.

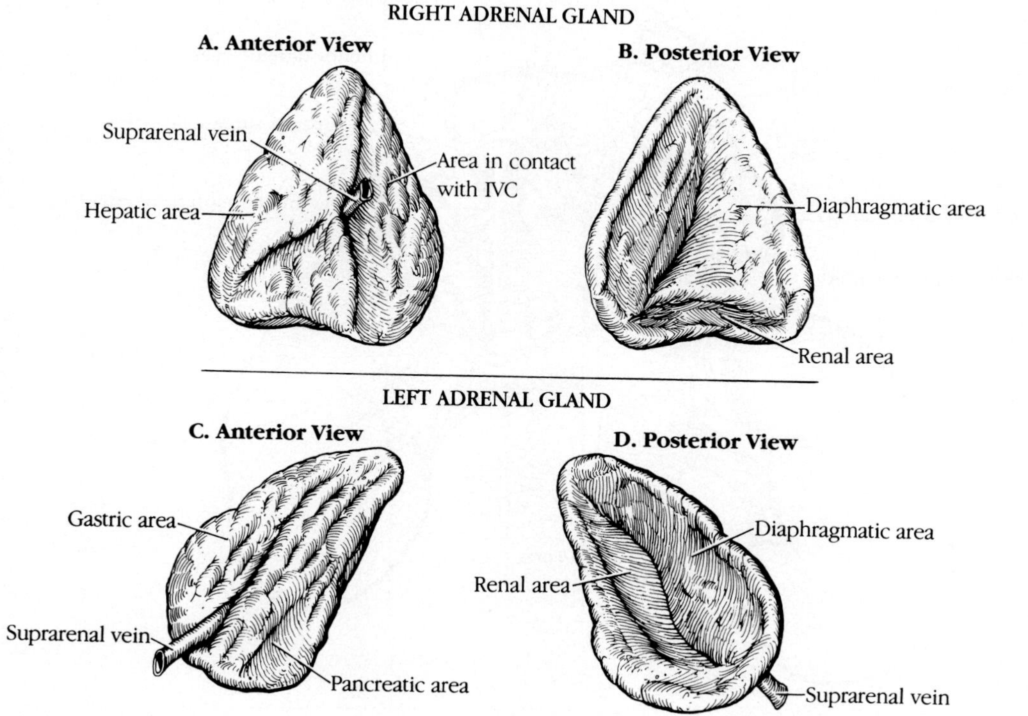

Figure 11-3. Topographical anatomy of the right and left adrenal glands.

Left Adrenal. Adapting to the medial border of the left kidney's superior surface, the left adrenal gland is elongated, crescentic, or semilunar.[17,31] Somewhat larger than the right one, it extends to the left renal hilus in 10% of normal persons and is frequently seen overlapping the abdominal aorta.[31]

The anterior portion can be separated into superior and inferior parts. The superior area is situated posterior to the peritoneal wall of the lesser sac and is covered by peritoneum of the omental bursa, which separates the gland from the cardiac portion of the stomach. The inferior area is not covered by peritoneum and lies posterior and lateral to the pancreas (Fig. 11-3C).[17,31] The splenic artery and vein course between the pancreas and the left adrenal gland.

The posterior surface is in close relationship to the splanchnic nerves.[17,31] It is divided into a medial and lateral area by a vertical ridge. The larger lateral area rests on the kidney, and the medial posterior area on the crus of the diaphragm (Fig. 11-3D).[17,31]

SYSTEMIC AND LYMPHATIC VESSELS

Similar to other endocrine glands, the adrenals are among the most vascular organs of the body.[31,39,43] Their vasculature is distinguished from other organs' in that the arteries and veins do not actually course together. The abundant arterial supply may contain as many as 50 to 60 small terminal arterioles, whereas the venous blood is channeled almost completely through a single large venous trunk.[31]

Arteries. Three arteries supply each gland: the superiorly located suprarenal branch of the inferior phrenic artery; the superior and medially located branch of the aorta; and the inferiorly located suprarenal branch of the renal artery (Fig. 11-4).[28,39,43]

These arteries are distinctively classified into three types: short capsular arterioles, intermediate

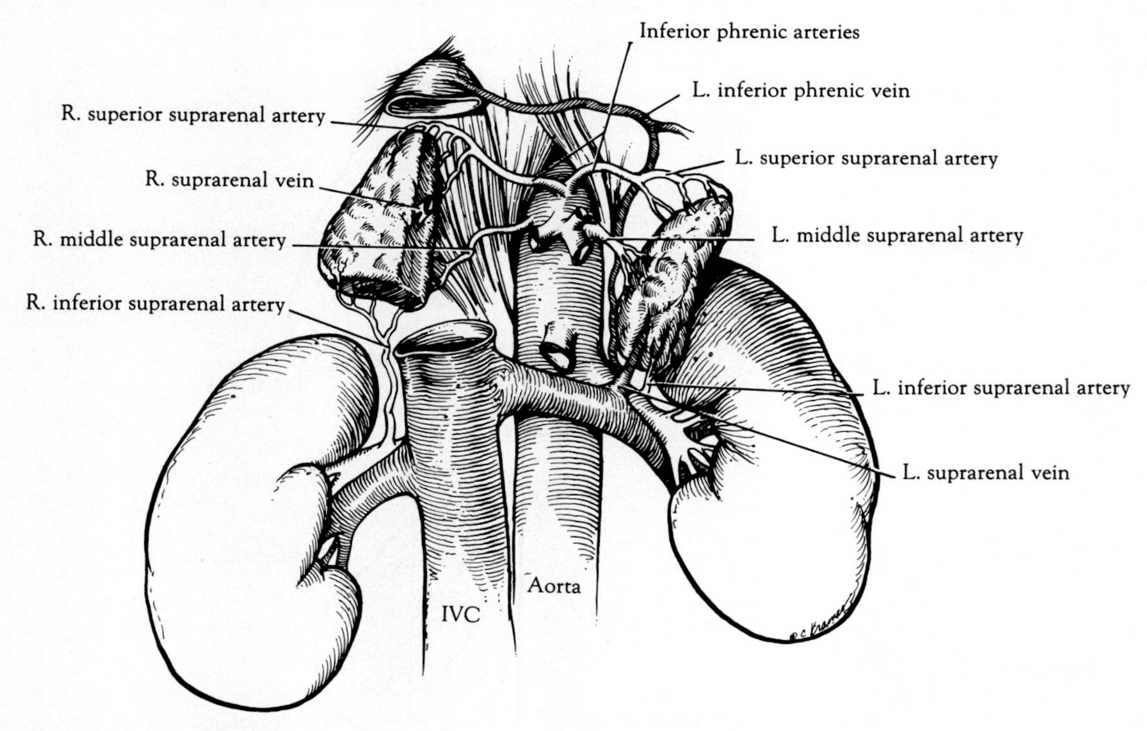

FIGURE 11-4. The adrenal vasculature.

cortical arteries (long branches that go through the cortex to the medulla), and the medullary sinusoids. Occasionally, a supplemental blood supply is furnished by branches of the spermatic or internal artery in males and the ovarian artery in females.[28,31,43]

Veins. The right gland empties directly into the inferior vena cava by way of the short (4 to 5 mm) suprarenal vein, which exits from the gland in an indentation or junction located on the anteromedial aspect between the upper and middle third. On the left side, inferior and medial to the gland, the left suprarenal vein drains directly into the left renal vein. Frequently, the left inferior phrenic vein and the left suprarenal vein join before emptying into the left renal vein (Fig. 11-4).[28,31,43]

Lymphatics. The lymphatic vessels accompany the suprarenal veins, drain first into the lumbar lymph nodes, which drain into the thoracic lymph nodes, returning lymph to the bloodstream.[28,40]

Physiology

The adrenals are endocrine glands essential to life. Just as their structure is unique, function and control of hormones for these two different glands, one inside the other, differs.[28,39]

CORTEX

The cortex makes up 90% of the gland. At approximately age 3 years, the cortex develops into three epithelial layers, each one evolving functionally into very specialized zones.[17,31,39,40] The zona glomerulosa, the outer layer directly beneath the connective tissue covering, makes up 15% of the cortex; the zona fasciculata, the middle layer, comprises 75% of the cortex; and the zona reticularis, the inner layer, accounts for the remaining 10% of the cortex (see Fig. 11-1).[3,17,31,39,40] Since these three layers have a mesodermal primordium similar to that of the gonads, they secrete steroid hormones.

Hormone secretion is often controlled by the negative-feedback mechanism. Low blood concentrations of a hormone trigger the hypothalamus to secrete a regulating factor, adrenocorticotropic hormone–releasing factor (ACTHRF), which triggers the anterior lobe of the pituitary to release adrenocorticotropic hormone (ACTH). As high blood concentrations of ACTH increase, adrenal hormone activity increases, producing a high concentration of that hormone in blood. This concentration inhibits ACTHRF, which inhibits ACTH, and ultimately hormone synthesis. When the blood concentration of the hormone is once again low, the cycle is repeated.[19,20,28,39,40,43] Adrenocortical hormone secretion, function, and regulation are summarized in Table 11-1.

MEDULLA

Originating from ectodermal cells, the medulla secretes catecholamine hormones, much like the posterior pituitary and thyroid glands. The medulla's chromaffin (pheochrome) cells, the hormone-producing portion, surround large blood-filled sinuses.[11,17,28,31,39]

Epinephrine (adrenalin) and norepinephrine (noradrenalin) are the two principal hormones synthesized by the medulla.[19,40,43] Epinephrine constitutes about 80% of the total secretion and its action is more important than that of norepinephrine.[19] Both hormones are sympathetic (that is, production is usually stimulated when any part of the sympathetic nervous system is stimulated), and the effects on target organs persist about 10 minutes longer than direct nerve stimulation.[19]

Adrenal nerve stimulation results in prompt discharge of medullary hormones without materially influencing cortical secretion.[28,43] Hormone secretion is controlled directly by the autonomic nervous system, and innervation by the preganglionic fibers allows the gland to respond to a stimulus.[19] Stress causes the hypothalamus to convey the message to the sympathetic preganglionic neurons to stimulate the chromaffin cells to increase output of epinephrine and norepinephrine.[17,19,40] The body responds by (1) accelerating the heart rate and constricting the vessels, causing increased blood pressure; (2) accelerating the rate of respiration and dilating the respiratory passage; (3) decreasing the rate of digestion, to make available more blood to the muscles, increasing the efficiency of muscle contraction; and (4) increasing blood sugar level for energy, thus stimulating cellular metabolism.[3,17,19,28,39,40,43] This physiologic response to stress is better known as the fight-or-flight response. Hypoglycemia may also stimulate medullary secretion

Table 11-1. Adrenal hormone secretion, function, and regulation[19,20,27,39,40,43]

Layer	Hormone	Function	Regulation
Zona glomerulosa	Three hormones classified as mineralocorticoids, but aldosterone is responsible for 95% of mineralocorticoid activity.	Regulate sodium and potassium levels, which affect the fluid and electrolyte homeostasis.	Complex process: dehydration, sodium deficiency, or hemorrhage contributes to one process, and elevated potassium levels contribute to a second process. ACTH has minor effect on secretion.
Zona fasciculata	Glucocorticoids, including cortisol or hydrocortisone (most abundant), cortisone, and corticosterone.	Major effect on metabolism of fats, proteins, and carbohydrates; encourages fat storage. When more energy is required, they assist in gluconeogenesis; helps resist both mental and physical stress. Hormones have an antiinflammatory effect and suppress immune responses.	High stress or low blood concentration (negative feedback mechanism).
Zona reticularis	Regardless of gender, secretes both male and female gonadocorticoids (estrogens and androgens).	Promotes normal development of bones and reproductive organs; affects secondary sex characteristics but not as much as hormones from ovaries and testes.	Low blood concentration (negative feedback mechanism).

of epinephrine and norepinephrine.[19,43] Like the glucocorticoids of the adrenal cortices, these hormones help the body resist stress; however, unlike the cortical hormones, the medullary hormones are not essential to life.[19]

Adrenal Function Tests

There are many different kinds of laboratory tests to evaluate adrenocortical function. They can be divided into two types: tests that determine the absolute values in serum and urine and tests that check the interdependency of the various hormones. Table 11-2 summarizes the significance of increased and decreased variance from normal laboratory values for various serum and urine tests.

The function of the medulla usually is not tested. With hypertension or pheochromocytoma, urine levels of catecholamine and/or vanillymandelic acid (VMA) may be elevated.[5]

Various tests are designed to determine the true functions and interdependency of the hypothalamus, pituitary, and adrenals. Included in this group are the ACTH stimulation test, the aldosterone stimulation and suppression tests, and the glucocorticoid suppression test.[7,25,42]

Sonographic Technique

Preparation

Usually, patients receive no preparatory instructions for ultrasonography of the adrenal glands, but when there is suspicion of a mass or metastases, or a need to sonographically image any retroperitoneal anatomy, it is recommended that the patient fast approximately 6 to 8 hours before the examination.

Patient Positions

A useful approach to evaluating the adrenals is to begin by placing the patient in the supine or decubitus position and scanning transversely before

TABLE 11-2. Tests of adrenal function[7,22,25,42]

SAMPLE	STEROID	VARIATION	CLINICAL IMPLICATIONS
Serum/urine	Aldosterone	Increase	Adenoma of the adrenal gland, adrenal gland hyperplasia, hemorrhage, low-sodium diet, excessive licorice consumption, stress, inadequate perfusion of kidney causing continual activity of the renin-angiotensin system (renin level would also be high), congestive heart failure, chronic obstructive lung disease, pregnancy, cirrhosis
		Decrease	Diabetes mellitus, high-sodium diet
Serum/urine	Cortisol	Increase	Pituitary tumor causing ACTH-dependent increase (Cushing's disease), Cushing's syndrome causing ACTH-independent increase, stress, long-term corticosteroid therapy
		Decrease	Addison's disease from primary hypofunction of the cortex or secondary to hypofunctioning of the pituitary gland, long-term administration of corticosteroids followed by withdrawal, iatrogenic adrenal insufficiency
Urine	17-Ketosteroids (17-KS)	Increase	Adrenogenital syndrome, cushing's syndrome
		Decrease	Addison's disease, Cushing's syndrome

scanning longitudinally.[23,27] While scanning, having the patient suspend inspiration may move the adrenal glands further inferiorly.[8] Various breathing excursions may be necessary before selecting the appropriate respiration excursion for optimal visualization of the right gland and then for the left one.

An appropriate transducer is selected for the patient's size and the depth of the adrenals,[27,47] as focal depth range may vary from 4 to 12 cm.[24] Enlarging the field size may improve visualization of small structures.[46] Scanning the patient in a prone position is uncommon, although this method is useful to show the spatial relationship between a large adrenal mass and the kidney.

Right Adrenal. For imaging the right adrenal, the liver and sometimes the right kidney are useful acoustic windows.[20] Successful utilization of the liver as an acoustic window depends on its size and attenuation characteristics.[47] Starting with transverse scans using an intercostal approach, the beam should be directed toward the IVC and perpendicular to the spine.[47] The entire right adrenal gland is evaluated by scanning from the renal hilus and proceeding superiorly (Fig. 11-5).

Longitudinal scanning of the right gland can be accomplished with several approaches (Fig. 11-6).[47] A higher success rate has been reported when utilizing the liver as an acoustic window and scanning the patient in a left lateral decubitus position.[20,47,48,50] The transducer is angled anterior to the inferior vena cava and posterior to the right kidney until the entire gland is visualized (Fig. 11-7).

Left Adrenal. The left adrenal gland is more difficult to locate and scan. Conventionally, the left adrenal has been imaged with the patient in the right decubitus position, using the spleen or left kidney as an acoustic window (Fig. 11-8).[20,23,24,47] Identifying the left adrenal and its alignment is first achieved in the transverse plane.

Longitudinal scans are easier to obtain with the patient in a right anterior oblique position using a left posterior oblique scanning plane. First the aorta is scanned through the left kidney or the spleen, until the axis of the left kidney and the position of the aorta are determined and the left adrenal gland is identified (Fig. 11-9A).[20,47] With the patient in the same position, the longitudinal plane is imaged. In imaging the left adrenal gland,

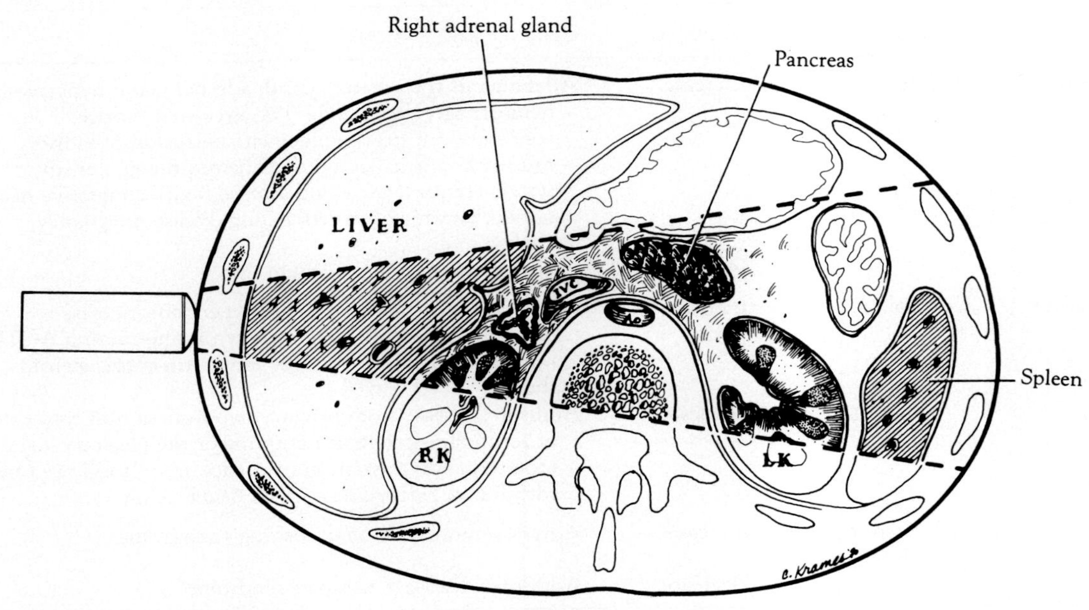

FIGURE 11-5. With the patient in a supine position, a series of transverse scans are imaged through the intercostal spaces of the right adrenal gland using the liver and kidney as acoustic windows. Generally the transducer is angled from posterior to superior (RK, right kidney; LK, left kidney).

the transducer may have to be oriented obliquely (Fig. 11-9B).[47]

Krebs and colleagues[23,24] have introduced a new approach to improved localization and delineation of the left adrenal gland. The patient is placed in a 45-degree left posterior oblique position, termed the cava-suprarenal line (CSL) position.[23,24] The transducer is placed on the patient's right side, allowing the acoustic beam to pass through a double vascular acoustic window, the inferior vena cava and the aorta (Fig. 11-10).[24] The protocol starts with transverse scans until the left adrenal gland is located; longitudinal views follow. With this position the success rate was 90%, compared to 60% in the same patient population using the conventional approach.[23,24]

PITFALLS

The size, location, and pathology of the adrenals and of surrounding structures impose significant limitations on sonographic visualization. Cirrhosis with fatty infiltration of the liver and obesity interfere with adequate penetration.[18] Shadowing from the ribs and narrow intercostal spaces may make this approach challenging.

Structures that converge in the area of the left adrenal gland can mimic the organ: the esophagogastric junction, stomach, splenic vessels, tail of the pancreas, medial lobulations of the spleen, or superior lobulations of the kidney.[20,46] A more posterolateral approach or the CSL position may be indicated.

The right adrenal gland may be obscured by gas and food in the second portion of the duodenum.[20] It is important to differentiate the crus of the diaphragm as a tubular structure located medial to the right adrenal, as it can be mistaken for a normal gland.[8,20,47] The right adrenal gland is usually displaced posteriorly when the retroperitoneal fat line is displaced by liver disease.[32,46]

(text continues on page 383)

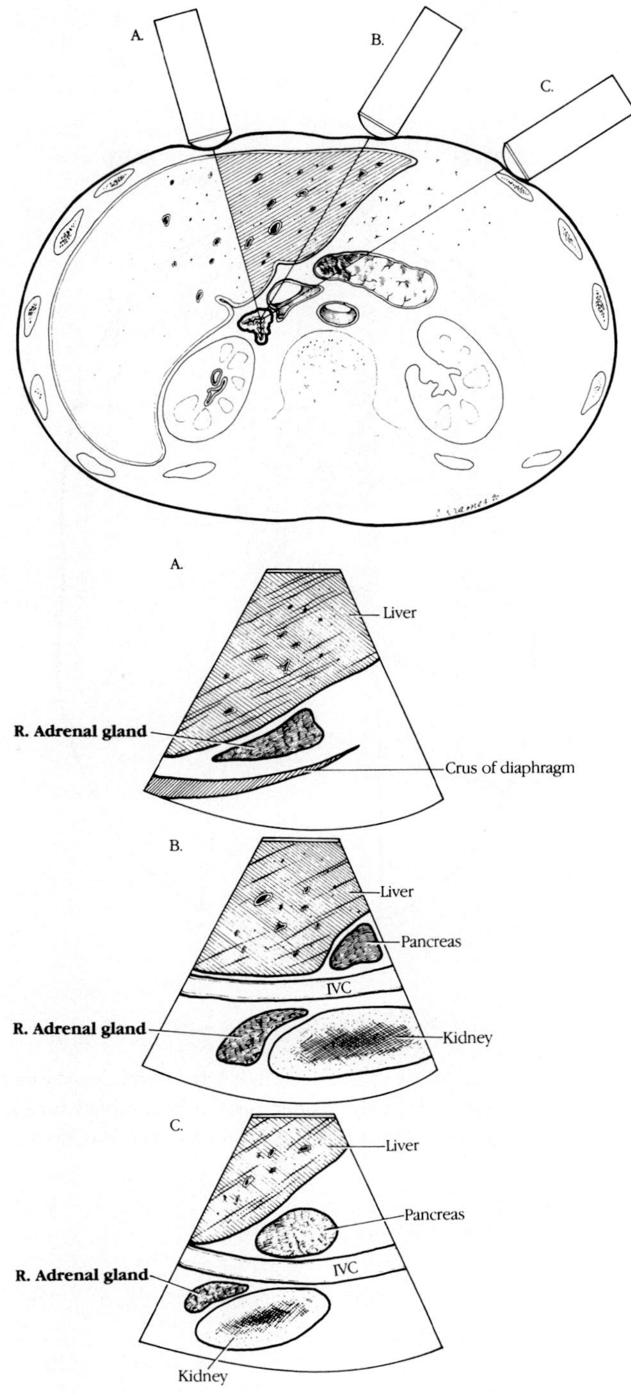

FIGURE 11-6. Longitudinal images of the right adrenal gland are obtained with the patient in a supine position using the liver as an acoustic window. Views A and B can be used on most patients, whereas view C requires that the left liver lobe be of moderate size.

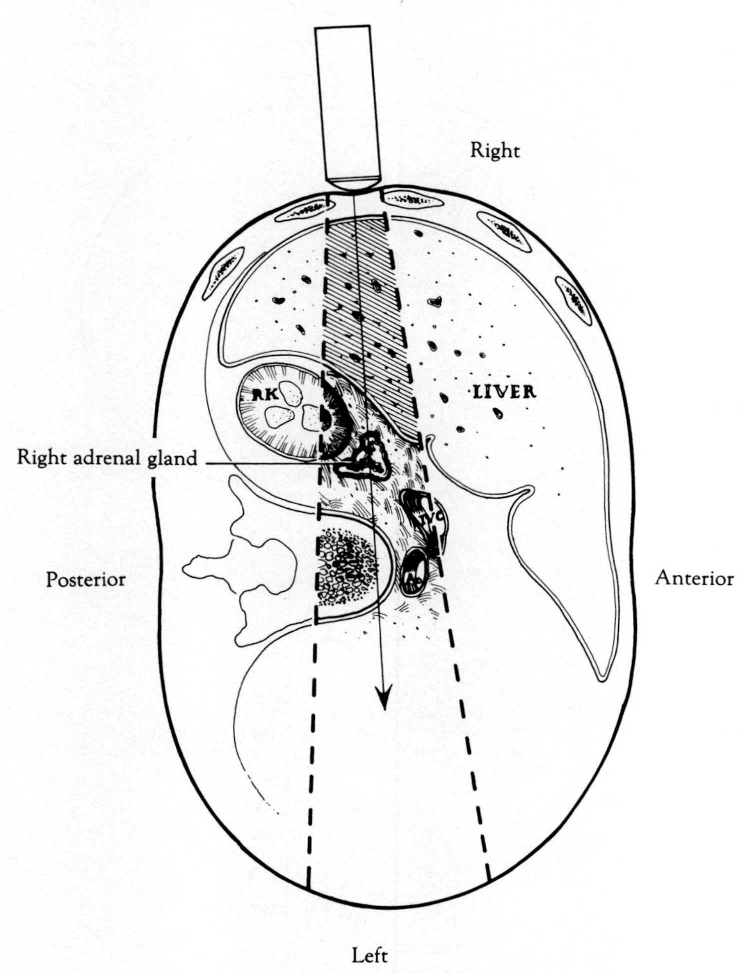

FIGURE 11-7. With the patient in a left lateral decubitus position, the right adrenal gland may be easier to visualize as the IVC moves forward and the aorta moves over the crus of the diaphragm (RK, right kidney; Ao, aorta).

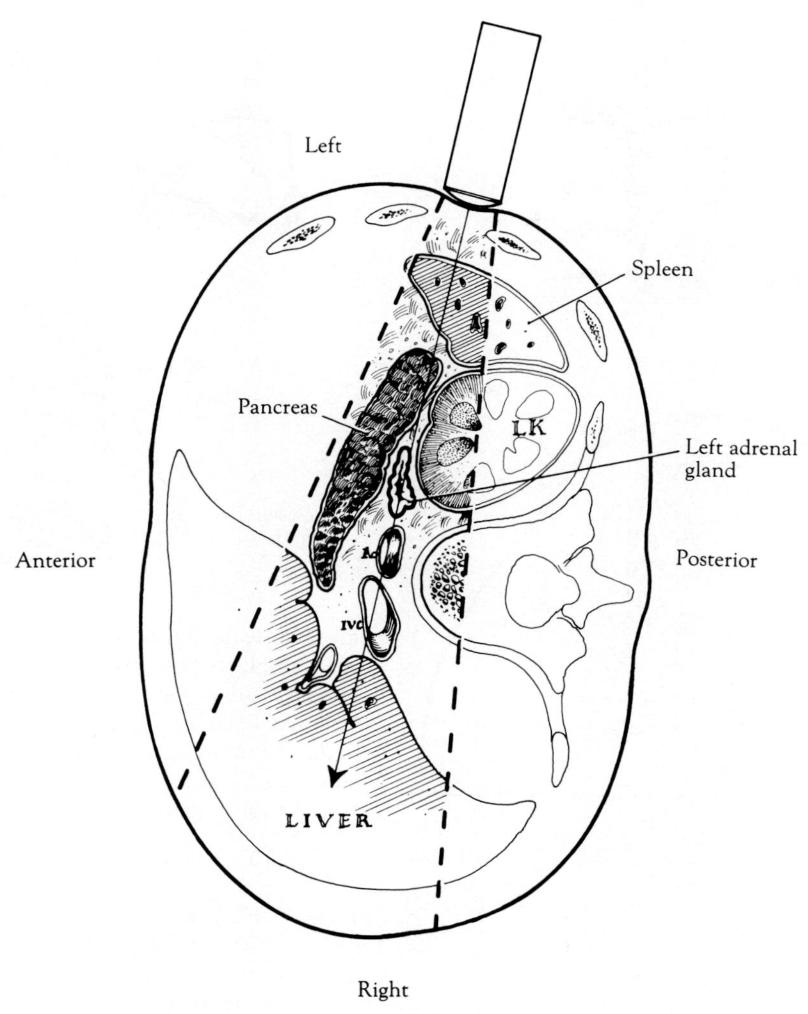

FIGURE 11-8. Using the spleen or the left kidney (LK) as an acoustic window, transverse images of the left adrenal gland can be made with the patient in a right lateral decubitus position (Ao, aorta; IVC, inferior vena cava).

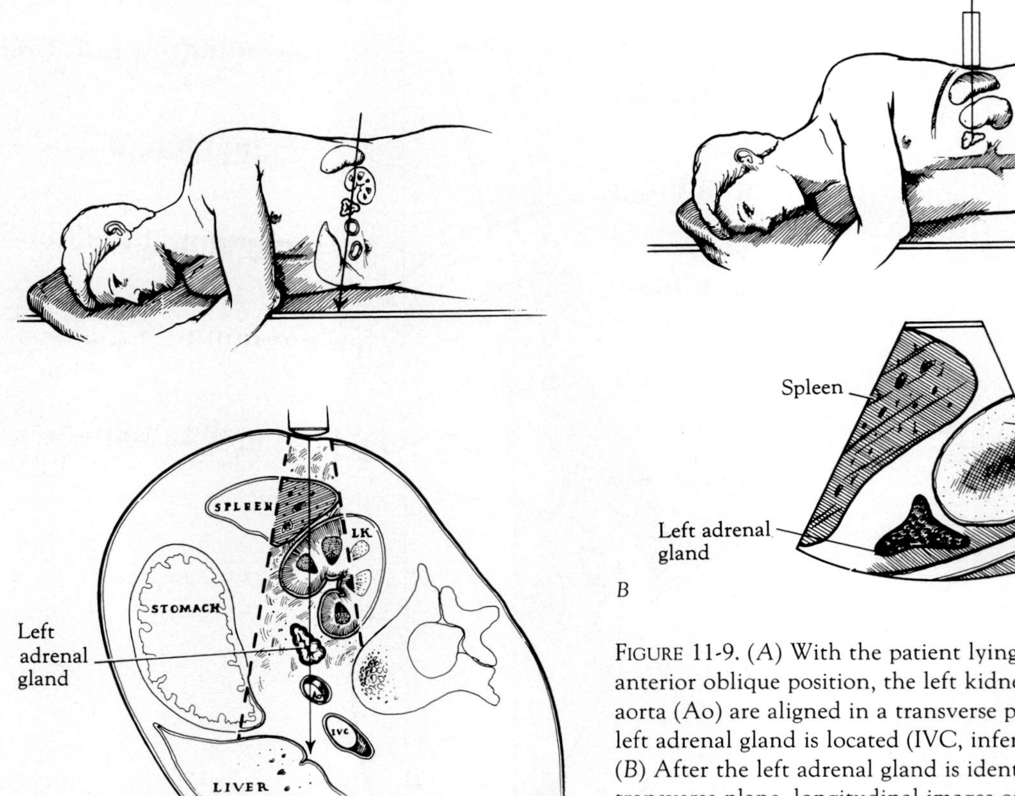

FIGURE 11-9. (*A*) With the patient lying in a right anterior oblique position, the left kidney (LK) and aorta (Ao) are aligned in a transverse plane until the left adrenal gland is located (IVC, inferior vena cava). (*B*) After the left adrenal gland is identified in the transverse plane, longitudinal images of the entire gland are easier to obtain.

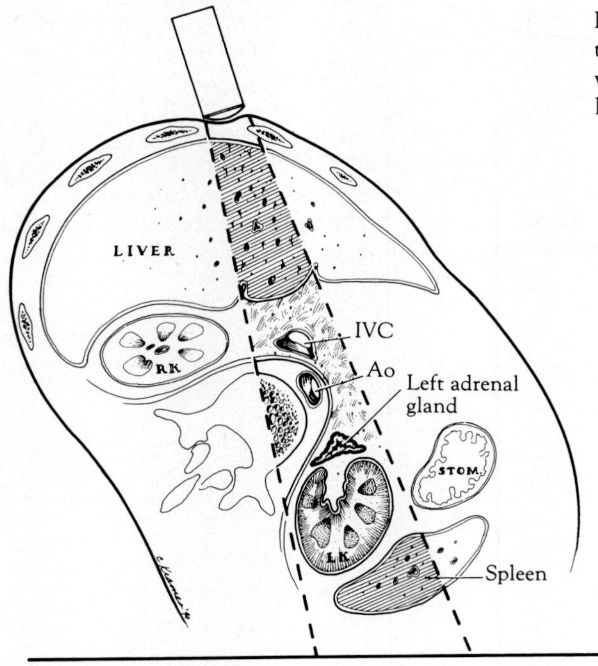

FIGURE 11-10. The cava-suprarenal line position uses the IVC and aorta (Ao) as a double vascular acoustic window for visualizing the left adrenal gland (RK, right kidney; LK, left kidney).[23,24]

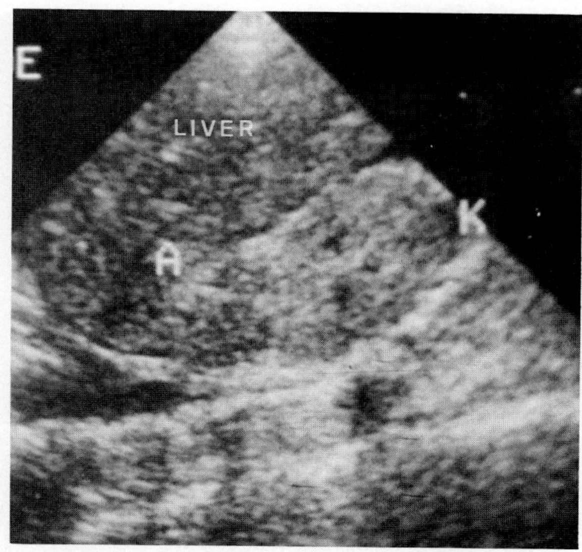

FIGURE 11-11. A normal right fetal adrenal gland (A) is visualized superior to the right kidney (K) in a longitudinal section.

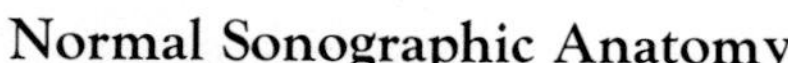

Normal Sonographic Anatomy

Fetal adrenal glands are quite large, and 90% of the time at least one can be imaged after 26 to 27 weeks' gestation (Fig. 11-11).[16,37] In adults, they are much smaller. The glands are generally located anterior, medial, and superior to the kidneys and vary in shape and configuration.[18,29,38] Size varies from 3 to 6 cm long, 2 to 4 cm wide, and 3 to 10 mm thick; the adult adrenals weigh 4 to 14 g.[17,20,29,31,47,48] The cortex and medulla are not distinguishable, as the normal internal texture appears homogeneous and hypoechoic.[29] In some patients, only highly echogenic fat can be identified.[18,29]

RIGHT ADRENAL

The right adrenal gland is identified superior to the kidney and lateral to the crus of the diaphragm.[29,48] On transverse sections, the gland is described as having a triangular, trapezoid or inverted Y or V shape, with the tail extending from the anteromedial aspect of the right kidney (Fig. 11-12).[29,49] In a longitudinal section scanning medial, the anteromedial ridge appears as a curvilinear or S-shaped structure and is visualized posterior to the IVC, slightly above or at the level of the portal vein.[20,29,48,49] Moving laterally in longitudinal sections, the anterior and posterior wings spread open and the gland takes on an inverted Y or V shape (Fig. 11-13).[49] The anterolateral portion is medial

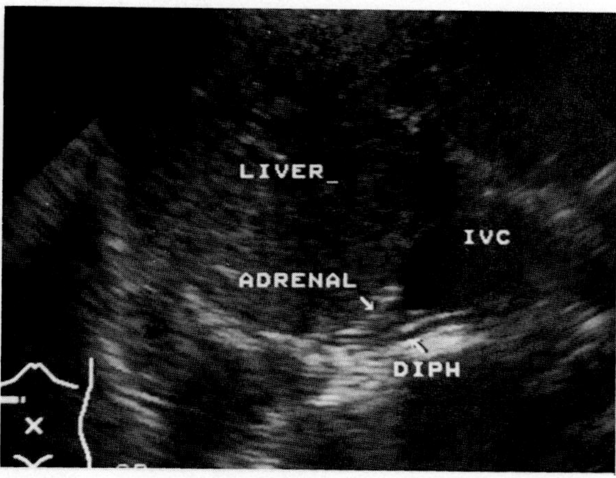

FIGURE 11-12. A transverse plane of the normal right adrenal gland demonstrates its relationship to the liver, IVC, and diaphragm (DIPH). (Courtesy Doug Amussen, Logan, UT.)

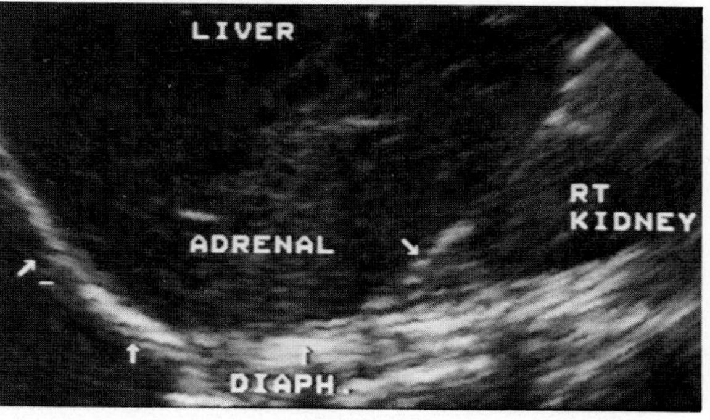

FIGURE 11-13. In longitudinal sections moving from lateral to medial, a normal V- or Y-shaped right adrenal gland is seen in relationship to the right kidney, liver, and diaphragm (DIAPH). (Courtesy Doug Amussen, Logan, UT.)

and posterior to the right lobe of the liver and posterior to the duodenum.[29]

Left Adrenal

Lateral to the crus of the diaphragm and lateral or slightly posterolateral to the aorta, the left adrenal gland is visualized superior to the kidney.[20,29,38,49] This gland is described as having a triangular or semilunar appearance (Fig. 11-14). Since the stomach lies posterior to the lesser omental sac (a potential space that is usually collapsed), the superior portion of the adrenal gland can appear directly behind the stomach.[49] The inferior portion of the gland lies posterior to the pancreas. The splenic artery and vein can be identified passing between the left adrenal gland and the pancreas, which is located anterior to the inferior portion of the left adrenal gland.[29,38,49] On longitudinal sections posterior to the pancreas, the left adrenal has a similar sonographic configuration to that of the right gland (Fig. 11-15).[49]

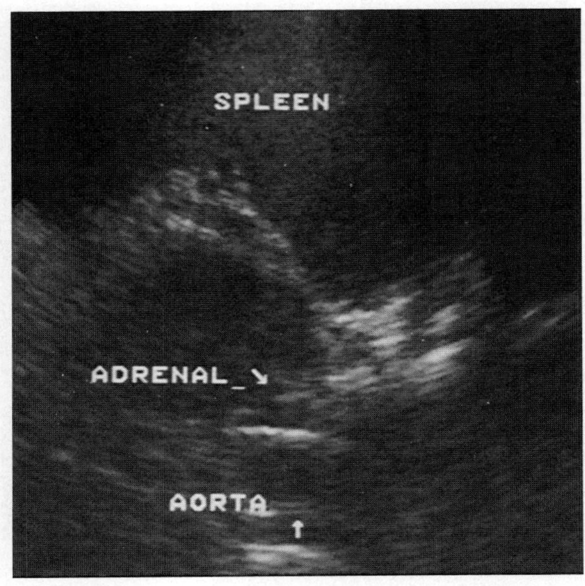

Figure 11-14. The normal left adrenal gland's triangular shape and its relationship to the aorta and spleen can be identified in this transverse section. (Courtesy Doug Amussen, Logan, UT.)

Pathology

In most cases of suspected adrenal disease, CT is the imaging modality of choice.[30] Better visualization of the adrenal areas is obtained with CT, particularly in patients with adequate retroperitoneal fat.[30] Ultrasonography provides an alternative for screening children from families with the multiple endocrine neoplasia (MEN) syndromes and for poor candidates for CT who have a paucity of retroperitoneal fat.[30] Indications for sonography include the presence of metastases; an adrenal hemorrhage, cyst, or tumor; and hypertrophy of the gland.

Since a mass may be encountered incidentally during routine abdominal or renal scanning, it is important to understand adrenal pathology and its clinical manifestations, to correlate laboratory values, and to identify normal and abnormal sonographic appearances. A change in the normal appearance of the gland's size and configuration serves as an indication of adrenal abnormalities. An increase in size can cause compression or displacement of surrounding structures. With right adrenal disease, the retroperitoneal fat line, inferior vena cava, and right renal vein may be displaced anteriorly while the right kidney is displaced posteriorly (Fig. 11-16).[32] An enlarged left adrenal gland may displace the splenic vein anteriorly and the left kidney inferiorly or posteriorly.[32] An adrenal mass should be differentiated from a renal mass by identifying an echo interface separating the mass from the upper pole of the kidney (Fig. 11-17).[29,49]

Metastatic Disease

Adrenal glands are the fourth most common site of metastases after lungs, liver, and bones.[29,30] Metastases to the adrenal glands occurs from squamous cell carcinoma of the lung (33%), breast carcinoma (30%), and lymphoma, melanoma, and carcinoma of the gastrointestinal tract, thyroid, pancrease, and kidney (37%).[29,30] Patients with bronchogenic carcinoma of the lung have adrenal metastases 33% of the time, and there is a 25% incidence of adrenal involvement in non-Hodgkin's lymphoma.[29]

Small adrenal masses (4 to 5 cm) characteristically are hypoechoic, round or oval, and are lo-

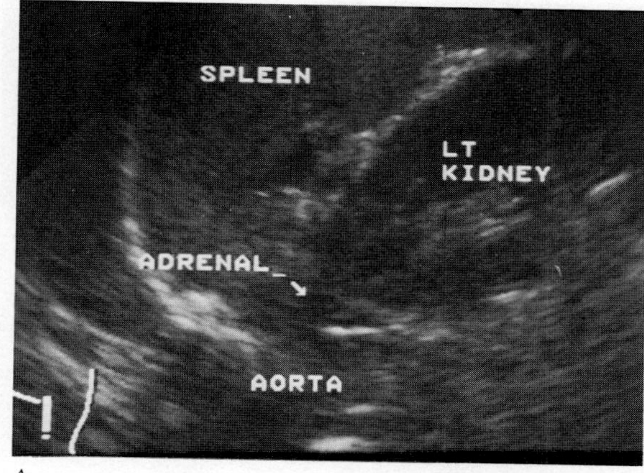

A

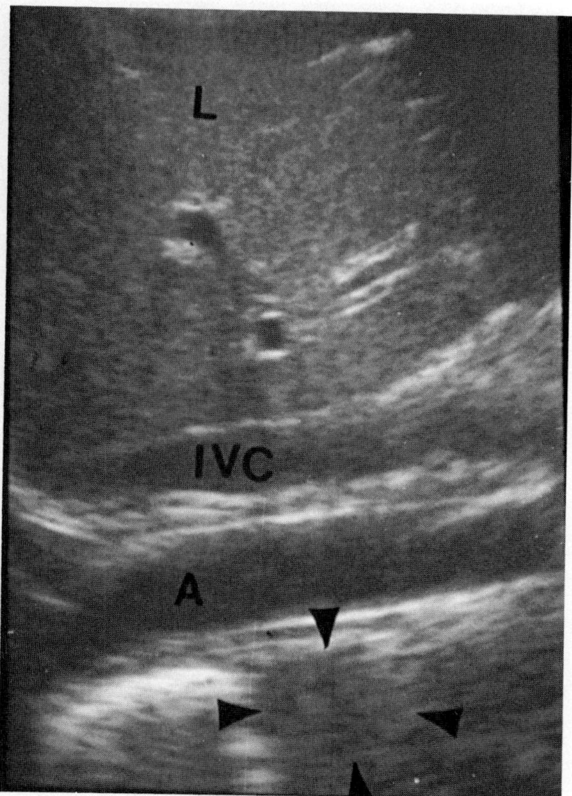

B

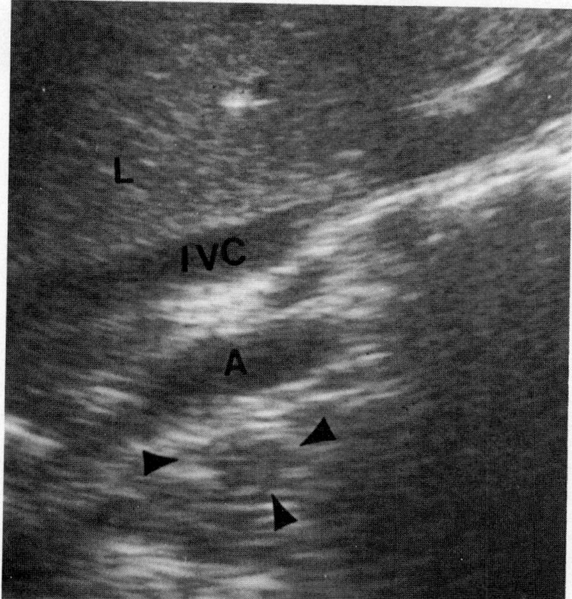

C

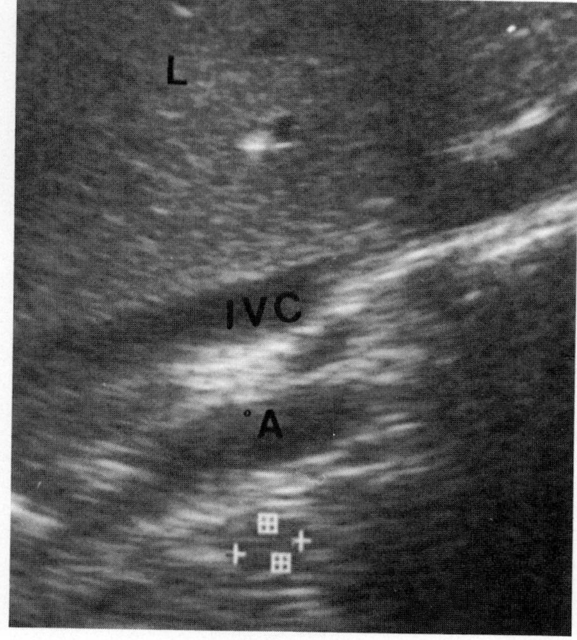

D

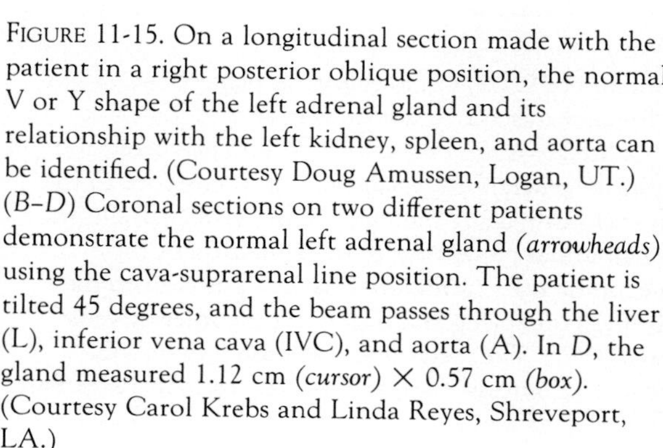

FIGURE 11-15. On a longitudinal section made with the patient in a right posterior oblique position, the normal V or Y shape of the left adrenal gland and its relationship with the left kidney, spleen, and aorta can be identified. (Courtesy Doug Amussen, Logan, UT.) (*B–D*) Coronal sections on two different patients demonstrate the normal left adrenal gland *(arrowheads)* using the cava-suprarenal line position. The patient is tilted 45 degrees, and the beam passes through the liver (L), inferior vena cava (IVC), and aorta (A). In *D*, the gland measured 1.12 cm *(cursor)* × 0.57 cm *(box)*. (Courtesy Carol Krebs and Linda Reyes, Shreveport, LA.)

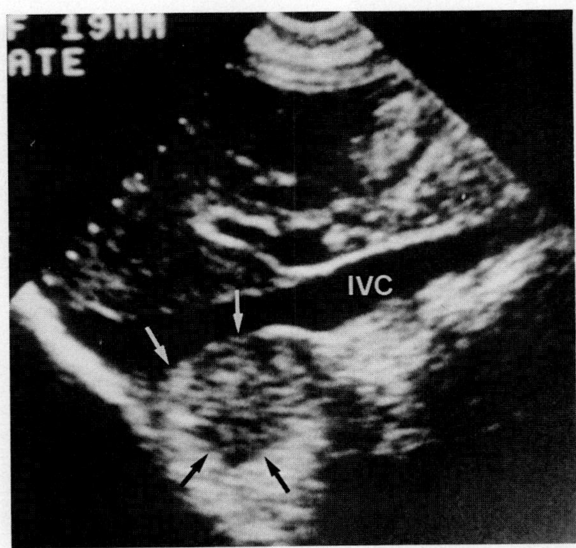

Figure 11-16. On a longitudinal scan through the liver, a right adrenal mass *(arrows)* is demonstrated indenting the posterior wall of the inferior vena cava (IVC).

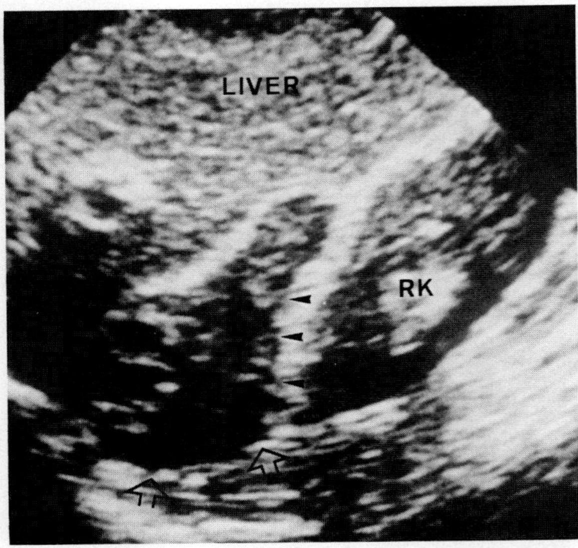

Figure 11-17. A longitudinal, coronal scan of a large right adrenal gland mass *(open arrows)* causing downward displacement of the right kidney (RK) is identified superior and separate from the upper pole of the kidney (RK) by an echo interface *(arrowheads)*.

cated anteromedial to the upper pole of the kidney (Fig. 11-18).[29,49,50] Larger masses may present with irregular margins and can indent the posterior wall of the IVC and displace the kidneys inferiorly (Fig. 11-19).[29,30] Hypoechoic and hyperechoic areas within these masses may represent necrosis and hemorrhage (Fig. 11-20); Table 11-3).[29] Only about half of the adrenal masses in patients with known primary tumors proved to be malignant on biopsy examination.[30] Therefore, a solitary nonfunctioning adrenal tumor should not be considered pathognomonic for metastatic disease without being correlated with other findings.[30] Percutaneous aspiration biopsy is capable of distinguishing metastases from an incidental adenoma or a primary adrenal carcinoma.[30]

Cysts

Relatively infrequent and usually asymptomatic, adrenal cysts may be incidental findings. The endothelial type may be subdivided into lymphangiomatous (41%) and angiomatous (3%); pseudocysts (40%) are secondary to hemorrhage into or around the gland; and epithelial cysts (6%) result from cystic degeneration of adenomas and parasitic cysts.[29,38]

Adrenal cysts demonstrate the characteristic sonographic cystic appearance. They appear as rounded, fluid-filled masses with thin, smooth walls. They may be unilocular or multilocular,

Figure 11-19. (*A*) On a transverse plane view, a right adrenal metastatic tumor measuring 8 × 7.5 cm is visualized as a solid mass with both hyperechoic and cystic degenerative areas *(arrowheads)* posterior to the liver (L) displacing the right kidney (RK). (*B*) On the longitudinal plane view of the same patient the metastatic mass *(arrowheads)* is seen posterior to the liver (L) indenting and displacing the inferior vena cava (IVC). The metastases are secondary to bone cancer. (Courtesy Tamara Salsgiver, Hill Air Force Base, UT.)

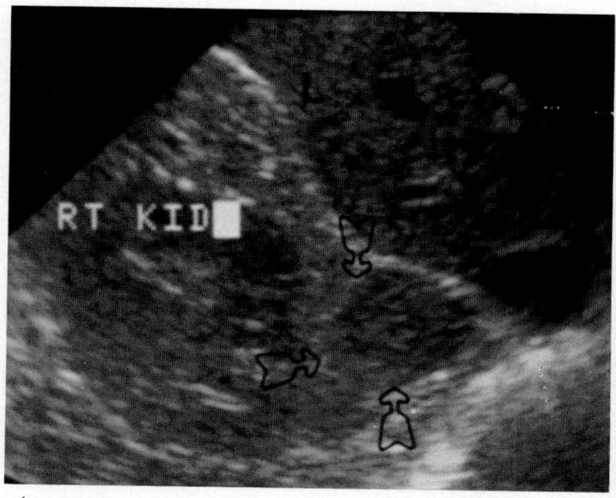

A

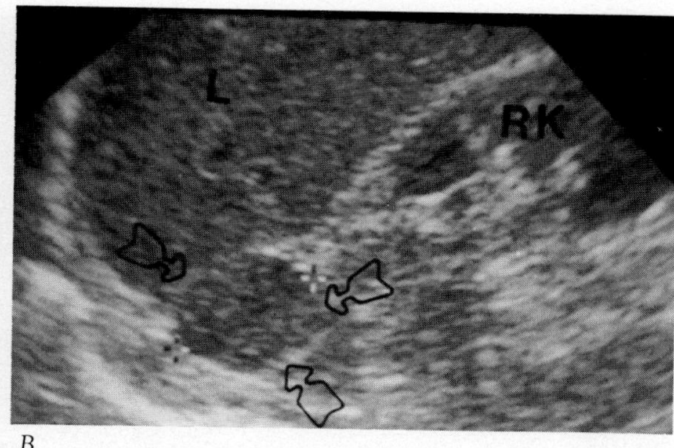

B

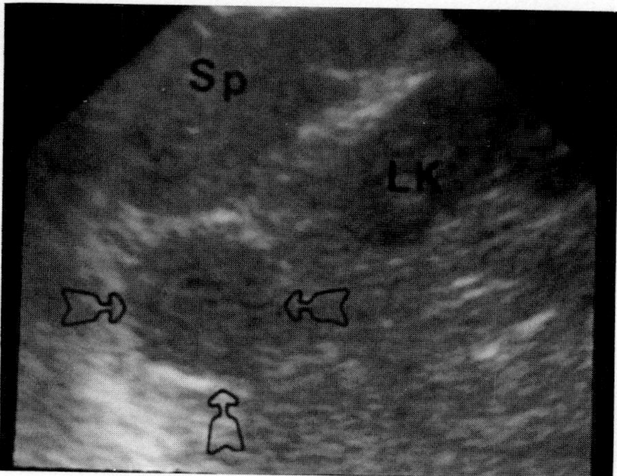

C

FIGURE 11-18. Solid masses *(open arrows)*, tumor metastases, are seen in both right and left adrenal gland. The right adrenal mass is identified posterior to the liver, medial to the right kidney, and lateral to the inferior vena cava (IVC). The left mass is identified inferior to the spleen (Sp) and medial to the left kidney (LK). (Courtesy John Guida, Portland, OR.)

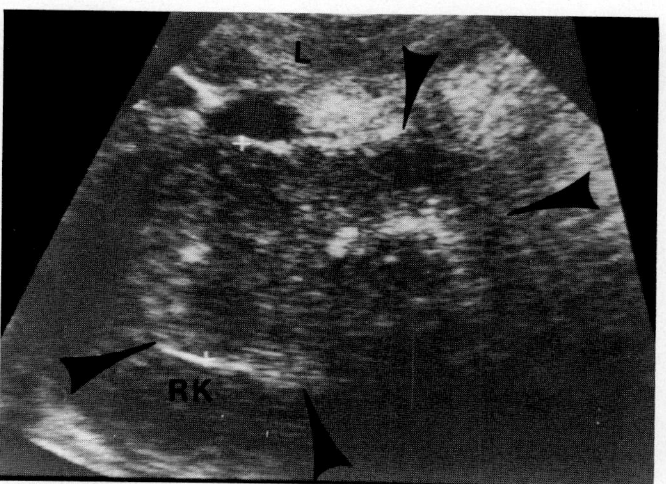

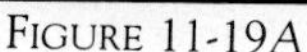

FIGURE 11-19*A*

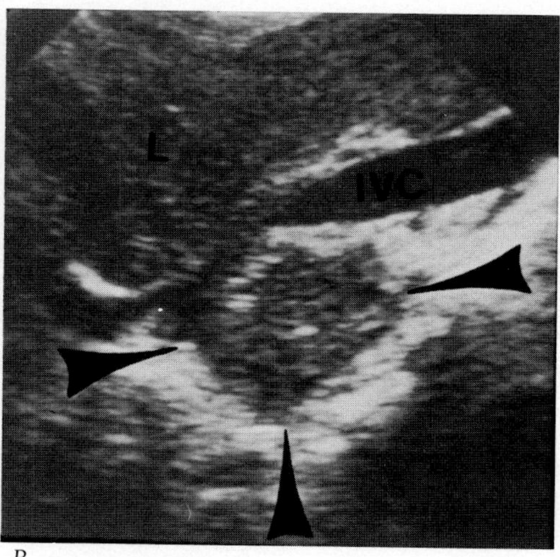

B

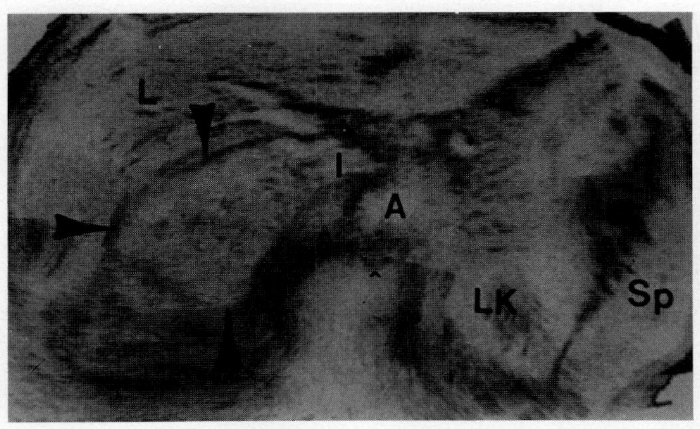

A

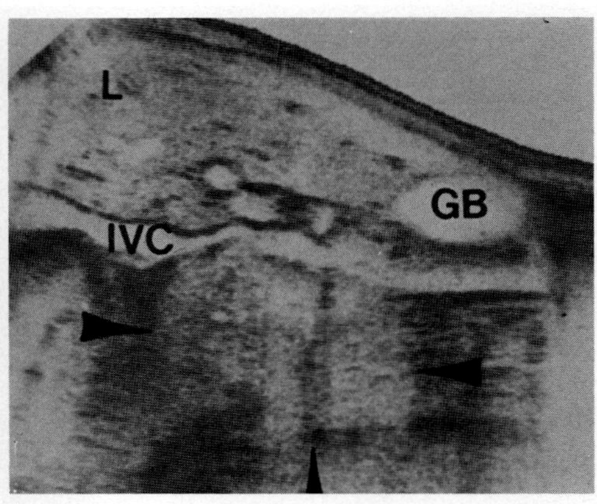

B

Figure 11-20. (*A*) A right adrenal metastatic tumor is visualized as a solid mass with both hyperechoic and cystic degenerative areas *(arrowheads)* on a transverse plane. Surrounding the aorta (A) and inferior vena cava (I) enlarged lymph nodes *(carets)* can be identified (L, liver; Sp, spleen; LK, left kidney). (*B*) On the longitudinal plane view of the same patient the metastatic mass *(arrowheads)* indents and displaces the inferior vena cava (IVC). The primary site is the lung (L, liver; GB, gallbladder). (Courtesy Cathy Carr-Hoefer, Corvallis, OR.)

Table 11-3. Adrenal gland pathology—general

Pathology	Cause	Sonographic Appearance
Metastatic disease	Develops from squamous cell carcinoma of the lung, breast, GI tract, thyroid, pancreas, kidney; lymphoma, melanoma	Small masses (4 to 5 cm); usually bilateral, solid, well-circumscribed, encased within the adrenal; located anteromedially; may have irregular margins and can indent IVC and displace kidney; necrosis (hypoechoic) or areas of hemorrhage (hyperechoic) may occur within the mass.
Cyst	Develops from hemorrhage, trauma, or idiopathic	Rounded, fluid-filled mass, with thin, smooth wall; unilocular or multilocular; calcifications may be present with acoustic shadowing affecting through-transmission; ring calcification has higher incidence of malignancy; hemorrhage with dense clot presents a thick, hyperechoic area in pseudocyst type.
Hemorrhage	Birth trauma or anoxia, systemic disease, anticoagulant therapy, metastases, adrenal trauma	Echo pattern variable, depending on age of hemorrhage; complex mass located anterosuperior to kidney may displace it; may shrink; calcifications if present appear as focal hyperechoic areas, with or without acoustic shadowing.

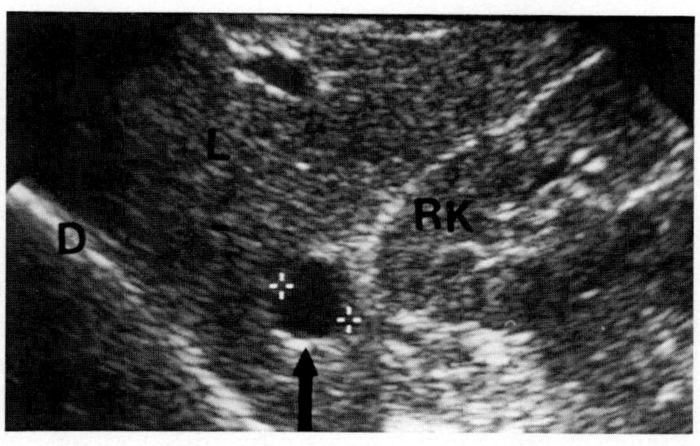

FIGURE 11-21. A right adrenal gland cyst (*arrow* and *cursors*) superior to the right kidney (RK) and posterior to the liver (L) can be identified in this longitudinal section (D, diaphragm). (Courtesy Cathy Carr-Hoefer, Corvallis, OR.)

small or large (Fig. 11-21).[29] Calcifications are found in 15% of cases, and dense clot retraction may persist, providing a thick, hyperechoic area in the pseudocystic variety.[29,38,49] Most adrenal cysts are benign, but adrenal cysts with a "ring" calcification are more often malignant.[49] The calicified cyst wall produces a thick, hyerechoic ring that may or may not cast an acoustic shadow (see Table 11-3).[49] For a purely cystic mass, percutaneous, fine-needle aspiration may be indicated to examine the contents or relieve symptoms associated with pressure.[29]

HEMORRHAGE

Hemorrhage of the adrenal gland is seen most often in newborns, especially after a difficult delivery in which fetal oxygen is diminished or cut off for some time (see Chapter 18). Hemorrhage can also be precipitated by meningococcal septicemia, anticoagulant therapy, adrenal vein thrombosis, adrenal metastases, or adrenal trauma.[21] The right side is often more involved in the hemorrhagic process, which is probably associated with right adrenal venous drainage directly off the IVC.

Depending on the stage of organization, the echo pattern of adrenal hemorrhage varies. The appearance can range from an anechoic to a hyperechoic suprarenal mass (Fig. 11-22).[12,29] With age, the mass may shrink, and calcifications can appear as focal hyperechoic areas with associated acoustic shadowing (see Table 11-3).[12]

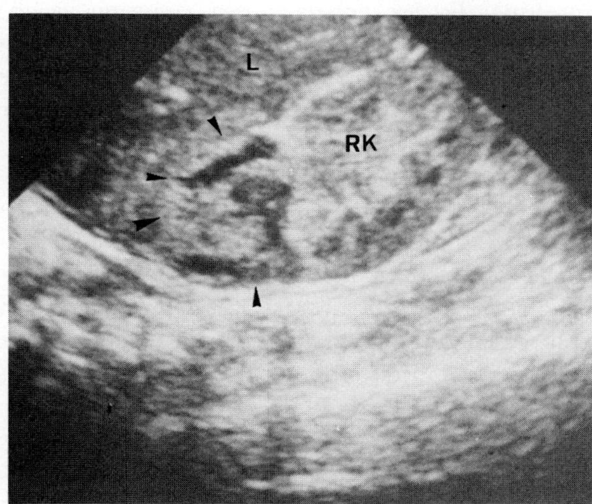

A

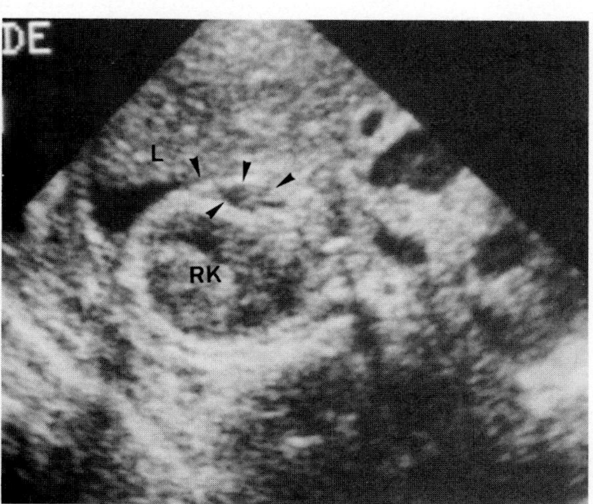

B

FIGURE 11-22. In both (*A*) longitudinal and (*B*) transverse plane views of an infant, a hemorrhage (*arrowheads*) is identified in the right adrenal gland posterior to the liver (L) and superior to the right kidney (RK).

Cortical Pathology

Adrenal cortex pathology can be divided into three categories: disorders that diminsh steroid output, disorders that increase steroid production, and lesions that have no functional effect. The representation of cortical disease contributes to an understanding of those that are evaluated with ultrasonography.

DEVELOPMENTAL ANOMALIES

The most important congenital disorders are the adrenocortical hyperplasias, which cause alterations and increases in steroid synthesis. These are discussed further with hyperadrenalism.

Congenital Hypoplasia. There are two types of congenital adrenal hypoplasia, the anencephalic type and the cytomegalic type. In both types, essential hormone production is altered.

In an anencephalic, usually stillborn, fetus, the adrenal gland consists of only a provisional cortex with no fetal zone.[36] The cause of the disorder is either cerebral, pituitary, or hypothalamic.

The cause of the cytomegalic type is unknown. An unusual adrenal cortex is made up histologically of large eosinophilic cells. Usually the gland weighs less than 1 g and is not identifiable by ultrasound. With early diagnosis, early replacement steroid therapy promotes long survival.[36]

Ectopy. Ectopic adrenal glands consist mainly of accessory cortical material and can occur anywhere from the diaphragm to the pelvis;[36] in the kidney, liver, retroperitoneal tissues, ovary, testis, and in the tissues accompanying the spermatic cord. The ectopia may have either cortical or cortical and medullary cellular components. On surgical resection, ectopic adrenal tissue is identified by its bright yellow color. Because of their location and size, they are not commonly identified by ultrasound.

HYPOADRENALISM (HYPOCORTICISM)

Hypoadrenalism or adrenocortical hypofunction may be caused by primary disorders of the cortex or by secondary failure in the elaboration of ACTH. The clinical manifestation—atrophic or necrotic destruction of the cortex—usually is not detectable by ultrasound, but complications such as hemorrhage can be identified.

Chronic Primary Hypoadrenalism (Addison's Disease). The chronic form of hypoadrenalism (Addison's disease) is the most common.[36] Insufficient secretion of adrenocortical hormones results from the insidious and profound atrophy of the adrenal glands.[4,36] Addison's disease is uncommon (four per 100,000); it becomes evident only when 90% of functioning adrenocortical cells have been destroyed.[34,36] The two major causes of adrenal destruction are idiopathic atrophy (80%) attributed to an autoimmune disorder and tuberculosis (20%).[4,31,36] Females are more often affected by the idiopathic atrophic type and males by the type caused by tuberculosis.[4]

Clinical symptoms depend on the degree of hormone deficiency.[31,36] Because of adrenal atrophy, steroid response is diminished or absent, causing an increase in the pituitary gland's production of ACTH.[18,36] Because ACTH has melanin-stimulating properties, about 98% of affected persons present with changes in skin color.[4] Other clinical manifestations include sodium and potassium retention, renal impairment, and decreases in blood volume, sugar, and lipids.[36] Symptoms can include fatigue, muscle weakness, hypotension, and gastrointestinal distress such as nausea, vomiting, weight loss, and diarrhea.[4,31,36] The disease may be managed by administration of steroids, but patients are vulnerable to all forms of stress, which may trigger hypoadrenal crisis and shock.[36]

When Addison's disease is caused by tuberculosis, the glands are enlarged, firm, and nodular, with a thick capsule. The sonographic appearance can range from a normal echoic appearance to hyperechoic with areas of necrosis. Small, irregular, and contracted adrenal glands that usually are not identified on ultrasound occur with idiopathic Addison's disease (Table 11-4).

Chronic Secondary Hypoadrenalism. Any disorder to the hypophyseal-thalamic axis that reduces the output of ACTH causes atrophy of the adrenal cortex and decreases secretion of cortisol and androgen.[4,36] The most common cause is abrupt cessation of exogenous steroid therapy.[4,21] Other causes include metastatic cancer, infection, infarction, and

Table 11-4. Disorders of the adrenal cortex

Disorder	Cause	Sonographic Appearance
Hypoadrenalism	Addison's disease caused by idiopathic atrophy of the adrenal cortex	Unable to identify
	Addison's disease caused by tuberculosis	Solid, enlarged, and nodular with hyperechoic capsule; may appear complex with areas of necrosis
	Waterhouse-Friderichsen syndrome	Hemorrhage may occur (see Table 11-3)
Aldosteronoma	Conn's disease	Hypoechoic, small (1 to 2 cm) round masses
Hyperplasia	Cushing's or Conn's disease, adrenogenital disease	Normal or diffusely enlarged; solid, cystic, or complex, with or without focal zones of necrosis within the gland

irradiation.[36] A syndrome of hypoadrenalism similar to Addison's disease results, except hyperpigmentation is absent with diminished ACTH.[4,21,36] The adrenal glands may be moderately to markedly shrunken, may appear leaflike, and become difficult to identify in the periadrenal fat.[36]

Acute Hypoadrenalism (Waterhouse-Friderichsen Syndrome). Massive destruction of the adrenals can occur at any age and in a variety of settings, causing acute adrenal insufficiency (addisonian or adrenal crisis).[36] The destruction occurs with either treated or undiagnosed Addison's disease or from a primary lesion in the adrenal gland itself, such as hemorrhage, infection, or infarction.[4,21,36] Immediate intervention, such as the administration of glucocorticoid therapy, is necessary or death will rapidly ensue.[4,21]

Hyperadrenalism (Hypercorticism)

With hyperadrenalism, the three types of corticosteroids elaborated by the adrenal cortex result in three distinctive, but sometimes overlapping clinical manifestations:[36] Cushing's syndrome, Conn's syndrome, or aldosteronism, and adrenogenital syndrome, or congenital adrenal hyperplasia.[4,21,36]

Cushing's Syndrome. In Cushing's syndrome, excessive glucose production results from hypersecretion of cortisol from the adrenal cortex.[4,34] The most common cause is treatment of nonendocrine disorders with long courses of potent glucocorticoid drugs such as prednisone and dexamethasone.[36] Three clinically similar forms of Cushing's disease result from glucocorticoid over-production: hypersecretion of ACTH by the anterior pituitary (Cushing's disease, 85% of cases), adrenal neoplasms (10%), and ectopic ACTH syndrome from adenocarcinoma, oat-cell carcinoma of the lung, or other malignant neoplasms (5%).[4,21,34,36] In children, tumors are the most common cause, and growth ceases if treatment is not begun before the epiphyses of the bones have sealed.[4,21,34]

With increased cortisol secretion, gluconeogenesis increases, resulting in elevated serum glucose levels.[4,18] Eventually, the islet cells of the pancreas are no longer able to produce sufficient amounts of insulin and diabetes mellitus results.[4,36] Protein loss occurs almost everywhere except in the liver.[4] This loss results in weakened muscles and elastic tissue, producing a protuberant abdomen and poor wound healing.[4,21,34] Humoral immunity is impaired, decreasing the threshold for infection.[4] With the loss of collagen in the skin, the tissues becomes very thin and susceptible to tearing and bruising. Red welts and striae are seen, mostly over the abdomen and thighs.[4] Owing to the melanin-stimulating properties of ACTH, hyperpigmentation may be seen.[19,36] Osteoporosis can result, causing weakness and fractures.[4,36] Hypertension is also evident in 99% of cases.[19,36]

Hyperaldosteronism. Primary hyperaldosteronism, or Conn's syndrome, is the result of excessive and uncontrolled secretion of the mineralocorticoid aldosterone.[4,34,36] It is uncommon, and in 90% of patients it results from a benign aldosterone-producing adrenal adenoma.[4,30,34] Rarely (10%), it results from carcinoma or cortical hyperplasia.

Secondary hyperaldosteronism is not a disease process but results from hypersecretion of aldosterone in response to stimulation of the renin-angiotensin system.[4,36] This occurs when almost any factor decreases the blood supply to the kidneys causing an increased plasma renin level and subsequent excessive aldosterone secretion.[4,36]

The clinical features of this disorder are a direct result of aldosterone's functions of conserving sodium and renal potassium wasting.[19,28,36,39] Hypernatremia (excess sodium in the blood) and hypokalemia (extreme potassium depletion in the blood) are the principal clinical manifestations.[4] The condition is suspected whenever a hypertensive patient exhibits concurrent hypokalemia.[4,36] Conservation of sodium leads to water retention, increasing the volume in the extracellular and vascular compartments causing arterial hypertension.[36] Potassium loss most commonly results in muscle cramps and weakness.[4,34,36] Because the kidneys are the primary site of sodium conservation, renal functional alterations occur.[4,34,36,43] The sonographic appearance of aldosteronoma is presented in Table 11-4 and is discussed in the section on cortical tumors.

Congenital Adrenal Hyperplasia—Adrenogenital Syndrome. Congenital adrenal hyperplasia encompasses at least six distinctive autosomal recessive syndromes, each characterized by a congenital deficiency of a specific enzyme involved in the biosynthesis of adrenal steroids.[4,21,36] With bilateral hyperplasia the enzyme deficiencies may also result from postpubertal adrenal hyperplasia, adrenal adenoma, or adrenal carcinoma.[4] The effect of the deficiencies impairs synthesis of cortisol and distorts other aspects of steroidogenesis.[36] In most cases, this increases levels of ACTH, leading to adrenal hyperplasia and subsequent overstimulation of the pathways of steroid hormone production, particularly those involving the production of adrenal androgens.[4,21,36] All of these syndromes are adrenogenital, representing an abnormal expression of androgen excess, and the ultimate result in most cases is the same, virilization.[4,21,25,36]

Newborn girls with congenital adrenal hyperplasia have ambiguous external genitalia resembling boys'.[21,36] Reconstructive surgery, if indicated, can be performed during the first 2 years of life to reduce the size of the clitoris, separate the labia, and exteriorize the vagina.[21] Internal female genitalia are normal.[4] Males are seldom diagnosed at birth unless they have enlarged genitalia, lose salt, or manifest adrenal crisis.[4,36]

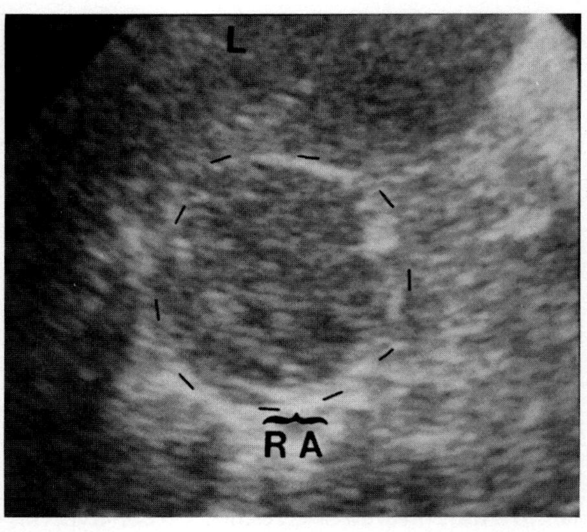

Figure 11-23. The right adrenal gland (RA) appears as a solid mass *(within dotted line)* on the transverse plane image of a 4-month-old girl displaying clinical signs and symptoms of hyperadrenalism (L, liver). (Courtesy Helen Johnson, Salt Lake City, UT.)

Age and sex of the affected person determine the nature and severity of the disorder when adrenogenital syndromes are caused by benign or malignant tumors.[4] Precocious sexual development and elevated plasma 17-hydroxyprogesterone levels aid in the diagnosis.[25,37] Early diagnosis is important, as the deficiency can often be controlled, allowing normal sexual and physical development.[36]

Hyperfunctioning adrenal glands can appear normal or diffusely enlarged but with normal shape.[15,30] With nodular hyperplasia, a solid, cystic, or complex mass, with or without focal zones of necrosis, may present in the adrenal gland (Fig. 11-23).[32] Since the sonographic appearance is used to describe and characterize and not to make tissue-specific diagnoses, correlation with the patient's clinical findings and laboratory values expedites interpretation of the sonographic study.

CORTICAL TUMORS

Adenomas. Adrenal adenomas are found at approximately 2% of adult autopsies.[36] An adenoma may be one part of the MEN syndromes.[36] Most are benign, poorly encapsulated, 1- to 5-cm diameter tumors, and are comprised of lipid-filled cells that do not secrete hormones.[36] Generally, a single nodule greater than 1 cm is considered an adenoma; whereas, multiple or bilateral nodules located either inside or oustide the capsule are considered expressions of nodular hyperplasia.[36] Administration of ACTH causes adrenal adenomas to grow in the same way it stimulates adrenal hyperplasia. Adenocarcinoma, however, is independent of the pituitary influence and does not respond to ACTH administration.[4,25]

An adenoma is sonographically difficult to detect because of its anatomic location and the presence of retroperitoneal fat.[38] Such masses appear small, round, and are frequently only 1.5 to 2 cm in diameter. Their hypoechoic sonographic appearance is similar to that of aldosteronomas.[18,38] Aldosteronomas also present sonographically as small, round, relatively anechoic masses. Adrenal adenoma is an incidental finding in almost 1% of adrenal CT studies.[30] Criteria used to support the diagnosis of an incidental adrenal adenoma include a small (less than 5 cm), round or oval mass, clear separation of the margins from adjacent structures, and no evidence of growth on serial examinations (Fig. 11-24), Table 11-5).[30]

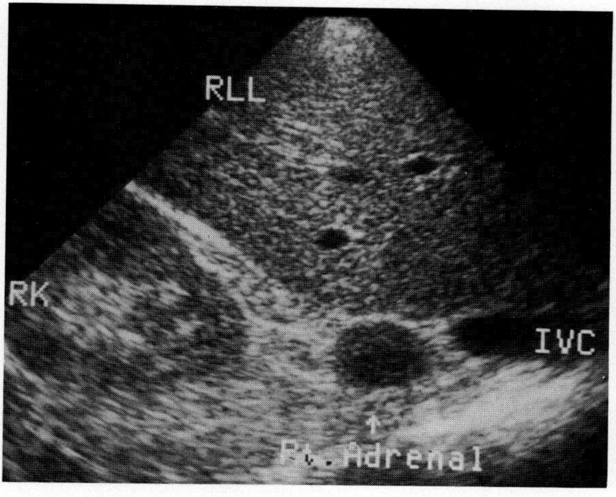

FIGURE 11-24. On a transverse plane, an adenoma measuring 2.9 cm is identified with a hypoechoic appearance relative to the right adrenal gland (RLL, right liver lobe; RK, right kidney; IVC, inferior vena cava). (Courtesy Cathy Carr-Hoefer, Corvallis, OR.)

Myelolipomas. Adrenal myelolipoma is a rare benign tumor of the adrenal cortex. Of uncertain cause, it is composed of mature adipose tissue with a variable proportion of hematopoietic elements resembling bone marrow.[6,9,10] Generally, myelolipomas are unilateral and hormonally inactive.[9] Before the advent of modern imaging techniques, most myelolipomas were found incidentally at postmortem examination, as they were asymptomatic.[28,33,44] Larger or bilateral lesions may become symptomatic, causing pain or endocrine dysfunction due to hemorrhage, necrosis, or pressure on adjacent structures.[6,9,10,33]

A combination of sonography, CT, and angiography can be fairly specific in the preoperative diagnosis of an adrenal myelolipoma.[6,9,10] Sonographically, the tumor is usually a well-defined, markedly

TABLE 11-5. Adrenal cortical tumors

TUMOR	SONOGRAPHIC APPEARANCE
Adenomas	Hypoechoic small (1.5 to 2 cm) round, encapsulated mass; clear separation of the margins from adjacent structures; may have calcifications
Myelolipomas	Hyperechoic, well-defined mass with interrupted posterior hemidiaphragm; if small, may blend with perirenal fat
Cancer	Hyperechoic, solid, larger masses; echo pattern varies with necrosis or hemorrhage; mass may invade vasculature and displace surrounding organs

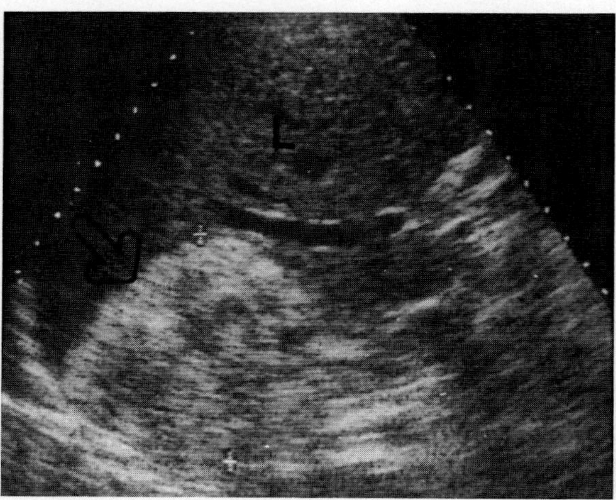

FIGURE 11-25. On a patient with a history of hemophilia, the transverse plane of the right adrenal gland, a well-defined and markedly hyperechoic myolipoma (*arrow* and *cursors*) measuring 8.1 cm is identified posterior to the liver (L). (Courtesy Cathy Carr-Hoefer, Corvallis, OR.)

hyperechoic mass demonstrating an interrupted, posteriorly displaced hemidiaphragm resulting from a propagation speed artifact caused by a lipomatous mass (Fig. 11-25, Table 11-5).[6,35] The ultrasound examination is useful in localizing the anatomic origin of these upper quadrant abnormalities, especially on the right side.[6,13] If it is detected sonographically, the differential diagnosis includes retroperitoneal lipoma, retroperitoneal liposarcoma, renal angiomyolipoma, lymphangioma, increased abdominal fat deposition, and retroperitoneal teratoma.[6,10,29] CT examination should follow, because it is capable of identifying the fatty nature of the mass.[10] On CT, a myelolipoma appears as a well-defined, fatty suprarenal mass with negative attenuation values compared to the avidly attenuating adrenal gland tissue, other tissue types, or hemorrhage.[6,45] If present, liposarcomas are nonhomogeneous, poorly defined, and infiltrative.[14,45] On angiography, a myelolipoma appears as an avascular mass in the adrenal gland rather than the kidney or liver.[6,9] Venography demonstrates displacement of veins around the tumor.[9]

Cancer. Cortical cancers, such as adenocarcinomas, produce steroids (90%) and are usually associated with one of the hyperadrenal syndromes; those that do not produce steroids are highly malignant.[29,36] Carcinomas are rare. They may appear to be encapsulated, and many exceed 20 cm diameter.[29,36] They may show zones of hemorrhage and necrosis.[36] Cortical cancers tend to invade the adrenal vein, inferior vena cava, and lymph nodes, and commonly metastasize to regional and periaortic nodes, with hematogenous spread to the lungs and other viscera.[29,36]

Cortical cancers are solid-looking masses, larger than most adrenal masses. The echogenic appearance varies with the presence and different degrees of hemorrhage and necrosis. Invasion of the mass to surrounding vasculature and displacement of normal tissue continuity and location help identify the mass (see Table 11-5).

Medullary Pathology

PHEOCHROMOCYTOMA

Pheochromocytomas are found in 0.5% to 1.0% of patients with hypertension.[29] Ninety percent originate in the medulla's epinephrine- or norepinephrine-producing chromaffin cells, and the remainder in the autonomic tissue.[2,4,29] Ninety percent are benign, 5% to 10% are malignant, and 3% to 5% are multiple.[4,29] The tumors are usually well-encapsulated and in some patients may be palpable.[4,34,40] They are highly vascular masses, and if rupture occurs, massive hemorrhage can be fatal.[4] This tumor occurs in both sexes, usually between ages 25 and 50 years, and children are rarely affected.[36] It is not uncommon for more than one family member to be affected or for pheochromocytoma to be associated with MEN syndromes.[4,30]

Symptoms include chronic or episodic hypertension (50% of cases), headaches, sweating, pallor, tachycardia, and accelerated basal metabolism.[4,32] In 14% of cases signs are typical or symptoms absent.[5] Benign and malignant pheochromocytomas have similar biochemical characteristics, such as elevated levels of urinary catecholamine and other metabolites (VMA).[4,5,29,30] Clinical manifestations, laboratory values, and metastases to liver, lymph nodes, lungs, or bones help establish a diagnosis of malignancy. The sustained elevation of catechol-

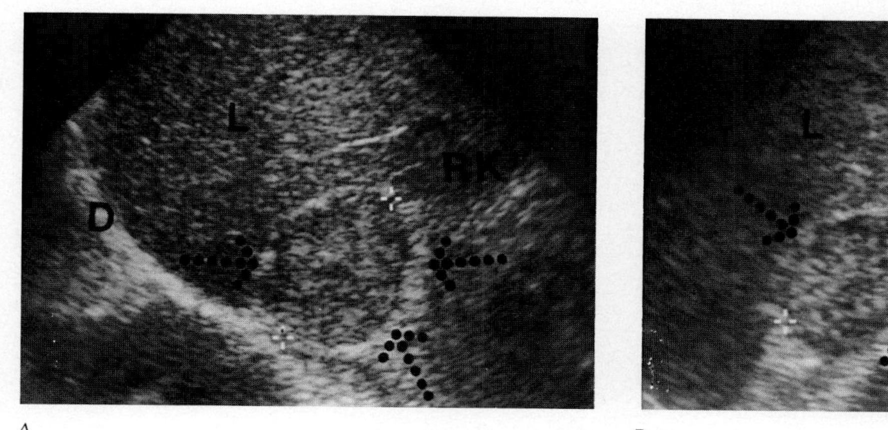

FIGURE 11-26. In the right adrenal gland, a pheochromocytoma (*arrows* and *cursors*) measures 4.2 cm in a longitudinal plane (*A*) and 4.0 cm in the transverse plane (*B*). The mass has both solid and cystic internal echoes and sharply marginated walls (L, liver; D, diaphragm; RK, right kidney). (Courtesy Cathy Carr-Hoefer, Corvallis, OR.)

TABLE 11-6. Tumors of the adrenal medulla

TUMOR	SONOGRAPHIC APPEARANCE
Pheochromocytoma	Hypoechoic, sharply marginated, with hyperechoic solid components of homogenous or heterogeneous echoes representing hemorrhage or necrosis; larger masses displace surrounding organs or indent vasculature; may be bilateral or external to the adrenal
Neuroblastoma	Generally affect children (see Chapter 18); hyperechoic, poorly defined borders; focal echogenic areas may be present due to calcifications; hypoechoic areas may be present due to necrosis; inferior and lateral displacement of kidney

amine secretion can lead to cardiomegaly, left ventricular failure, cardiomyopathy, and ultimately, death due to heart failure.[4] Generally, treatment is surgical removal of the gland and epinephrine and norepinephrine substitution therapy.

Pheochromocytomas may appear sharply marginated and quite large, with purely solid components of homogeneous (hemorrhage) or heterogeneous (necrosis) echoes (Fig. 11-26).[29] Larger masses may displace surrounding organs or indent vasculature (Table 11-6).[38] CT has replaced all previous imaging modalities as the initial examination for detection and localization by indicating the presence of a soft-tissue mass, but magnetic resonance imaging (MRI) may identify the type of tumor.[30]

NEUROBLASTOMA

Neuroblastoma is a highly malignant tumor of the adrenal medulla generally found in children (see Table 11-6 and Chapter 18).

Other Imaging Procedures

RADIOGRAPHY

With advances in sectional imaging technology, radiographic examinations are no longer the procedure of choice for the adrenal gland, but incidental findings may indicate adrenal gland pathology. Calcifications may be visualized on an abdominal radiograph of kidneys, ureters, and bladder, which is the "scout study" prior to excretory urography, intravenous pyelography (IVP), or nephrotomography. (Tomography eliminates obscuring overlying structures.) Visualizing calcifications is not specific, as they occur in 10% of adrenal tumors and 15% of adrenal cysts. In adrenal cysts, calcifications are usually located at the periphery and appear more curvilinear.[30] Approximately 70 to 80% of adrenal masses can be detected by combined IVP and tomography, relying on both the delineation of the mass and demonstration of the degree to which it impinges on the kidney. Small adrenal masses, such as aldosteronomas and extraadrenal pheochromocytomas, are difficult to demonstrate with these modalities.[1,30]

Angiography is specific for the demonstration of vascular adrenal masses,[6,9] and for defining the vascular supply to the tumor, useful information for the surgeon. Angiography may not be specific, though, in differentiating neoplasms from hyperplasia or delineating hypovascular lesions.[1] Venography demonstrates the displacement of veins around the tumor.[9] Venography with venous sampling is 100% accurate in detecting hyperfunction.[1] The risks of angiography, venography, and venous sampling include intraadrenal hemorrhage with pain, infarction, and possibly Addison's disease.[1]

RADIONUCLIDE STUDIES

In the past, the usefulness of adrenal scintigraphy has been limited because scans must be performed 2 to 14 days after intravenous administration of iodine-131-labeled cholesterol derivatives.[1] Now, metaiodobenzylguanadine (^{131}I-MIGA) offers a new potential for localizing adrenal medullary lesions and the more elusive extraadrenal pheochromocytomas.[30]

COMPUTED TOMOGRAPHY

Computed tomography is the single best imaging modality for evaluating most cases of suspected adrenal disease. CT is better than ultrasound in detecting normal adrenal glands, especially in obese patients.[38] Several adrenal lesions have inherent tissue characteristics that permit a more precise diagnosis.[30]

MAGNETIC RESONANCE IMAGING

On MRI, adenomas produce weak signals, pheochromocytomas strong ones, and carcinomas intermediate signals.[30] Initial indications are that MRI is equal to CT in the identification of a variety of adrenal abnormalities. Continued research in MRI applications, examination cost, and machine availability will determine its place in future adrenal gland protocols.

Conclusion

With the improved flexibility and maneuverability of real-time systems, imaging the adrenal glands is more successful. Much depends on patient size, perirenal fat, bowel gas, pathology, and the persistence and expertise of the sonographer. While other imaging procedures may be the examination of choice, noninvasive ultrasound is an excellent alternative method for adrenal gland evaluation.

References

1. Abrams HL, Siegelman SS, Adams DF, et al: Computed tomography versus ultrasound of the adrenal gland: A prospective study. Radiology 1982, 143:121–128.
2. Anderhub B: Manual of Abdominal Sonography. Baltimore, University Park Press, 1983.
3. Anthony CP, Thibodeau GA: Textbook of Anatomy and Physiology, 10th ed. St. Louis, CV Mosby, 1979.
4. Bullock BL, Rosendahl PP: Pathophysiology: Adaptations and Alterations in Function, 2nd ed. Glenview, IL, Scott, Foresman, 1988.
5. Casola G, Nicolet V, vanSonnenberg E, et al: Unsuspected pheochromocytoma: Risk of blood-pressure alterations during percutaneous adrenal biopsy. Radiology 1986, 159:733–735.
6. Cintron E, Quntero EC, Perez MR, et al: Computed tomography, sonographic, and radiographic findings in adrenal myelolipoma. Urology 1984, 23:608–610.
7. Corbet JV: Laboratory Tests and Diagnostic Procedures with Nursing Diagnosis, 2nd ed. Norwalk, CT, Appleton and Lange, 1987.
8. Craig M: Pocket Guide to Ultrasound Measurements. Philadelphia, JB Lippincott, 1988.
9. Del Gaudio A, Solidoro G: Myelolipoma of the ad-

renal gland: Report of two cases with a review of the literature. Surgery 1986, 99:293–301.

10. Dieckmann KP, Hamm B, Pickartz H, et al: Adrenal myelolipoma: Clinical radiologic, and histologic features. Urology 1987, 29:1–7.
11. England MA: Color Atlas of Life Before Birth: Normal Fetal Development. Chicago, Year Book Medical Publishers, 1983.
12. Fleischer AC: Renal and urological sonography. *In* Fleisher AC, James AE Jr (eds): Diagnostic Sonography: Principles and Clinical Applications. Philadelphia, WB Saunders, 1989.
13. Frick MP, Feinberg SB: Deceptions in localizing extrahepatic right upper quadrant abdominal masses by CT. AJR 1982, 139:501–510.
14. Friedman AC, Hartman MD, Sherman J, et al: Computed tomography of abdominal fatty masses. Radiology 1981, 139:415–429.
15. Ghiacy S, Dubbins PA, Baumer H: Ultrasound demonstration of congenital adrenal hyperplasia. J Clin Ultrasound 1985, 13:419–420.
16. Goldstein RB, Callen PW: Ultrasound evaluation of the fetal thorax and abdomen. *In* Callen PW (ed): Ultrasonography in Obstetrics and Gynecology, 2nd ed. Philadelphia, WB Saunders, 1988.
17. Gray H: Gray's Anatomy: Anatomy of the Human Body, 29th ed, (American Edition, edited by Charles Mayo Goss). Philadelphia, Lea & Febiger, 1973.
18. Gunther RW, Kelbel C, Lenner V: Real-time ultrasound of normal adrenal glands and small tumors. J Clin Ultrasound 1984, 12:211–217.
19. Guyton AC: Textbook of Medical Physiology, 6th ed. Philadelphia, WB Saunders, 1981.
20. Hagen-Ansert SL: Textbook of Diagnostic Ultrasonography, 3rd ed. St. Louis, CV Mosby, 1989.
21. Hurwitz LS, Porth CM: Alterations in endocrine control of growth and metabolism. *In* Porth CM: Pathophysiology: Concepts of Altered Health States. Philadelphia, JB Lippincott, 1986.
22. Jacobs D, Kastgen B, Demott WT, et al: Laboratory Test Handbook with DRG Index. St. Louis, CV Mosby, 1984.
23. Krebs CA, Eisenberg RL: Ultrasound Imaging of the Adrenal Glands. Radiol Tech 1985, 56:421–423.
24. Krebs CA, Eisenberg RL, Ratcliff S, et al: Cava-suprarenal line: New position for sonographic imaging of the left adrenal gland. J Clin Ultrasound 1986, 14:535–539.
25. Lamb JA: Laboratory Tests for Clinical Nursing. Bowie, MD, RJ Brady, Prentice-Hall, 1984.
26. McDonnel WY: Myelolipoma of adrenal. Arch Pathol 1956, 61:416–419.
27. Marchal G, Gelin J, Verbeken E, et al: High-resolution real-time sonography of the adrenal glands: A routine examination? J Ultrasound Med 1986, 5:65–68.
28. Marieb EN: Human Anatomy and Physiology. Redwood City, CA, Benjamin/Cummings, 1989.
29. Mittelstaedt CA: Abdominal Ultrasound. New York, Churchill Livingstone, 1987.
30. Mitty HA: Adrenal disease. *In* Eisenberg RL (ed): Diagnostic Imaging: An Algorithmic Approach. Philadelphia, JB Lippincott, 1988.
31. Netter FH: The CIBA Collection of Medical Illustrations, vol 4, Endocrine System and Selected Metabolic Diseases. NY, The Case-Hoyt Corporation, 1965.
32. Odwin CS, Dubinsky T, Fleischer AC: Ultrasonography Examination Review and Study Guide. Norwalk, CT, Appleton and Lange, 1987.
33. Plaut A: Myelolipoma in the adrenal cortex (myeloadipose structures). Am J Pathol 1958, 34:487–502.
34. Price SA, Wilson LM: Pathophysiology: Clinical Concepts of Disease Processes, 2nd ed. New York, McGraw-Hill, 1982.
35. Richman TS, Taylor JK, Kremkau FW: Propagation speed artifact in fatty tumor (myeloleioma): Significance for tissue differential diagnosis. J Ultrasound Med 1983, 2:45–47.
36. Robbins SL, Cotran RS: Pathologic Basis of Diseases, 2nd ed. Philadelphia, WB Saunders, 1979.
37. Rosenberg ER, Bowie JD, Andreoti RF, et al: Sonographic evaluation of fetal adrenal glands. AJR 1982, 139:1145–1147.
38. Sarti DA: Diagnostic Ultrasound: Text & Cases, 2nd ed. Chicago, Year Book Medical Publishers, 1987.
39. Seeley RR, Stephens TD, Tate P: Anatomy and Physiology. St. Louis, Times Mirror/Mosby College Publishing, 1989.
40. Spence AP, Mason EB: Human Anatomy and Physiology. Menlo Park, CA, Benjamin/Cummings, 1987.
41. Thomas CL (ed): Taber's Cyclopedic Medical Dictionary, 16th ed. Philadelphia, FA Davis, 1989.
42. Tilkian SO, Conover MB, Tilkian AG: Clinical Implications of Laboratory Tests, 3rd ed. St. Louis, CV Mosby, 1983.
43. Tortora GJ, Anagnastakos NP: Principles of Anatomy and Physiology, 5th ed. New York, Harper and Row, 1987.
44. Vick CW, Zeman RK, Mannes E, et al: Adrenal myelolipoma: CT and ultrasound findings. Urol Radiol 1984, 6:7–13.
45. Waligore MP, Stephens DH, Soule EH, et al: Lipomatous tumors of the abdominal cavity. AJR 1981, 137:539–545.

46. Wheelock IL: Adrenals. *In* Sanders RC: Clinical Sonography: A Practical Guide. Boston, Little, Brown, 1984.
47. Worthen NJ: Adrenal sonography. *In* Sarti DA (ed): Diagnostic Ultrasound: Text & Cases, 2nd ed. Chicago, Year Book Medical Publishers, 1987.
48. Yeh HC: Sonography of the adrenal glands: Normal glands and small masses. AJR 1980, 135:1167–1177.
49. Yeh HC: Ultrasound and CT of the adrenals. Semin Ultrasound 1982, 3:97–113.
50. Yeh HC, Mitty HA, Rose J, et al: Ultrasonography of adrenal masses: Usual features. Radiology 1978, 127:467–474.

CHAPTER 12

Retroperitoneum and Lymphatic System

JIM BAUN

Gross Anatomy of the Retroperitoneum

The retroperitoneum is the potential abdominal space that lies behind the parietal peritoneum. The parietal peritoneum is the outermost of two membranes that enclose most of the intraabdominal contents—intestines, liver, head of the pancreas, spleen, and pelvic organs. The other membrane, the visceral peritoneum, lies in direct apposition to the parietal membrane, thus forming a potential space. The area lying behind the peritoneal membranes is referred to as the retroperitoneum and is bounded anteriorly by the posterior parietal peritoneum and posteriorly by the psoas and quadratus lumborum muscles, the spine and the transversalis fascia. It extends from the diaphragm superiorly to the pelvic floor inferiorly. The kidneys, adrenals, great vessels, pancreas, duodenal sweep, and the ascending and descending colon are contained within the retroperitoneum, as are abdominal lymph nodes and somatic nerves (Fig. 12-1).[42,48]

Within the retroperitoneum, and important in the accurate sonographic assessment of retroperitoneal pathology, are three potential spaces or compartments: anterior pararenal, perirenal, and posterior pararenal. The boundaries of the pararenal space are defined by the anterior and posterior renal fascia (Gerota's fascia), which is a sheet of fibrous tissue surrounding the kidney and associated adipose tissue. Bound to the renal capsule by many trabeculae, the renal fascia serves to hold the kidney in place. It is sealed medially, laterally, and superiorly by blending with adjacent abdominal fascial planes (Fig. 12-2). Inferiorly, the renal fascia extends approximately 8 cm beyond the lower pole of the kidney before fusing.[41]

The anterior pararenal space lies between the posterior parietal peritoneum and the anterior renal fascia and contains the pancreas, retroperitoneal duodenum, and the ascending and descending colon. The perirenal space contains the kidney itself as well as the renal vessels, the adrenal gland, and perinephric fat. The aorta and inferior vena cava (IVC) are also located in the perirenal space, and their connective tissue sheaths fuse with the renal fascia.[46] The pararenal space occupies the area between the anterior and posterior renal fascia. The posterior pararenal space lies between the posterior renal fascia and the transversalis fascia. It contains fat, which extends laterally as the preperitoneal fat line.[49]

Gross Anatomy of the Lymphatics

The lymphatic system consists of small-caliber vessels and functioning bean-shaped nodes. Architecturally similar to the vascular system, lymph vessels are found throughout the body. Lymph capillaries collect excess interstitial water, electrolytes, and colloids for filtration in the nodes and return the filtrate to the bloodstream. Physiologically, the role

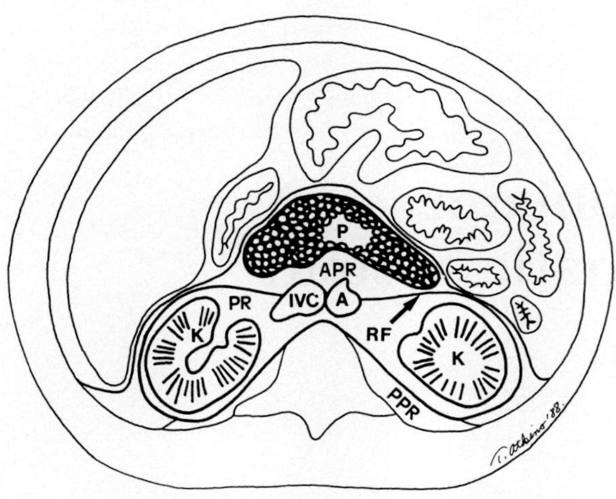

Figure 12-1. Cross-sectional schematic drawing of retroperitoneum (P, pancreas; IVC, inferior vena cava; A, aorta; K, kidney; RF, renal fascia; APR, anterior pararenal space; PR, perirenal space; PPR, posterior pararenal space).

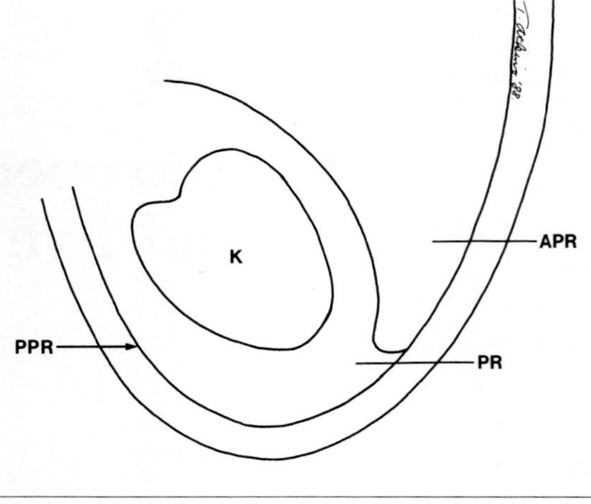

Figure 12-2. Schematic representation of retroperitoneal compartments (K, kidney; APR, anterior pararenal space; PR, perirenal space; PPR, posterior pararenal space).

of the lymphatic system is varied. First, by returning excess interstitial fluid to the bloodstream, homeostasis (internal fluid balance) is maintained. Second, lymph vessels located around the small intestine aid in digestion by absorbing fatty acids. While the preponderance of fatty acids is absorbed through the mucosal cells of the intestinal mucosa and is thus directed through the portal venous system to the liver, some bypass this normal route by spilling into the lymphatic channels. The nodes themselves serve other vital physiologic functions, such as the production of lymphocytes essential in the proper function of the immune response and filtration of lymph fluid. Serving as filters, the nodes remove invading organisms and debris from infected areas and protect the rest of the body against infection. Nodes involved in this activity are generally enlarged and tender.

Deep Abdominal (Parietal) Nodes

In the retroperitoneum and along the course of the prevertebral vasculature lie groups of small, irregularly shaped lymph nodes. Connected to each other by lymphatic channels, these nodes can lie anywhere in the retroperitoneum, although they usually follow the course of the principal blood vessels. Generally classified as parietal nodes, they are grouped according to the arterial vessel with which they are associated. In the upper retroperitoneum, aggregations can be found around three unpaired vascular branches: inferior mesenteric, superior mesenteric, and celiac. Groups found in the lower retroperitoneum include the external, common, and internal iliac, and epigastric (Fig. 12-3).

Nodes are positioned 360 degrees around the aorta and inferior vena cava. Those that lie posterior to the main vessels provide the most reliable indicator of lymphadenopathy since they frequently displace the aorta or IVC anteriorly.[51] The deep abdominal lymphatic system drains many organs in the abdomen and pelvis. The adrenal glands and kidneys drain through connecting channels into paraaortic nodes; the testicles and ovaries drain into more inferiorly placed nodes near the aortic bifurcation. While the main collecting channels of the lymphatic system begin in the abdomen, the various pathways eventually anastomose to empty into the inferior vena cava at the level of the eleventh thoracic vertebra.

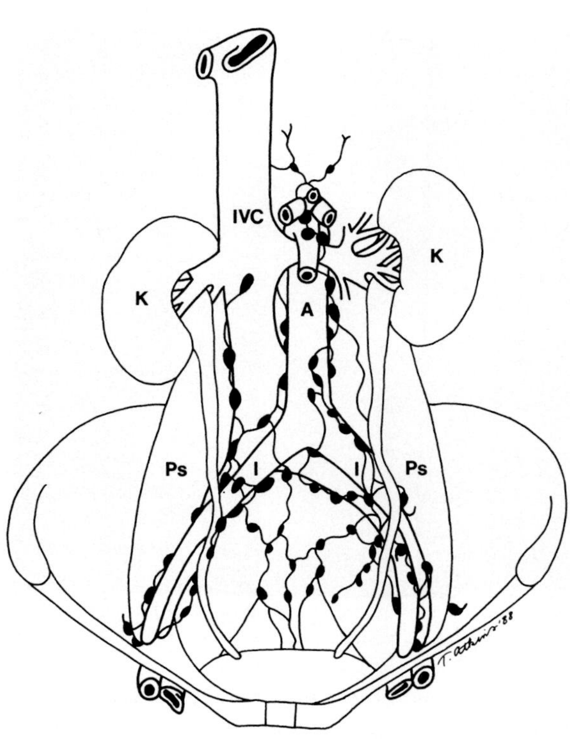

Figure 12-3. Schematic representation of deep abdominal parietal lymph nodes following the course of major blood vessels (IVC, inferior vena cava; A, aorta; K, kidney; Ps, psoas muscle; I, common iliac arteries).

Superficial Abdominal (Visceral) Nodes

Following the course of the visceral vasculature are groups of nodes classified as superficial. As with the parietal groups, these nodes can lie anywhere in the peritoneal cavity but most frequently follow the course of associated blood vessels. The most common groups are gastric, hepatic, pancreatic, splenic, and various groups associated with branches of the colic artery.

Sonographic Examination Techniques

Retroperitoneum

Since the retroperitoneal compartments are potential spaces, frequently they are not identified as discrete structures on routine abdominal sonography.[29] Only when fluid collections or other pathologic processes distort normal anatomic relationships can the various sections be easily seen. Using the appropriate scanning planes, however, the location of various compartments can be identified in relation to normal adjacent anatomic structures. The most important sonographic landmark in evaluation of the retroperitoneal compartments is the perirenal fat and the surrounding renal (Gerota's) fascia. Perirenal fat, which is generally hyperechoic relative to the associated kidney, sits within the perirenal space. The exact amount and configuration of fat varies from patient to patient. The renal fascia forms the anterior and posterior boundaries of the perirenal space and can be seen in average or large patients as a high-level linear reflector surrounding the perirenal fat (Fig. 12-4). In cases where the renal fascia is clearly defined, the retroperitoneal compartments can be seen (Fig. 12-5).

In clinical practice, however, the presence of intestinal gas, thick musculature, or excessive fatty layers frequently precludes adequate sonographic evaluation of the normal compartments. Sagittal and transverse scans are attempted along generally accepted anatomic planes. When intestinal gas or the bony thorax interferes, additional views should

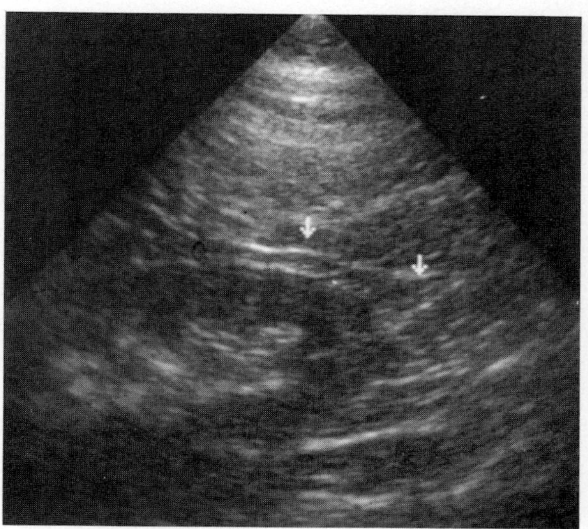

Figure 12-4. Sagittal sonogram demonstrates Gerota's fascia *(arrows)*.

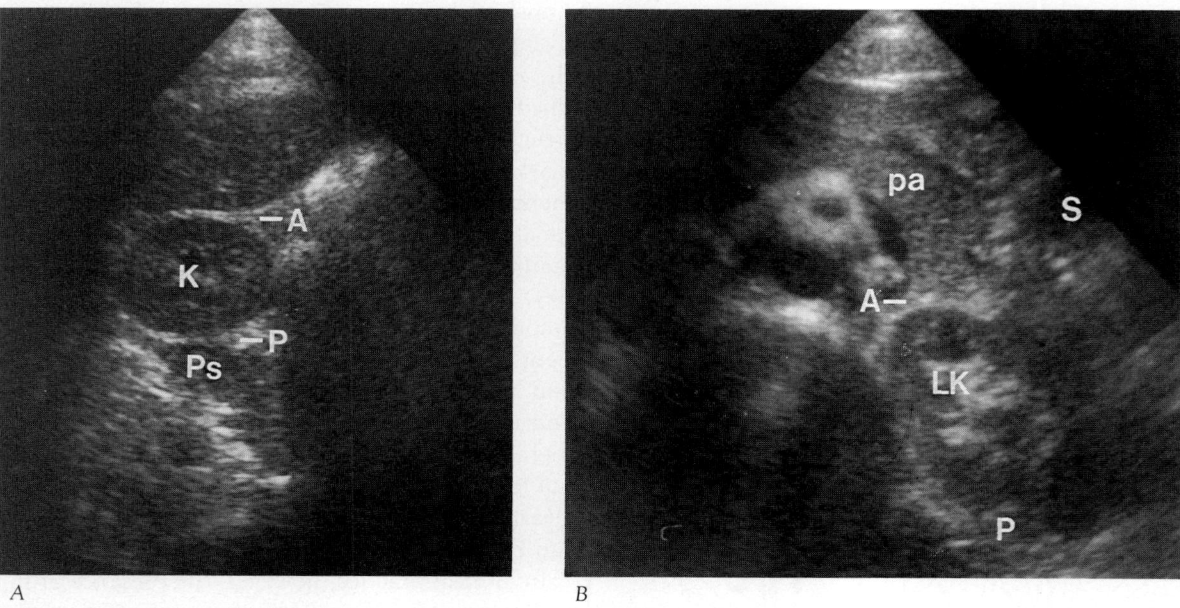

FIGURE 12-5. (*A*) Transverse sonogram demonstrates right retroperitoneal compartments (A, anterior pararenal space; P, posterior pararenal space; Ps, psoas major; K, right kidney). (*B*) Transverse sonogram demonstrates left retroperitoneal compartments (pa, pancreas; LK, left kidney; S, stomach; A, anterior pararenal space; P, posterior pararenal space).

be obtained. Manual compression of gas-filled bowel loops may aid in imaging, as may altering patient position. A right lateral decubitus position may cause the stomach to move slightly toward the right side, affording an acoustic window in the left upper quadrant. Lateral intercostal scanning with a real-time sector transducer affords the best approach to imaging the upper compartments, especially when the left-sided spleen or the right-sided liver can be used as an acoustic window. When the area of concern is the posterior pararenal space, an approach through the back muscles may demonstrate this compartment. With the patient lying prone, the transducer is aligned in an intercostal space and rocked laterally.[32,37,47]

The normal lymphatic structures in the retroperitoneum are not seen on routine abdominal sonography. As a rule of thumb, if lymph nodes are imaged, they are enlarged and probably involved by a pathologic process.

INDICATIONS

Diagnostic ultrasonography can be an effective method of evaluating the retroperitoneum; however, because of the limitations imposed by bowel gas, incisions, and patient habitus, it is usually used as an adjunct to other imaging modalities. Computed tomography (CT) is the imaging method of choice for evaluating the retroperitoneum. Because of its ability to precisely and consistently demonstrate fascial planes and the relationship of pathologic entities deep in the abdomen it is generally preferred over ultrasonogrphy.[5]

Sonography is indicated as a follow-up modality in cases where retroperitoneal disease has been detected and can be adequately evaluated. Pathologic processes that displace or compress bowel loops are especially suited to sonographic examination. Because they cannot displace the musculoskeletal structures of the back, most solid tumors grow anteriorly and eventually can be palpated from the front. The major advantages of sonography include portability, low cost, and the nonionizing acoustic beam. For these reasons it may be the modality of choice for examining children, very ill patients who cannot be transported for CT or magnetic resonance imaging (MRI), and thin patients. The resolution of known abscesses and hematomas may also be followed with sonography, as may the response of solid tumors to therapy. Fine-needle biopsy of retroperitoneal masses and aspiration or drainage procedures may be performed with sonographic guidance.[16,18,21,52]

Preparation

To minimize intestinal gas, the patient should be instructed to refrain from eating or drinking for 8 to 12 hours before the examination. Barium studies and CT contrast examinations should be deferred until the sonogram is completed. Endoscopic procedures should also be performed after ultrasound, because they introduce air into the alimentary tract.

Pathology

As discussed in this chapter, the retroperitoneal spaces do not contain specific organs, so pathologic changes in these areas are the result of disease elsewhere. The organs most frequently associated with retroperitoneal manifestations are the pancreas, kidneys, and colon. Additionally, lymphatic involvement in either an inflammatory or neoplastic process may produce alterations in the appearance of the retroperitoneum. From an imaging perspective, retroperitoneal pathology may be classified as either cystic or solid. Each is considered below.

Solid Masses

Solid masses found in the retroperitoneum are usually metastatic and most frequently involve the lymph nodes. Although primary tumors do occur in the retroperitoneum, they are rare. The role of ultrasonography in evaluating retroperitoneal adenopathy is limited. Sonography can detect the presence of solid masses and, in cases where intestinal gas or overlying bony structures do not obscure retroperitoneal imaging, may demonstrate the relationship of these masses to normal structures. The exact histologic nature of solid masses cannot, however, be definitively ascertained by sonography alone. When solid lesions are noted, the patient should be referred for additional diagnostic testing. CT with thin-needle biopsy is the modality of choice for evaluating solid masses in the retroperitoneum.

Lymphatic Masses

Well-circumscribed, hypoechoic masses adjacent to the abdominal aorta may be assumed to be lymph nodes, especially in patients with a history of primary neoplastic or lymphatic disease. Patterns of nodal disease vary according to number of nodes involved, the extent of involvement, and the type and location of the primary pathologic process. Various appearances have been reported: single paraaortic masses, symmetric paraaortic masses, and mantles.[17] Usually they are well-circumscribed, hypoechoic areas adjacent to the abdominal aorta. They may be seen displacing visceral or mesenteric vessels, compressing the inferior vena cava, or distorting the appearance of normal anatomic structures (Fig. 12-6).[2,26,31]

Anterior displacement of the aorta by enlarged lymph nodes has been called the "floating aorta sign" on CT studies,[22] and obliteration of the echogenic anterior wall of the abdominal aorta creates a "sonographic silhouette" sign.[8] Both signs are sensitive indicators of retroperitoneal lymphadenopathy. Additionally, the normal configuration of any of the mesenteric vessels may be altered by adjacent nodes, especially at the origin of the superior mesenteric artery or the celiac axis. When scanning for suspected lymphadenopathy, it is essential that the renal, hepatic, and splenic hili be imaged carefully. A major pitfall in the sonographic recognition of enlarged nodes is the presence of normal structures that may mimic disease. The crus of the diaphragm in the upper abdomen and the testicular vein in the left renal space have been misinterpreted as lymphatic masses.[51]

Primary Neoplasms

Primary neoplasms of the retroperitoneum are rare, comprising only 0.16 to 0.20% of all malignancies,[1,43] but 10 to 20% of all soft tissue tumors are retroperitoneal in origin and carry a questionable prognosis.[3,4] Early diagnosis is important, since the likelihood of metastatic invasion increases as the

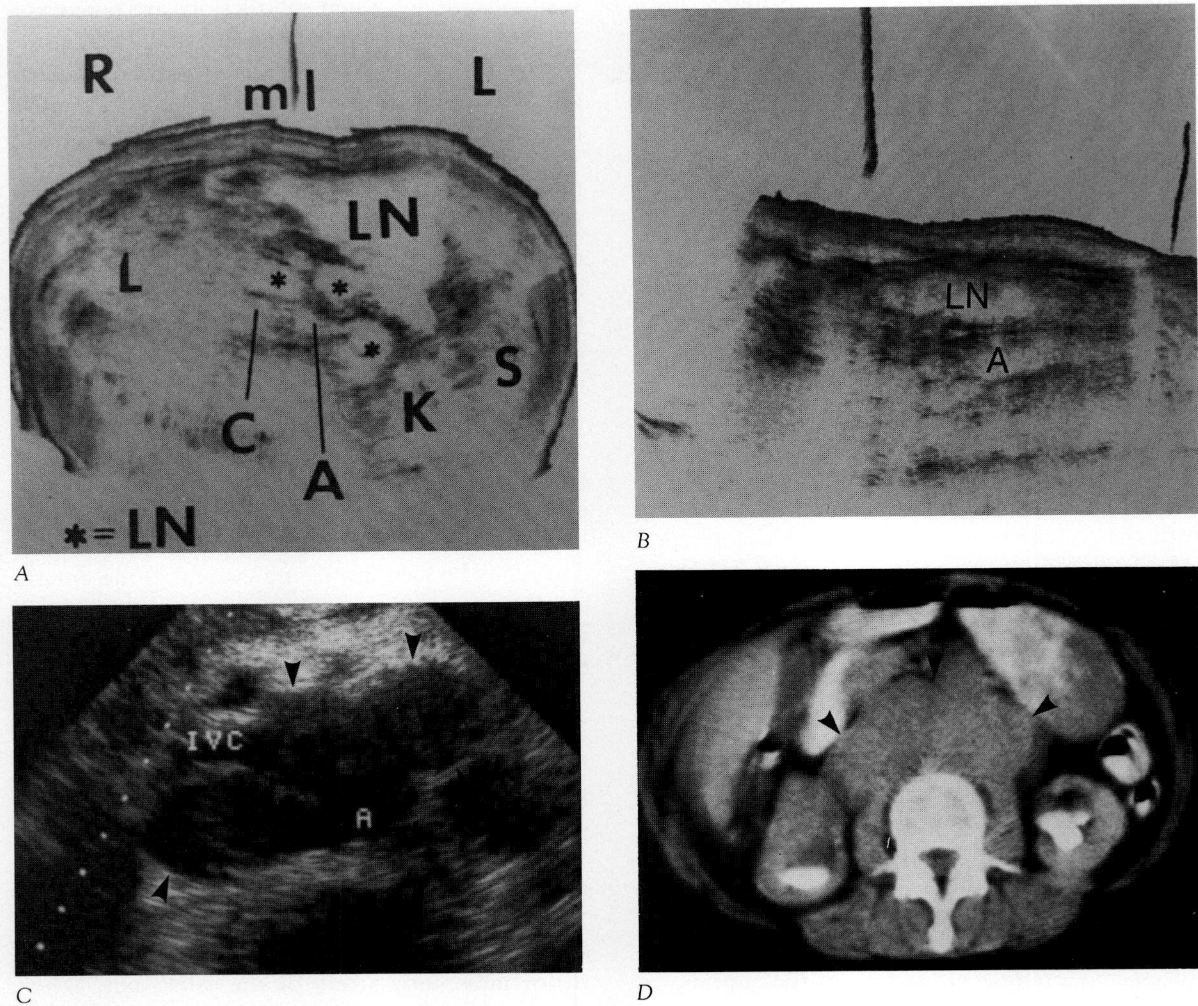

A B C D

Figure 12-6. (*A*) Transverse static B-scan of paraaortic lymphadenopathy demonstrates the relationship between the nodes and surrounding vessels (*, lymph nodes; ml, midline; K, kidney; A, aorta; C, inferior vena cava; S, spleen; L, liver). (*B*) Sagittal sonogram in a different patient demonstrates paraaortic lymphadenopathy with a mantle appearance (A, aorta; LN, lymphadenopathic tissue). (*C*) Sonographic demonstration of primary retroperitoneal lymphoma (IVC, inferior vena cava; A, aorta; *arrowheads,* mass). (*D*) CT image of primary retroperitoneal lymphoma *(arrowheads).*

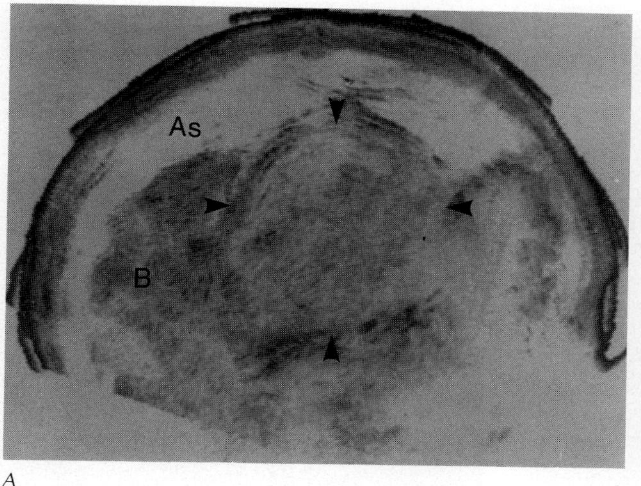

A

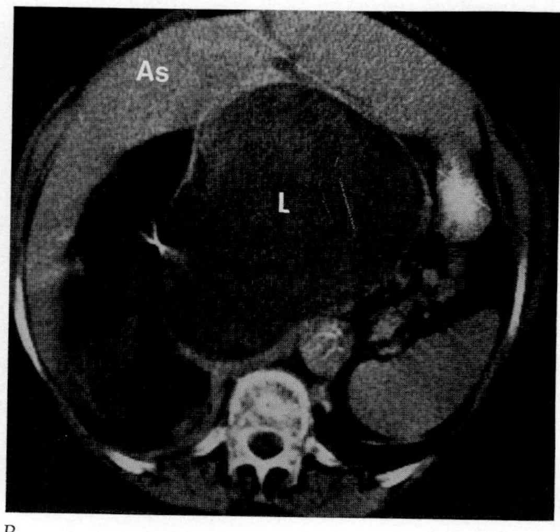

B

FIGURE 12-7. (*A*) Transverse sonogram of a densely echogenic retroperitoneal liposarcoma *(arrowheads)* (As, ascites; B, bowel loops). (*B*) CT image of same patient (As, ascites; L, liposarcoma).

tumors grow larger. While sonography cannot define the histologic character of retroperitoneal solid masses, it frequently can detect them and can prompt further diagnostic procedures.

Liposarcomas, the most common type of soft tissue tumor, are malignant tumors that can occur in fatty tissue anywhere in the body but are most frequently seen in the extremities and retroperitoneal tissues.[13] They tend to infiltrate surrounding tissues and may metastasize, although this occurs later in the disease process and is usually less widespread than with fibrosarcomas. One remarkable characteristic of retroperitoneal liposarcomas is the immense size some of them attain before being diagnosed. Tumors weighing 20 pounds or more are not rare.[39] The histologic composition of liposarcomas varies, but the presence of large amounts of fat in all of these tumors renders them hyperechoic on sonographic examination (Fig. 12-7).

Leiomyosarcomas are malignant tumors of smooth muscle origin that most frequently occur in the uterus and gastrointestinal tract. Unlike their benign counterpart, the leiomyoma, leiomyosarcomas grow rapidly and eventually invade surrounding tissues and venous structures. Metastasis to the lungs is common in untreated cases. Sonographically, these lesions present a mixed echo texture depending on the nature of the gross pathologic structure. Internal necrosis and hemorrhage produce fluid-filled areas within the well-circumscribed mass (Fig. 12-8). Erosion of adjacent visceral walls may result in gas being present within the mass (Fig. 12-8).

Other solid tumors of the retroperitoneum include benign lipomas, sarcomas, fibromas, and myxomas, as well as malignant myxosarcomas and fibrosarcomas (Fig. 12-9). Because solid masses cannot displace the musculoskeletal structures of the back, clinical detection may be delayed. Frequently the tumor must reach sufficient size so as to displace intraperitoneal contents before it can be palpated anteriorly. When the mass is finally detected, it is quite large and may have been present for as long as 20 years or more.[12,14] Typically, the patient presents with a large, protruding abdomen or complains of increasing abdominal girth, weight loss, or abdominal pain. If the tumor has spread to the intestinal tract, symptoms such as nausea, vomiting, anorexia, diarrhea, and altered bowel habits may develop.[50] Involvement of the kidneys or ure-

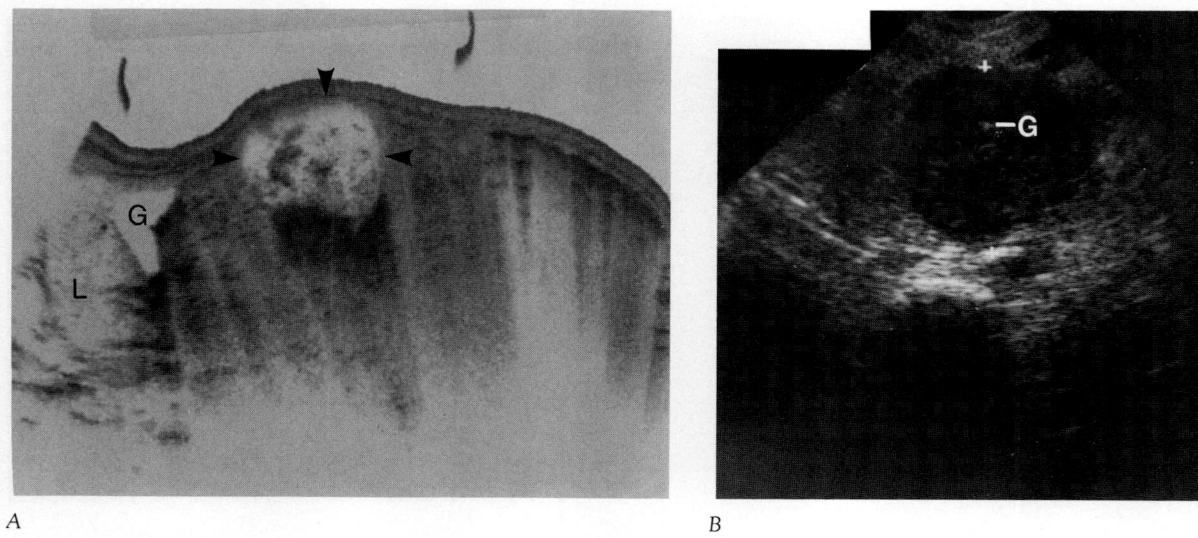

FIGURE 12-8. (*A*) Retroperitoneal leiomyosarcoma *(arrowheads)* with internal necrosis (G, gallbladder; L, liver). (*B*) Retroperitoneal leiomyosarcoma contains gas (G), indicating erosion of adjacent bowel.

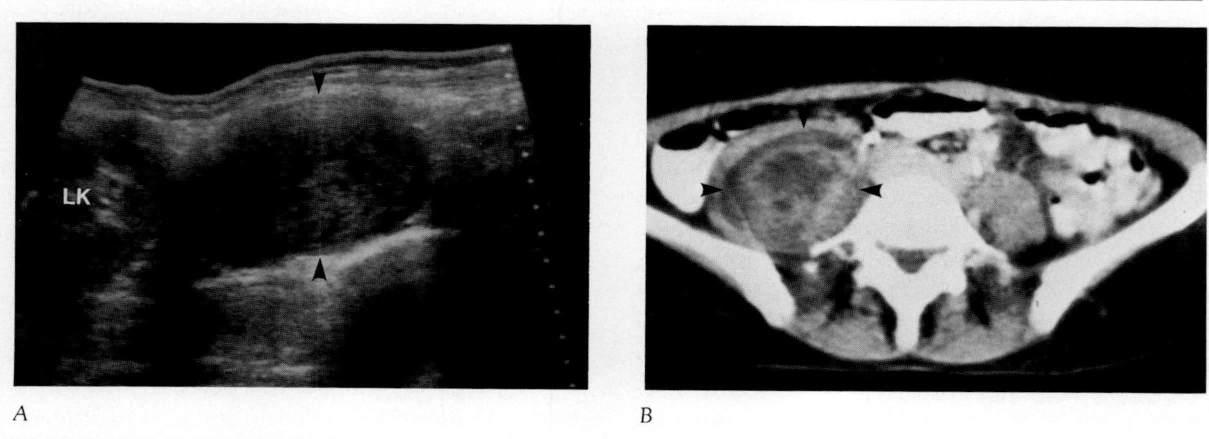

FIGURE 12-9. (*A*) Retroperitoneal sarcoma (arrowheads) demonstrated on sagittal scan to the left of midline (LK, left kidney). (*B*) CT of same patient (*arrowheads,* mass).

ters, either by direct invasion or mechanical compression, may lead to hydronephrosis and subsequent pyelonephritis and uremia. As noted above, primary tumors are rare in the retroperitoneum. When a solid lesion is noted on sonographic examination, the patient should be referred for further imaging or needle biopsy of the suspicious area.[9,15,28,35]

Retroperitoneal Fibrosis

The cause of retroperitoneal fibrosis is not known. It has been attributed to low-grade infections, tuberculosis, brucellosis, and regional enteritis. It has also been noted in patients taking methysergide for migraines. Pathologically, the disease consists of a fibrous mass sitting anterior to the sacral promontory and extending laterally around the ureters. It may be seen as far superiorly as the lower pole of the kidneys. The major clinical sequela is ureteral obstruction. Sonographically, retroperitoneal fibrosis looks similar to lymphadenopathy. A mass may be seen enveloping the abdominal aorta, although elevation from the spine usually is not present. Unilateral or bilateral hydronephrosis may be present. The primary difference in sonographic appearance between retroperitoneal fibrosis and paraaortic lymphadenopathy is that renal fascia is less echogenic and smaller than paraaortic adenopathy.[15,23,34]

Cystic Masses

A variety of fluid collections can present sonographically as cystic retroperitoneal masses. These include abscesses, hematomas, urinomas, and lymphoceles. Because they can all have the same sonographic appearance, it is impossible to differentiate the pathologic process on the basis of ultrasound alone, however, correlation of sonographic findings with the patient's clinical history can frequently provide a presumptive diagnosis. Fine-needle aspiration of suspicious areas provides the clinician more specific information on the nature of the mass. Identifying the compartments within which the collection is localized may help narrow the diagnostic possibilities.

The anterior pararenal space is the most common site of retroperitoneal infections.[40] Since the appendix frequently occupies a retrocecal position and lies outside the peritoneal cavity and since portions of the duodenum and colon also border the anterior pararenal space, perforation by trauma, inflammation, or as a sequela of bowel disease can lead to retroperitoneal infection. The inflammatory response to microbes in the otherwise sterile retroperitoneal space includes the secretion of serous fluids and, ultimately, accumulation of pus. When the volume of inflammatory material reaches a certain point, it can be demonstrated sonographically. In cases of pancreatitis, digestive enzymes are extravasated and cause an inflammatory response in the anterior pararenal space. Typically this develops into a pseudocyst.[10,20] As the cell walls within the pancreas are destroyed by proteolytic digestive enzymes, additional enzymes are released into the interstitial spaces, precipitating further destruction of pancreatic parenchyma. Necrosis of blood vessel walls may also cause hemorrhage into the anterior pararenal space, increasing the fluid content. In some cases, the tissue-dissolving capabilities of the pancreatic enzymes cause further spread of the fluid into the posterior pararenal space.[10,25,33]

Fluid collections within the perirenal space or contained within Gerota's fascia are generally associated with renal abnormalities. Nephritis with subsequent abscess formation, rupture of a renal artery aneurysm, or bleeding from a renal neoplasm may all create a perinephric fluid collection (Fig. 12-10). These conditions are discussed in chapters 3 and 9. Sonographically, the fluid collection is contained within the borders of the renal fascia and does not demonstrate significant movement with alterations in patient position.

The posterior pararenal space is bounded anteriorly by the posterior renal fascia and posteriorly by the transversalis fascia. Since it does not contain any specific organs, alterations in anatomic appearance are due solely to processes that originate outside this space. Hemorrhage from trauma or ruptured vessels may dissect along the posterior pararenal space. Postoperative infections from aortic grafts may produce abscess collections, and leaking anastomoses may allow blood to collect there. The most common cause of posterior pararenal fluid collections is aortic disease.[6,19,38,44]

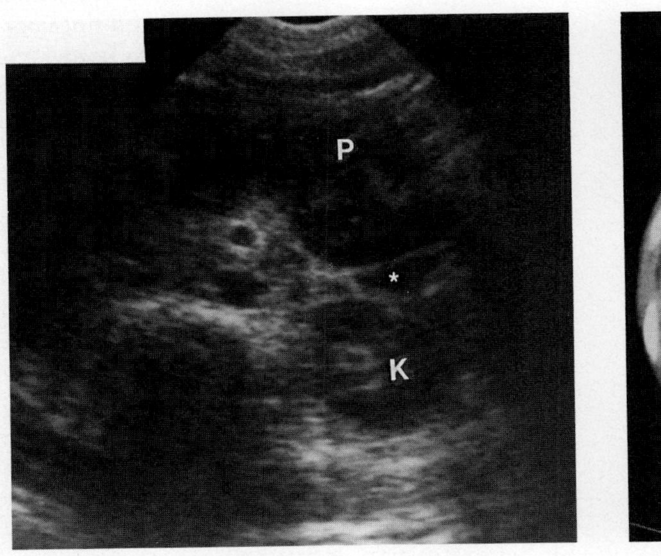

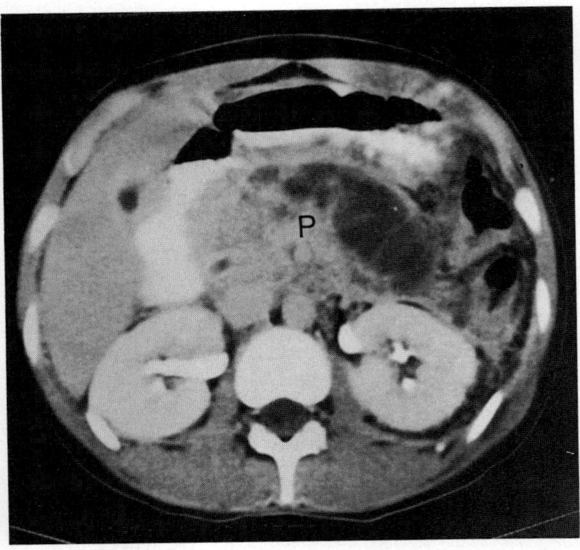

Figure 12-10. (*A*) Transverse sonogram through left upper quadrant demonstrates a large pancreatic pseudocyst (P) and a small amount of free anterior pararenal fluid (*; K, left kidney). (*B*) CT scan of same patient demonstrates extent of pseudocyst (P).

Hematomas

Bleeding into the retroperitoneum may be the result of trauma, hemophilia, malignant invasion, surgery, or anticoagulant therapy. It may also occur spontaneously. Depending on the stage of organization of the hemorrhage, the sonographic appearance can vary from purely cystic with smooth borders and no internal echoes to a solid structure with rough borders and high-level echoes (Fig. 12-11). It is impossible to differentiate such a mass from an abscess with ultrasonography alone, although a strong clinical suspicion of retroperitoneal bleeding combined with a positive sonogram may be sufficient to render a diagnosis. Fine-needle aspiration may provide the answer if nonclotting blood is obtained. CT is recommended as the primary screening modality for detection of retroperitoneal hematomas. If left untreated, continued bleeding may be life threatening, and ultrasound may not be adequate to make an accurate and timely diagnosis.

Abscesses

Fluid-filled inflammatory masses in the retroperitoneum may be imaged with ultrasound.[11] Clinically, the patient presents with an elevated white blood cell count, fever, and, depending on the location, point tenderness. Unfortunately, abdominal abscesses are often difficult to diagnose by clinical examination alone. Localizing signs may not be present, and in some cases fever is the only presenting symptom. In patients who recently had an operation or who have a history of an inflammatory process in the pancreas, colon, or duodenum, retroperitoneal abscess may be suspected. Recent perforation of the gastrointestinal tract lends strong suspicion to the diagnosis of retroperitoneal abscess.

The sonographic appearance of abscesses varies with the size, age, and internal composition of the mass. Generally they appear as ill-defined, poorly marginated, hypoechoic lesions with low to mid-level internal echoes (Fig. 12-12). Occasionally, a

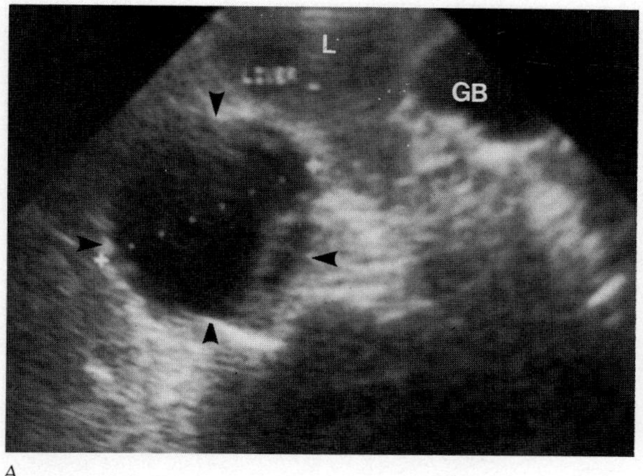

A

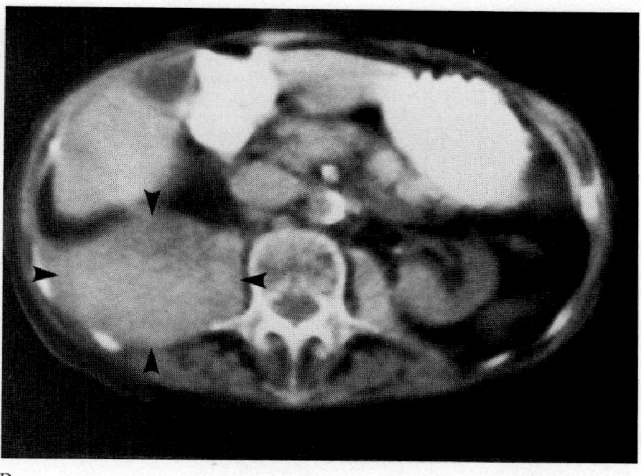

B

FIGURE 12-11. (*A*) Transverse sonogram though right upper quadrant demonstrates postoperative hematoma (*arrowheads;* GB, gallbladder; L, liver). (*B*) CT scan of same patient (*arrowheads,* hematoma).

highly echogenic appearance may be due to the presence of gas bubbles in the abscess.[30] Since ultrasound is an accurate method of detecting fluid collections, it should be the modality of choice for investigating suspected retroperitoneal abscesses, especially in young women and children.[20,27]

URINOMAS AND LYMPHOCELES

Usually associated with renal transplants, collections of sterile urine (urinomas) or lymph (lymphoceles) may be detected in the retroperitoneum. The specific clinical and sonographic considerations are discussed in Chapter 9.

ACQUIRED IMMUNODEFICIENCY SYNDROME

Acquired immunodeficiency syndrome (AIDS) is a disease characterized by viral destruction of the cellular immune response and subsequent development of a plethora of infectious and neoplastic processes. The human immunodeficiency virus (HIV) enters the body only by intimate contact with body fluids of an infected person. Unprotected sexual activity and sharing nonsterile needles by intravenous drug users are the most common methods of transmission. Although there have been reports of transmission to health care workers, these cases are rare and occur only when there is a breach of basic infection control procedures. All needles used in venipuncture should be discarded without being recapped; gloves should be worn when direct contact with body fluids such as urine, feces, semen, and blood is possible. Infection control professionals in the San Francisco Bay area, an area with a large population of AIDS patients, recommend that sonographers routinely wear gloves when scanning patients. Masks and gowns are not required unless the patient is incontinent or combative secondary to AIDS-induced dementia.

The pathologic manifestations of AIDS are many and varied. The virus destroys T lymphocytes, thereby incapacitating the immune system. With the body's defenses diminished or completely destroyed, a host of normally nonpathogenic organisms can invade without challenge. Pathologically, the manifestations of AIDS can be divided into three categories: structural changes associated with depletion of lymphoid tissue, unusual neoplasms, and opportunistic infections.

Opportunistic infections occur because the body's defenses are suppressed or nonfunctional. Bacteria, viruses, fungi, and protozoa enter the body

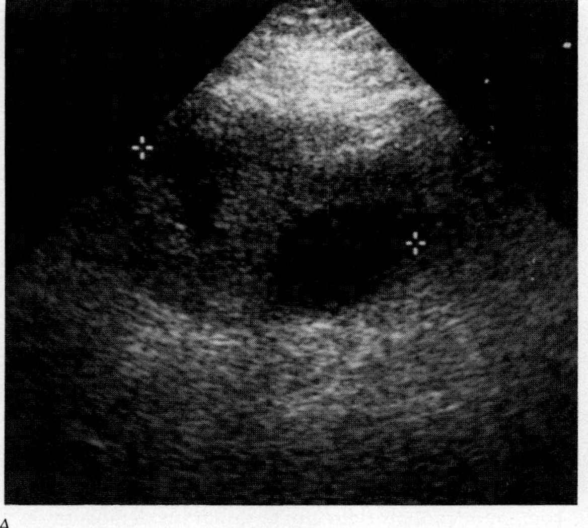

A

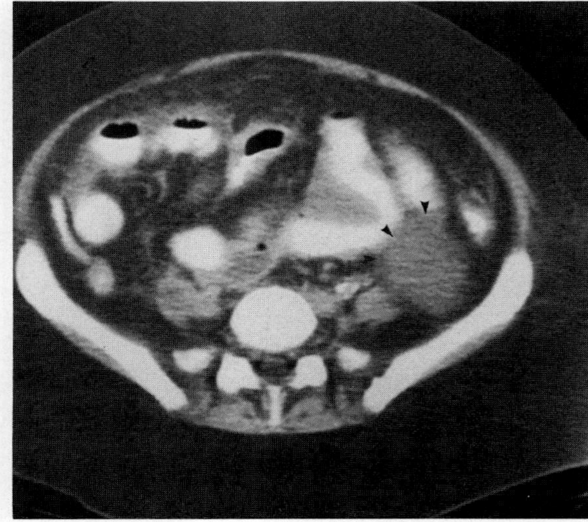

B

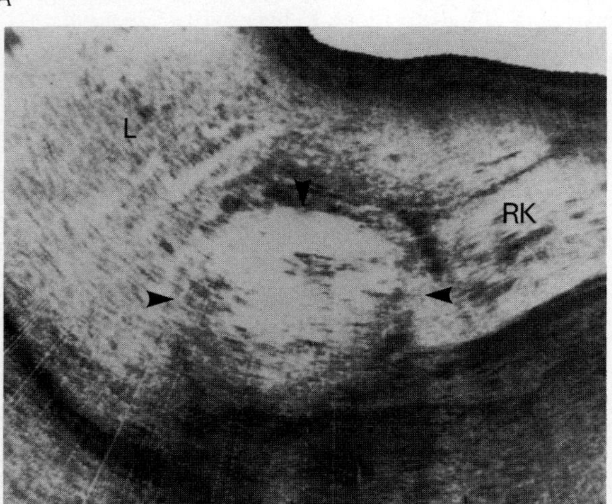

C

FIGURE 12-12. (*A*) Sagittal section through the left flank demonstrates a well-circumscribed abscess (*cursors*). (*B*) CT of same patient (*arrowheads*, abscess). (C) Chronic perinephric space abscess (*arrowheads*; RK, right kidney; L, liver).

and reproduce without resistance, causing fulminant infections. In AIDS patients, these opportunistic infections are difficult to treat and almost always recur. The infection can be localized to a specific organ or broadly disseminated. The most frequent sites of opportunistic infection are the lungs, central nervous system, and gastrointestinal tract.[24] Ubiquitous organisms that occur normally in the environment and present little, if any, threat to immunocompetent persons become devastating pathogens in patients with AIDS. *Pneumocystis carinii*, *Mycobacterium avium-intracellulare* (MAI), *Toxoplasma gondii*, and *Candida* organisms are examples of opportunistic pathogens. *Pneumocystis* infection invades the intraalveolar spaces and causes a pneumonia that accounts for 56% of all AIDS-related deaths;[45] *Cryptococcus* and *Toxoplasma* organisms frequently invade the CNS, causing a multitude of neurologic syndromes; cytomegalovirus and herpes simplex virus (HSV) have been isolated as infectious agents in numerous central nervous system and cutaneous conditions. The esophagus can be

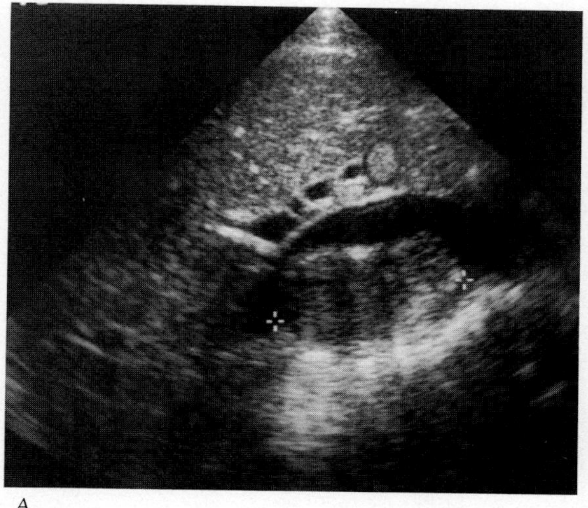

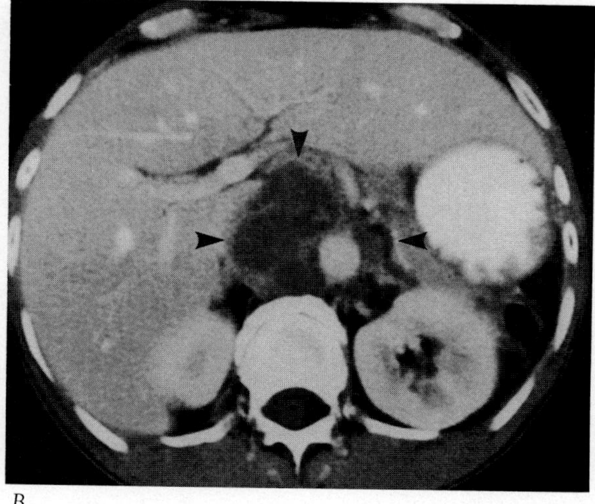

FIGURE 12-13. (*A*) Sonographic demonstration of MAI abscess (*cursors*) in the retroperitoneum of a patient with AIDS. (*B*) CT scan of same patient (*arrowheads*, mass).

infected by HSV or *Candida*, resulting in ulcerative esophagitis; *Cryptosporidium* and *Salmonella* organisms may invade the bowel, causing fulminant, life-threatening diarrhea. MAI has been found to be broadly disseminated in AIDS patients and is frequently implicated in systemic abscess formation (Fig. 12-13). In summary, a large number of normally innocuous organisms may be isolated as pathogens in symptomatic AIDS patients. These organisms are not a hazard to immunocompetent persons, but to those with an immune deficiency they are frequently deadly.

Unusual neoplasms that occur in AIDS include Kaposi's sarcoma, non-Hodgkin's (B-cell) lymphoma, oat cell carcinoma, and a number of extremely rare malignancies related to papillomavirus infections. Kaposi's sarcoma is the most common malignancy of AIDS patients. While it commonly involves the skin, spleen, and lymphatics, it can also be found in the upper and lower gastrointestinal tract and in the lungs. Non-Hodgkin's lymphoma is the second most common AIDS-related neoplasm. Typically, the disease is broadly disseminated and lesions can be found in multiple extranodal locations, including bone marrow, central nervous system, gastrointestinal tract, and a variety of other locations.[36] A plethora of other malignancies have been reported with AIDS, an important clinical point for sonographers to remember.

Sonographic Considerations. Sonographic evaluation of the abdomen in AIDS patients may help detect or localize infectious or neoplastic processes. The retroperitoneum should be examined for evidence of fluid collections that may represent abscess formation and for evidence of adenopathy. Laboratory data are frequently abnormal in AIDS patients, so specific tests may not provide clues about which organ system to evaluate. A thorough examination of intraperitoneal structures, as well as retroperitoneal spaces, should be performed.

References

1. Armstrong JR, Cohn L: Primary malignant retroperitoneal tumors. Am J Surg 1965, 110:937–951.
2. Asher W, Freimanis AK: Echographic diagnosis of retroperitoneal lymph node enlargement. AJR 1969, 105:438–445.

3. Binder SC, Katz B, Sheridan B: Retroperitoneal liposarcoma. Ann Surg 1978, 187:257–266.
4. Brasch JW, Moon AB: Primary retroperitoneal tumors. Surg Clin North Am 1967, 47:663–682.
5. Braschо DJ, Durant JR, Green LE: The accuracy of retroperitoneal ultrasonography in Hodgkin's disease and non-Hodgkin's lymphoma. Radiology 1977, 125:485–487.
6. Breiman RS, Korobkin M: Overview. *In* Margulis AR, Burhenne HJ (eds): Alimentary Tract Radiology, 3rd ed. St. Louis, CV Mosby, 1983.
7. Burney BT, Klatte EC: Ultrasound and computed tomography of the abdomen in the staging and management of testicular carcinoma. Radiology 1979, 132:415–419.
8. Carroll B: The retroperitoneum. *In* Sarti DA (ed): Diagnostic Ultrasound: Text and Cases, 2nd ed. Chicago, Year Book Medical Publishers, 1987.
9. Cooperburg PL: Ultrasonography. *In* Margullis AR, Burhenne HJ (eds): Alimentary Tract Radiology, 3rd ed. St. Louis, CV Mosby, 1983.
10. Donovan PJ, Sanders RC, Siegelman SS: Collections of fluid after pancreatitis: Evaluation by computed tomography and ultrasonography. Radiol Clin North Am 1982, 20:653–665.
11. Doust BO, Zuiros F, Stewart JM: Ultrasonic distinction of abscesses from other intraabdominal fluid collections. Radiology 1977, 125:213–220.
12. Enterline HT, Culberson JD, Rochlin DB, et al: Liposarcoma: A clinical and pathological study of 53 cases. Cancer 1960, 13:932–941.
13. Enzinger FM, Weiss SW: Soft Tissue Tumors, 2nd ed. St. Louis, CV Mosby, 1988.
14. Enzinger FM, Winslow DJ: Liposarcoma: A study of 103 cases. Virchows Arch 1962, 335:367–374.
15. Fagan CJ, Larrieu AJ, Amparo GE: Retroperitoneal fibrosis: Ultrasound and CT features. AJR 1979, 133:239–243.
16. Ferrucci JT: Diagnosis of abdominal malignancies by radiologic fine-needle aspiration biopsy. AJR 1980, 34:323–329.
17. Freimanis AK: Echography of retroperitoneal organs. Proceedings of the American Roentgen Ray Society, San Francisco, 1981.
18. Gerzhof SG, Robbins AH, Birkett DH, et al: Percutaneous catheter drainage of abdominal abscesses guided by ultrasound and computed tomography. AJR 1979, 133:1–8.
19. Gomes MN, Hakkal HG, Schellinger D: Ultrasonography and CT scanning. A comparative study of abdominal aortic aneurysms. Comput Tomogr 1978, 2:99–105.
20. Gonzales AC, Bradley EL, Clements JL Jr: Pseudocyst formation in acute pancreatitis—ultrasonographic evaluation of 99 cases. AJR 1976, 127:315–317.
21. Gronvall J, Gronvill S, Hegedus V: Ultrasound-guided drainage of fluid-containing masses using angiographic catheter techniques. AJR 1977, 129:997–1002.
22. Havrilla TR, Reich NE, Haaga JR: The floating aorta in computerized tomography: A sign of retroperitoneal pathology. Comput Axial Tomogr 1977, 1:234–236.
23. Jacobson JB, Redman HC: Ultrasound findings in a case of retroperitoneal fibrosis. Radiology 1974, 113:423–424.
24. Jaffe ES, Macher AM, Katz DA: Pathology of AIDS. *In* Broder S (ed): AIDS, Modern Concepts and Therapeutic Challenges. New York, Marcel Dekker, 1987.
25. Jeffrey BL, Laing FC, Wing VW: Extrapancreatic spread in acute pancreatitis: New observations with real-time US. Radiology 1986, 159:707–711.
26. Karp W, Hafstrom LO, Jonsson PE: Retroperitoneal sarcoma: Ultrasonographic and angiographic evaluation. Br J Radiol 1980, 53:525–531.
27. Knochell JQ, Koehler JQ, Lee TG, et al: Diagnosis of abdominal abscesses with computed tomography, ultrasound, and I11 in leukocyte scans. Radiology 1980, 137:425–432.
28. Kobayashi T, Takatani O, Kimaur E: Echographic patterns of malignant lymphoma. J Clin Ultrasound 1977, 4:181–187.
29. Korobkin M, Callen PW, Fisch AE: Computed tomography of the pelvis and retroperitoneum. Radiol Clin N Am 1979, 17:301–319.
30. Kressel HY, Filly RA: Ultrasonographic appearance of gas-containing abscesses in the abdomen. AJR 1978, 130:71–73.
31. Kurtz AB, Rubin C, Goldberg BB: Ultrasound diagnosis of masses elevating the inferior vena cava. AJR 1979, 132:401–406.
32. Laing FC, Jacobs RP: Value of ultrasonography in the detection of retroperitoneal inflammatory masses. Radiology 1977, 123:169–178.
33. Lawson TL: Acute pancreatitis and its complications. Computed tomography and sonography. Radiol Clin North Am 1983, 21:495–513.
34. Leopold GR, Asher WM: Echographic diagnosis of extraorgan retroperitoneal space lesions by B-scan ultrasonography. Radiology 1972, 103:133–139.
35. Lepor H, Walsh PC: Idiopathic retroperitoneal fibrosis. J Urol 1979, 122:1–9.
36. Levine AM, Gill PS, Rasheed S: AIDS-related malig-

nant B-cell lymphomas. *In* Broder S (ed): AIDS: Modern Concepts and Therapeutic Challenges. New York, Marcel Dekker, 1989.
37. McCullough DL, Leopold GR: Diagnosis of retroperitoneal fluid collections by ultrasonography: A series of surgically proved cases. J Urol 1976, 115:656–659.
38. Maklad NF, Doust BD, Baum JK: Ultrasonic diagnosis of postoperative intraabdominal abscesses. Radiology 1974, 113:417–422.
39. Manlove CH, Lawler KM: Retroperitoneal liposarcoma. Minnesota Med 1985, 68:581–585.
40. Meyers M: Retroperitoneum. *In* Margulis AR, Burhenne HJ (eds): Alimentary Tract Radiology, 3rd ed. St. Louis, CV Mosby, 1983.
41. Meyers MA: Dynamic Radiology of the Abdomen. New York, Springer-Verlag, 1976.
42. Miller MA, Leavell LC. Anatomy and Physiology, 16th ed. New York, Macmillan, 1972.
43. Pack GT, Tabah EJ: Collective review. Primary retroperitoneal tumors: A study of 120 cases. Surg Gynecol Obst 1954, 99:313–317.
44. Raskin MM, Cunningham JB: Comparison of CT and ultrasound for abdominal aortic aneurysm: A preliminary study. CT 1978, 2:381–385.
45. Riven BE, Monroe JM, Hubschman BP, et al: AIDS outcome: A first follow-up. N Engl J Med 1984, 311:857.
46. Sample DA: The retroperitoneum: Cases. *In* Sarti DA (ed): Diagnostic Ultrasound: Text and Cases, 2nd ed. Chicago, Year Book Medical Publishers, 1987.
47. Schmoller H, Kunit G, Frick J: Ultrasonic diagnosis of the retroperitoneal space. Urology 1979, 5:113–117.
48. Thornbury JR: Perirenal anatomy: Normal and abnormal. Radiol Clin North Am 1979, 17:321–331.
49. Weill FS, Perriguey G, Rohmer P: Sonographic study of the juxtarenal retroperitoneal compartments. J Ultrasound Med 1982, 1:307–310.
50. Wist E, Solheim P, Jacobsen AB, et al: Primary retroperitoneal sarcomas: A review of 36 cases. Acta Radiol 1985, 24:305–310.
51. Zelch MG, Haaga JR: Clinical comparison of computed tomography and lymphangiography for detection of retroperitoneal lymphadenopathy. Radiol Clin North Am 1979, 17:157–168.
52. Zornova J, Jonsson K, Wallace S, et al: Fine-needle aspiration biopsy of retroperitoneal lymph nodes and abdominal masses: An updated report. Radiology 1977, 125:87–88.

PART TWO

Pediatric Abdominal Sonography

CHAPTER 13

Abdominopelvic Cavity

LAURA NEWREN

Prevertebral Vessel Evaluation

Real-time sonography is a simple, noninvasive technique used to evaluate the prevertebral vessels in neonates. Ultrasound is an excellent choice of imaging to evaluate neonatal vessels because it allows bedside examination. Critically ill infants who are sensitive to stress (i.e., transport, temperature changes) can easily and safely be examined with a portable ultrasound unit.

SONOGRAPHIC TECHNIQUES

Although anatomically they are similar to adults, neonates and children require a different scanning approach. Using multiple planes on the neonate, the full length of the great vessels can easily be evaluated from the level of the diaphragm to the bifurcation without any particular patient preparation. Although it is not impossible to evaluate the adult aorta from the left flank,[30] it is not as easy to accomplish as in neonates.

TECHNICAL CONSIDERATIONS

Patients in the neonatal intensive care unit are often intubated, so if it is necessary to tilt the patient to one side or the other, it is advisable to seek the aid of a caregiver. For scanning neonates, a 7.5-MHz transducer produces the best detail, while a 5-MHz transducer produces the best possible detail with adequate penetration. Depending on which great vessel is to be evaluated, it may be necessary to turn the patient to the appropriate side. The left posterior oblique (LPO) or left lateral decubitus (LLD) position is better for evaluating the inferior vena cava (IVC), as the vessel is nearer to the transducer placed on the right lateral abdomen. Each position is described in Chapter 1. The LPO position permits use of the liver and right kidney as the sonographic window, thus avoiding bowel gas. In the right posterior oblique (RPO) or right lateral decubitus (RLD) position, the aorta lies nearer the transducer placed on the left lateral abdomen. This approach has been used successfully in other laboratories.[9]

A secondary imaging modality, duplex Doppler, should also be used to evaluate aortic and right and left iliac arterial flow. Although the angle may not be truly parallel to the flow of the arteries, it would be possible to detect decreased flow or adequate flow in each vessel. If the acoustic beam is directed from the left flank, the flow in the left iliac artery should move toward the transducer, or above the baseline. Flow in the right iliac artery should move away from the transducer, or below the baseline. Similar techniques are useful for evaluating the inferior vena cava and its bifurcation.

ROUTINE EXAMINATION

The routine examination of the abdominal great vessels should include longitudinal sections from the coronal plane and longitudinal and transverse sections from anterior to posterior with the patient lying supine. Scanning longitudinally from the co-

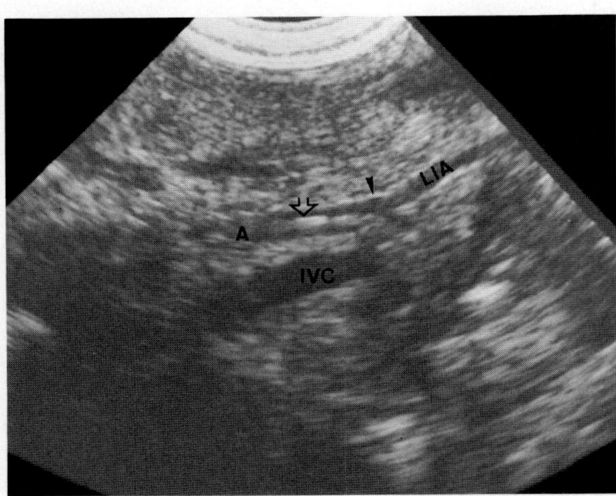

Figure 13-1. A longitudinal section made in the coronal plane demonstrates a catheter *(open arrow)* in the abdominal aorta (A), the aorta's bifurcation *(arrowhead)*, the left iliac artery (LIA), and the inferior vena cava (IVC).

ronal plane, the transducer can be manipulated anteroposterior, rotating or tilting the transducer to optimize the image of the inferior vena cava to include the length of the IVC from the diaphragm to the bifurcation (Fig. 13-1). The abdominal aortic approach from the left flank also permits aortic visualization from the level of the diaphragm to its bifurcation and identification of the right and left iliac arteries. Usually the renal arteries may also be identified (Fig. 13-2). In supine transverse sections, the great vessels can be identified by scanning from the level of the diaphragm and inferiorly until bowel gas interferes. Pressing firmly but carefully on the abdomen often moves the sound-attenuating bowel, restoring the images of the great vessels. To prevent vascular compromise, care must be taken not to press too hard on the abdominal aorta and IVC.

Normal Anatomy

The liver and kidney may be seen using the LPO patient position; with the left flank approach (RPO patient position), the left kidney, stomach, and spleen may be seen.[9] In the coronal longitudinal plane, the transducer parallels the great vessels, producing long, linear, anechoic, tubelike structures with bright walls.

Congenital Anomalies

Coarctation of the Abdominal Aorta

Hypoplasia or coarctation of the abdominal aorta is a rare congenital defect. Although 98% of coarctations are located in the proximal descending thoracic aorta, only 2% of them actually affect the abdominal aorta (Fig. 13-3). Renal artery stenosis is a feature of more than half of these cases. Congenital abdominal coarctation can occur any time in embryonic development. The earlier it occurs, the more obvious the manifestations. Acquired coarctation of the abdominal aorta has been associated with hypercalcemia,[6,28,33] neurofibromatosis,[2,3,10,18,28] tuberous sclerosis,[28,33] rubella,[25,26,28] and Turner's syndrome.[25,28] Children present with severe hypertension, headaches, and fatigue, whereas infants exhibit failure to thrive.[6] An interrupted abdominal aorta produces vascular compromise such as cyanotic limbs, mottled and discolored limbs, and decreased femoral pulses. The extreme consequences of untreated severe hypertension can be fatal by age 30.[2,15] Although the neonatal and pediatric

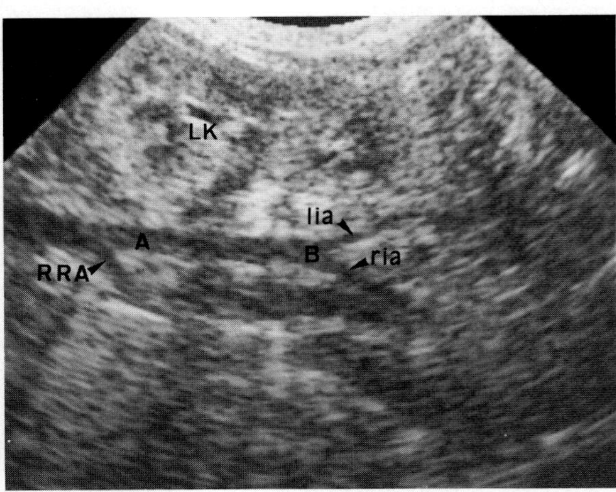

Figure 13-2. The aorta (A), right renal artery (RRA), bifurcation (B), and the right (ria) and the left (lia) iliac arteries are visualized on this longitudinal, coronal scanning plane (LK, left kidney).

great vessels can be easily evaluated with ultrasound, a complementary tool, the aortogram, should also be included (Fig. 13-4).

Inferior Vena Cava

When scanning the inferior vena cava and the aorta, the sonographer must note both position and relation of the two vessels. In the normal relationship, the IVC is on the right side, receiving the hepatic veins as it enters the right atrium. An IVC on the patient's left side is diagnositc of situs inversus. Besides an abnormal relationship of IVC and aorta, the IVC can also be interrupted, in which case it drains via an azygous continuation,[12,16,31] which may lie either left or right of the spine (Fig. 13-5). The hemiazygous continuation lies farther posterior than the aorta (Fig. 13-6).[12] Another abnormal vessel that may be imaged in the long axis plane is an anomalous venous connection associated with total anomalous pulmonary venous return, which connects to the ductus venosus. It crosses between the aorta and IVC. Displacement or distortion of the IVC or the aorta should alert the sonographer that other anomalies may be present.[9] (Congenital heart disease is discussed in detail in Volume II of this series.) Sonographers must be cognizant of the fact that unusual presentations of the aortic or IVC and anomalous vessels in the lower abdomen may indicate complex congenital heart disease.

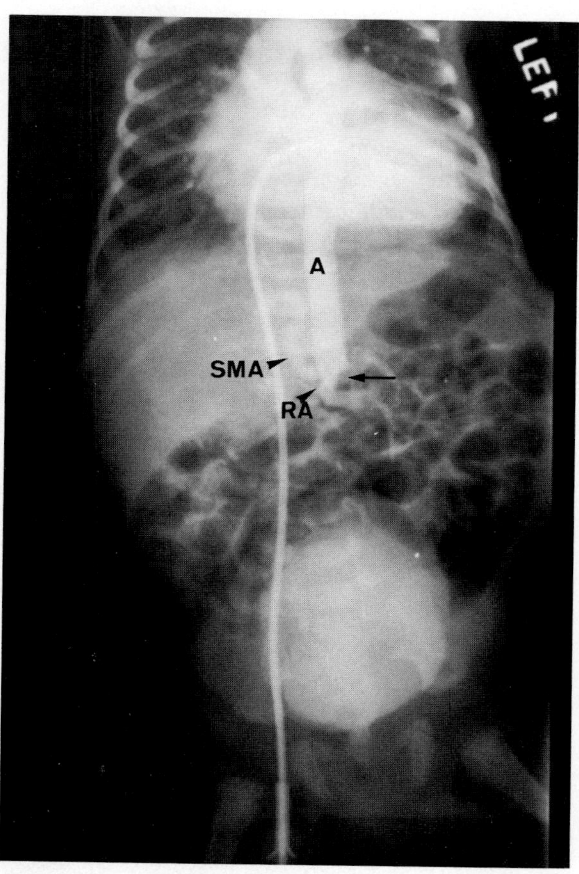

Figure 13-4. An aortogram of the patient in Figure 13-3 shows the interrupted *(arrow)* abdominal aorta (*A*) and the collateral circulation of the superior mesenteric artery (SMA) and renal artery (RA).

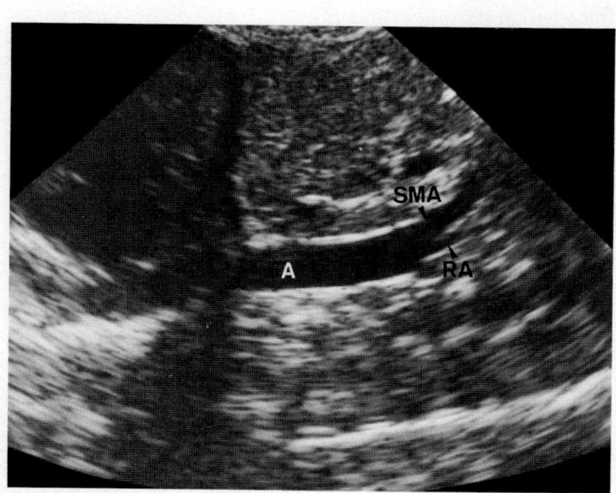

Figure 13-3. Coarctation of the abdominal aorta (*A*) is demonstrated on this longitudinal section with the interruption of the abdominal aorta and collateral circulation of the superior mesenteric artery (SMA) and renal artery (RA).

Acquired Disorders

Abdominal Aorta in the Neonate

The most common reason for evaluating the aorta in the neonate is for aortic thrombus, a well-recognized complication of indwelling umbilical artery catheters (UAC).[24] Clinical signs of aortic thrombus include (1) absence of femoral pulses, (2) hematuria, and (3) signs of vascular compromise such as, extremity blanching, cyanosis, hypertension, or necrotizing enterocolitis. Several factors have been found to increase the frequency of aortic thrombus (1) weight of 1500 g or less, (2) use of a No. 3.5 French catheter on smaller infants, (3) use of No. 5.0 French catheters on patients heavier than 1500 g, (4) infusing calcium salts, and (5) catheterization above the renal artery. A catheter in place more than 7 days showed no evidence of increased risk.

The UAC appears within the aorta as two bright parallel lines with an anechoic center (Fig. 13-7). The clot formation at the tip of the catheter appears as an irregular echo-dense border pattern (Fig. 13-8). The clot may be long and thick, and is termed extensive if it fills 40% of the aorta in a cross-sectional view, goes to the level of the renal artery or iliac artery, or causes proximal dilatation. One study concluded that leaving the catheter in the aorta after the clot was detected neither increased the size of the clot nor increased the symptoms.[30] However, ultrasound can alert clinicians that the UAC is above the renal artery and should

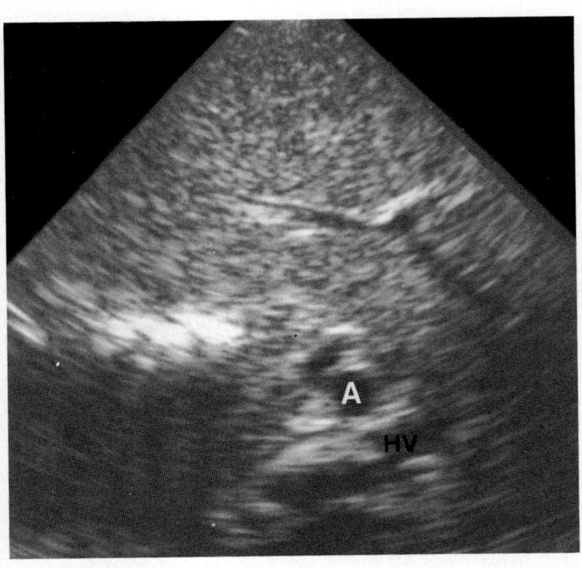

Figure 13-5. In this transverse scan low in the abdomen, the aorta (A) is demonstrated on the left side. The interrupted inferior vena cava is not seen but drains through a hemiazygous (HV) continuation.

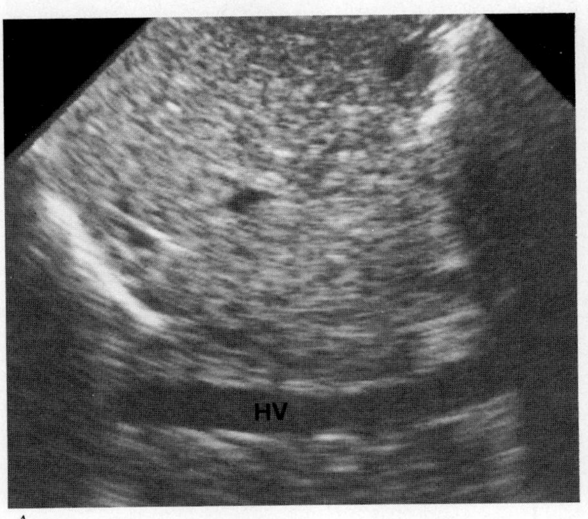

A

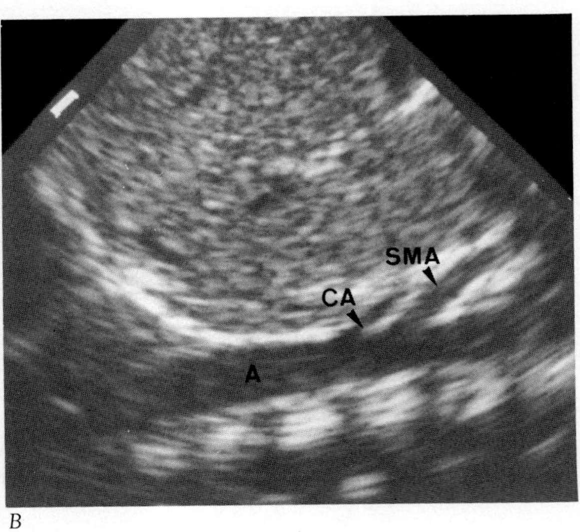

B

Figure 13-6. (*A*) This longitudinal section (the same patient as in Figure 5) is slightly left of the midline and demonstrates the hemiazygous vein (HV) continuation. (*B*) The hemiazygous vein continuation in *A* is farther posterior than the normal aorta (A) in this longitudinal scan. (CA, celiac artery; SMA superior mesenteric artery).

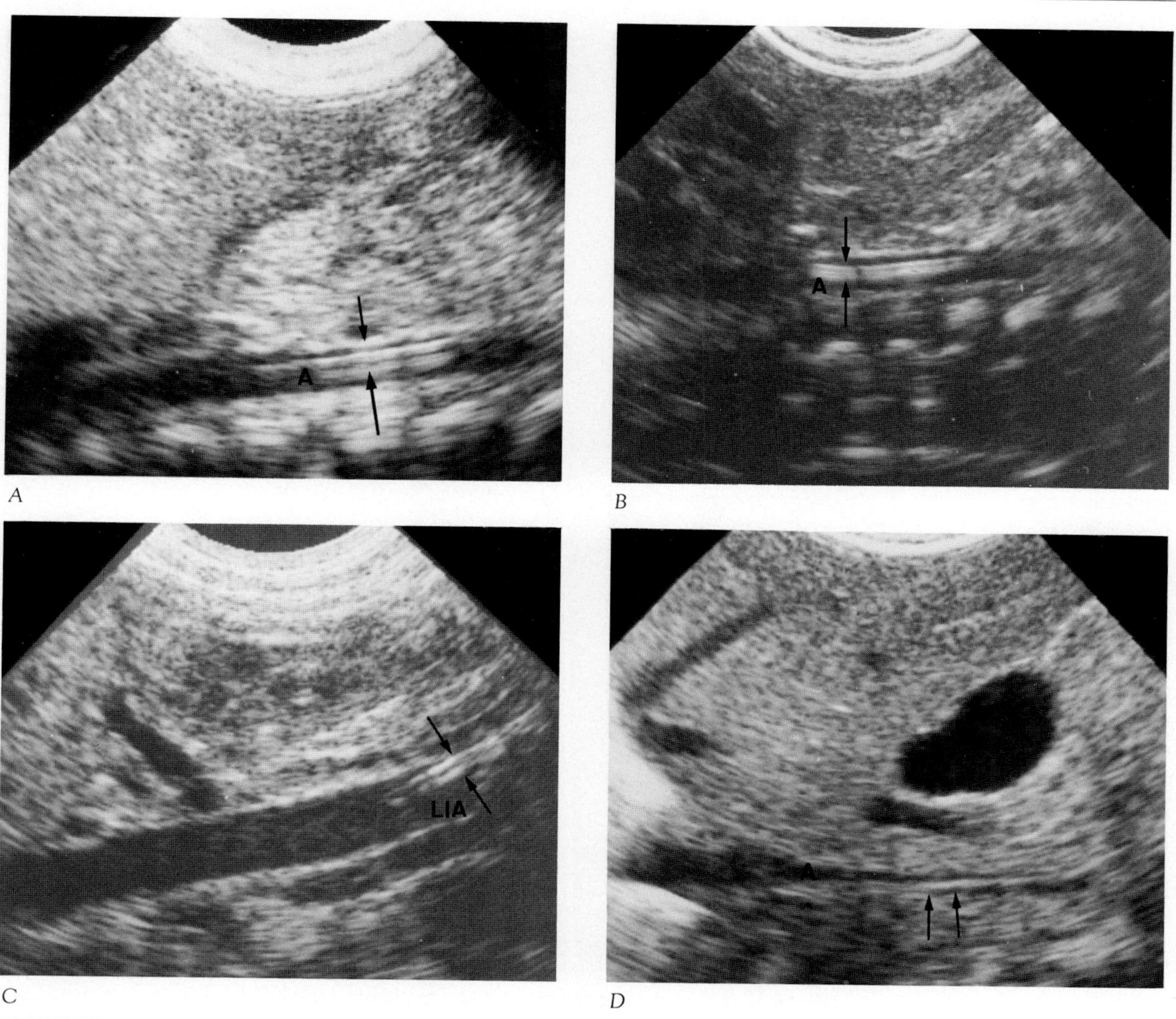

FIGURE 13-7. (*A, B,*) An indwelling umbilical artery catheter is visualized as two parallel lines *(arrows)* with an anechoic center representing the catheter lumen on these longitudinal sections in the abdominal aorta (A). (C) This indwelling umbilical artery catheter *(arrows)* is visualized on the longitudinal section in the left iliac artery (LIA). (*D*) After removal of the umbilical artery catheter, a fibrinous sheath *(arrow)* can develop, as identified on this longitudinal section of the abdominal aorta (A).

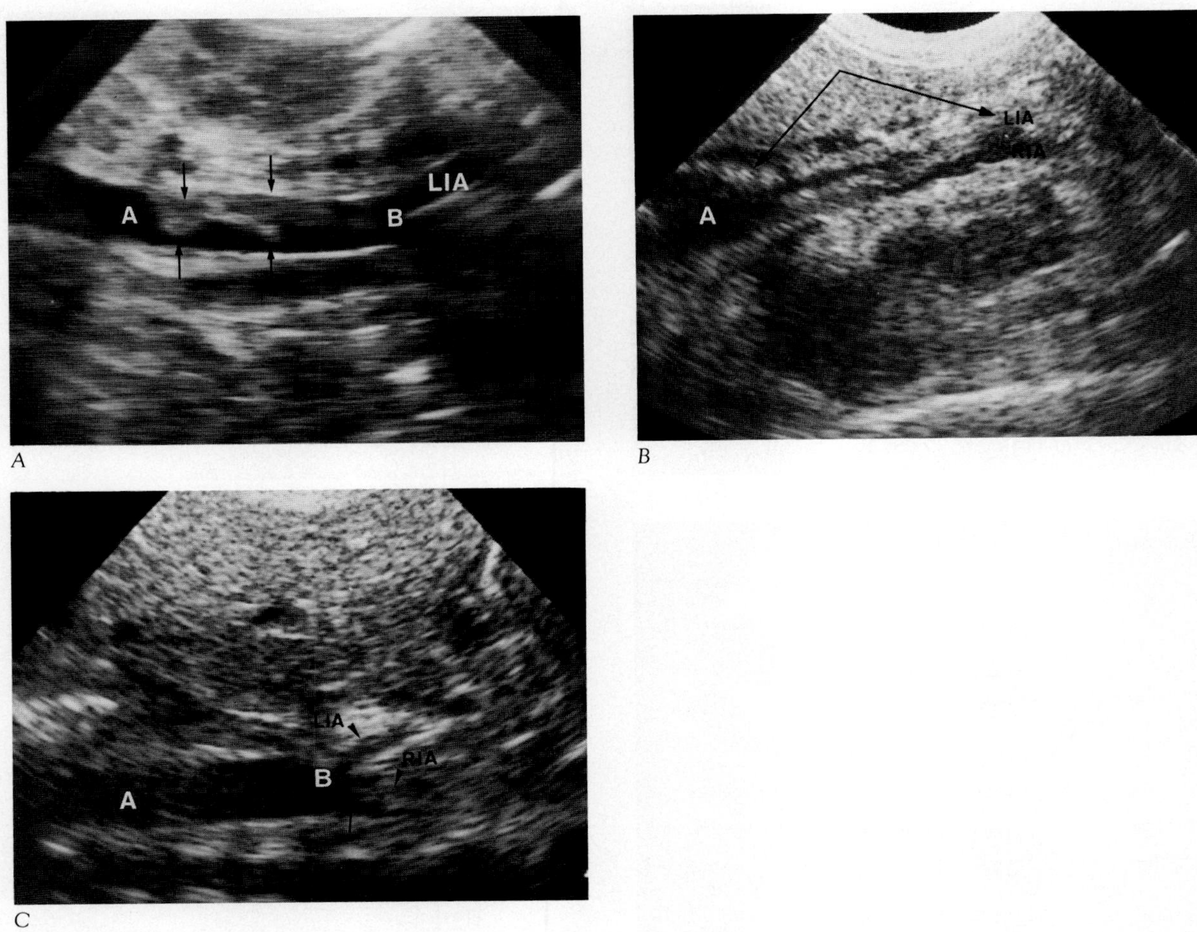

Figure 13-8. (*A*) A longitudinal section made over the left flank area demonstrates a thrombus *(arrows)* in the abdominal aorta (A; b, bifurcation; LIA, left iliac artery). (*B*) A thrombus *(arrows)* in the abdominal aorta (A) is visualized extending and occluding the left iliac artery (LIA) on this longitudinal section made over the left flank area (RIA, right iliac artery). (C) A thrombus *(arrow)* is identified in the right iliac artery (RIA) on a longitudinal section made over the flank area (A, abdominal aorta; B, bifurcation; LIA, left iliac artery).

be pulled back. There are several courses of treatment for clot in the UAC. If the neonatalogist elects to do nothing after removing the catheter, spontaneous regression of the thrombus may take place. Other choices are urokinase or streptokinase or surgical embolectomy. The long-term outcomes of unresolved thrombus include renal dysfunction, hypertension, limb anomalies, and growth disturbances.[30]

In any patient with signs suggestive of thrombus (pale, mottled extremities or decreased femoral pulses) the bladder should be evaluated. If the bladder remains extremely full after an attempt to empty it by pressing on the lower abdomen just above the symphysis pubis (Crede's method), it is possible that the skin color will return to normal and the femoral pulses will get stronger.[14]

INFERIOR VENA CAVA

The inferior vena cava can be a site of thrombus or calcifications in neonates (Fig. 13-9). Children can have tumor invasion into the IVC, such as Wilms' tumor (Fig. 13-10A).

Extension of renal carcinoma into the IVC has been well-documented.[7] Extension can occur from the right kidney, adrenal gland (neuroblastoma), retroperitoneum (sarcoma), and from hepatocellular carcinomas, teratomas, and lymphomas. It is important to evaluate the extension of the tumor into the hepatic veins or right atrium and to seek evidence of tumor invasion of the wall of the IVC. Tumor extension appears similar to the solid texture of the tumor itself. Case studies have reported IVC enlargement with a distended and bulging anterior wall without alteration of the posterior wall. The vessel did not lose its normal respiratory variation. The differential diagnosis includes simple thrombus.[7] Although ultrasound is the best modality for evaluating cephalad extension of IVC tumor invasion, IVC wall invasion is best demonstrated by CT (Fig. 13-10B–D). Neither ultrasound nor CT can distinguish between neoplastic tissue and a blood clot within the thrombus.[7]

Pelvic Cavity

Sonography is the preferred method of evaluating the pediatric pelvis because it is fast, accurate, painless, and noninvasive.[17,19,21]

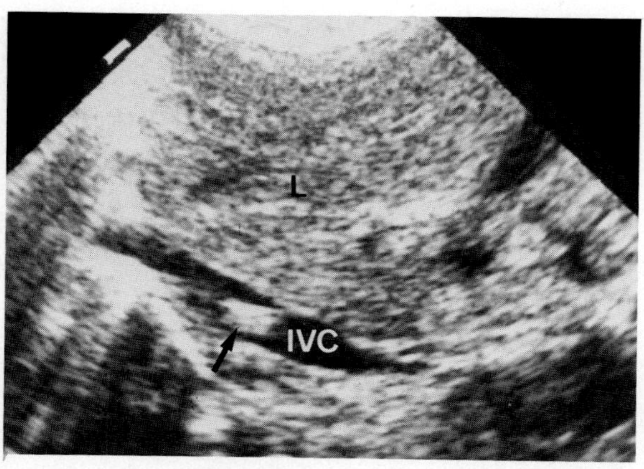

FIGURE 13-9. A clot *(arrow)* is visualized on a longitudinal section of the inferior vena cava (IVC) posterior to the liver (L).

PATIENT PREPARATION

As in studies of the adult pelvis, a full urinary bladder is used as an acoustic window. It is not always possible to get full cooperation from the patient in filling the bladder. With bottle-fed infants, this can usually be accomplished by feeding the infant before, after, and during the examination. The sonographer usually can capture the necessary images before the patient voids spontaneously. If it is necessary to fill the bladder, the patient can be catheterized. A young child can be given three full glasses of fluid a half hour before the examination and instructed not to void.

SCANNING TECHNIQUE

The pediatric pelvis should be examined with the highest-frequency transducer that allows adequate depth penetration. As with adult patients, the pediatric patient is scanned in the supine position. Scans should be obtained from multiple planes, both transverse and longitudinal.

Uterus. Normally the neonatal uterus is larger and more easily identified than the prepubertal uterus, owing to residual maternal hormone.[8,17,22] The endometrial cavity appears as a thin and highly echogenic reflector (Fig. 13-11). The myometrium is homogeneous with a medium-level echo pattern.

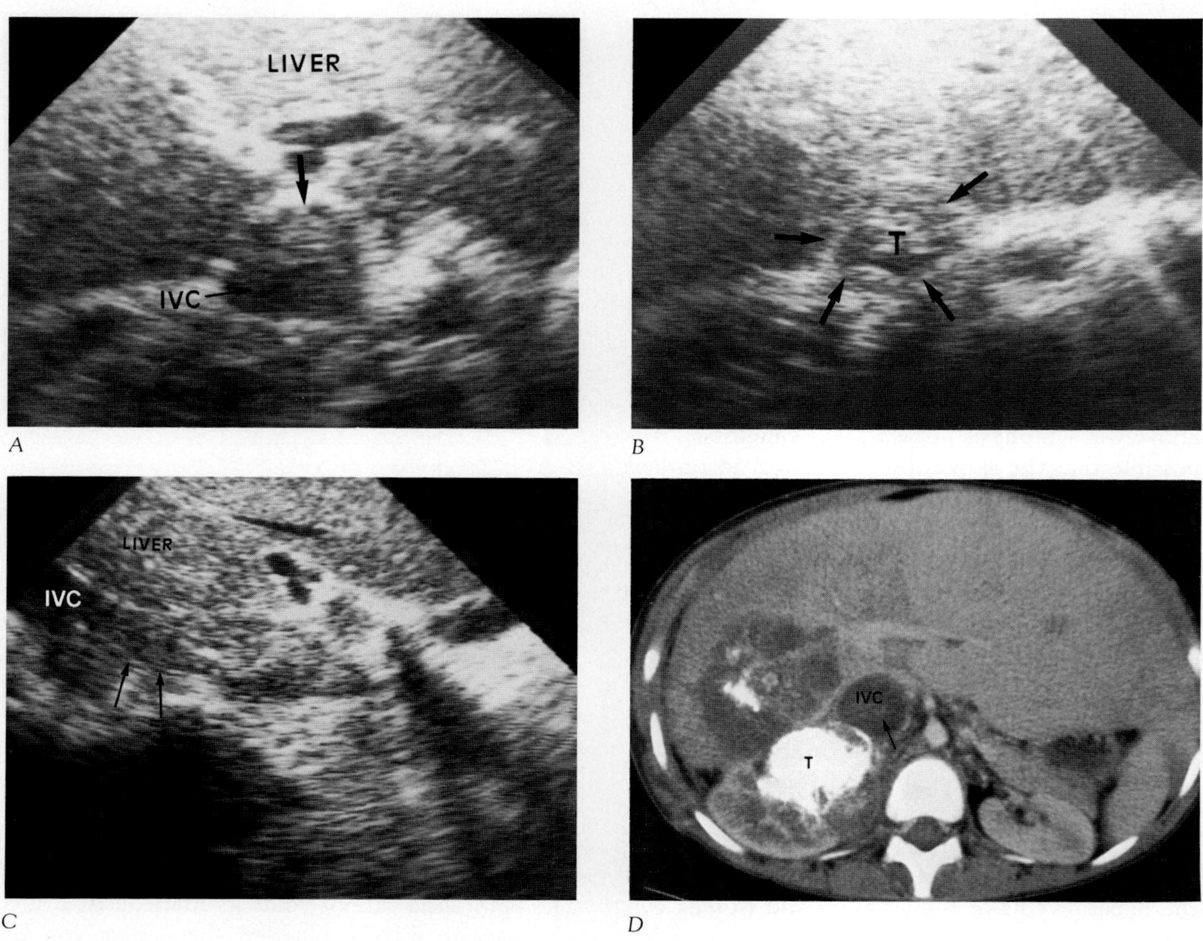

Figure 13-10. (*A*) Tumor invasion *(arrow)* is seen on this transverse view of the inferior vena cava (IVC). (*B*) Tumor invasion (T) is seen on this transverse section through the inferior vena cava *(arrows)*. (C) The cephalad extension of a tumor *(arrows)* into the inferior vena cava (IVC) is seen on this longitudinal section. (*D*) On a transverse computed tomographic image, the tumor (T) extension is visualized in the lumen *(arrow)* of the inferior vena cava (IVC).

The size of the prepubertal uterus ranges from 2 to 3.3 cm.[19] It is suggested that from ages 2 to 7 years the mean uterine length is 2.5 cm, at 10 years of age it is 3.5 cm, and at 11 years 4.2 cm (see Volume I for more details).

Ovaries. According to one study, 85% of girls younger than 7 months have cysts in their ovaries. Other studies, however, have reported difficulty in identifying the ovaries in neonates.[32] Such difficulties may be related to size, as neonatal ovaries range from 0.5 to 1.5 cm long and 0.3 to 0.4 cm thick.[17]

Hydrometrocolpos. Hydrometrocolpos occurs in 1 of 30,000 live births, and accounts for 15% of abdominal masses in girls.[13] It is due to obstruction of the

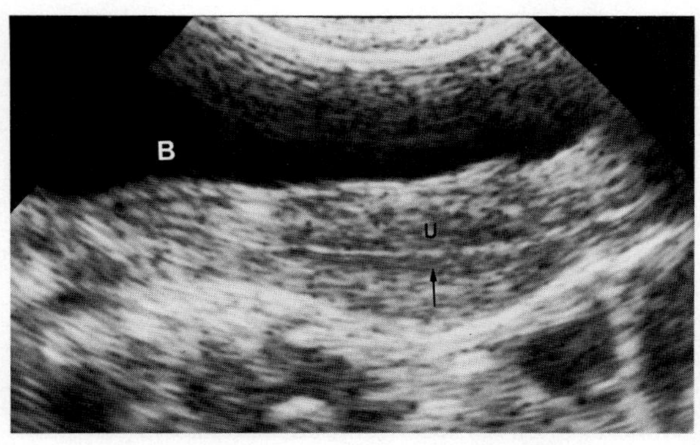

FIGURE 13-11. A longitudinal scan demonstrates the normal appearance of the neonatal uterus (U) with the endometrial cavity *(arrow)* appearing as a thin and highly echogenic reflector (B, bladder).

genitourinary tract and the accumulation of mucous secretions secondary to the stimulation of maternal estrogen (Fig. 13-12). It can cause hydronephrosis, bowel obstruction, and lower extremity edema. The neonate with hydrometrocolpos may have other more serious anomalies, such as imperforate anus, rectouterine or rectovaginal fistula, unilateral renal agenesis, hypoplasia of the vagina, or polycystic kidneys. It is important for the sonographer to search for associated malformations.

The differential diagnosis includes urachal cyst, mesenteric cyst, ovarian cyst or tumor, intestinal duplication, anterior myelomeningocele, and presacral teratoma.[13]

Endocrine Disorders. In girls precocious puberty is generally defined as the onset of puberty before age 9 years. The patient presents with premature breast enlargement, pubic hair, or menstruation. Making the diagnosis of precocious puberty is essential for proper treatment. Because a manual pelvic examination of a young child can be difficult, ultrasound offers a noninvasive alternative for evaluting the size of the ovaries. The patient's height may be compromised by premature closure of the epiphyses of the long bones. Gonadal enlargement is characteristic of true sexual precocity. The uterus is measured for length and width in the sagittal plane. Ovarian volume is calculated from measurements of width, thickness, and length. According to Sample,[11] normal ovaries are measured using the formula 0.5 × width × thickness × length. Data from Sample[11] established normal volume ranges

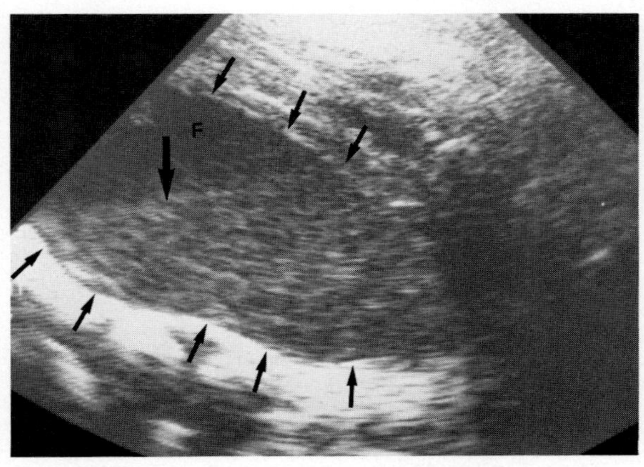

A

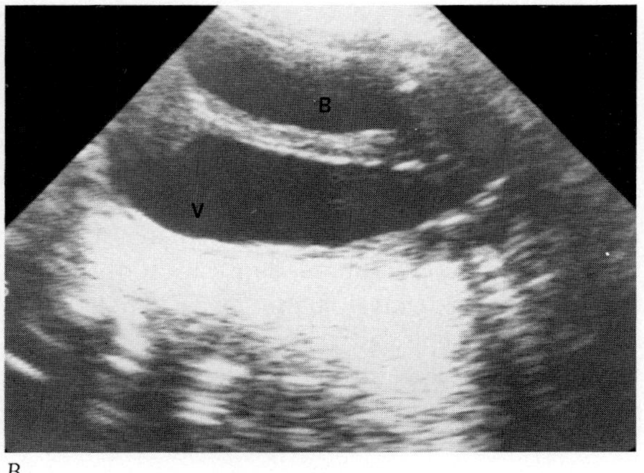

B

FIGURE 13-12. (*A*) On a patient with hydrometrocolpos, a distended vagina *(black arrows)* with a fluid (F)-debris level *(larger black arrow)* is visualized in a longitudinal section. (*B*) On the same patient after drainage, a longitudinal section demonstrates a distended, anechoic vagina (V) posterior to the bladder (B).

for ovaries prepubertal less than 0.9 cm^3, postpubertal, 1.8 to 5.7 cm^3. Normal uterine size before puberty is 2 to 3.3 cm long, 0.5 to 1 cm thick; postpubertal length is 5 to 8 cm and thickness 1.6 to 3 cm.

In true precocious puberty, ovaries are well above normal prepubertal size and in the range of normal size for postpubertal girls. Numerous tiny cysts may also be seen.

Adrenal glands must be scanned to exclude enlarged adrenal cortex due to adrenogenital syndrome or adrenal tumors, which can also produce abnormal secondary sexual characteristics.

Sacrococcygeal Teratomas. Although sacrococcygeal teratomas (SCT) are rare (one in 40,000 live births), they are the most common congenital tumor of newborns.[12,16,20,27] Arising from the region of the coccyx, they may protrude or involve the abdomen and lower pelvis, displacing the bladder. SCT occurs more often in girls, but is more often malignant in boys. It may be visualized sonographically and suspected before birth if the mother is examined to determine why there is a discrepancy between the gestational dates and the uterine size,[23,29] but usually it is diagnosed at birth. An SCT detected late is more likely to be malignant.

The SCT usually appears as an encapsulated echogenic mass but may contain cystic areas (Fig. 13-13). In addition to solid and cystic components, calcifications may also be present in both benign and malignant types. Studies indicate that solid tumors are usually malignant.

Associated anomalies include hydronephrosis and Potter's syndrome but probably no other major organ anomalies. The differential diagnosis includes lipoma, neuroblastoma, hemangioma, soft tissue tumors, bone tumors, duplication of the rectum, and anterior myelomeningocele. The latter is usually more cephalad than SCT. The treatment includes coccygectomy to ensure against recurrences.[30,31]

Anterior Sacromeningocele. Anterior sacromeningoceles (ASM) are extremely rare. Sonographically they look similar to sacrococcygeal teratomas, having the characteristic solid component, cystic, and complex texture. ASMs have been categorized. Type I is mostly external; type II is external but displaces and invades pelvic structures; type III has a larger pelvic component that profoundly displaces or invades surrounding structures; and type IV is presacral with no external portion and displaces the rectum, and if large enough, the bladder anteriorly. An ASM can cause obstruction of the urinary tract, bladder, and rectum. The differential diagnosis includes neuroblastoma, abscess, chordoma, rectal duplication, and anterior myelomeningocele.[5]

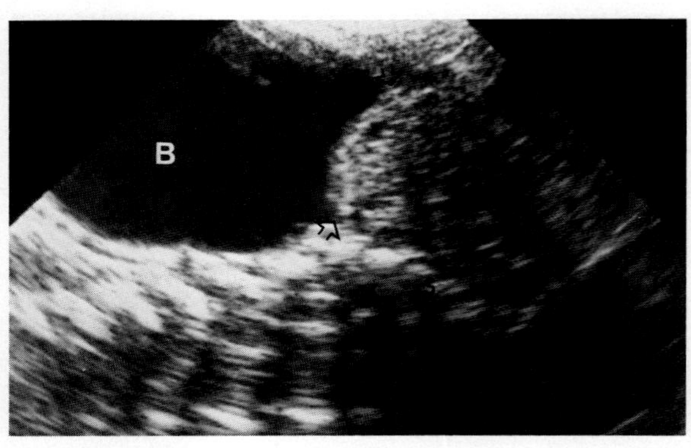

Figure 13-13. A longitudinal section in a female patient demonstrates a presacral sacrococcygeal teratoma (*arrows*) anterior to the sacrum (S) and indenting the bladder (B).

Conclusion

Ultrasound offers an alternative for evaluating abdominopelvic structures. It is an excellent choice because today's real-time units are simple to use, flexible, and portable, providing a noninvasive imaging modality especially suitable for critically ill neonates.

References

1. Adler DD, Blane CE, Silver TM, et al: Splenic trauma in the pediatric patient: The integrated roles of ultrasound and CT. Presented at the Radiologic Society of North American's Scientific Assembly and Annual Meeting, Washington, DC, November 1984.
2. Bjork VO, Intanti F: Coarctation of abdominal aorta with right renal artery stenosis. Ann Surg 1964, 170:54–60.

3. Bloor K, Williams RT: Neurofibromatosis and coarctation of the abdominal aorta with right renal artery involvement. Br J Surg 1963, 50:811–813.
4. Braly BD: Neonatal arterial thrombosis and embolism. Surgery 1965, 58:869–873.
5. De Klerk JJ, McCusker I, Loubser JS: Anterior sacral meningoceles. S Afr Med J 1978, 54:361–365.
6. Derrick JR, Cooley RN: Obstruction by calcium plaques of the descending aorta in an 18-year-old girl. Am Surg 1964, 30:153–157.
7. Didier D, Racle A, Etievent JP, et al: Tumor thrombus of the inferior vena cava secondary to malignant abdominal neoplasms: US and CT evaluation. Radiology 1987, 162:83–89.
8. Forest MG: Function of the ovary in the neonate and infant. Eur J Obstet Gynecol Reprod Biol 1979, 9:145–160.
9. Grunebaum M, Ziv N, Kornreich L: The sonographic evaluation of the great vessels' interspace in the pediatric retroperitoneum. Pediatr Radiol 1986, 16:384–387.
10. Halpern N, Currarino G: Vascular lesions causing hypertension in neurofibromatosis. N Engl J Med 1965, 273:248–252.
11. Hayden CK, Swischuk LE: Pediatric Ultrasonography. Baltimore, Williams & Wilkins, 1987.
12. Huhta JC: Pediatric Imaging, Ultrasound of the Chest. Philadelphia, Lea & Febiger, 1986.
13. Janus C, Godine L: Newborn with hydrometrocolpos and ambiguous genitalia: Clinical significance. J Clin Ultrasound 1986, 14:739–741.
14. Kushner DC, Chin JK, Cleveland RH: Neonatal aortoiliac compression caused by a distended bladder. AJR 1986, 146:1273–1275.
15. Lewis III VD, Meranze SG, McLean GK, et al: The midaortic syndrome: Diagnosis and treatment. Radiology 1988, 167:111–113.
16. Moss AJ, Adams FH: Heart Disease in Infants, Children, and Adolescents. Baltimore, Williams & Wilkins, 1977.
17. Nussbaum AR, Sanders RC, Jones MD: Neonatal uterine morphology as seen on real-time US. Radiology 1986, 160:641–643.
18. Robicsek, F, Daugherty HK, Cook JW, et al: Coarctation of the abdominal aorta with stricture of the major vessels. Surgery 1980, 87:545–548.
19. Sample WF, Lippe BM, Gyepes MT: Gray-scale ultrasonography of the normal female pelvis. Radiology 1977, 125:477–483.
20. Schey WL, Shkolnik A, White H: Clinical and radiographic considerations of sacrococcygeal teratomas: An analysis of 26 new cases and review of the literature. Radiology 1977, 125:189–195.
21. Schneider M, Grossman H: Sonography of the female child's reproductive system. Pediatr Ann 1980, 9:180–186.
22. Sedin G, Bergquist C, Lindgren PG: Ovarian hyperstimulation syndrome in preterm infants. Pediatr Res 1985, 19:548–552.
23. Seed JW, Mittelstaedt CA, Cefalo RC: Prenatal diagnosis of sacrococcygeal teratoma. J Clin Ultrasound 1982, 10:193–195.
24. Seibert JJ, Taylor BJ, Williamson SL: Sonographic detection of neonatal umbilical artery thrombosis: Clinical correlation. AJR 1987, 148:965–968.
25. Siassi B, Klyman G, Emmanoulides GC: Hypoplasia of the abdominal aorta associated with the rubella syndrome. Am J Dis Child 1970, 120:476–479.
26. Simpson JW, Nora JJ, Singer DB, et al: Multiple valvular sclerosis in Turner phenotypes and rubella syndrome. Am J Cardiol 1969, 23:94–97.
27. Sheth S, Nussbaum AR, Sanders RC, et al: Prenatal diagnosis of sacrococcygeal teratoma: Sonographic-pathologic correlation. Radiology 1988, 169:131–136.
28. Smith SH, Kelly DR: Coarctation of the abdominal aorta in a child: Morphometric analysis of the arterial lesion. Pediatr Pathol 1986, 5:363–371.
29. Stauffer RA: Sacrococcygeal teratoma. Med Ultrasound 1981, 5:119–120.
30. Steiner E, Rubens D, Weiss SL, et al: Sonographic examination of the abdominal aorta through the left flank: A prospective study. J Ultrasound Med 1986, 5:499–502.
31. Vaughan TJ, Hawkins IF Jr, Elliott LP: Diagnosis of polysplenia syndrome. Radiology 1971, 101:511–518.
32. Venta LA, Ramilo JL, Yousefsadeh DK: Sonography of the normal, prepubertal, and polycystic ovary: Potential diagnositc pitfall. Am J Dis Child 1987, 141:400.
33. Wiest JW, Traverso LW, Dainko EA, et al: Atrophic coarctation of the abdominal aorta. Ann Surg 1980, 191:224–227.

CHAPTER 14

Liver and Biliary System

JOYCE LUKKEN

The liver and biliary tree and its corresponding landmarks are the same in infants and children as in adults but smaller. It is important that the sonographic instrumentation afford high resolution to detect small ducts, vessels, and pathology.

A 7.5-MHz short-focus transducer is good for infants and a 5-MHz medium-focus for children. For very premature infants, the sonographer may consider a 10-MHz transducer for optimal resolution.

It is important to image all of the "adult" landmarks in an infant's or child's abdomen. Special attention should be paid to the position and size of the gallbladder, portal vein, portal vein bifurcation, hepatic artery, common bile duct, hepatic veins, and liver. Measurements should be recorded.

Ideally, the liver and biliary tree are best viewed with the patient in a fasting state. Since infants are fed every 3 to 4 hours, the examination should be performed just before a feeding. Children aged 1 to 3 years are best examined 4 hours after fasting, and older children after 8 hours' fasting. Special precautions should be taken to keep infants warm by placing blankets over all but the scanning surface and using warm gel.

Establishing a protocol of longitudinal, coronal, and transverse views is important to ensure consistency from one patient to the next, though special attention can be paid to differences such as position of anatomy, pathology, and size.

The normal liver appears as a smooth-outlined, homogeneous organ, usually situated in the right upper quadrant of the abdomen. It is divided into a large right lobe in the right side of the abdomen, a smaller left lobe extending across the midline, a caudate or Spigelian lobe situated on the posterior superior surface of the right lobe, and a quadrate lobe on the posterior-inferior surface of the right lobe. The right and left lobes are divided by the falciform ligament, which is sometimes seen easily on scans of infants and children. The liver is supplied by the hepatic artery arising from the celiac artery and is drained by the hepatic veins, which empty into the inferior vena cava near the diaphragm.

The blood supply to the liver is of a dual type, additional blood from the digestive system is carried to the liver via the convergence of the superior mesenteric vein and the splenic vein, which forms the portal vein. The portal vein enters the liver at the porta hepatis, where it quickly branches left and right into each lobe of the liver. The major vessels of the liver provide important visual landmarks.

Congenital Anomalies

HEMANGIOMAS

Hemangiomas of the liver are rare[34,76,101] congenital[26,34] anomalies arising from an arteriovenous malformation (AVM) forming blood-filled spaces. They are the most common vascular liver tumor in infancy[12,21,56,69] and are either cavernous (blood-

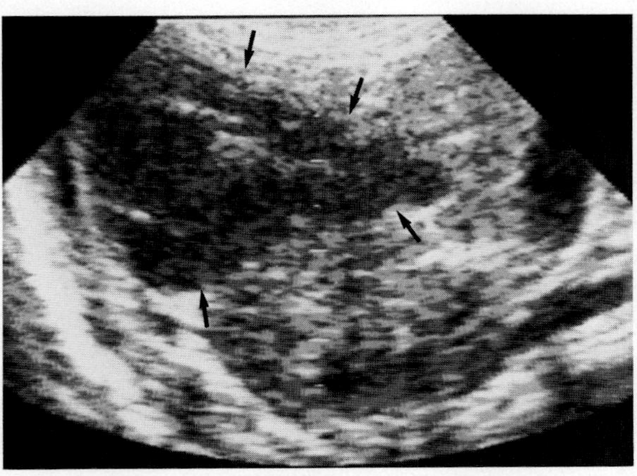

FIGURE 14-1. A large hypoechoic mass (*arrows*) in the right lobe of the liver is visualized on this transverse plane in a 5-day-old infant. The final diagnosis was cavernous hemangioma.

filled spaces lined with a single layer of endothelial cells) or hemangioendotheliomas (lining or endothelium is multilayered or hypertrophic with primitive or infantile cells) (Fig. 14-1).[21,69,74]

Hemangiomas may or may not be present at birth but usually become evident about age 2 months,[3,26,56] or they may be found incidentally.[34] They are more common in females.[11,12,21,26,47,74] A clinical symptom arising from suspected liver hemangiomas is hepatomegaly with or without accompanying abdominal distention due to hepatomegaly.[69] They cease to grow and then undergo spontaneous involution.[7,26,64,95,101,103]

After enlarging but before regression, the infant may experience a number of complications, including fatal rupture of the hemangioma, anemia[21] due to platelet trapping,[26] hepatic dysfunction due to portal hypertension,[21] intravascular coagulation,[56] intestinal bleeding, bowel obstruction, obstructive jaundice,[21] and irreversible congestive heart failure.[15,95]

Typical sonographic findings are of a well-defined hyperechoic area within the liver.[11,12,107] The hemangioma's hyperechoic appearance results from the multiple interfaces between the walls of the blood-filled sinuses.[11] Less frequently, the mass is hypoechoic and may mimic a collection of simple cysts.[11,12,21] It can also appear complex, demonstrating irregular walls and hypoechoic to anechoic areas, possibly due to necrosis (Figs. 14-2, 14-3). The presence of calcifications or fibrotic changes within the mass produces a hyperechoic pattern with posterior acoustic shadowing.[11,2156,97,105]

On unenhanced computed tomography (CT), hemangiomas usually appear as well-defined, low-density masses.[11,12,21,47,56] Areas of high as well as low density or calcifications due to fibrosis and thrombosis may be seen.[11,56] On enhanced CT scans, contrast accumulation along the periphery of the mass is early, with variable delayed central enhancement.[11,12,21,97]

Hemangiomas appear on magnetic resonance images (MRI) as homogeneous spherical masses with well-defined, smooth borders. Precontrast images show areas of diminished attenuation.[73] Bolus dynamic imaging shows peripheral enhancement, and delayed scans, complete filling with high signal intensity.[73] These masses also have a long T2 relaxation time, which produces a bright appearance.[12] On T1-weighted images, the hemangioma appears to be less bright or as bright as the surrounding liver tissue.[12] It is important to note that some liver metastases also have a prolonged T2 relaxation time, similar to that of hemangiomas.[11]

Radiographically, congestive heart failure or cardiomegaly can be demonstrated. A discrete abdominal mass or hepatomegaly, with or without accompanying calcifications, can be seen.[21,56]

In angiography, the larger masses quickly fill with contrast, producing a "cotton wool" or cloud-like appearance.[11,47,107] Smaller hemangiomas have more of a circular or C shape, with an unopacified center.[11,47,97] Contrast stain can persist as long as 30 seconds after the initial injection.[11,21,47,69] In large masses the hepatic artery and its branches appear enlarged,[11,47] whereas in small masses they appear normal sized.[11] The aorta can appear narrowed just distal to the celiac origin.[65]

An important factor in differentiating a metastatic lesion from a hemangioma is that metastatic lesions demonstrate increased flow in the perfusion phase but not increased delayed activity.[11] Richly vascular hepatocellular carcinomas may show increased perfusion but also demonstrate decreased activity on delayed images. Technetium^{99m}–sulfur colloid is nonspecific as it demonstrates a focal cold

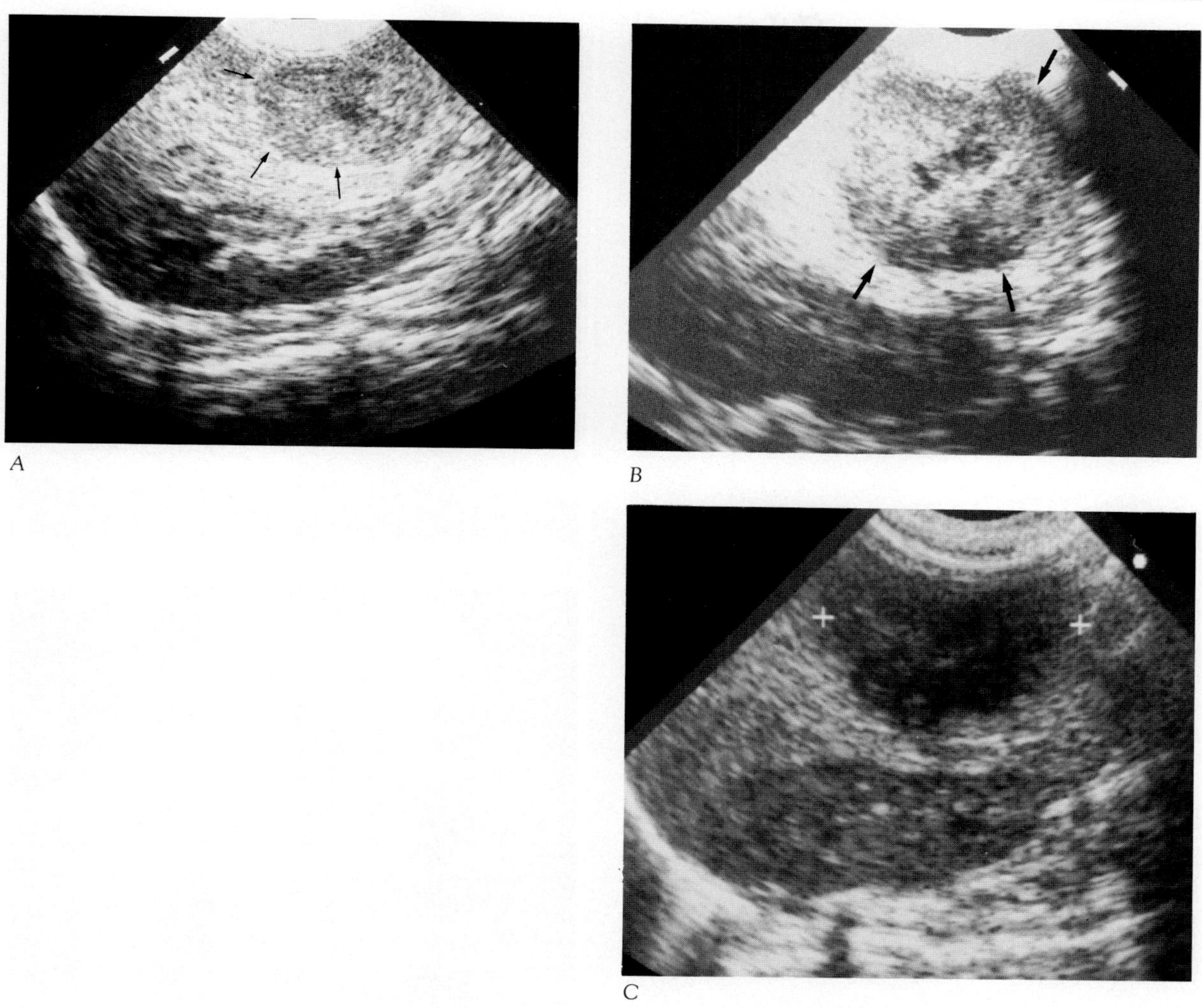

FIGURE 14-2. (*A*) In the longitudinal plane view of a 3-month-old patient, a hemangioma's borders appear well-circumscribed *(arrows)* while the center of the mass appears more sonolucent, perhaps because of necrosis. (*B*) In the same patient 1 month later, the hemangioma's walls *(arrows)* are more irregular and necrosis is increasing within the mass, as seen on a longitudinal image plane. (*C*) In the same patient 2 months later, a transverse plane visualizes the mass *(cursors)* as almost completely sonolucent with very irregular walls.

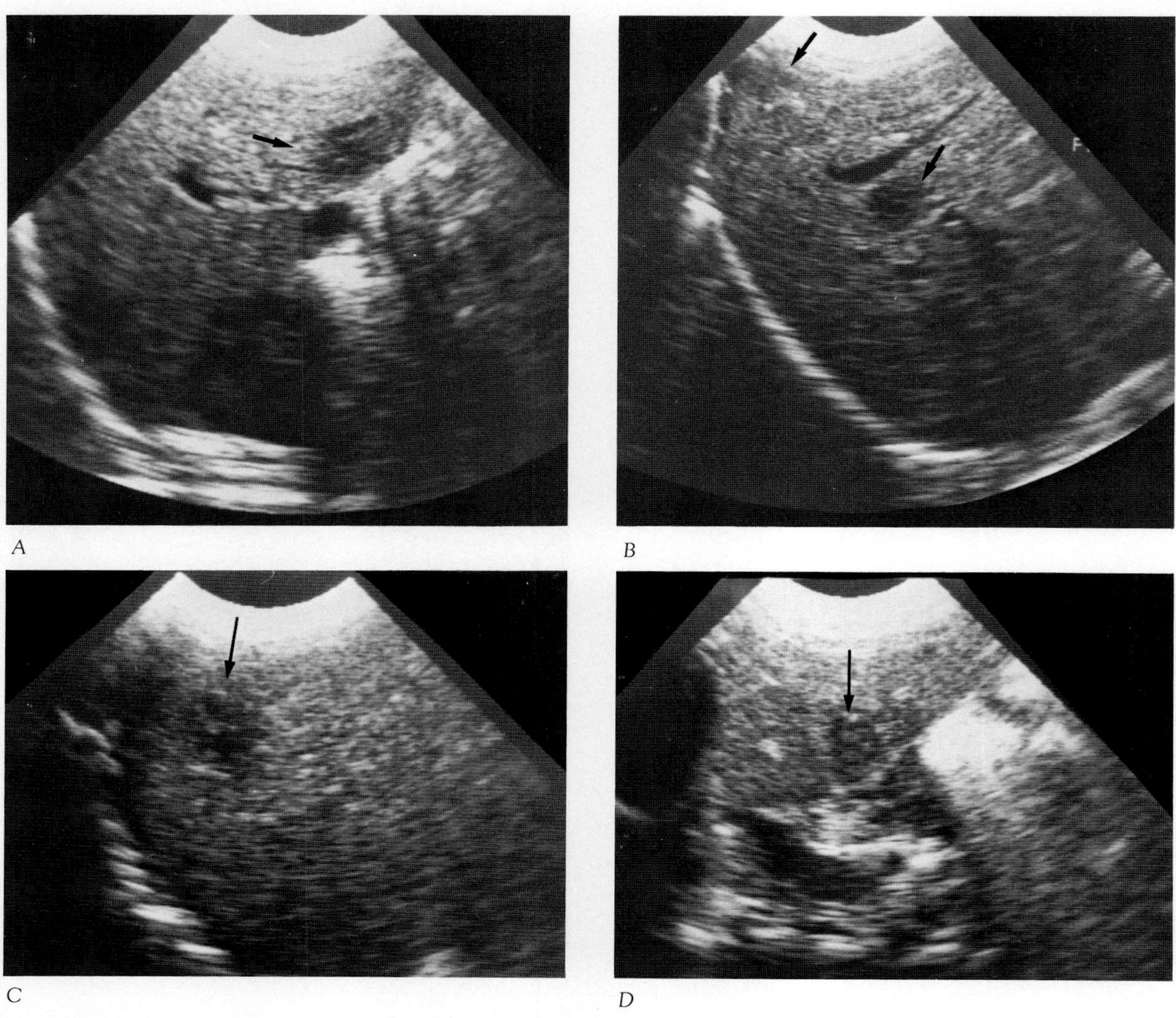

FIGURE 14-3. Multiple hemangiomas *(arrows)* with mixed echogenicity and irregular walls may mimic abscesses.

lesion, but a ^{99m}Tc-labeled red blood cell scan can be specific with increased flow to the lesion during the perfusion phase and increased activity on delayed images.[11]

Needle biopsy for confirmation of hemangiomas is a dangerous procedure that can result in fatal hemorrhage.[11,47,97] It is usually used as a last resort when a diagnosis cannot be reached by other means.[11] Some institutions have reported the safety of fine-needle biopsy for confirmation of diagnosis.[11,12] The cytologic diagnostic criteria include the presence of benign epithelial cells, fresh blood from the mass, and no malignant cells.[11]

The treatment of hemangioma varies with the size of the mass. Most hemangiomas undergo spontaneous involution and regression.[21,26,64,95,101] When a large hemangioma threatens the patient's health, aggressive procedures are instigated. A lobectomy[7] or resection of the tumor[15,21,74,76] is sometimes performed, but if the patient is experiencing congestive heart failure, hepatic artery ligation[15,25,64,74,76,95,101] or embolization[15,76,95] is performed. In many cases, the lesion is also very responsive to steroid therapy[15,64,76,95,101] and radiation therapy.

The differential diagnosis includes angiomatous tumors, hepatoblastoma, hepatoma and metastatic neuroblastoma,[21] cysts, abscesses, and focal nodular hyperplasia (Fig. 14-4).[56]

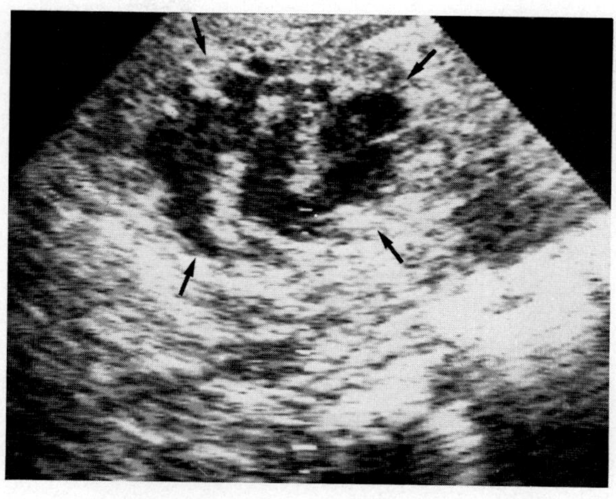

FIGURE 14-4. In a 4-year-old child thought to have a cavernous hemangioma *(arrows)* of the liver, a hemangiosarcoma was diagnosed.

MESENCHYMAL HAMARTOMA

Mesenchymal or fibrous hamartoma is a rare congenital anomaly[27,31,84] arising from the connective tissue or mesenchyme of the portal tracts.[14,81,96] It is usually situated within the right liver lobe, as opposed to the left, but can also attach to the liver by a pedicle. The tumor is seen in males more than females.[14,81,96]

The lesion usually presents within the first 2 years of life; painless abdominal swelling is the first clinical symptom.[27,36,81,84,96] Congestive heart failure has also been noted in patients with mesenchymal hamartoma.[3] Patients can experience respiratory distress from this large fluid-filled lesion if fluid accumulation has been rapid.

Sonographically mesenchymal hamartoma is sometimes mistaken for hemangioma; however, while it frequently reveals internal septations demonstrating a complex appearance, it is avascular.[81] These septations have been noted to be strands of hepatocytes, bile duct elements, or mesenchyme separating multiple cysts.[36,65,84,96]

Abdominal radiographs can show calcifications and overall hepatic enlargement with possible displacement of one or both kidneys, depending on the size of the mass.[3,14] Barium studies can show displacement of bowel gas, and chest radiographs can demonstrate an elevated diaphragm.[81]

Angiographically, mesenchymal hamartoma can display varying degrees of peripheral hypervascularity but are generally avascular internally.[96] Fine vascularity of the septa surrounding the cysts can also be seen.[81] On CT, hamartomas display well-defined margins but are centrally homogeneous and produce low attenuation. Septations may also be seen.[96] On sulfur colloid scintigraphy, hamartomas show no uptake,[81] and tagging the red blood cells can demonstrate a hypervascular ring around the mass.[96]

Prognosis of mesenchymal hamartoma is excellent. Resection is usually all that is required,[81] although in patients with respiratory distress, percutaneous drainage of the mass is performed prior to surgery.

The differential diagnosis of mesenchymal hamartoma includes mesenchymoma, hemangiomas, parasitic or congenital cysts, teratomas, biliary cystadenoma,[84] and choledochal cyst.

Abscesses

Abscesses in the liver of infants usually result from neonatal infection from the umbilicus or mesentery or from surgery. With a neonatal infection, an abscess can form in the ductus venosus as well. It has also been noted that transplacental (in utero) infections can cause calcifications of the fetal liver. These patients usually present with hepatic dysfunction as well as hepatomegaly.[90] Calcifications in the liver of neonates can also result from trauma from fluid infusion through umbilical vein catheters not properly positioned in the inferior vena cava.[1]

Childhood abscesses can be caused by Crohn's disease, abdominal surgery, chronic granulomatous

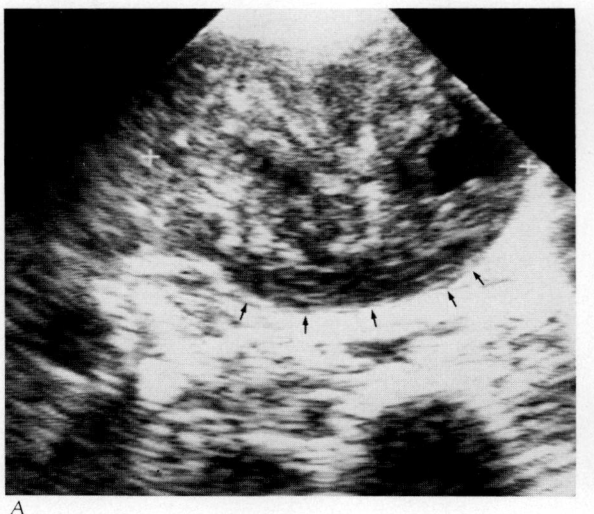

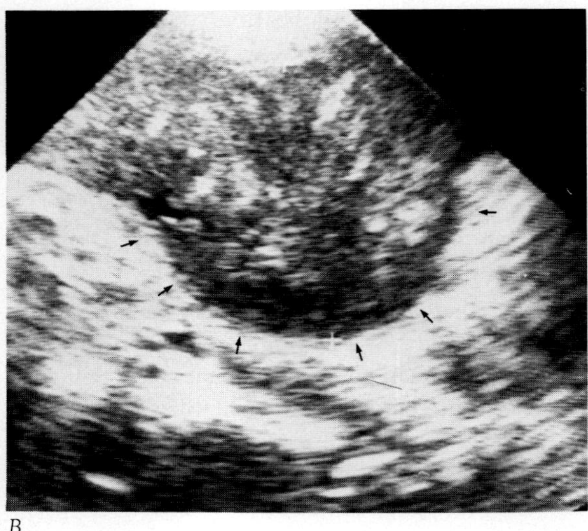

FIGURE 14-5. A liver abscess in the left liver lobe is visualized on transverse (*A*) and longitudinal (*B*) planes of a 5½-year-old patient after appendectomy. The abscess appears to have sharp margins *(arrows)* but echogenicity within is mixed. After a drainage tube was inserted, the patient improved and was discharged.

disease, trauma, polycythemia, perforated viscus, *Candida* organisms,[57,67] and hematopoietic malignancies (Fig. 14-5).[60,66,71,77,93]

Intrahepatic abscesses in infants present sonographically as in older patients and vary from discretely marginated, hypoechoic structures with good sound transmission to complex hyperechoic masses with poorly defined margins (Fig. 14-6). Shadowing may be present with air in the lesion.[66,71] The mass may also present with a bullseye appearance—a central hyperechoic area surrounded by a more anechoic one.[57,66,67] In the cases of transplacental infection with calcifications, a bright, hyperechoic lesion with posterior shadowing can be seen.

Both technetium^{99m}-sulfur colloid and gallium scintigraphy of anaerobic abscesses show cold or focal voids, usually along the periphery of the liver.[66] Unenhanced CT can show focal areas of low density compared with surrounding liver tissue.[66,67,93] Angiographically, abscesses are typically radiolucent owing to the avascularity. The surrounding compressed parenchyma may produce a stain, giving the abscess a peripheral rim.[57]

The differential diagnosis includes abscesses, hepatic hemorrhage, hepatoblastoma, small cell carcinoma, hepatocellular carcinoma, and hepatic metastases.

Cysts

Liver cysts in infants and children are either simple congenital cysts or parasitic cysts. Congenital liver cysts are relatively rare[83] but do occur and can range in size from small to large. The patients are generally asymptomatic unless the lesion is large enough to impair function. They may be palpated on physical examination or found incidentally on an imaging examination.

Sonographically, simple congenital liver cysts appear as smooth-walled, anechoic lesions demonstrating good posterior enhancement.[37,83]

Hydatid echinococcal cysts or parasitic cysts are usually associated with exposure to livestock and farming. A number of authors have classified these lesions into four groups according to their sonographic appearance.[8,33,55] The first classification is similar to simple nonparasitic cysts with well-de-

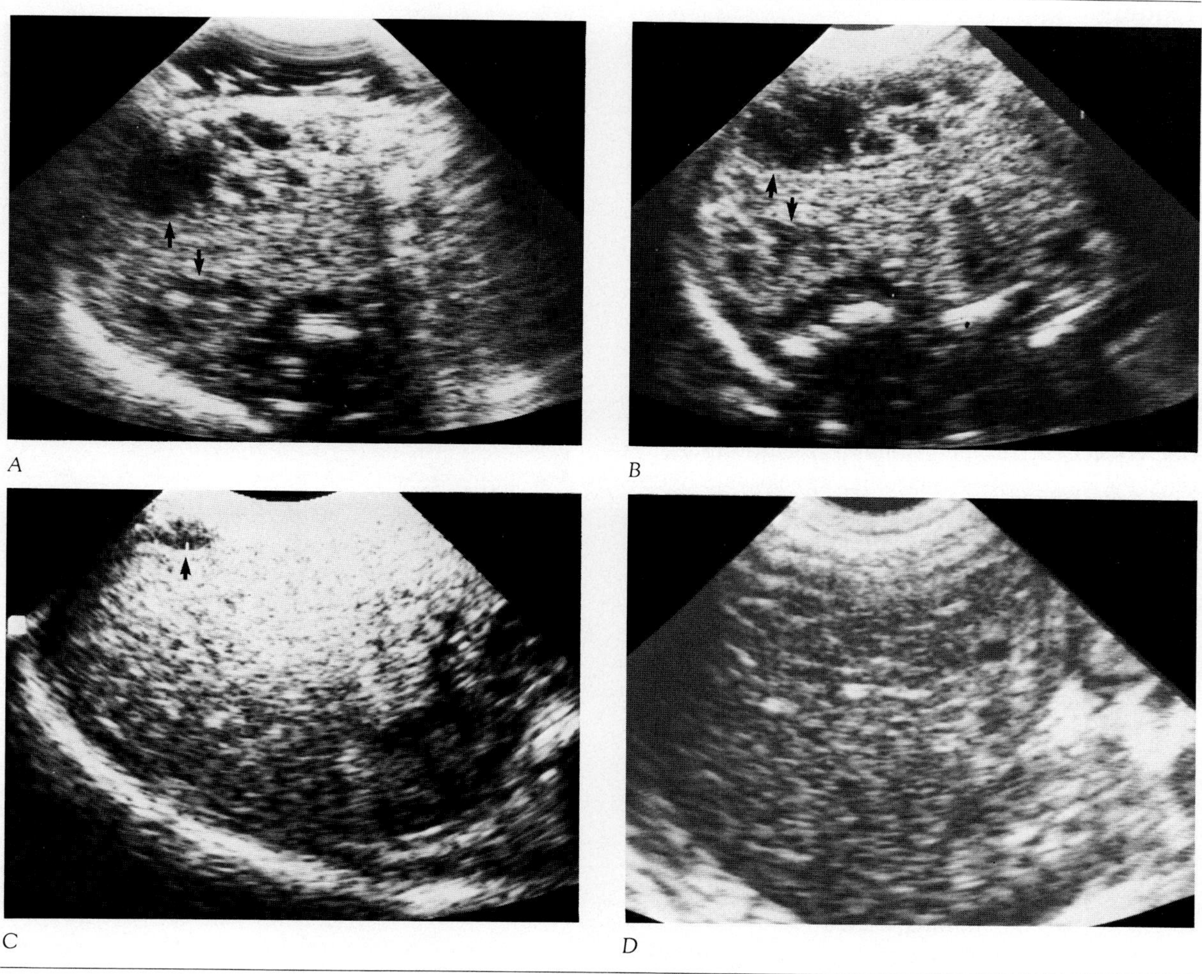

FIGURE 14-6. (*A*) Transverse and (*B*) longitudinal planes in a 3-week-old infant demonstrate liver abscesses *(arrows)* with mixed echogenicity and irregular walls. (C) One and one half months later, the longitudinal plane view demonstrates that one of the abscesses is resolving. (*D*) In the same patient 2 years later, the two abscesses are completely resolved, as demonstrated on this transverse plane.

fined borders.[8,33] Sand has also been noted in some of these cysts, and layering can be detected by rolling the patient on one side.[55] The second classification usually demonstrates some wall degeneration. The contour is still well-defined, but the shape of the lesion is somewhat flat. The border may appear to be separating into layers, more commonly called a split wall.[8,33] The third classification is typified by the appearance of septa within the cyst.[8,33,55] The fourth classification generally demonstrates more of a mixed or complex internal hyperechoic pattern, which may or may not contain calcifications.[8,33,55]

Depending on the size and location of the lesions, the patient could experience infection, impaired liver function due to biliary obstruction, or other complications due to obstruction or compression of abdominal vasculature.[8,33,55]

Trauma

Trauma to the liver can be treated by surgery (laparotomy, hemihepatectomy) or conservatively, depending on the size of the injury and the physical stability of the patient. Once the patient is stabilized, the healing process is observed by follow-up ultrasound examinations, liver isotope scans, or CT.[20]

Sonographically, liver trauma is presented by hepatomegaly, intrahepatic hematomas if bleeding is present,[20] and bilomas (a collection of bile associated with the laceration of one or more bile ducts). Bilomas appear as anechoic collections with irregular borders in the liver, or if injury is extensive the bile collects in the peritoneum, resembling ascites (Fig. 14-7). Initially hematomas appear as a hyperechoic mass in the liver with irregular borders, but over time they become more anechoic as the hematoma liquefies. Eventually, the resolving hematoma can develop calcifications. This would present as bright, hyperechoic areas with posterior shadowing.

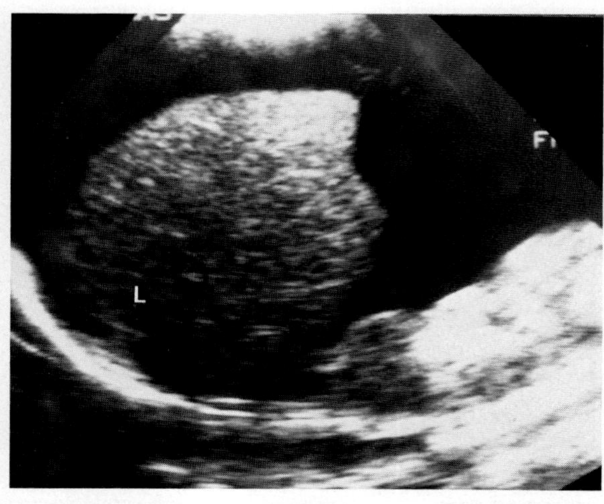

Figure 14-7. The longitudinal plane demonstrates a large fluid (Fl) collection mimicking ascites in a 3-month-old infant with a massive biloma produced by a lacerated common bile duct (L, liver).

CT shows liver hematomas with irregular borders and lower attenuation than surrounding liver tissue. CT has been used in the past to determine if surgical intervention was needed by defining the extent of the injury.[13]

The differential diagnosis of liver trauma includes hemangioma, congenital or parasitic liver cysts, hematoma, biloma, hamartoma, malignant conditions that cause extensive ascites, polycystic liver disease, abscess, focal nodular hyperplasia, and hepatoblastoma.

Hepatitis

Hepatitis is, quite simply, inflammatory disease of the liver. It is commonly divided into two groups: infectious hepatitis (type A), which is transmitted in contaminated material or blood products, and serum hepatitis (type B), which is transmitted in blood products, parenterally or by intimate contact. A third group, non A–non B hepatitis, resembles type B in that it is transmitted by blood transfusions, but more than one virus is probably responsible. Type A most often affects children and young adults.[86]

The clinical symptoms vary, depending on the stage of the disease. The patient can experience abdominal swelling (hepatomegaly) with pain, nausea, fever, chills, jaundice, fatigue, or loss of appetite. An important point to remember is that the clinical symptoms of infectious mononucleosis (IM), jaundice, hepatosplenomegaly, fever, fatigue, sore throat, and lymphadenopathy closely resemble those of acute viral hepatitis (AVH). An important difference with IM is that the spleen is usually larger than in AVH.[46]

Sonographically, acute viral hepatitis appears as diffuse enlargement of the liver. Depending on the stage of the disease, the appearance of the liver can range from normal to increasingly hyperechoic. As the patient recovers, the size and echogenicity return to normal; however, with chronic hepatitis, where the disease is ongoing, the size of the liver may decrease but echogenicity and attenuation increase as normal liver tissue is destroyed and replaced by fibrosis and nodular regeneration, which then leads to cirrhosis. Liver biopsy is helpful for detecting cirrhosis (Fig. 14-8).[35]

Congenital Syphilitic Hepatitis

Congenital syphilitic hepatitis is a multisystem disease that infants contract from their mother. Clin-

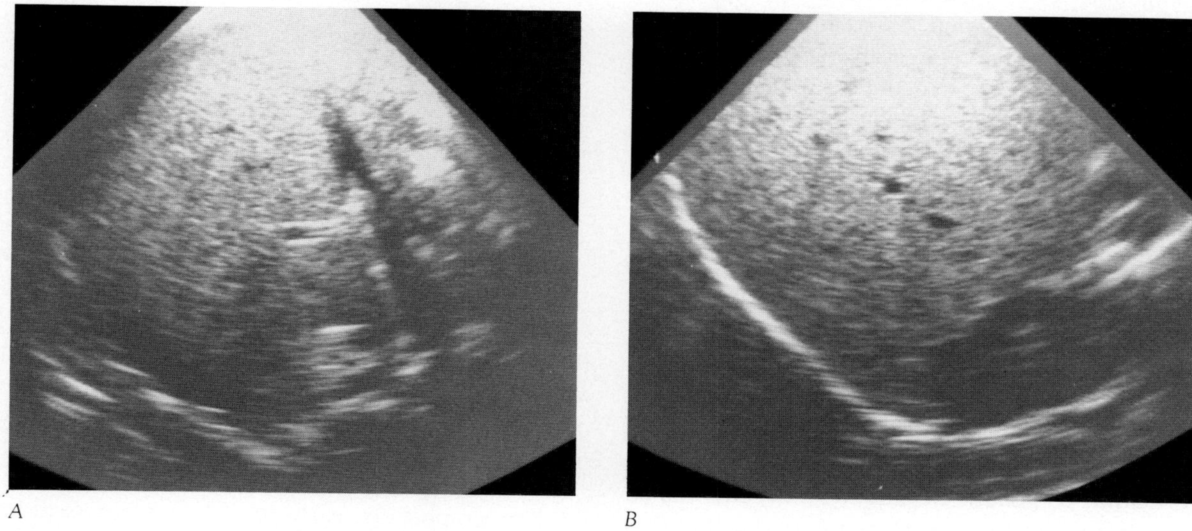

FIGURE 14-8. An enlarged liver with increased echogenicity is visualized on transverse (*A*) and longitudinal (*B*) plane views of a 4-month-old patient suffering from neonatal hepatitis.

ical signs and symptoms are rare in the neonatal period but present within the first 3 months of life[17]: hepatosplenomegaly, erythematous body rash,[17] fever,[31] low birth weight, anemia, jaundice, thrombocytopenia, nonimmune hydrops, Parrot's pseudoparalysis, and sometimes respiratory distress.[17] Although now the disease is usually confirmed by serologic tests, the imaging findings are important. Since this condition is multisystemic, it is important to correlate all the findings of the various imaging studies. Laboratory values may include decreased hemoglobulin concentration and decreased platelet count.[17]

Sonographically, the liver and spleen may appear diffusely enlarged but with normal tissue,[31] or cirrhosis can be present with slightly hyperechoic tissue and increased attenuation of the acoustic beam. Angiographically, the vessels may appear small and thin but without displacement.[31]

Scintigraphy shows no radiocolloid uptake in the liver or very little. Uptake will be dramatically increased in the enlarged spleen and in lungs and bone marrow.[31] Radiography of the long bones can demonstrate periosteal elevation along the shafts with metaphyseal irregularities. This is considered a typical finding in congenital syphilis. Treatment for the disease is penicillin. Subsequent sonograms and radionuclide images appear more normal,[31] but the prognosis is poor if nonimmune hydrops is present.[17]

The differential diagnosis of congenital syphilitic hepatitis includes acute viral hepatitis, hematologic disease, biliary atresia, and benign or malignant liver masses.

PELIOSIS HEPATIS

Peliosis hepatis is a rare angiomatous[99] complication developed by patients exposed to copper sulfate, corticosteroids,[94,100] androgenic-anabolic steroids,[91,94,99,100] contraceptive steroids,[99,101] azathioprine,[54,99,100] prednisone,[99] arsenic,[23,94] thorium dioxide,[100] vinyl chloride,[94,100] chemotherapy,[54,99] radiation therapy,[99] and contrast agents such as Thorotrast.[94,99] It has also been noted in patients suffering from toxic oil syndrome,[100] endocarditis,[99,100] tuberculosis,[54,89,94,99,100] leprosy, liver abscess, retroperitoneal abscess,[99] marasmus, acquired immunodeficiency syndrome (AIDS),[89,94,100] diabetes,[94,100] malignancies,[89,94,100] Waldenstrom's macroglobulinemia, multiple myeloma,[100] systemic light-chain deposition disease, sprue, necrotizing vasculitis,[94] hypervitaminosis A, Fanconi's anemia,[89,91] and hepatic focal nodular hyperplasia.[80] It can be seen in renal or cardiac allograft recipients and in patients receiving hemodialysis long term.[100]

Biopsy is needed for definitive diagnosis.[99] Ultrastructurally, this disease consists of increased dilatation of the space of Disse.[89,94] These blood-filled sinusoids are lined with normal or atrophic hepatocytes.[54,100] Microscopically, they are brownish blue lesions of varying size.[99] The name was derived from the Greek word *pelios,* meaning black and blue.[99]

Three mechanisms have been proposed for the formation of peliosis hepatis[89,99,100]: (1) the dilated sinusoids are due to a primary injury that weakens the wall; (2) the dilated sinusoids are a result of increased pressure because of partial or complete obstruction of the sinusoids themselves or between the central veins and the sinusoids; and (3) there may be a direct lesion of the barrier between the sinusoid, such as hepatocellular necrosis.

The clinical presentation may include hepatomegaly, liver failure[54,91] with abnormal liver function tests, hypertension, intraperitoneal bleeding,[54] pain, and jaundice.[91] Patients suffering from Fanconi's anemia and taking anabolic steroids are more susceptible to cancer. It is possible that hepatocellular carcinoma (HCC) may be present with peliosis hepatis, which would be detected by α-fetoprotein in the blood.[43,91]

Sonographically, focal hyperechoic areas can be noted within the liver. Angiographically, multiple prominent contrast accumulations can be seen in the parenchymal and venous stages.[94] CT can show a low-density liver suggestive of fatty infiltration if the disease is mild, and successive scans demonstrate multiple focal defects, which can resolve as the patient recovers.[94]

Prognosis for peliosis hepatis varies, as it is a complication of a wide spectrum of disorders. If it is drug induced and the drug is withdrawn, it may regress. If malignancy or infection is the cause, that should be treated. In cases of abscess, regression was noted upon drainage of the infection.[91]

The differential diagnosis of peliosis hepatis includes polycystic liver disease, Budd-Chiari syndrome, hemangioma, hematoma, and metastatic carcinoma.

Toxic Hepatitis

Toxic hepatitis is a complication in patients undergoing chemotherapy or radiation therapy in which the portals involve liver parenchyma. Not only can intra- or extrahepatic malignant neoplasms disrupt metabolic processes or arterial or portal blood flow or cause hormonal imbalances, all of which can harm the liver, but the very agents, drugs or radiation therapy, used to destroy the malignancy can also injure it. It is thought that long-term chemotherapy or radiation therapy can produce hepatic fibrosis, which in turn can develop into hepatocellular carcinoma.[67]

Sonographically, early toxic hepatitis resembles AVH with hepatomegaly, which may or may not be associated with increased echogenicity. As it progresses with long-term cancer therapy, the liver's size decreases and fatty infiltrates develop into hepatic fibrosis with increased echogenicity and increased attenuation of the acoustic beam. This hepatic fibrosis can then develop into secondary hepatocellular carcinoma[67] with accompanying liver dysfunction. Splenomegaly may also be present.

Technetium^{99m}–sulfur colloid scintigraphy shows a small liver with irregular uptake and a considerable shift to the spleen and bone marrow. Children who are also suffering from jaundice brought on by chemotherapy exhibit decreased hepatic-gastrointestinal tract transit time.[67]

CT shows a small liver with irregular margins and a dilated portal vein with accompanying splenomegaly. As fatty infiltration progresses, liver size increases and the density may decrease.[67]

Chronic Disease

Fatty Metamorphosis of the Liver

Fatty infiltration of the liver is caused by chronic hepatic injury and results from an accumulation of abnormal amounts of triglycerides and lipids in the hepatocytes.[40,42] In children it is caused by malnutrition, malignancies, tyrosinemia, hyperalimentation, cystic fibrosis, Reye syndrome, glycogen storage disease, malabsorption syndrome, high-dose

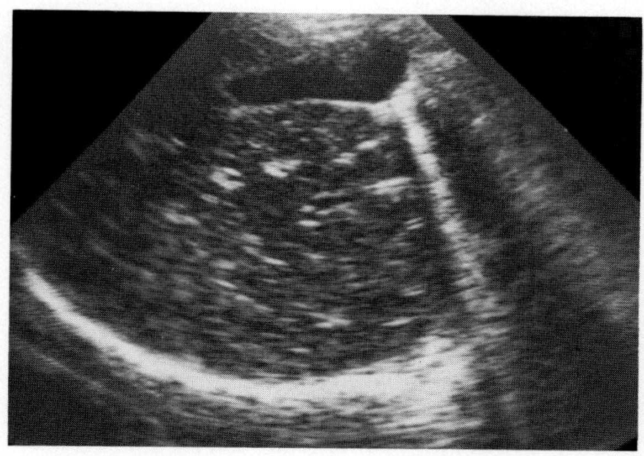

FIGURE 14-9. The appearance of fatty liver metamorphosis is the result of the echogenic fatty interfaces noted on this plane of the right liver lobe of a patient who experienced sudden weight loss. The liver's size and vasculature appeared normal.

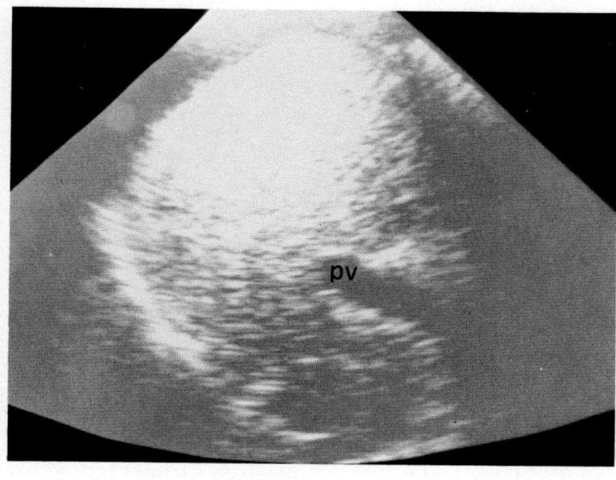

FIGURE 14-10. The liver appears small with increased echogenicity and a dilated portal vein (pv) on this transverse plane in a 6½-year-old child with cirrhosis.

steroid therapy, acute hepatitis,[40,42,67,107] general obesity, kwashiorkor, Cushing's syndrome, galactosemia, fructose intolerance, familial hyperlipidemia, abetalipoproteinemia, diabetic ketoacidosis, exposure to liver toxins,[40,42,67,107] and chronic granulomatous disease.[20]

Sonographically, the liver appears enlarged and more hyperechoic due to the multifat and nonfat interfaces within the hepatocytes (Fig. 14-9). Attenuation is increased, and there is a corresponding decrease in the demonstration of vasculature.[42,67]

On unenhanced CT, the early phase of fatty infiltration shows equal density of liver and spleen. As the infiltration progresses, the density of the liver can decrease quickly and it shows focal areas that resemble metastases.[67]

CIRRHOSIS AND PORTAL HYPERTENSION

Cirrhosis is the nodular regeneration or fibrosis of normal hepatocytes that have been damaged. It is brought on by chronic disease of the liver and results in severely impaired liver function. Advanced cirrhosis is associated with jaundice, portal hypertension, ascites, central nervous system disorders, and eventually, death.

Laboratory tests show elevations of aspartate aminotransferase (AST, also known as serum glutamic oxaloacetic transaminase or SGOT), alanine aminotransferase (ALT, also known as serum glutamic pyruvic transaminase, SGPT), lactic dehydrogenase (LDH), with increased direct and indirect bilirubin values if the patient is jaundiced.

Sonographically, the liver appears smaller than normal, with a bright hyperechoic parenchymal pattern and increased attenuation of the acoustic beam (Fig. 14-10).[38] Advanced portal hypertension is also seen when the portal vein dilates due to reduced blood flow in the liver. Portal vein thrombosis may also be seen (Fig. 14-11).[67] Both the splenic vein and the spleen are enlarged. Ascites may also be present.[38]

CT may show dilatation of the splenic and portal vein and splenomegaly with decreased density. The liver may show increased density and decreased size.

Gallium and technetium^{99m}-IDA scintigraphy show decreased uptake in the liver, or none. Technetium^{99m}-sulfur colloid scans also show decreased activity in the liver, with increased activity in the spleen and a shift to lungs and bone marrow.[67]

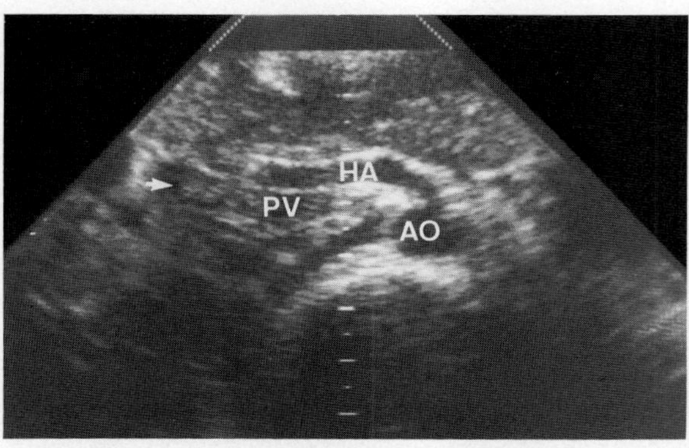

FIGURE 14-11. The echogenic material *(arrow)* represents a clot in this patient with portal vein (pv) thrombosis (ao, aorta; ha, hepatic artery).

Benign Neoplasms

Hepatic tumors account for a third of all abdominal masses of children, and malignant tumors are ten times more common than benign ones. With malignancy the α-fetoprotein level is elevated. An important factor for sonographically differentiating malignant from benign tumors in children is that malignancies often invade or amputate vessels, whereas benign masses displace them. Careful scrutiny of the vascular channels (i.e., portal and hepatic veins) is in order. Often, angiography can confirm or rule out the presence of a malignancy.[14]

FOCAL NODULAR HYPOPLASIA

Focal nodular hypoplasia is an uncommon, hypervascular, nonencapsulated, benign tumor[59,104] containing bile duct elements, hepatocytes, Kupffer cells, fibrous connective tissue, and reticuloendothelial cells. It is most often an incidental finding,[62] typically located superficially on the right lobe of the liver, but it may also be found in the lateral border of the left lobe. Typically the tumor has a stellate (star-shaped) configuration,[36] owing to the presence of arterioles, venules, and bile ducts in the fibrous strands that radiate from the center of the mass.[5,9,59,62,80,103,104] Patients may present with vague abdominal pain associated with abdominal distention,[11] although laboratory values are usually normal.[62,103,104]

Because the lesions are benign, treatment is conservative and surgical resection usually is not required unless size causes complications. In cases of pedunculation where torsion or infarction is a possibility, resection may be necessary.[5,62,80] Some institutions suggest embolization as a possible alternative in treatment.[62,78]

Sonographic findings are variable.[104] The mass usually appears as a homogeneous, isoechoic lesion,[5] sometimes with a focal scar.[103] There may be internal hypoechoic or hyperechoic areas as a result of necrosis and hemorrhage, but this is the exception rather than the rule.

On unenhanced CT the mass appears homogeneous, producing somewhat decreased attenuation.[103] Enhanced CT shows the mass as more isodense or hyperdense than the surrounding normal liver tissue.[80,103]

Scintigraphy is the most helpful imaging modality for diagnosis.[5,9,80,104] Because focal nodular hypoplasia contains Kupffer cells, uptake of technetium^{99m}–labeled sulfur colloid is greater than in normal liver tissue.[62,103] This finding is unique for focal nodular hypoplasia and should differentiate it from other hepatic lesions.[5,59,80]

Arteriography shows this lesion to be hypervascular[36,62] at times, with large feeding vessels.[5,103] These vessels arise centrally and radiate peripherally in most cases.[80] The vessels in the mass can be tortuous, and the capillary phase is usually prolonged.[5,59,62] The differential diagnosis includes adenoma, angiomatous tumors, hepatoblastoma, and hepatoma.

HEPATIC ADENOMAS

Liver adenomas in infants and children are vascular tumors[30] and are usually secondary to a metabolic condition called type I glycogen storage disease (von Gierke's disease), in which glucose is not processed properly and, so, is continually stored within the hepatocytes. Hepatic adenomas do not contain Kupffer cells.[10,41,103,104]

Clinically, the disorder is usually manifested by hepatomegaly[10,41] (due to accompanying fatty infiltration) and the onset of abdominal pain, but it may produce no symptoms.[103] In the cases of von Gierke's disease, the mass usually has an increased malignant potential,[10,41,104] so resection is the preferred treatment.[103] Generally, with this tumor, results of liver function tests are normal.[103]

Sonographically, the mass appears solid, with

sharp, encapsulated margins that can appear heterogeneous with the presence of hemorrhage and necrosis.[10,103] Sometimes the mass may exhibit a hypoechoic rim.[10] Diffuse increased echogenicity may also be seen in the surrounding liver tissue, due to fatty infiltration.

On angiography, the mass appears hypervascular, with occasional hypovascular areas due to necrosis or hemorrhage.[103] The feeding artery may be enlarged, or peripheral hypovascularity may be seen.[104] On precontrast CT the mass appears hypodense.[103] Postcontrast scans show areas of hypodensity, hyperdensity, and isodensity.[103,104] Radionuclide imaging shows focal defects on technetium^{99m}–sulfur colloid liver and spleen scans.[103,104]

Malignant Neoplasms

TUMORS

The primary malignant liver tumors of childhood are hepatoblastoma, hepatic cell carcinoma or hepatoma, small cell sarcoma, and congenital neuroblastoma. Sonographically, they are usually represented by a single solid, homogeneous, hyperechoic mass, and less frequently by multiple hyperechoic lesions.[20,65] Occasionally a hypoechoic rim or halo is also seen with malignancies, and infrequently the malignancy may appear isoechoic. After chemotherapy, the lesion changes, and it can present a marbled or complex appearance.[14]

HEPATOBLASTOMA

Hepatoblastoma is the most common liver mass in children younger than 5 years. Usually it occurs in the first 3 years of life, predominantly in boys. Microscopically, it is classified as an epithelial (with different stages of maturity) or mixed (with mesenchymal and epithelial elements) mass. Epithelial tumors are subdivided into embryonal and fetal ones, the latter having a better prognosis. It is usually situated in the right lobe of the liver, although diffuse involvement of the liver has been noted, as has left or multilobe involvement.[22]

Clinically, patients usually present with hepatomegaly or a palpable abdominal mass. There can be accompanying fever, weight loss, nausea, vomiting, jaundice,[65] anemia, leukocytosis, adenopathy, and fractures due to bone metastases from the mass. Laboratory values include elevation of α-fetoprotein.[72]

Sonographically, a hepatoblastoma appears as a solitary multinodular mass with a heterogenous hyperechoic pattern. Anechoic foci may also be present, representing necrosis or hemorrhage (Figs. 14-12 to 14-14). Dense or coarse calcifications with posterior shadowing are also common.[22]

Radiographically, a soft tissue mass with calcifi-

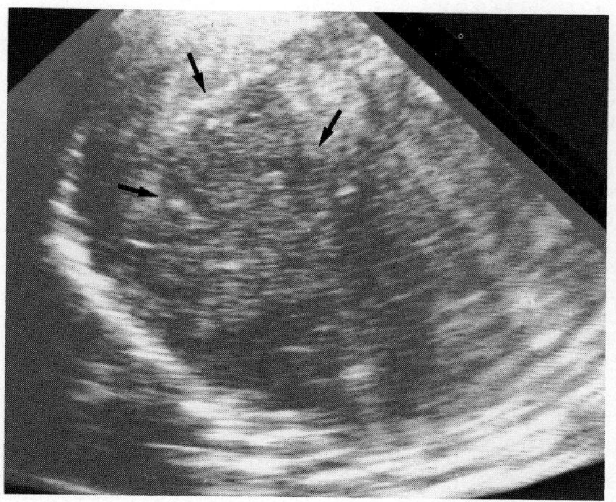

A

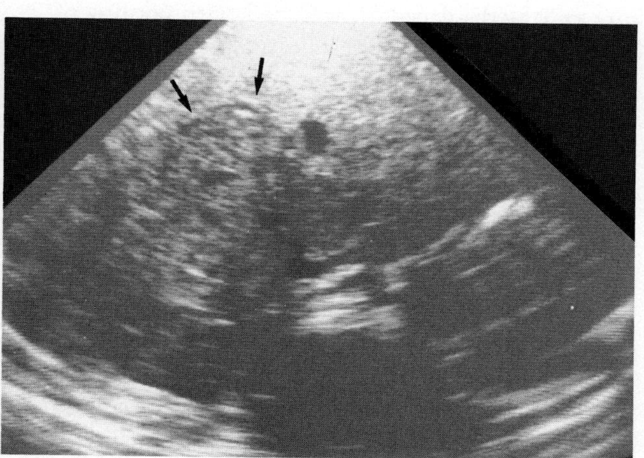

B

FIGURE 14-12. In a 3-year-old, a hepatoblastoma is visualized on the longitudinal plane view with irregular borders *(arrows)* and mixed echogenicity.

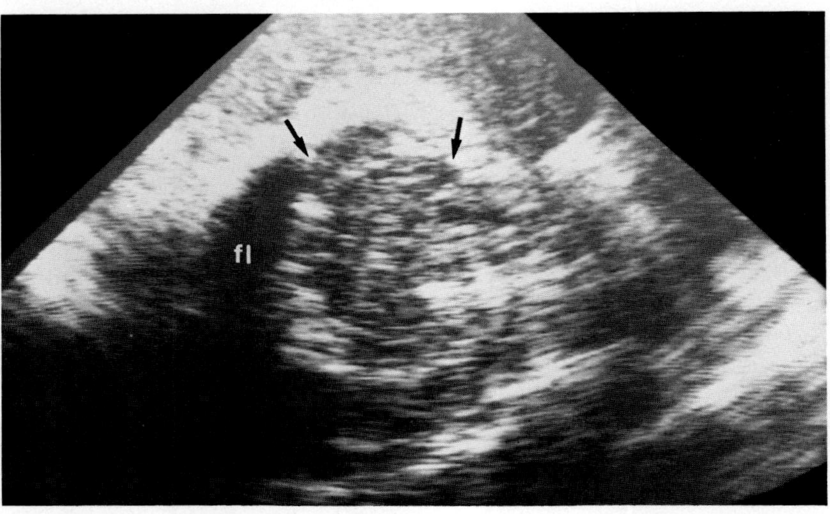

FIGURE 14-13. In a 10-year-old, a hepatoblastoma *(arrows)* has a mixed echogenic appearance with a large fluid (fl) area partially surrounding the mass.

cation can be detected in the right upper quadrant.[22,65] Excretory urography often shows displaced or compressed kidney.[22] An upper gastrointestinal series can show displacement of bowel by the mass.[65]

Angiographically, the mass usually presents as a hypervascular lesion, and it is possible that hypovascular areas may also be detected. The vasculature may be displaced or stretched, with pooling of the contrast material.[22,65,69] It can also appear to be amputated or invaded by the mass.[14,65]

Precontrast CT scans show hepatoblastoma to be of lower attenuation than surrounding liver tissue. The margins may be sharply or poorly delineated. Lower-density areas represent necrosis or hemorrhage. On enhanced CT these masses are enhanced slightly, if at all. A rim of enhancement may appear, representing surrounding liver tissue that was compressed. Septations may also be noted on CT.[22]

Gallium scans can show dramatically increased uptake in the mass, and technetium–sulfur colloid scans demonstrate a filling defect. Hepatic scintiangiography may also show an early transient perfusion period with central focal defects representing necrosis or hemorrhage in cases of hepatoblastoma.[22]

T1-weighted MRI demonstrates hypointense lesions with central hyperintense areas due to hemorrhage. On corresponding T2-weighted images, the areas are inhomogeneous and hyperintense.[22] The differential diagnosis includes hepatoblastoma, hepatocellular carcinoma, infantile hemangioendothelioma, and mesenchymal hamartoma.[22]

HEPATOCELLULAR CARCINOMA

In children, hepatocellular carcinoma or hepatoma is usually the result of long-term liver insult, as from chronic cirrhosis, long-term anabolic steroid therapy, chronic hepatitis B viral infection, or a diet rich in aflatoxin. Pathologically, these lesions have characteristics that differentiate them from other hepatic lesions: daughter nodules, hepatic or portal tumor thrombosis, septa, and pseudocapsules. This tumor can be well-encapsulated or not encapsulated.[45]

Clinically, the patient may present with sudden liver failure due to invasion of the tumor or thrombosis in the portal or hepatic veins, hepatomegaly, gastrointestinal bleeding, ascites, and hypoglycemia. Laboratory values include elevated α-fetoprotein.

Sonographically, the tumor generally presents as

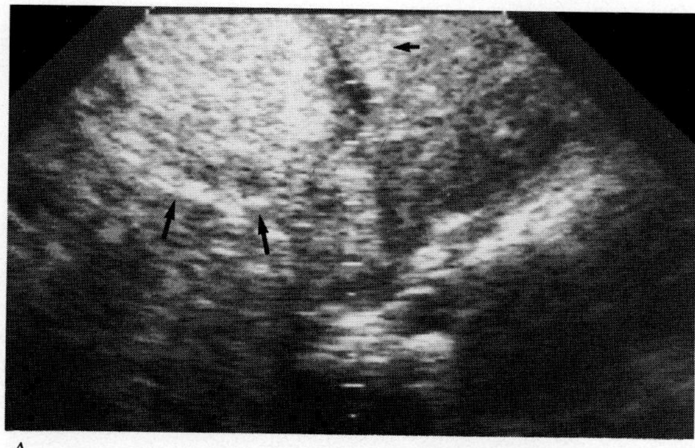
A

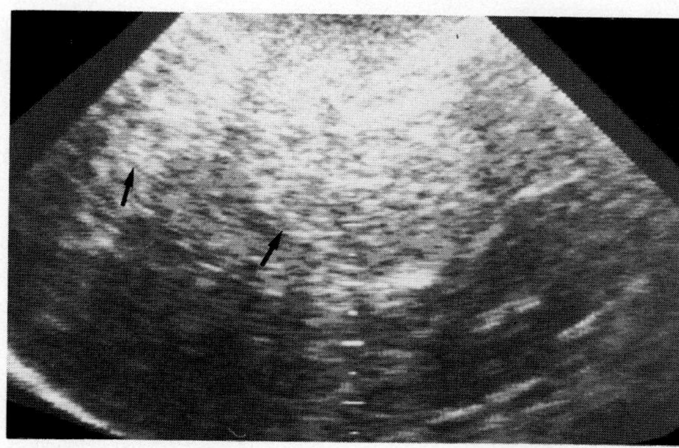
B

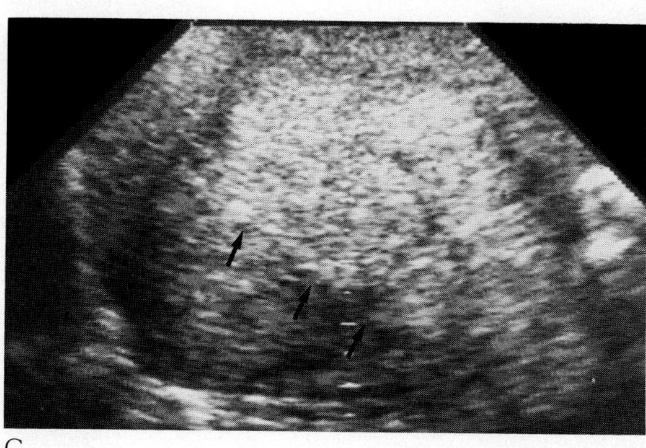
C

FIGURE 14-14. The hepatoblastoma *(arrows)* demonstrated in these liver sonograms has very irregular walls and appears very echogenic.

a solid hyperechoic mass.[65] It can have well-defined or ill-defined borders.[45] There may be anechoic areas within the mass, representing necrosis or hemorrhage, usually as a result of chemotherapy or radiation therapy. Other authors report that the small tumors begin as hypoechoic lesions and as they enlarge become isoechoic and then finally hyperechoic.[92] An anechoic or hypoechoic halo or rim may also be seen.[14] Tumor thrombi are frequently seen in the portal and hepatic veins and inferior vena cava and should be documented if present.[45]

Radiographs of the abdomen generally show a soft tissue mass in the right upper quadrant with some possible bowel and organ displacement.[65]

Angiographically, hepatocellular carcinoma or hepatoma in infants and children can appear similar to that in adults.[69] The examination can show initial vessel enlargement followed by tapering or invasion of the mass and contrast pooling.[14,65,69]

Radionuclide scanning shows a transient early increase in the perfusion stage due to the vascularity.[30] Focal defects may be seen that are due to necrosis and hemorrhage. Although hepatomas are generally vascular, avascular hepatocellular focal defects have also been documented with scintigraphy.[43]

MRI can show low intensity of the pseudocapsule and zone of vessels on T1-weighted images. On T2-weighted images they may appear double layered.[45] The mass may also have high signal intensity on T2-weighted images.[73] Areas of isointensity may also be present, representing focal necrosis, hemorrhage, or fatty degeneration.[73]

The prognosis for hepatocellular carcinoma depends on its features and the general condition of the patient. A well-encapsulated mass is easier to resect than a poorly encapsulated hepatoma.[73] Cirrhosis patients who develop hepatocellular carcinoma usually die. The differential diagnosis includes hepatoblastoma, abscess, focal nodular hyperplasia, adenoma, hemangiosarcoma, and hemangioendothelioma.

SMALL CELL SARCOMA

Small cell sarcoma is a rare malignant lesion of the liver arising from the mesenchyme. It has a lobulated appearance, contains multiple cystic spaces, and is the fourth most common primary pediatric liver tumor following hepatoblastoma, infantile hemangioendothelioma, and hepatocellular carcinoma.[82]

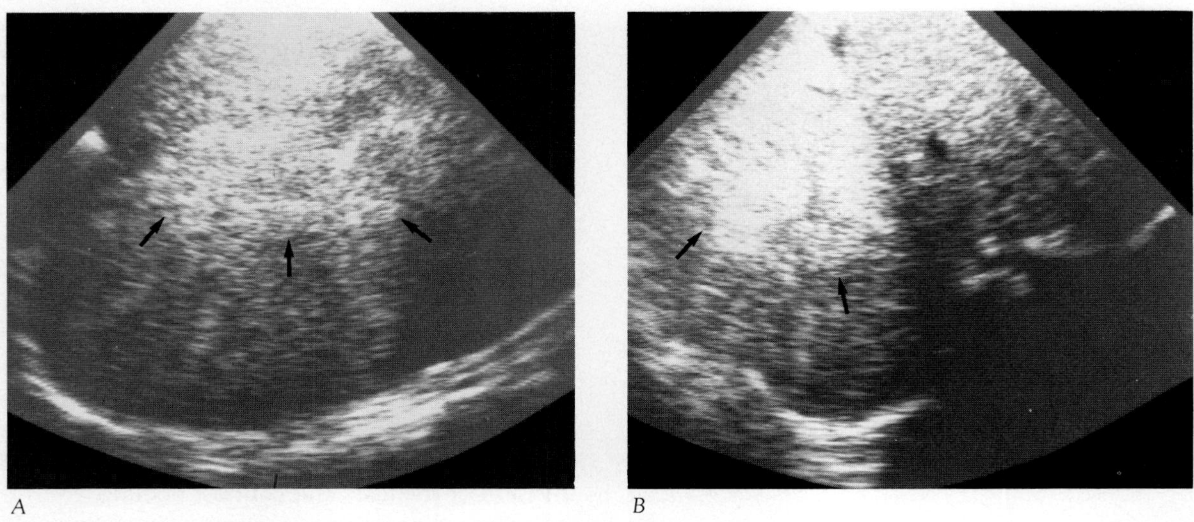

Figure 14-15. On longitudinal (*A*) and transverse (*B*) plane views of a 3-year-old patient, a yolk sac tumor *(arrows)* is visualized as echogenic with irregular borders.

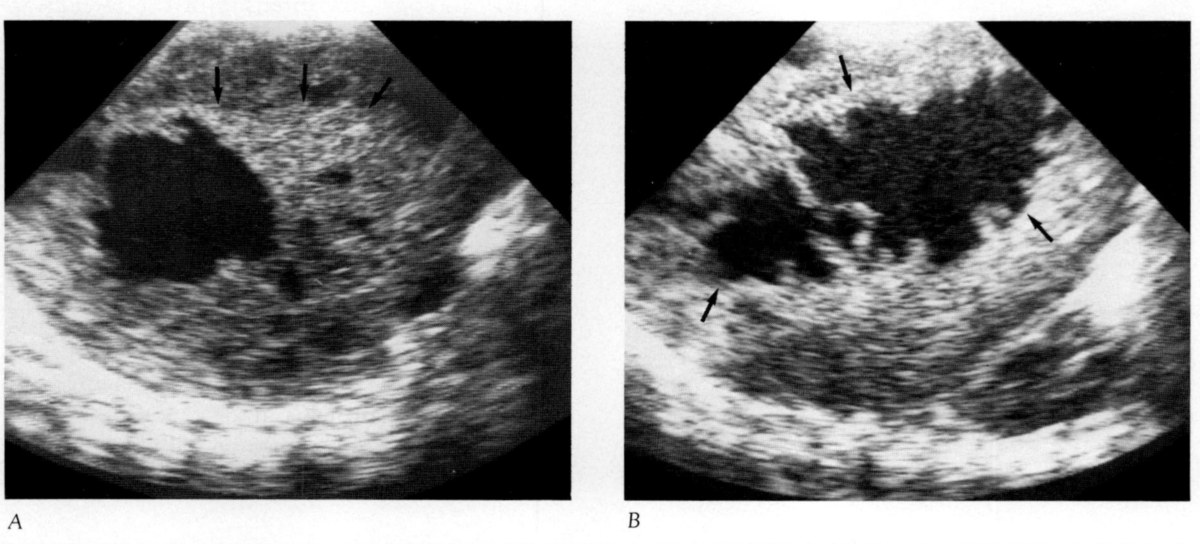

Figure 14-16. On sonograms of a 1-year-old child with embryonål carcinoma of epithelial origin in the right liver lobe the mass has irregular borders *(arrows)* and multiple cystic areas.

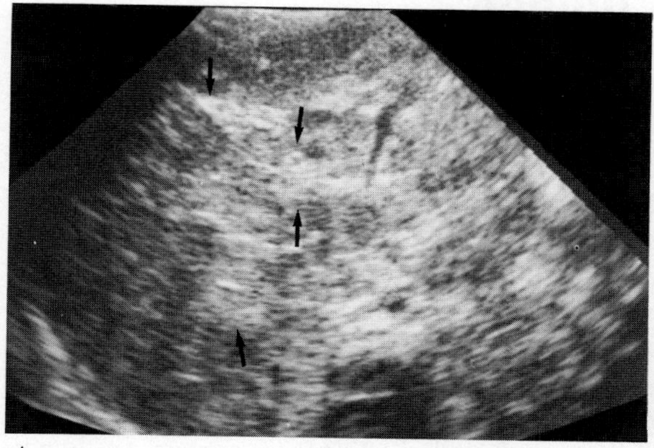

A

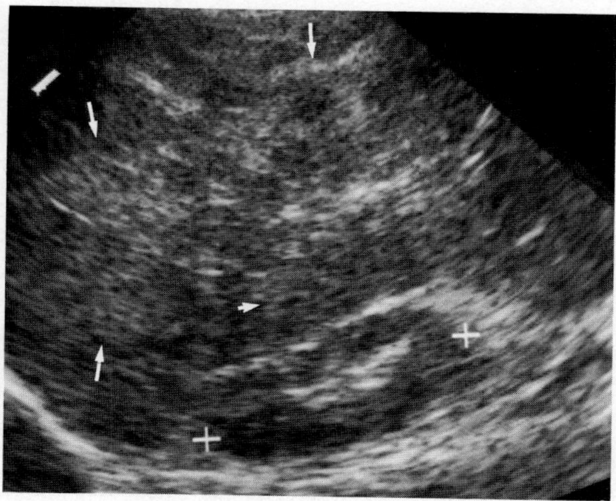

B

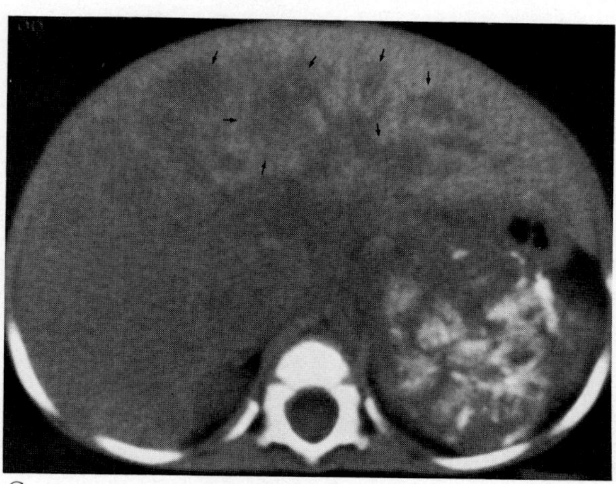

C

Figure 14-17. (*A*, *B*) Hepatic metastasis is demonstrated sonographically with multiple diffuse echogenic areas, giving the liver a mottled or heterogeneous appearance *(arrows)*. (C) On CT examination of the same patient, hepatic metastases appears as hypodense areas *(arrows)* within the normal homogeneous liver tissue.

Sonographically, small cell sarcoma usually presents as a single hyperechoic mass containing anechoic areas, which represent the cystic spaces,[82] but it can also appear homogeneous and hyperechoic or as a complex lesion with anechoic areas as well as calcifications producing posterior shadowing (Figs. 14-15, 14-16).[82]

Metastases

In children liver metastases can originate in neuroblastomas, rhabdomyosarcomas, primary gastrointestinal malignancies, and infrequently Wilms' tumor. Metastasis to the liver from a right adrenal neuroblastoma is called Pepper's syndrome.

Children's liver metastases are sonographically similar to those of adults. They appear as multiple hyperechoic focal areas compared to surrounding liver tissue (Fig. 14-17). These secondary tumors may also appear complex, owing to necrosis, hemorrhage, or involution from chemotherapy or radiation therapy. If the metastatic lesions are small, they can appear homogeneous with surrounding liver tissue and consequently can be missed.[44]

Gallbladder and Biliary Tree

Although gallbladder disease is rare in children,[39] it can occur. In a fasting child, the gallbladder should appear as a thin-walled, well-defined structure, completely echo free internally. Table 14-1 demonstrates normal pediatric gallbladder and biliary tract measurements.[58]

GALLBLADDER PATHOLOGY

Cholecystitis. In children, as in adults, a gallbladder wall thickness of 2 to 5 mm suggests disease and 5 mm and greater is considered indicative of disease.[18,39,75,104]

Acute or chronic cholecystitis or a thickened gallbladder wall in children has a number of causes: hypoalbuminemia, acute viral hepatitis, heart failure, renal failure, gallbladder carcinoma, ascites, multiple myeloma, portal node lymphatic obstruction, insufficient fasting time prior to scan,[18,39,48,58,75] and nonperpendicular scanning angle.[75] Cholelithiasis and adenomyomatosis can also mimic a thickened gallbladder wall. Clinically the patients can present with right upper quadrant pain, fever, and vomiting.[39] The differential diagnosis includes cholecystitis, abdominal abscesses of the right upper quadrant, pancreatitis, appendicitis, and peptic ulcer disease.[39]

Sonographically, in a diseased state the gallbladder wall is usually thickened and has a highly reflective, irregular wall. An accompanying anechoic area around the wall is usually due to either infection of the wall itself or a disease process in surrounding liver tissue (Fig. 14-18).[18,39,48,58,75] At times sludge can be seen in the gallbladder owing to stasis.[39] Sludge produces low-level echoes that move as the patient changes position.

Cholelithiasis. Cholelithiasis is the presence of one or more calculi or stones in the gallbladder, cystic duct, or common bile duct. Situated in the cystic duct or common bile duct, they often cause biliary obstruction (Figs. 14-19, 14-20). It was once thought that cholelithiasis rarely occurred in children, but their incidence has increased with the increase in infant hyperalimentation therapy and total parenteral nutrition (TPN)[63] and in pediatric patients taking Lasix for congenital heart disease.

Sonographically, gallstones appear as hyperechoic, rounded areas within the gallbladder. The stones also produce the typical posterior shadowing and move with positional changes of the child as they do in adults (Fig. 14-21). If the child has fasted for a reasonable period of time but the gallbladder is not sufficiently distended by the fast, a stone in the cystic duct cannot be ruled out and that area must be explored further (Fig. 14-19). Gallbladder sludge is also associated with cystic fibrosis and TPN. The cause is thought to be bile stasis in the gallbladder, and it is probably a precursor of gallstones.[23,63]

The sonographic appearance of gallbladder sludge can appear as sand-like or hyperechoic, nonshadowing areas within the gallbladder. The material forms layers and moves when the patient changes position.

Hydropic Gallbladder. Hydropic gallbladder—one dramatically enlarged—develops in children who

TABLE 14-1. Sonographic measurements of the normal pediatric gallbladder and biliary tree

Age Range (yr)	AP Diameter (cm)		Coronal Diameter (cm)		Length (cm)		Wall Thickness (mm)		Common Hepatic Duct Size (mm)		Right Portal Vein Size (mm)	
	Mean	Range	Mean	Range	Mean	Range	Mean	Range	Mean	Range	Mean	Range
0–1 (8 patients)	0.9	0.5–1.2	0.9	0.7–1.4	2.5	1.3–3.4	1.7	1.0–3.0	1.3	1.0–2.0	3.8	3.0–5.0
2–5 (10 patients)	1.7	1.4–2.3	1.8	1.0–3.9	4.2	2.9–5.2	2.0	None	1.7	1.0–3.0	4.8	3.0–7.0
6–8 (11 patients)	1.8	1.0–2.4	2.0	1.2–3.0	5.6	4.4–7.4	2.2	2.0–3.0	2.0	None	5.7	6.0–9.0
9–11 (12 patients)	1.9	1.2–3.2	2.0	1.0–3.6	5.5	3.4–6.5	2.0	1.0–3.0	1.8	1.0–3.0	6.8	4.0–9.0
12–16 (10 patients)	2.0	1.3–2.8	2.1	1.6–3.0	6.1	3.8–8.0	2.0	1.0–3.0	2.2	1.0–4.0	7.8	6.0–10.0

(From McGahan JP, Phillips HE, Cox KL: Sonography of the normal pediatric gallbladder and biliary tract. Radiology 1982, 144:873–875.)

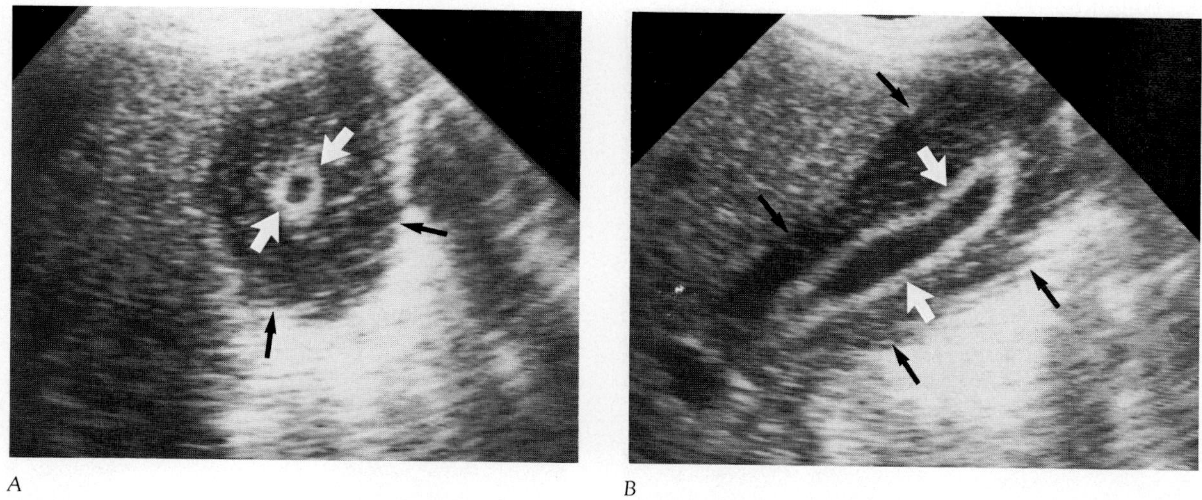

FIGURE 14-18. A highly reflective gallbladder wall *(white arrows)* is seen in a patient with cholecystitis. The anechoic area *(black arrows)* surrounding the gallbladder can represent either the diseased gallbladder wall itself or surrounding liver infection secondary to the gallbladder disease.

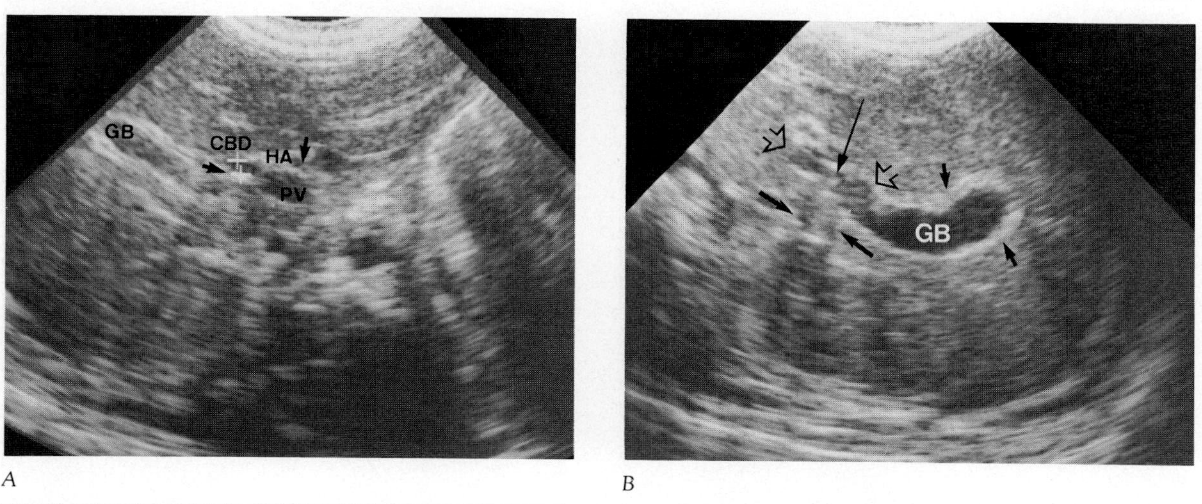

FIGURE 14-19. (*A*) Enlargement of the common bile duct (CBD) is seen in a patient with obstruction (GB, gallbladder; PV, portal vein; HA, hepatic artery). (*B*) In the same patient, the gallbladder (GB) wall appears thickened *(small black arrows)*. A calculus *(long arrow)* casting a subtle acoustic shadow *(large black arrows)* is identified obstructing the enlarged, tortuous cystic duct *(open arrows)*.

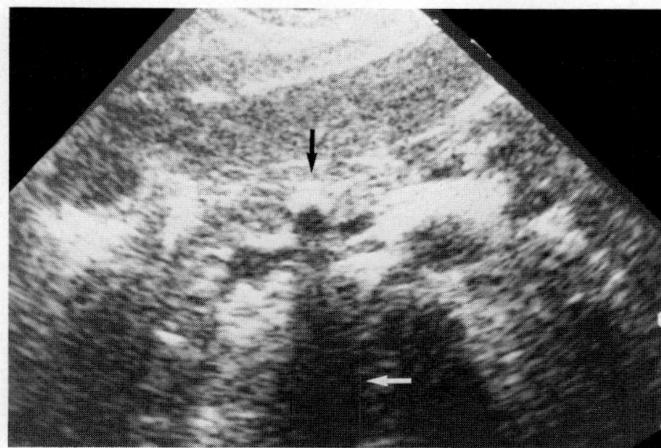

FIGURE 14-20. In a 10-year-old girl with a history of abdominal pain and increased total bilirubin value, a common bile duct calculus *(black arrow)* is identified sonographically as having the typical posterior acoustic shadowing *(white arrow)*. The position of the calculus was confirmed at surgery.

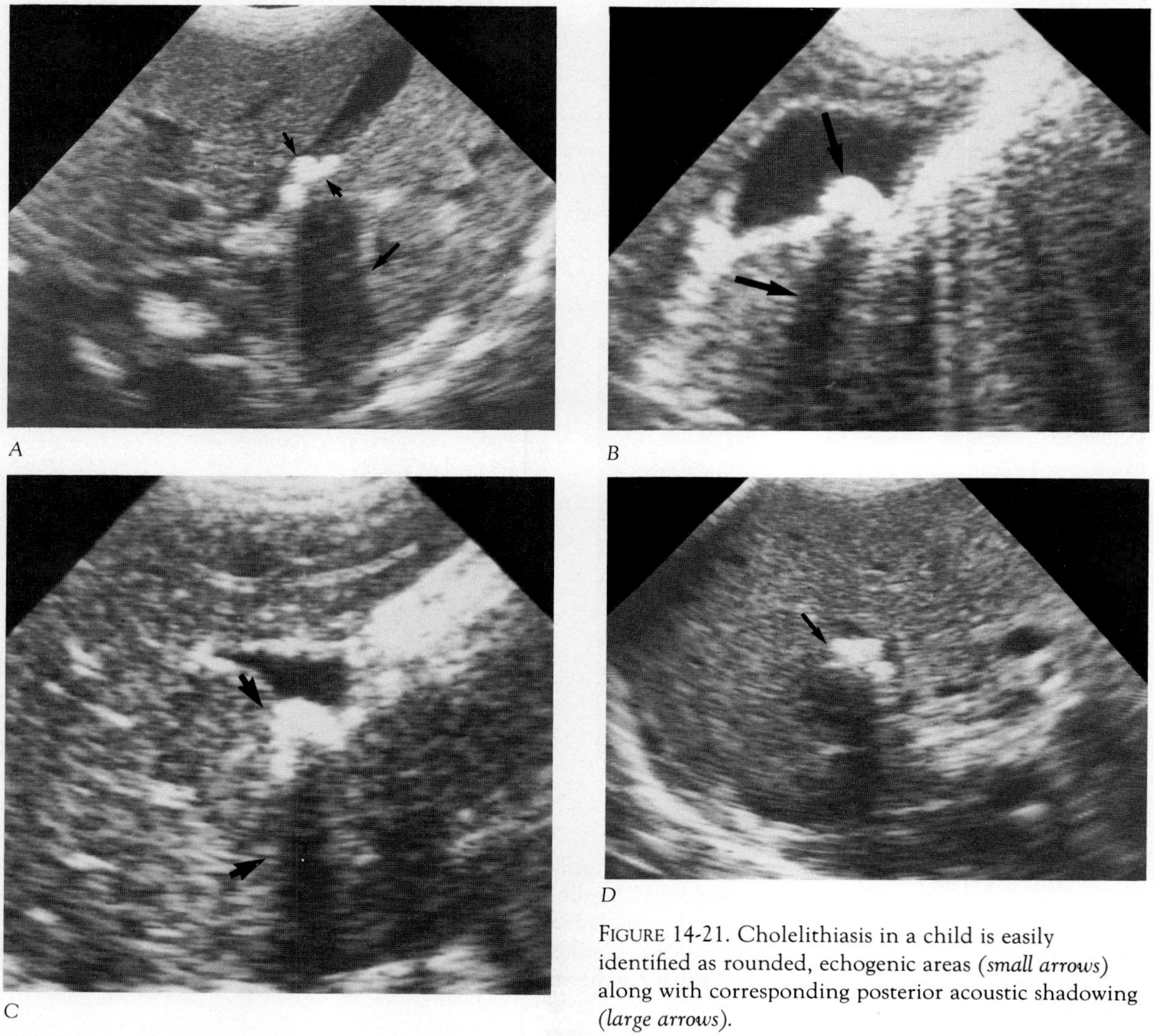

A

B

C

D

FIGURE 14-21. Cholelithiasis in a child is easily identified as rounded, echogenic areas *(small arrows)* along with corresponding posterior acoustic shadowing *(large arrows)*.

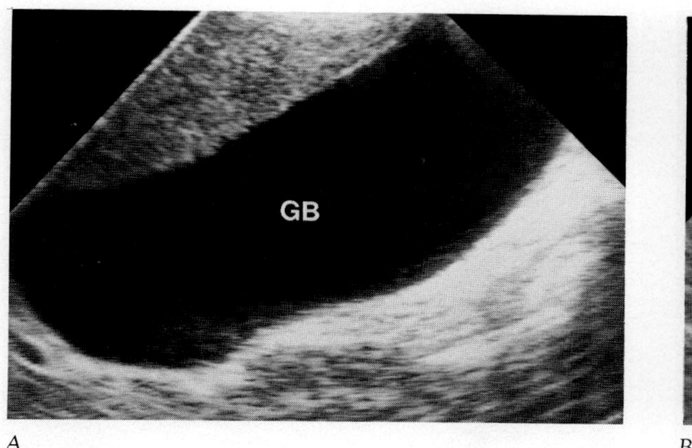

A

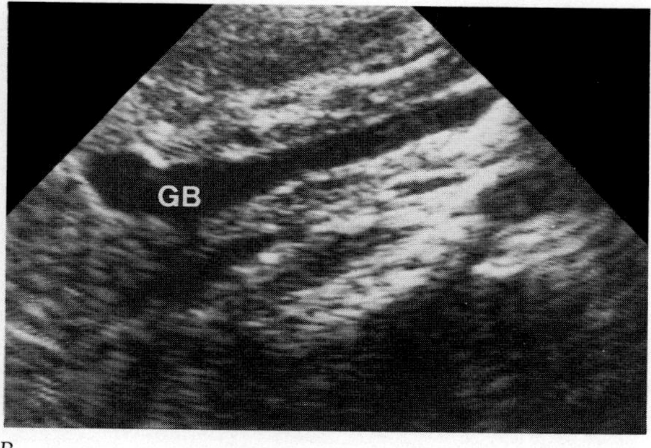

B

Figure 14-22. (*A*) A severely hydropic gallbladder (GB) is seen in a patient suffering from Kawasaki's disease. (*B*) In the same patient after a fatty meal, contraction of the hydropic gallbladder (GB) is identified. Normally, hydropic gallbladder does not contract very well.

receive TPN[61] or hyperalimentation therapy[16,19,58] and in association with diseases such as Kawasaki's, or mucocutaneous lymph node syndrome, leptospirosis,[58] typhoid fever, ascariasis, *Salmonella, Pseudomonas,* or group B streptococcal sepsis, congestive heart failure, shock, chronic biliary tract obstruction,[16] upper respiratory tract infection, and gastroenteritis.[19] Clinically, patients may present with right upper quadrant pain, fever, dehydration, and abdominal distention.[19]

Sonographically, the gallbladder is highly dilated with or without internal sludge or gallstone echoes. Such a gallbladder generally does not contract well following a fatty meal (Fig. 14-22).

Pathology

Nonobstructive Biliary Dilatation. Nonobstructive biliary dilatation, also known as Caroli's disease or communicating cavernous ectasia of the biliary tract, is associated with congenital hepatic fibrosis (CHF) and with autosomal recessive polycystic kidney disease (RPKD) (Fig. 14-23).[49,61] It is thought that the embryonic formation of the intrahepatic bile duct is stopped or slowed down.[61] Complications of this disease are chronic inflammation of the bile ducts and stones in the ducts.[61]

Sonographically, the intrahepatic ducts appear segmental and irregularly dilated, probably owing to bulbar protrusion and bridge formation of the duct walls. Small portal branches may also be seen passing through these dilated bile ducts.[61]

Obstructive Biliary Dilatation. It is worthwhile to note that any intrahepatic mass, whether it is benign or a primary malignancy, has the capacity to cause biliary obstruction, depending on its size and position. It is equally important to understand that extrahepatic masses such as pancreatic tumors, neuroblastomas, Wilms' tumor, and metastases to the liver from an extrahepatic primary tumor also can cause biliary dilatation by obstructing the common bile duct. It is important to determine if biliary obstruction is intrahepatic or extrahepatic (Fig. 14-24).

Biliary Rhabdomyosarcoma. Biliary rhabdomyosarcoma is a rare soft tissue tumor occurring in children, usually between ages 1 and 5 years.[4,24,32,87,106] It arises in the biliary tract and produces obstruction. It is the second most common cause of obstructive jaundice: in older children after choledochal cyst[24,106] and in neonates after biliary atresia.[24] The tumor appears lobulated and is usually situated in the hilus of the liver. It invades the intra- or extra-

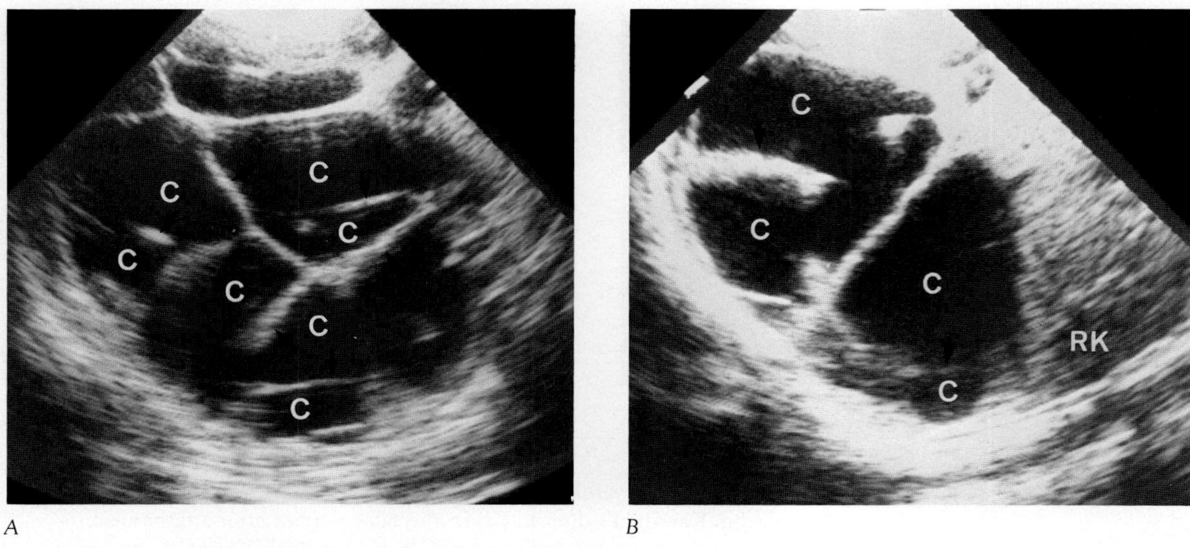

FIGURE 14-23. (*A* and *B*) Polycystic liver disease is demonstrated in a 2-week-old patient with familial, autosomal recessive polycystic kidney disease. Note the multiple cystic (C) areas separated by the walls *(arrows)* of the cysts (RK, right kidney).

hepatic ducts[4,32] with lacunar polypoid projections causing obstruction.[4,24] Occasionally, the tumor can be discovered in the right lobe of the liver.[32]

Clinical signs are increasing abdominal girth,[32,87] jaundice,[4] pain, and weight loss.[4,24,87,106] Usually these clinical symptoms are confused with infectious hepatitis.[24,87] Laboratory values may include elevated total serum bilirubin, a marked increase in alkaline phosphatase, and normal or mildly elevated AST (SGOT). There may also be a moderate increase in the white blood cell count, owing to subsequent cholangitis.[87] Unlike hepatoblastoma or hepatocellular carcinoma, biliary rhabdomyosarcoma may not increase the α-fetoprotein level.[32] Biopsy and histologic examination are definitive for diagnosis.

Sonographically, rhabdomyosarcoma is predominantly solid,[106] with hyperechoic formations in the bile duct.[4] With biliary rhabdomyosarcoma there is no posterior shadowing as is commonly seen with stones.[4] There may be cystic spaces representing intrahepatic radicles of the bile ducts.[44] There may also be focal areas of necrosis and hemorrhage in the mass.[24] Usually, dilated bile ducts surround the mass.

CT can demonstrate the extent and the vascular relationships of the mass[73] for the surgeon.[87] The attenuation of the tumor is lower than that of the surrounding liver tissue.[32] CT also allows visualization of hepatic metastases or adenopathy associated with the mass.[4]

Opacification of the bile ducts—by direct puncture of the gallbladder, percutaneous cholangiography, or retrograde endoscopic catheterization of the bile papilla—accurately shows extension of the mass.[4]

Surgical excision is a must, although complete excision is almost impossible.[32] Since these tumors are very chemosensitive,[4] the favored method of treatment is surgery with adjuvant chemotherapy and radiation therapy.[4,32,87,106] Rhabdomyosarcomas tend to recur quickly, so prognosis is poor.[4,106]

The differential diagnosis includes benign and malignant lesions[24,87]: choledochal cyst, infectious hepatitis, recurrent cholestasis,[24,87] gallstones, lymphoma, neuroblastoma, pancreatic pseudocysts,

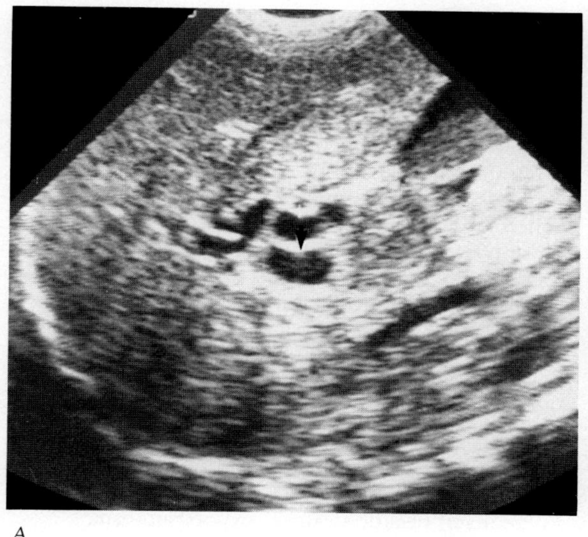

A

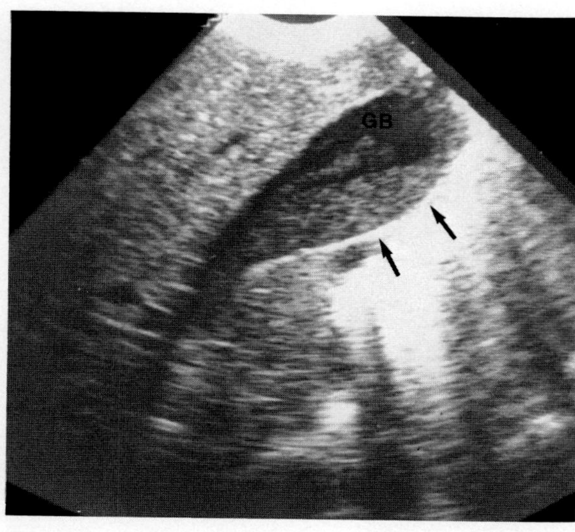

B

FIGURE 14-24. (*A*) A longitudinal plane view demonstrates a biliary duct obstruction *(arrow)* secondary to recurrent neuroblastoma in a 3½-year-old patient. (*B*) Sludge *(arrows)* in the gallbladder (GB) due to stasis is identified in the same patient.

hepatic hemangioma, enteric duplication cysts, hepatoblastoma, hepatocellular carcinoma, hemangioendothelioma, focal nodular hypoplasia, hepatic adenoma, and mixed mesenchymal sarcomas.[106]

CONGENITAL ANOMALIES

Gallbladder Duplication. A second gallbladder is a congenital anomaly. It is usually discovered as an incidental finding on a routine scan, but either or both may be involved with a disease such as cholecystitis or cholelithiasis. Sonographically, it is best to view two cystic ducts entering the common bile duct in order to definitively diagnose gallbladder duplication (Fig. 14-25). Oral cholecystography may not be reliable for diagnosis of a duplicated gallbladder as either one might not be visualized if obstructive disease is present.[28]

The differential diagnosis includes a tortuous gallbladder with a fold in the fundus, body, or neck, pericholecystic fluid, gallbladder diverticulum, phrygian cap, focal adenomyomatosis, Ladd bands dividing the gallbladder,[28] choledochal cyst, biloma, and congenital or parasitic liver cysts.

Biliary Atresia. Conjugated hyperbilirubinemia in the newborn has two major causes, diseases of the liver such as hepatitis and biliary tract abnormalities such as atresia.[29] Other considerations are listed in Table 14-2.[70] The manifestations of biliary atresia can range from total absence of the biliary tree to a rudimentary gallbladder and cystic duct or a visibly patent gallbladder, cystic duct, and common bile duct. In the most common form, the usual intra- and extrahepatic ducts near the porta hepatis are absent. Biliary atresia is suspected when there is persistent neonatal jaundice and infectious causes have been excluded.[38,102]

Some patients with biliary atresia also have other congenital anomalies, such as anomalous origin of the hepatic artery, azygous continuation of the inferior vena cava, polysplenia, bilaterally bilobed lungs, preduodenal portal veins, abdominal malrotation, and visceral situs anomalies.[2]

It is important to make sure that the patient is fasting appropriately for age, to ensure visualization of the gallbladder. If an atretic gallbladder is seen prior to feeding, it should also be checked postprandially to see if the size has changed. If it is

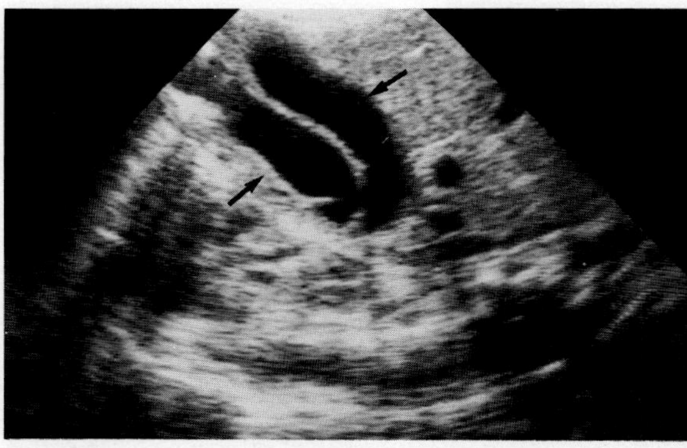

A

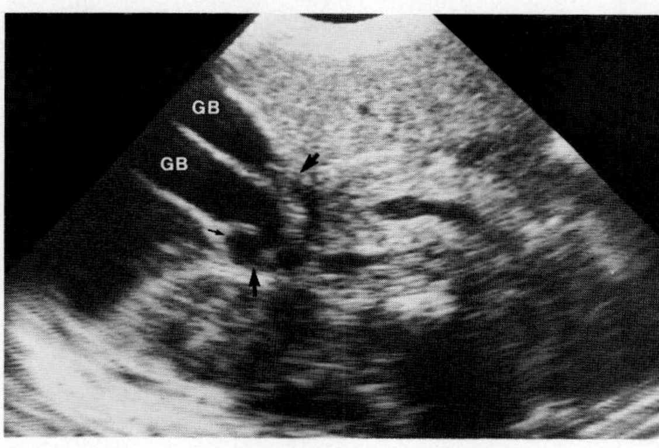

B

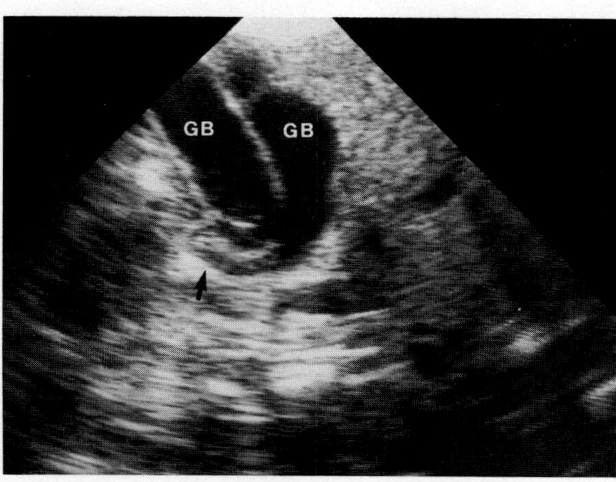

C

FIGURE 14-25. Two separate gallbladders *(arrows)* are visualized. (*B,C*) On a longitudinal plane, two separate cystic ducts *(large arrows)* are also visualized, arising from each gallbladder (GB) and converging at a distal point *(small arrow)*.

TABLE 14-2. Causes of conjugated hyperbilirubinemia in infancy

Structural defects
- Bile duct abnormalities: Biliary atresia, spontaneous perforation of bile duct, choledochal cyst, bile duct stenosis, biliary hypoplasia syndromes, choledocholithiasis, cholangiolitis
- Polycystic disease
- Vascular lesions: Venoocclusive disease, poor perfusion syndromes, hemangioendothelioma, lymphatic defects
- Chromosomal abnormalities

Metabolic disorders
- α-I-antitrypsin deficiency, galactosemia, fructosemia, tyrosinemia, cystic fibrosis, Niemann-Pick disease, neurovisceral storage disease (with ophthalmoplegia), Gaucher's disease, Wolman's disease, Zellweger's syndrome, Dubin-Johnson syndrome, trihydroxycoprostatic acidemia (THCA), familial neonatal hepatic steatosis, hypopituitarism, hypothyroidism

Infections
- Bacterial infections (particularly *E. coli*), listeriosis, syphilis, toxoplasmosis, hepatitis B, cytomegalovirus, rubella, herpes simplex, coxsackie B virus, and varicella zoster, adenovirus, echovirus and reo virus

Posthemolytic disorders

Toxic or deficiency disorders
- Intravenous nutrition, drugs

Familial syndromes

Neonatal hepatic necrosis

Idiopathic

(From Mowat AP: Liver: Conjugated hyperbilirubinemia in infancy. *In* Rudolph AM, Hoffman JIE (eds): Pediatric, 17th ed. Norwalk, CT, Appleton-Century-Crofts, 1982.)

not connected to the biliary system, there should be no change in its size.[16,38]

Sonographically, the gallbladder, cystic duct, common bile ducts, and intrahepatic bile ducts may be seen incompletely, depending on the degree of atresia. If a rudimentary gallbladder is seen, a fasting measurement of less than 1.5 cm suggests atresia.[38] The accompanying hepatomegaly produces an image of the liver as somewhat diffusely hyperechoic, as in cirrhosis, with increased attenuation. Splenomegaly and ascites may be associated (Fig. 14-26).[38]

Surgical interventions include the Kasai procedure to develop a communication between the duodenum and the gallbladder, common bile duct, or

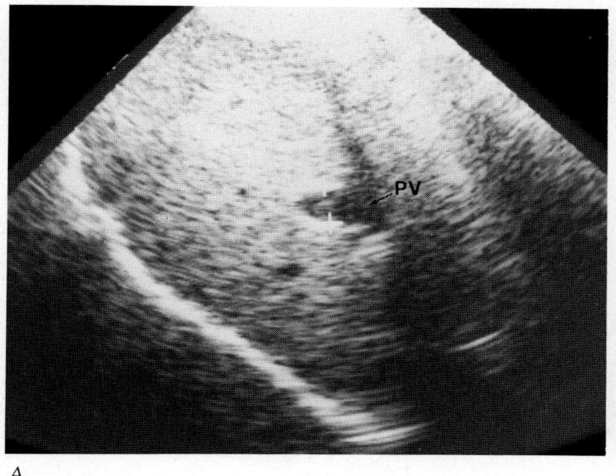

A

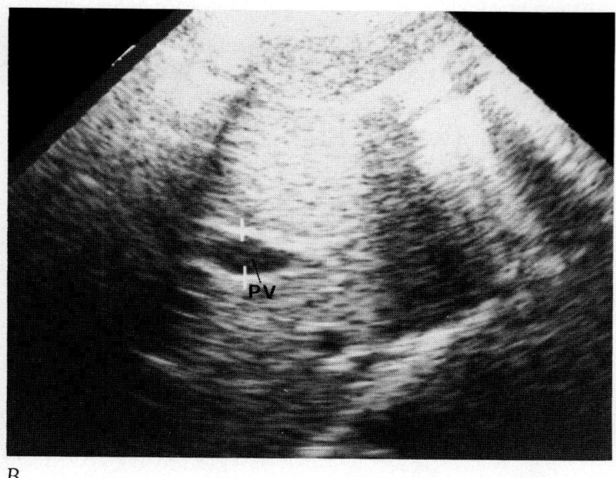

B

FIGURE 14-26. Liver sonogram in a 2-month-old patient suffering from persistent jaundice demonstrates a portal vein (PV), but a gallbladder could not be visualized. The diagnosis was biliary atresia.

liver, to promote drainage of the bile into the duodenum[102] and liver transplantation.

Choledochal Cyst. Congenital cystic dilatation of the common bile duct is commonly called choledochal cyst.[51,53,98] It is a rare congenital anomaly found predominantly in females.[6,50,53,68] Usually detected within the first decade of life,[51,79] choledochal cyst most often affects the common bile duct, but it can involve the intrahepatic ducts as well. The exact cause is uncertain, but currently it is thought to be either eccentric epithelial proliferation or anomalous arrangement of the pancreatobiliary ducts.[50]

A theory of Yotuyanagi postulates that inequalities of epithelial proliferation during the stage of epithelial occlusion result in the varying sizes of the proximal and distal common bile duct in the recanalization stage.[98] If intraductal pressure increases owing to stenosis (either inherent or acquired), the proximal choledochus usually enlarges into a cystic dilatation. Without an increase in intraductal pressure, only the proximal common bile duct remains enlarged.[98] Intrahepatic duct enlargement or dilatation is also frequently associated with congenital dilatation of the common bile duct.[72,98]

According to Babbitt's theory, the formation of the function of the pancreatic and biliary ducts varies, with two types predominating[50,52,53,85]: (1) the pancreatic duct joins the common bile duct at a right angle, forming a long common segment (Fig. 14-27A,B) or (2) the common bile duct joins the pancreatic duct at a right angle, forming a long common segment (Fig. 14-27C).

Because the pressure is higher in the pancreatic duct than in the common bile duct[53] it is thought that the loss of normal sphincter control at the pancreatobiliary junction permits the regurgitation of pancreatic juices into the biliary tree. It is possible that this regurgitation, along with a lack of uniformity in the construction of the duct wall itself, could explain the location and degree of dilatation. Complications of this anomaly include inflammation, cholangitis, fibrosis, choledochal cyst, cirrhosis, pancreatitis,[85] intrahepatic lithiasis,[98] abscess, and thrombosis of the portal vein.[51]

Authors have divided choledochal cysts into two main types.[6,52,53] Concentric or fusiform dilatation is most common in infants and children (Fig. 14-28A).[50,52,53] If the intrahepatic ducts are also dilated, usually only the distal third of the duct is involved and the peripheral intrahepatic ducts are not necessarily affected as they are in Caroli's disease (Fig.

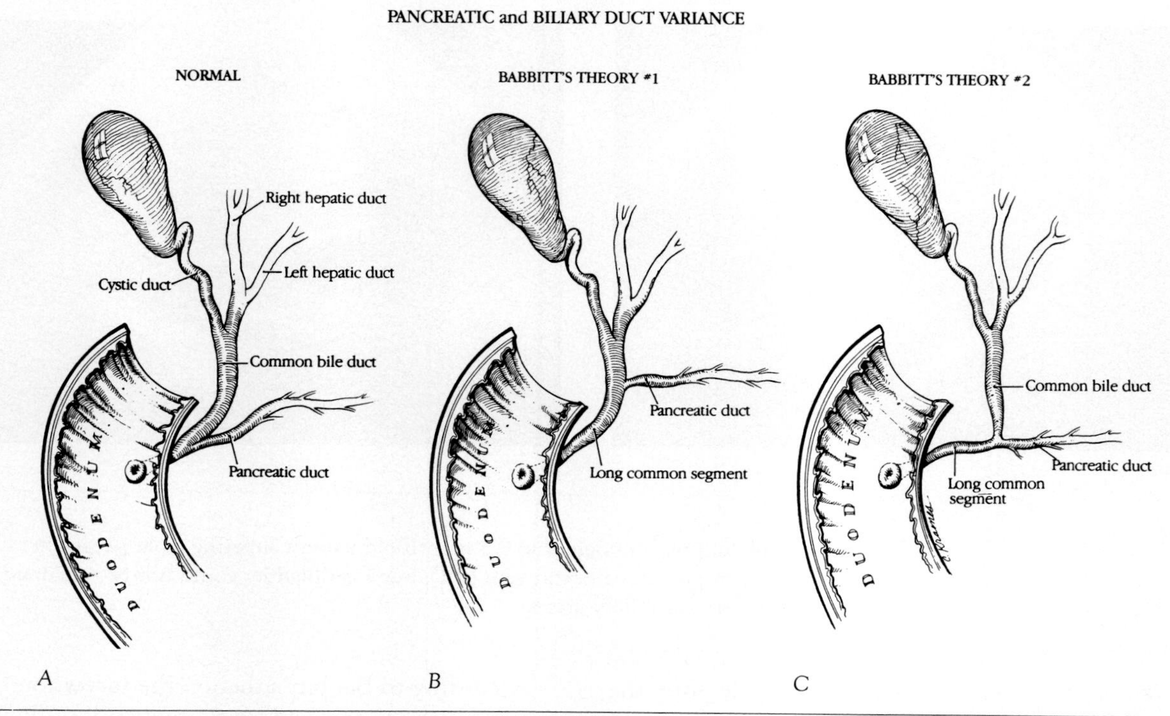

FIGURE 14-27. Normal anatomy (*A*) and two predominant types of variation in which (*B*) the pancreatic duct joins the common bile duct at a right angle or (*C*) the common bile duct joins the pancreatic duct at a right angle, in each case forming a long common segment.

14-28B).[61] Eccentric or rosary common bile duct diverticula, the second most common sort, can present as a solitary diverticulum or multiple ones (Fig. 14-29), with or without dilatation of the intrahepatic duct as in type 1.[50,52] Congenital choledochocele presents as a cystic dilatation of the intraduodenal portion of the common bile duct (Fig. 14-30). Although the cause is not known for certain it is believed to be the result of a stricture at the ampulla of Vater. This lesion is not considered to be a true choledochal cyst, and is generally asymptomatic,[50] however it is reported in the literature.[6,52] Clinical manifestations may include upper abdominal mass, pain, jaundice, fever, and vomiting, though not all of these may be present. Pain is the most common symptom.

Sonographically, a type I choledochal cyst presents as a fusiform dilatation of the common bile duct (Fig. 14-31). The right, left, and common bile duct may be seen entering the cyst and the gallbladder is demonstrated as a separate cystic structure. A type II choledochal cyst demonstrates one or more diverticulae or fluid-filled structures near or coming off the common bile duct. Either type may show intrahepatic duct dilatation.[50] If pancreatitis is present, the pancreas appears diffusely enlarged, probably owing either to pancreatic duct obstruction or stasis of bile in the pancreatic duct.

Radiographically, a choledochal cyst can manifest itself in many ways. An upper gastrointestinal series shows the stomach (usually displaced anterolaterally to the left),[6] a displaced or compressed duodenum,[85] and in the case of choledochocele, a filling defect in the duodenum near the am-

TYPE I CHOLEDOCHAL CYSTS
Common bile duct
Pancreatic duct
DUODENUM
Right hepatic duct
Left hepatic duct
Common bile duct
Pancreatic duct
DUODENUM
A CONCENTRIC DILATATION
B FUSIFORM DILATATION

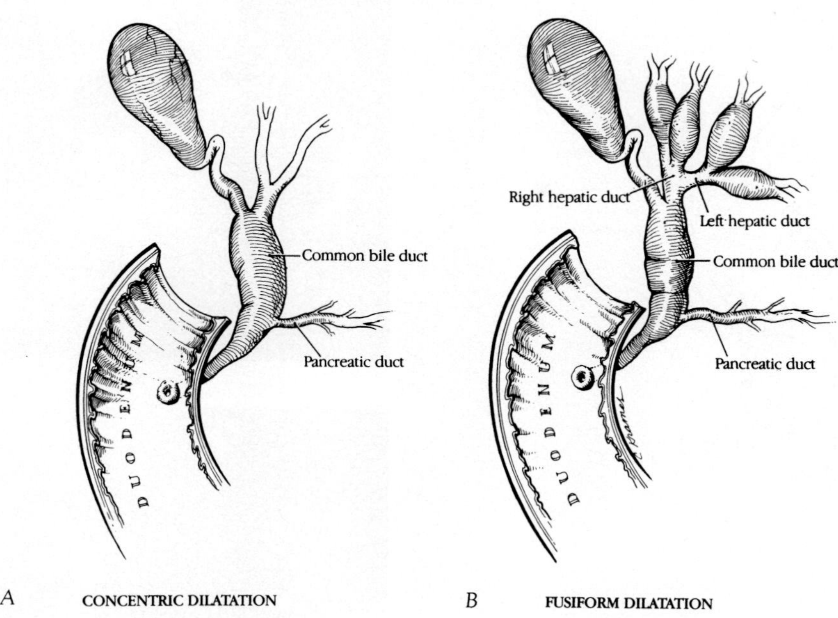

FIGURE 14-28. (*A*) Type 1 concentric dilatation, (*B*) type 1 fusiform dilatation.

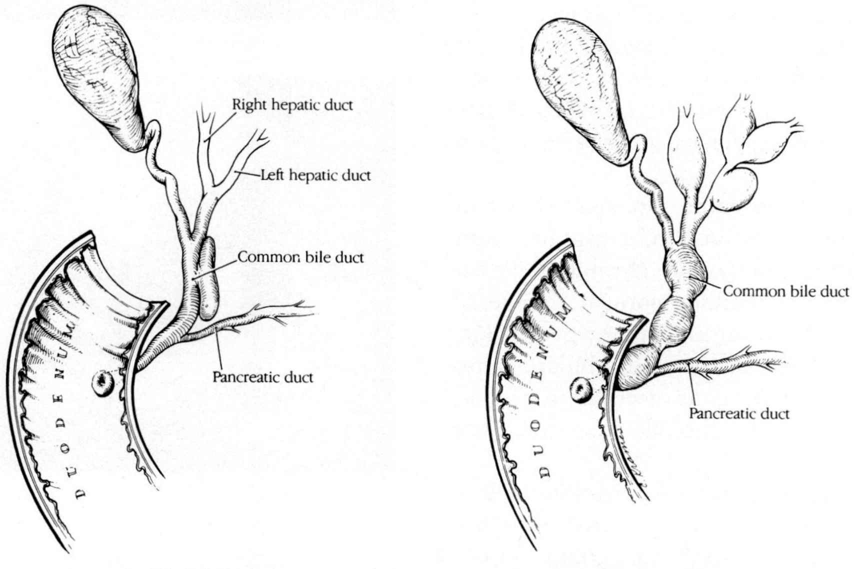

TYPE II CHOLEDOCHAL CYSTS
Right hepatic duct
Left hepatic duct
Common bile duct
Pancreatic duct
DUODENUM
Common bile duct
Pancreatic duct
DUODENUM
A ECCENTRIC DIVERTICULUM
B ROSARY DIVERTICULA

FIGURE 14-29. (*A*) Type 2 eccentric common bile duct diverticulum, (*B*) type 2 rosary common bile duct diverticulum.

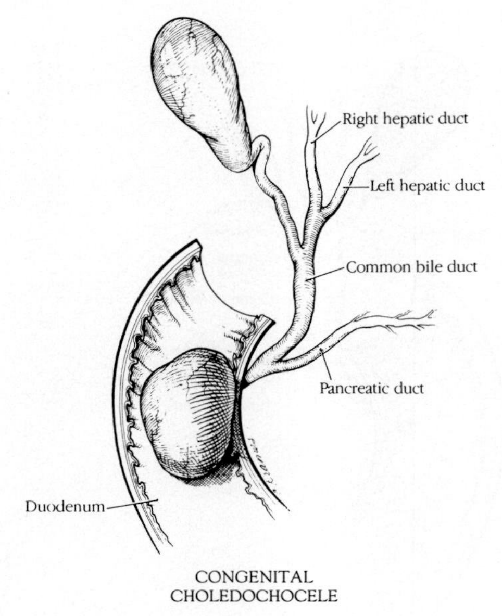

FIGURE 14-30. Congenital choledochocele.

pulla.[6,79,85] Plain radiographs usually show displacement of gas shadows in the stomach, duodenum, and colon.[6] Other studies, such as excretory urography, can also show a mass effect,[79] whereas arteriograms may show displacement of the hepatic and celiac arteries.

Complications of untreated choledochal cyst include chronic biliary obstruction,[6] portal hypertension,[6] portal vein thrombosis,[51] chronic cholangitis,[6,51,98] cirrhosis,[6,51,85] carcinomatous changes,[6,85] biliary rupture with resulting biliary peritonitis,[6] hepatic abscess,[51,85] pancreatitis,[85] and biliary stones (Fig. 14-32).[85,98] The treatment of choice for a choledochal cyst is usually choledochocystojejunostomy.[51]

The differential diagnosis of congenital dilatation of the common bile duct is extensive, including gallbladder duplication,[68] malignant hepatic neoplasm,[88] hemangioma, hematoma,[88] congenital or parasitic liver cyst,[88] Caroli's disease,[98] mesenteric[50,88] or omental cyst, renal or adrenal cyst, abscess, fluid-filled bowel, hepatic artery aneurysm,[50,68] and pancreatic pseudocysts.[50,68,79]

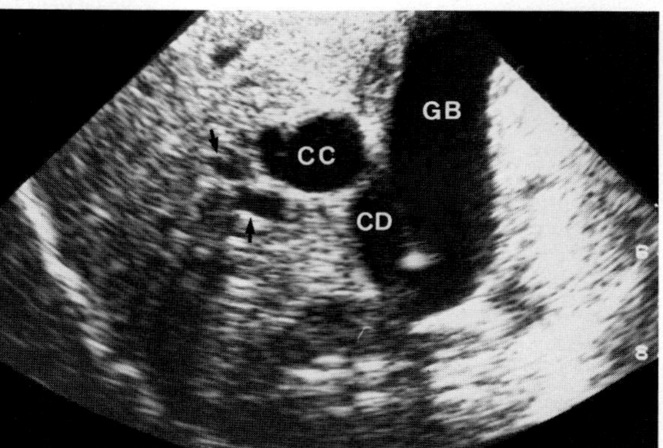

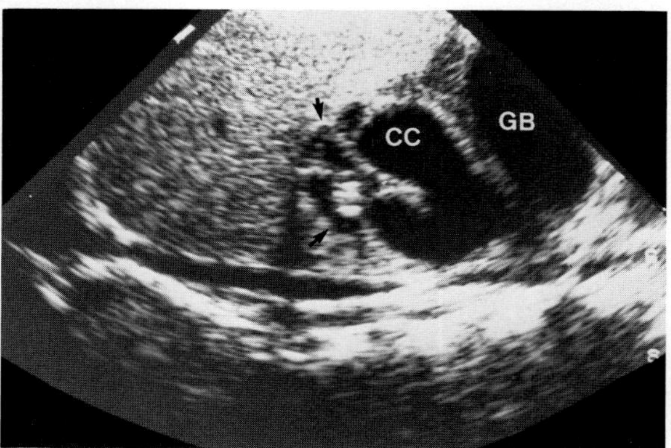

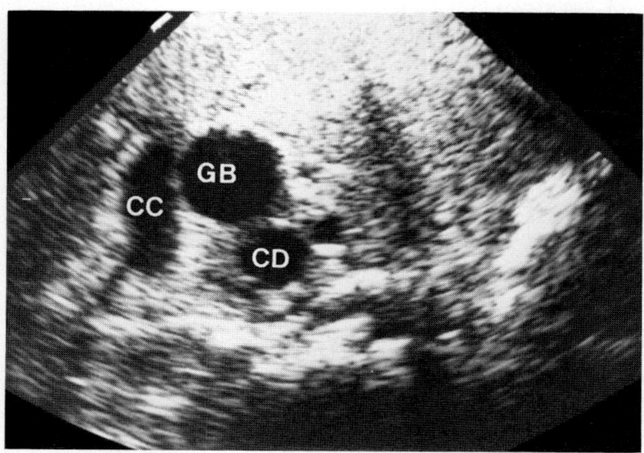

FIGURE 14-31. In a 1-year-old patient, a choledochal cyst (CC) is demonstrated with dilated intrahepatic ducts *(arrows)*, which were easily visualized and were thought to be caused by the cyst. This diagnosis was confirmed by histological examination. The patient also had a markedly dilated cystic duct (CD; GB, gallbladder).

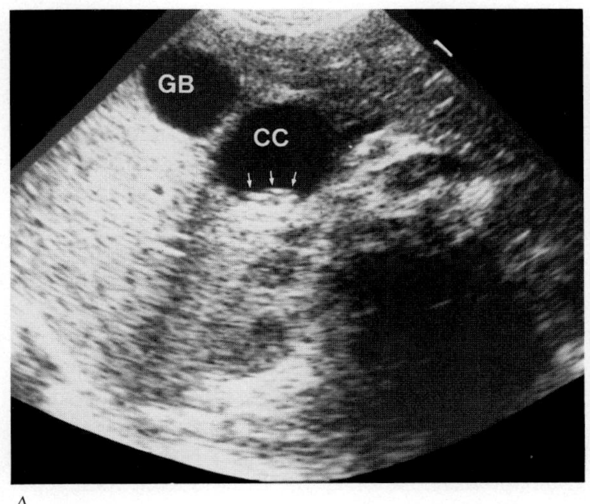

A

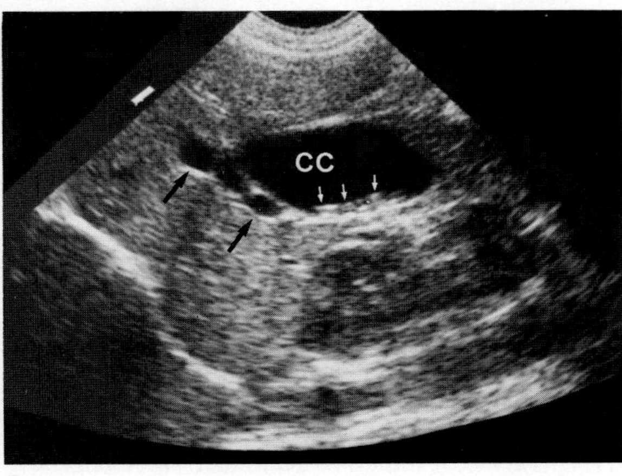

B

FIGURE 14-32. (*A*) A transverse plane view demonstrates a choledochal cyst (CC) in a 6-year-old child. The cyst also contained sludge *(arrows)*, which could be mistaken for a gallbladder (GB) with stones. (*B*) A longitudinal plane view demonstrates a choledochal cyst (CC) containing sludge *(white arrows)*, and dilated ducts *(black arrows)* were also visualized.

Acknowledgments

I acknowledge and thank Peggy Kaul for her patience in pulling sonographic examinations, Val Kemp for typing the manuscript, Dr. Richard Jaffe for his valuable advice and direction, Dr. Barbara Reid for her patient answers to my incessant questions, and Diane Kawamura for giving me the opportunity to be involved in this project.

References

1. Ablow RC, Effman EL: Hepatic calcifications associated with umbilical vein catheterization in the newborn infant. AJR 1972, 114:380–385.
2. Abramson SJ, Berdon WE, Altman RP, et al: Biliary atresia and noncardiac polysplenic syndrome: US and surgical considerations. Radiology 1987, 163:377–379.
3. Abramson SJ, Lack EE, Teele RL: Benign vascular tumors of the liver in infants: Sonographic appearance. AJR 1982, 138:629–632.
4. Arnaud O, Moscq M, Asquier E, et al: Embryonal rhabdomyosarcoma of the biliary tree in children: A case report. Pediatr Radiol 1987, 17:250–251.
5. Atkinson GO, Kodroff M, Sones PJ, et al: Focal nodular hyperplasia of the liver in children: A report three new cases. Radiology 1980, 137:171–174.
6. Bass EM, Cremin BJ: Choledochal cysts: A clinical and radiological evaluation of 21 cases. Pediatr Radiol 1976, 5:81–85.
7. Berdon WE, Baker DH: Giant hepatic hemangioma with cardiac failure in the newborn infant. Value of high-dosage intravenous urography and umbilical angiography. Radiology 1969, 92:1523–1528.
8. Bezzi M, Teggi A, De Rosa F, et al: Abnormal hydatid disease: US findings during medical treatment. Radiology 1987, 162:91–95.
9. Biersack HJ, Thelen M, Torres JF, et al: Focal nodular hyperplasia of the liver as established by ^{99m}-Tc-sulfur colloid and HIDA scintigraphy. Radiology 1980, 137:187–190.
10. Bowerman RA, Samuels BI, Silver TM: Ultrasonographic features of hepatic adenomas in type I glycogen storage disease. J Ultrasound Med 1983, 2:51–54.
11. Brant WE, Floyd JL, Jackson DE, et al: The radiological evaluation of hepatic cavernous hemangioma. JAMA 1987, 257:2471–2474.
12. Bree RL, Schwab RE, Glazer GM, et al: The varied

appearance of hepatic cavernous hemangiomas with sonography, computed tomography, magnetic resonance imaging and scintigraphy. RadioGraphis 1987, 7:1153–1175.

13. Brick SH, Taylor GA, Potter BM, et al: Hepatic and splenic injury in children: Role of CT in the decision for laparotomy. Radiology 1987, 165:643–646.
14. Brunelle F, Chaumont P: Hepatic tumors in children: Ultrasonic differentiation of malignant benign lesions. Radiology 1984, 150:695–699.
15. Burrows PE, Rosenberg HC, Chuang HS: Diffuse hepatic hemangiomas: Percutaneous transcatheter embolization with detachable silicone balloons. Radiology 1985, 156:85–88.
16. Carroll BA, Oppenheimer DA, Muller HH: High-frequency real-time ultrasound of the neonatal biliary system. Radiology 1982, 145:437–440.
17. Chawla V, Pandit PB, Nkrumah FK: Congenital syphilis in the newborn. Arch Dis Child 1988, 63:1393–1394.
18. Cohan RH, Mahony BS, Bowie JD, et al: Striated intramural gallbladder lucencies on US studies: Predictors of acute cholecystitis. Radiology 1987, 164:31–35.
19. Cohen EK, Stringer DA, Smith CR, et al: Hydrops of the gallbladder in typhoid fever as demonstrated by sonography. J Clin Ultrasound 1986, 14:633–635.
20. Cywes S, Rode H, Miller AJW: Blunt liver trauma in children: Nonoperative management. J Pediatr Surg 1985, 20:14–18.
21. Dachman AH, Lichtenstein JE, Friedman AC, et al: Infantile hemangioendothelioma of the liver: A radiologic-pathologic-clinical correlation. AJR 1983, 140:1091–1096.
22. Dachman AH, Pakter RL, Ros PR, et al: Hepatoblastoma: Radiologic-pathologic correlation in 50 cases. Radiology 1987, 164:15–19.
23. Davies C, Daneman A, Stringer DA: Inspissated bile in a neonate with cystic fibrosis. J Ultrasound Med 1986, 5:335–337.
24. Davis GL, Kissane JM, Ishak KG: Embryonal rhabdomyosarcoma (sarcoma botryoides) of the biliary tree. Report of five cases and a review of the literature. Cancer 1969, 2:333–342.
25. Day DL, Letourneau JG, Allan BT, et al: Hepatic regenerating nodules in hereditary tyrosinemia. AJR 1987, 149:391–393.
26. DeLorimier AA, Simpson EB, Baum RS, et al: Hepatic artery ligation for hepatic hemangiomatosis. N Engl J Med 1967, 277:333–336.
27. Foucar E, Williamson RA, Yiu-Chiu V, et al: Mesenchymal hamartoma of the liver identified by fetal sonography. AJR 1983, 140:970–972.
28. Garfield HD, Lyons EA, Levi CS: Sonographic findings in double gallbladder with cholelithiasis of both lobes. J Ultrasound Med 1988, 7:589–591.
29. Gartner L, Arian IM: Liver: Hyperbilirubinemia. *In* Rudolph AM, Hoffman JIE (eds): Pediatrics, 17th ed. Norwalk, CT, Appleton-Century-Crofts, 1982.
30. Gates GF, Miller JH, Stanley P: Scintiangiography of hepatic masses in childhood. JAMA 1978, 239:2667–2670.
31. Gates GF, Stanley P, Gwinn JL, et al: Congenital syphilitic hepatitis: A radionuclide study. Radiology 1978, 128:163–164.
32. Geoffray A, Couanet D, Ontagne JP, et al: Ultrasonography and computed tomography for diagnosis and follow-up of biliary duct rhabdomyosarcomas in children. Pediatr Radiol 1987, 17:127–131.
33. Gharbi HA, Hassine W, Brauner MW, et al: Ultrasound examination of the hydatid liver. Radiology 1981, 139:459–463.
34. Gibney RG, Hendin AP, Copperberg PL: Sonographically detected hepatic hemangiomas: Absence of change over time. AJR 1987, 149:953–957.
35. Giorgio A, Amoroso P, Fico P, et al: Ultrasound evaluation of uncomplicated and complicated acute viral hepatitis. J Clin Ultrasound 1986, 14:675–679.
36. Goldstein HM, Neiman HL, Mena E, et al: Angiographic findings in benign liver cell tumors. Radiology 1974, 110:339–343.
37. Gonzalez LR, Marcos J, Illanas M, et al: Radiologic aspects of hepatic echinococcosis: Value of the intravenous viscerogram and computed tomography. Radiology 1979, 130:21–27.
38. Green D, Carroll BA: Ultrasonography in the jaundiced infant: A new approach. J Ultrasound Med 1986, 5:323–329.
39. Greenberg M, Kanarloo H, Cochran ST, et al: The ultrasonographic diagnosis of cholecystitis and cholelithiasis in children. Radiology 1980, 137:745–749.
40. Griscom NT, Capitanio MA, Wagoner ML, et al: The visibly fatty liver. Radiology 1975, 117:385–389.
41. Grossman H, Ram PC, Coleman RA, et al: Hepatic ultrasonography in type I glycogen storage disease (von Gierke disease). Radiology 1981, 141:753–756.
42. Henschke CI, Goldman H, Teele RL: The hyperechogenic liver in children: Cause and sonographic appearance. AJR 1982, 138:841–846.
43. Holder LE, Gnarra DJ, Lampkin BC, et al: Hepatoma associated with anabolic steroid therapy. AJR 1975, 124:638–642.
44. Holm J, Jacobsen B: Accuracy of dynamic ultrasonography in the diagnosis of malignant liver lesions. J Ultrasound Med 1986, 5:1–4.
45. Itoh K, Nishimura K, Togashi K, et al: Hepatocel-

lular carcinoma: MR imaging. Radiology 1987, 164:21–25.
46. Ishibashi H, Okumura Y, Higuchi N, et al: Differentiation of mononucleosis from hepatitis by sonographic measurement of spleen size. J Clin Ultrasound 1987, 15:313–316.
47. Johnson CM, Sheedy II PF, Stanson AW, et al: Computed tomography and angiography of cavernous hemangiomas of the liver. Radiology 1981, 138:115–121.
48. Juttner HU, Ralls PW, Quinn MF, et al: Thickening of the gallbladder wall in acute hepatitis: Ultrasound demonstration. Radiology 1982, 142:465–466.
49. Kaiser JA, Mall JC, Salmen BJ, et al: Diagnosis of Caroli disease by computed tomography: Report of two cases. Radiology 1979, 132:661–664.
50. Kangarloo H, Sarti DA, Sample WF, et al: Ultrasonographic spectrum of choledochal cysts in children. Pediatr Radiol 1980, 9:15–18.
51. Karjoo M, Bishop HC, Borns P, et al: Choledochal cyst presenting as recurrent pancreatitis. Pediatrics 1973, 51:289–291.
52. Kimura K, Ohto M, Ono T, et al: Congenital cystic dilatation of the common bile duct: Relationship to anomalous pancreaticobiliary ductal union. AJR 1977, 128:571–577.
53. Komi N, Udaka H, Ikeda N, et al: Congenital dilatation of the biliary tract: New classification and study with particular reference to anomalous arrangements of the pancreaticobiliary ducts. Gastroenterol Jap 1977, 12:291–304.
54. Larrey D, Freneaux E, Berson A, et al: Peliosis hepatis inducted by 6-thioguanine administration. Gut 1988, 29:1265–1269.
55. Lewall DB, McCorkell SJ: Hepatic echinococcal cysts: Sonographic appearance and classification. Radiology 1985, 155:773–775.
56. Lucaya J, Enriquez G, Amat L, et al: Computed tomography of infantile hepatic hemangioendothelioma. AJR 1985, 144:821–826.
57. Mahmud F, Baxter JA, Shah NR: Multiple liver abscesses with vascular blush in total body opacification. AJR 1979, 133:1180–1182.
58. McGahan JP, Phillips HE, Cox KL: Sonography of the normal pediatric gallbladder and biliary tract. Radiology 1982, 144:873–875.
59. McLoughlin MJ, Colapinto RF, Gilday DL, et al: Focal nodular hyperplasia of the liver. Angiography and radioisotope scanning. Radiology 1973, 107:257–263.
60. Mallory GK: The liver and biliary tract. *In* Robbins SL (ed): Textbook of Pathology with Clinical Application, 2nd ed. Philadelphia, WB Saunders, 1964.
61. Marchal GJ, Desmet VJ, Proesmans WC, et al: Caroli disease: High-frequency US and pathologic findings. Radiology 1986, 158:507–511.
62. Markowitz RI, Harcke HT, Ritchie WGM, et al: Focal nodular hyperplasia of the liver in a child with sickle cell anemia. AJR 1980, 134:594–597.
63. Matos C, Avni EF, Van Gansbeke D, et al: Total parenteral nutrition (TPN) and gallbladder diseases in neonates. Sonographic assessment. J Ultrasound Med 1987, 6:243–248.
64. Miller JH: Technetium-99m–labeled red blood cells in the evaluation of hemangiomas of the liver in infants and children. J Nucl Med 1987, 28:1412–1418.
65. Miller JH, Gates GF, Stanley P: The radiologic investigation of hepatic tumors in childhood. Radiology 1977, 123:451–458.
66. Miller JH, Greenfield LD, Wald BR: Candidiasis of the liver and spleen in childhood. Radiology 1982, 142:375–380.
67. Miller JH, Weinberg K: Liver and spleen. *In* Miller JH (ed): Imaging in Pediatric Oncology. Baltimore, Williams & Wilkins, 1985.
68. Morgan CL, Trought WX, Oddson TA, et al: Type II choledochal cyst: Ultrasonographic appearance. Radiology 1979, 132:130.
69. Moss AA, Clark RE, Palubinskas AJ, et al: Angiographic appearance of benign and malignant hepatic tumors in infants and children. AJR 1971, 113:61–69.
70. Mowat AP: Liver: Conjugated hyperbilirubinemia in infancy. *In* Rudolph AM, Hoffman JIE (eds): Pediatrics, 17th ed. Norwalk, CT, Appleton-Century-Crofts, 1982.
71. Newlin N, Silver TM, Stuck KJ, et al: Ultrasonic features of pyogenic liver abscesses. Radiology 1981, 139:155–159.
72. Ohi R, Koike N, Matsumoto Y, et al: Changes of intrahepatic bile duct dilatation after surgery for congenital dilatation of the bile duct. J Pediatr Surg 1985, 20:138–142.
73. Ohtomo K, Itai U, Yoshikawa K, et al: Hepatic tumors: Dynamic MR imaging. Radiology 1987, 163:27–31.
74. Pantoja E: Angiography in liver hemangioma. AJR 1968, 104:874–879.
75. Patriquin HB, DiPietro M, Barber FE: Sonography of thickened gallbladder wall: Causes in children. AJR 1983, 141:57–60.
76. Pereyra R, Andrassy RJ, Mahour GH: Management of massive hepatic hemangiomas in infants and children: A review of 13 cases. Pediatrics 1982, 70:254–258.
77. Preimesberger KF, Goldberg ME: Acute liver abscess in chronic granulomatous disease of child-

hood. Radiology 1974, 110:147–150.

78. Pueyo I, Guzman A, Fernandez F, et al: Liver abscess complicating embolization of focal nodular hyperplasia. AJR 1979, 133:740–742.
79. Reuter K, Raptopoulos VD, Catelmo N, et al: The diagnosis of choledochal cyst by ultrasound. Radiology 1980, 136:437–438.
80. Rogers JV, Mack LA, Freeny PC, et al: Hepatic focal nodular hyperplasia: Angiography, CT, sonography and scintigraphy. AJR 1981, 137:983–990.
81. Ros PR, Goodman ZD, Ishak KG, et al: Mesenchymal hamartoma of the liver: Radiologic-pathologic correlation. Radiology 1986, 158:619–624.
82. Ros PR, Olmsted WW, Dachman AH, et al: Undifferentiated (embryonal) sarcoma of the liver: Radiologic-pathologic correlation. Radiology 1986, 161:141–145.
83. Rosch J, Mayer BS, Campbell JR, et al: "Vascular" benign liver cyst in children: Report of two cases. Radiology 1978, 126:747–750.
84. Rosenbaum DM, Mindell HJ: Ultrasonographic findings in mesenchymal hamartoma of the liver. Radiology 1981, 138:425–427.
85. Rosenfield N, Griscom NT: Choledochal cysts: Roentgenographic findings. Radiology 1975, 114:113–119.
86. Rosoff L: New developments in viral hepatitis. Bull Mason Clin 1985–1986, 39:157–166.
87. Ruymann FD, Raney RB, Crist WM, et al: Rhabdomyosarcoma of the biliary tree in childhood. A report from the intergroup rhabdomyosarcoma study. Cancer 1985, 56:575–580.
88. Schey WL, Pinsky WM, Lischutz HS, et al: Hepatic duct diverticulum simulating a choledochal cyst. AJR 1977, 128:318–320.
89. Scoazec J-Y, Marche C, Girard P-M, et al: Peliosis hepatis and sinusoidal dilatation during infection by the human immunodeficiency virus (HIV). An ultrastructural study. Am J Pathol 1988, 131:38–47.
90. Shackelford GD, Kirks DR: Neonatal hepatic calcification secondary to transplacental infection. Radiology 1977, 122:753–757.
91. Shapiro P, Ikeda RM, Ruebner BH, et al: Multiple hepatic tumors and peliosis hepatis in Fanconi's anemia treated with androgens. Am J Dis Child 1977, 131:1104–1106.
92. Sheu JC, Sung JL, Chen DS, et al: Ultrasonography of small hepatic tumors using high-resolution linear-array real-time instruments. Radiology 1984, 150:797–802.
93. Shirkhoda A, Lopez-Berestein G, Holbert JM, et al: Hepatosplenic fungal infection: CT and pathologic evaluation after treatment with liposomal amphotericin B[1]. Radiology 1986, 159:349–353.
94. Simon DM, Krause R, Galambos JT: Peliosis hepatis in a patient with marasmus. Gastroenterology 1988, 95:805–809.
95. Stanley P, Grinnell VS, Stanton RE, et al: Therapeutic embolization of infantile hepatic hemangioma with polyvinyl alcohol. AJR 1983, 141:1047–1051.
96. Stanley P, Hall TR, Woolley MM, et al: Mesenchymal hamartomas of the liver in childhood: Sonographic and CT findings. AJR 1986, 147:1035–1038.
97. Takayasu K, Moriyama N, Shima Y, et al: Atypical radiographic findings in hepatic cavernous hemangioma: Correlation with histologic features. AJR 1986, 146:1149–1153.
98. Tsuchida Y, Ishida M: Dilatation of the intrahepatic bile ducts in congenital cystic dilatation of the common bile duct. Surgery 1971, 69:776–780.
99. Van Schil P, Mortelmans L, Schoofs E, et al: Peliosis hepatis associated with liver and retroperitoneal abscesses. Digestion 1988, 41:55–60.
100. Voinchet O, Degott C, Scozaec J-Y: Peliosis hepatis, nodular regenerative hyperplasia of the liver, and light-chain deposition in a patient with Waldenström's macroglobulinemia. Gastroenterology 1988, 95:482–486.
101. Vorse HB, Smith EI, Luckstead EF, et al: Hepatic hemangiomatosis of infancy. Am J Dis Child 1983, 137:672–673.
102. Weinberger E, Blumhagen JD, Odell JM: Gallbladder contraction in biliary atresia. AJR 1987, 149:401–402.
103. Welch TJ, Sheedy PF, Johnson CM, et al: Radiographic characteristics of benign liver tumors: Focal nodular hyperplasia and hepatic adenoma. Radiographics 1985, 5:673–682.
104. Welch TJ, Sheedy II PF, Johnson CM, et al: Focular nodular hyperplasia and hepatic adenoma: Comparison of the angiography, CT, US and scintigraphy. Radiology 1985, 156:593–595.
105. Wiener WN, Parulekar SG: Scintigraphy and ultrasonography of hepatic hemangioma. Radiology 1979, 132:149–152.
106. Williams AG, Sheward SE: Ultrasound appearance of biliary rhabdomyosarcoma. J Clin Ultrasound 1988, 14:63–65.
107. Yousefzadeh DK, Lupetin AR, Jackson JH: The radiographic signs of fatty liver. Radiology 1979, 131:351–355.

CHAPTER 15

Pancreas

LORIANN D. FORBUSH

Sonography is currently the diagnostic procedure of choice for the examination of children with symptoms of pancreatic disease.[24] Real-time ultrasound of the pancreas in infants and children is easily performed, and in most cases successful. In a large study by Coleman and coworkers, the entire gland was adequately visualized in more than 86% of cases.[6] The pancreas is more easily seen in children because most are lean and have a large left hepatic lobe, which serves as an excellent sonic window for visualizing the pancreas.[28] Sonography affords the ability to image from multiple directions and to follow the course of the common bile duct accurately. Because it is free of the hazards of ionizing radiation, it is the study of choice for children. Less expensive than computed tomography (CT), sonography affords bedside imaging of critically ill patients. The drawbacks of pancreatic sonography include technically unsatisfactory studies due to obesity or excessive bowel gas, and limited scanning surfaces when surgical dressings or ostomy sites are present.[1]

Sonographic Technique

Relevant clinical laboratory tests for the pancreas are presented in Chapter 6.

Patient Preparation

Various sonographic studies have been undertaken to determine the most valuable technique for examining the pancreas. It is well-known that visualization can be limited by bowel gas in the mid-abdomen. Because gas is a major culprit, it is helpful to have the patient fast.[16] A general time guideline for fasting in pediatric patients is 3 hours for infants younger than 1 year, 6 hours for patients 1 to 5 years, and 12 hours for patients older than 5 years. Some investigators have found that instead of a strict fast, hydration is useful for producing high-quality examinations. Other investigators have used glucagon to reduce peristaltic activity.[4] Presently, no single technical procedure is universally accepted. An adequate study is most dependent on clearly visualizing patient anatomy.[20]

Scanning Techniques

Except for the smaller size of most of the abdominal organs in children, the anatomic features as visualized with sonography are similar to those in adults. Most infants and children can cooperate long enough for the examination to be completed if they are handled with the appropriate combination of patience and firmness.[10]

Standard Examination

A standard examination of the pancreas includes transverse and longitudinal scans of the supine patient. The transverse scans may require some initial survey to determine the exact position of the gland, as it generally lies oblique in the middle portion of the body, with the head lower then the body and tail.[1] Longitudinal scans should be oriented to the true longitudinal axis of the pancreas, as determined by the transverse scans. It is not uncommon to examine the patient in different positions (i.e., prone, upright, decubitus) in order to adequately visualize the pancreas.[22] This is particularly important in the presence of disease, as the scan must demonstrate the lesion's relationship to surrounding pancreatic structure and adjacent organs. Another helpful technique is to use the water-filled duodenum to outline the pancreas. The patient is given approximately 16 ounces of water, and the progress of the water into the duodenum is checked periodically by the sonographer. When the duodenum is appropriately distended, the patient is repositioned until the water-filled duodenum outlines the area of the pancreas that is of interest. A fluid-filled stomach may also be helpful to outline the pancreatic tail. This technique however, has several drawbacks: (1) many patients suffer severe nausea and large amounts of water may induce vomiting; (2) fluid filling is contraindicated for fasting patients receiving intravenous fluid; and, (3) this method can be very time consuming.

TECHNICAL CONSIDERATIONS

During pancreatic sonography, the gain control is usually at settings comparable to those used for scanning the liver. Determination of the normal pancreatic sonographic pattern is based on a comparison to the liver parenchymal pattern.[1] In children the normal pancreatic parenchyma is relatively homogeneous, with even, high- and medium-level echo distribution. This is in contrast to the irregular echo texture, or "cobblestone" appearance, considered normal for adults.[13] The normal pancreas is similar to or more echogenic than the liver parenchyma. Vascular structures abound in this area and should have a clearly echo-free pattern and not be filled in by a too high gain setting. The transducer frequency selections should be made to obtain the highest resolution with adequate penetration.[1]

Normal Anatomy

A sonographic pancreatic study should pay particular attention to surrounding vascular landmarks, to the gland's shape and size, and to delineation of the pancreatic duct.[24]

Attention to the surrounding vascular landmarks may be necessary to identify this rather small structure.[1] Primary vascular landmarks include (1) the splenic vein, which can be seen lying inferior and posterior to the tail of the pancreas (transverse scans) and running left to right from the splenic hilus to the portal vein confluence; (2) the superior mesenteric vein, located posterior to the junction of the head and body of the pancreas and best seen on the sagittal scans; (3) the inferior vena cava, which passes posterior and slightly to the right of the pancreatic head; and, (4) the superior mesenteric artery, which travels inferiorly along the posterior aspect at the junction of the head and body of the pancreas and anterior to the uncinate process. (Figs. 15-1, 15-2).

Weil and colleagues established four categories for the shape of the pancreas: (1) similar-sized head and tail separated by a thin body; (2) uniform thickness of head, body, and tail; (3) disproportionate amount of tissue in the head; and, (4) disproportionate amount of tissue in the tail. In children, the pancreatic head and tail are usually similar in size and are separated by a thinner body.[30]

Sonographic studies should also give specific attention to the pancreas' size. The maximum anteroposterior (AP) diameters of the head, body, and tail are measured on transverse images obtained by

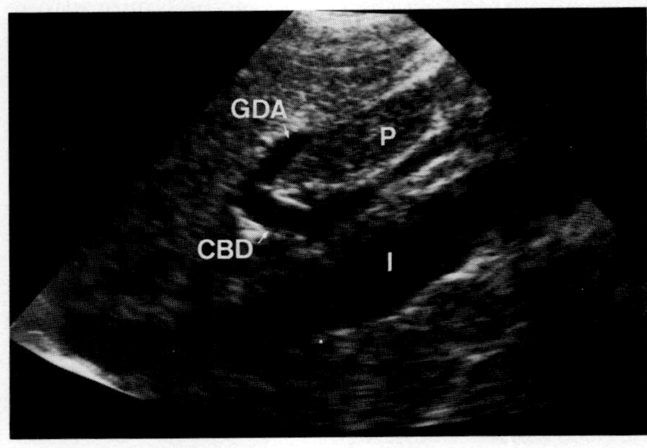

FIGURE 15-1. Longitudinal sonogram of a normal pancreas (P) and surrounding vasculature, gastroduodenal artery (GDA), common bile duct (CBD), and inferior vena cava (I).

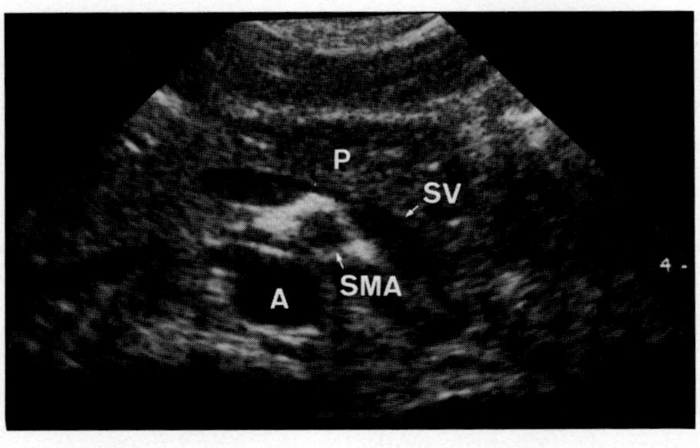

FIGURE 15-2. Transverse sonogram of a normal pancreas (P), aorta (A), superior mesenteric artery (SMA), and splenic vein (SV).

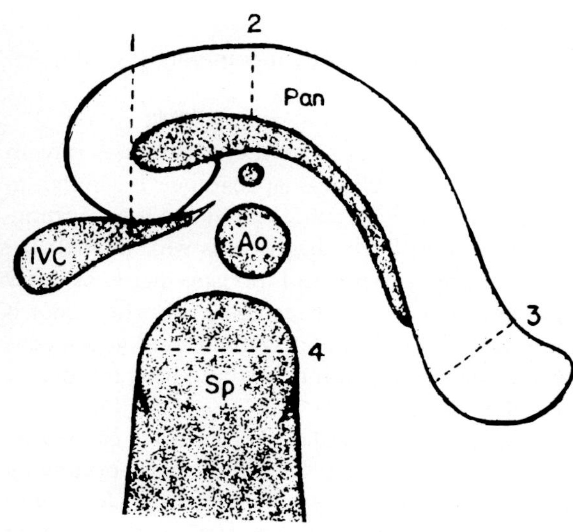

FIGURE 15-3. Diagram of a normal child's pancreas: 1, maximum AP diameter of the head of the pancreas; 2, maximum AP diameter of the body; 3, maximum AP diameter of the tail; 4, widest transverse dimension of the lumbar vertebral body (IVC, inferior vena cava; A, aorta; Pan, pancreas; S, spine). (From Siegel MJ, Martin KW, Worthington JL: Normal and abnormal pancreas in children: US studies. Radiology 1987, 165:15–18.)

angling the transducer to visualize more parenchyma (Fig. 15-3). The entire gland can usually be seen in one image if it is oriented transversely across the abdomen, but often it lies oblique to some degree, with the tail more craniad than the head and body, in which case it may be necessary to obtain several images to demonstrate the entire gland.

Pancreatic measurements can be compared with the patient's age and classified into one of five categories: younger than 1 month, 1 month to 1 year, 1 to 5 years, 5 to 10 years, and 10 to 19 years. In a study by Siegel and coworkers, the correlation of pancreatic dimensions with age was equivalent to or higher than the correlation with height, weight, or body surface area. Because age is more easily determined, it has been used to construct the normal tables. Mean pancreatic dimensions as a function of age are shown in Table 15-1.

The pancreatic duct is not always seen in normal patients. Usually appearing as a single echogenic line less than 1 mm, it can be located in the pancreatic body in a plane cephalad to the splenic vein.[24]

TABLE 15-1. Normal dimensions of the pancreas as a function of age

		MAXIMUM ANTEROPOSTERIOR DIMENSIONS OF PANCREAS (cm ± 1 STANDARD DEVIATION)		
PATIENT AGE	PATIENTS (N)	HEAD	BODY	TAIL
<1 mo	15	1.0 ± 0.4	0.6 ± 0.2	1.0 ± 0.4
1 mo–1 yr	23	1.5 ± 0.5	0.8 ± 0.3	1.2 ± 0.4
1–5 yr	49	1.7 ± 0.3	1.0 ± 0.2	1.8 ± 0.4
5–10 yr	69	1.6 ± 0.4	1.0 ± 0.3	1.8 ± 0.4
10–19 yr	117	2.0 ± 0.5	1.1 ± 0.3	2.0 ± 0.4

(Data from Siegel MJ, Martin KW, Worthington JL: Normal and abnormal pancreas in children: US studies. Radiology 1987, 165:15–18.)

Abnormal Findings

Tumors

Pancreatic neoplasms are uncommon in young persons.[14]

Carcinoma. Carcinoma of the pancreas is rare in children but its clinical appearance is similar to that in adults.[13] Pancreatic carcinoma is a nonfunctioning tumor. Early diagnosis is very difficult because of the variety and nonspecificity of early signs and symptoms.[26] Because of this, the tumor is often large by the time it is discovered and metastasis to the liver, lymph nodes, and lung frequently is already established.[13]

Sonographic appearance. Pancreatic carcinoma usually appears as a localized, space-occupying lesion[31] that is hypoechoic in comparison to the homogeneous texture of the normal pancreas. Focal enlargement is also an important sonographic clue. Lesions smaller than 2 cm are often difficult to detect, especially if they create only minor acoustic alterations.[5] Although identifying the primary pancreatic tumor is critically important, in many cases, ultrasound can provide additional information about the relative stage of the patient's disease. This can be accomplished by identifying changes in the upper abdominal organs and blood vessels as a result of local invasion and regional dissemination by the tumor. Ultrasound or CT can identify the mass, but the final diagnosis is usually made histologically.[22]

Islet Cell Tumors. Approximately two thirds of islet cell tumors are functional, producing a hormone that provokes the clinical suspicion of tumor early in the course of disease. Because of this, most islet cell tumors are usually quite small when first detected. The diagnosis is usually made by analyzing serum hormone levels. Therefore, in these cases, diagnostic imaging is used to localize rather than to diagnose.

The remaining third of islet cell tumors are nonfunctional. Owing to lack of hormone secretion, they remain silent until they grow large enough to produce a palpable mass that obstructs the biliary system or the gastrointestinal tract.

Sonographic appearance. Sonographically an islet cell tumor is a well-circumscribed, anechoic mass. It is important to search for metastatic disease, which may be the only reliable sign of malignancy. Sonography can be uniquely helpful in identifying the islet cell tumors in the operating room when all other modalities have failed. Direct pancreatic scanning can aid in tumor localization.[5]

Insulinomas. Insulinoma, another tumor that occurs in childhood, is round, firm, and encapsulated and 75% of the time is located in the body or tail of the pancreas. Ectopic adenomas are rare, and most are benign.[26]

Sonographic appearance. Insulinomas appear as relatively anechoic well-circumscribed masses.[20]

Lymphoma. Lymphoma of the pancreas is a rare neoplasm that accounts for only 0.16% of pancreatic malignancies.[2] The involvement of the pancreas in a lymphatic process is usually secondary to primary lymph node disease.[23] The neoplasm can be located anywhere in the pancreas, and symptoms depend on anatomic location.

The diagnosis of pancreatic lymphoma should be considered in several clinical situations: when a pancreatic mass develops in a patient known to have disseminated lymphoma, when fine-needle aspiration biopsy of a pancreatic mass reveals lymphocytes without evidence of carcinoma, and when a pancreatic mass is associated with chylous ascites.[9]

Sonographic appearance. Focal infiltration of the pancreas in lymphoma appears sonographically as large, solitary, hypoechoic space-occupying lesions. Differential diagnosis is facilitated by the presence of paraaortic lymphomas, and the fact that the underlying disease is usually obvious at the time the pancreatic lesions are demonstrated (Figs. 15-4–15-6).[31]

Fine-Needle Aspiration

Ultrasound-guided fine-needle aspiration biopsy is a simple and reliable method of establishing or excluding malignancy in intraabdominal mass lesions.[11] Indications for this procedure are the presence of one or more sonographically demonstrated masses and the need to establish whether they are malignant or benign.[18] Fine-needle aspiration is somewhat less successful with pancreatic tumors than with other tumors. Reported results vary widely: sensitivity ranges between 63% and 100%. The lower success rate may be due to the fact that

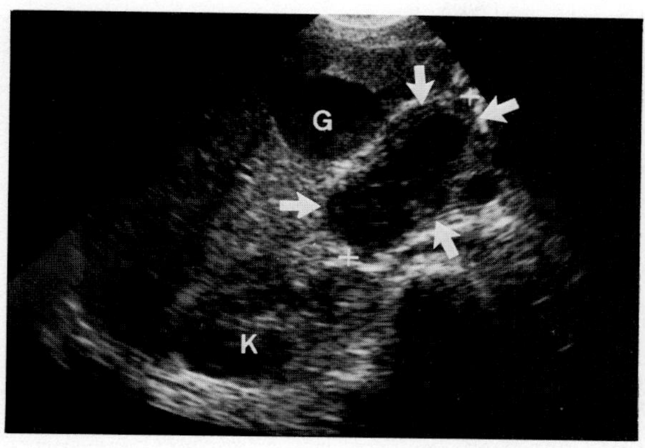

FIGURE 15-4. Transverse sonogram of pancreatic lymphoma (*arrows*), gallbladder (G), and kidney (K).

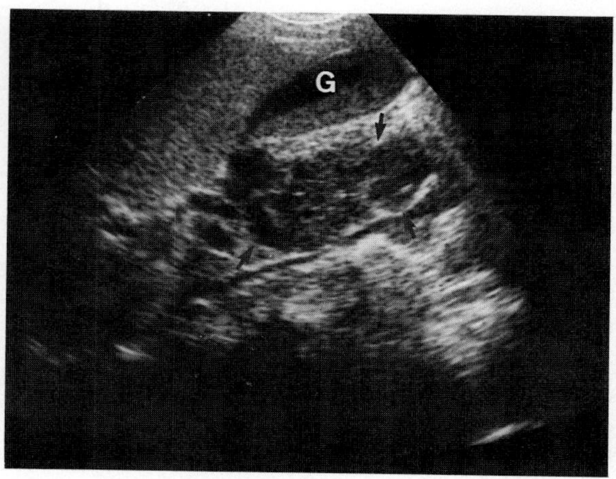

FIGURE 15-5. Longitudinal sonogram of the patient in Figure 15-4 demonstrates the lymphoma (*arrows*) and gallbladder (G).

the tumors are often masked by associated pancreatitis; many tumors are small, and in some cases, the mass may not be visualized and its presence must be inferred from duct strictures.[12]

Using sonographic guidance to perform fine-needle aspiration biopsy allows the needle to be directed precisely into the tumor and away from major blood vessels or the dilated pancreatic duct.[25] Many real-time ultrasound machines are equipped with a built-in guidance system (for a more detailed description of equipment and technique, see Chapter 20). A needle is inserted through a guide attached to the transducer, making it visible along a fixed path that is superimposed on the real-time image. When the lesion is large or contains necrotic or cystic areas, it is important that the samples be taken from several solid areas as well as the rim. Like all invasive procedures, needle aspiration biopsy carries a certain amount of risk, although with fine needles the risk is small.[18]

Some investigators have found that dual sonography and fluoroscopy during fine-needle aspiration biopsy provide complementary information. Sonographic imaging demonstrates the mass boundaries and also the internal composition of the tumor and guides sampling to the appropriate areas. Fluoroscopy, combined with the duct opacification, accurately identifies stricture position and clearly and continuously shows needle tip position. Combining the two modalities minimizes guidance errors.[12]

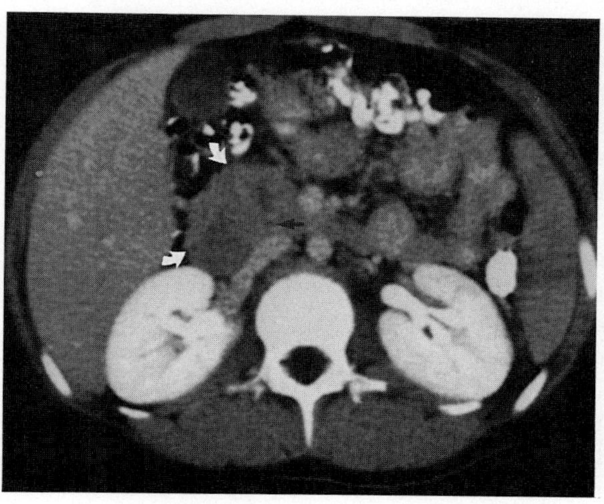

FIGURE 15-6. CT of patient presented in Figure 15-4 and 15-5 demonstrates lymphoma (*arrows*).

TRUE PANCREATIC CYSTS

True pancreatic cysts are fluid-filled structures circumscribed by an epithelial lining. The cysts range in size from microscopic to 3 to 5 cm. They can be congenital or acquired.

Congenital Cysts. Congenital cysts of the pancreas are uncommon but can occur singly or in groups.[1] The cysts associated with polycystic renal disease are small and asymptomatic.[14] Congenital cysts also include dermoid cysts and fibrocystic disease.

Cystic fibrosis is a common inherited metabolic disorder of Caucasian children. The estimated incidence is approximately 1 in 2000 births.[10] Cystic fibrosis affects the exocrine glands in the lungs and gastrointestinal tract, which produce abnormal, highly viscous mucous.[15] Secretions precipitate or coagulate in small pancreatic ducts to form obstructive eosinophilic concretions. Fluid collects proximal to the obstruction and intrapancreatic pressure increases. Proximal distension of the ducts and acini leads to their degeneration and replacement by small cysts. Eventually, normal function is compromised and pancreatic insufficiency results.[19] Late changes include atrophy of glandular elements and replacement of the altered architecture by fibrosis.[13] The patient usually presents to the ultrasound laboratory with a previous diagnosis of cystic fibrosis; pancreatic involvement occurs later than pulmonary manifestations.

Ultrasound is a useful tool for evaluating the degree of pancreatic involvement. Sonographic abnormalities have been reported in 95% of patients older than 5 years. Increased echogenicity and decreased size are the most frequent findings.[7,19,21,33] It is postulated that inspissated mucus plugs account for the hyperechogenicity, although chronic fibrotic changes associated with concurrent chronic pancreatitis may contribute to the changes noted.

Acquired Cysts. There are three classes of acquired cysts: retention, parasitic, and neoplastic cysts. A retention cyst is a distension of the pancreatic duct, usually caused by pancreatitis. Parasitic cysts of the pancreas have not been reported in the United States[1] but are most common in countries where sheep and cattle grazing is carried out with the help of dogs. Increased worldwide travel and immigration have resulted in dissemination of many diseases that formerly were confined to large but localized endemic areas. Cysts begin as microscopic lesions and take 5 or more years to reach massive size. Most grow at a rate of 0.25 to 1.00 cm per year and remain asymptomatic for 5 to 10 years. After the cysts are present about 6 months, daughter cells develop within them, arising from the germinal epithelium. Vascular thrombosis and infarction can occur when the cysts impinge on blood vessels. Cysts may rupture, and escaping fluid can produce a massive anaphylactic reaction.[17]

Cystic neoplasms are divided into two groups, microcystic adenomas and macrocystic adenomas. The former are benign and contain cysts that produce glycogen. Macrocystic adenomas, measuring larger than 2 cm in diameter, have malignant potential. Both of these cystic neoplasms are most common in adult women.

Sonographic appearance. The sonographic appearance of polycystic and retention cysts is similar to that of other cystic structures. The cyst usually appears as an anechoic mass devoid of internal echoes. The walls appear fairly sharp, with prominent through-transmission deep to the mass, indicating the cyst's fluid content.[20] Dermoid cysts have a large range of sonographic appearances, from totally anechoic to echogenic, depending on the internal component distribution.[10]

In patients with cystic fibrosis, the most dramatic feature is a striking increase in the echogenicity of the pancreas. In some younger patients, it has been reported that small cystic degenerations could be observed in the pancreatic tail. The echogenicity of the pancreas reportedly becomes more obvious with increasing patient age. A secondary finding is a decrease in pancreatic diameter in all parts of the organ.[27]

The sonographic findings associated with parasitic cysts include discrete simple cysts (with or without calcification), multiple cysts (the daughter cysts appear dense early on), honeycomb cysts (fluid collection with septa), and solid-looking cysts. Most types of cysts have an oval or spherical shape and regular walls.[17] Cystic neoplasms usually appear as anechoic masses with easily visible internal septations.[5]

PANCREATITIS

Pancreatitis is significantly less common in children than in adults but is not all that rare. Pediatric pancreatitis may have a variety of causes: (1)

trauma (blunt abdominal trauma secondary to childhood accident, motor vehicle accidents, and child abuse); (2) infection (usually viral, such as mumps or mononucleosis); (3) toxicity (secondary to such drugs as prednisone and L-asparaginase); (4) heredity (an autosomal dominant disorder beginning in childhood); and (5) idiopathic. The most common of these is blunt abdominal trauma.[13] To distinguish between the possible causes of pancreatitis it is important to obtain a detailed patient history.[26]

Acute Pancreatitis. Acute pancreatic inflammation causes the escape of pancreatic enzymes from the acinar cells into surrounding tissues.[1] Acute pancreatitis can usually be diagnosed with combined clinical and laboratory information without requiring pancreatic imaging.[29] However, diagnostic imaging may be necessary when a wide variety of clinical symptoms, possible causes, and complications cause confusion. The examination may be ordered to explain abdominal pain or elevated enzyme levels.[5] The use of sonography enables earlier diagnosis of acute pancreatitis in children with acute or chronic pain.[26] Diagnostic imaging is also useful in defining the extent of the disease in the patient with suspected complications such as necrotizing pancreatitis, hemorrhagic pancreatitis, pseudocyst formation, and superimposed infection.[29]

Sonographic appearance. The primary sonographic appearance in acute pancreatitis is of an enlarged, edematous gland that is less echogenic than the liver parenchyma (Figs. 15-7–15-9). These characteristics are most obvious during the first hours after an acute attack.[1] A dilated pancreatic duct is another indication of pancreatitis.[24] The pancreas' size and echo pattern usually return to normal as the disease resolves. The entire pancreas is usually involved, but sometimes only portions are affected,

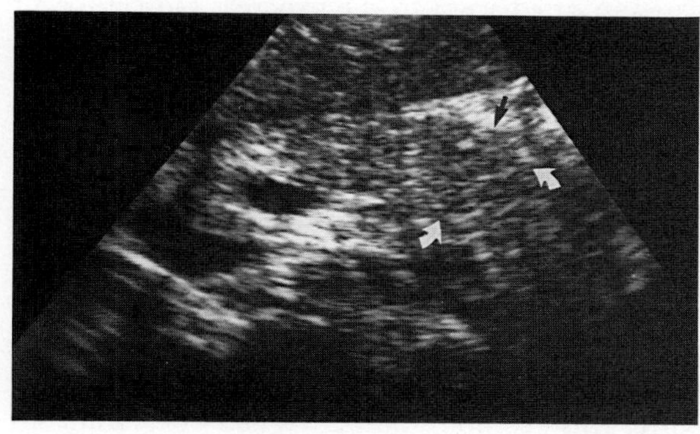

FIGURE 15-7. Transverse sonogram of an enlarged edematous pancreatic tail *(arrows)* on a patient with pancreatitis.

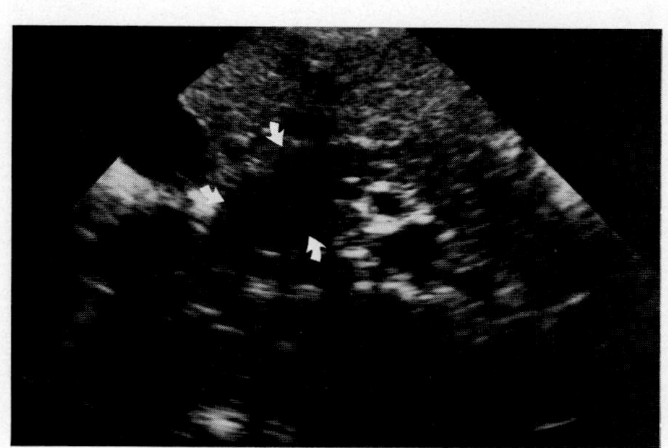

FIGURE 15-8. Transverse sonogram of an enlarged pancreatic head *(arrows)* in a patient with pancreatitis.

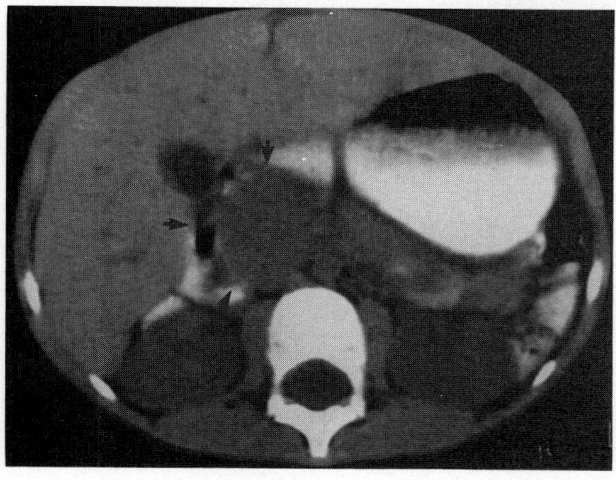

FIGURE 15-9. CT scan of patient in Figure 15-8 demonstrates an enlarged pancreatic head *(arrows)*.

particularly in pancreatitis caused by trauma.[1] Follow-up examinations may help to establish the diagnosis of pancreatitis by showing the pancreas' shrinking.[24]

Complications of Acute Pancreatitis. After an episode of acute pancreatitis, a range of pathologic changes may develop in the gland and peripancreatic region.[32]

Pseudocysts. The best-known complication of pancreatitis is pseudocyst formation. Pseudocysts can cause pain, bowel or biliary obstruction, and can become infected.[5] Pseudocysts are usually located in or adjacent to the pancreas but can occur anywhere in the abdomen or pelvis. Occasionally, pseudocysts may even extend into the mediastinum.[10] Serial examinations are useful for monitoring enlargement and regression of pseudocysts. The majority of pseudocysts resolve spontaneously within 4 to 12 weeks, but those that develop mature, fibrous capsules are unlikely to be reabsorbed spontaneously. Recurrent abdominal pain, elevated serum amylase, and intermittent nausea and vomiting are common clinical symptoms consistent with this complication.[26] When percutaneous drainage of the pseudocyst is indicated, sonographic guidance may be used.

Percutaneous external drainage (PED) is usually performed in the radiology department under sterile conditions with intravenous sedation. The puncture is performed with an 18- or 20-gauge plastic-sheathed catheter, and the aspirate is sent for appropriate laboratory analysis. After the liquid has been aspirated, the initial catheter is removed and a pigtail catheter is inserted and left in place through which contrast medium is injected into the pseudocyst to identify any possible communication with the duct of Wirsung. The patient receives extended intravenous broad-spectrum antibiotics for approximately 10 to 14 days. The catheter is removed when no further drainage occurs and disappearance of the cavity has been confirmed by ultrasound, CT, and fistulogram. Because children's pseudocysts often have a different pathogenesis, they may resolve more rapidly than the more common adult pancreatitis of biliary or alcoholic origin. Children's pseudocysts are less likely to recur following PED.[3] PED often eliminates the need for surgery. Therefore, it is helpful to use sonography for follow-up assessment after PED to monitor possible reaccumulation of fluid in the pseudocyst (Figs. 15-10, 15-11).

SONOGRAPHIC APPEARANCE. Pseudocysts are usually anechoic masses, with a sharp back wall and increased through-transmission. They may be single or multiple (Figs. 15-12–15-14).[5] Pseudocysts

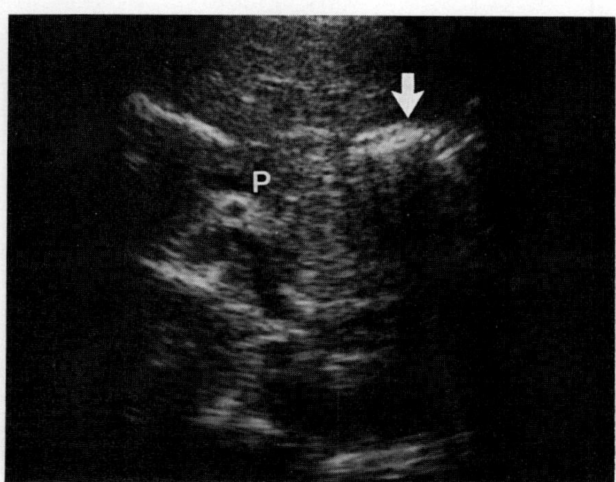

FIGURE 15-10. Transverse sonogram of the pancreas after pseudocyst drainage demonstrating the catheter *(arrows)* and pancreas (P).

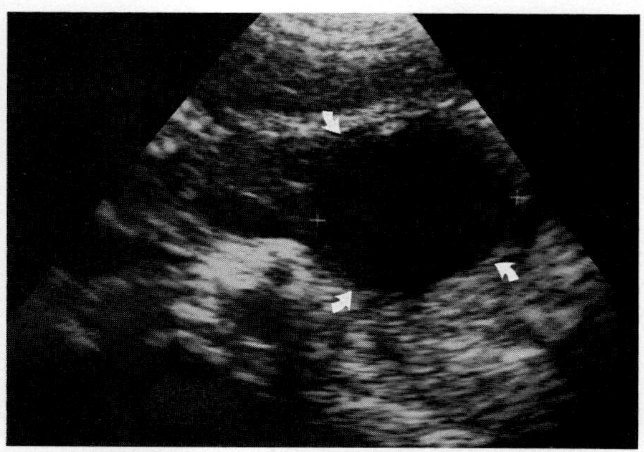

FIGURE 15-11. Transverse sonogram of reaccumulation of fluid in the pseudocyst *(arrows)* in the patient in Figure 15-10.

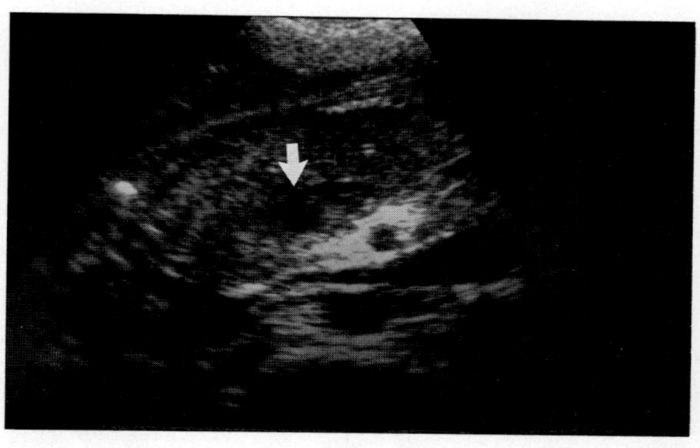

FIGURE 15-12. Transverse sonogram of a very small pseudocyst (*arrow*).

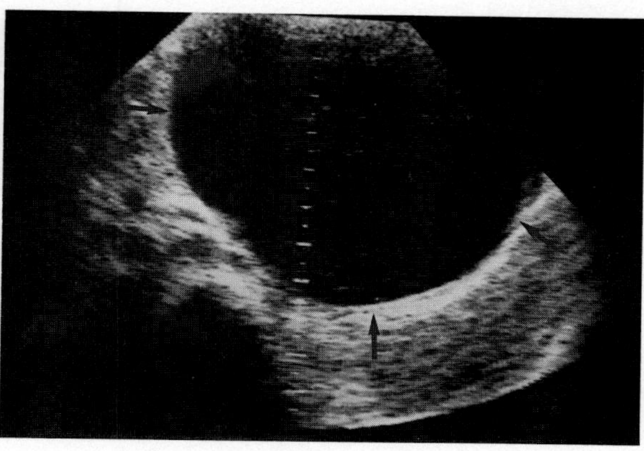

FIGURE 15-13. Transverse sonogram of a large single pseudocyst (*arrows*).

sometimes contain internal echoes emanating from pus and cellular debris.[10]

Hemorrhage. Intrapancreatic hemorrhage with acute pancreatitis results from disruption of one or more pancreatic blood vessels. This is uncommon, but is a potentially lethal complication that may produce large pancreatic hematoma.[32]

SONOGRAPHIC APPEARANCE. Sonographically, hemorrhagic pancreatitis appears as an inhomogeneous mass. Initially, acute hemorrhage into the pancreas may appear anechoic, but it becomes moderately echogenic as organization occurs.[10]

Phlegmon. A phlegmon is a solid inflammatory mass that may develop following acute pancreatitis. Comprised of necrotic tissue mixed with inflammatory exudate and tissue edema,[26] phlegmons may resolve spontaneously whenever the necrotic process is not progressive. With more severe episodes of acute pancreatitis, a necrotizing process may predominate and provoke further complications.[32] The patient is also at risk for developing a pancreatic abscess by bacterial seeding into necrotic tissue.[26]

SONOGRAPHIC APPEARANCE. A phlegmon appears as an anechoic mass in the pancreatic bed. Clinical history plus sonographic findings usually leads to the correct diagnosis (Figs. 15-15, 15-16).[20]

Abscess. Abscess formation is more likely to occur in severe cases of pancreatitis with extensive necrosis. Marked by spiking fevers, chills, and a recurrence of abdominal pain 10 to 14 days after the initial episode, drainage is required in all cases, since untreated, mortality is usually 100%.[26]

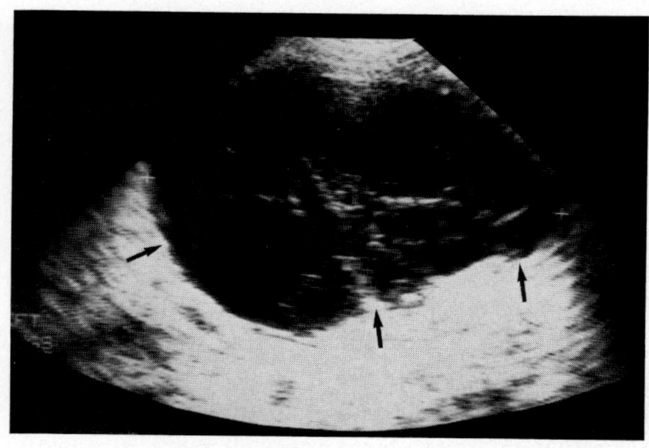

FIGURE 15-14. Longitudinal sonogram of a large septate pseudocyst (*arrows*).

Pancreatic abscesses can arise from different sources. A pancreatic phlegmon may develop into an abscess when the necrotic pancreatic and peripancreatic tissues are invaded by infection. An abscess can also occur in a pseudocyst in much the same way. Terminology can be confusing here because the infected pseudocyst is sometimes considered a different entity and not called an abscess.

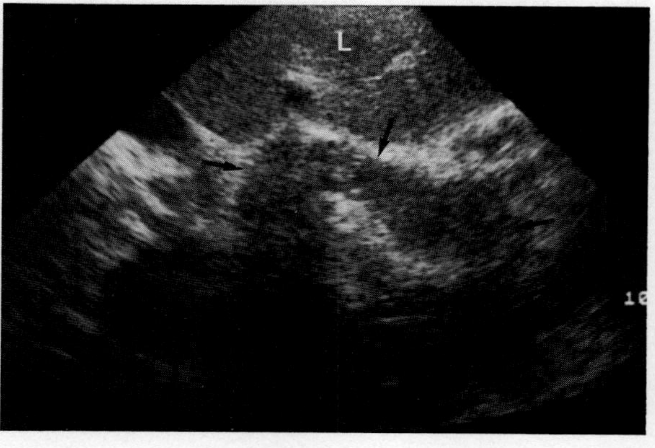

Figure 15-15. Transverse sonogram of a pancreatic phlegmon *(arrows)* and the liver (L).

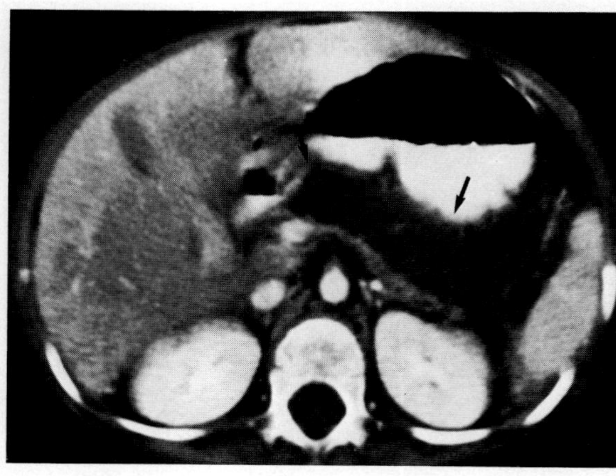

Figure 15-16. CT of the patient in Figure 15-15 demonstrates a pancreatic phlegmon *(arrows)*.

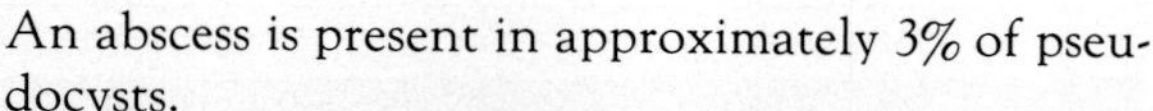

An abscess is present in approximately 3% of pseudocysts.

Air can be a notable diagnostic criterion for pancreatic inflammation. Air appears within abscesses in 30% to 60% of cases. Air within the pancreatic bed can be produced by a pancreatic abscess with gas-forming organisms or from a fistulous communication with a hollow viscus. The most common site for pancreaticoenteric fistula is the transverse colon at the splenic flexure. Fistulization is considered an ominous finding because it can facilitate seeding and may contribute to a secondary abscess.[5]

Sonographic appearance. Pancreatic abscess usually appears as a large anechoic mass in the pancreatic bed. Because pancreatic abscess cannot be differentiated sonographically from other anechoic pancreatic masses, it is important to combine the clinical history with the sonographic findings to make the correct diagnosis. The sonographic appearance of the abscess varies with the amount of suppurative material and debris. Abscess walls are usually thick, irregular, and echogenic. When air bubbles are present, the pancreatic area appears highly echogenic with occasional shadowing. The air may obscure visualization on sonograms.[20]

Chronic Pancreatitis. Chronic pancreatitis, or chronic relapsing pancreatitis, is a clinical condition caused by repeated attacks of acute pancreatitis, which cause fibrosis and destruction of pancreatic cells. In the late stages of the disease, pancreatic tissue fibrosis causes alternating areas of stricture and dilatation in the main duct system. In very late stages, calcifications can occur in the duct system.[1]

A majority of the childhood cases of chronic relapsing pancreatitis have a definite familial clustering pattern and represent examples of the disease called hereditary pancreatitis. Familial cases have an autosomal dominant inheritance pattern with complete penetrance but variable expressivity. More than 200 cases of proved or suspected hereditary pancreatitis have been reported. The likelihood that patients with "hereditary pancreatitis" will develop pancreatic carcinoma is increased, particularly for those with pancreatic calcifications.[26]

Sonographic appearance. Sonographically, in early stages of chronic pancreatitis, the pancreas is less echogenic than the normal liver parenchyma. This appearance is similar to that of acute pancreatitis. In advanced stages of chronic pancreatitis, the pancreas shrinks, develops irregular borders, and is more echogenic than usual with fibrosis. Calcifications and dilated ducts may also be present. The calcifications may be so pronounced and cause so much acoustic shadowing that pancreatic identification is difficult (Figs. 15-17–15-19).[1]

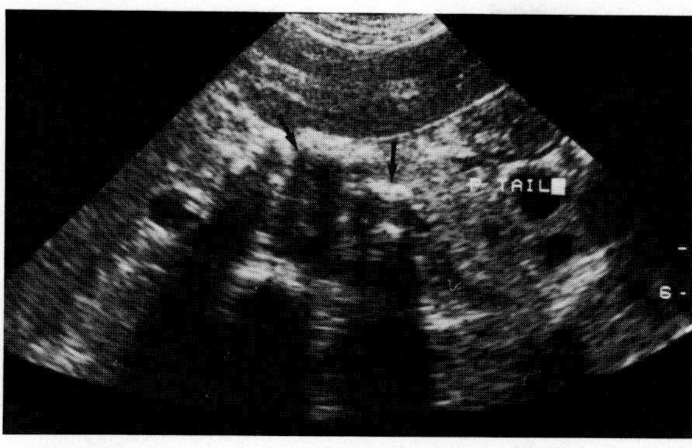

FIGURE 15-17. Transverse sonogram demonstrates pancreatic calcifications *(arrows)* in a patient with chronic pancreatitis.

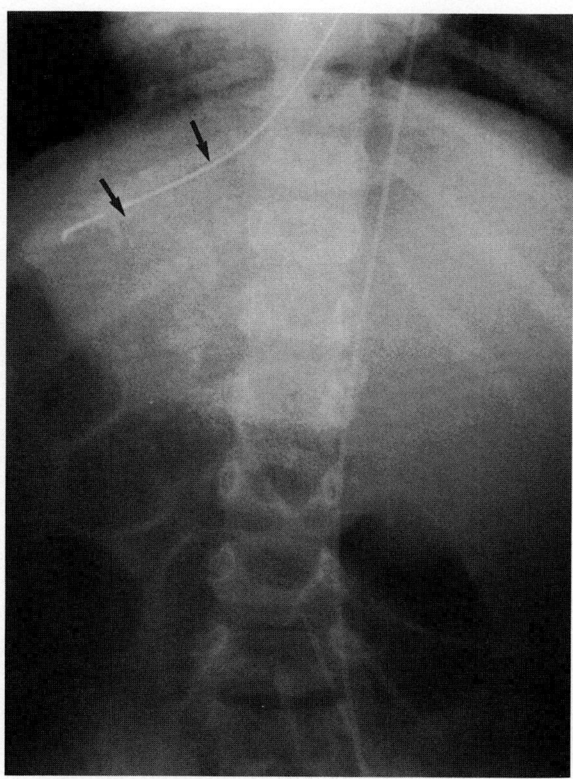

FIGURE 15-18. Abdominal radiograph of pancreatic calcifications *(arrows)* in the patient presented in Figure 15-17 with chronic pancreatitis.

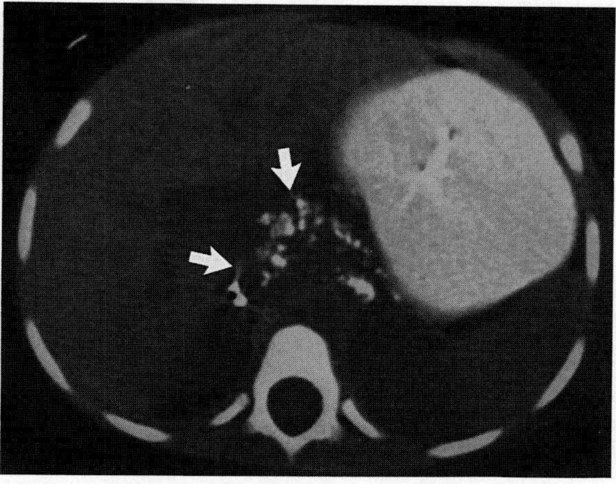

FIGURE 15-19. CT scan demonstrating pancreatic calcifications *(arrows)* on the same patient presented in Figures 15-17 and 15-18 with chronic pancreatitis.

Related Imaging Procedures

No single study always provides all necessary diagnostic information and appropriate utilization of each modality requires an understanding of its strengths and weaknesses.[29]

ABDOMINAL AND UPPER GASTROINTESTINAL RADIOGRAPHY

An abdominal radiograph may detect pancreatic calcifications or a mass in the pancreatic bed. Barium studies are more useful for identifying disease in the pancreatic head than in the body or tail. Such lesions may cause widening of the duodenal loop and displacement of the stomach or loops of bowel. These studies provide limited diagnostic results, and with the introduction of sonography and CT, their importance has decreased.[8]

COMPUTED TOMOGRAPHY

CT is excellent at detecting lesions of the pancreas.[5] High-resolution CT has a reported accuracy rate of nearly 100% for pancreatic carcinoma detection and 96% for acute and chronic pancreatitis. The advantages of CT include a more complete abdominal examination, which is not limited to bowel gas, clearer definition of anatomic relationships, and fewer unsatisfactory examinations.[29] The disadvantages of CT include ionizing radiation, difficulty in imaging the pancreas in a thin patient, and the necessity for transporting the patient to the CT suite.[1] It is very uncommon to have an inadequate pancreatic CT study unless the patient cannot tolerate swallowing contrast material or cannot tolerate a bolus of intravenous contrast material given during dynamic study.

ENDOSCOPIC RETROGRADE CHOLANGIOPANCREATOGRAPHY

Endoscopic retrograde cholangiopancreatography (ERCP) is best used as a secondary procedure when results of ultrasound or CT studies are ambiguous or technically inadequate.[5] ERCP is very helpful in evaluating subtle changes of the pancreatic duct and side branches. ERCP is considerably more expensive and invasive than sonography or CT[29] and must be performed by an experienced gastroenterologist. Successful cannulation of the pancreatic duct may be anatomically difficult.[5]

ARTERIOGRAPHY

The primary function of arteriography is to differentiate benign from malignant disease or tumors of the pancreas. With the widespread use of ultrasound, CT, and ERCP, the importance of arteriography has decreased, but it is still used to determine the resectability of pancreatic malignancies. Arteriographic indications that a tumor is not resectable include hepatic metastases, invasion or occlusion of the portal or superior mesenteric veins, and encasement in tumor of the celiac, superior mesenteric, hepatic, gastric, or intestinal arteries. Arteriography is also helpful in demonstrating small, highly vascular tumors that affect pancreatic endocrine function.[1] The major disadvantages of arteriography are its invasive nature and its ionizing radiation.

MAGNETIC RESONANCE IMAGING

Magnetic resonance imaging (MRI) is more useful for evaluating secondary changes, including liver metastases, biliary obstruction, and peripancreatic vessels. The quality of the pancreatic MRI images is limited by poor spatial resolution, suboptimal gastrointestinal contrast, and respiratory motion. A sparsity of retroperitoneal fat makes it difficult to distinguish bowel from pancreas on MRI. CT provides better spatial resolution than MRI and demonstrates abdominal contour as well as cystic spaces. The current role of MRI in evaluation of the pancreas is limited, but hopefully, new improvements in technology will lead to new advances in this area.[5]

References

1. Anderhub B: Manual of Abdominal Sonography. Baltimore, University Park Press, 1983.
2. Baylor SM: Cross-classification of survival characteristics of 5,000 cases of cancer of the pancreas. J Surg Oncol 1973, 4:355–358.
3. Bass J, Dilorenzo M, Desjardins JG: Blunt pancreatic injuries in children: The role of percutaneous external drainage in the treatment of pancreatic pseudocysts. J Pediatr Surg 1988, 23:721–724.
4. Bowie JD, MacMahon H: Improved techniques in pancreatic sonography. Semin Ultrasound 1980, 1:170–177.
5. Clark LR, Jaffe MH, Choyke PL, et al: Pancreatic imaging. Radiol Clin North Am 1985, 23:489–499.
6. Coleman BG, Arger PH, Rosenberg HK, et al: Grayscale sonographic assessment of pancreatitis in children. Radiology 1983, 146:145–150.
7. Daneman A, Gaskin K, Martin DJ, et al: Pancreatic changes in cystic fibrosis: CT and sonographic appearances. AJR 1983, 141:653–655.
8. Eisenberg R, Amberg J: Critical Diagnostic Pathway in Radiology: An Algorithmic Approach. Philadelphia, JB Lippincott, 1981.
9. Fischer MG, Kabakow G: Lymphoma of the pancreas. Mt Sinai J Med 1987, 54:423–426.
10. Fleisher AC, James AE Jr: Introduction to Diagnostic Sonography. New York, John Wiley & Sons, 1980.
11. Frable WJ: Fine-needle aspiration biopsy: A review. Human Pathol 1983, 14:9–28.
12. Hall-Craggs MA, Lees WR: Fine-needle aspiration biopsy: Pancreatic and biliary tumors. AJR 1986, 147(2):399–403.
13. Hayden KC Jr, Swischuk LE: Pediatric Ultrasonography. Baltimore, Williams & Wilkins, 1987.
14. Kissane JM: Pathology of infancy and childhood, 2nd ed. St. Louis, CV Mosby, 1975.
15. Kopleman H, Durie P, Gaskin K, et al: Pancreatic fluid secretion and protein hyperconcentration in cystic fibrosis. N Engl J Med 1985, 312:329–334.
16. McHugo JM, McKeown C, Brown MT, et al: Ultrasound findings in children with cystic fibrosis. Br J Radiology 1987, 60:137–141.
17. Mittelsteadt CA: Abdominal Ultrasound. New York, Churchill Livingstone, 1987.

18. Mok PM, Yeong ML: Ultrasound-guided fine-needle biopsy of abdominal mass lesions. NZ Med J 1986, 99:111–113.
19. Park RW, Grand RJ: Gastrointestinal manifestations of cystic fibrosis: A review. Gastroenterology 1981, 81:1143–1161.
20. Sarti D: Diagnostic Ultrasound: Text and Cases, 2nd ed. Chicago, Year Book Medical Publishers, 1987.
21. Schulman MH, Teele RL, Ataude AP, et al: Pancreatic cystosis in cystic fibrosis. Radiology 1986, 158:629–631.
22. Shawker TH, Garra BS, Hill MC, et al: The spectrum of sonographic findings in pancreatic carcinoma. J Ultrasound Med 1986, 5:169–177.
23. Shtamler B, Bickel A, Manor E: Primary lymphoma of the head of the pancreas. J Surg Oncol 1988, 38:48–51.
24. Siegel MJ, Martin KW, Worthington JL: Normal and abnormal pancreas in children: US studies. Radiology 1987, 165:15–18.
25. Sigel B, Machi J, Ramos JR: The role of imaging ultrasound during pancreatic surgery. Ann Surg 1984, 200:486–493.
26. Silverman A, Roy CC: Pediatric Clinical Gastroenterology, 3rd ed. St. Louis, CV Mosby, 1983.
27. Swobodnik W, Wolf A, Wechsler JG, et al: Ultrasound characteristics of the pancreas in children with cystic fibrosis. J Clin Ultrasound 1985, 13:469–474.
28. Teele RL: The pancreas, spleen, mesentery, and gastrointestinal tract. *In* Haller JO, Sneider M (eds): Ultrasound in Pediatrics. Chicago, Year Book Medical Publishers, 1980.
29. Van Dyke JA, Stanley RJ, Berland LL: Pancreatic Imaging. Ann Intern Med 1985, 102:212–217.
30. Weil F, Schraub A, Eisencher A, et al: Ultrasonography of the normal pancreas. Radiology 1977, 123:417–423.
31. Wernecke K, Peters PE, Galanski M: Pancreatic metastases: US evaluation. Radiology 1986, 160:399–402.
32. White EM, Wittenberg J, Mueller PR, et al: Pancreatic necrosis: CT manifestations. Radiology 1986, 160:399–402.
33. Wilson-Sharp RC, Irving HC, Brown RC, et al: Ultrasonography of the pancreas, liver, and biliary system in cystic fibrosis. Arch Dis Child 1984, 59:923–926.

CHAPTER 16

Gastrointestinal Tract

Barbara S. Reid

In most pediatric institutions, ultrasound is the examination of choice for pyloric stenosis and is useful in a gasless abdomen to locate and identify intraluminal or extraluminal fluid.[29] It has also been used to investigate clinical questions such as appendicitis and intussusception. Except for these specific indications, imaging of the gastrointestinal tract is not generally performed in children.[37] Bowel findings are usually incidental findings at abdominal examination for pain or palpable mass.

Stomach

Gastric Wall Thickness

Normal gastric mucosa measures some 2.5 to 3.5 mm (Table 16-1). The gastric wall's thickness can be assessed with the patient lying in the supine and right lateral decubitus positions before and after ingestion of fluid. For such a study, the child should fast (Fig. 16-1). With abnormalities associated with stomach wall thickening, the measurements and configuration remain unchanged when water is ingested.

A variety of abnormalities—eosinophilic gastritis, gastric ulcer, lymphoid hyperplasia, gastric hamartoma—have been reported to cause gastric wall thickening of 5 to 15 mm. In children with gastric ulcer disease, the thickening occurs in the anteropyloric mucosa. Moderate or generalized thickening up to 5 mm was present with lymphoid hyperplasia, varioliform gastritis, and Crohn's disease involving the stomach. The greatest amount of thickening (up to 10 mm) occurred in children with chronic granulomatous disease.[5,19,24,39]

Gastritis

Gastritis is an infrequent problem in children. As it is difficult to diagnose radiographically, the diagnosis is most often made by endoscopy. Lymphoid hyperplasia affecting the stomach is very rare in children and would be associated with lymphoid hyperplasia of the colon and rectum. Crohn's disease rarely affects the stomach of children. Children with chronic granulomatous disease of childhood or other neutropenic conditions appear to have the greatest amount of thickening of the stomach wall.

Pyloric Stenosis

Pyloric stenosis occurs with enlargement of the pyloric muscle, the channel between the stomach and the duodenum. Affected children present with vomiting between age 1 week and 6 months and may present with dehydration and vigorous gastric peristalsis, particularly during feeding. There is a higher incidence in males. An epigastric, olive-shaped, firm muscular tumor may be palpated by experienced observers. If such a tumor cannot be palpated, a sonographic examination is indicated.

It is preferred that children not take oral feedings for 2 to 3 hours before the examination, though feeding is not a contraindication to the ex-

TABLE 16-1. Gastric wall thickness

	NORMAL (mm)	ABNORMAL (mm)
Stomach	<2.5–3.5	5–15
Duodenum	<2–3	<3.5–4

amination. The patients are scanned in both the supine and right decubitus position. The transverse plane view demonstrates the long axis of the pylorus and the sagittal plane its transverse axis.

To identify the pylorus, scans should be made in the transverse plane, descending along the lesser curvature of the stomach through the left lobe of the liver, just to the right of the midline. The antrum of the stomach appears just anterior and to the left of the lumbar spine in the transverse plane and the pylorus is continuous with the stomach. If the tumor or pylorus is not well-visualized, the patient may drink some water to display the gastric lumen.

The mass presents a doughnut sign: an anechoic to hypoechoic muscle mass with a central lumen of increased echogenicity (Fig. 16-2A). Measurements should be made from the antrum of the stomach to the most distal portion of the identifiable channel (Fig. 16-2B–D). Various parameters have been published by several investigators: muscle thickness from the central lumen to the external muscle wall, muscle length from the gastric antrum, and total diameter of the pylorus (Table 16-2). In pyloric stenosis, the pyloric diameter should be 1.5 cm or greater, its muscle length should be 2 cm or greater and thickness at least 4 mm.

DUODENUM

Since sonography has been used to detect pyloric stenosis in vomiting children, other gastric outlet obstructions have been identified; specifically, malrotation with and without volvulus and duodenal stenosis. Sonographic examination through a fluid-filled stomach provides superb imaging.

The duodenum is best examined in the transverse and sagittal planes while the patient lies supine or in the right decubitus position.[8] With real-time instruments, fluid is seen in the first and second portions of the duodenum but does not pass beyond. The duodenum is noticeably dilated. In older children, duodenal and jejunal hematomas also have been associated with the fluid-filled bowel lumen and is indicative of a hematoma in the bowel wall. With congenital atresia, stenosis, or malrotation, the duodenal wall is not necessarily abnormally thickened but the lumen is markedly distended (Fig. 16-3).[18,23,34]

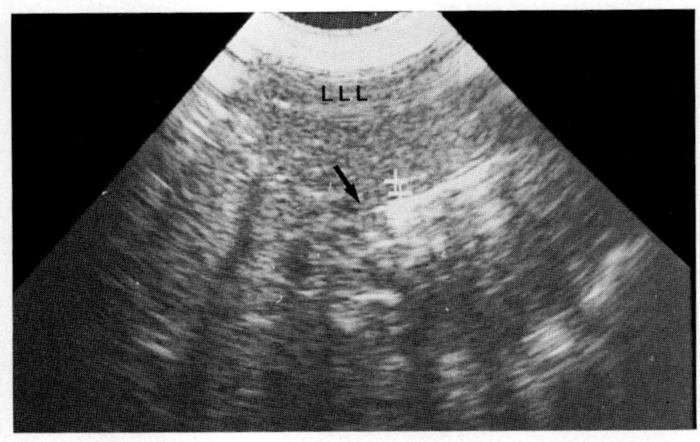

FIGURE 16-1. A transverse section scanned through the left liver lobe (LLL) demonstrates an infant's stomach with a normal gastric mucosal measurement of 1.5 mm (*cursors; arrow*, duodenum).

DIAGNOSTIC CONSIDERATIONS

False negative results have occurred, and there have been reports of false positive results in children with antral spasm. In the normal child, fluid and air can be seen passing through the pylorus, but this has also been described in early pyloric stenosis. Muscle hypertrophy may be eccentric, either the anterior or posterior wall having unequal thickness. The duodenum is usually collapsed or does not appear to be an individual structure in pyloric stenosis, but with obstruction of the duodenum, such as annular pancreas, duodenal web, or duodenal atresia, there is usually an obvious fluid-filled duodenum terminating abruptly with little or no bowel gas or fluid present in the remainder of the bowel.

A midgut malrotation may have a somewhat similar appearance. The clue to correct diagnosis is identification of the superior mesenteric artery, which usually runs inferior to the body of the pancreas. With malrotation and volvulus, the superior

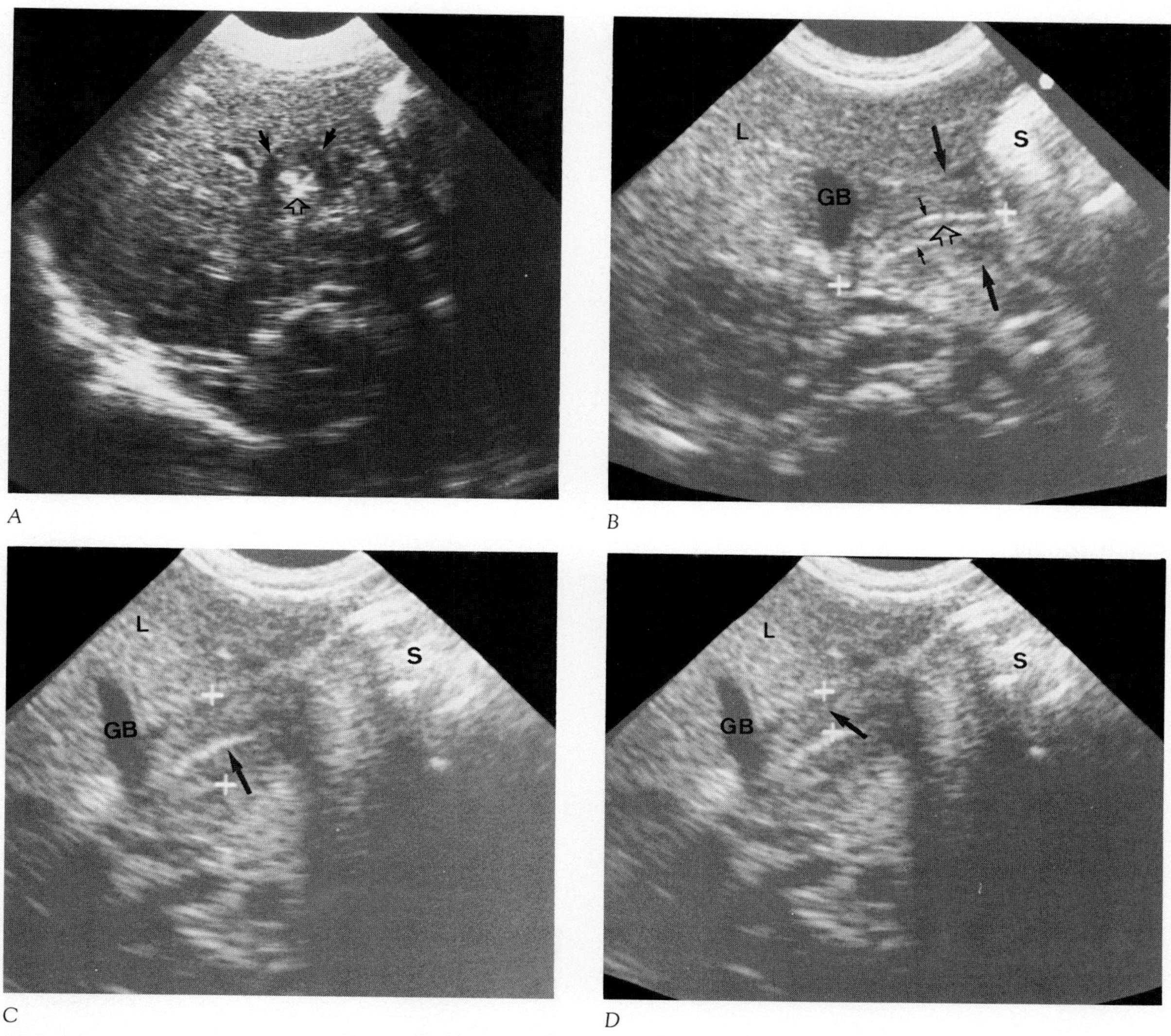

Figure 16-2. (*A*) On a sagittal section through the liver, pyloric stenosis presents as an anechoic to hypoechoic muscle mass *(arrows)* with a hyperechoic central lumen *(open arrows)*. This is the doughnut sign. (*B*) On a transverse section of a 10-day-old male infant who presented with vomiting, pyloric stenosis is identified. There is enlargement of the pyloric muscle diameter *(large arrows)* surrounding the hyperechoic lumen representing the opposing mucosal surface *(small arrows)* and the hypoechoic pyloric channel *(open arrow; cursors,* linear extent of the pyloric channel; GB, gallbladder). (C) Pyloric stenosis is represented by an enlarged diameter of the pyloric muscle *(cursors)* surrounding the hyperechoic lumen representing opposing mucosal surfaces *(arrow;* GB, gallbladder). (*D*) Pyloric stenosis presents as hypertrophic diameter of the pyloric muscle *(cursors)* surrounding the hyperechoic lumen, which represents the opposing mucosal surfaces *(arrow)* on this sonogram (GB, gallbladder).

TABLE 16-2. Abnormal sonographic measurements of the pylorus

AUTHOR (YEAR)	AP DIAMETER (cm)	LENGTH (cm)	MUSCLE THICKNESS (mm)
Grignon[14] (1984)	>1.5	>2	>4
Mollitt[30] (1987)	>1.3	>1.7	>4
Haller[16] (1986)	≥1.5	≥1.8	>4
Blumhagen[3] (1988)	—	≥1.4	≥3.5
Cohen[7] (1987)	>1.5	1.8	>3
Keller[22] (1987)	>1.4	>1.6	>4.0

mesenteric artery is pulled to the right side to lie anterior to the inferior vena cava or to the right of the aorta.

Small Bowel

Normal bowel appears as a very thin, hypoechoic rim around an echogenic centrum of variable width. In the term infant, the lumen of the colon segment should not exceed 18 mm diameter, and the internal diameter of the small bowel loop should not exceed 7 mm (Fig. 16-4).[32] During the ultrasound study, decreased small bowel motility can be appreciated and documented. Real-time scanning reveals the movement of the intestinal content to be very irregular or may show complete paralysis, with passive particle movements related only to breathing.[28]

The target or bullseye pattern—a discrete round or oval abnormality with dense central echoes and an anechoic periphery—is a characteristic sonographic feature of stomach and bowel abnormalities. The target pattern has been described in cases of malignant tumors but also in Crohn's disease, intramural hematoma, pancreatitis, and radiation enteritis.[11]

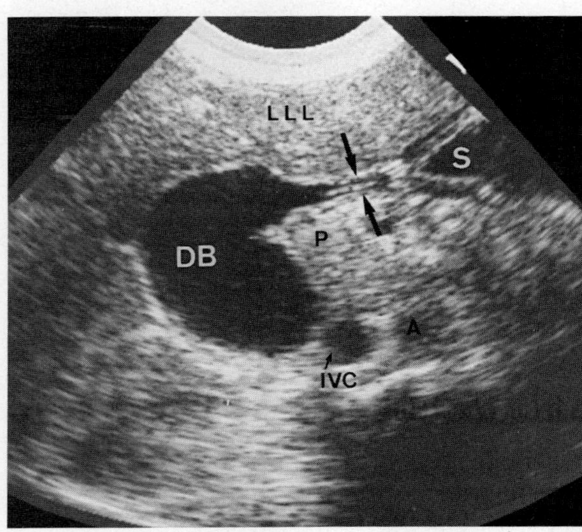

FIGURE 16-3. In this 3-week-old infant with Down's syndrome, congenital heart disease, and duodenal atresia, a markedly distended duodenal bulb (DB) can be identified distal to the normal stomach (S; *arrows*, normal pyloric canal; LLL, left liver lobe; IVC, inferior vena cava; a, aorta).

INTUSSUSCEPTION

Intussusception is the telescoping of bowel. The proximal loop of bowel telescopes into the lumen of the adjacent distal portion (Fig. 16-5A, B). If the diagnosis is made early, the intussusception can easily be reduced by hydrostatic pressure before complications, such as bowel obstruction, perforation, peritonitis, and vascular compromise (which in turn leads to edema of the bowel wall and gangrene), occur.

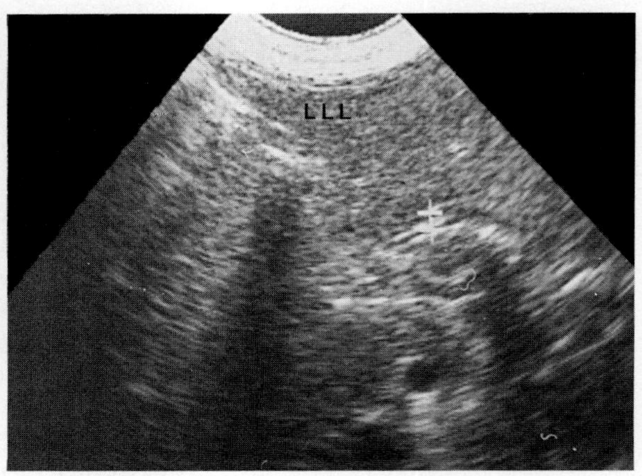

FIGURE 16-4. A transverse section of an infant's normal small bowel wall measures 1.9 mm (*cursors;* LLL, left liver lobe).

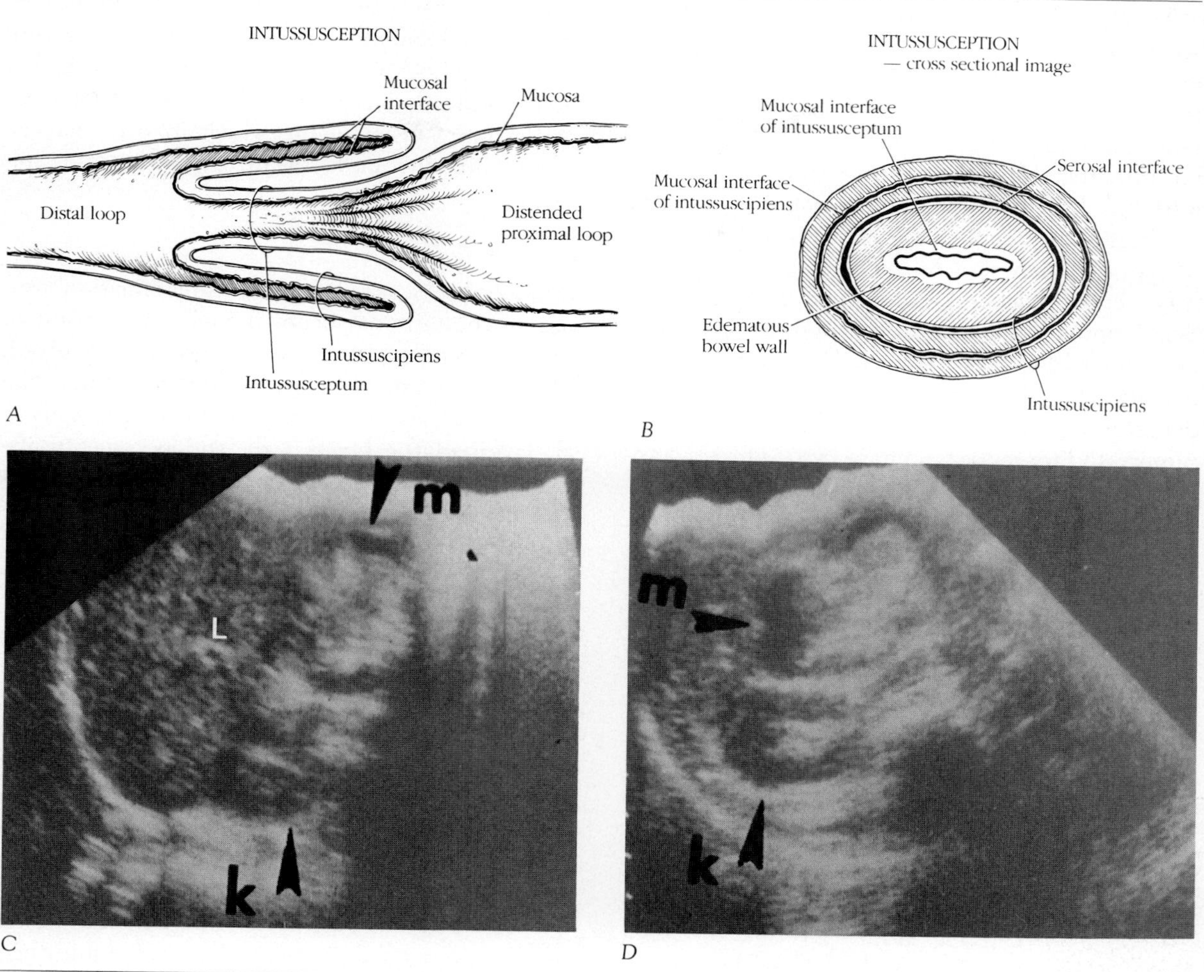

FIGURE 16-5. (*A*) An illustration of intussusception caused by the proximal bowel loop telescoping into the lumen of the adjacent distal portion. (*B*) A cross-sectional illustration of intussusception. (C) In this sagittal section, the hypoechoic border, hyperechoic middle, and anechoic center echo appearance of an ileocolic intussusception (*arrowhead,* m) presents the recognizable target pattern, doughnut sign, or the pseudokidney appearance (k, *arrowhead,* normal right kidney). (*D*) On a transverse section in the same patient, a better comparison can be made of the intussusception's pseudokidney appearance (m, *arrowhead*) with the normal right kidney (k, *arrowhead*).

Ninety percent of intussusceptions in children are ileocolic and typically occur between ages 3 months and 3 years. The child has a history of intermittent colicky abdominal pain, distension, vomiting, and possibly an abdominal mass and rectal bleeding. Intussusception is rare in the first month of life. In children older than 3 years, there is a higher incidence of a lead point for the intussusception, such as a Meckel's diverticulum or a small bowel mass or tumor such as lymphoma. Small bowel intussusception has been described postoperatively, and may be a cause of early postoperative bowel obstruction in children. The incidence is higher for children who have undergone surgery and for those who have cystic fibrosis,[31] appendicitis, or Henoch-Schönlein purpura.[2,27]

If intussusception is suspected, a barium enema can be not only diagnostic but therapeutic. In many pediatric hospitals intussusceptions are now reduced with either hydrostatic pressure under ultrasound guidance or fluoroscopy and retrograde flow of air or barium.[15,42]

Since sonography is now used as a screening procedure for patients with an abdominal mass as well as for children with vomiting and since the presentation of an intussusception often is not typical, there is a sonographic pattern of intussusception that should be recognized. This is the so-called target pattern otherwise known as the doughnut sign, or the pseudokidney appearance in the long axis.[11,40] The intussuscipiens (the distal bowel into which the intussusceptum or proximal bowel herniates) does not usually suffer vascular compromise and so is not edematous but normally thin. As the intussusceptum becomes edematous, it compresses the bowel lumen, creating a hypoechoic ring with increased central echogenicity. Depending on the imaging plane, fluid may be present centrally in the obstructed bowel lumen (Fig. 16-5C, D).

Without clinical correlation, the target sign may be nonspecific, as other bowel disease can create this picture; specifically, any process involving the bowel wall, and certainly in adults the target sign is typical of carcinoma. Target patterns have been described in children with Henoch-Schönlein purpura and Burkitt's lymphoma. The target pattern has many variations, and the pattern may change in the presence of antegrade or retrograde flow of contrast material.[1]

Patients with ileoileocolic intussusception, or ileum into ileum into colon, show a three-ring sign. The very echogenic center is surrounded by the hyperechoic intussusceptum with intervening mucosa of the more distal ileum, which in turn may be edematous, surrounded again by the intussuscipiens.[6]

Crohn's Disease

Crohn's disease is an idiopathic inflammation, usually in the terminal ileum though any portion of the gastrointestinal tract can become involved. The most common nonspecific inflammation of the small bowel, it starts in the submucosa, spreads to all layers of the bowel wall, and becomes transmural. This disease usually occurs in young adults and affects principally the ileum, and to a lesser extent the colon, but it can also affect the entire bowel, including jejunum, duodenum, and stomach.

The sonographic criteria include the nonspecific bullseye or target lesion phenomena with the hypoechoic wall if the lumen is viewed transversely; when the lumen is viewed in the long axis, it has the pseudokidney appearance, although this more often appears to be a more elongated tubular structure, sometimes with a narrowed lumen and sometimes with a normal lumen (Fig. 16-6). These appearances correlate with involvement of the entire wall at the time of diagnosis. The segment of bowel has been described as aperistaltic with diminished compressibility and decreased mobility. Wall thickness is similar to adults', at least 4 or 5 mm.[10,25,43]

Any child with neutropenia or immune deficiency can experience infections of the bowel wall such as those described in patients with leukemia and typhlitis. The sonographic appearance is similar, so the clinical history is important in making a diagnosis.

Meconium Peritonitis

Meconium peritonitis is a sterile irritative peritonitis caused by prenatal or perinatal bowel perforation accompanied by spilling of the ingested amniotic fluid into the peritoneal cavity. The underlying bowel disorders that lead to this may be small bowel or ileal atresia, meconium ileus, volvulus, internal hernia, intussusception, congenital bands, Meckel's diverticulum, vascular insuffi-

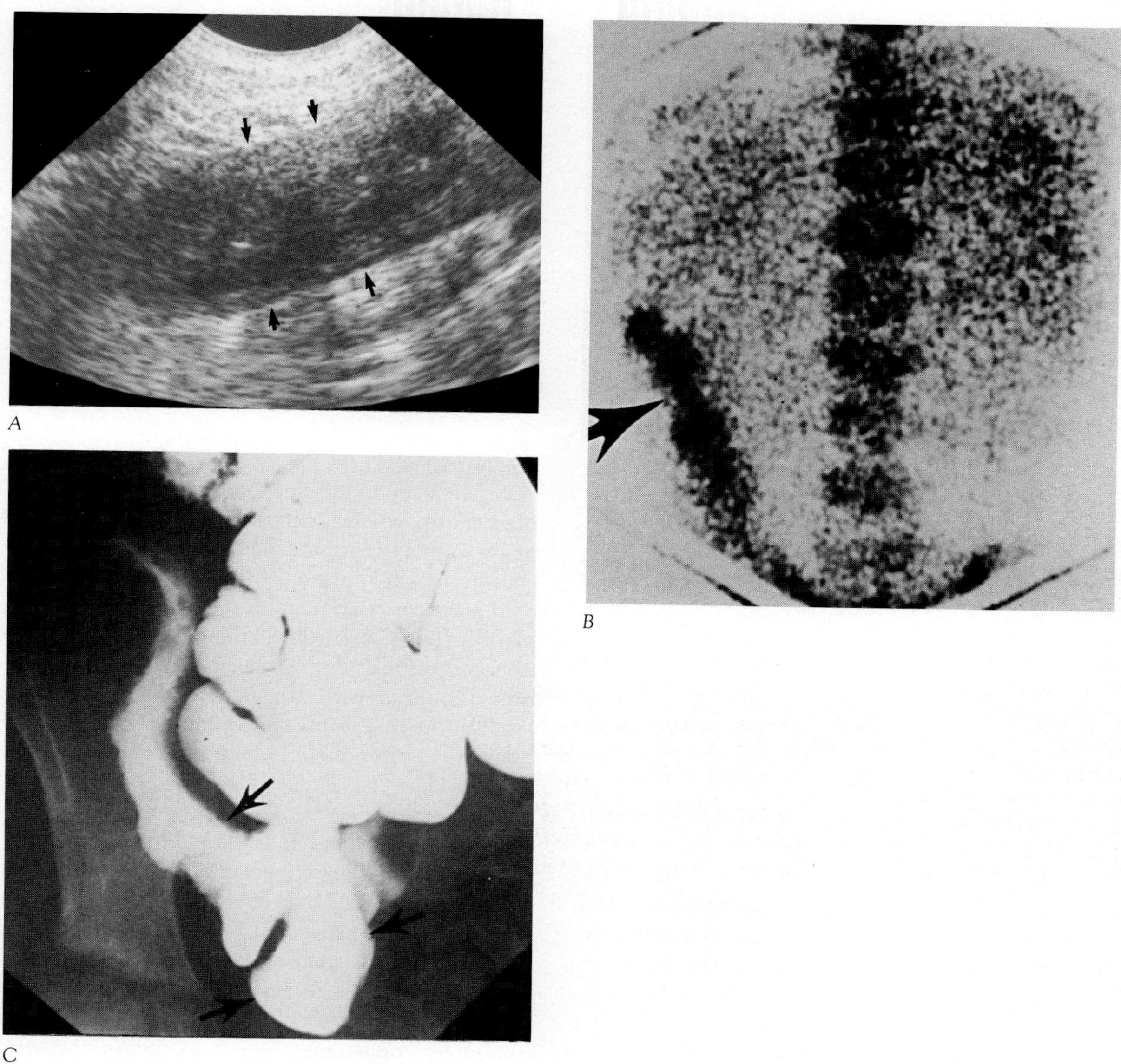

FIGURE 16-6. (*A*) A sagittal section of the right lower quadrant demonstrates a thickened, hypoechoic terminal ileum wall *(arrows)* with fluid in the middle in a 9-year-old boy with Crohn's disease who presented with fever and failure to thrive. (*B*) A radionuclide examination of the same patient shows gallium uptake in the right lower quadrant, which confirms the inflammation of the terminal ileum *(arrow)*. (C) A small bowel barium study performed on the same patient also demonstrates a narrow aperistaltic terminal ileum *(arrow)* consistent with Crohn's disease.

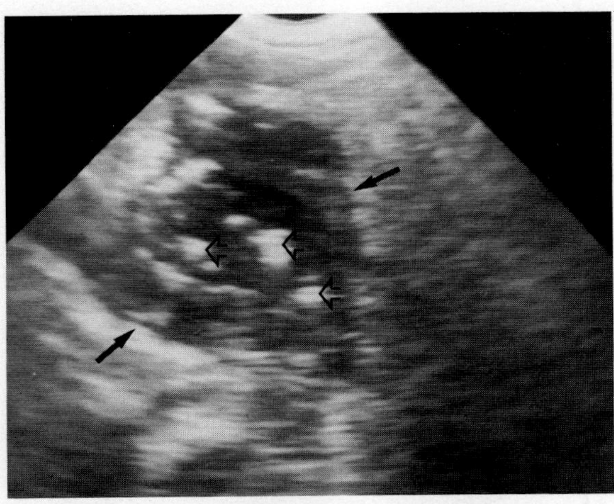

Figure 16-7. An encapsulated meconium cyst *(black arrows)* presents both an anechoic and a hypoechoic pattern, with hyperechoic spots *(open arrows)* representing air bubbles.

ciency, and other unknown causes. As many as 40% of infants with neonatal meconium peritonitis have cystic fibrosis. The diagnosis of meconium peritonitis has been made in utero.[9,13,44]

Sonographically, hyperechoic regions appear in the abdomen, which may demonstrate acoustic shadowing secondary to calcification. The meconium perforation may become encapsulated and form a meconium cyst, which presents sonographically as an anechoic cystic mass in the abdomen (Fig. 16-7).

Large Bowel

Normally, the large bowel is filled with air and feces and is not well-visualized. In a neonate who has not been fed, the meconium-filled colon is easily seen in the pelvis (Fig. 16-8A, B). In infants and older children a sonographically identifiable colon is usually abnormal (Fig. 16-8C, D).

Gasless Abdomen

The diagnosis of gasless abdomen is made from a plain radiograph. The clinical reasons may be multiple. Sonography is valuable in evaluating the gasless abdomen for identification of obstruction, fluid-filled loops of bowel, ascites, necrotizing enterocolitis, or peritonitis (Fig. 16-9).

Ascites

Ascites may be secondary to hematologic diseases such as immune hydrops in the newborn, liver failure in the older child, or bowel perforation, obstructive uropathy, cardiovascular diseases, intrauterine or extrauterine infection, biliary peritonitis, and chylous ascites (Fig. 16-10). Diffuse echogenic ascites may be due to peritonitis. Echogenic ascites may also be indicative of active intraperitoneal bleeding or may be associated with meconium.

Obstruction

Persistence of fluid-filled loops of bowel suggests obstruction, whereas persistence of echogenic loops of bowel may represent malabsorption or delayed transit. In the normal child, the bowel changes configuration relatively quickly during active normal peristalsis. A C-shaped dilated, fluid-filled loop of bowel is consistent with a closed loop of obstruction. Children with ascites secondary to protein loss also have a thickened bowel wall, as do children with ascites due to infection in the bowel wall (Fig. 16-11).

Hirschsprung's Disease

Hirschsprung's disease (aganglionic megacolon) is a congenital disorder that is much more frequent in males than in females and is often associated with other anomalies, such as Down's syndrome. It is usually manifested in early infancy and has been diagnosed inutero.[41] Hirschsprung's disease is caused by congenital absence of parasympathetic ganglion cells in the submucosal and intramuscular plexuses; the bowel becomes enormously dilated and there is no peristaltic action in the aganglionic area. The aganglionic segment remains contracted without reciprocal relaxation and produces a functional obstruction. The area most frequently affected is the rectosigmoid.

The clinical manifestations depend on the length of aganglionosis or bowel distension. When the disease is manifest in early infancy, the patient presents with abdominal distension, constipation,

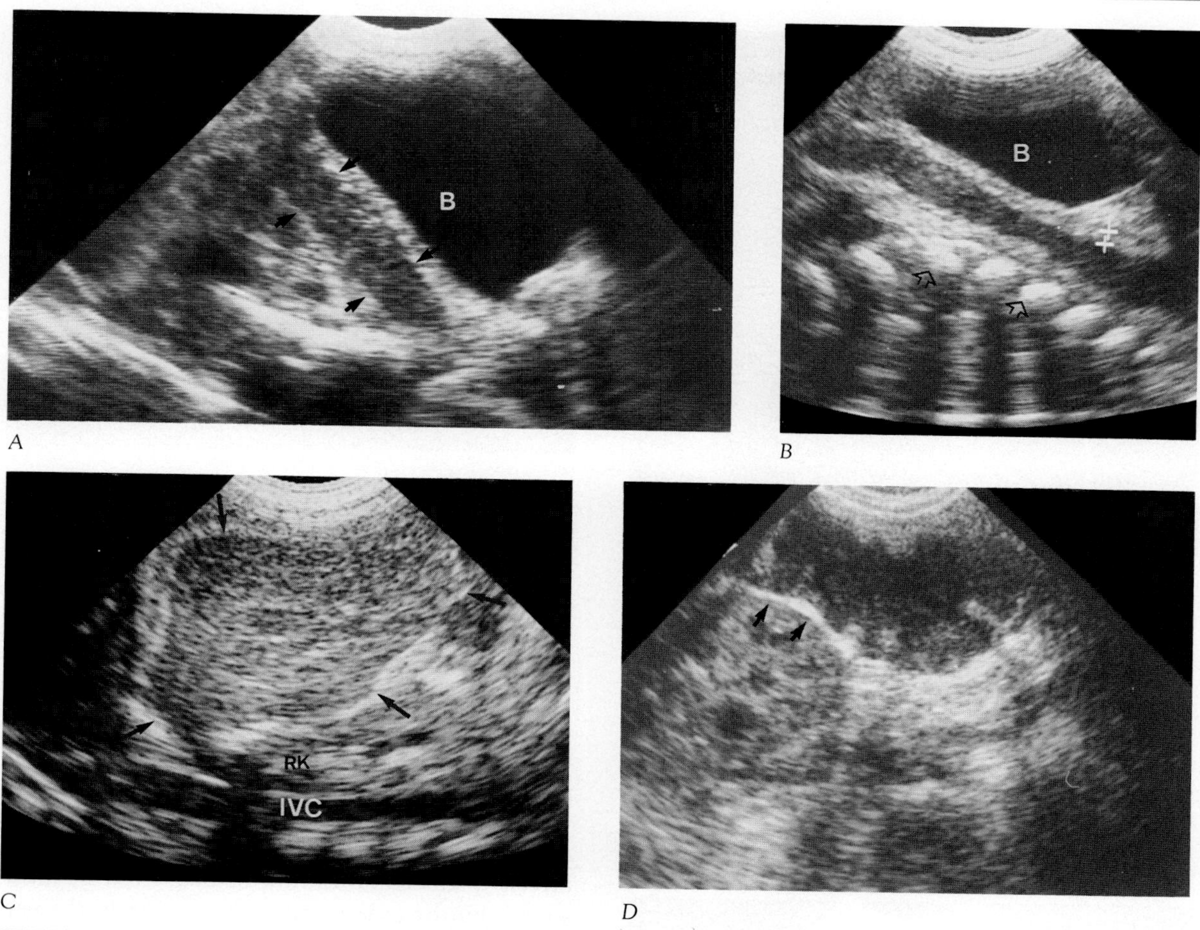

Figure 16-8. (*A*) The normal, meconium-filled rectum *(arrows)* can be identified posterior to the urinary bladder on this sagittal section made on a neonate who had not passed meconium owing to complications of prematurity. (*B*) A sagittal section demonstrates a meconium-filled rectum *(arrows)*, normal bowel wall measuring 1.8 mm *(cursors)* distal to the urinary bladder (B), and a normal spine *(open arrows)*. This neonate had a sonographically identifiable imperforate anus and a perineal fistula that allowed the rectum to remain filled with meconium. (C) A sagittal section demonstrates a normal infeior vena cava (IVC) and right kidney (RK) posterior to a hyperechoic mass *(arrows)*, which represents a dilated, meconium-filled colon. The infant patient had colon atresia distal to the mass. (*D*) The abnormal thick wall *(arrows)* of the descending colon was spastic on this child with Henoch-Schönlein purpura. There is hemorrhage in the wall.

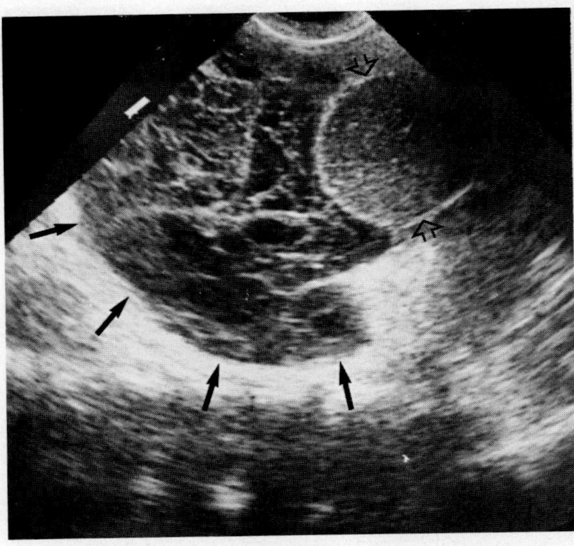

Figure 16-9. Sonographically, this section demonstrates a large heterogenous collection of fluid *(black arrows)* in the right flank of a 2-week-old infant who presented in septic shock with a protuberant gasless abdomen. The ascites represents blood and pus. A dilated bowel loop *(open arrows)* filled with water fecal material is also identified.

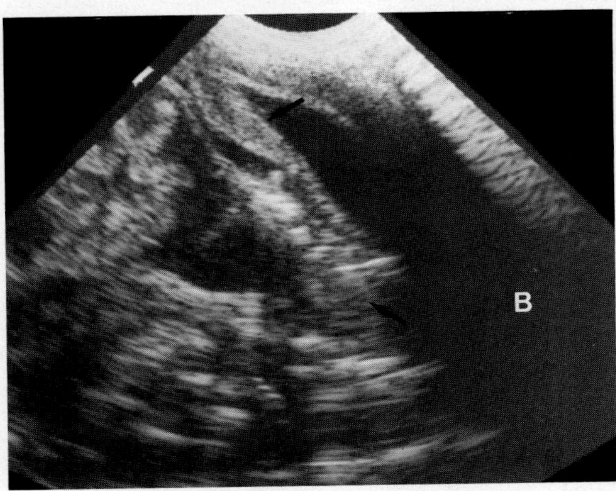

Figure 16-10. Superior and posterior to an incompletely filled urinary bladder, ascites surrounds collapsed bowel *(arrows)* on this section through the pelvis.

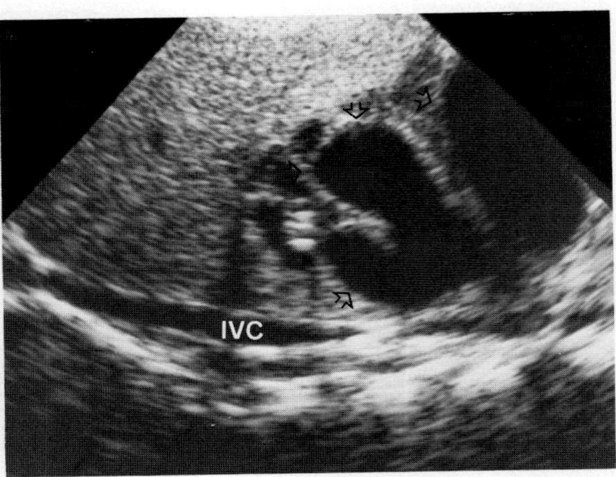

Figure 16-11. Fluid-filled loops of bowel *(open arrows)* and thickened bowel wall *(arrows)* are visualized anterior to the inferior vena cava (IVC) on a sagittal section made on an infant with severe colitis.

and vomiting and often appears malnourished and anemic. Hirschsprung's disease can be suggested by ultrasonography if the transition zone can be seen high in the sigmoid colon. Imperforate anus and atrecia of the colon cannot be diagnosed by ultrasound, but by examining the patient from the perineal surface, the distance from the anus to the colon lumen can be measured.[33]

Appendicitis

Appendicitis may occur in any age group, but young adults are most often affected. It is almost always associated with obstruction of the appendiceal lumen and has generally been considered a clinical diagnosis characterized by fever, leukocytosis, and periumbilical pain.

High-resolution real-time ultrasonography employing graded compression can be used to evaluate for clinically suspected acute appendicitis—in adults or children.[21,36] The examination is initiated by scanning transversely in the right midabdomen at about the level of the umbilicus, continuing caudad, with gradually increasing compression and then followed by reducing and then increasing the

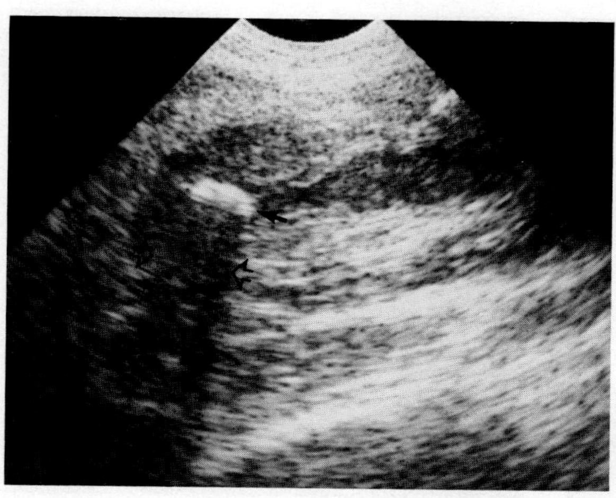

Figure 16-12. A hyperechoic appendicolith *(arrow)* can be identified with an associated acoustic shadowing artifact *(open arrows)*.

pressure of the transducer. This action allows assessment of the compressibility of normal bowel. Normal cecum and terminal ileum are easily compressed with only moderate pressure. The inflamed appendix is most often visualized at the base of the cecal tip during maximum graded compression.

There are two important limitations to ultrasound scanning; a noncompressible appendix with thickening can resolve spontaneously. Thickening from Crohn's disease may be located in the appendix only and can be misleading. The findings may be inconclusive owing to massive ascites or exquisite tenderness. An abnormal appendix contains a hypoechoic thickened wall with central hyperechoic mucosa, similar to other bowel lesions (Fig. 16-12). Finally, a hypoechoic solid mass or a hypoechoic cystic mass may surround the appendix.[26]

Bowel Masses

Bowel enteric and colon duplications are unusual. They can occur anywhere in the abdomen but are usually associated with the terminal ileum. Duplications can also be calcified.[17,20]

Lymphangiomas contain cystic fluid, and sometimes septa of varying thickness and number. The cysts are soft and can be displaced by adjacent organs or other loops of bowel. Lymphangiomas can arise as extraperitoneal masses and appear similar to free ascites fluid in the abdomen; but changing the subject's position produces changes only in the lymphangioma, and there is not evidence of ascites (Fig. 16-13A, B). Because of their very large size and clear fluid content, lymphangiomas may be confused with ovarian tumors or pancreatic pseudocysts; however, lymphomatous masses usually are not truly cystic.[4] For imaging such lesions, computed tomography (CT) and magnetic resonance imaging (MRI) are preferred, particularly when the masses are extensive.[38]

Another cause of cystic masses in the peritoneal cavity may be cerebrospinal fluid collections in patients with known ventriculoperitoneal shunts. Often the shunt is difficult to identify. These cysts are often under some pressure and displace bowel.

Hemangiomas, especially if there is a lymphangiomatous component, can be recognized as multiseptate masses. A pure hemangioma is usually very small and is not identifiable by ultrasound.

The most common malignant tumor of the bowel in children is non-Hodgkin's lymphoma. These lesions are usually hypoechoic, with a brightly echogenic lumen. They may be eccentric and are usually larger or more extensive than the usual target sign, and the hypoechoic mass is usually eccentric.[35]

Other more unusual tumors of adults can also be seen in children, such as leiomyosarcoma (Fig. 16-13C, D).

Blunt Abdominal Trauma

While ultrasonography can be useful for evaluating renal and perirenal abnormalities, CT is an excellent imaging modality for detecting injuries to intraabdominal organs, especially in an acutely injured child or one with head trauma and possibly occult intraabdominal injuries. Sonography is useful for detecting free peritoneal fluid[12] and for evaluating the pancreas after blunt trauma.

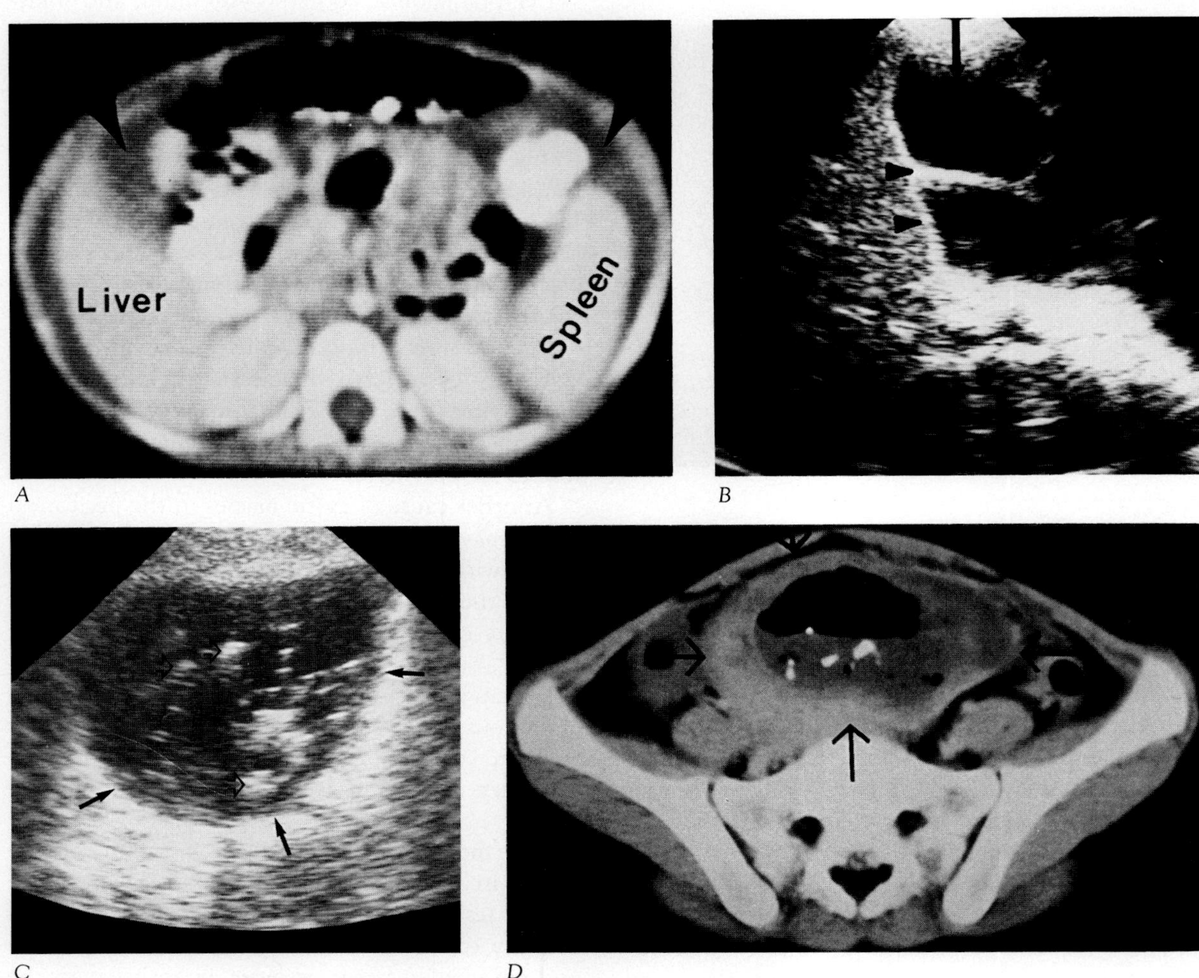

Figure 16-13. (*A*) On a transverse CT section, the large volume of fluid *(arrows)* in the peritoneal cavity was felt to be ascites in this 2-year-old girl who presented with a protuberant abdomen. (*B*) In the same patient, the sonographic appearance of this multiloculated *(arrowheads)* fluid *(arrow)* seen on this sagittal section is more representative of lymphangioma, as it does not surround the bowel as would ascites. (*C*) On this transverse section of the pelvis of a patient with leiomyosarcoma of the ileum, a thin-walled, cyst-filled mass *(arrows)* contains hyperechoic debris *(open arrows)*. (*D*) CT section through this leiomyosarcoma *(arrows)* demonstrates air, fluid, and barium.

References

1. Alzen G, Funke G, Truong S: Pitfalls in the diagnosis of intussusception. J Clin Ultrasound 1989, 17:481–488.
2. Bisset III GS, Kirks DR: Intussusception in infants and children: Diagnosis and therapy. Radiology 1988, 168:141–145.
3. Blumhagen JD, Maclin L, Krauter D: Sonographic diagnosis of hypertrophic pyloric stenosis. AJR 1988, 150:1367–1370.
4. Blumhagen JD, Wood BJ, Rosenbaum DM: Sonographic evaluation of abdominal lymphangiomas in children. J Ultrasound Med 1987, 6:487–495.
5. Bowen III A, Gibson MD: Chronic granulomatous disease with gastric antral narrowing. Pediatr Radiol 1980, 10:119–120.
6. Bowerman RA, Silver TM, Jaffe MH: Real-time ultrasound diagnosis of intussusception in children. Radiology 1982, 143:527–529.
7. Cohen HL, Schechter S, Mestel AL, et al: Ultrasonic "double track" sign in hypertrophic pyloric stenosis. J Ultrasound Med 1987, 6:139–143.
8. Cohen HL, Haller JO, Mestel AL, et al: Neonatal duodenum: Fluid-aided US examination. Radiology 1987, 164:805–809.
9. Dillard JP, Edwards DK, Leopold GR: Meconium peritonitis masquerading as fetal hydrops. J Ultrasound Med 1987, 6:49–51.
10. Dinkel E, Dittrich M, Peters H, et al: Real-time ultrasound in Crohn's disease: Characteristic features and clinical implications. Pediatr Radiol 1986, 16:8–12.
11. Fakhry JR, Berk RN: The "target" pattern: Characteristic sonographic feature of stomach and bowel abnormalities. AJR 1981, 137:969–972.
12. Filiatrault D, Longpre D, Patriquis H, et al: Investigation of blunt abdominal trauma: A practical approach using ultrasound as the initial diagnositc modaility. Pediatr Radiol 1987, 17:373–379.
13. Foster MA, Nyberg DA, Mahony BS, et al: Meconium peritonitis: Prenatal sonographic findings and their clinical significance. Radiology 1987, 165:661–665.
14. Grignon A, Filiatrault D, Patriquin H, et al: Ecographie de la stenose du pylore. J Canad Assoc Radiol 1984, 35:271–275.
15. Gu L, Alton DJ, Daneman A, et al: Intussusception reduction in children by rectal insufflation of air. AJR 1988, 150:1345–1348.
16. Haller JO, Cohen HL: Hypertrophic pyloric stenosis: Diagnosis using US. Radiology 1986, 161:335–339.
17. Haller JO, Schneider M, Kassner EG, et al: Sonographic evaluation of mesenteric and omental masses in children. AJR 1978, 130:269–274.
18. Hayashi K, Futagawa S, Kozaki S, et al: Ultrasound and CT diagnosis of intramural duodenal hematoma. Pediatr Radiol 1988, 18:167–168.
19. Hayden Jr CK, Swischuk LE, Rytting JE: Gastric ulcer disease in infants: US findings. Radiology 1987, 164:131–134.
20. Jeffrey RB Jr, Laing FC, Townsend RR: Acute appendicitis: Sonographic criteria based on 250 cases. Radiology 1988, 167:327–329.
21. Kangarloo H, Sample WF, Hansen G, et al: Ultrasonic evaluation of abdominal gastrointestinal tract duplication in children. Radiology 1979, 131:191–194.
22. Keller H, Waldmann D, Greiner P: Comparison of preoperative sonography with intraoperative findings in congenital hypertrophic pyloric stenosis. J Pediatr Surg 1987, 22:950–952.
23. Kleinman PK, Brill PW, Winchester P: Resolving duodenal-jejunal hematoma in abused children. Radiology 1986, 160:747–750.
24. Kopen PA, McAlister WH: Upper gastrointestinal and ultrasound examinations of gastric antral involvement in chronic granulomatous disease. Pediatr Radiol 1984, 14:91–93.
25. Limberg B: Diagnosis of acute ulcerative colitis and colonic Crohn's disease by colonic sonography. J Clin Ultrasound 1989, 17:25–31.
26. Machan L, Pon MS, Wood BJ, et al: The "coffee-bean" sign in periappendiceal and peridiverticular abscess. J Ultrasound Med 1987, 6:373–375.
27. Martinez-Frontanilla LA, Silver L, Meagher DP Jr: Intussusception in Henoch-Schönlein purpura: Diagnosis with ultrasound. J Pediatr Surg 1988, 23:375–376.
28. Meiser G, Meissner K: Ileus and intestinal obstruction—ultrasonographic findings as a guideline to therapy. Hepatogastroenterology 1987, 34:194–199.
29. Miller JH, Kemberling CR: Ultrasound scanning of the gastrointestinal tract in children: Subject review. Radiology 1984, 152:671–677.
30. Mollitt DL, Golladay S, Williamson S, et al: Ultrasonography in the diagnosis of pyloric stenosis. Southern Med J 1987, 80:47–50.
31. Mulvihill DM: Ultrasound findings of chronic intussusception in a patient with cystic fibrosis. J Ultrasound Med 1988, 7:353–355.
32. Nyberg DA, Mack LA, Patten RM, et al: Fetal bowel—normal sonographic findings. J Ultrasound Med 1987, 6:3–6.
33. Oppenheimer DA: Sonography of imperforate anus. Radiology 1983, 148:127–128.
34. Orel SG, Nussbaum AR, Sheth S, et al: Duodenal hematoma in child abuse: Sonographic detection. AJR 1988, 151:147–149.

35. Parker LA, Vincent LM, Ryan FP, et al: Primary lymphomas of the ascending colon: Sonographic demonstration. J Clin Ultrasound 1986, 14:221–223.
36. Puylaert JBCM: Mesenteric adenitis and acute terminal ileitis: US evaluation using graded compression. Radiology 1986, 161:691–695.
37. Seibert JJ, Williamson SL, Golladay ES: The distended gasless abdomen: A fertile field for ultrasound. J Ultrasound Med 1986, 5:301–308.
38. Siegel MJ, Glazer HS, St Amour TE, et al: Lymphangiomas in children: MR imaging. Radiology 1989, 170:467–470.
39. Stringer DA, Daneman A, Brunelle F, et al: Sonography of the normal and abnormal stomach (excluding hypertrophic pyloric stenosis) in children. J Ultrasound Med 1986, 5:183–188.
40. Swischuk LE, Hayden CK, Boulden T: Intussusception: Indications for ultrasonography and an explanation of the doughnut and pseudokidney signs. Pediatr Radiol 1985, 15:388–391.
41. Vermesh M, Mayden KL, Confino E, et al: Prenatal sonographic diagnosis of Hirschsprung's disease. J Ultrasound Med 1986, 5:37–39.
42. Wang G-D, Liu S-J: Enema reduction of intussusception by hydrostatic pressure under ultrasound guidance: A report of 377 cases. J Pediatr Surg 1988, 23:814–818.
43. Worlicek H, Lutz H, Heyder N, et al: Ultrasound findings in Crohn's disease and ulcerative colitis: A prospective study. J Clin Ultrasound 1987, 15:153–163.
44. Wu C-C: Sonographic findings of generalized meconium peritonitis presenting as neonatal ascites. J Clin Ultrasound 1988, 16:48–51.

CHAPTER 17

Urinary Tract

BARBARA S. REID

Ultrasonography has become one of the most important means of evaluating the pediatric urinary tract, for several reasons. Besides not exposing the child to ionizing radiation, there are no contrast reactions. The procedure is tolerated very well by patients and parents. For infants particularly, ultrasound is preferred over excretory urography because poor concentration results in poor nephrograms.

A common indication for ultrasonographic examination of infants and children is suspected renal anomalies suggested by clinical findings such as vertebral, cardiac or colon abnormalities. Findings at prenatal ultrasonography may also raise the question of renal anomalies.[7,20,21,36] For older infants and young children, the most common reasons for referral are work-up for a urinary tract infection, enuresis, diuresis, or, less commonly, masses. Some of the other current clinical indications for genitourinary ultrasonography include possible obstructive uropathy, ambiguous genitalia, neonatal ascites, anasarca, renal failure, localization for renal biopsy, evaluation of a renal allograft, anomalies of the bladder, assessment of bladder volume, urachal remnant, precocious puberty, pelvic tumors, pelvic abscesses, and pregnancy.

Sonographic Technique

For evaluation of the kidneys, no preparation is necessary although hydration is preferred. Patients need not fast, since the kidneys can be imaged from either the posterior surface (prone sagittal or transverse scan planes) or from the patient's side (coronal planes).

Most pediatric patients are evaluated in the supine or prone position, but scanning children requires a certain amount of flexibility. They have been scanned in the sitting position, decubitus positions, or held in a parent's arms, across their shoulders, or on the lap. Since children may be unable or unwilling to hold their breath or obey simple instructions, the sonographer must be prepared to scan from multiple planes or through ribs in order to visualize all portions of the kidney. As part of the kidney examination, visualizing the ureters is very important, particularly if there is evidence of hydronephrosis. The bladder should also be examined as part of the evaluation of the urinary tract.

For babies or young infants, a 10-mHz transducer affords exquisite resolution and detail of the kidney. Since the kidney is very close to the posterior skin surface (0.5 to 3 cm) in young infants, a 10-MHz transducer can easily provide excellent detail. A 7.5-MHz transducer is useful for scanning young children and older, thin children, providing excellent kidney detail. Either an annular-array or a linear-array transducer may be used. Since the kidneys are close to the skin surface, a standoff device such as a Gelfoam block may be especially valuable for measuring kidney length. A standoff allows ir-

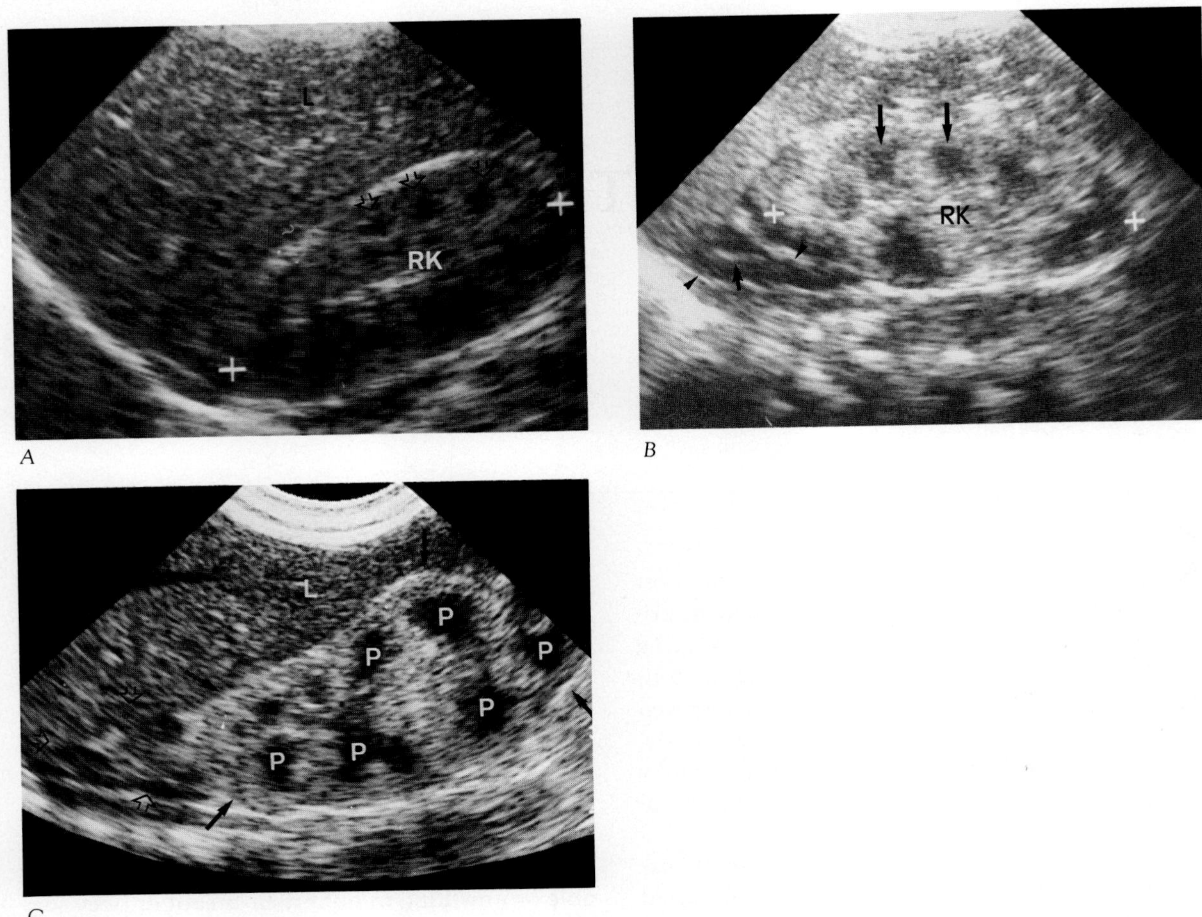

Figure 17-1. (*A*) The normal neonatal right kidney (RK) is seen in a sagittal section with hypoechoic pyramids (*open arrows*) evenly spaced in the kidney. The renal echogenicity is similar to the liver. (*B*) A sagittal section through a newborn's right kidney (RK, *cursors*) demonstrates the normal sonographic appearance. The pyramids appear hypoechoic to anechoic (*arrows*), and the echogenicity of the kidney is greater than that of the adjacent liver. The normal adrenal gland (*arrowheads*) appears hypoechoic with a dense central echo (*short arrow*). (*C*) On a 38-week-old infant, compared to the liver, the normal right kidney (*black arrows*) is hyperechoic, with normally aligned pyramids (P). The normal adrenal gland (*open arrows*) lacks cortical demarcation.

ritable children to be scanned without stimulating the child while manipulating the transducer.

Normal Kidneys

With modern high-resolution systems, the renal pyramids or medulla of a normal newborn or infant can be identified as hypoechoic, triangular or rectangular structures. Sonographers unfamiliar with children have mistaken them for renal cysts. The renal pyramids show symmetric alignment within the kidney periphery.[7] In 70% of kidneys, a compound renal pyramid or a normal hypoechoic medullary region occurs in the upper pole (50%), lower pole (30%), or middle region (20%).[31] Compound calyces are a conglomerate of calyces that come to one infundibulum and are associated with compound pyramids. Sonographically, these fused medullary pyramids appear as an irregular, hypoechoic area. They are not associated with evidence of renal, pelvic, infundibular, or calyceal dilatation (Fig. 17-1). If obstruction exists or other renal anomalies are present, the renal pyramids may be compressed and poorly visualized.

Table 17-1 summarizes the normal infant and pediatric renal echo patterns.[9,23,28,31] In older children, however, increased echogenicity in the cortex, although nonspecific, may indicate parenchymal disease.[26] Causes of increased echogenicity are the same as for adults. Specific pediatric conditions include leukemia, progressive glomerulonephritis, nephrotic syndrome, renal artery stenosis, and chronic infection.[4,35]

Standard measurements of renal size have been published,[10,24,37,55,61] and are related to the length of the kidney for age and also to the child's weight and body surface area. These measurements are particularly useful for examining children who may have a diffuse process such as infection or leukemia.

Comparative measurements should be made to determine appropriate growth in children with chronic infection. Also, in children the renal vein may be unusually prominent, including the intrahilar portion and sinus portion. It can be distinguished from structures of the collecting system by following the course of the vein or by identifying flow pattens with Doppler instrumentation. Fetal lobulations are present in most premature infants and in many newborns and infants. By approximately 1 year of age, fetal lobulations should not be as evident, although in some children they persist as a normal variant. Fetal lobulation may be confused with scarring, but the pyelonephritic scar is usually opposite a clubbed calyx whereas fetal lobulation is usually seen between the renal pyramids or calyces.

TABLE 17-1. Normal pediatric renal echo pattern[9,23,28,31]

AGE	RENAL STRUCTURE	ECHO PATTERN
Newborn	Cortex	More echoic than liver and spleen
	Sinus	Poorly defined because of paucity of fat in infants
6–8 wk	Cortex	Isoechoic to liver and spleen
2–6 mo	Cortex	Hypoechoic to liver and spleen
>6 mo	Cortex	Hypoechoic to renal sinus

There is a great deal of variation in the size of kidneys. Large kidneys, by defintion, are 2 standard deviations (SD) *larger than* the mean. Small kidneys are 2 SD *smaller than* the mean. An abnormality may be bilateral or unilateral, symmetric or asymmetric. There are a multitude of causes for an increase or decrease in the size of the kidneys (Tables 17-2, and 17-3).

Congenital Anomalies

AGENESIS

Bilateral renal agenesis is associated with an unusually small amount of amniotic fluid. Renal agenesis is associated with Potter's syndrome, features of which include abnormal facies with a small mandible and low-set ears. Affected infants also have pulmonary hypoplasia and frequently are stillborn or survive only for a very short time. They may live longer with ventilatory support, but they die of renal failure. In cases of renal agenesis, the adrenal glands are usually well-developed: they can measure up to 3 cm in length and lie in the renal fossa (Fig. 17-2), so they must not be mistaken for the kidneys. It is very important to use the highest-res-

Table 17-2. Causes of enlarged kidneys

Bilateral Enlargement
Congenital: Duplication, cystic disease, storage disease, generalized visceromegaly, systemic infection
Acute: Pyelonephritis, glomerular nephritis
Neoplastic: Nephroblastomatosis, bilateral Wilms' tumor, leukemia, lymphoma, tuberous sclerosis or hamartoma
Vascular: Renal vein thrombosis, acute tubular necrosis, hemolytic uremia, sickle cell anemia
Obstructive: Congenital or acquired
Unilateral Enlargement
Congenital: Duplication, cystic disease, cross-fused ectopia, horseshoe kidney
Infectious: Acute pyelonephritis, abscess
Neoplastic: Mesoblastic nephroma, Wilms' tumor, angiomyelolipoma or hamartoma, sarcoma, lymphoma
Vascular: Renal vein thrombosis, transplant complication (rejection or tubular necrosis)
Traumatic: Contusion, hematoma
Obstructive: Congenital, acquired

Table 17-3. Causes of small kidneys

Bilateral
Congenital: Aplasia, hypoplasia
Infectious: Chronic pyelonephritis, reflux nephropathy with infarction
Vascular: Real vein thrombosis, arterial occlusion (intrinsic or extrinsic)
Atrophic: Chronic obstruction, chronic recurrent infarction, chronic failure, dysplasia
Unilateral
Congenital: Agenesis, hypoplasia
Infectious: Chronic, chronic reflux with infarction
Vascular: Venous thrombosis, arterial obstruction (acquired or congenital)
Atrophic: Chronic obstruction, chronic infection and infarction, dysplasia

olution transducer available to achieve good definition of the adrenal glands and kidneys. With total renal agenesis the bladder is also absent. Unilateral renal agenesis is more common and may be asymptomatic, in which case it may be detected only incidentally. Renal hypoplasia probably is due to renal infarction, possibly occurring in utero but more likely postpartum. It may result from unsuspected chronic atrophic pyelonephritis, unsuspected reflux nephritis, an anoxic insult, or decreased blood flow due to a vascular problem.

Hydronephrosis

Hydronephrosis is dilatation of the collecting system of the urinary tract, specifically of the renal calyces, the renal pelves and the ureters. It is the most common renal mass in infants and children. In infants, the most frequent site of obstruction is at the ureteropelvic junction.[66] With hydronephrosis, there should be recognizable renal parenchyma surrounding the dilated collecting system (Fig. 17-3A). In some cases no parenchyma is recognizable. Great care must be used to identify the ureter, which may be dilated as well.

Distal ureteral obstructions are the next most common cause of hydronephrosis.[5,42] In cases of bilateral hydronephrosis, obviously the obstruction is going to be located distally, in the bladder or urethra. The bladder must be examined for obstructing masses such as dilated distal ureters that distend its outlet. These are called ureteroceles. A thick-walled small bladder with distension of the posterior urethra, such as has been described in posterior urethral valves, can obstruct the ureters.[19] A thick-walled bladder indicates chronic obstruction.

The third most common cause of hydronephrosis is duplication of the collecting system (Fig. 17-3B). These lesions are recognized by dilatation of the upper pole calyx and a separate dilated ureter, which often can be followed to the level of the bladder. When it appears in the bladder lumen it is known as ureterocele (Fig. 17-3C–E). There may be dilatation, but to a lesser degree in the lower pole, either due to reflux or obstruction by the ectopic ureter. Unobstructed duplicated kidneys may be difficult to image in uncooperative children. The finding of infolding of cortical tissue into the

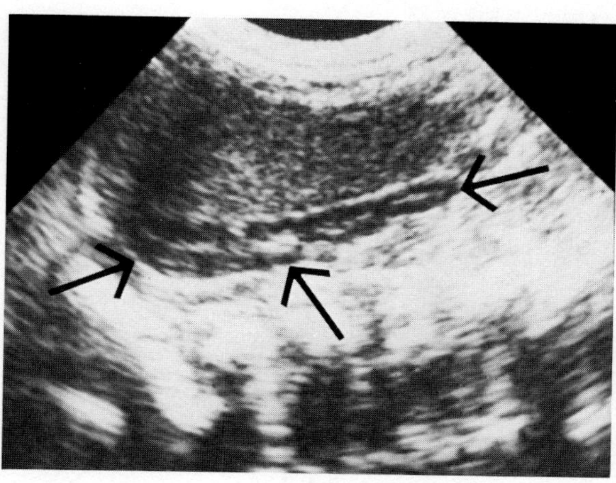

FIGURE 17-2. An abnormally long left adrenal gland *(arrows)* is identified on this sagittal scan. No defininte renal tissue could be definitively demonstrated in this patient, who died with renal agenesis.

medulla of the kidney as well as a slight discrepancy in the length of the kidneys should be clues to existence of a duplication.[60] Kidney duplication is often bilateral.

If an obstructed dilated collecting system is identified, a voiding cystourethrogram is the examination of choice to determine whether reflux or outlet obstruction is responsible (Fig. 17-3F–I). Reflux may occur with a variety of obstructive bladder lesions, such as prune belly syndrome (absence of the abdominal musculature, undescended testicles, and dilated bladder with hydroureter) or neurogenic bladder with sphincter spasm. Many infants with prune belly syndrome have small, cystic, dysplastic kidneys, but some have hydronephrotic kidneys. They may also have posterior urethral valves as well as abnormal musculature and lack of contractility of the bladder and ureteral walls.

An obstructed kidney, from whatever cause, is an important indication for radionuclide scanning. Even with severely impaired function, radionuclide activity can be detected in an obstructed kidney (Fig. 17-3I). Notably, multicystic dysplastic kidneys exhibit no function on radionuclide scanning, and this is a significant finding. Diuretic-augmented radionuclide scanning can in some cases differentiate significant obstruction from insignificant obstruction due to poorly functioning nonobstructive hydronephrotic systems.

CYSTIC DYSPLASTIC KIDNEYS

There are several classifications of cystic renal disease, based on pathologic or radiographic findings.[3,32,43,49] Sonographically it may be difficult to differentiate many of the cystic diseases without a family history. Dysplastic kidneys may be small or large without cysts or have small cysts or very large ones. The cysts may involve only a portion of one kidney or both kidneys.

MULTICYSTIC KIDNEY

Multicystic kidney, probably the most common cystic dysplasia, is difficult to differentiate from hydronephrosis, but the distinction is important because multicystic dysplasia is a nonsurgical mass whereas surgical correction of the obstruction may be in order to salvage a hydronephrotic kidney.[48,51,58,62,64] A multicystic kidney develops from a complete ureteral obstruction in utero. Terminal tubules become cysts, and as these cysts develop they do not communicate and are eventually joined together by small connective tissue cords. There may be mutliple cysts of varying sizes or a dominant or single cyst (Fig. 17-4). Multicystic kidneys may be bilateral, but this condition is inconsistent with life and affected infants have a similar presentation to patients with renal aplasia, with Potter's syndrome and respiratory difficulties.

A multicystic kidney may present as a very large mass at birth, as a progressive or decreasing cystic flank mass in utero, or as an unidentifiable kidney at a later age. A distal ureter is present in multicystic disease, whereas with agenesis no ureter is present. The disorganized cysts do not communicate with the blind ureter, which is otherwise present. Reflux may occur into the blind ureter. Unilateral multicystic kidney disease may be associated with ureteropelvic junction obstruction in the opposite kidney (Table 17-4).[34]

HYPOPLASIA AND DYSPLASIA

Hypoplasia—a small but otherwise normal kidney—most often results from atrophy secondary to

(text continues on page 496)

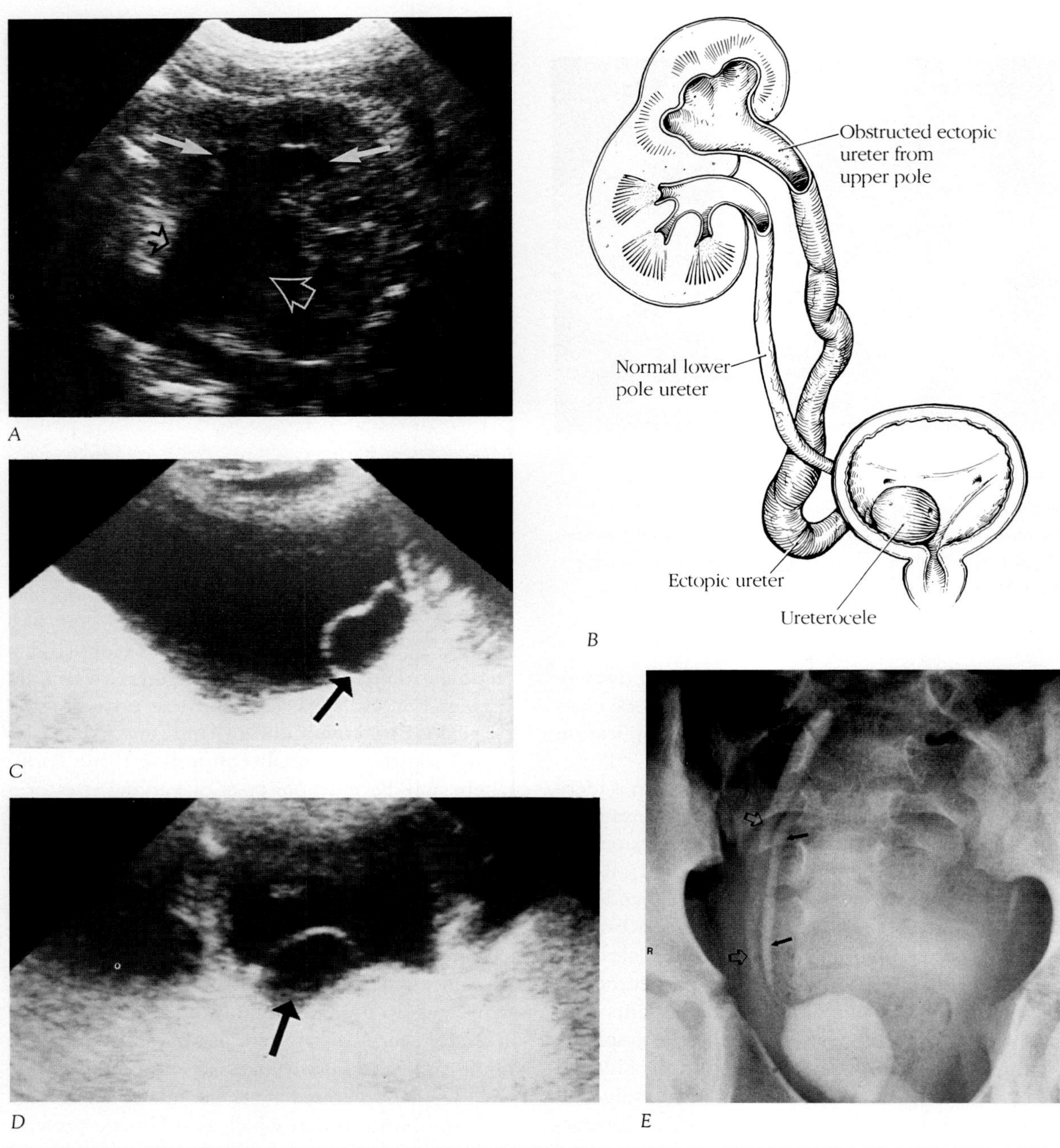

FIGURE 17-3. (*A*) With hydronephrosis, the calyces *(black arrows)* are seen communicating with the renal pelvis *(open arrows)*. This can be differentiated from multicystic kidneys, in which the cysts do not communicate. (*B*) A duplicated collecting system is illustrated, with an ectopic ureter from the upper pole ending in a ureterocele in the bladder. (C) A sagittal section of the bladder demonstrates a ureterocele *(arrow)*. (*D*) On a transverse bladder section in the same patient, the ureterocele *(arrow)* is again identified. (*E*) The excretory urogram demonstrates a duplex collecting system with the normal lower pole (*open arrows*) draining into the bladder and the obstructed upper pole *(black arrows)* ending in a ureterocele.

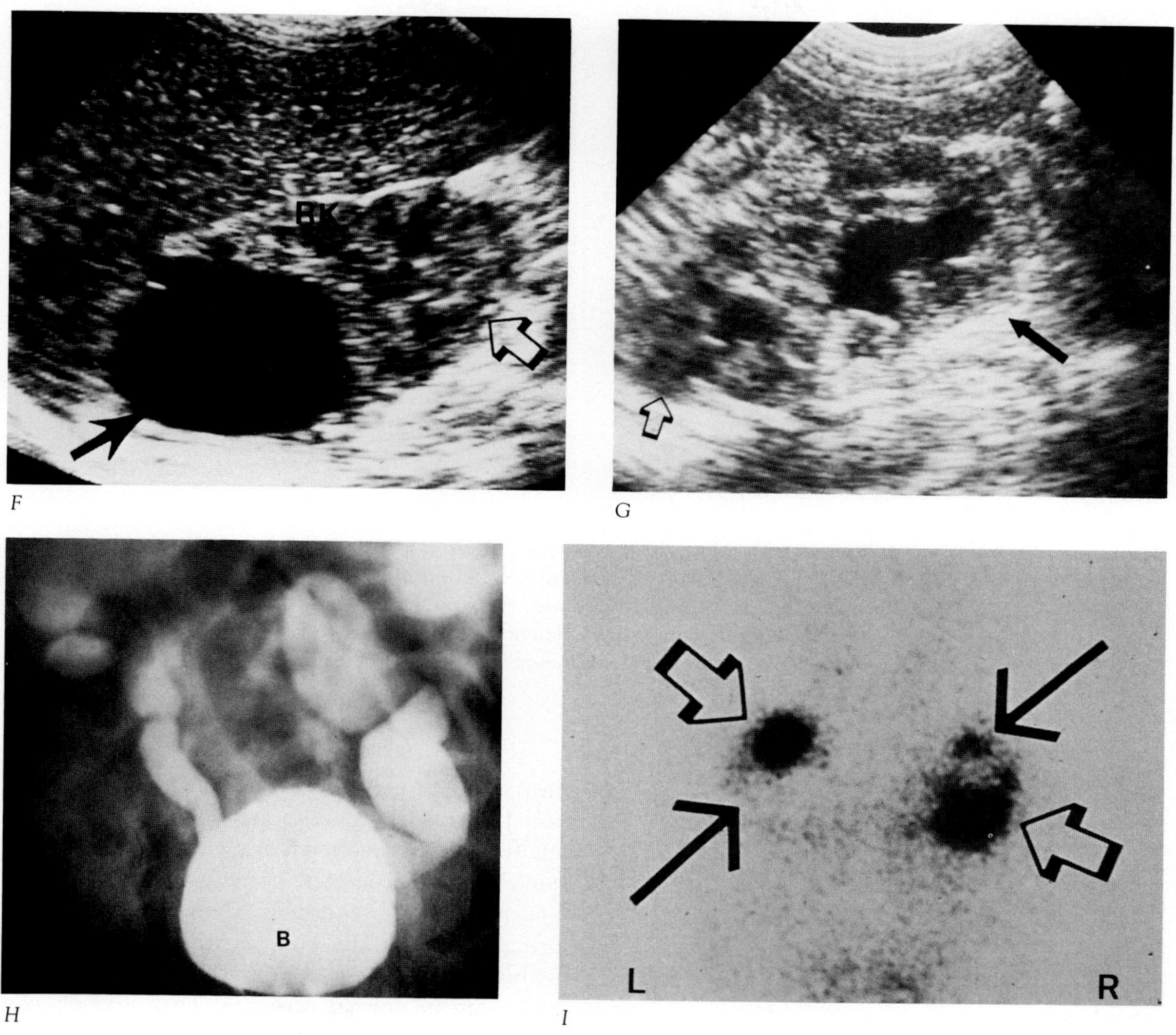

FIGURE 17-3 *(continued)*. *(F)* In a male patient, the sagittal section view of a duplex right kidney (RK) demonstrates normal lower pole parenchyma *(open arrow)* and an obstructed upper pole calyx *(arrow)* with no visible parenchyma. (G) A sagittal section of the duplex left kidney of the same patient demonstrates mild dilatation of the upper pole *(open arrow)* and a dilated lower pole *(arrow)* with good visualization of parenchyma. *(H)* Bilateral lower pole reflux with greater reflux on the left than the right is seen on the voiding cystourethrogram examination performed on this patient (B, bladder). *(I)* The radionuclide scan in this patient shows on left (L), the normally functioning left upper pole *(open arrow)* with decreased function in the left lower pole *(arrow)* due to reflux. On right (R), upper pole *(arrow)* is decreased function and the right lower pole *(open arrow)* has normal function.

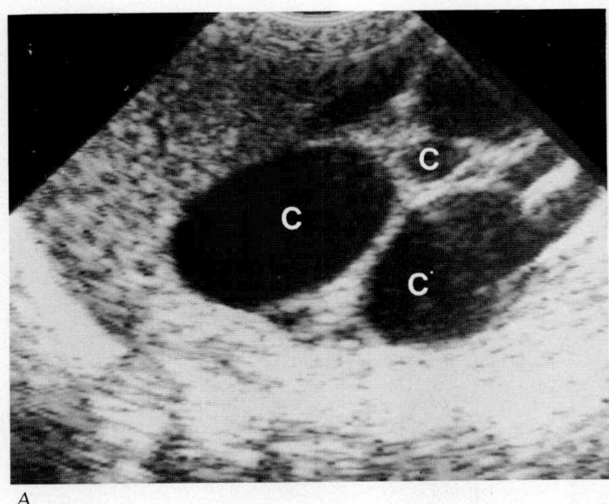

A

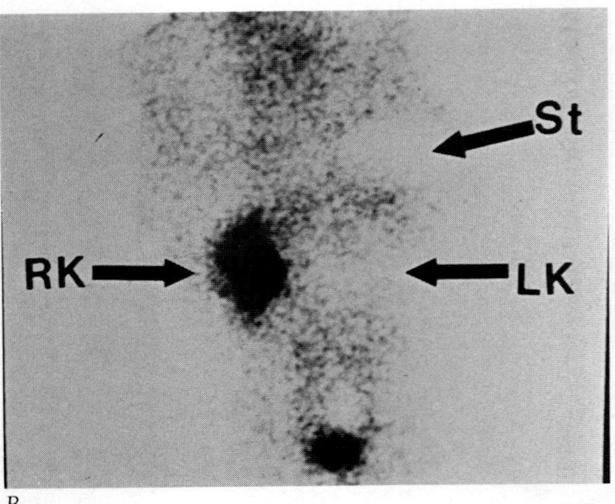

B

FIGURE 17-4. (*A*) On this sagittal section of a multicystic right kidney, no normal renal parenchyma can be identified but multiple cysts (C) of various sizes are seen, which do not communicate with the renal pelvis. (*B*) A radionuclide examination shows normal right kidney function (RK) but no renal function in the left kidney space (LK) in a patient diagnosed with left multicystic kidney disease (St, stomach).

TABLE 17-4. Ultrasonographic differentiation of hydronephrosis and multicystic disease*

FEATURE	MULTICYSTIC KIDNEY	HYDRONEPHROTIC KIDNEY
Reniform	2	4
Lobular	4	1
Parenchyma present	1	3
Continuity between cysts	1	1
Separated sinus	1	4
Interfaces	4	1
Largest cyst medial	1	4
Largest cyst peripheral	4	0
Single cyst	2	1

*Reliability of findings, 1 (least) to 4 (most).

infection and infarction or from vascular occlusions with infarction. Dysplastic kidneys, on the other hand, may be large or small, and all are anatomically abnormal. Dysplasia is associated with urinary tract malformations in 90% of the cases, usually obstruction. Dysplasia occurs with other malformations such as an obstructed ureter, ureterocele with hydroureter, posterior urethral valves, and prune belly syndrome. The patient may have urinary ascites.[1] The kidneys are often small and without the corticomedullary junction and pyramids seen in normal neonates. They may or may not have visible cysts.[22] The renal pelves may be small or dilated, and the ureter may be dilated for some distance. Caliectasis (dilatation of the renal calyx) often is not present. Congenital megacalyces and infundibular stenosis may be the same entity. Affected infants demonstrate asymptomatic hydrocaliectasis without obstruction, which is a radionuclide finding. The calyces are dilated, but the renal pelvis is of normal size and the kidneys may appear small and hyperechoic.[15,35]

INFANTILE POLYCYSTIC KIDNEY DISEASE

Infantile polycystic kidney disease or autosomal recessive polycystic kidney disease (ARPKD) is usually present at birth as symmetrically enlarged kid-

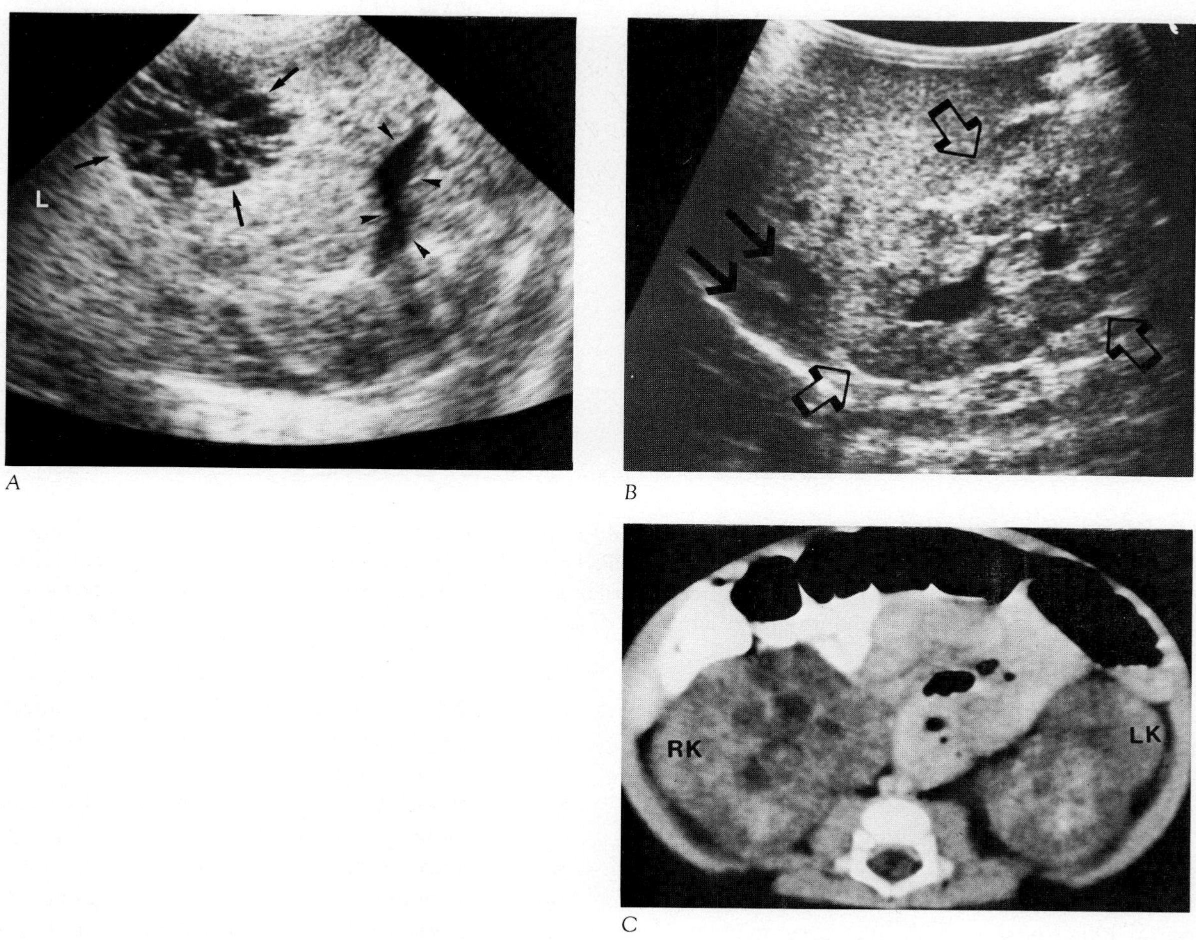

Figure 17-5. (*A*) Dilated ectatic tubules *(arrows)* are identified in the right kidney of an infant with infantile polycystic kidney disease (ARPKD). Compared to the liver, the large kidneys are echogenic, perhaps owing to multiple interfaces of renal tubules, some of which dilate to form visible cysts. Also seen is a stretched, deformed adjacent calyx *(arrowheads)*. (*B*) On a 6-month-old girl with hypertension and ARPKD, bilateral hyperechoic and enlarged kidneys were identified. The left kidney measured 7.8 cm, and this sagittal section of the right kidney *(open arrows)* is greater than 8 cm. Liver cysts *(arrows)* are also seen. (C) CT demonstrates the enlarged right (RK) and left (LK) infantile polycystic kidneys of the patient shown in *B*. Decreased renal function is evidenced by the lack of contrast medium in both kidneys.

neys. Although this condition is described as a cystic disease, the cysts result from tubular dilatation and are microscopic. These cysts cause the pyramids or medulla of the kidney to reflect multiple bright echoes. At birth, cortical echogenicity is increased, but with time the thin cortex becomes anechoic. It is the medullary portion of the kidney that enlarges and causes stretching of the calyces and renal pelvis (Fig. 17-5).

Congenital hepatic fibrosis is associated with

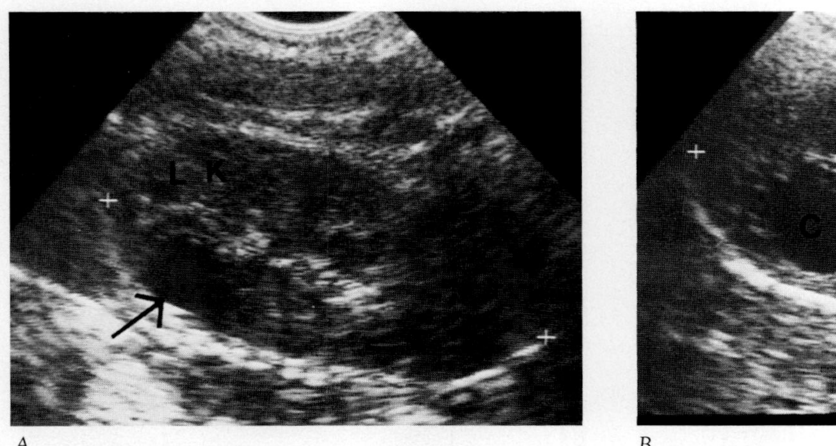

FIGURE 17-6. (*A*) A sagittal section of the left kidney (LK) measures 6.4 cm on a 3-month-old boy with ADPKD. Large *(arrow)* and small cysts are demonstrated. (*B*) In the same patient the right kidney (RK) measures 6.6 cm, the upper limit for a 3-month-old. A large cyst (C) is also seen. The patient's mother has ADPKD.

ARPKD. All patients who survive with recessive polycystic kidney disease eventually develop congenital hepatic fibrosis, although not all patients with congenital hepatic fibrosis have ARPKD. These patients may have adult polycystic disease or dysplastic kidneys. Children with less extensive renal involvement present with liver disease or portal hypertension. The liver cysts may be visualized without a microscope.[11,44,53,59] Within a given family the presentation may vary, some members developed liver failure and others renal failure.

ADULT POLYCYSTIC KIDNEY DISEASE

Adult polycystic kidney disease or autosomal dominant polycystic kidney disease (ADPKD) may occur in the neonatal period.[52] ADPKD may affect one or both kidneys (Fig. 17-6). Cysts described in the liver, pancreas, and lung in adults have not been described at this time in neonates. The cysts in neonates may range from 0.1 to 5 mm and can be difficult to visualize by ultrasound.[65] The most common sonographic finding in the neonate is renal enlargement. Of cases described in the literature, only 50% had recognizable cysts at presentation.[54] When visible, the cysts appear to be more cortical. Probably the best way to separate ADPKD from ARPKD is by history or by screening of the rest of the family. There is a 75% chance that other members of the family have the disease (Table 17-5).

TABLE 17-5. Sonographic comparison of ARPKD, ADPKD, and GKD

DISEASE	BILATERAL	RENAL SIZE	CYSTS	INHERITANCE
Autosomal recessive polycystic kidney disease	+	Very large	Rare	Autosomal recessive
Autosomal dominant polycystic kidney disease	+	Variable	Rare	Autosomal dominant
Glomerulocystic kidney disease	+	Normal to huge	Variable	Sporadic

MEDULLARY CYSTIC DISEASE

Medullary cystic disease, which has not been described in children, usually presents as a salt-losing metabolic dysfunction in young adults.

GLOMERULAR CYSTIC DISEASE

Glomerular cystic disease is hard to separate from ADPKD, ARPKD, and the hamartomas of tuberous sclerosis. At birth, the kidneys may be large and hyperechogenic. With age, they become relatively smaller and their echogenicity may decrease. The cysts described are usually in the renal cortex and are usually microscopic, but some may be macroscopic. Although the cortical echogenicity appears to resolve, there is persistent loss of the corticomedullary junction. Patients do not develop renal failure but may develop significant hepatic fibrosis and portal hypertension. The glomerular cystic disease may be associated with syndromes such as cerebral hepatorenal or Zellweger's syndrome, short-rib polydactyly, onofacial digital syndrome, renal-retinal dysplasia, Conradi's disease, Turner's syndrome, von Hippel-Lindau disease, trisomy D or E, inflammatory cysts from tuberculosis or other abscesses, and tuberous sclerosis (Fig. 17-7).[13,39,41,68]

Tumors

WILMS' TUMOR

Wilms' tumor is the second most common solid abdominal tumor of children after neuroblastoma. It most often presents as a palpable mass but may cause nonspecific symptoms such as pain, fever, malaise, and weight loss. The patient may also present with hematuria or hypertension. The peak age is 3 to 4 years, but adult and infant cases have been detected on sonography as solid masses, and they may arise from the area of the renal sinus, displacing and distorting the kidney. The masses may be of mixed echogenicity and may fill the pelvicalyceal system, or they may arise on a stalk from a single portion of the renal parenchyma. The mass may distort or displace the collecting system, causing obstruction. Anechoic or cystic spaces may be seen within the mass, which probably represents necrosis or hemorrhage but could be a remnant of functioning calyx or infundibulum trapped in the mass (Fig. 17-8A, B).

Wilms' tumor may involve retroperitoneal nodes. It is also one of the pediatric tumors that frequently invades the inferior vena cava and may extend into the heart. Therefore, these structures should be carefully examined as part of the evalu-

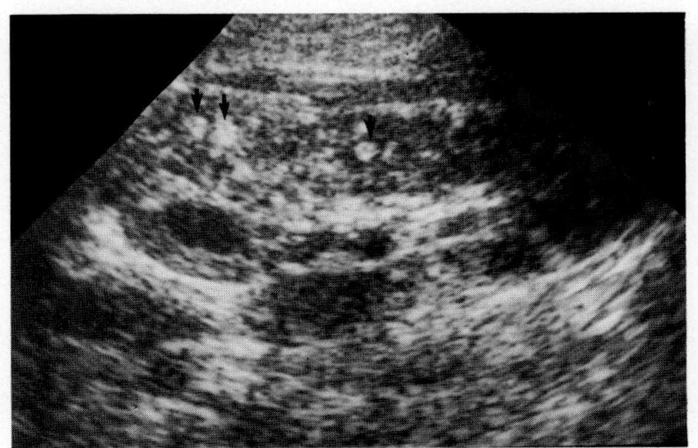

A

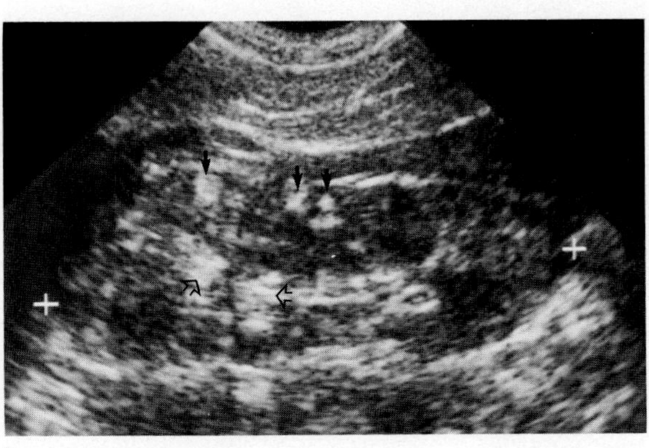

B

FIGURE 17-7. (*A*) Multiple hyperechoic foci *(arrows)* are identified in the renal cortex on this longitudinal section in a patient with tuberous sclerosis. (*B*) Multiple hyperechoic foci *(arrows)* in the renal cortex represent tuberous sclerosis and a hyperechoic focus in the kidney *(open arrows)* represents an angiomyolipoma on this sagittal section.

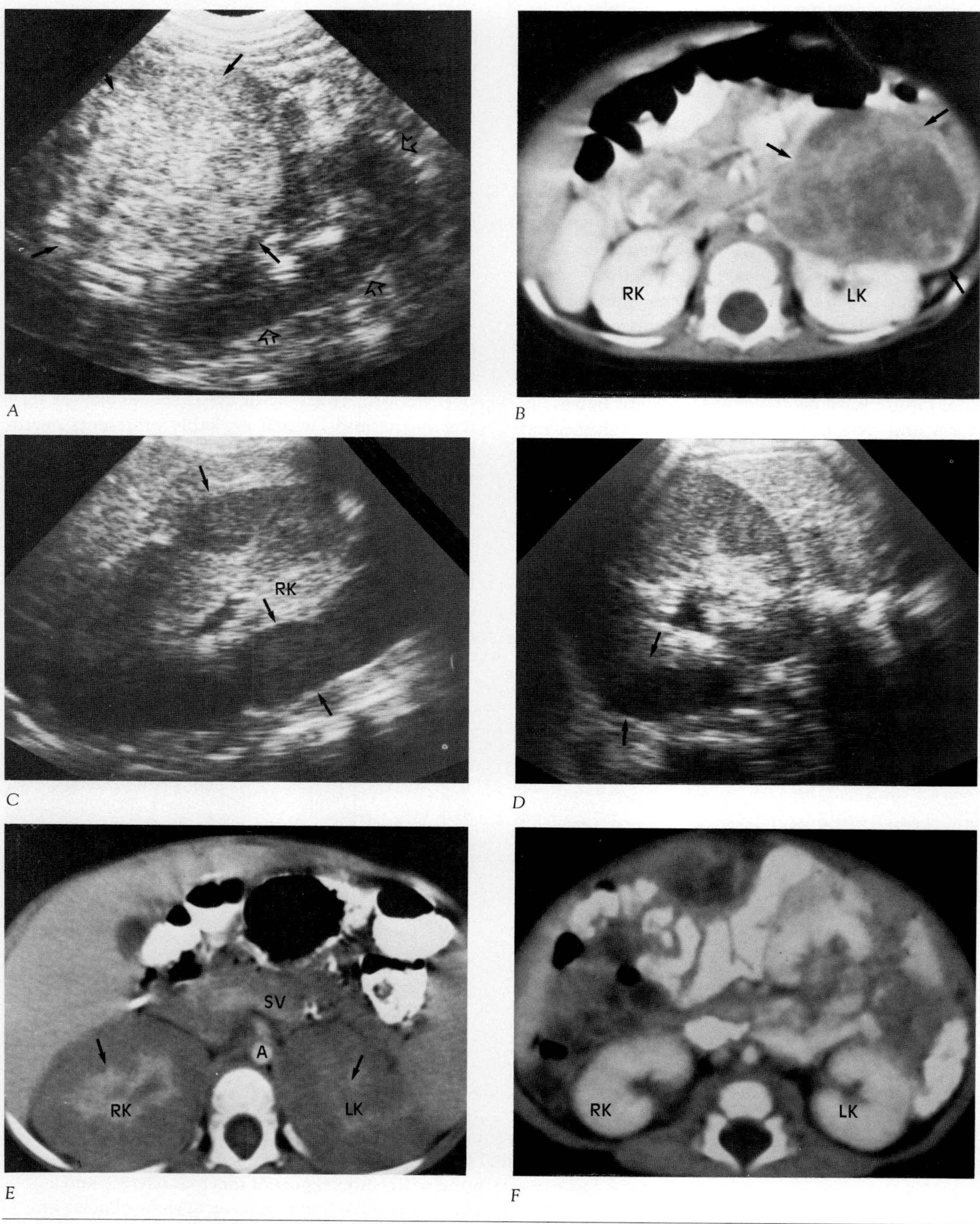

A B C D E F

ation of renal tumors.[30] Wilms' tumor may be bilateral.

Multicystic nephroblastoma, a cystic variant of Wilms', presents as multiple thin-walled cysts or as septation within cysts. Normal renal parenchyma may be present elsewhere. The presence of multiple cysts aids in the specific diagnosis of a multicystic nephroblastoma.

Nephroblastomatosis, or nodular renal blastoma, is a precursor of Wilms' tumor and can be confused with it on histologic examination. Nephroblastomatosis presents in infants or children younger than 2 years as bilateral flank masses. The diffuse process involves the subcapsular portion of the kidney. This entity can be identified on ultrasound as a thick rim of hypoechoic subcapsular tissue with irregular central contours and smooth outer margins. These findings on ultrasound and computed tomograpy (CT) are very specific (Fig. 17-8C–F).[14,56,67]

MESOBLASTIC NEPHROMA

Mesoblastic nephroma is a unilateral or bilateral benign tumor composed of connective tissue, which can replace most of the renal parenchyma. Other names are fetal renal hamartoma, mesenchymal hamartoma of infancy, and benign Wilms' tumor. They present in neonates, whereas Wilms' tumors are most common in children older than 2 years and in older children and adults. Mesoblastic nephroma is the most common solid intrarenal mass of neonates. If the tumor is unilateral, it may be removed, as Wilms' tumor would be; if bilateral, radiation and chemotherapy may be prescribed. Sonographically they resemble Wilms' tumor (Fig. 17-9).[16,25]

Renal cell carcinomas have been reported in children, and for this reason hematuria in a child should probably be evaluated with excretory urography if ultrasound findings are normal.

All of the aforementioned tumors can be recognized as arising from the kidney. Neuroblastoma, which often arises from the adrenal gland immediately adjacent to the upper pole of the kidney, may invade the renal capsule, making it very difficult to distinguish from a primary renal tumor. Usually, however, neuroblastomas cross the midline, encroaching and surrounding the great vessels rather than invading them.

Acquired Disease

INFECTION

Ultrasonography may be used for evaluating pyelonephritis or infection of the upper urinary tract, as in adults. The most common finding is enlargement of the kidneys.[12,46,47] The microabscesses described at histologic examination that may affect the kidney cannot be resolved by ultrasound and

FIGURE 17-8. (*A*) Wilms' tumor (*arrows*) is identified arising from the upper pole of the kidney (*open arrows*). The mass is usually hyperechoic, although cystic spaces or more hamartomatous tissue may be present as hypoechoic areas. (*B*) On a CT section, the right kidney (RK) is normal but the left kidney (LK) is compressed in the midportion by a large, nonenhancing Wilms' tumor (*arrows*). At this level, this appearance cannot be differentiated from normal renal tissue compressed by an extrarenal tumor, such as neuroblastoma. (C) On a sagittal section of the right kidney (RK) in a neonate with nephroblastomastosis, the lobulated hypoechoic cortex (*arrows*) appears thick and the pyramids are not discernible. (*D*) A transverse axial section of the right kidney (RK) on the same patient demonstrates the typical sonographic appearance of nephroblastomatosis, with a thick hypoechoic cortex (*arrows*) in infants with enlarged kidneys. (*E*) CT through the right (RK) and left (LK) kidneys of an infant with nephroblastomatosis demonstrates enlarged and lobulated renal tissue. The thick renal cortex accounts for most of the enlargement. Contrast is present in the aorta (A), splenic vein (SV), and the renal hilus (*arrows*) but not in the cortex as it would be in normal infants. (*F*) CT after treatment for nephroblastomatosis demonstrates normal renal contrast enhancement in both the right (RK) and left (LK) kidneys.

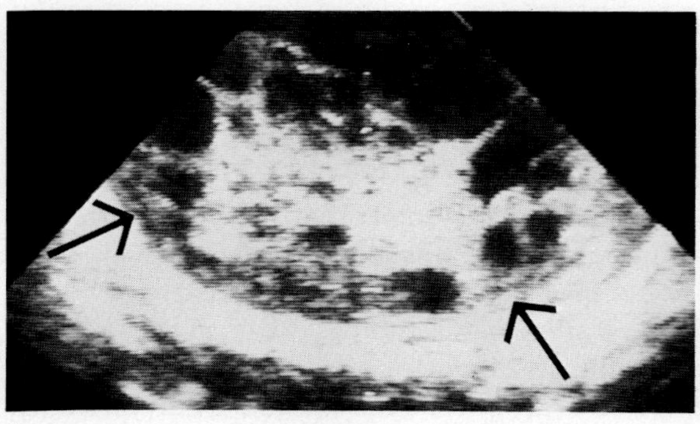
A

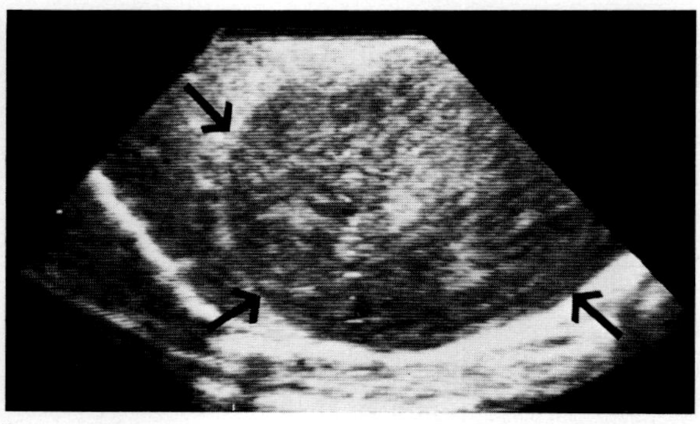
B

FIGURE 17-9. (*A*) Cystic mesoblastic nephroma can be identified as a hyperechoic mass with multiple cysts on this sagittal section of the left kidney *(arrows)*. The normal kidney shape is maintained. (*B*) On this sagittal section of the right kidney *(arrows)*, cystic mesoblastic nephroma can be identified as a solid mass. The reniform shape is maintained but normal renal parenchyma is replaced with a heterogeneous hyperechoic tissue.

rarely present as renal enlargement. Renal abscesses have been described on ultrasonography.[27,63] Mild scarring of a kidney due to chronic infection is a difficult specific sonographic diagnosis to make because the scars may be very small and difficult to image. Second, the calyces do not become dilated. Significant cortical scarring, of course, is easy to identify.[33] In children with continuous lower urinary tract infections, baseline renal measurements may be important to follow over a period of time, to make sure the kidneys are growing properly. Ultrasound is also a useful screening tool to seek anatomic causes of infection, specifically obstruction (Fig. 17-10).

NEPHROCALCINOSIS

Nephrocalcinosis is the deposit of calcium in the kidney. It usually affects both kidneys with focal echogenicity, with or without acoustic shadowing. Nephrocalcinosis can occur in children with hyperparathyroidism, renal tubular acidosis, hypercalcemia, and particularly those infants receiving long-term furosemide or lasix for chronic lung or heart disease. Sonography in children at risk for nephrocalcinosis may identify hyperechoic pyramids (Figure 17-11A). This could also represent sloughed papilla, blood clots, fungus balls, cellular debris, or proteinuria. Children at risk for urolithiasis because of urinary stasis or infection may have echogenic calculi in the ureter or bladder.

RENAL VASCULAR DISEASE

Renal vascular problems in children are usually the result of trauma or other underlying conditions such as nephrotic syndrome. Another cause of renal artery problems can be umbilical artery catheterization that produces clot formation or emboli in infants' renal arteries, and ultimately, hypoplasia of the kidneys. In small infants it can be difficult to detect actual renal vein thrombosis, as it often occurs in the small vein, but diffuse enlargement and increased echogenicity of the kidneys can be seen.[45,57]

TRAUMA

Renal trauma is unusual in infants but may be related to a birth injury.[40] The cause of a flank mass in a newborn is more often adrenal than renal parenchymal hemorrhage. Sonographically, the hemorrhage has mixed echogenicity, and the mass or flank fluid may be seen extending subcapsularly into the peritoneal cavity (Fig. 17-11B). For imaging renal trauma in a child CT is the modality of choice.[6,8]

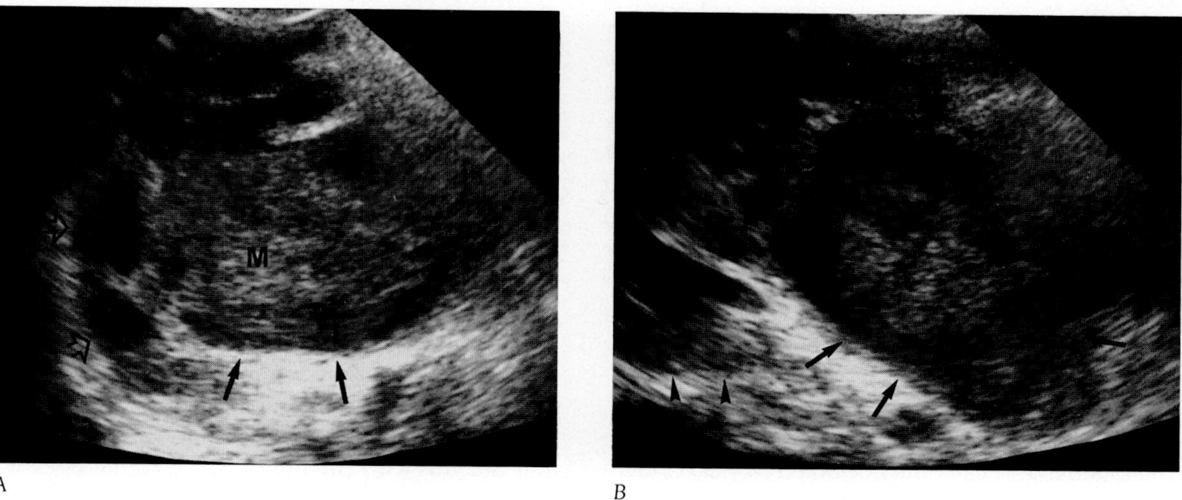

FIGURE 17-10. (*A*) A transverse section through the right kidney demonstrates a hyperechoic mass (M, *arrows*), compressed hyperechoic renal parenchyma, and dilated calyces (*open arrows*). The central mass is a pus-filled renal pelvis. (*B*) A longitudinal section made on a patient in the prone position with ureteropelvic junction (UPJ) obstruction demonstrates a pus-filled, enlarged renal pelvis (*arrows*) with a hypoechoic space posterior (*open arrows*), which represents urine surrounding pus that has settled to the dependent portion of the dilated pelvis (*arrowheads*, renal parenchyma).

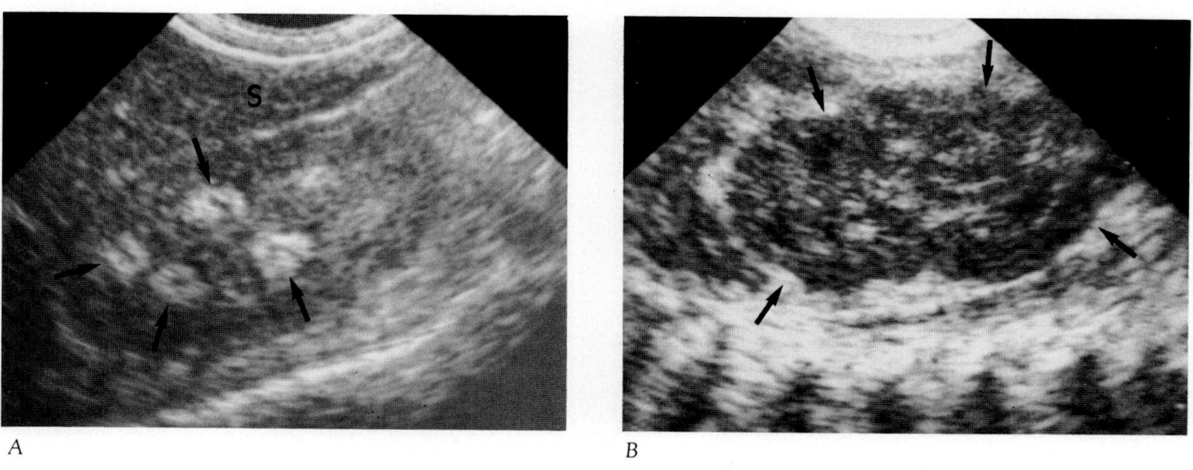

FIGURE 17-11. (*A*) This longitudinal section of an infant's left kidney has the same echoic pattern as the spleen, and hyperechoic nodules (*arrows*) in the area of the renal pyramids with anechoic centers are demonstrated. (*B*) On a coronal section, the hyperechoic left kidney (*arrows*) of a 4-month-old is seen to have lost the normal pyramids. At autopsy 24 hours later, diffuse interstitial hemorrhage was confirmed.

Bladder

In the infants, the bladder is an abdominal rather than a pelvic organ, and frequently it is difficult to evaluate because the mere pressure of the transducer on the abdomen causes the bladder to evacuate. When it is necessary for an infant's bladder to be full, a Foley catheter can be used to fill it and the inflated balloon to keep it full. It is unusual to see a very distended bladder in a normal neonate unless the mother received drugs during labor or delivery, which could affect the infant's nervous system for several hours, or the infant is receiving drugs that would inhibit voiding. Bladder distension may be caused by neurogenic disease or a pelvic mass. Cystic pelvic masses can be confused with the bladder and care must be taken to clearly identify the bladder.

Congenital Anomalies

Urachal Abnormalities. The urachus is a tubular structure continuous with the anterior dome of the bladder and extending outside the peritoneum to the umbilicus superiorly. Normally during the fourth and fifth months of gestation, the urachus narrows to small-caliber tube. The normal urachus is either completely obliterated and fibrotic at or before birth, or it seals off in the neonatal period. In a few infants the urachus persists. It may persist as a cord from the umbilicus to the superior aspect of the bladder, producing an anterior superior vesical diverticulum, which is usually continuous with the bladder. It may remain an open structure (patent urachus) between the umbilicus and the bladder, but usually only in cases of bladder outlet obstruction where the urachus decompresses the otherwise obstructed bladder. Such patients may exhibit an abdominal mass after the umbilical cord is clamped at birth. Sometimes the urachus persists in continuity with the umbilicus but not with the bladder; sometimes it is continuous with the bladder but not with the umbilicus. Urachal cysts may present as palpable midline abdominal masses but more often the patient has an infection (Fig. 17-12).[2,29]

Ultrasonography is useful for evaluating urachal cyst. The bladder is tethered anteriorly. Masses are continuous with the bladder, and the echo pattern is cystic or, if infected, mixed.

The posterior urethral valve syndrome is another congenital urethral abnormality. The valve

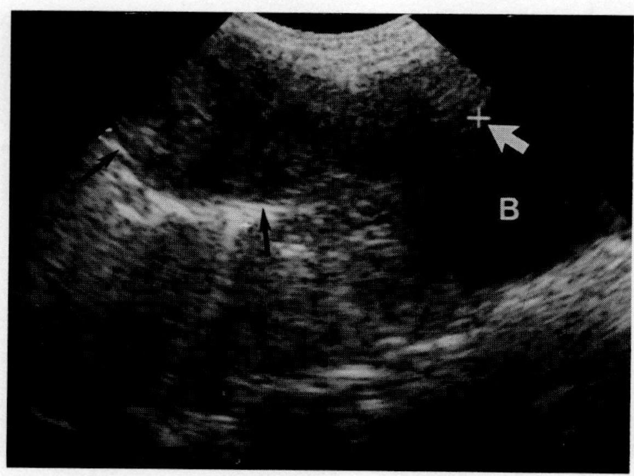

A

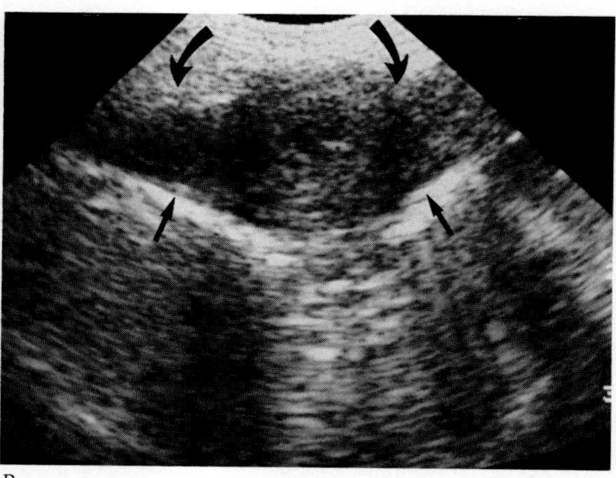

B

Figure 17-12. (*A*) A sagittal section of the pelvis in a 3-month-old demonstrates a hyperechoic mass (*arrows*) arising from the superior anterior surface of the urinary bladder (B) typical of an infected urachal cyst. (*B*) A transverse section in the midline on the same patient demonstrates that the mass appears outside the peritoneal reflection (*straight arrows*) with edema in the abdominal wall (*curved arrows*).

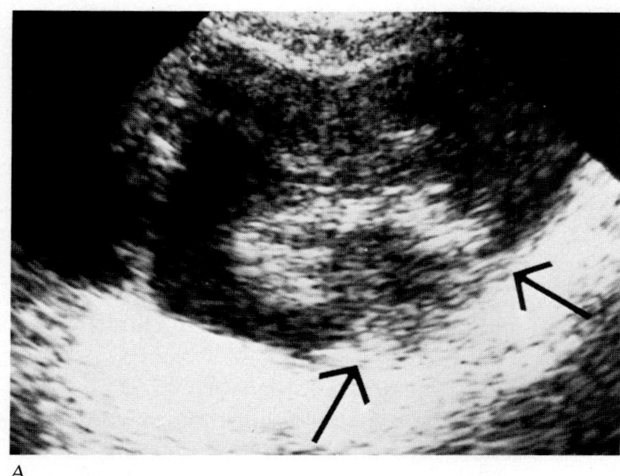
A

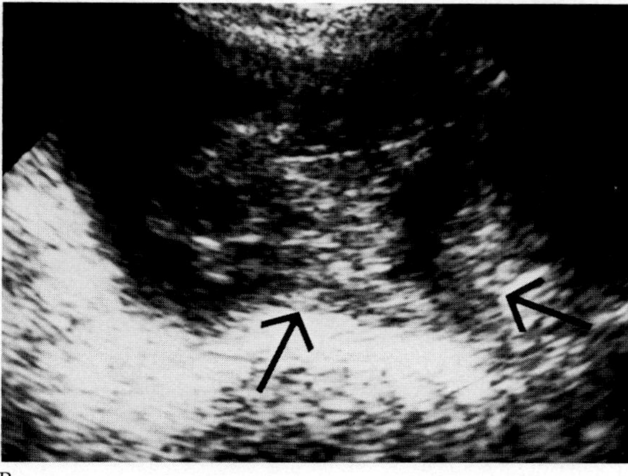
B

FIGURE 17-13. (*A*) A transverse section in the right pelvic region of this 6-year-old boy demonstrates a mass (rhabdomyosarcoma, *arrows*) arising from the posterior inferior bladder wall. (*B*) A sagittal section in the midline of the same patient demonstrates the mass (*arrows*) arising from the posterior inferior bladder wall.

is a thin membrane positioned across the membranous portion of the penile urethra in boys. With secondary changes in the bladder, ureters, or kidneys, it can obstruct voiding as previously described. On ultrasonography, the bladder may have a thick wall and dilatation of the posterior urethra can be identified. The ureters are tortuous and dilated, and the kidneys have varying degrees of dysplasia. Children with prune belly syndrome may have posterior urethral valves with hydroureteronephrosis and renal dysplasia, but the bladder is usually very large and flaccid.

TUMORS

Rhabdomyosarcomas. Rhabdomyosarcomas often involve or arise from the bladder, prostate, uterus, or vagina of children. Depending on the point of origin, they may cause various changes in the urinary tract.[17] Sonographically, rhabdomyosarcomas are of mixed echogenicity and associated with thickening of the bladder wall, or they are seen as a mass posterior and inferior to the bladder. Masses within the bladder are often immovable blood clots that are adherent to the thick wall (Fig. 17-13).[17] The bladder may also be obstructed by sacrococcygeal teratoma (see Chapter 13).

INFECTION

Cystitis, the most common urinary tract infection of children, is ten times more common in girls than in boys. In children with chronic cystitis, the bladder wall may be thickened, measuring more than 0.3 cm. Usually, cystitis produces diffuse thickening of the bladder wall, which can be a nonspecific finding. Bladder calculi in children are extremely unusual unless there is urinary stasis in the bladder. Children with active urinary tract bleeding may show clots or blood in the bladder. Bladder perforation and trauma are best evaluated by cystography.

References

1. Avni EF, Thoua Y, Van Gansbeke D, et al: Development of the hypodysplastic kidney: Contribution of antenatal US diagnosis. Radiology 1987, 164:123–125.
2. Bauer SB, Retik AB: Urachal anomalies and related umbilical disorders. Urol Clins North Am 1978, 5:195–211.
3. Bernstein J: The classification of renal cysts. Nephron 1973, 11:91–100.
4. Brenbridge AN, Chevalier RL, Kaiser DL: Increased renal cortical echogenicity in pediatric renal disease:

histopathologic correlations. J Clin Ultrasound 1986, 14:595–600.

5. Brown T, Mandell J, Lebowitz RL: Neonatal hydronephrosis in the era of sonography. AJR 1987, 148:959–964.
6. Cass AS, Luxenberg M, Gleich P, et al: Clinical indications for radiographic evaluation of blunt renal trauma. J Urol 1986, 136:370–372.
7. Chevalier RL, Campbell F, Brenbridge ANA: Nephrosonography and renal scintigraphy in evaluation of newborns with renomegaly. Urology 1984, 24:96–103.
8. Colombani PM, Buck JR, Dudgeon DL, et al: One-year experience in a regional pediatric trauma center. J Pediatri Surg 1985, 20:8–13.
9. Cramer BC, Jequier S, de Chadarevian JP: Factors associated with renal parenchymal echogenicity in the newborn. J Ultrasound Med 1986, 5:633–638.
10. Currarino G, Williams B, Dana K: Kidney length correlated with age: Normal values in children. Radiology 1984, 150:703–704.
11. Davies CH, Stringer DA, Whyte H, et al: Congenital hepatic fibrosis with saccular dilatation of intrahepatic bile ducts and infantile polycystic kidneys. Pediatr Radiol 1986, 16:302–305.
12. Dinkel E, Orth S, Dittrich M, et al: Renal sonography in the differentiation of upper from lower urinary tract infection. AJR 1986, 146:775–780.
13. Fitch SJ, Stapleton FB: Ultrasonographic features of glomerulocystic disease in infancy: Similarity to infantile polycystic kidney disease. Pediatr Radiol 1986 16:400–402.
14. Franken EA, Yiu-Chiu V, Smith WL, et al: Nephroblastomatosis: Clinicopathological significance and imaging characteristics. AJR 1982, 138:950–952.
15. Garvia CJ, Taylor KJW, Weiss RM: Congenital megacalyces: Ultrasound appearance. J Ultrasound Med 1987, 6:163–165.
16. Geirsson RT, Ricketts NEM, Taylor DJ, et al: Prenatal appearance of mesoblastic nephroma associated with polyhydramnios. J Clin Ultrasound 1985, 13:488–490.
17. Geoffray A, Counant D, Montagne JP, et al: Ultrasonography and computed tomography for diagnosis and follow-up of pelvic rhabdomyosarcomas in children. Pediatr Radiol 1987, 17:132–136.
18. Gilsanz V, Fernal W, Reid BS, et al: Nephrolithiasis in premature infants. Radiology 1985, 154:107–110.
19. Gilsanz V, Miller JH, Reid BS: Ultrasonic characteristics of posterior urethral valves. Radiology 1982, 145:143–145.
20. Grignon A, Filiatrault D, Homsy Y, et al: Ureteropelvic junction stenosis: Antenatal ultrasonographic diagnosis, postnatal investigation and follow-up. Radiology 1986, 160:649–651.
21. Grignon A, Filion R, Filiatrault D, et al: Urinary tract dilatation in utero: Classification and clinical applications. Radiology 1986, 160:645–647.
22. Gordillo R, Vilaro M, Sherman NH, et al: Circumscribed renal mass in dysplastic kidney. Pseudomass vs. tumor. J Ultrasound Med 1987, 6:613–617.
23. Haller JO, Berdon WE, Friedman AP: Increased renal cortical echogencity: A normal finding in neonates and infants. Radiology 1982, 142:173–174.
24. Han BK, Babcock DS: Sonographic measurements and appearance of normal kidneys in children. AJR 1985, 145:611–616.
25. Hartman DS, Lesar MSL, Madewell JE, et al: Mesoblastic nephroma: Radiologic-pathologic correlation of 20 cases. AJR 1981, 136:69–74.
26. Hayden CK Jr, Santa-Cruz FR, Amparo EG, et al: Ultrasonographic evaluation of the renal parenchyma in infancy and childhood. Radiology 1984, 152:413–417.
27. Hoddick W, Jeffrey RB, Goldberg HI, et al: CT and sonography of severe renal and perirenal infections. AJR 1983, 140:517–520.
28. Hricak H, Slovis TL, Callen CW, et al: Neonatal kidneys sonographic anatomic correlation. Radiology 1983, 147:669–702.
29. Jarzylo SV, Challis TW, Bruce WA: Urachal abnormalities. J Canad Assoc Radiol 1965, 16:175–180.
30. Johnson KM, Horvath LJ, Caisie G, et al: Wilms tumor occurring as a botryoid renal pelvicalyceal mass. Radiology 1987, 163:385–386.
31. Jones BE, Hoffer FA, Teele RL, et al: The compound renal pyramid. A normal hypoechoic region on the pediatric sonogram. J Ultrasound Med 1987, 6:515–518.
32. Kaariainen H, Jaaskelainen J, Kivisaari L, et al: Dominant and recessive polycystic kidney disease in children: Classification by intravenous pyleography, ultrasound, and computed tomography. Pediatr Radiol 1988, 18:45–50.
33. Kay CJ, Rosenfield AT, Taylor KJW, et al: Ultrasonic characteristics of chronic atrophic pyelonephritis. AJR 1979, 132:47–49.
34. Kleiner B, Filly RA, Mack L, et al: Multicystic dysplastic kidney: Observations of contralateral disease in the fetal population. Radiology 1986, 161:27–29.
35. Krensky AM, Reddish JM, Teele RL: Causes of increased renal echogenicity in pediatric patients. Pediatrics 1983, 72:840–846.
36. Laing FC, Burke VD, Wing VW, et al: Postpartum evaluation of fetal hydronephrosis: Optimal timing for follow-up sonography. Radiology 1984, 154:423–424.
37. Lawson TL, Foley WD, Berland LL, et al: Ultrasonic

evaluation of fetal kidneys. Radiology 1981, 138:153–156.

38. Lucaya J, Enriquez G, Delgado R, et al: Infundibulopelvic stenosis in children. AJR 1984, 142:471–474.
39. Luisiri A, Sotelo-Avila C, Silberstein MJ, et al: Sonography of the Zellweger syndrome. J Ultrasound Med 1988, 7:169–173.
40. Newman B, Smith S: Unusual renal mass in a newborn infant. Radiology 1987, 163:193–194.
41. McAlister WH, Siegel MJ, Shackelford G, et al: Glomerulocystic kidney. AJR 1979, 133:536–538.
42. McGrath MA, Estroff J, Lebowitz RL: The coexistence of obstruction at the ureteropelvic and ureterovesical junctions. AJR 1987, 149:403–406.
43. Mellins HZ: Cystic dilatations of the upper urinary tract: A radiologist's development model. Radiology 1984, 153:291–301.
44. Melson GL, Shackelford GD, Cole BR, et al: The spectrum of sonographic findings in infantile polycystic kidney disease with urographic and clinical correlations. J Clin Ultrasound 1985, 13:113–119.
45. Metreweli C, Pearson R: Echographic diagnosis of neonatal renal venous thrombosis. Pediatr Radiol 1984, 14:105–108.
46. Morehouse HT, Weiner SN, Hoffman JC: Imaging in inflammatory disease of the kidney. AJR 1984, 143:135–141.
47. Morehouse HT, Weiner SN, Hoffman-Tretin JC: Inflammatory disease of the kidney. Semin Ultrasound CT, MR 1986, 7:246–258.
48. Nussbaum AR, Hartman DS, Whitley N: Multicystic dysplasia and crossed renal ectopia. AJR 1987, 149:407–410.
49. Osathanondh V, Potter EL: Pathogenesis of polycystic kidneys. Survey of results of microdissection. Arch Pathol 1984, 77:510–513.
50. Patriquin H, Robitaille P: Renal calcium deposition in children. AJR 1986, 146:1253–1256.
51. Pedicelli G, Jequier S, Bowel A'D, et al: Multicystic dysplastic kidneys: Spontaneous regression demonstrated with US. Radiology 1986, 161:23–26.
52. Porch P, Noe HN, Stapleton FB: Unilateral presentation of adult-type polycystic kidney disease in children. J Urology 1986, 135:744–746.
53. Premkumar A, Berdon WE, Levy J, et al: The emergence of hepatid fibrosis and portal hypertension in infants and children with autosomal recessive polycystic kidney disease. Initial and follow-up sonographic and radiographic findings. Pediatr Radiol 1988, 18:123–129.
54. Pretorius DH, Lee ME, Manco-Johnson ML, et al: Diagnosis of autosomal dominant polycystic kidney disease in utero and in the young infant. J Ultrasound Med 1987, 6:249–255.
55. Rosenbaum DM, Korngold E, Teele RL: Sonographic assessment of renal length in normal children. AJR 1984, 142:467–469.
56. Rosenberg ER, Trought WS, Kirks DR, et al: Ultrasonic diagnosis of renal vein thrombosis in neonates. AJR 1980, 134:35–38.
57. Rosenfeld NS, Shimkin P, Bearden W, et al: Wilms tumor arising from spontaneously regressing nephroblastomatosis. AJR 1980, 135:381–384.
58. Sanders RC, Hartman DS: The sonographic distinction between neonatal multicystic kidney and hydronephrosis. Radiology 1984, 151:621–625.
59. Sanders RC, Nussbaum AR, Solez K: Renal dysplasia: Sonographic findings. Radiology 1988, 167:623–626.
60. Schaffer RM, Shih YH, Becker JA: Sonographic identification of collecting system duplications. J Clin Ultrasound 1983, 11:309–312.
61. Schlesinger AE, Hedlund GL, Pierson WP, et al: Normal standards for kidney length in premature infants: Determination with ultrasound. Radiology 1987, 164:127–129.
62. Stuck KJ, Koff SA, Silver TM: Ultrasonic features of multicystic dysplastic kidney: Expanded diagnostic criteria. Radiology 1982, 143:217–221.
63. Sty JR, Wells RG, Sharshak RJ, et al: Imaging in acute renal infection in children. AJR 1987, 148:471–477.
64. Vinocur L, Slovis TL, Perlmutter AD, et al: Follow-up studies of multicystic dysplastic kidneys. Radiology 1988, 167:311–315.
65. Walker FC Jr, Loney LC, Root ER, et al: Diagnostic evaluation of adult polycystic kidney disease in childhood. AJR 1984, 142:1273–1277.
66. Wolfson BJ, Gainey MA, Faerber EN, et al: Renal masses in children. An integrated imaging approach to diagnosis. Urol Clin North Am 1985, 12:755–769.
67. Wood BP, Muurahainen N, Anderson VM, et al: Multicystic nephroblastoma: Ultrasound diagnosis (with a pathologic-anatomic commentary). Pediatr Radiol 1982, 12:43–46.
68. Worthington JL, Shackelford GD, Bole BR, et al: Sonographically detectable cysts in polycystic kidney disease in newborn and young infants. Pediatr Radiol 1988, 18:287–293.

CHAPTER 18

Adrenal Glands

LORIANN D. FORBUSH

Sonography is the preferred imaging modality for visualizing the adrenal glands of children.[26] Diagnostic ultrasound is particularly useful in the examination of the neonatal adrenals: it has been reported to be possible to image 97% of right adrenal glands and 83% of left ones.[8] Improvements in visualization of the normal neonatal adrenal glands by sonography are due to several factors: (1) the neonatal adrenals are proportionally larger than adult glands (about one third the size of the kidney at birth, as opposed to one thirteenth in adults); (2) newborn infants' sparsity of perirenal fat affords better image resolution than the abundance of areolar fatty tissue surrounding the adult gland; and (3) the neonatal adrenal glands are closer to the skin surface, which permits use of higher-frequency transducers for sharper resolution of small structures.[19] In older infants and children, normal adrenal glands are sometimes difficult to identify, especially the left one. Adrenal sonography provides an opportunity to image from several directions, avoids the negative effects of ionizing radiation, is less expensive than computed tomography (CT), and can be performed at the bedside of a critically ill patient.[1] The drawbacks of adrenal sonography include technically unsatisfactory studies resulting from the small size of the gland in older children, obesity, and overlying bowel gas.[19]

Sonographic Technique

PATIENT PREPARATION

Adrenal visualization may be limited because of attenuation by bowel gas. Since air is a major culprit, it may be helpful to examine the patient after fasting[17] using an approximate time line of 3 hours for patients younger than 1 year; 6 hours for patients 1 to 5 years; and 12 hours for older children.

Techniques. The accuracy of adrenal sonographic visualization varies greatly, depending on what technique is used and on the experience and skill of the operator.[15] The age of the patient is also an important factor, because the adrenal glands of neonates and young infants are larger and more easily identified.[10] It is not uncommon to examine the patient in different positions until the entire gland can be visualized. Various techniques have been developed to provide optimal visualization. The adrenal glands may be demonstrated by scanning from the flanks in sagittal, coronal, and transverse projections. These projections are useful for avoiding overlying bowel.

The use of various decubitus and oblique views may aid visualization.[19] A combination of transverse and longitudinal oblique scans has been reported to be very accurate in identifying adrenal disease. When the patient lies in the decubitus position, the kidney falls forward and the adrenal gland may come into the scanning plane. However, because the gland is a complicated, folded piece of tissue, a single scan may demonstrate only part of it. For a complete adrenal evaluation, the sonographer should scan anterior as well as posterior to the gland, until is it imaged entirely.[27]

Another helpful technique in left adrenal gland visualization is the cava-suprarenal line (CSL) position, in which the patient lies in a 45-degree left posterior oblique position while transverse scans are made from the right side to localize the left adrenal gland. The patient's position is then adjusted so that the acoustic beam lines up and passes through the inferior vena cava (IVC) and aorta. The left adrenal gland is then visualized. Sagittal views are obtained by using the IVC and aorta as a double window for transmission.[15]

Yeh found that transverse scanning afforded the single best view of the adrenal glands. He noted that, with special attention to its exact anatomic location, the entire gland can be delineated by serial, closely spaced anterior transverse scans. The left adrenal gland is more difficult to visualize than the right one because of nearby stomach or bowel gas interference. This difficulty may be overcome by scanning through the intercostal spaces near the posterior axillary line. In difficult cases, it may be helpful to elevate the patient's left side, so that the adrenal area can be scanned through the spleen and kidney and behind the stomach gas bubble.[27]

Technical Considerations. During adrenal scanning the gain control setting should be comparable to that used for studying the liver. The normal adrenal glands have about the same echogenicity as the normal liver. The transducer should be selected to provide the highest available resolution with adequate penetration.[1]

Normal Anatomy

The use of adjacent structural landmarks facilitates accurate localization of the adrenal glands. These paired retroperitoneal structures are located within the perirenal space. The right adrenal gland lies over the kidney between the right crus of the diaphragm and the liver, posterior to the IVC. Any mass in the right adrenal area must be differentiated from a renal, hepatic, or a retrocaval lymph node mass.

Imaging the left adrenal gland may be more difficult because of the numerous structures located in the left upper quadrant. The left adrenal lies anterior to the upper pole of the left kidney but lateral to the left crus of the diaphragm and posterior to the pancreatic tail. The esophagogastric junction is superior to the left gland and the fourth portion of the duodenum, inferior to it. It is important not to mistake the spleen, the splenic vessels, or the left renal vessels for the adrenal gland. These structures are usually distinguishable by their differing sonographic textures and contours, although masses originating in any of these structures can be mistaken for left adrenal masses or vice versa. A collapsed stomach or the duodenum can also be differentiated from the adrenal by the presence of "bright" central mucosal echoes and the real-time demonstration of peristalsis. The patient can drink water to demonstrate the stomach if there is any question. The spleen varies in size and location and may have lobulations (accessory spleens). Such findings can cause confusion and lead to misdiagnosis of an enlarged left adrenal gland.[26] Abdominal vessels can be identified by observing their pulsations and using Doppler instrumentation to detect blood flow.

The typical sonographic appearance of the adrenal gland is a Y- or V-shaped structure on longitudinal scans[20] (Fig. 18-1) and curvilinear on transverse scans.[19] It has two parts: the medulla, which is sonographically visualized as a thin, echogenic central area, and the cortex, which appears as a thicker, anechoic zone surrounding the medulla.[16] The newborn's adrenal cortex is relatively thick because it is composed of two layers: a thick fetal zone that occupies approximately 80% of the gland, and a thin peripheral zone that will become the adult cortex. After birth, the fetal zone undergoes involution, gradually shrinking, and takes on a more typical adult appearance as it is replaced by connective tissues by 1 year of age.[19,22]

Sonographic studies should note the adrenals' size. In an extensive study of normal neonates, Oppenheimer and coworkers found the normal adrenal length to range between 0.9 to 3.6 cm and the width between 0.2 and 0.5 cm. Their study found no statistically significant difference in the size of

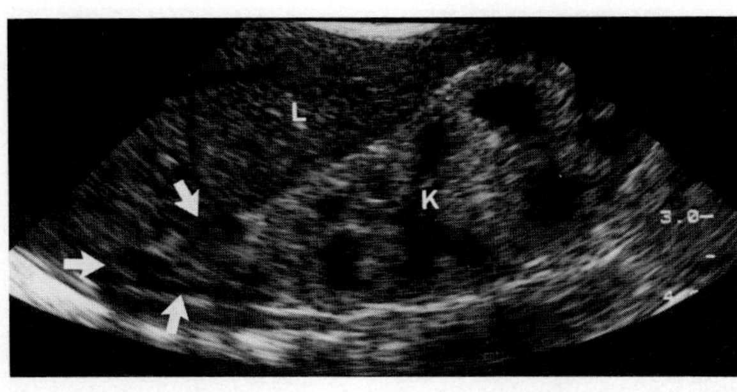

FIGURE 18-1. Longitudinal sonogram demonstrates the normal right adrenal gland *(arrows)*, kidney (K), and liver (L) in a newborn infant.

right and left adrenals. It is important to note that with renal agenesis the adrenal gland is large and occupies the renal fossa. It may lose its typical Y or V shape but should not be mistaken for the kidney or another mass.[10]

Abnormal Findings

TUMORS

Sonography can document the presence of adrenal masses, but it cannot differentiate tumor types.[26] Masses are usually more readily visualized than the normal gland.[27] The sonographic appearance must be correlated with clinical and laboratory data to determine the type of lesion.[26] Adrenal masses usually appear as sonographically discrete lesions superior and medial to the upper pole of the kidney. A large mass may compress and deform the kidney, producing the appearance of tumor invasion. The most important feature for differentiating adrenal and renal masses is an interface or demarcation between the mass and the kidney. An adrenal mass shows such a demarcation, whereas a renal mass does not.[28]

Neuroblastoma. The most common adrenal tumors of childhood are the complex of neuroblastomas, which include ganglioneuromas, ganglioneuroblastomas, and neuroblastomas. All of these tumors are of neural crest origin, but the ganglioneuroma is considered less malignant and actually is a mature neuroblastoma.[10] Neuroblastoma is a tumor of infancy.[2,13] Half the reported cases appear in the first year of life. Uncommon after age 8 years, neuroblastoma almost never occurs in adults.[14] It is important to note that these lesions can also arise from sympathetic ganglia in the lower abdomen, presacral region, chest, and even the neck and nasopharynx.[10] In the first year of life, almost all neuroblastomas involve the adrenal gland. The older the patient, the more likely is the tumor to arise outside the adrenal gland.[14] The prognosis for neuroblastoma is usually better in neonates and young infants than in older infants or children.[23]

Neuroblastoma is well known to have an unpredictable course.[6] Ordinarily, staging is based on the local extent of the lesion and the presence or absence of metastases. In most cases, patients with neuroblastoma present with advanced disease, having a large abdominal mass or signs of metastases. Unlike Wilms' tumor, most neuroblastomas are not "clean" lesions; usually they spread rapidly beyond the confines of the adrenal gland, often crossing the midline in the abdomen and sometimes extending into the chest. Calcification is a common finding in neuroblastoma, and calcifications frequently are irregular and visible in the primary tumor or its metastases.[10]

Sonographic appearance. Sonographically, neuroblastoma is highly echogenic, with poorly defined borders (Figs. 18-2, 18-3). When tumor calcification is present, focal echogenic areas can be seen producing acoustic shadowing (Figs. 18-4, 18-5). Hypoechoic areas within the neoplasm may result from necrosis.[20] In the classic case of neuroblastoma arising from the adrenal gland, sonography clearly demonstrates the relationship of the tumor to the kidney, with its typical downward and outward displacement. Extraadrenal lesions exhibit a variety of configurations and relationships between the kidney and other organs.[10] Sonographic evaluation of neuroblastoma occurring in the chest and paraspinal area has obvious limitations.[25] In these and other cases CT more clearly demonstrates the extent and borders of the mass. Because of this, even though sonography may originally make the diagnosis, CT is generally necessary to provide precise tumor mapping. Magnetic resonance imaging (MRI) also provides similar information which is

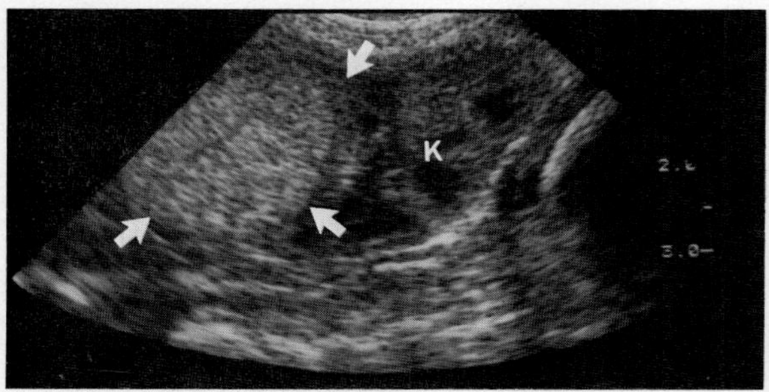

FIGURE 18-2. Longitudinal sonogram shows neuroblastoma *(arrows)* displacing the right kidney (K) downward.

important for both the initial diagnosis and post-treatment follow-up.[10]

To maximize the amount of information obtained from each study, the sonographer must direct the search by attempting to differentiate the neuroblastoma from other abdominal masses, to define the margins of the tumor, and to identify any signs of metastatic disease. It may not be possible on the basis of the sonographic study alone to differentiate neuroblastoma from other solid tumors, such as Wilms' tumor or lymphoma, seen often in the abdomen. When the normal renal parencymal pattern is distorted, Wilms' tumor is suspected. However, Wilms' tumor may sometimes arise in an exophytic fashion from the kidney, and evidence of extrarenal origin may suggest neuroblastoma. Wilms' tumors are surrounded by a capsule or pseudocapsule, whereas neuroblastomas usually have ill-defined borders. Like Wilms' tumor, neuroblastoma can metastasize to almost any organ.[6] In a neonate with a suprarenal mass, adrenal hemorrhage should be distinguished from necrotic neuroblastoma. The adrenal hemorrhage should show a characteristic pattern of resolution over a short time.[25]

Adrenocortical Carcinoma. In children, adrenal gland tumors other than neuroblastoma are quite rare. The most common of these is the congenital adrenocortical carcinoma, which can produce virilizing symptoms or be linked with fetal alcohol syndrome or congenital hemihypertrophy.[23] These lesions tend to be highly malignant and locally invasive. Adrenocortical carcinoma is more common in adults than in children.[10]

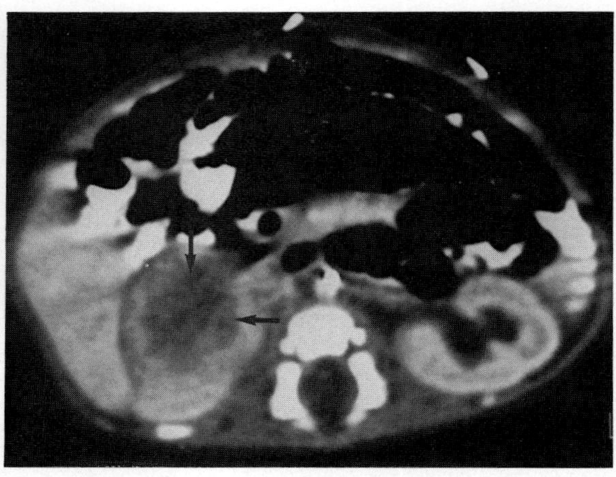

FIGURE 18-3. A neuroblastoma *(arrows)* is demonstrated on CT in the patient in Figure 18-2.

Sonographic appearancce. Sonographically, adrenocortical carcinoma has a moderately echogenic, complex pattern.[4] The heterogeneous pattern probably represents areas of hemorrhage and necrosis dispersed throughout the tumor.[10] Diagnostic imaging is an important tool for defining the extent of the primary tumor and determining the presence or absence of metastatic disease. Vascular extension is characteristic of adrenocortical carcinoma, and sonography can clearly demonstrate tumor extension into the IVC, hepatic veins, and right atrium. Metastasis in the retroperitoneum can also be visualized.[4]

Pheochromocytoma. Pheochromocytomas are rare, functioning tumors that originate in chromaffin tissue. Fewer than 5% of all pheochromocytomas affect children,[11] but most of those occur in the adrenal medulla. Pheochromocytomas may also be found in aberrant tissue along the sympathetic chain, the thorax, the paraaortic area, the aortic bifurcation, the retroperitoneum, and the bladder. Multiple pheochromocytomas are sometimes

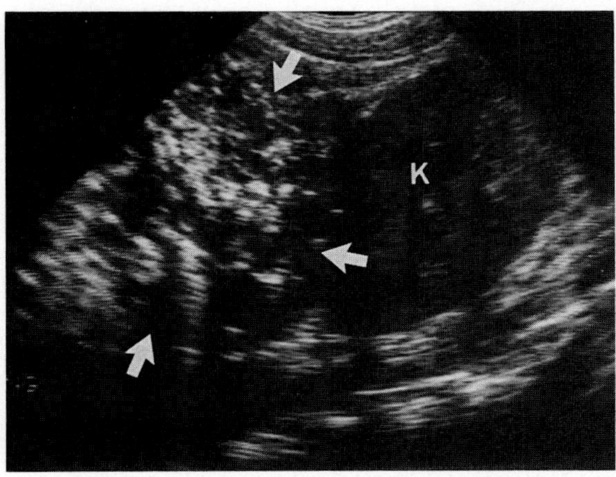

Figure 18-4. Longitudinal sonogram shows a neuroblastoma *(arrows)* compressing the left kidney (K).

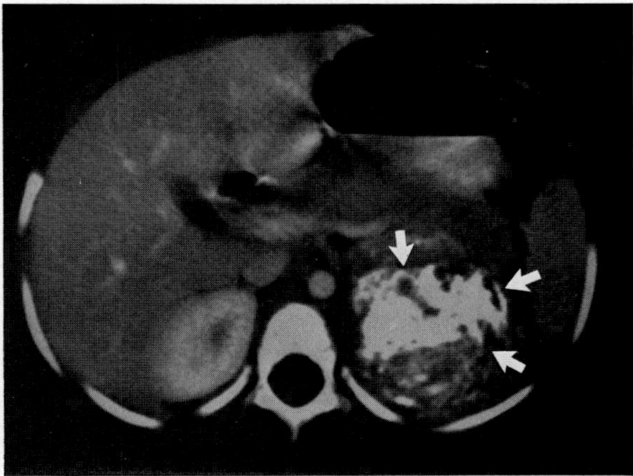

Figure 18-5. CT of the patient in Figure 18-4 shows the neuroblastoma *(arrows)*.

found in children, so it is important to search for a second and even a third lesion. In approximately 10% of pediatric cases, other family members are similarly affected, so careful examination of the child's immediate family is in order.[12] Clinically, the diagnosis of pheochromocytoma is made by determination of urinary catecholamine excretion. Clinical symptoms include hypertension, headaches, palpitations, and diaphoresis.[9]

Sonographic appearance. Sonographically, pheochromocytomas usually appear as small to moderate-sized, homogeneous masses containing low-level internal echoes.[12,26] Tumors several centimeters in diameter are uncommon.[12] When the lesions are large, they often contain areas of hemorrhage and necrosis, which result in a heterogeneous sonographic appearance (Fig. 18-6).[26] Pheochromocytomas are almost always sharply encapsulated, producing a sharp, echogenic wall.[12] Extraadrenal masses are difficult to image sonographically and are often obscured by bowel gas.[26]

Metastases. Many neoplasms can metastasize to the adrenal gland, most commonly tumors of the lung or breast and melanomas. Although metastases to the adrenal gland rarely cause clinical symptoms,

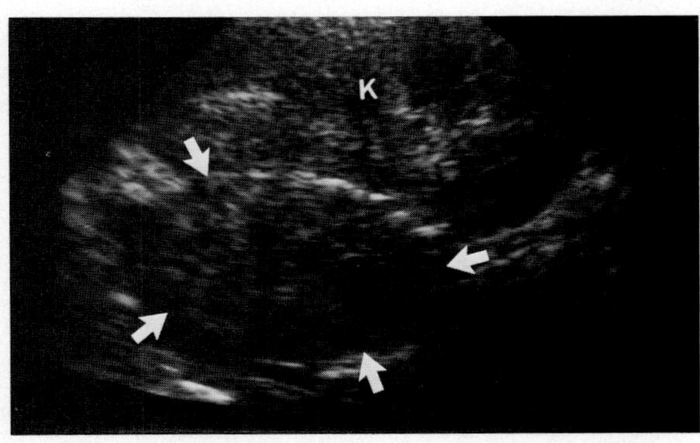

Figure 18-6. Longitudinal sonogram shows a heterogenous pheochromocytoma *(arrows)* adjacent to the left kidney (K).

sonography is helpful for examining patients with known primary tumors for progressions of metastatic adrenal disease.[26] Such tumors are often bilateral and large.[1]

Sonographic appearance. Sonographically, adrenal metastasis is nonspecific and may look identical to a primary adrenal tumor. Metastases appear solid, with varying degrees of echogenicity.[26] Bilateral masses heighten the suspicion of adrenal origin.[1]

Cysts

Adrenal cysts are rare.[26] They are usually unilateral, asymptomatic lesions that may be large and may cause hypertension.[1] Adrenal cysts may occur secondary to hemorrhage or may be true cysts, such as retention cysts, cystic adenomas, or angiomatous cysts. Malignancies associated with adrenal cysts have not been reported.[26]

Sonographic appearance. Sonographically, adrenal cysts usually appear as anechoic structures in the adrenal area that demonstrate well-defined walls and posterior acoustic enhancement.[12] Typically, they displace the kidney inferiorly and present a definite interface with the upper pole of the kidney. Some adrenal cysts contain debris and have irregular borders, for example adrenal pseudocysts and hemorrhagic cysts.[1] Adrenal cysts can simulate, and must be distinguished from, renal cysts, hydronephrosis, and splenic or pancreatic pseudocysts.[26]

Hemorrhage

Adrenal hemorrhage may result from prematurity, neonatal sepsis or hypoxia, or birth trauma inflicted on the rapidly involuting adrenal gland, particularly in large infants of diabetic mothers. Often, more than one factor is responsible.[23] Adrenal hemorrhage is most frequently identified between the second and seventh days of life.[11] Clinically, there may be a palpable mass and anemia.[20] Jaundice may occur because of the resorption of excessive hemoglobin from massive hemorrhage.[23] The symptoms vary, depending on the degree of bleeding.[12] Most infants are not particularly ill from the initial hemorrhage,[23] but with massive hemorrhage complete exsanguination of the infant can result.[10] An uncommon complication of adrenal hemorrhage is adrenal insufficiency.[23]

Sonographic appearance. Sonographically, the appearance of adrenal hemorrhage depends on the age of the hemorrhage. Initially, hemorrhage appears as an echogenic mass in the suprarenal area. As it liquifies the mass becomes progressively more sonolucent, so that eventually, a suprarenal anechoic, cystlike structure is visualized (Fig. 18-7A, B).[10] The diagnosis of adrenal hemorrhage may be established if sonography is repeated at 3- to 5-day intervals to observe the appearance of the mass as it changes from solid to cystic.[11]

In most cases, the enlarged, hemorrhagic adrenal gland shrinks very rapidly and calcifications may become visible within a few weeks or months. Initially the calcifications outline the enlarged anechoic adrenal gland in a rimlike fashion. With time, as the adrenal gland becomes progressively smaller, the calcifications become more compact and eventually, conform to the triangular configuration of the normal gland. Calcifications may be found incidentally on abdominal radiography or sonography. Documentation of adrenal hemor-

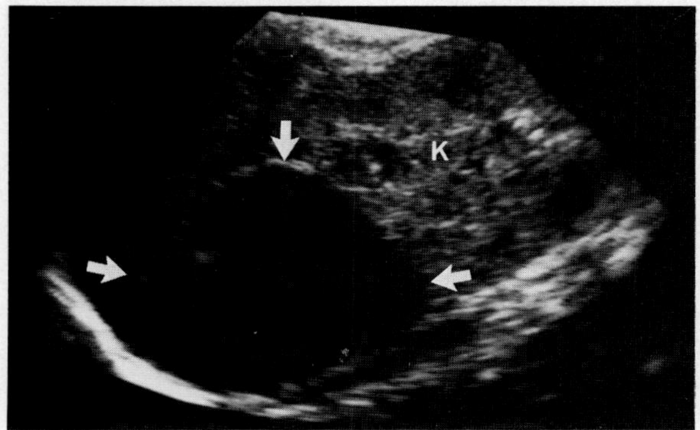

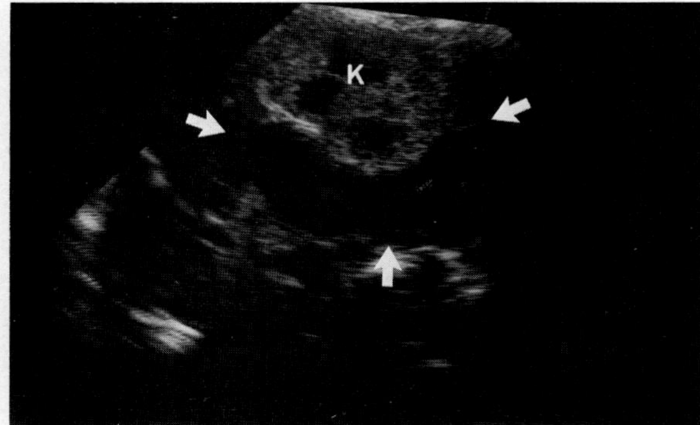

Figure 18-7. (*A*) Longitudinal sonogram demonstrates a liquefied adrenal hemorrhage *(arrows)* above the right kidney (K). (*B*) Transverse sonogram shows a liquefied adrenal hemorrhage *(arrows)* and the upper pole of the kidney (K).

rhage is uncommon is these cases, but calcifications are assumed to be evidence of this. The calcified glands are echogenic.[10]

Hypertrophy

In patients with renal agenesis or severe renal hypoplasia (Potter's syndrome) or ectopia of the kidney, the adrenal glands may become enlarged or hypertrophic or may assume an unusual shape.[20]

Sonographic appearance. In cases of renal agenesis, ectopia, or hypoplasia, it is important to recognize the characteristic sonographic appearance of the neonatal adrenals.[19] When normal renal tissue is absent, the adrenal gland preserves its typical echogenic medulla and hypoechoic cortex but enlarges, losing its characteristis Y or V shape and assuming a more elliptic shape (Fig. 18-8).[16] The distinctive appearance of the adrenal medulla and cortex should not be mistaken for the kidney.[19]

An enlarged adrenal gland without an adjacent kidney does not necessarily indicate renal agenesis, as the kidney may merely be ectopic. Whenever enlarged adrenal glands are identified, a careful search should be made for renal tissue elsewhere in the abdomen or pelvis. Because renal agenesis is accompanied by Potter's syndrome and pulmonary hypoplasia, it is important to identify affected fetuses and neonates, because of direct therapeutic implications. The sonographic appearance of an elongated and thickened adrenal is probably the result of lack of pressure from the kidney against the developing adrenal.[16]

Abscess

Adrenal abscesses are rare in children,[10] as the adrenals are relatively resistant to ordinary bacterial infection, although pyogenic abscesses can develop in the cortex with bacteremia, staphylococcal infections being the most common ones. The adrenal gland may also be involved by disseminated granulomatous disease. Before 1946, adrenal tuberculosis accounted for nearly 90% of reported Addison's disease cases in childhood. Since that time, histoplasmosis has become the most common childhood granulomatous disease of the adrenal gland. Infection of the adrenal gland by other fungi, particularly *Candida (Monilia)* or *Aspergillus*, may occur in terminal stages of leukemia or other hematopoietic diseases.[14] Clincially, abscesses are characterized by fever, chills, and abdominal pain.[21]

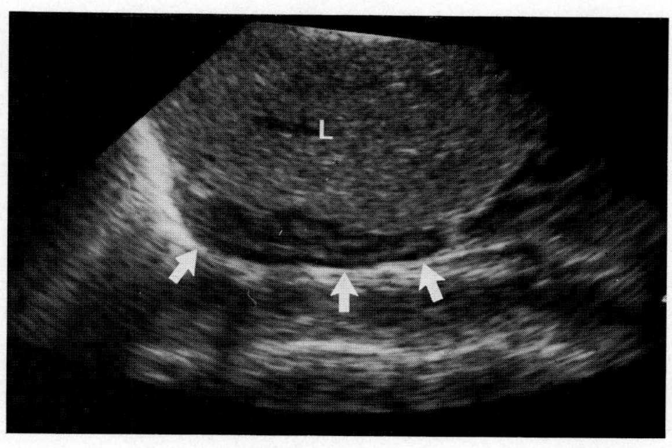

Figure 18-8. In a longitudinal sonogram through the right upper quadrant in a patient with renal agenesis, the adrenal gland *(arrows)* preserves its typical echogenic medulla and hypoechoic cortex but not its characteristic shape (L, liver).

Sonograpic appearance. Sonographically, an adrenal abscess is identified as a relatively anechoic suprarenal mass, sometimes containing echogenic debris.[10] It is important to correlate the clinical history with the sonographic findings to make the correct diagnosis.[26] Abscesses are usually unilateral, although bilateral ones have been documented.[10]

Congenital Adrenal Hyperplasia

Congenital adrenal hyperplasia (CAH) is an inborn error of the metabolism involving a deficiency of one of several enzymes necessary for normal steroid biosynthesis. It is transmitted as an autosomal recessive trait; the incidence is about one in 50 births in the United States.[11] The diagnosis of CAH depends on specific biochemical tests.

Sonographic appearance. Sonographically, congenital adrenal hyperplasia is demonstrated by increased adrenal size. The adrenal glands become markedly enlarged, with preservation of the characteristic anechoic cortex and echogenic medulla. The enlargement involves the cortex predominantly, without obvious medullary enlargement except in length. Sonography is used in CAH to directly determine the adrenal gland enlargement to monitor the response to treatment, to reduce the likelihood of overtreatment and oversuppression and their effects on growth and maturation.[8]

Related Imaging Procedures

Because no single procedure always provides all the necessary diagnostic information, the appropriate use of each modality requires an understanding of its strengths and weaknesses.[24]

Intravenous Pyelography

Intravenous pyelography (IVP) may demonstrate medial displacement by a superior pole renal mass, which may indicate the presence of an adrenal tumor, particularly if it distorts the normal position of the adjacent kidney. It is difficult to obtain adequate visualization in the presence of severe hypertension. An IVP provides limited diagnostic information, and its importance has decreased with the introduction of sonography and CT. It also has the disadvantage of using ionizing radiation and injected radiopaque contrast medium.

Computed Tomography

High-resolution CT can accurately image the normal adrenal glands as well as tumors or masses, particularly in obese patients.[1] It has been suggested that CT is the most important modality for assessment of primary and metastatic disease at the time of diagnosis and for follow-up.[4] The advantages of CT are that it provides a more complete abdominal examination that is not limited by bowel gas, clearer definition of anatomic relationships, and very few unsatisfactory examinations.[24] Disadvantages of CT include its ionizing radiation, opaque contrast material, relative expense, and limitation to imaging suite.[1]

Arteriography

Arteriography is the method of choice for accurate demonstration of an adrenal mass and its vascular supply. The principal disadvantages of arteriography are its invasiveness and its ionizing radiation. During the injection, care must also be taken to prevent adrenergic shock in patients with hypertension or hormone overproduction.[1]

Magnetic Resonance Imaging

Magnetic resonance imaging (MRI) demonstrates excellent soft tissue contrast and is very helpful in differentiating among several diagnostic possibilities. It is effective in diagnosing adrenal hemorrhage,[3] adrenal cortical carcinoma, metastases, pheochromocytoma (particularly ectopic lesions),[5] and neuroblastoma, including staging (in children beyond the neonatal period). MRI of the abdomen may be less helpful than CT because physiologic motion artifacts—respiration, cardiac pulsations, peristalsis—may limit image quality. It also has the disadvantages of being relatively expensive and not portable for bedside examinations.[3]

References

1. Anderhub B: Manual of Abdominal Sonography. Baltimore, University Park Press, 1983.
2. Atkinson GO, Zaatari GS, Lorezo RL, et al: Cystic neuroblastoma in infants: Radiographic and pathologic features. AJR 1985, 146:113–117.
3. Brill PW, Jagannath A, Winchester P, et al: Adrenal hemorrhage and renal vein thrombosis in the newborn: MR imaging. Radiology 1989, 170:95–98.
4. Davies RP, Lam AH: Adrenocortical neoplasm in children. J Ultrasound Med 1987, 6:325–328.
5. Doppman JL, Reinig JW, Dwyer AJ, et al: Differentiation of adrenal masses by magnetic resonance imaging. Surgery 1987, 102:1018–1026.
6. Filliatrault D, Hoyoux C, Benoit P, et al: Renal metastases from neuroblastoma. Pediatr Radiol 1987, 17:137–138.
7. Fleisher AC, James AE Jr: Introduction to Diagnostic Sonography. New York, John Wiley & Sons, 1980.
8. Ghiacy S, Dubbins PA, Baumer H: Ultrasound demonstration of congenital adrenal hyperplasia. Clin Ultrasound 1985, 13:419–420.
9. Havlik RJ, Cahow CE, Kinder BK: Advances in the diagnosis and treatment of pheochromocytoma. Arch Surg 1988, 123:626–629.
10. Hayden KC Jr, Swischuk LE: Pediatric Ultrasonography. Baltimore, Williams & Wilkins, 1987.
11. Hung W, August GP, Glasgow AM: Pediatric Endocrinology. New York, Medical Examination Publishers, 1983.
12. Johnson CD, Baker ME, Dunnick NR: CT demonstration of adrenal pseudocyst. J Comput Assist Tomogr 1985, 9:817–819.
13. Kirks DR, Conrad MR, Dammert W: Left adrenal neuroblastoma with normal conventional radiologic

studies: Value of grey-scale ultrasonography. South Med J 1980, 73:389-91.

14. Kissane JM: Pathology of Infancy and Childhood, 2nd ed. St. Louis, CV Mosby, 1975.
15. Krebs CA, Eisenberg RL, Ratcliff S, et al: Cava-suprarenal line: New position for sonographic imaging of the left adrenal gland. J Clin Ultrasound 1986, 14:535–539.
16. McGahan JP, Myracle MR: Adrenal hypertrophy: Possible pitfall in the sonographic diagnosis of renal agenesis. J Ultrasound Med 1986, 5:265–268.
17. McHugo JM, McKeown C, Brown MT, et al: Ultrasound findings in children with cystic fibrosis. Br J Radiol 1987, 60:137–141.
18. Mittelstaedt CA, Volberg FM, Merten DF, et al: The sonographic diagnosis of neonatal adrenal hemorrhage. Radiology 1979, 131:453–457.
19. Oppenheimer DA, Carroll BA, Yousem S: Sonography of the normal neonatal adrenal gland. Radiology 1983, 146:157–160.
20. Shkolnik A: Applications of ultrasound in the neonatal abdomen. Radiol Clin North Am 1985, 23:141–145.
21. Silverman A, Roy CC: Pediatric Clinical Gastroenterology, 3rd ed. St. Louis, CV Mosby, 1983.
22. Silverman PR, Carroll BA, Moskowitz PS: Adrenal sonography in renal agenesis and dysplasia. AJR 1980, 134:600–602.
23. Swischuk LE: Radiology of the Newborn and Young Infant. Baltimore, MD, Waverly Press, 1979.
24. Van Dyke JA, Stanley RJ, Berland LL: Pancreatic imaging. Ann Intern Med 1985, 102:212–217.
25. White SJ, Stuck KF, Blane CE, et al: Sonography of neuroblastoma. AJR 1983, 141:465–468.
26. Worthen NJ: Adrenal sonography. *In* Sarti D (ed): Diagnostic ultrasound: Text and Cases, 2nd ed. Chicago, Year Book Medical Publishers, 1987.
27. Yeh HC: Sonography of the adrenal glands: Normal glands and small masses. AJR 1980, 135:1167–1177.
28. Yeh HC, Mitty HA, Rose J, et al: Ultrasonography of adrenal masses: Usual features. Radiology 1978, 127:467–474.

PART THREE
Superficial Structures

CHAPTER **19**

Thyroid, Parathyroids, and Neck

JERRY PEARSON

A wide array of lesions can affect the thyroid, parathyroid glands, and the neck. Many can be accurately diagnosed by clinical signs and symptoms and laboratory data. Radionuclide imaging can also contribute valuable information. Sonography may be used to ascertain the internal consistency of a mass detected on physical examination, to characterize the internal contents of a "cold" nodule found on a radionuclide scan, or to seek suspected nodules that are impalpable and cannot otherwise be imaged.

Thyroid Gland

ANATOMY

The thyroid is an endocrine gland located in the anterior aspect of the neck (Fig. 19-1). During fetal development it migrates to this position from the foramen cecum located at the base of the tongue. Generally, the thyroid is composed of two lobes connected by an isthmus. In 15 to 30% of persons, there may be an additional pyramidal lobe, which extends superiorly from the isthmus.[19] The superior border of the lateral lobes begins at approximately the thyroid cartilage (Adam's apple) and extends inferiorly (see Fig. 19-1). Although its size varies, the normal lateral lobe should measure approximately 5 to 6 cm in its longest axis and 2 cm in height and width.[21] The right lobe is often larger than the left. The normal gland has a firm, rubbery texture on physical examination.[17]

The normal thyroid demonstrates low to medium-level echoes with a very homogeneous pattern (Fig. 19-2, 19-3). In addition, many landmarks help define its position. On cross-sectional views, the common carotid artery and internal jugular vein, located within the carotid sheath, form the posterior lateral border of the gland. These structures are easily distinguished from the thyroid, owing to their echogenic walls and anechoic centers (Figs. 19-3 to 19-7). The common carotid artery is located medial to the jugular vein. In this view, the thyroid appears somewhat circular. The longus colli muscle forms the posterior border of the gland, and it appears as a low-level echogenic structure posterior to the gland. On the transverse view, it appears circular (see Fig. 19-5). The trachea forms the medial border and appears hyperechoic with posterior shadowing from the air it contains. The group of muscles that form the anterolateral border of the gland, collectively called the strap muscles, are the sternothyroid, sternohyoid, and omohyoid muscles (see Fig. 19-4). The sternothyroid muscle is located directly superficial to the thyroid gland, and the sternohyoid and omohyoid lie on that muscle's anterior and lateral borders, respectively. Another important muscle of the neck, the sternocleidomastoid, is located lateral to the omohyoid and more superficial. The most superficial muscle, which surrounds the neck, is the very thin platysma. It is difficult to image, as it tends to blend in with the skin and be obscured.

(text continues on page 525)

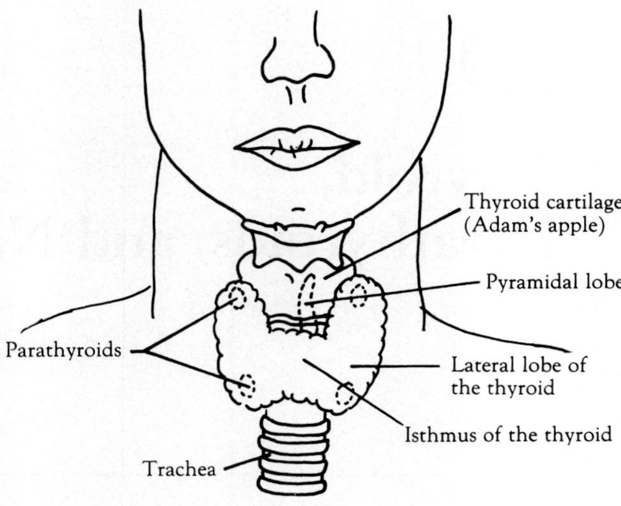

FIGURE 19-1. Anterior view of the neck demonstrates the normal position of the thyroid. Note the pyramidal lobe extending upward from the isthmus.

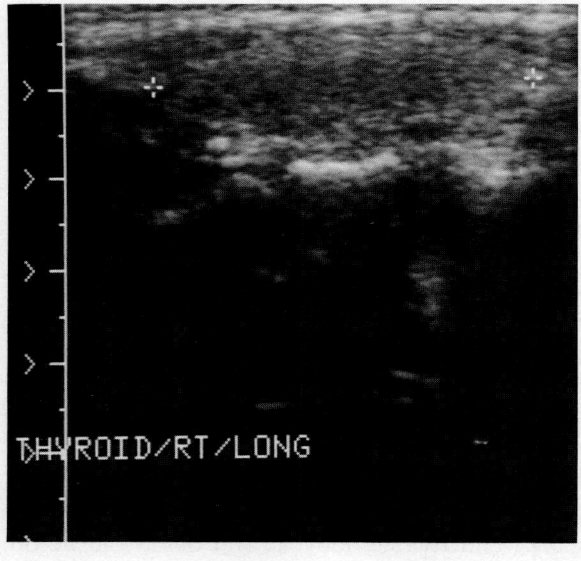

FIGURE 19-2. Longitudinal view of the right lateral lobe of the thyroid (*cursor*) demonstrates the homogeneous pattern of the gland.

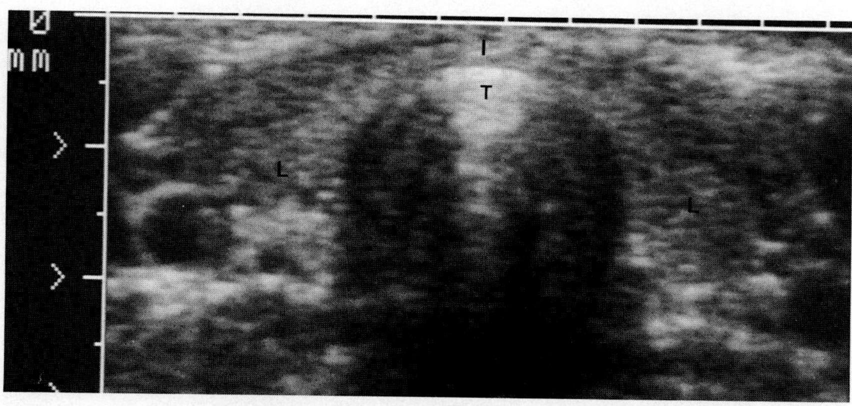

FIGURE 19-3. Transverse view of the thyroid demonstrates a homogeneous pattern (T, trachea; I, isthmus; L, lateral lobes of the thyroid).

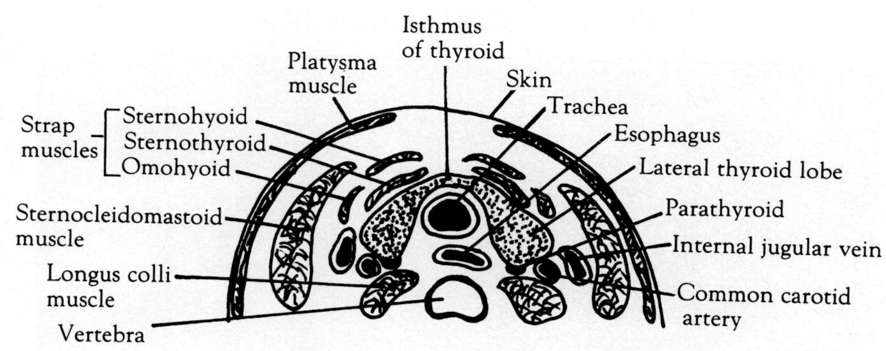

FIGURE 19-4. Cross-sectional diagram shows the relationship of the thyroid, parathyroids, vasculature, and musculature.

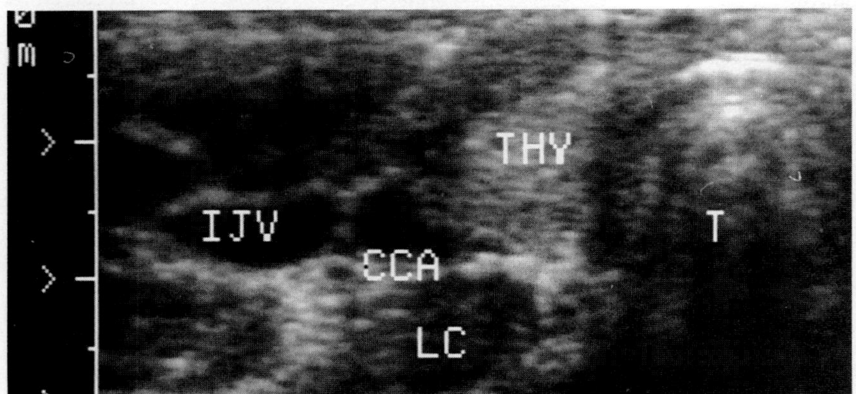

FIGURE 19-5. Transverse view of the hyperechoic trachea (T), right lateral lobe of the thyroid (THY), internal jugular vein (IJV), common carotid artery (CCA), and longus colli muscle (LC). Note the homogeneous pattern of the thyroid.

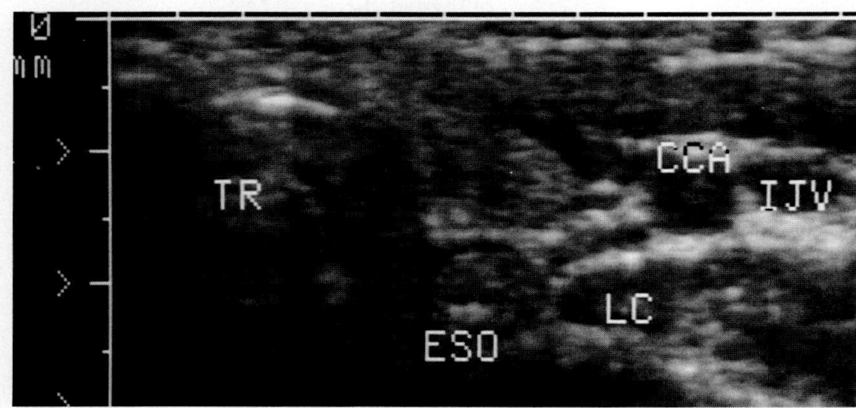

FIGURE 19-6. Transverse view demonstrates the homogeneous left lateral lobe of the thyroid. The esophagus (ESO) appears as a circular structure with a hyperechoic center, located slightly to the left of the trachea (TR). The sonolucent, circular longus colli (LC) muscle is located lateral to the esophagus. Note the common carotid artery (CCA) and internal jugular vein (IJV).

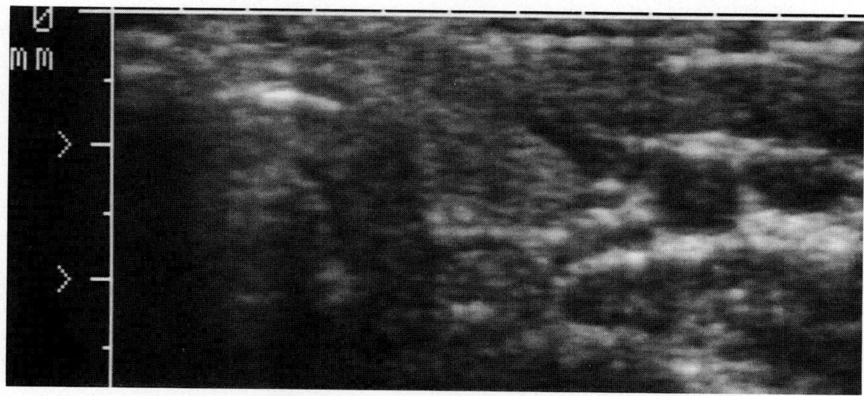

Figure 19-7. The image is identical to Figure 19-6, but the labels are deleted to allow optimal visualization of the structures.

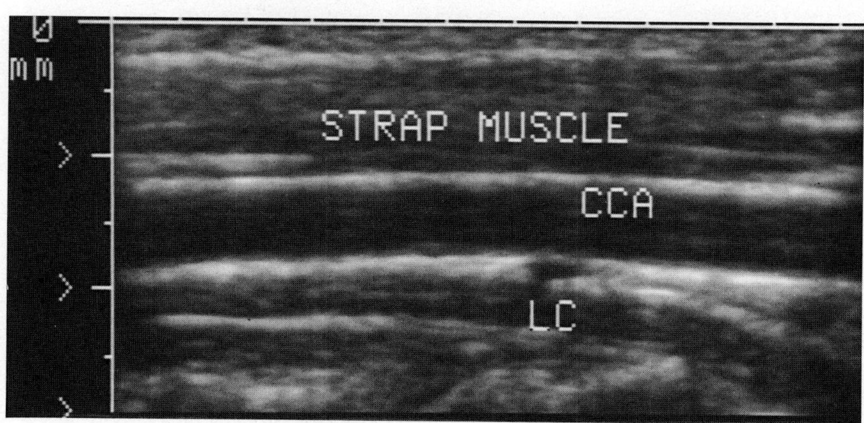

Figure 19-8. In a longitudinal section obtained lateral to the lateral lobe of the thyroid, a strap muscle is seen in the anterior aspect. The common carotid artery (CCA) lies posterior to the strap muscle and anterior to a small section of the longus colli muscle (LC).

Scanning laterally in the sagittal and parasagittal (longitudinal) planes, one visualizes the jugular vein or common carotid artery posteriorly (Fig. 19-8). As scanning movement is directed medially, the longus colli muscle, located posteriorly, becomes visible as a low-level echogenic structure (Figs. 19-9, 19-10). The hyperechoic trachea comes into view next as the most medial structure (Fig. 19-11).

Anatomic Variants

Failure of thyroid migration in utero may result in an ectopic thyroid, which, though rare, may lie at the base of the tongue (lingual), directly underneath the tongue (sublingual), superior to the hyoid bone (suprahyoid or prelaryngeal), or posterior to the sternum (substernal).[11,23] A case has been reported where remnants were found within

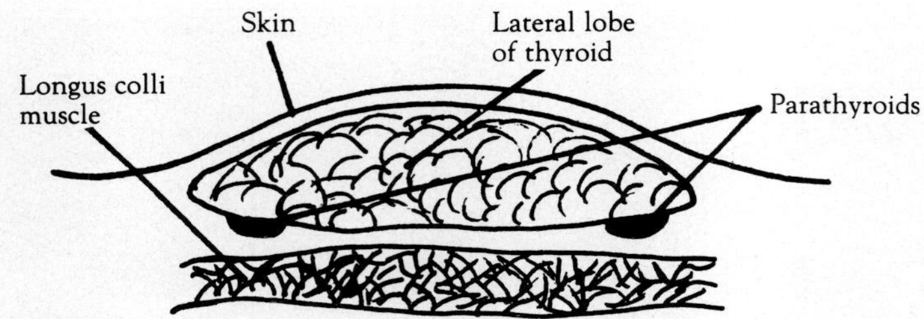

FIGURE 19-9. Structures as they would appear from a longitudinal section taken in the center of a lateral lobe of the thyroid (slightly medial to the image in Figure 19-8).

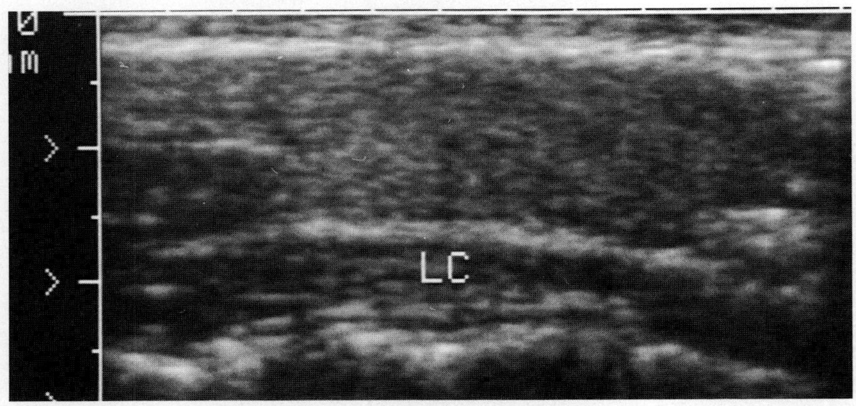

FIGURE 19-10. On a longitudinal section medial to Figure 19-8 homogeneous thyroid tissue is located anterior to the longus colli muscle (LC), which has a low-level echogenic appearance. This corresponds with the longitudinal section drawing in Figure 19-9.

the myocardium.[8] The lingual, followed by the substernal locus, are the most common sites of ectopic thyroid (Fig. 19-12).[1] It should also be noted that partial or complete development may not occur with each lobe. This most commonly affects the isthmus.[3,11]

PHYSIOLOGY

The thyroid is critical in controlling the body's growth and its basal metabolic rate (BMR) because two thyroid hormones, triiodothyronine (T_3) and thyroxine (T_4) are produced by the follicular cells. T_3 and T_4 increase protein synthesis and oxygen consumption of most body tissues.[22] The thyroid requires iodine to produce its hormones. In the United States, a sufficient amount of iodine is generally acquired in the diet.

The thyroid is regulated by thyroid-stimulating hormone (TSH) produced by the pituitary gland, via a negative-feedback mechanism. In negative feedback, the amounts of free circulating T_3 and T_4 are monitored by the body. When the levels increase to a specific point, the pituitary ceases to produce TSH, and the thyroid, no longer stimulated, slows or stops production of its hormones. When T_3 and T_4 levels decline and the pituitary senses

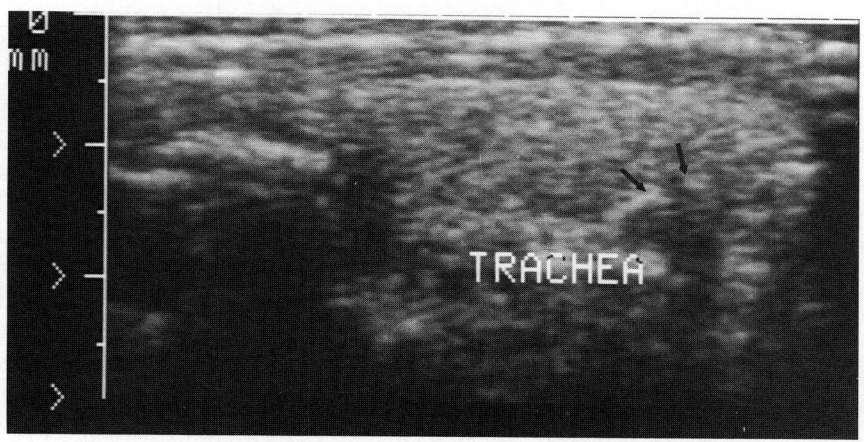

Figure 19-11. Oblique section of the longitudinal plane taken medial to Figure 19-10 shows the trachea (*arrows*) beginning to come into view.

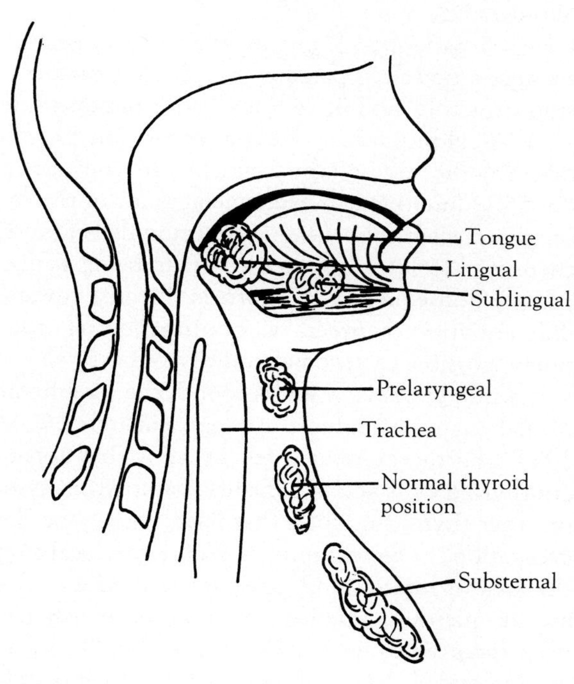

Figure 19-12. Common sites of ectopic thyroid.

that more of the thyroid hormones are needed, it begins to secrete TSH again.[22] The thyroid produces another hormone from its parafollicular cells, calcitonin, which aids the parathyroid glands in regulating short-term calcium utilization.[2]

Laboratory Tests

Numerous laboratory tests can be utilized to help diagnose thyroid disease, and interpreting different tests can be a complex undertaking.[6]

One important test of thyroid hormone levels is the radioimmunoassay (RIA), although it does not accurately measure the levels of physiologically active thyroid hormones.[2,17] The RIA measures the total amount (bound and unbound) of T_3 and T_4, but only the free (unbound) fractions of the hormones are physiologically active. The majority of both hormones (more than 99%) circulates through the body bound to three proteins: thyroxine-binding globulin (TBG), thyroxine-binding prealbumin (TBPA), and albumin. Many conditions can affect the level of these proteins, thus affecting the RIA measurement, although free (physiologically active) levels may be normal.[17,22] A more recent method that is used to measure the level of thyroid hormones is a T_3 resin uptake test along with the RIA. In conjunction with the RIA, it provides a more accurate estimate of free T_3 and T_4. In addition, a new immunoradiometric assay (IRMA) has been shown to measure TSH more accurately than previous tests.[17,22]

EXAMINATION TECHNIQUE

No patient preparation is required for a satisfactory sonographic examination of the thyroid, but the sonographer should know the location of any nodule that was palpated or imaged on a radionuclide scan. Also, the patient can be advised not to eat or drink for an hour before the examination in order to be more comfortable while lying flat with the neck extended. This prevents gastric reflux and eructation. The patient should lie in the supine position with a pillow or rolled towel under the upper shoulder area (Fig. 19-13) to facilitate extension of the neck and allow easier access to the thyroid.

The scanning protocol consists of multiple transverse, sagittal, parasagittal, and oblique views at 0.5 to 1 cm intervals. To ensure the entire gland has been imaged, the following anatomic landmarks should be demonstrated: the jugular vein and common carotid artery located laterally, the trachea located in the midline, the muscles in the anterolateral neck, and the longus colli muscle located posteriorly. The isthmus should also be shown clearly, anterior to the trachea.

The highest-frequency transducer that allows adequate penetration should be used. Typically, this is a 7.5- or 10-MHz transducer with a short focal lenth; however, in a patient with a broad neck or a lesion deep within the neck a transducer with a medium focal length may increase diagnostic accuracy. If a sonographer does not have access to a transducer with the appropriate focal length, a gel pad may be utilized to place the area of interest within the focal zone of the available transducer. The sonographer should carefully adjust the gain settings to demonstrate the gland with low to medium echogenicity. The near field should not contain excessive echoes that could obscure a lesion.

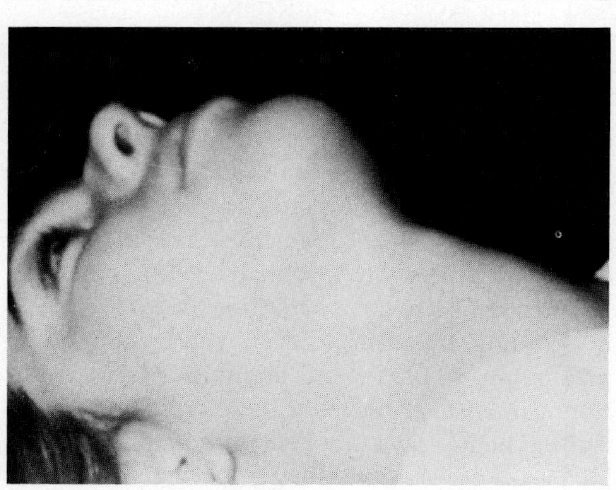

FIGURE 19-13. Proper patient position for a sonographic examination of the thyroid, parathyroids, and neck.

It may be difficult to distinguish whether a mass is cystic or solid.[2,24,25] The presence of posterior enhancement may be difficult to demonstrate when the amount of thyroid tissue posterior to a cyst is small. Furthermore, the air-filled echogenic trachea may obscure posterior enhancement in that area. Numerous scanning angles may be necessary to obtain the most precise information possible about the internal consistency of a mass.

THYROID DISEASE

Cysts. A patient is often referred for sonography because a nodule is palpated on physical examination or a cold nodule is found on a radionuclide scan. A cold nodule is one that is not able to trap (absorb) the radiopharmaceutical. (In contrast, a "hot" nodule traps an excessive amount of the radiopharmaceutical.) When a cold nodule is found, there is a 15% to 25% chance of its being malignant.[21] Consequently, concern is directed toward differentiating between a nonfunctioning adenoma, possible carcinoma, and thyroid cyst.[1,24]

If a purely cystic lesion is found, the likelihood of malignancy is reduced to approximately 7% to 19%.[5,17] Furthermore, it is felt by some that apparent thyroid cysts are, in actuality, parathyroid cysts or other thyroid nodules that have undergone degeneration.[5,21] Sonography is useful for localizing the area of interest and guiding the needle to the area in question. Fine-needle aspiration biopsy has been reported to have a 97% success rate,[15] so it is recommended that such lesions be biopsied or followed closely.

The sonographic appearance of a thyroid cyst should be the same as that of any other cyst located in the body. It should be circular or oval with discrete margins, contain no internal echoes, and produce posterior enhancement (Fig. 19-14).

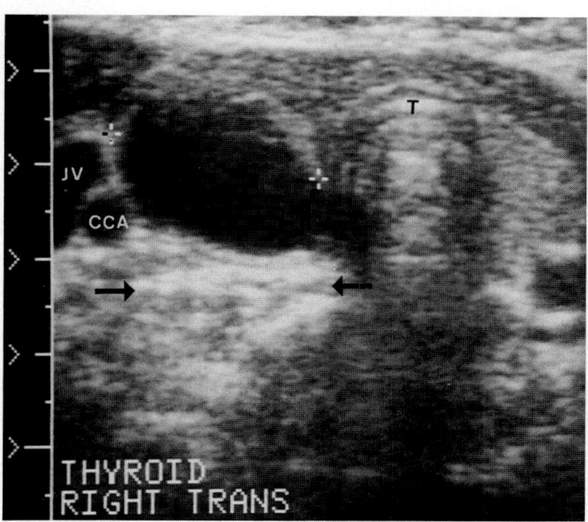

Figure 19-14. Transverse view of a well-circumscribed, circular, anechoic structure (*cursor*) located on the posterior aspect of the right lateral lobe of the thyroid with good posterior enhancement (*arrows*). Although this structure meets the criteria of a thyroid cyst, it was diagnosed sonographically as cystic degeneration of an adenoma because other small nodules were present in the left lateral lobe. The patient continues to be followed (T, trachea; cca, common carotid artery; JV, internal jugular vein).

Adenomas. Adenomas may have many histologic types: embryonal, fetal, colloid, follicular, papillary, and hyperplastic.[1,11] Sonography cannot differentiate between cell types.

Adenomas are one of the most common solid nodules of the thyroid.[3] They usually occur as a single nodule in young adults,[16] though they can be multiple.[24] Patients often present with a mass in the anterior neck. Pain may be present if the mass is large enough to cause pressure or if hemorrhage has taken place. Although adenomas usually appear hot on radionuclide scans, they can also appear cold. Sonography is often utilized to evaluate the contents of cold nodules.[1] Furthermore, the inability of nuclear medicine to detect nodules smaller than 1 to 2 cm[21] makes sonography valuable, especially since the likelihood of malignancy is decreased if more than one nodule is present.[11,22,24]

The sonographic appearance of adenomas varies widely. It may be a cystic, complex, or solid pattern, depending on the amount of degeneration. The most common appearance is of a solitary, well-circumscribed oval or circular, hypoechoic, isoechoic, or hyperechoic mass when compared to the normal thyroid tissue. (Figs. 19-15, 19-16)[2,3] In the past it was felt that the halo sign, a hypoechoic ring measuring 2 to 3 mm, was specific to the adenoma,

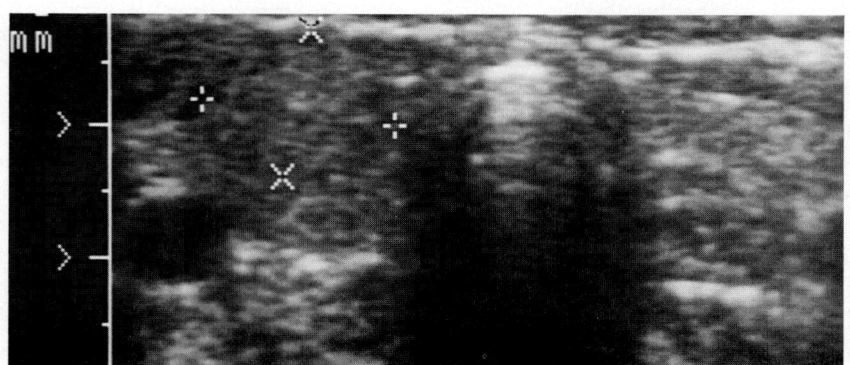

Figure 19-15. In this transverse section, a well-defined, isoechoic nodule (X, *cursor*) is displayed in the right lateral lobe of a patient with a history of a right thyroid nodule. Findings on radionuclide scan were normal. Although this lesion meets the sonographic criteria for an adenoma, malignancy could not be ruled out. Biopsy revealed a degenerating nodule.

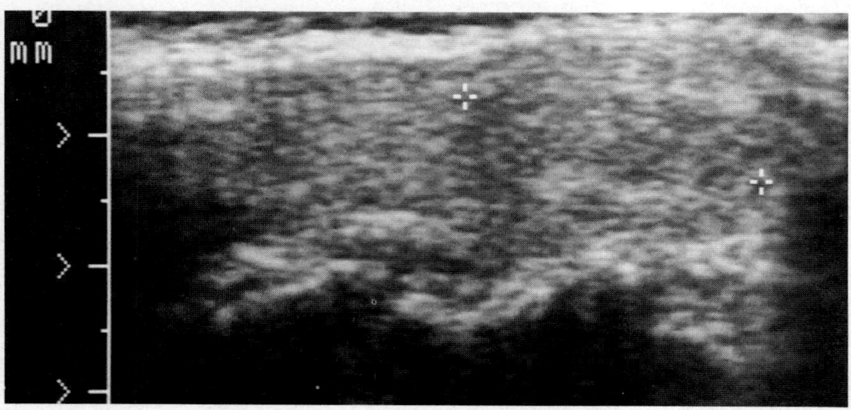

FIGURE 19-16. A longitudinal section of the solid, isoechoic, well-defined nodule (*cursor*) in Figure 19-15.

and it was taken as evidence of that lesion. It has since been shown that the halo sign also occurs in malignancies.[13,17] Although carcinoma of the thyroid is rare,[3,16] all solitary masses are considered potential carcinomas, especially if they register as a cold nodule on radionuclide imaging. Therefore, biopsy should be considered.

Multinodular Goiter. Multinodular goiter, also called nontoxic diffuse goiter or nontoxic nodular goiter, is the most common cause of thyroid enlargement.[21,22] Fortunately, fewer than 6% are malignant.[21]

The goiter (enlarged thyroid gland) can be caused by decreased iodine intake, ingesting substances that decrease TSH production, or by defects of hormone production within the gland itself.[22] When this happens, the pituitary increases production of TSH and the thyroid gland enlarges in an attempt to produce more hormone.

Goiters usually present as a painless neck mass, though there may be pain if the mass causes pressure or if hemorrhage has occurred. Thyroid hormone levels are generally normal (euthyroid).

The sonographic appearance usually consists of an enlarged, heterogeneous gland containing few to several different-sized nodules. Many cystic areas are often demonstrated, owing to degeneration and hemorrhage (Figs. 19-17 to 19-19).

Although goiters are usually considered benign, rapid growth of the gland or ensuing hoarseness are possible signs of malignancy.[3] If the underlying cause of the goiter cannot be identified, the patient is usually treated by thyroid hormone replacement.

Graves' Disease. Graves' disease is recognized by many other names: diffuse hyperthyroidism, diffuse toxic goiter, and thyrotoxicosis.[12,22] The cause is thought to be autoimmune: the body produces antibodies against its own tissues. Women of childbearing age are the most likely candidates for this systemic disease. The ratio of females to males is 8:1.[11,16]

Graves' disease has specific clinical signs and symptoms. The patient has an enlarged thyroid gland (goiter) and accompanying hyperthyroidism (which can be diagnosed by elevated thyroid hormone levels), intolerance to heat, increased respiratory and heart rate, tremors, weight loss, and generalized nervousness.[17] In brief, the patient's BMR is significantly accelerated. Equally important, Graves' disease patients often demonstrate exophthalmos—prominent, bulging eyes with eyelid retraction. Although other causes of hyperthyroidism, such as toxic (hyperfunctioning) adenoma of the thyroid, can cause most of the signs and symptoms mentioned above, exophthalmos is specific to Graves' disease.[17] Patients with Graves' disease can

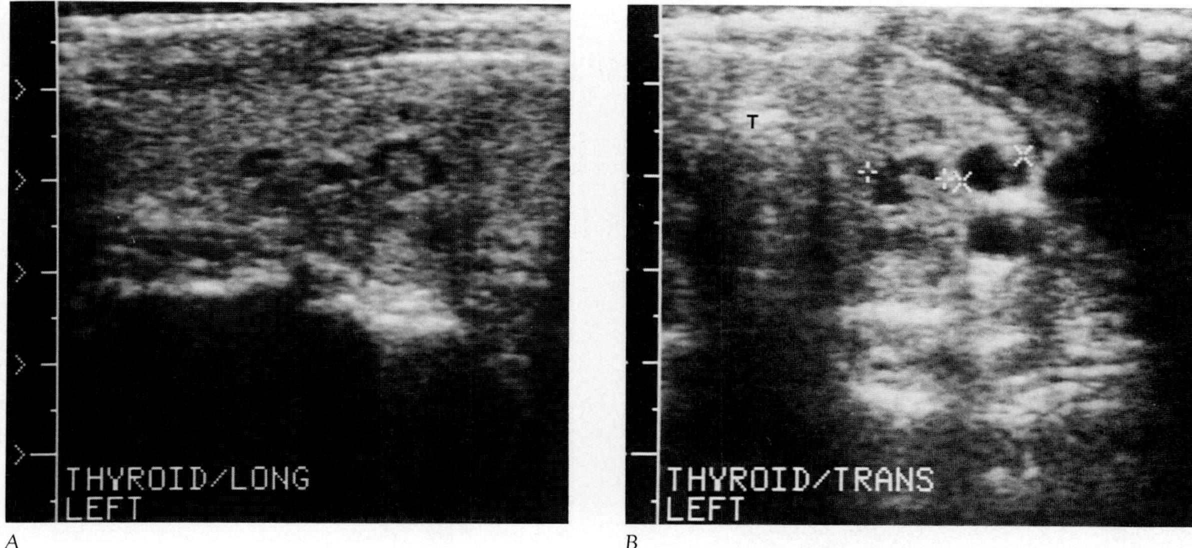

FIGURE 19-17. (*A*) A longitudinal and (*B*) transverse views of the left lateral lobe of the thyroid of a 39-year-old woman with a history of breast carcinoma. A heterogeneous echo pattern with multiple areas of cystic degeneration (X, *cursor*) are seen. Findings were essentially unchanged from a study performed in 1985, when multinodular goiter was sonographically diagnosed. Malignancy, however, could not be ruled out (T, trachea).

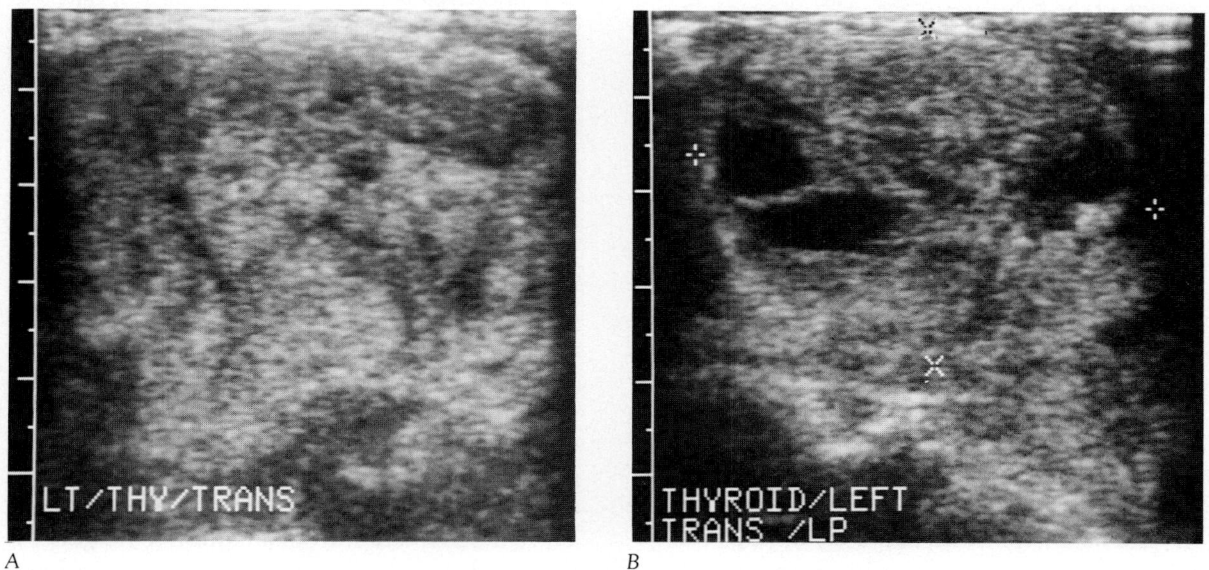

FIGURE 19-18. (*A*) A 73-year-old woman presented with an asymptomatic left neck mass. This transverse view of the upper pole of the left lateral lobe of the thyroid demonstrates a diffusely heterogeneous echo pattern, the common appearance of a multinodular goiter that has not yet undergone cystic degeneration. (*B*) In a transverse view of the lower pole of the left lateral lobe of the thyroid of the same patient, the mass (X, *cursor*) contains areas of cystic degeneration. The sonographic diagnosis was multinodular goiter with areas of cystic degeneration.

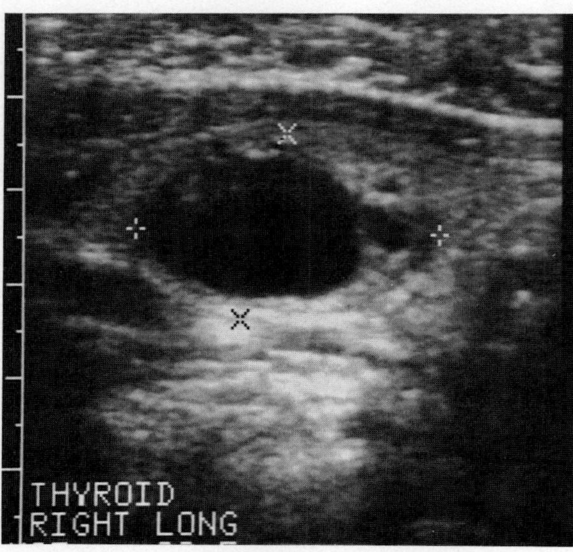

FIGURE 19-19. A sagittal section of the right lateral lobe of the thyroid of a 47-year-old woman with possible hyperthyroidism. A complex, predominantly cystic nodule (X, *cursor*) was demonstrated in the middle portion of the right lateral lobe. Also, the left lobe contained multiple small nodules. This was diagnosed sonographically as multinodular goiter with cystic degeneration. This patient continues to be followed.

develop menstrual irregularities and myxedema, which appears similar to thickening of the skin located on the lower extremities and forearms. A bruit or thrill can often be heard over the gland, indicating increased vascularity.[11,16,17] Ralls and colleagues documented increased vascular flow with color-flow Doppler instrumentation. They described what is referred to as a "thyroid inferno," many areas of increased blood flow throughout the thyroid parenchyma seen diffusely during both systole and diastole.[14] This phenomenon did not occur in normal patients or in patients with other documented types of thyroid disease.

Although gray-scale sonography is not routinely indicated in Graves' disease, on sonography the gland appears enlarged and hypoechoic.[3] The disease is often controlled with medication.

Hashimoto's Thyroiditis. Hashimoto's (or chronic) thyroiditis is a progressive disease that most frequently affects women 10 to 50 years of age and is thought to be autoimmune.[11,22] Concurrent genetic disorders or a family history of thyroid disorders is often associated with this disease.[11,22] The clinical signs and symptoms are usually gradual in onset—enlargement of the thyroid gland with normal (euthyroid) or decreased function (hypothyroidism).[16,22]

Common physical symptoms of hypothyroidism can include intolerance to cold, weakness, eyelid and facial droop, coarse, dry, or scaly skin, weight gain, and intellectual impairment with a gradual personality change.[16,17,22] The disease is generally diagnosed by physical signs and symptoms and laboratory data (detectable thyroid antibodies, increased TSH, decreased T_3 and possibly decreased T_4.[21,22] The sonographic appearance is usually indistinguishable from that of a multinodular goiter.[3,21] Once again, it should be emphasized that this is a clinical diagnosis.

Acute and Subacute Thyroiditis. Acute thyroiditis, also known as acute diffuse, acute nonsuppurative, or pseudotubercular thyroiditis, should be suspected when a patient presents with firm, painful thyroid enlargement associated with fever and malaise.[11,16] Often the pain radiates to the jaw or ear. Subacute thyroiditis, more commonly known as De Quervain's or granulomatous thyroiditis, has basically the same clinical signs and symptoms as acute thryoiditis.[1,11,16] In contrast to the acute form, subacute thyroiditis is generally self-limiting, lasting only several weeks.[11,22] The agent of acute and subacute thyroiditis is suspected to be a virus.[11,16]

Although the diagnosis is usually a clinical one, the sonographic appearance of these conditions is most often a diffusely enlarged, hypoechoic thyroid gland.[3] A patient with subacute thyroiditis, however, may have hypo- and hyperechoic nodules.[3] Thus, differentiation from a multinodular goiter is not possible by sonography, and clinical signs and symptoms must be considered. Treatment of these conditions is usually medication.

Thyroid Carcinoma. Thyroid cancer is rare, being responsible for approximately 0.5% of all cancer deaths.[3,16,22] Although attempts can be made sonographically to classify thyroid lesions as malignant or benign, results are inadequate at best.[5] Carcinoma has been reported in 21% of solid nodules, 12% of cystic-solid nodules, and 7% to 19% of cystic nodules.[517]

Patient history, clinical data, and laboratory data are necessary to formulate a diagnosis of malignancy. On the whole, features that should suggest carcinoma are an asymptomatic or pressure-related, painful lump in the neck; vocal cord paralysis due to tumor invasion; a solitary nodule; a cold nodule on a radionuclide scan; a history of radiation exposure to the head, neck, or chest; or rapid enlargement of a mass or preexisting goiter.[3,16,22] Carcinoma of the thyroid most often affects young persons: 34.9% of all patients are younger than 40 years old at diagnosis.[9] Women are more often affected (ratio 2 to 4.5:1).[9,16] Examiners should be most suspicious of thyroid carcinoma when a young patient has a solitary nodule that is cold on radionuclide scan and solid on sonography. Although the sonographic appearance of thyroid carcinoma varies widely, it is most often reported as a hypoechoic mass (Fig. 19-20).[3,20,21] Sonography, however, cannot discriminate between benign and malignant lesions.

Reviewing the literature on thyroid carcinoma can be quite confusing as there are many types. The term adenocarcinoma may be used to refer to any suspicious nodule. A specific histologic diagnosis should be pursued by biopsy to help the clinician choose the best medical management. Adenocarcinoma originates from two different types of thyroid cells, follicular and parafollicular. Tumors that arise from the follicular cell can be subclassified as papillary, follicular, and anaplastic. Anaplastic tumors can be further subdivided into small cell, giant cell, and spindle cell types (Table 19-1).[16] The parafollicular cells gives rise to medullary carcinoma. Papillary, follicular, and medullary carcinoma comprise approximately 90% of thyroid cancers.[20]

Papillary carcinoma. Papillary carcinoma is the most common malignant tumor of the thyroid gland, comprising 50% to 70% of all thyroid cancers.[11,16,19] It occurs most often in young adults, es-

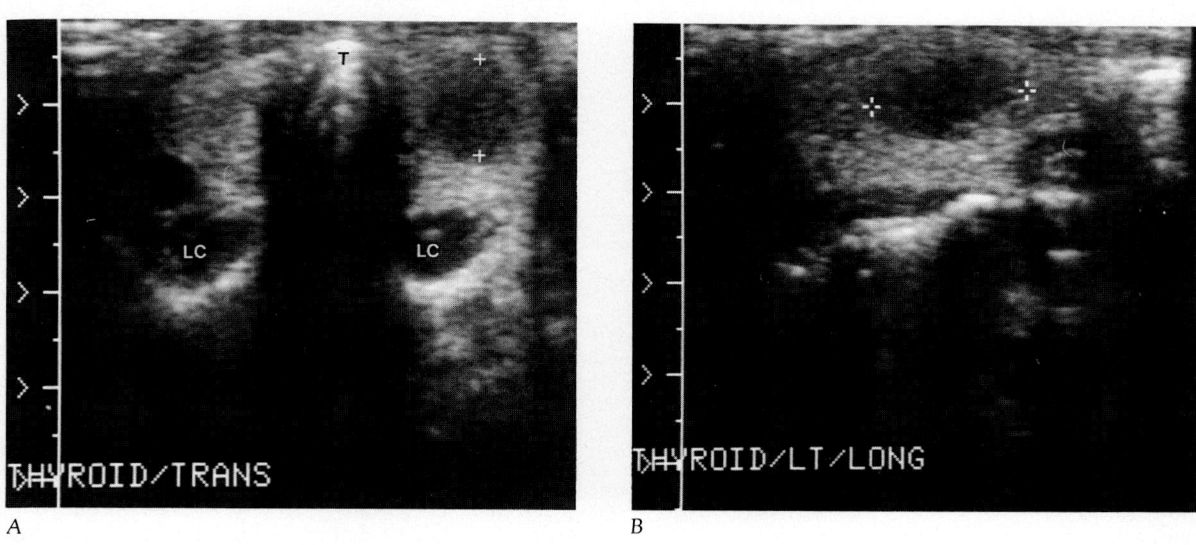

FIGURE 19-20. (*A*) A transverse section of the thyroid in a 15-year-old girl with multiple small suprasternal masses and a breast mass identified histologically as carcinoma. Also, lymphadenopathy was noted. A hypoechoic solid nodule (*cursor*) in the middle portion of the left lateral lobe was diagnosed as adenocarcinoma (LC, longus colli muscle; T, trachea). (*B*) A longitudinal section of the same solid, hypoechoic nodule (+).

TABLE 19-1. Classification of thyroid carcinoma by cell type

Classification
Follicular Cell
Papillary: 50%–70%
Follicular: 12%–20%
Anaplastic: 15%
Small cell
Giant cell
Spindle cell
Parafollicular Cell
Medullary: 10%

pecially in women during their childbearing years.[11,22] This tumor is generally the least aggressive and malignant of the thyroid carcinomas; although it can be very aggressive in children younger than 7 years and adults older than 50.[11] Papillary carcinoma metastasizes frequently to the cervical and upper mediastinal lymph nodes, less frequently to the lungs, and rarely to bone and brain.[11,16,22] The treatment varies, and may consist of a thyroid lobectomy or radical neck dissection, both followed by medication.[11,22]

Follicular carcinoma. Follicular carcinoma, the next most common thyroid carcinoma, accounts for approximately 12% to 20% of all thyroid carcinomas and is most common in women 20 to 40 years old.[11,16] Follicular carcinoma is more malignant than papillary and it frequently metastasizes to the lymph nodes, with lung and skeletal metastasis late in the disease.[11] The treatment is consistent with that of papillary carcinoma.

Medullary carcinoma. Medullary carcinoma accounts for only some 10% of thyroid carcinomas.[3,16] It often appears in genetic syndromes along with other tumors of the endocrine glands; the adrenal and parathyroid glands are frequently involved.[16,22] It can metastasize to the lymphatics, lungs, and bones.[22] The treatment is compatible with treatment for the other thyroid carcinomas, but other endocrine tumors must also be excised.

Anaplastic carcinoma. Anaplastic carcinoma accounts for fewer than 15% of thyroid carcinomas.[3,11,16] It generally affects persons 60 to 80 years old and is the most lethal form: most patients survive less than 12 months after diagnosis.[11,16,22] It often presents as a rapidly growing, painful neck tumor.

Lymphoma. Lymphoma of the thyroid is another uncommon thyroid tumor most often seen in older persons.[3,19] It is rare in persons younger than 40 years.[12] Clinical signs, symptoms, and treatment are often similar to those of other thyroid carcinomas.[12] Although the prognosis is not outstanding, the survival rate has been increasing.[13,19]

Metastatic lesions. Metastatic disease to the thyroid most often originates as breast carcinoma, followed by bronchogenic and renal carcinoma.[11]

Parathyroid Glands

ANATOMY

Although the number may vary, there are normally four parathyroid glands, located on the posteromedial aspect of the lateral lobes of the thyroid (see Fig. 19-1, 19-4). Generally, the glands are located on the superior and inferior aspects of the thyroid gland (see Figs. 19-1, 19-4, 19-9). Their size may vary but they should not exceed 5 mm in the longest axis. Normal parathyroid glands usually cannot be demonstrated sonographically because of their small size and tendency to blend in with normal thyroid tissue.[3]

PHYSIOLOGY

The parathyroid glands play a critical role in calcium metabolism and regulation by producing parathyroid hormone (PTH), which acts most intensely on the skeletal and renal systems. PTH is responsible for maintaining serum calcium levels by influencing resorption of calcium and phosphorus by the bones and by increasing or decreasing the rate of tubular reabsorption of these minerals in the kidneys.[22] When the serum calcium level is low, PTH is secreted to act upon its target organs to increase the calcium level. If the level falls too low (hypocalcemia), several neurologic, muscular, and cardiovascular effects may occur, such as numbness or tingling of the lips, tongue, fingers, or feet: unexplained dementia, depression, or psychosis; muscle aches or spasms; and electrocardiographic (EKG) changes.[22] If calcium levels become too high (hypercalcemia), the renal, skeletal, and gastrointestinal system are most often affected.[22] The clinical manifestations of hypercalcemia may include polyuria, nocturia, polydipsia, nephrolithiasis, and urolithiasis; osteitis and bone cyst forma-

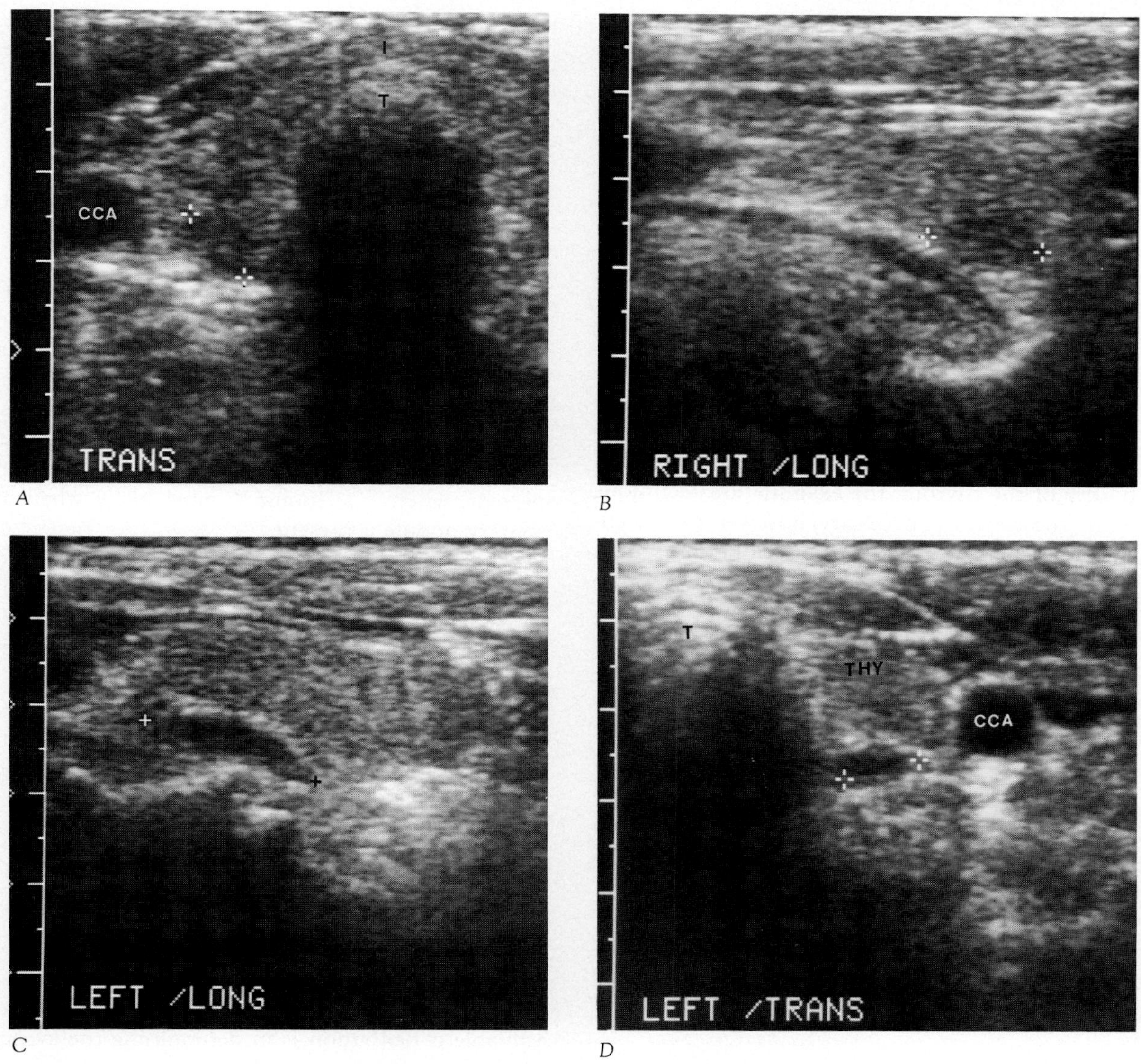

FIGURE 19-21. (A) Transverse and (*B*) longitudinal sections of the posterior inferior pole of the right lateral lobe of the thyroid of a 75-year-old man with hyperparathyroidism. A small, hypoechoic nodule (*cursor*) is demonstrated, which was diagnosed sonographically as a parathyroid adenoma. This was confirmed at surgery and symptoms resolved after parathyroidectomy (T, trachea; I, isthmus; CCA, common carotid artery). (C) Longitudinal and (*D*) transverse sections of the left superior posterior aspect of the thyroid from the same patient demonstrate a 13-mm hypoechoic nodule (*cursor*) that was also diagnosed sonographically as a parathyroid adenoma. Parathyroid hyperplasia should also be considered in the differential diagnosis. Adenoma was confirmed at surgery (T, trachea; THY, left lateral lobe of the thyroid; CCA, common carotid artery).

tion; EKG changes, constipation, anorexia, abdominal pain, ileus, and nausea and vomiting. Shock, renal failure, and death may result from severe hypercalcemia.[22]

LABORATORY TESTS

The most widely used measurement of parathyroid function is the serum PTH level. RIAs can also be implemented to ascertain PTH levels. Calcium and phosphorus levels can be measured during urinalysis.

SONOGRAPHIC TECHNIQUE

Preparation for a parathyroid examination is the same as that for a thyroid examination, and because the parathyroids lie on the posteromedial border of the thyroid, the examination technique is also the same. It is necessary, however, to concentrate on the area where the parathyroids most often are located, the posteromedial aspect of the thyroid. On cross section, one should concentrate on the area medial to the carotid artery, posterior to the lateral lobe of thyroid, and anterior to the longus colli muscle (Fig. 19-4). Sonographers must be careful not to mistake the minor neurovascular bundle (containing the recurrent laryngeal nerve and inferior thyroid artery) located posteriorly and just slightly medial to the lateral thyroid lobes, for a parathyroid adenoma. The examiner should be conscious of the esophagus, which often appears between the left lateral thyroid lobe and the trachea (see Figs. 19-5–19-7). Furthermore, the posteriorly located longus colli muscle may be mistaken for parathyroid disease.

PARATHYROID DISEASE

Evidence of parathyroid disease is often sought in patients who present with signs and symptoms of hyperparathyroidism, although such signs and symptoms are numeorus. Hypercalcemia, diagnosed from laboratory data, is the predominant finding.[22] Hypoparathyroidism is most often due to another underlying disease and generally is not a result of a primary parathyroid lesion.[22] The most frequent causes of primary hyperparathyroidism are adenomas, parathyroid hyperplasia, and carcinoma.[3,21]

Adenomas. Solitary adenomas are responsible for approximately 80% of cases of primary hyperparathyroidsm and multiple adenomas for 4.5%.[3,21] The most typical sonographic appearance of an adenoma is a well-circumscribed nodule located at the posteromedial border of the thyroid gland. Although its echogenicity can vary, it is commonly homogeneous and hypoechoic compared to normal thyroid tissue (Figs. 19-21A–D).[3,21]

Hyperplasia. Parathyroid hyperplasia accounts for approximately 13.5% to 18% of primary hyperparathyroidism. There is usually hyperplasia of more than one gland, but sonographically it cannot be differentiated from adenoma. Although adenomas may be multiple, parathyroid hyperplasia is the most likely diagnosis when multiple nodules are present, whereas adenoma is most likely when a solitary nodule is present.[3]

Carcinoma. Parathyroid carcinoma is responsible for fewer than 2% of cases of primary hyperparathyroidism.[3,21] While the sonographic appearance often cannot be differentiated from that of an adenoma or parathyroid hyperplasia, more attenuation may be present than is normally seen with other disorders.[3] If malignancy is suspected, a biopsy is indicated to reach an accurate diagnoses.

Disease of the Neck

The neck is often the site of disease, but sonography, is not a useful tool except to evaluate the thyroid and parathyroid glands. Sonography's most valuable contribution is in determining the cystic or solid nature of a mass. Also, sonography can ascertain the location and size of the mass. Among the cystic entities visible by sonography are thyroglossal duct cyst, branchial cleft cyst, cystic hygroma, cystic teratoma, hematoma, and abscess. The solid lesions for which sonography is diagnostically most helpful generally involve lymph nodes.

CYSTIC MASSES

Thyroglossal Duct Cyst. The thyroglossal duct extends from the base of the tongue to the isthmus of the thyroid. Normally, it atrophies and is absent in adults, though if this does not occur, a cyst may form. This entity most often appears as a mass in the anterior aspect of the neck, and the diagnosis is suggested if the mass is located superior to the thyroid and in the midline. It may or may not cause discomfort.

The sonographic appearance may be completely cystic or may vary depending on whether hemorrhage, debris, or colloid material is present in the cyst. If fever or pain is present, abscess is a possibility. Carcinoma can also appear totally cystic.[2,19]

Branchial Cleft Cyst. Branchial cleft cyst, often called lateral cervical cyst, typically appears as a mass lying directly below the angle of the mandible and anterior to the sternocleidomastoid muscle.[10] It originates from the branchial cleft, a remnant of embryonic development that may extend from the pharyngeal cavity to the anterior neck or auricle.[10,19,24] The most common sonographic appearance of a branchial cleft cyst is a cystic mass in the previously described location, but solid components may be present if infection or hemorrhage has occurred.[19] Depending on the clinical history, abscess may be part of the differential diagnosis.

Cystic Hygroma. Cystic hygromas, also called lymphangiomas, often appear in conjunction with Turner's syndrome, and it is thought that the associated webbed neck may be secondary to a reabsorbed cystic hygroma.[7,18] These benign, congenital masses can occur at many sites, but the neck is the most common one (80%).[7] Although they are often located in the anterior or lateral aspect of the neck, the posterior neck is the most frequent site.

Sonographically, cystic hygroma is a thin-walled, multilocular or septate mass.[7,18] Although branchial cleft cysts may appear in the same location, they are generally much smaller and are acquired later in life.

Cystic Teratoma. Teratomas are most common in the sacral area, and then in the cervical region,[2,18] usually on the anterior aspect. They can cause respiratory compromise. The sonographic appearance may be cystic, mixed, or solid.[7] Often, teratomas contain calcifications that produce acoustic shadowing.[7,18]

Hematoma. Neck hematomas may develop after trauma or surgery. Because hematoma in the neck region may appear cystic, solid, or complex, depending on the degree of coagulation, the clinical history is very important to narrow the differential diagnoses. Abscess merits serious consideration if signs and symptoms of infection are present.

Abscess. Neck abscesses are relatively uncommon and most often occur in three spaces: submandibular, retropharyngeal, and lateral pharyngeal. The submandibular space is basically the floor of the mouth, and abscesses can form here following dental work or disease.[4] Sonographic evaluation of this area is not common.

The retropharyngeal space is located posterior to the pharynx and anterior to the vertebral column and extends from the base of the skull to the posterior mediastinum. Abscesses in this area often follow upper respiratory tract infections in children and tuberculous infections in adults.[4] This area is not well-suited to sonographic evaluation.

The most common location for an abscess is in the lateral or parapharyngeal space; fortunately, this space does lend itself to sonographic evaluation.[4] The parapharyngeal space comes into contact with the retropharyngeal space and lies lateral to the trachea (pharynx).[4] Tonsillitis and complications of tonsillectomy account for 90% of cases.[4] Following tooth extraction, adults more often develop abscesses in this area than children.[4] Abscesses generally produce fever, white blood cell elevation, and tenderness. Their sonographic appearance varies much, but they often appear as a complex mass with jagged margins. Clinical history and laboratory data are extremely helpful in diagnosing neck abscesses.

SOLID MASSES

Lymph Node Disease. Benign lymphadenopathy can be caused by several conditions: tuberculosis, cat-scratch disease, syphilis, mononucleosis, and other nonspecific viral and bacterial infections.[4] The most common mass in the cervical area of children is cervical lymphadenitis, which commonly follows an upper respiratory tract infection (Fig. 19-22).[4]

Metastatic lesions to the lymph nodes cannot be differentiated from benign lymphadenopathy and may take origin in lung, breast, gastrointestinal

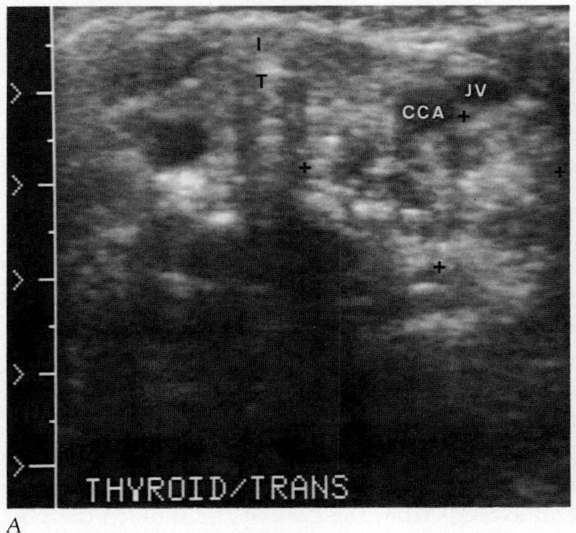

A

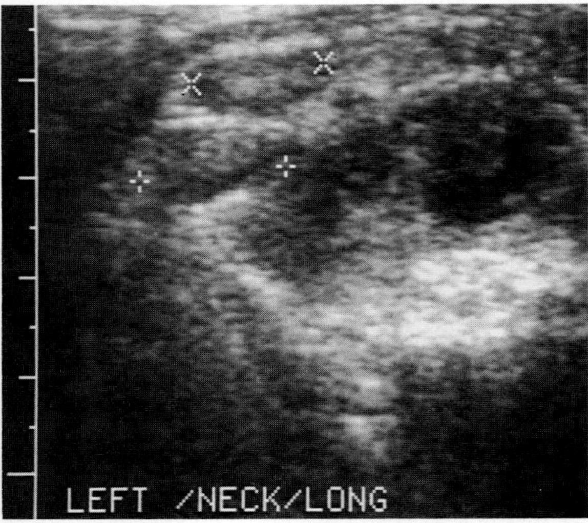

B

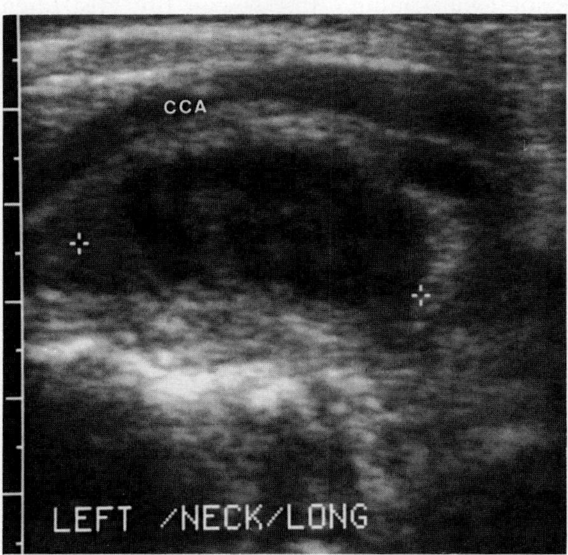

C

Figure 19-22. (*A*) Transverse scan of the neck of a 19-month-old boy who presented with a left neck mass of 3 weeks' duration. The patient had a temperature of 104° F and the white blood cell count was elevated. The scan reveals a heterogeneous mass (*cursor*) in the left neck that displaces the common carotid artery (CCA) and jugular vein (JV) anteriorly. This was sonographically diagnosed as evolving cervical lymphadenitis. Needle aspiration provided very little fluid. Surgery confirmed necrotic suppurative lymph nodes (lymphadenitis; I, isthmus; T, trachea). (*B*) Longitudinal section of the same mass. The nodules (*cursor*, X) were felt to represent lymph nodes because of their location, size, echogenicity, and clinical signs and symptoms. (C) Longitudinal section of the same mass. The nodule (*cursor*) anteriorly displaces the common carotid artery (cca).

tract, pancreas, or other head and neck primary tumors (Fig. 19-23).[4]

Hodgkin's disease and lymphomas are typically seen in young adults; however, they are the most common malignant lymph node tumors of children. Although lymphoma may occur at any age, Hodgkin's disease peaks between ages 5 and 9 years.[4] In children younger than 3 years it is rare.[4] Rhabdomyosarcoma is the most common solid head and neck tumor of children between 1 and 5 years,[4] although they often develop in areas that are not accessible to sonographic evaluation.[4]

The sonographic appearance of lymphadenopathy is consistent, with single or multiple, well-circumscribed, circular or oval, hypoechoic nodules (Figs. 19-22, 19-23).[19] Sonography is helpful for differentiating the masses from the thyroid gland. A complete clinical history and histologic laboratory data are crucial for distinguishing benign from malignant lesions.

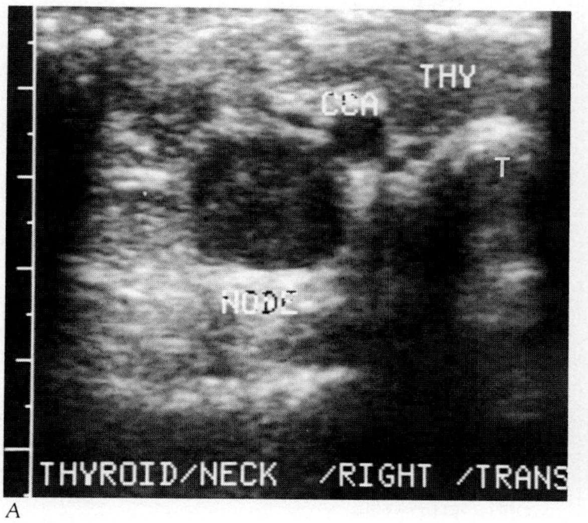

A

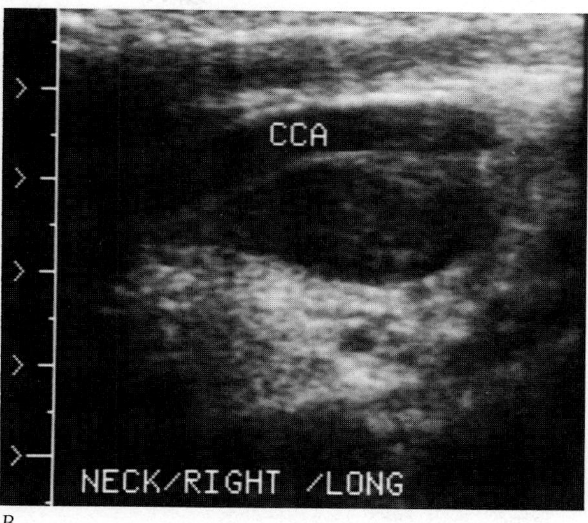

B

FIGURE 19-23. (*A*) A 39-year-old woman presented with adenopathy and liver metastasis from an occult primary tumor. This transverse image of the right neck demonstrates a solid, hypoechoic nodule, which was diagnosed sonographically as cervical lymphadenopathy. The nodule has displaced the common carotid artery (CCA) anteriorly. It was proven at biopsy to be adenocarcinoma (T, trachea; THY, right lateral lobe of the thyroid). (*B*) On a longitudinal section of the nodule (NODE), note the correlation of the displacement of the common carotid artery (CCA).

Conclusion

Ultrasonography of the thyroid, parathryoids, and neck can often demonstrate the internal contents and location of a mass and narrow the differential diagnosis. Furthermore, sonography can define the number of nodules, which aid in arriving at a diagnosis. Because ultrasonography is not histologically specific, correlating the sonographic results with available clinical signs, symptoms, and laboratory data is crucial for an accurate diagnosis.

Acknowledgments

I would like to take this opportunity to thank Laura Pearson for providing the drawings used in this chapter. Also, I would like to thank Lynn Reyes, BS, RDMS, and Nancy Sawyer, RDMS for their assistance during the literature review and image acquisition phases of this project.

References

1. Ackerman LV, Rosai J: Surgical Pathology, 5th ed. St. Louis, CV Mosby, 1974.
2. Anderhub B: Manual of Abdominal Sonography. Baltimore, University Park Press, 1983.
3. Cole-Beuglet C: Ultrasonography of thyroid, parathyroid, and neck masses. *In* Sarti DA (ed): Diagnostic Ultrasound: Text and Cases, 2nd ed. Chicago, Year Book Medical Publishers, 1987.
4. Damion J, Hybels RL: The neck mass 2. Inflammatory and neoplastic causes. Postgrad Med 1987, 81:97–103.
5. Evans DM: Diagnostic discriminants of thyroid cancer. Am J Surg 1987, 153:569–570.
6. Fallis G: Hashimoto's thyroiditis: An unusual sequela. J Fam Pract 1987, 25:399–401.
7. Goldstein RB, Callen PW: Ultrasound evaluation of the fetal thorax and abdomen. *In* Callen PW (ed): Ultrasonography in Obstetrics and Gynecology, 2nd ed. Philadelphia, WB Saunders, 1988.
8. Greco LP, Ottino GM, Avonto L, et al: Ectopic thy-

roid remnants within the myocardium: An unusual case of right ventricular mass. Am Heart J 1988, 115:195–198.
9. Hoffman E: Carcinoma of the thyroid: Review of 303 cases. South Med J 1987, 80:741–752.
10. Moore KL: Clinically Oriented Anatomy, 2nd ed. Baltimore, Williams & Wilkins, 1985.
11. Netter FH: The Ciba Collection of Medical Illustrations: Vol 4, Endocrine System and Selected Metabolic Diseases. Summit, NJ, Ciba Pharmaceutical Company, 1985.
12. Oertel JE, Heffess CS: Lymphoma of the thyroid and related disorders. Semin Oncol 1987, 14:333–342.
13. Propper RA, Skolnick ML, Weinstein BJ, et al: The nonspecificity of the thyroid sign. J Clin Ultrasound 1980, 8:129–132.
14. Ralls PW, Mayekawa DS, Lee KP, et al: Color-flow Doppler sonography in Graves disease: "Thyroid inferno." AJR 1988, 150:781–784.
15. Rizzato G, Solbiati L, Croce F, et al: Aspiration biopsy of superficial lesions: Ultrasonic guidance with a linear-array probe. AJR 1987, 148:623–625.
16. Robbins SL, Angell M, Kumar V: Basic Pathology, 3rd ed. Philadelphia, WB Saunders, 1981.
17. Sakiyama R: Common thyroid disorders. Am Fam Phys 1988, 38:227–238.
18. Sanders RC, James EA: The Principles and Practice of Ultrasonography in Obstetrics and Gynecology, 3rd ed. Norwalk, CT, Appleton-Century-Crofts, 1985.
19. Schorzman L: High-resolution ultrasonography of superficial structures. *In* Hagen SA (ed): Textbook of Diagnostic Ultrasonography, 2nd ed. St. Louis, CV Mosby, 1983.
20. Simeone JR, Daniels GH, Hall DA, et al: Sonography in the follow-up of 100 patients with thyroid carcinoma. AJR 1987, 148:45–49.
21. Simeone JR, Mueller PR: The thyroid and parathyroid glands. *In* Taylor KJ (ed): Atlas of Ultrasonography, 2nd ed. New York, Churchill Livingstone, 1985.
22. Berkow R (ed): The Merck Manual, 15th ed. Rathway, NJ, Merck Sharp & Dome, 1987.
23. Walling AD: Ectopic thyroid tissue. Am Fam Phys 1987, 36:147–150.
24. Wheelock IR, Sanders PC: Neck mass. *In* Sanders RC (ed): Clinical Sonography, A Practical Guide. Boston, Little, Brown, 1984.
25. Woestyn J, Afschrift M, Schelstraete K, et al: Demonstration of nodules in the normal thyroid by echocardiography. Br J Radiol 1985, 58:1179–1182.

CHAPTER 20

Breast

CATHERINE CARR-HOEFER

Ultrasonography is a useful complement to mammography and physical examination in the evaluation of breast disease. Sonography provides a noninvasive, tomographic display of the breast without ionizing radiation.

Overall, mammography surpasses other imaging modalities in the detection and diagnosis of breast malignancy. It is the only method proven effective in screening asymptomatic patients for minimal breast cancer.[1,10,16,19,41] Quality mammography is capable of detecting microcalcifications, which may be the first sign of a developing malignancy. Early cancer detection and treatment improves long-term survival by decreasing the incidence of lymph node involvement and metastasis to distant sites.[1,21,48]

Although mammography is the most common imaging tool used to evaluate the breast, it has some diagnostic limitations. Mammography cannot detect all breast masses. Detection of lesions is high in a translucent, fatty breast but is compromised in a radiopaque, dense breast. Occasionally, superimposition of a local area of normal tissues can create a pseudomass, which is hard to differentiate from a real lesion. Mammography alone cannot consistently determine whether a mass is cystic or solid. Additionally, radiographic features of some breast malignancies are similar to those of benign masses, so the level of diagnostic confidence is reduced.[19]

For these reasons, adjunctive tests may be necessary to evaluate certain breasts. When used in addition to mammography or physical examination, sonography can often improve diagnostic accuracy and assist in appropriate patient management.

Clinical Role of Breast Sonography

Table 20-1 summarizes the advantages, applications, and indications for sonographic evaluation of the breast.[5,10,16,18,26,27,30,44,48,62,65] The principal diagnostic feature of sonography is its ability to differentiate between cystic and solid lesions, thus allowing further characterization of palpable or radiographically indeterminate breast masses. Unlike mammography, sonography detects masses best in echogenic, dense breasts but is less effective in hypoechoic, fatty breasts. In order to be recognized, a lesion must have different imaging features than those from adjacent tissues. Most breast masses are hypoechoic or anechoic and are best seen against the echogenic background provided by parenchymal tissue. Sonography, therefore, can help evaluate the patient with radiographically dense breasts for masses and may serve as the primary nonionizing imaging modality to evaluate symptomatic patients who are young, pregnant, or lactating. For patients with equivocal physical or mammographic findings, sonography can help determine whether a mass actually exists before aspiration biopsy is considered.

Since sonography allows tomographic imaging of

TABLE 20-1. Clinical role of sonographic breast evaluation

Advantages
- Noninvasive, painless
- No ionizing radiation
- Tomographic display
- Good patient acceptance
- Imaging near chest wall

Applications
- Complementary to mammography, physical examination (not a screening device for early-stage cancer)

Indications
- Differentiation of cystic from solid masses, whether palpable or mammographically indeterminate
- Evaluation of "radiographic dense" breast
- Evaluation of pregnant or lactating breast
- Initial examination of "young breasts" (before age 30 years)
- Verification of presence of mass when mammographic or physical findings are equivocal: asymmetric superimposition of structures, mass seen on only one mammographic view, palpable mass not seen on mammogram
- Evaluation of inflammatory processes
- Evaluation of augmented breast
- Evaluation of traumatic breast
- Evaluation of irradiated breast
- Evaluation of male breast
- Guidance during needle aspiration biopsy procedures
- Serial evaluation of benign processes

the breast without painful compression, it is useful in examining patients with breast trauma, inflammatory changes, augmentation mammoplasty, or postirradiation changes. Sonography is helpful in evaluating the male breast for abnormal glandular changes or masses. Mammography is often difficult to perform on these patients.

High-resolution, real-time sonography can assist fine-needle placement during cyst aspiration or biopsy procedures, affording direct visualization of the needle tip as it approaches and enters the mass. Evacuation of cystic lesions can be observed and confirmed.

Although sonography is useful in a number of clinical settings, its limitations must be recognized. It cannot be used as a screening examination for breast cancer, since it seldom detects microcalcifications and can miss small solid masses, especially in fatty breasts.[5,16,22,32,35,42] When strict criteria are followed, sonography can reliably distinguish cystic from solid masses, but differentiation between benign and malignant solid masses is less reliable when imaging patterns are similar.[6,10,26,30,40]

Anatomy

The breasts, or mammary glands, are paired, dome-shaped structures lying along the anterior chest wall adjacent to the axilla. These modified skin glands are composed of fatty, glandular, and fibrous connective tissue.[18,19,21,29,50,52] Figure 20-1 illustrates the major anatomic components of the adult female breast. The glandular tissue is positioned within layers of superficial and deep fascia. Posterior to the breast and deep fascial plane lie the pectoralis major and -minor muscles. Although the breast slides easily over these muscles, the gland itself is firmly attached to the skin by fibrous connective tissue bands known as Cooper's ligaments.[51] These suspensory ligaments extend radially from the deep fascial plane to the skin, enclosing fat lobules and providing support to the glandular structures of the breast. A portion of mammary tissue may extend into the region of the axilla, forming the axillary tail of Spence.

The nipple is a round, fibromuscular papilla projecting from the center of the breast. Inversion can be a normal variant. The areola, a small circular area of pigmented skin surrounding the nipple, contains numerous sebaceous glands (Montgomery's glands) that appear as small nodules beneath the skin.

The functional fibroglandular tissue of the breast is called the parenchyma. The function of the gland is to produce and to secrete milk. The parenchymal layer contains 15 to 20 overlapping segments, called lobes, which are arranged in a radial fashion. Each lobe divides into 20 to 40 small sections called lobules.[29] During pregnancy, numerous microscopic saclike secretory glands called acini form within the lobules at the ends of the ducts. The acini produce milk in the lactating breast and involute or disappear after lactation ceases.[18] An intricate network of lactiferous ducts drains the acini, lobules, and lobes. One major collecting duct empties each lobe. The main collecting duct from each lobe converges radially toward the nipple, enlarging just beneath the areola. This focal area of enlargement is called the ampulla or lactiferous sinus. Some of the main ducts may join

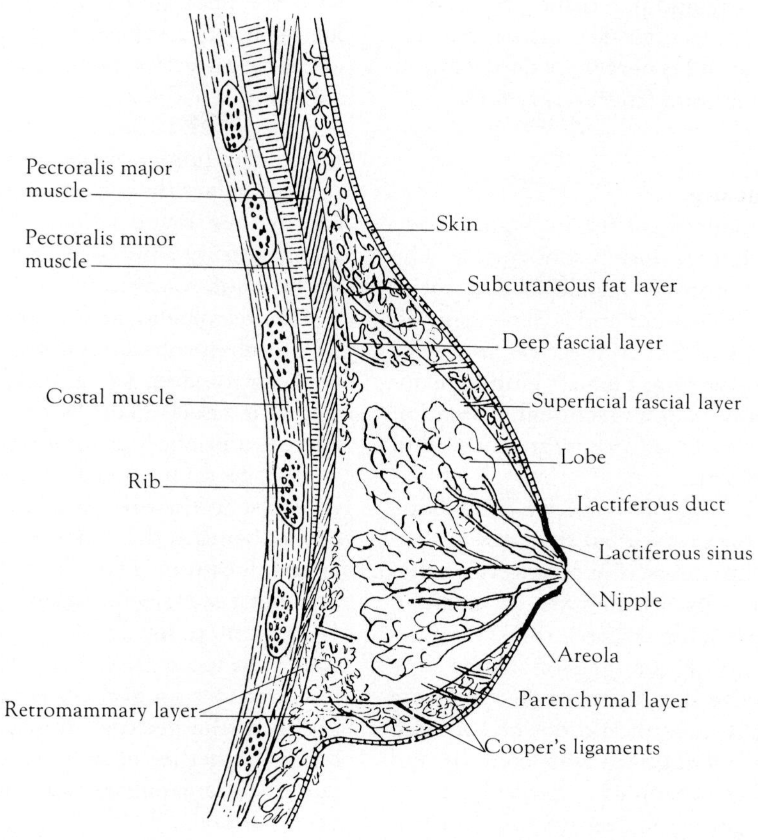

FIGURE 20-1. Major anatomic components of the female breast and chest wall.

at the sinus level before exiting through tiny openings at the summit of the nipple. The majority of the glandular tissue lies in the upper outer quadrant of the breast and beneath the areola.

Stroma serve as the supporting elements of the breast and consist of fat and connective tissue. Adipose tissue is found beneath the skin and glandular tissue and fills out the spaces between the lobes and lobules. The connective tissue septa of Cooper's ligaments enclose and separate the fat, lobes, and lobules. A layer of specialized connective tissue covers the ducts.[19,21]

The primary arterial blood supply to the breast is from branches of the internal mammary and lateral thoracic arteries, and to a lesser extent the intercostal arteries.[19,21,50] Arterial anastomoses are found beneath the areola.

Venous drainage is through superficial and deep networks.[2,19,21] Venous anastomosis may occur in a circular pattern around the base of the areola. Deep veins follow the path of the arteries to drain the breast.

Lymph vessels originate in the connective tissues and lactiferous ducts and communicate with the subareolar plexus.[52] Numerous lymphatics lie under the skin. Lymph vessels follow venous drainage of the breast to the axilla. The majority of lymph drains into the pectoral group of the axillary lymph nodes. Other sites of termination include the supraclavicular, subclavicular, parasternal, and intramammary nodes. Some lymph vessels may drain to the opposite breast and to the abdominal nodes.[50]

The nerves of the breast are located along the

skin and within the glandular tissue.[2] Superficial sensory nerves join the cervical, brachial, and intercostal nerves. Glandular nerves are derived from branches of the intercostal (thoracic) nerves.

Sonographic Anatomy

The anatomic components of the breast are easily demonstrated by high-resolution sonography. The appearance of the normal female breast varies widely from patient to patient and is dependent on the relative amounts of fat, connective, and glandular tissue in the scanning plane.[26] Unlike mammography, sonography allows sectional evaluation of the breast, one "slice" at a time, from the skin surface to the chest wall.

The skin is seen as a highly reflective band along the surface of the breast. Normal thickness is usually 2 to 3 mm.[55] The skin may appear as two echogenic lines separated by a thin layer of medium-level echoes, especially when thickening is present.[10,31] When using compression bands or a standoff device on the skin, echoes reflecting from the surface of such devices should not be confused with the skin line. Changes in skin contour and thickness may indicate neoplastic, postsurgical, or inflammatory changes at or deep to the skin surface.

The nipple, which is composed of dense connective tissue, displays a homogeneous texture of medium-level echoes. Attenuation of the sound beam by the nipple and connective tissues surrounding the subareolar ducts leads to nipple shadowing.[5,11,26] During scanning, air pockets around the nipple accentuate shadowing. Compression techniques or extra scanning gel reduce nipple shadowing, allowing better evaluation of the subareolar region.

The subcutaneous fat layer lies between the skin and the parenchymal (fibroglandular) tissue. It does not extend beneath the nipple. Sonographically, fat appears less echogenic than other breast tissues. Cooper's ligaments are imaged as thin, echogenic, curvilinear tissue strands encasing the hypoechoic fat lobules. At times, streaks of acoustic shadowing are seen at oblique interfaces from these dense ligaments, possibly caused by refraction of the sound beam.[5]

The parenchyma is imaged as a homogeneous, moderately echogenic layer of tissue beneath the nipple and subcutaneous fat. This pattern varies with the amount of fat interspersed in the glandular tissue. The superficial and deep fascial planes appear as reflective lines encasing the glandular tissue. Fluid-filled ducts may be seen radiating from the nipple and into the breast core. Sonography images the lumen of the duct, whereas, mammography displays the lumen, epithelial lining, and the collagenous tissue surrounding it.[11,26] Generally, ducts measure 2 mm or less, but they may be larger at the lactiferous sinus.[11,21]

The retromammary layer contains smaller fat lobules than those found beneath the skin and lies between the deep fascial plane and pectoralis muscle. This fascial plane is highly reflective and appears as a bright line anterior to the pectoral fascia.

The pectoralis major muscle lies immediately posterior to the breast. The pectoralis minor muscle lies beneath the major muscle in a more superolateral location. These muscles are best seen on transverse scans, where they appear as linear bands of medium- to low-level echoes parallel to the chest wall. The pectoral fascial planes produce bright, linear echoes on both sides of the muscles. Recognition of the pectoral muscles is important to determine whether deep-lying masses are intramammary, extramammary, or invading through the pectoral fascia.[26,31]

Occasionally, normal lymph glands can be seen, especially in the axillary portion of the breast near the pectoral layers. A normal lymph node typically measures less than 5 mm and appears as a flat, oval, hypoechoic, solid mass. The center of the node may be hyperechoic if internal adipose tissue is present.[54]

Deep to the pectoral muscles are the ribs and intercostal muscles of the thoracic cage. Laterally, the bone of the ribs attenuates the sound beam, resulting in acoustic shadowing. Medially, the cartilage appears as oval structures containing low-level echoes. These features are best seen on sagittal scans. Care must be taken not to mistake the cartilaginous portions of the ribs for a mass.

Variations in Normal Patterns

The proportionate amount of fat and glandular tissue in the breast depends on the patient's age, parity, and whether she is premenopausal or postmenopausal, pregnant or lactating, or obese.[18,21,26,55] The prepubertal breast is small and fatty. Early-de-

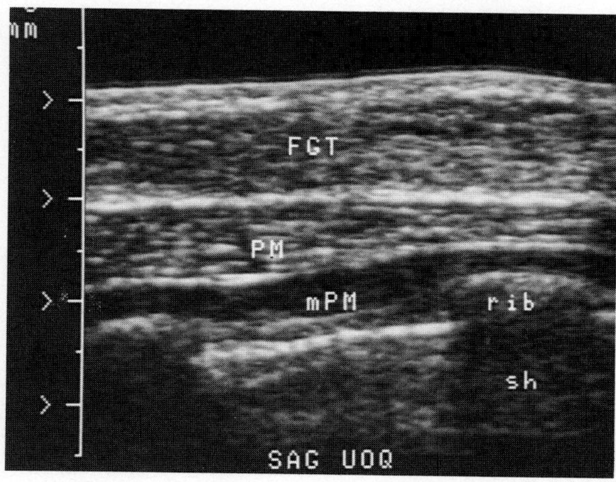

FIGURE 20-2. Normal young adult breast. Real-time image displays minimal subcutaneous fat. The parenchyma, or fibroglandular tissue (FGT), fills the breast. The major pectoral muscle (PM) and minor pectoral muscle (mPM) are seen. A rib is noted casting an acoustic shadow.

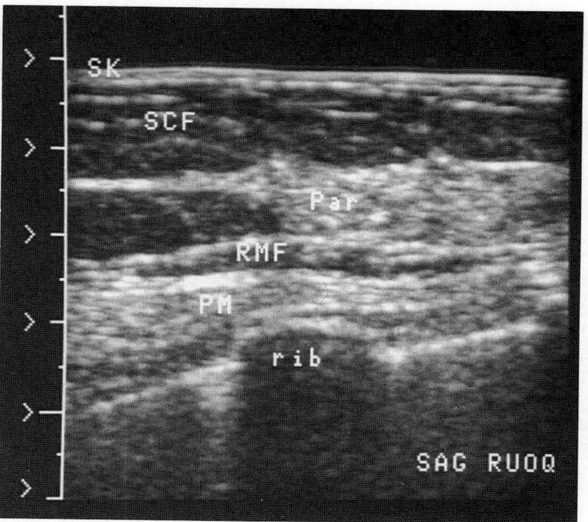

FIGURE 20-3. Normal adult breast. Real-time image demonstrates the skin (SK), subcutaneous fat (SCF), parenchymal tissue (Par), retromammary fat (RMF), pectoral muscle (PM), and rib shadowing (rib). The amount of fat and parenchymal tissue is evenly distributed. A standoff gel pad was placed between the linear-array probe and the skin to better image the anterior breast.

veloping parenchyma is demonstrated as a small echogenic mass of tissue beneath the nipple in an otherwise fatty breast. After puberty, the adolescent breast becomes increasingly glandular and the amount of surrounding fat diminishes. Sonographically, the parenchyma has a very fine, uniform, echogenic texture. The cone-shaped glandular tissue is surrounded by a thin, weakly echogenic layer of fat.

The adult breast has the greatest range of appearances. Characteristically, the young nulliparous female breast is densely glandular, with little internal or surrounding fat (Fig. 20-2). With increasing age and number of pregnancies, fatty replacement of the parenchyma occurs. Additional fat is deposited in the subcutaneous and retromammary layers (Fig. 20-3). Fat lobules in the parenchyma appear moderately hypoechoic compared to the echogenic glandular tissue and may resemble a mass. Around menopause, parenchymal tissue may diminish to the point where it is mainly seen beneath the nipple and in the upper outer quadrant. The postmenopausal breast may show complete or nearly complete fatty replacement as the lobules and ducts atrophy.[19] Cooper's ligaments are easily seen encasing the fat lobules (Fig. 20-4). However, older, nulliparous women may retain considerable amounts of glandular tissue.

In the pregnant or lactating breast, the expanding glandular tissue practically fills the breast, compressing the surrounding fat. The overall texture of the parenchyma is finely echogenic. Duct dilatation may be marked during late pregnancy and lactation.

Developmental Anomalies

Developmental anomalies of the breast are uncommon. Some are associated with abnormal endocrine gland development or dysfunction and may not become apparent until puberty. An accessory nipple (polythelia) is the most common congenital breast anomaly. Accessory breast (polymastia) is rare. Either anomaly can occur anywhere along the milk line.[19,29,51] Underdevelopment (hypoplasia) or excessive growth (hypertrophy) of the breast tissue

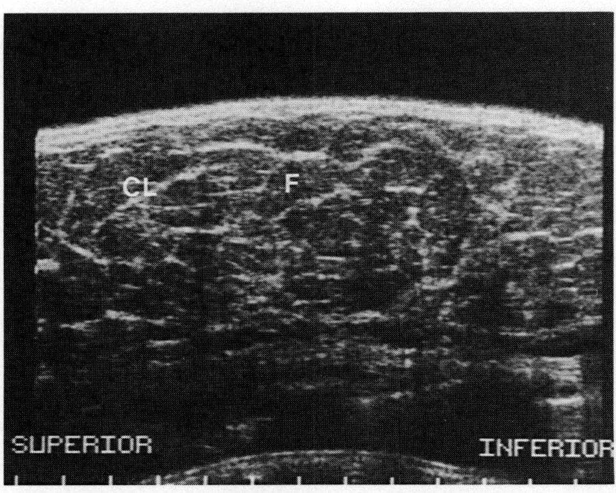

Figure 20-4. Postmenopausal fatty breast. Supine water-path linear scan demonstrates complete fatty replacement (F). Cooper's ligaments (CL) and the connective tissues are seen as thin, echogenic lines encasing the hypoechoic fat lobules. (Courtesy Margaret Washburn, MD, Sedro Woolley, WA.)

may affect one or both breasts. Complete failure of the breast tissue to develop is called amastia.[19] This rare condition is typically accompanied by congenital absence of the nipple (athelia) and is usually associated with underdevelopment of the pectoral muscle.[29] Amazia refers to absence of the breast tissue with presence of the nipple.

Between age 6 and 8 years, growth of one breast occasionally occurs before the other. By age 9, however, both breasts are comparable in size and development. This normal variant, referred to as unilateral early ripening, should not be mistaken for pathology and does not necessitate biopsy.[18,26]

If development of both breasts occurs before 8 years of age, precocious puberty is suspected.[51] Other possible sonographic signs of precocious puberty may include ovarian enlargement with possible cystic change, a large-for-age uterus, and adrenal tumor.

Instrumentation and Scanning Technique

Before the ultrasound examination begins, the patient's history is obtained, the mammogram is reviewed, and the breast is examined. A worksheet is used to record the patient's history and to mark the location of palpable masses, biopsy scars, and other changes in the skin, nipple, and breast contour (Fig. 20-5). After the examination, any lesions are drawn on the worksheet and described.

Proper equipment set-up, transducer selection, patient positioning, and scanning technique are essential to produce quality images. The time gain compensation (TGC), overall gain, and focal zone should be selected to display an image that clearly demonstrates all breast tissue from the skin line to the chest wall. Table 20-2 lists the advantages and disadvantages of breast ultrasound systems, many of which are discussed in the literature.[4,6,16,22,24,26,31,35,37,43]

Hand-Held, High-Resolution Real-Time Systems

High frequency, real-time imaging provides excellent detail of superficial structures and is the most common form of breast sonography. Commercially available small-parts transducers operate at frequencies of 5 to 10 MHz and have excellent axial and lateral resolution. These probes can be added to most existing real-time systems.

High-resolution, real-time sonography provides a rapid, safe, low-cost method for differentiating cysts from solid masses as well as allowing visual needle guidance during aspiration and biopsy procedures.

Several types of real-time probes are designed specifically to evaluate superficial structures. They are available in sector, linear, or convex array displays. Depending on probe design, beam focusing is fixed or variable. Biopsy attachments are available with some probes. Split-screen capabilities of many newer systems allow linear scans to be "pieced together," to show the boundaries of a large mass and the position of a mass relative to the nipple.

Using an acoustic standoff device between the transducer and the breast allows visualization of the skin line, eliminates near field artifacts, and optimizes beam focusing.[66] If the transducer does not have an internal or attachable acoustic standoff, a water bag or gel pad can be placed between the probe and skin surface when desired. Several commercially available gel-type standoff pads come in

BREAST ULTRASOUND

Pt. Name: ______________________ Age: ________ Date: ____________

Dr. ______________________ I.D. # ____________

PREVIOUS MAMMOGRAMS
Date: Findings:

PREVIOUS SONOGRAMS
Date: Findings:

HISTORY
Complaint/Duration (Palpable mass, tenderness, nipple discharge or inversion, skin changes, etc.):

LMP: Menarche: Menopause:
Hysterectomy: Oophorectomy:

Medications: Hormones:
Birth Control Pills:
Other:

FAMILY HX. OF BREAST CANCER (circle)
Mother Grandmother Sister Daughter Aunt

PREVIOUS SURGERY (side, location, date)
Biopsy:
Lumpectomy: Rad. Rx.
Mastectomy:
Findings:

ULTRASOUND FINDINGS:

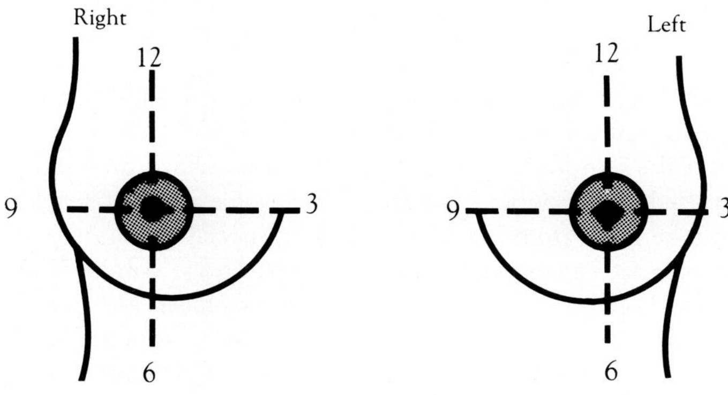

FIGURE 20-5. Example of breast sonography worksheet.

TABLE 20-2. Advantages and disadvantages of breast ultrasound systems

<table>
<tr><th rowspan="2"></th><th rowspan="2">HAND-HELD, REAL-TIME SYSTEMS</th><th colspan="2">AUTOMATED SYSTEMS</th></tr>
<tr><th>SUPINE</th><th>PRONE</th></tr>
<tr><td rowspan="2">Advantages</td><td rowspan="2">Contact scanning over palpable mass
Improved resolution with higher frequencies
Lower cost
Use of existing systems
Flexible scanning planes
Supine positioning allows palpation and evaluates for mass compressibility
Rapid mass evaluation
Continuous needle visualization during needle guidance procedures
Patient can sit during examination</td><td colspan="2">Reproducible, systematic survey of whole breast
Less operator variability
Standardized labelling
Increased probability of recording nonpalpable masses</td></tr>
<tr><td>Supine accessibility
Compressed breast allows use of higher frequencies, better resolution
Multifrequency selection
Biplane imaging</td><td>Prone imaging allows realistic demonstration of skin, nipple, and breast contour
Dual review station</td></tr>
<tr><td rowspan="2">Disadvantages</td><td rowspan="2">Less reproducible
Less systematic labelling
Limited field of view
More operator variability
Need standoff to image skin
May miss nonpalpable mass if examination is incomplete</td><td>Frequent repositioning of water-bag
Loss of normal skin contour
No continuous imaging during needle guidance procedures</td><td>Lower frequencies due to water path
Requires additional scanning with compression to penetrate many breasts and to reduce nipple shadowing
Not suitable for guidance procedures</td></tr>
<tr><td colspan="2">No direct palpation while scanning
Higher cost, large equipment requires more space
No real-time capability</td></tr>
</table>

thicknesses of 1, 2, or 4 cm.[3,17,38] For best results, the thickness of the standoff should be at least the same amount as the depth of the structure of interest. If the standoff is too thin, reverberation artifacts appear within the breast at distances equal to the standoff's thickness. If the standoff is too thick, the focal zone will be shifted out of optimal range. Acoustic standoffs should be made from low-attenuating materials with impedance values matched to soft tissue to reduce artifacts.

Scan Procedure. The patient lies supine or slightly oblique with a Styrofoam support elevating the side of the body to be examined (Fig. 20-6A). The adjacent arm is extended to the side with the hand placed near or under the head. The breast should appear flattened with the nipple centered. Warm gel is applied to the skin.

Scan Protocol. Ideally, the entire breast is surveyed methodically. The skin overlying palpable masses is marked. Each quadrant is scanned in sagittal and transverse planes or radially in a clockwise direction; special attention is paid to areas of concern.

The entire volume and adjacent tissues of each detected mass are carefully scanned in various planes and beam angles. Radial scans help to follow ductal structures and to show the position of masses relative to the nipple. Masses are measured and their positions are noted. When questionable areas of architectural change are noted, images are made of the other breast for comparison.

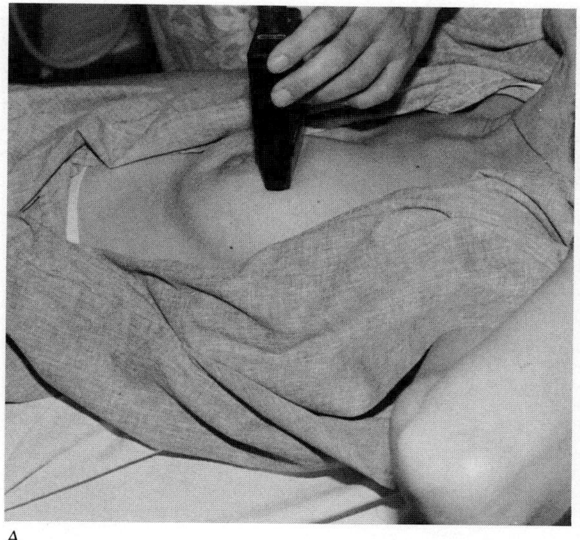

A

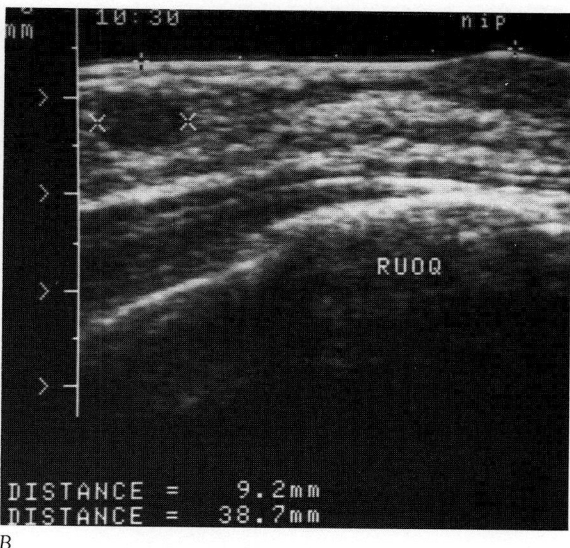

B

FIGURE 20-6. (*A*) Hand-held, real-time position. (*B*) Real-time labelling. Linear-array supine scan of a 9-mm solid mass (X cursor) located in the right upper outer quadrant (RUOQ) at the 10:30 radial position. The center of the mass is 7 mm beneath the skin and 39 mm (+ cursor) from the center of the nipple. A standoff pad was used between the probe and the skin to better visualize this anterior mass.

Multiple representative images are made of each quadrant and mass. Images are clearly labelled by position and scan plane, and hard copies are made.

Labelling methods commonly used include the quadrant or the clock method. With the quadrant method, a transverse scan of the upper outer quadrant of the left breast would be denoted as TV-LUOQ. A sagittal scan of the lower inner quadrant of the right breast would be denoted SAG-RLIQ. With the clock method, a lesion directly lateral to the nipple in the left breast would be marked (L) 3:00; whereas, a lesion lateral to the nipple in the right breast would be marked (R) 9:00. For more precision, the distance from the nipple to the lesion is noted (Fig. 20-6B).

Many new systems can display a small schematic diagram of the breast on the viewing monitor next to the sonographic image for documentation of scan plane information. On systems without body marker capability, small labels showing a diagram of the breast can be affixed to the hard copy of the ultrasound image. The location of the mass and scan plane can be drawn on the label and placed next to the corresponding image. Such labels can be purchased (MammoGraphic Labels) for use on mammograms or sonograms.

Ultrasound Craniocaudad Position. With the patient supine, it is occasionally difficult to be sure whether a mass seen by sonography is the same mass demonstrated by mammography, especially in larger-breasted women. By rescanning the breast in a position simulating the radiographic craniocaudad (C-C) position, the location of the mass can be more precisely compared with the mammographic image.

The patient is seated. The lower surface of the breast is raised and placed on an examination table or tray so that the nipple is parallel to the tabletop (Fig. 20-7). For limited scanning, the patient can simply place her hand under the breast and lift it to obtain a similar projection. The C-C position

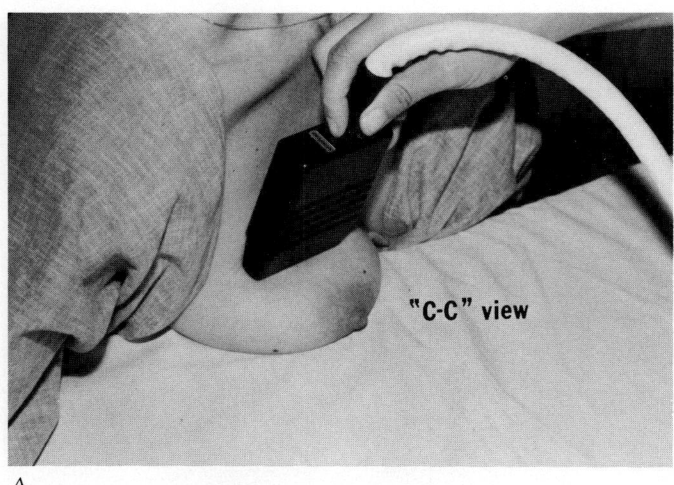

A

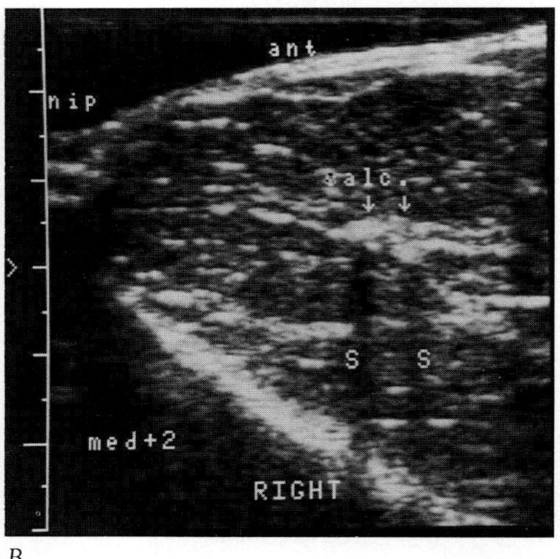

B

FIGURE 20-7. (*A*) Real-time view made with patient in C-C position. (*B*) Real-time C-C view on a woman with large, fatty breasts. Sonography revealed bright echoes with distal shadowing near the path of a previous biopsy. By positioning the patient in a position similar to the one used to make the radiographic view, the location of these calcifications was easily compared to the mammogram. Final diagnosis was calcified fat necrosis.

can be used during aspiration or biopsy procedures, allowing needle placement parallel to the chest wall and providing greater tissue stability when needling masses in a large breast.

AUTOMATED WHOLE-BREAST SYSTEMS

Supine Water-Bag Scanner. A specially designed static B-mode scanner utilizing a single motor-driven transducer that moves rapidly across the confines of a water bag can produce systematic, reproducible, linear scans of the breast while the patient lies supine (Fig. 20-8A).

Current systems feature a multifrequency transducer, which operates at selective, true center frequencies of 3.5, 4.5, 6.5 and 7.5 MHz.[43] This transducer is made from a piezoelectric polymer called polyvinylidene fluoride-trifluoroethylene (PVDF-TrFE), which has acoustic impedance properties closer to those of water and soft tissues than traditional ceramic crystals. At higher frequencies, the reflectivity of fat is increased and hypoechoic lesions are better seen.[35]

The Mylar water bag provides an acoustic standoff between the skin and the transducer, compresses the breast for more uniform penetration, and flattens the skin for optimal sound beam incidence.[26,28] When filled with degassed, distilled water, the scanning dimensions of the bag are approximately 13 × 4.5 cm.[43]

Scan procedure. The patient lies supine or slightly oblique with a sponge beneath the side of the body to be examined. The adjacent arm is extended near the head. Palpable masses are marked on the skin so the outline will be visible through the transparent bag.[27] A thin layer of mineral oil is brushed on the skin. The water-bag assembly is lowered manually over the breast and positioned to optimize compression, angle of incidence, and focal beam placement.[26] The height for the fixed-focus transducer is raised or lowered in the water bag to further optimize beam focusing. Frequency selection is based on the breast's size, texture, and the depth of the area of interest.

Scan protocol. Longitudinal and/or transverse scans are obtained at 3- to 5-mm intervals through the entire breast. Areas of interest are reexamined

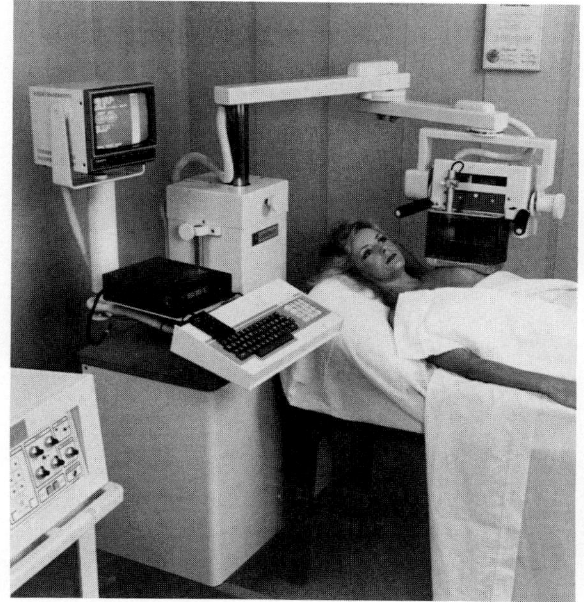
A

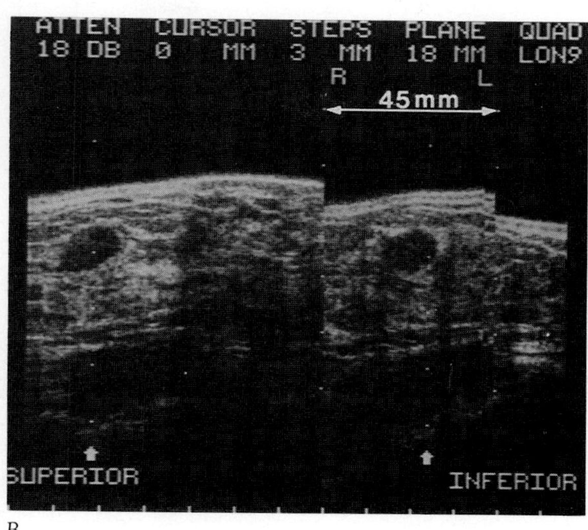

B

FIGURE 20-8. (*A*) Supine water-bag whole-breast scanner. A Mylar water bag is attached to an articulated scan arm assembly. A large, multifrequency transducer moves across the confines of the water bag to produce automated, linear scans of the compressed breast. (Courtesy Labsonics, Inc., Mooresville, IN.) (*B*) Biplane image of a fibroadenoma imaged with an automated supine breast scanner. The initial sagittal scan revealed a well-defined solid mass. An electronic cursor was placed over the lesion on the monitor. A 45-mm transverse scan was made at the level of the cursor. The resultant image showed the transverse scan overlaid on the sagittal image for easy correlation. (Courtesy Margaret Washburn, MD, Sedro Woolley, WA.)

at intervals of 1 mm.[26,35] Biplane imaging allows a suspected area to be imaged and displayed in two perpendicular planes on the same image without moving the water bag (see Fig. 20-8B).[43] When needed, added oblique or radial scans can be obtained by changing the angle or rotation of the water-bag assembly. Any changes in architecture are compared by scanning both breasts. The entire examination is videotaped and hard copies are made of selected images.

Prone Water-Path Scanner. Dedicated prone water-path breast scanners are no longer manufactured, but some systems are still in clinical use.

The patient lies prone on a specially designed examination bed containing a partially exposed water tank (Fig. 20-9A). One breast at a time is immersed in the warmed water bath. Sonographic examination of the breast in the natural hanging position allows accurate demonstration of the skin, nipple, and breast contour.

Four large, fixed-focus, 4.5-MHz transducers are mounted on a curved scanning arm located at the base of the tank (Fig. 20-9B).[26] The scanning arm is raised or lowered in the tank to achieve proper beam focusing in the breast. The transducers can operate singly, in pairs, or jointly to produce single-pass or compound scans in longitudinal, transverse, rotational, and oblique planes.[4,21,26,44]

To evaluate abnormal or underpenetrated

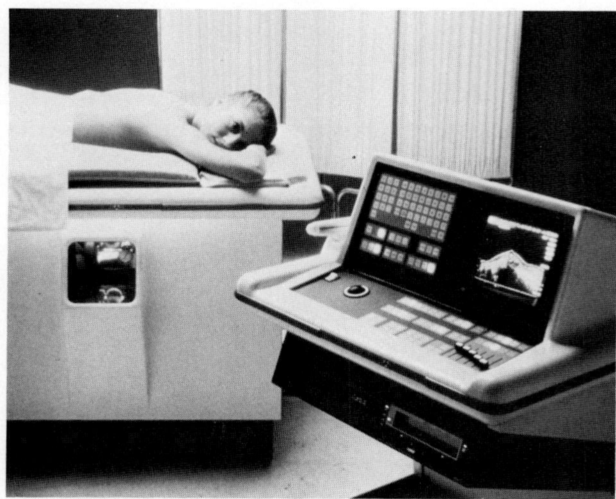

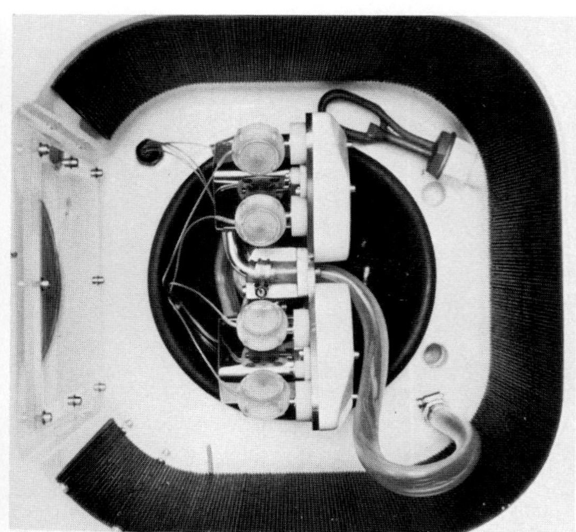

FIGURE 20-9. (*A*) Prone water-bath whole-breast scanner. One breast at a time is immersed in a water bath. A specialized examination bed houses the water bath and four transducers. Console permits operation of the automated system. (Courtesy Ausonics Corporation, Milwaukee, WI.) (*B*) Overview of the four large-aperture transducers mounted on a curved scanning arm located at the base of the water tank examination bed. (Courtesy Ausonics Corporation, Milwaukee, WI.)

regions of the breast, the breast is rescanned after applying a compression band made of a thin polyethylene membrane or nonattenuating mesh.[19]

Breast Disease

When a mass is demonstrated by sonography, its imaging characteristics must be carefully examined. Evaluation is made of the lesion's size, shape, border definition, internal echogenicity, and the degree of distal sound beam enhancement or attenuation. Tissues around the mass are studied for signs of secondary architectural changes. Position of the mass in the breast can often give a clue to its origin. At times, no definite mass is seen and only an area of localized or diffuse tissue distortion is noted. Knowledge of the patient's age, history, and physical and mammographic findings is helpful before making a diagnosis.

The accuracy of sonography in the detection and diagnosis of breast disease depends on several factors. Sensitivity and specificity vary with the technical quality of the examination, the experience of the interpreter, the "imaging pattern" or texture of the breast, and the type and stage of the disease. A knowledge of the potential pitfalls of breast sonography is necessary to avoid misdiagnosis. Many of these pitfalls are listed in Table 20-3.[5,16,28,32]

BENIGN FLUID-FILLED MASSES

Cysts. Cysts, the most common breast lesions, are almost always benign. They are usually associated with a variety of conditions of epithelial origin, collectively termed fibrocystic disease. Cysts occur most often in menstruating women between ages 35 and 50 years.[5,19,29] Generally, they subside after menopause, but postmenopausal women who take estrogen,[55] blood pressure medications, steroids, or digitalis may develop cysts.[29,44]

Theoretically, these localized areas of duct dilatation occur at the terminal portion of the lobular ducts. Intrinsic or extrinsic processes, such as intraductal hyperplasia or fibrosis, may obstruct the duct causing secretions to accumulate and form a

TABLE 20-3. Potential pitfalls of sonographic breast evaluation

Technical
- Improper transducer frequency selection: too low, reduced resolution; too high, reduced penetration
- Improper TGC and gain settings: too low, missed echoes in solid mass, reduced penetration; too high, false echoes in cystic mass
- Improper focal zone placement: suboptimal delineation of structures, suboptimal demonstration of transmission characteristics
- Artifact production: reverberation from use of standoff, acoustic shadowing from "nonpathologic" sources (nipple, Cooper's ligaments, air between offset and skin, etc.), false echoes from excessive gain, defocusing
- Limited resolution: unable to routinely image microcalcifications
- Improper positioning: suboptimal angle of incidence to skin, mass; improper amount of compression

Diagnostic
- Isoechoic mass in fatty breast may be missed
- Fat lobule can simulate mass
- Well-marginated cancer can mimic benign solid mass
- Well-marginated cellular cancer can mimic cyst
- Attenuating benign mass can mimic cancer
- Microcalcifications not routinely seen
- Cysts do not always demonstrate beam enhancement
- Mass underlying attenuating tissues may be missed
- Rib can be mistaken for intramammary mass

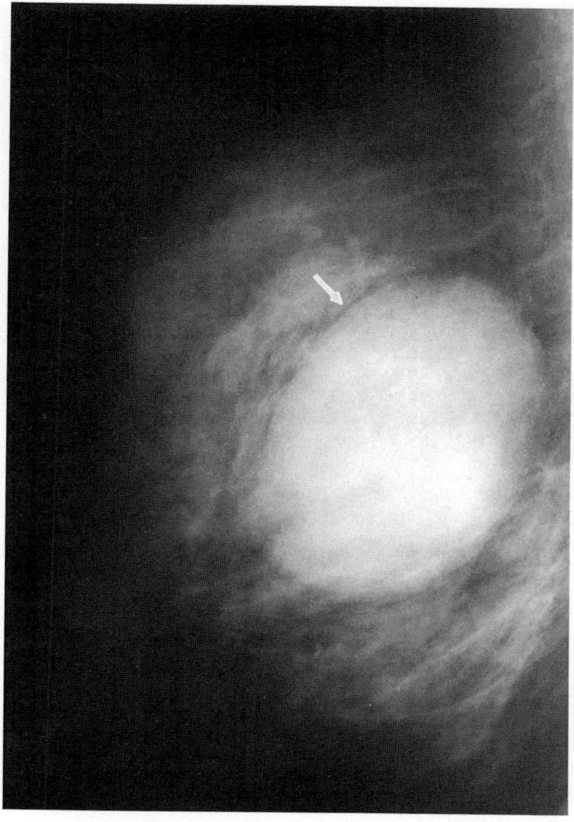

FIGURE 20-10. Mammographic image of a benign cystic mass. Margins of the mass are smooth and well-defined. A thin rim of fat (halo sign) is seen around the mass (*arrow*).

cyst.[63] Secretion and reabsorption of fluid by the cyst contributes to their variability in size.[2]

Cysts may be single or multiple, unilocular or multilocular. They occur in one or both breasts and range in size from a millimeter to several centimeters. Their size may change at different times in the menstrual cycle.[33] High-resolution sonography is extremely proficient at detecting breast cysts; the reported accuracy rate is approximately 98%.[5,10,44,55]

Signs and symptoms. Symptoms include pain, tenderness, and palpable mass. Tenderness is common before menstruation, especially with cystic enlargement. On physical examination, cysts are soft or firm, round or oval, smooth, and freely mobile.

Mammographic features. Cysts appear as circular or oval masses with smooth, well-defined margins. As they displace neighboring tissue, these low-density lesions are encircled by a thin, lucent rim of fat referred to as the halo-sign (Fig. 20-10).[19,21,64] When calcified, they have a thin, eggshell appearance.

Sonographic features. The main application of breast sonography is accurate diagnosis of true simple cysts (Figs. 20-11, 20-12).

DIAGNOSTIC CRITERIA OF SIMPLE CYST
Shape: Round or oval
Borders: Smooth, well-defined walls
Internal echoes: Absent, anechoic
Distal echoes: Posterior enhancement—variable
Associated findings: Lateral refractive edge shadowing—variable

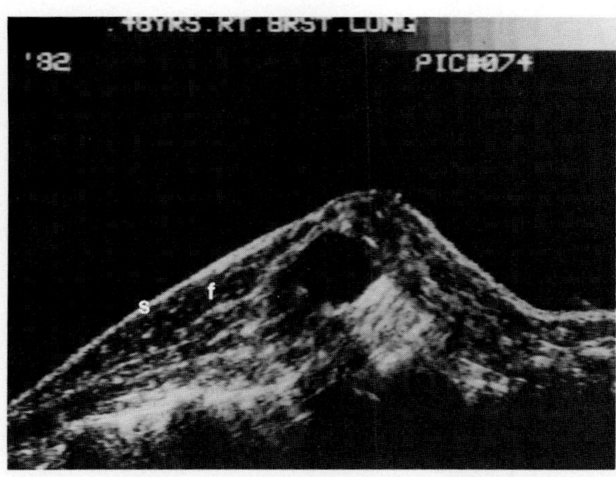

FIGURE 20-11. Simple cyst. Prone, water-path sonogram of a 48-year-old woman demonstrating a rounded, well-marginated anechoic mass with sound enhancement distal to the lesion. The skin (s) and fatty tissue (f) are well seen. (Courtesy Ausonics Corporation, Milwaukee, WI.)

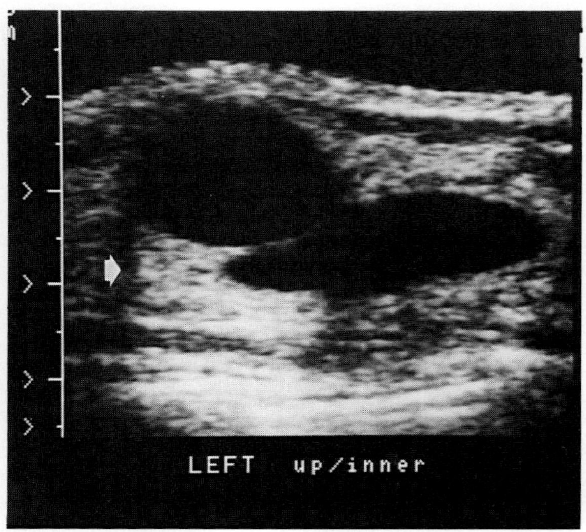

FIGURE 20-12. Cyst characteristics. Some variability can be seen in the imaging characteristics of simple cysts. This real-time image shows two cysts, both anechoic with thin, smooth walls. One is rounded; the other oval. The anterior cyst shows typical edge shadowing and sound beam enhancement *(arrow)*; the posterior cyst shows no sound enhancement.

In patients with fibrocystic disease, sonography may demonstrate a variety of changes in the breast. The parenchyma may be more echogenic than normal, showing areas of attenuation shadowing secondary to stromal hyperplasia and fibrosis.[19,44,46] Ducts may be prominent, and cysts, when seen, may be numerous and have thickened walls. The glandular tissue may have a basket-weave appearance.[24]

Complicated cysts. Hemorrhagic or infected cysts may have fine internal echoes or display a more complex pattern with wall thickening. Sonography following recently failed cyst aspiration may be deceptive if there is hemorrhage into or around the cyst. When a cyst is calcified, acoustic shadowing may obscure complete demonstration of the wall.

Scanning tips. Appropriate equipment settings and scanning technique are critical to ensure diagnostic accuracy. Artifactual echoes within a cyst may result if gain settings are too high or the TGC is improperly set. A true simple cyst should be echo-free at normal gain and retain a crisp back wall at low gain. Wall margins and distal sound enhancement are best seen when the cyst is within the focal zone; however, enhancement may not be seen, especially if the cyst is located posteriorly or surrounded by fibrous tissue.[6,26,55] The type of cyst fluid may also affect the degree of beam transmission. Reverberation artifacts from use of an acoustic standoff are eliminated by changing the thickness of the standoff, changing the beam incidence, or scanning without the standoff (Fig. 20-13). Applying transducer pressure shows the compressibility or tension of the cyst. Angulation of the sound beam allows all walls to be visualized, helping to rule out an intracystic mass.

Differential diagnosis. When all the criteria of a cyst are fulfilled, the diagnosis of a benign simple cyst can be made with a high level of confidence. If any evidence of wall irregularities or internal echoes is present within what appears to be a fluid-filled mass, other conditions must be considered, which are discussed in the remainder of this section. Occasionally, homogeneous cellular tumors such as medullary carcinoma appear anechoic at normal gain settings and mimic a cyst.

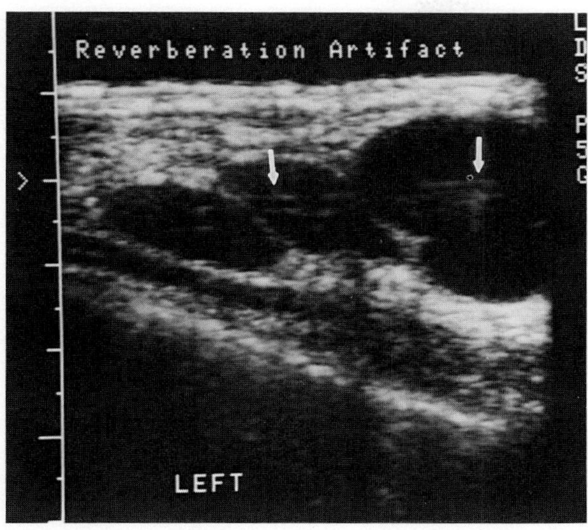

Figure 20-13. Reverberation artifacts *(arrows)* are projected within cystic lesions when a thin standoff pad is placed between skin and transducer.

Treatment. When a fluid-filled mass does not meet all the criteria of a simple cyst, aspiration with fluid analysis is recommended.[26] Pneumocystography allows further inspection of cyst walls. Recurrent or atypical cysts may require excision.[9] Aspiration of simple cysts is indicated when they are symptomatic or interfere with mammography or physical examination. Monitoring asymptomatic patients with serial ultrasound examinations may obviate more traumatic intervention.

Galactocele. A galactocele is a milky cyst caused by obstruction of a lactiferous duct in the pregnant or lactating woman.[2,5] Mastitis may result, leading to abscess formation. A galactocele may persist after the lactation period, undergo oily transformation, and become an oil cyst.[2]

Signs and symptoms. Palpation may be difficult in enlarged, lactating breasts. The presenting mass is usually firm, and tenderness may be associated with mastitis.

Mammographic features. The mass appears as a cyst containing radiolucent material.[19] Radiolucency varies with the lipid content.

Sonographic features.[2,5,10,26]

DIAGNOSTIC CRITERIA OF A GALACTOCELE

Shape: Round or oval
Borders: Well-defined margins, smooth walls
Internal echoes: Anechoic or fine, low-level echoes
Distal echoes: Posterior enhancement—variable
Associated findings: Lateral refractive shadowing—variable

The echogenicity of the mass depends on the amount of fat present. The lactating breast may show prominent glandular tissue and ductal enlargement.

Differential diagnosis. Depending on the amount of internal echoes, a simple cyst, oil cyst, hemorrhagic cyst, or infected cyst may have similar imaging features.

Treatment. Resolution of the galactocele is usually spontaneous but aspiration using a low-gauge needle is often curative.[2]

Sebaceous Cysts. Sebaceous or epidermal cysts may grow large enough to be seen by mammography and sonography. These skin appendage tumors contain sebum, an oily material, which accounts for their sonographic appearance. The subcutaneous location is a clue to their origin.[19]

Mammographic features. On mammography, sebaceous cysts are round, homogeneous, cystlike masses under the skin (Fig. 20-14A).[19]

Sonographic features. (Fig. 20-14B).

DIAGNOSTIC CRITERIA OF SEBACEOUS CYST

Shape: Round
Borders: Well-defined, smooth
Internal echoes: Medium- to low-level echoes of uniform distribution or anechoic
Distal echoes: Posterior enhancement—variable
Associated findings: Lateral refractive shadowing—variable, occasionally may calcify

Differential diagnosis. Other discrete subcutaneous masses secondary to trauma, infection, or apocrine gland hyperplasia[19] can mimic sebaceous cysts on sonography.

Intracystic Papilloma. Intracystic papillomas are uncommon lesions that usually affect older women. The papilloma grows from a fibrovascular stalk into the lumen of a serous or hemorrhagic cyst.[19,21]

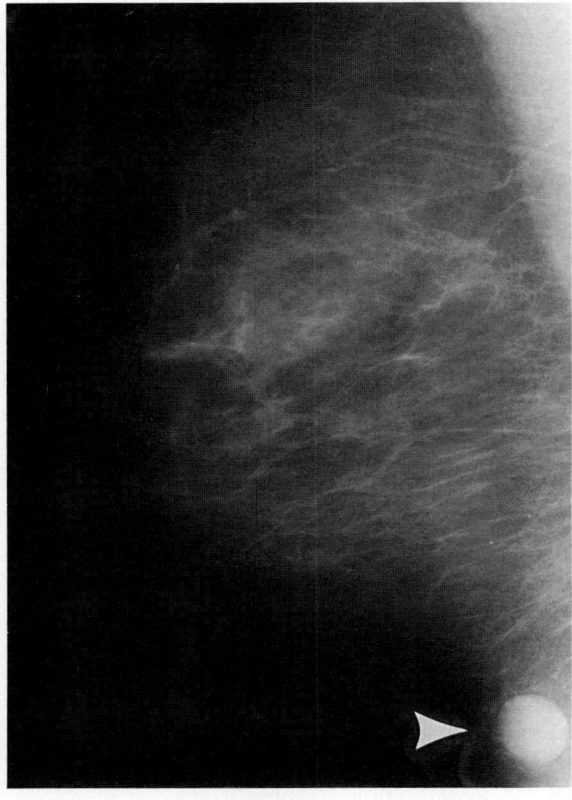

A

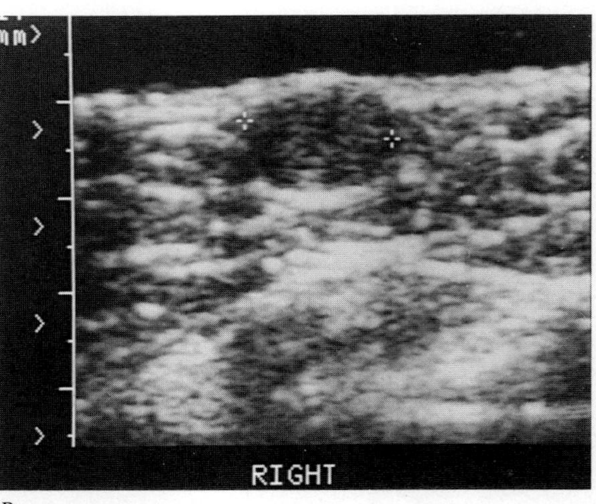

B

FIGURE 20-14. (*A*) Sebaceous cyst. Mammographic image reveals a round, radiodense lesion *(arrow)* with a thin, lucent rim located under the skin, just inferior to the fatty breast. (*B*) Sebaceous cyst. Real-time image of a palpable mass located just inferior to the breast under the skin. The 1.5-cm lesion *(cursor)* was well-marginated, containing medium-level echoes. No acoustic beam enhancement or attenuation was noted. A cross-section through the excised mass revealed greasy material consistent with a sebaceous cyst.

The cyst results from blockage of the duct by the ingrowing, soft tissue mass. These complex lesions are usually small but may grow to several centimeters. Larger masses are more likely to undergo hemorrhagic or malignant changes.[52]

Signs and symptoms. The patient may present with bloody nipple discharge and/or a mildly tender breast lump.[52]

Mammographic features. The solid component of these radiodense lesions may not be detected by mammography. Cyst aspiration with pneumocystography allows evaluation of the cyst walls.

Sonographic features. When a cystic lesion is identified, careful evaluation of all the walls is necessary to exclude an intracavitary lesion (Fig. 20-15).

DIAGNOSTIC CRITERIA OF INTRACYSTIC PAPILLOMA

Shape: Round or oval

Borders: Well-defined, usually smooth

Internal echoes: Echogenic soft tissue mass extending into anechoic cyst or cyst with low-level echoes

Distal echoes: Posterior enhancement behind fluid

Associated findings: Lateral refractive sign—variable; wall thickening due to hemorrhage

Differential diagnosis. Intracystic carcinoma cannot be ruled out on the basis of sonography alone,[26] but extension of the soft tissue mass beyond the cyst wall suggests malignancy (Fig. 20-16). The differential also includes complex lesions such as a hemorrhagic cyst with clot and necrotic tumor.

Treatment. Excisional biopsy is required to rule out malignancy. If aspiration biopsy is elected, both the fluid and soft tissue components of the lesion should be sampled and evaluated.[56]

Abscess. Abscesses develop in a small percentage of patients with acute mastitis. Mastitis, or inflamma-

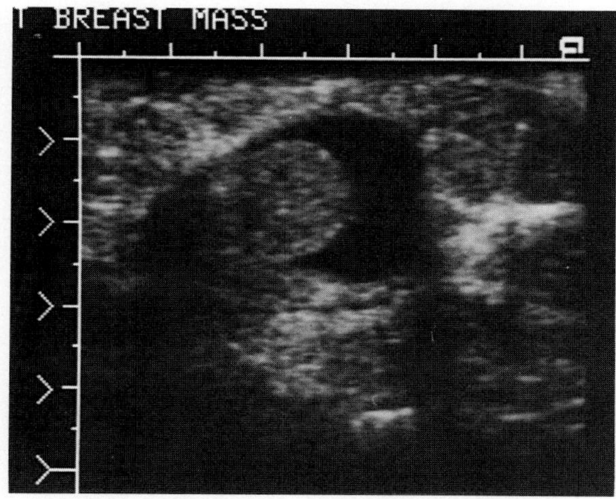

FIGURE 20-15. Intracystic papilloma. Real-time linear-array scan demonstrates a smooth-walled soft tissue mass projecting into a cystic mass. Aspiration biopsy determined the mass to be benign. (Courtesy University of Alabama at Birmingham and Acuson Corporation, Mountain View, CA.)

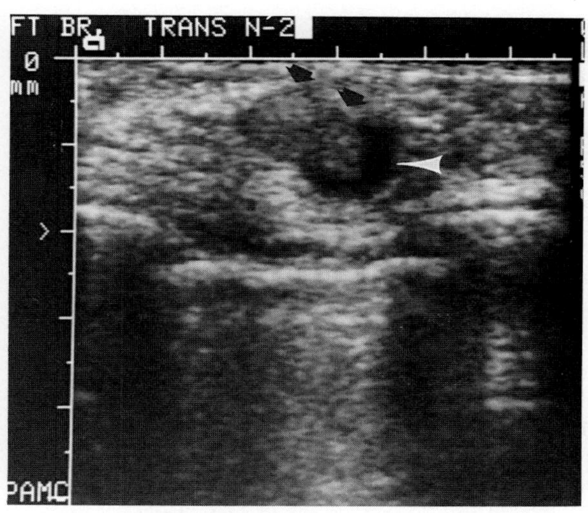

FIGURE 20-16. Intracystic carcinoma. Real-time image shows a soft-tissue mass *(black arrows)* extending out of the confines of a cystic lesion *(white arrow)*. Biopsy proved the mass to be malignant. (Courtesy Portland Adventist Medical Center, Portland, OR.)

tion of the breast, presents most often in lactating women but can affect women of any age. The condition may be diffuse or localized.[10] Abscesses have various causes. Bacteria may enter the lactiferous ducts through a skin wound or a cracked nipple.[19,51] Obstructed lactiferous ducts are susceptible to infection. If unrestricted, infection may spread by way of the blood and lymph vessels to other parts of the breast. Most often abscesses form beneath the nipple (subareolar), or they may develop under the skin (subcutaneous), within the gland (intramammary), or deep to the gland in front of the pectoral muscles (retromammary).[52]

Signs and symptoms.[21,33] Acute mastitis presents with varying degrees of fever, pain, skin reddening, and thickening. A mass may be palpable. Axillary nodes may be enlarged and tender. Nipple discharge, when present, may be purulent. Nipple retraction may be seen in older patients with chronic mastitis.

Mammographic features. The mammographic findings of abscess vary from those of an infected cyst to a retractive mass with surrounding edema. At times, differentiation from infiltrating or inflammatory carcinoma is difficult. Microcalcifications, however, are not characteristic of abscess.[18]

Sonographic features.[26,44,55] The sonographic appearance varies with the stage and distribution of the inflammatory process. Initial findings may include duct dilatation and some increased echogenicity and attenuation of the affected tissues. Later, an organized abscess may form, displaying varying amounts of liquefaction and necrosis (Figs. 20-17, 20-18).

DIAGNOSTIC CRITERIA OF ABSCESS

Shape: Round, oval, or irregular

Borders: Variable margination, usually thick, irregular wall

Internal echoes: Nonuniform internal echoes, possible septations, seldom anechoic

Distal echoes: Enhancement varies with fluid content

Associated findings: Variable; skin thickening, surrounding edema or increased echoes, thickening of Cooper's ligaments

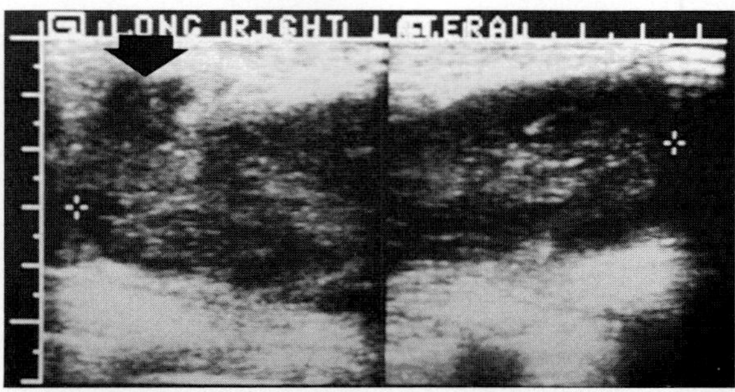

FIGURE 20-17. Abscess. Sonogram of a 32-year-old lactating woman. The breast was enlarged, tender, reddened, and hot to the touch. The complex mass, revealed by sonography, measured 10 cm long. A portion of the abscess was noted tipping toward the skin surface *(arrow)*. Two days later, the abscess broke through the skin surface. (Courtesy Harvard Diagnostic Center, Roseburg, OR.)

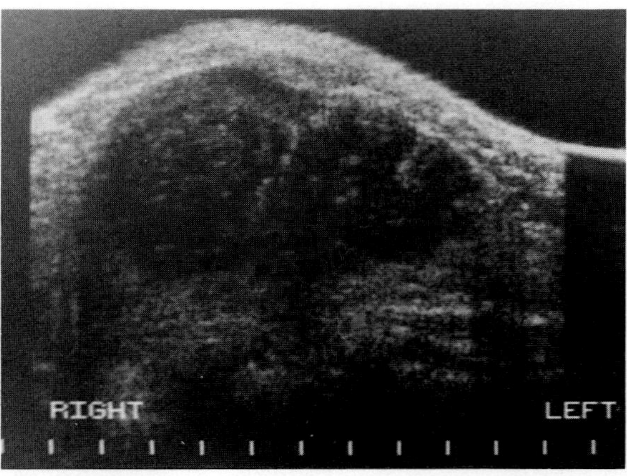

FIGURE 20-18. Abscess. Sagittal scan made with an automated supine scanner on a 20-year-old woman complaining of left breast tenderness and a palpable mass. The left breast was enlarged and hard on palpation. Sonography revealed a large, moderately well-marginated mass containing nonuniform low-level echoes. Needle aspiration was performed with a resultant diagnosis of staphylococcal abscess. (Courtesy Margaret Washburn, MD, Sedro Woolley, WA.)

Differential diagnosis. Depending on the stage of the process, inflammatory change can mimic a hematoma, infected galactocele, degenerating mass, or even cancer. Clinical correlation is important. Skin retraction and fibrosis may indicate residual change from a serious abscess. Inflammatory response to a rapidly growing infiltrating carcinoma should be considered, especially in older patients and possibly in lactating ones.[10,51]

Treatment. With proper antibiotic treatment, most inflammatory processes resolve spontaneously. Sonography is useful to follow their involution. Needle drainage, aspiration, or excisional biopsy is recommended for masses that do not respond to treatment or to rule out carcinoma.[26]

Hematoma. Hematomas usually result from breast trauma, either direct or secondary to aspiration or surgical procedures. Nontraumatic hematomas may develop in patients with a history of blood disorders or anticoagulant treatment.[2]

Signs and symptoms. Bruising and some skin thickening are external signs of hemorrhage. Tenderness is present in varying degrees. A palpable mass following biopsy or trauma suggests a hematoma.

Mammographic features. The appearance of hemorrhage varies from mild changes of increased density and skin thickening to an opaque hemorrhagic cyst or a more sclerotic, retractive mass.[2]

Sonographic features.[10,44,55] Imaging patterns of hemorrhage depend on the extent, the duration, and the organization of the bleed. Mild skin thickening and altered echogenicity of subcutaneous fat or other affected tissues may be present. The appearance of an organizing hematoma depends on the degree of liquefaction and the amount of clotted blood present (Figs. 20-19, 20-20).

DIAGNOSTIC CRITERIA OF HEMATOMA

Shape: Round, oval, or irregular

Borders: Variable wall margination, irregular, thickened walls

Internal echoes: Nonuniform distribution of low- to high-level echoes, possible sediment layer

Distal echoes: Variable enhancement

Associated findings: Localized skin thickening

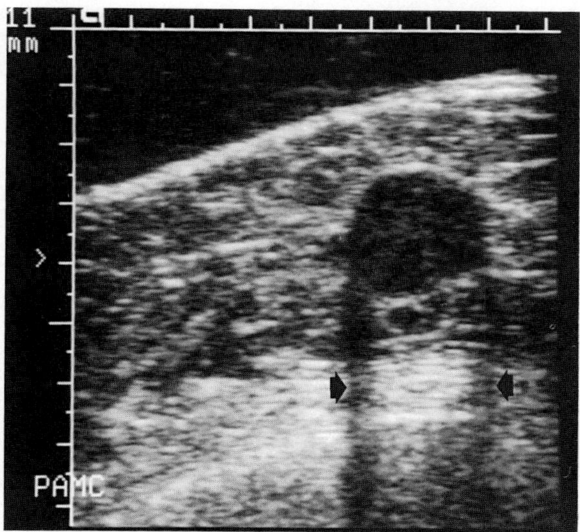

FIGURE 20-19. Organized hematoma within a large cystic duct. Hand-held, real-time sonogram of a woman with recent history of breast trauma revealed a localized, well-marginated, complex mass containing low-level echoes. Lateral refractive shadowing is seen *(arrows)*. (Courtesy Portland Adventist Medical Center, Portland, OR.)

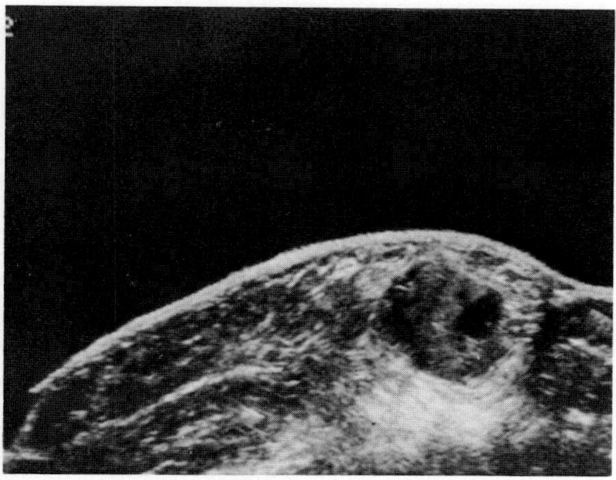

FIGURE 20-20. Localized hematoma in a 42-year-old woman with clinically apparent mass and history of breast trauma 2 weeks prior to examination. Prone, water-path sonogram demonstrates a well-delineated, complex mass containing nonuniform medium-level echoes and a focal anechoic area. Aspiration yielded bloody fluid. The mass slowly resolved. (From Egan R: Breast Imaging: Diagnosis and Morphology of Breast Disease. Philadelphia, WB Saunders, 1988.)

Tissues generally return to normal. Hemorrhage, however, occasionally leaves residual changes, including thickened Cooper's ligaments[10] and increased tissue echogenicity with attenuation shadowing secondary to scarring.

Differential diagnosis. Various imaging patterns of hemorrhage can simulate inflammatory or malignant changes. Clinical correlation and subsequent remission of ultrasound findings leads to an accurate diagnosis. Hemorrhage into a simple cyst can occur.

Treatment. Serial sonograms can follow resolution of a hematoma and assess residual changes. With a large hemorrhage, it may take several months before tissues return to normal.[55]

Ductal Ectasia. Ductal ectasia refers to overall dilatation of the lactiferous ducts that occurs around menopause. The subareolar ducts fill with cellular and fatty debris.[9] If complicated by infection, an abscess may develop. Ductal ectasia is thought to be the end result of previous periductal inflammation and secondary fibrosis.[29] Shortening of the ducts from fibrosis can cause nipple inversion and simulate malignant change. Women who have nursed for long periods may develop ductal ectasia.

Signs and symptoms. A thick, sticky nipple discharge is the primary feature. Subareolar nodularity[44] and nipple inversion are possible. Pain, if present, may be intermittent.

Mammographic features. Ducts seen on mammography include the lumen, wall, and periductal structures.[26] Dilated ducts appear as wormy, tubular structures extending from the nipple and producing a triangular density beneath the areola.[19,55]

Sonographic features. Ducts imaged on ultrasound represent their true lumen. Dilated, tubular, fluid-filled structures seen converging toward the nipple represent the ectatic ducts (Fig. 20-21).

Differential diagnosis. Generalized ductal ectasia is usually bilateral. If a single duct is dilated and

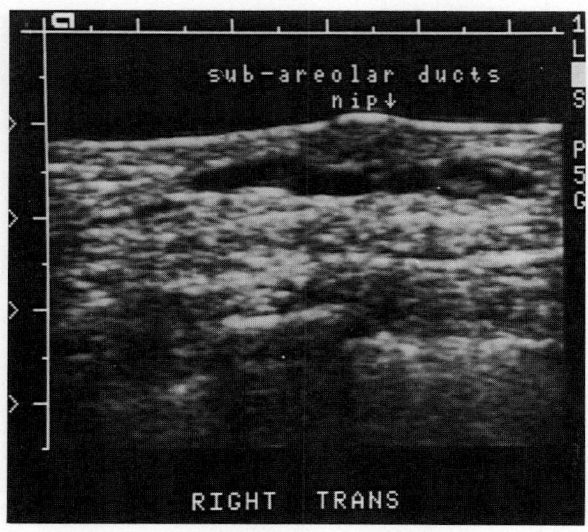

Figure 20-21. Ductal ectasia. Hand-held, real-time sonogram reveals dilated subareolar ducts in a 70-year-old woman. Findings were bilateral.

bloody nipple discharge is present, an obstructing mass such as papilloma should be suspected.

Benign Solid Masses

The sonographic criteria for a benign solid mass include round or oval shape, smooth, defined borders, uniform low- or medium-level internal echoes, intermediate or strong boundary echoes, and minimal, if any, attenuation of the sound beam.[10,11,19,26,44] Some solid masses show distal enhancement when they attenuate less sound than adjacent tissues. Rather than causing invasive changes, benign masses displace adjacent tissues as they grow. Occasionally, a benign-appearing solid lesion may prove to be a well-marginated cancer. For this reason, any suspicious solid breast mass requires fine-needle or excisional biopsy for histologic diagnosis.[6,10,30,61]

Fibroadenoma. Fibroadenomas are common, benign, solid tumors composed of a proliferation of connective and epithelial tissues. The incidence rate is higher in patients 15–40 years of age and in black women.[9,19] In older patients, fibroadenomas may undergo involution, hyalinization, and calcification. These circumscribed lesions may be small or grow to fill most of the breast. Since fibroadenomas are hormonally influenced, they can grow rapidly during pregnancy and undergo infarction.[29] Fibroadenomas may be single or multiple, unilateral or bilateral.

Signs and symptoms.[21,33] When palpable, these masses are non-tender, discrete, firm or rubbery, possibly lobulated, and movable.

Mammographic features.[9,19,64] This low-density radiopaque mass is circumscribed, smooth or lobulated, and may show a distinctive notch. A thin halo of fat around the mass suggests its benign nature. Coarse calcifications help distinguish older lesions. Mammographic distinction from a cyst is not always possible.

Sonographic features (Figs. 20-22, 20-23).

DIAGNOSTIC CRITERIA OF FIBROADENOMA

Shape: Round, oval, or lobulated
Borders: Smooth, well-defined walls
Internal echoes: Uniform, low- to medium-level echoes
Distal echoes: Minimal or no attenuation; mild enhancement possible
Associated findings: Lateral refractive shadow; if calcified, echogenic wall with distal shadowing; possible skin bulging

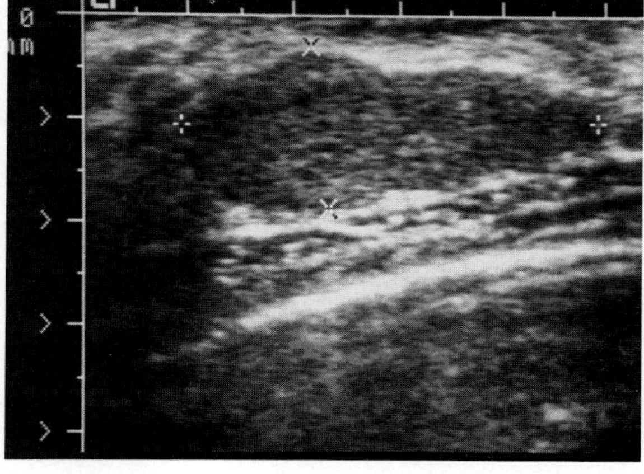

Figure 20-22. Fibroadenoma. Real-time image displays a 4-cm lobulated, well-marginated solid mass in a 28-year-old woman.

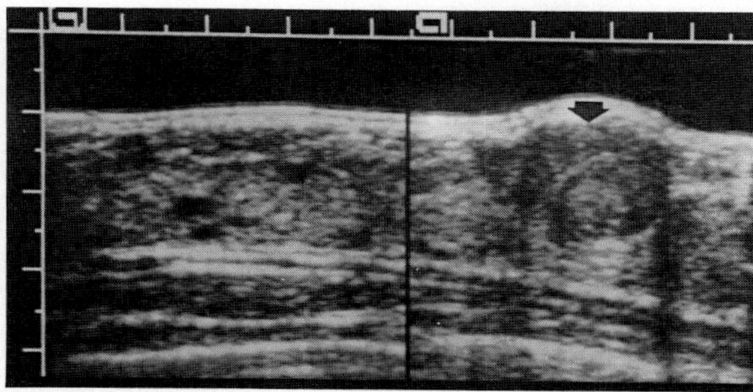

FIGURE 20-23. Fibroadenoma. Real-time sonogram of a 29-year-old woman who presented with a nontender, palpable mass. Dual-mode image was made with a 5-MHz linear-array probe. The transducer was offset from the skin with a 2-cm gel standoff pad. A solid mass with refractive edge shadowing was seen bulging the skin as the breast was compressed. Excisional biopsy proved the suspected diagnosis of benign fibroadenoma.

Differential diagnosis. Depending on the patient's age and functional status, a rapidly growing, large, solid mass suggests juvenile or giant fibroadenoma, cystosarcoma phylloides, adenolipoma, or lactating adenoma. Tubular adenomas present in young patients but are slow-growing epithelial tumors (Fig. 20-24).[29] Other benign solid masses and marginated carcinomas that can mimic fibroadenomas are discussed in the remainder of this section. Additionally, entrapped mammary fat lobules, focal areas of fibrosis, or nodular sclerosing adenosis can present as solid lesions (Fig. 20-25). A degenerating fibroadenoma displaying a heterogeneous texture, irregular margins, and acoustic shadowing can mimic carcinoma.

Intraductal Papilloma. Papillomas are benign epithelial tumors that grow from the lining of the breast ducts.[9,55] Although most lesions are very small; some grow to several centimeters. These polypoid lesions may be solitary or multiple, within one or many ducts. A solitary papilloma usually occurs beneath the areola. Multiple papillomas (papillomatosis) are more peripherally located. An intraductal papilloma develops most often between the ages of 30 and 55 years.[59] Papillomatosis is less com-

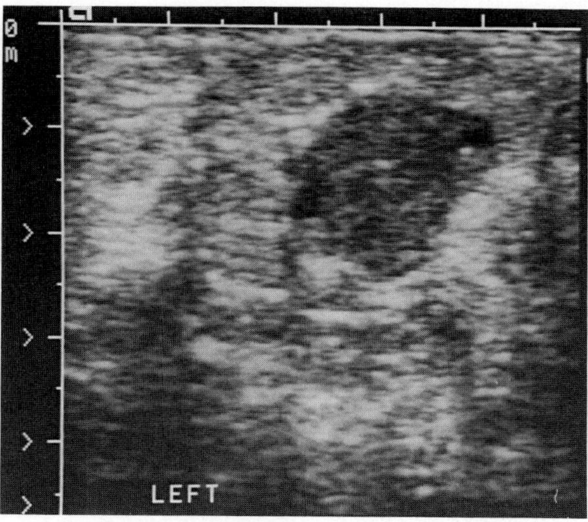

FIGURE 20-24. Tubular adenoma. Real-time sonogram of a 17-year-old girl with a palpable, mobile mass that had been present for 2 years by history. Ultrasonography revealed a solid, lobulated lesion with small sonolucent regions near the periphery. Excisional biopsy and histologic examination diagnosed a mixed tubular adenoma with focally cellular stroma.

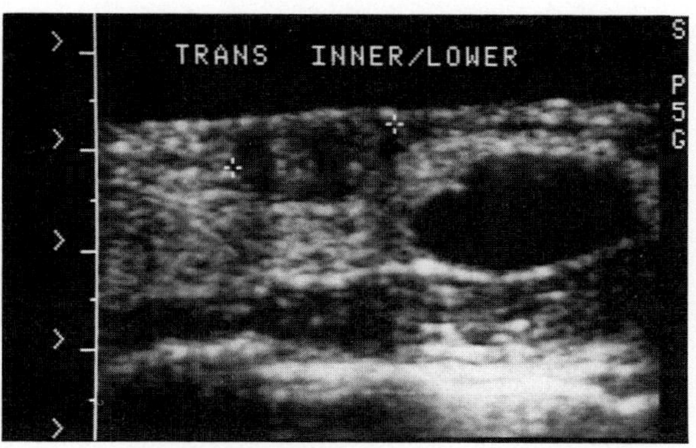

FIGURE 20-25. Sclerosing adenosis. Real-time image demonstrates a solid and a cystic mass in a 45-year-old woman. The anterior solid mass was palpable. Scattered calcifications were noted on mammography. The biopsy specimen revealed the solid mass to be nodular sclerosing adenosis. The cyst was aspirated. In this case, sclerosing adenosis resembled fibroadenoma on sonography.

mon and occurs in young and older women. Malignant degeneration is rare.

Signs and symptoms. The patient may be asymptomatic or may complain of persistent, often bloody, nipple discharge from a single duct. Subareolar masses may be palpable.

Mammographic features.[7] A solitary papilloma images as a high-density, circumscribed lesion with a raspberry appearance best seen by ductography. Calcifications are not common.

Sonographic features. A very small papilloma may escape detection. The only clue to its presence may be localized dilatation, especially of a solitary duct.[26,55] Occasionally, the duct dilates enough to allow visualization of a portion of the mass. A large papilloma may appear as a discrete, solid mass with imaging characteristics similar to those of fibroadenoma. Dilatation of multiple ducts in the peripheral gland suggests papillomatosis.[19,26] Juvenile papillomatosis may present as an ill-defined, heterogeneous mass with rounded, relatively echo-free areas near its outer margins.[36]

Differential diagnosis. Sonography cannot reliably differentiate papillomas from other benign solid masses, papillary carcinoma, or other well-marginated malignancies without ductal enlargement. Infarcted papillomas, often accompanied by architectural distortion of adjacent tissues, may simulate invasive carcinoma.[29]

Cystosarcoma Phylloides. Cystosarcoma phylloides is an uncommon tumor composed of epithelial and predominantly fibrous tissue. Histologically, this solid mass contains narrow, cystlike clefts within a stroma of uniform cellularity.[14,19,29] The lesions most often develop in women in their forties and fifties, later than is typical for fibroadenoma. Tumors are usually unilateral and can grow to huge proportions, sometimes suddenly. Although it is usually benign, cystosarcoma phylloides can undergo malignant transformation and has the potential to metastasize.[14,19,21,29] Recurrence is possible if excision is not complete.

Signs and symptoms. The palpable mass is discrete, non-tender, and mobile. A large mass may bulge and stretch the skin.

Mammographic features.[19,21,33] Findings include a radiopaque, circumscribed mass, which may be indistinguishable from fibroadenoma or lobulated

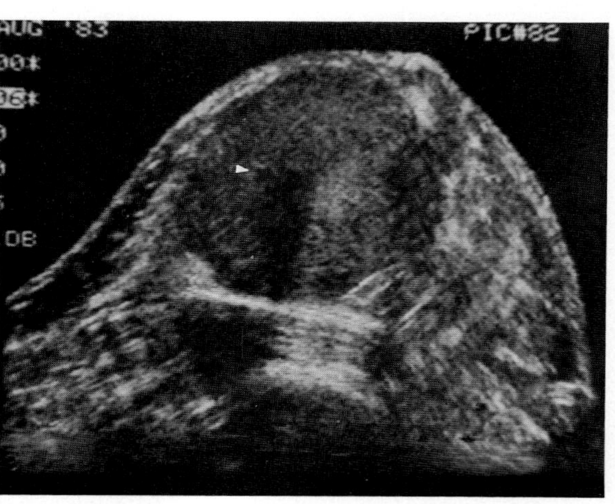

FIGURE 20-26. Cystosarcoma phylloides. Prone water-path scan of a large, well-circumscribed solid mass. The small central sonolucency *(arrow)* may represent a cystic cleft. (Courtesy Ausonics Corporation, Milwaukee, WI.)

cyst. Calcification is not typical. Veins may be enlarged.

Sonographic features (Fig. 20-26).[14,26,44] The demonstration of cystic spaces, especially within a large, solid lesion, suggests the diagnosis of cystosarcoma phylloides.

DIAGNOSTIC CRITERIA OF CYSTOSARCOMA PHYLLOIDES

Shape: Round, oval, or lobulated
Borders: Well-marginated
Internal echoes: Low- to medium-level echoes; possible internal cystic areas
Distal echoes: Variable enhancement
Associated findings: Skin bulging possible

Differential diagnosis. Benign and malignant cystosarcoma phylloides cannot reliably be distinguished by sonography. Depending on the history, the possibilities include fibroadenoma and its variants (e.g., giant, juvenile, adenolipoma) or lactating adenoma, medullary carcinoma, or degenerating tumor.

Lipoma. True lipomas are nodules of mature adipose tissue surrounded by a thin connective tissue capsule.[2,29] These extraglandular, benign fatty tumors are secondary to atrophy[26] and occur more frequently in middle-aged or older women. Adenolipomas are encapsulated tumors containing fatty, fibrous, and epithelial elements. They are considered a variant of fibroadenoma, are intraglandular, and can grow large.[19,44]

Signs and symptoms. If palpable, a lipoma is typically soft and compressible, as compared to a more fibrous mass.

Mammographic features.[7,21,64] A lipoma images as a well-circumscribed radiolucent mass that displaces the tissue around it. No calcification is seen. An adenolipoma appears as a discrete lesion with a combination of radiolucent and low-density components surrounded by a halo.

Sonographic features (Fig. 20-27).[19,21]

DIAGNOSTIC CRITERIA OF LIPOMA

Shape: Round or oval

Borders: Relatively well-defined, smooth wall

Internal echoes: Pattern similar to fat; low-level echoes

Distal echoes: Mild enhancement or none

Associated findings: Compressible

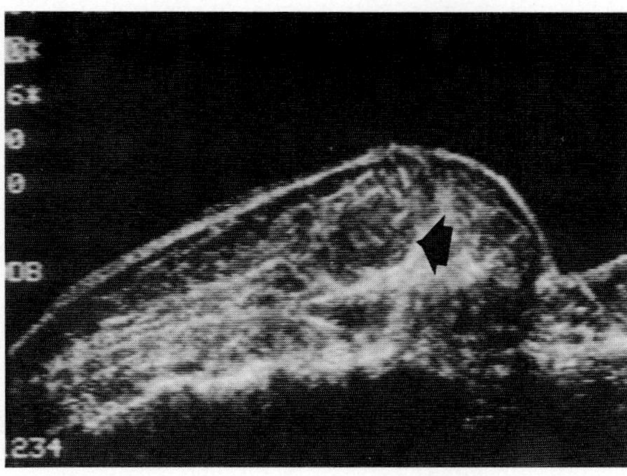

FIGURE 20-27. Lipoma. Sagittal, prone water-path scan of a rounded solid mass *(arrow)* containing low- and medium-level echoes. No attenuation shadowing was seen. The mass had a texture similar to that of other breast fat. (Courtesy Ausonics Corporation, Milwaukee, WI.)

Lipomas may be difficult to delineate in a fatty breast. Fibroadenolipomas have a less uniform pattern, containing both hyperechoic and hypoechoic regions reflective of the fibrous, epithelial, and fatty components. Fibroangiolipomas may be very echogenic.[55]

Differential diagnosis. Sonographically, lipomas can mimic fibroadenomas, entrapped intramammary fat lobules, or another fatty mass. Mammographic findings aid in the diagnosis. Liposarcomatous degeneration is rare.[55]

Fat Necrosis. Fat necrosis is uncommon and usually is secondary to breast trauma. It develops mostly in older, obese women.[29] Findings can closely resemble those of cancer on physical, radiographic, and sonographic examination.

Local trauma, surgery, or inflammation can cause hemorrhage and liquefaction of a focal area of fat.[55] Subsequently, the necrotic fat may form a dense, fibrous scar or an oily cyst and ultimately may calcify. Fat necrosis is usually subareolar or subcutaneous.[19] Changes may persist for years or regress spontaneously.

Signs and symptoms.[29] When located superficially, fat necrosis can cause skin fixation, retraction, and nipple inversion.

Mammographic features.[7,64] The appearance varies from that of a circumscribed, radiolucent cyst to that of a spiculated lesion. Calcification may be present.

Sonographic features.[10,19,21,44] Findings vary. Traumatic fat necrosis can present as a complex cystic mass or as an irregular hypoechoic or hyperechoic mass with attenuation shadowing (Figs. 20-27B, 20-28). Distortion of the skin, Cooper's ligaments, or surrounding tissues may be seen.

Differential diagnosis. Differentiation of fat necrosis from invasive duct carcinoma, radial scar, hyperplastic fibrosis, and the residual effects of an abscess or hematoma is achieved by biopsy and microscopic analysis.

Malignant Masses

Risk factors for breast cancer are well-documented.[9,19,21,32,40,61] Besides sex and increasing age, two major risk factors are personal or family history of breast cancer and personal history of biopsy-proven atypical hyperplasia. Most malignan-

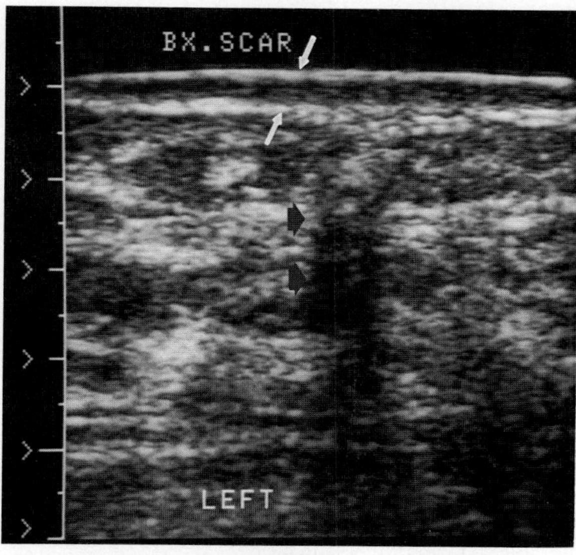

FIGURE 20-28. Traumatic fat necrosis. Real-time sonogram of a 58-year-old woman 1 year after excisional biopsy of a benign breast mass. Follow-up mammography revealed a small, spiculated mass at the site of the previous biopsy. Sonography demonstrated 5 mm skin thickening at the level of the biopsy scar *(white arrows)* and an ill-defined area of architectural change with focal distal shadowing *(black arrows)*.

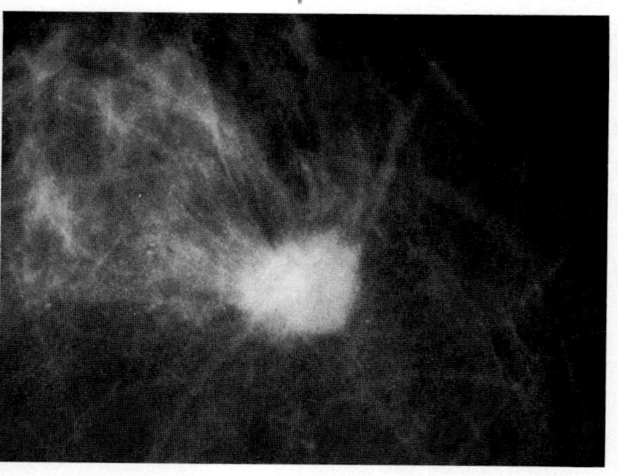

FIGURE 20-29. Mammographic image of a malignant breast mass shows spiculated margins, central microcalcifications, and thickened connective tissue strands.

cies invade rather than displace neighboring tissue.[19,44] Signs of invasion include architectural distortion affecting any level of the breast: skin, subcutaneous fat, Cooper's ligaments, tissues bordering the mass, retromammary space. Axillary lymph nodes may be enlarged and occasionally are imaged. Any suspicious mass, especially in an older woman, requires biopsy and histologic evaluation for a definitive diagnosis.

Poorly Marginated Carcinoma. Invasive ductal carcinomas are the most common breast malignancies. When a cancer invades neighboring tissues, the borders become irregular and ill-defined. Tissues adjacent to the tumor may undergo reactive fibrosis (desmoplasia), edema, and retraction.[19,44,55] Cancers that exhibit this scirrhous pattern include infiltrating types of most ductal, comedo, and lobular carcinomas.[26,44] In a pregnant or lactating woman invasive carcinoma can grow rapidly.

Signs and symptoms. When palpable, the mass is usually hard, fixed, and painless. Location is usually in the upper outer quadrant. Secondary skin, nipple, and breast contour changes may be visible.

Mammographic features.[19] (Scirrhous Type). The principal sign of cancer is an asymmetric, very dense mass with spiculated margins (Fig. 20-29). Associated clustered microcalcifications are common. Thickened trabeculae, increased vascularity, and other secondary changes may be seen.

Sonographic features.[11,13,19,21,26,28,44,53] Most invasive cancers detectable by sonography display certain primary characteristics. Secondary findings vary greatly in presentation and are not always seen (Figs. 20-30 to 20-33).

DIAGNOSTIC CRITERIA OF INVASIVE CARCINOMA

Primary findings

Shape: Variable
Borders: Irregular, ill-defined
Boundary echoes: Anterior wall—intermediate to strong; posterior wall—weak to absent
Internal echoes: Low-level, nonuniform distribution
Attenuation: Moderate to marked

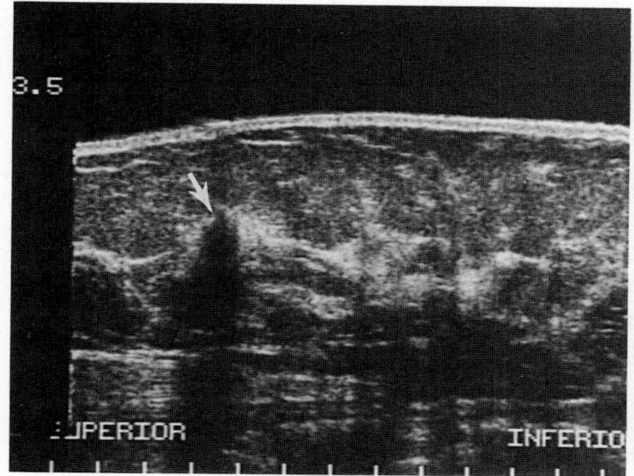

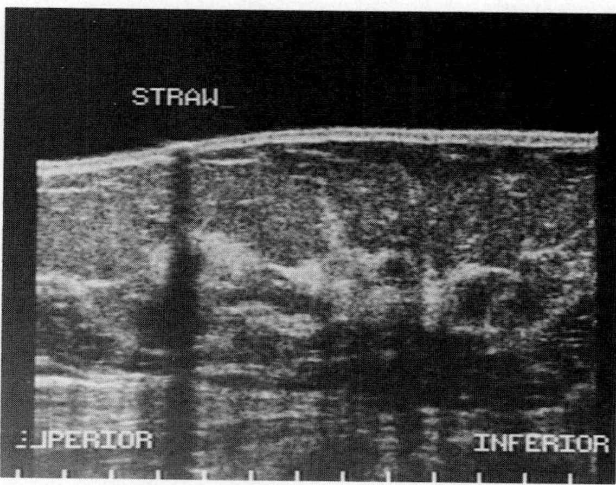

Figure 20-30. (*A*) Invasive ductal carcinoma, scirrhous type. Sagittal sonogram produced by an automated supine scanner on a woman with a family history of breast cancer revealed a focal area of pronounced acoustic shadowing. Some increased echoes were noted in surrounding tissues. Findings were highly suspicious for malignancy. (Courtesy Margaret Washburn, MD, Sedro Woolley, WA.) (*B*) Localization of previously shown suspicious mass by placing a thin straw between the skin and water-bag. On repeat scanning, the area shows the position of the straw in relation to the mass.

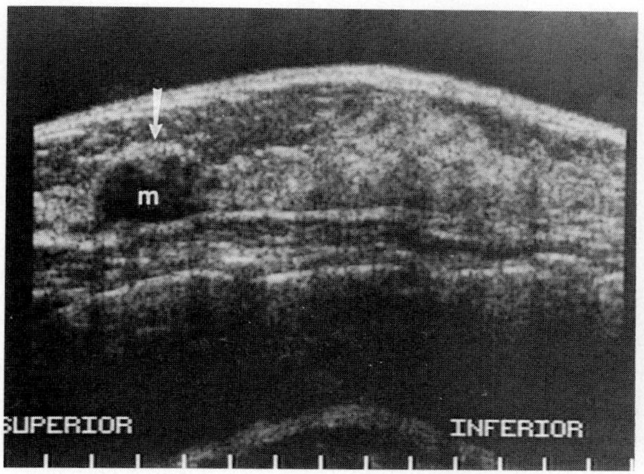

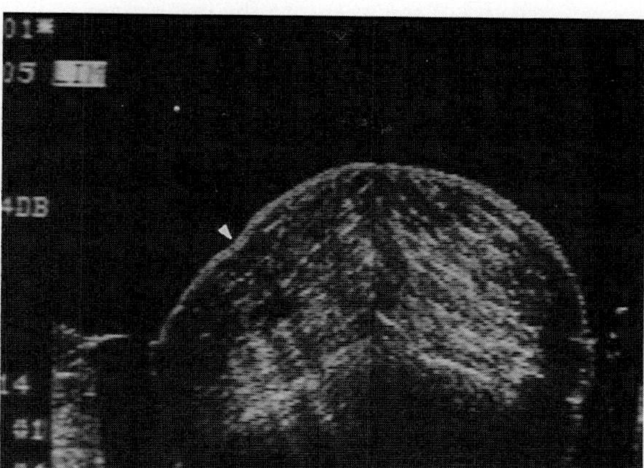

Figure 20-31. Invasive carcinoma. Automated supine scan of a 35-year-old woman displays a hypoechoic mass with slightly irregular margins. Increased echoes at the anterior portion of the mass suggested reactive fibrosis (*white arrow*). Faint shadowing was noted from only small portions of the mass. (Courtesy Margaret Washburn, MD, Sedro Woolley, WA.)

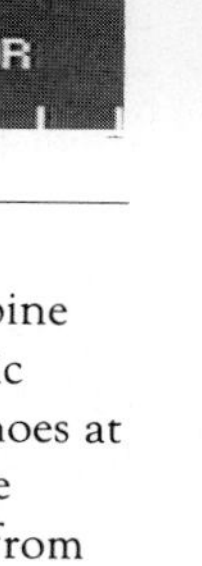

Figure 20-32. Small infiltrative carcinoma. Prone immersion scan demonstrates subtle skin dimpling secondary to an underlying malignancy. (Courtesy Ausonics Corporation, Milwaukee, WI and University of Madison, Madison, WI.)

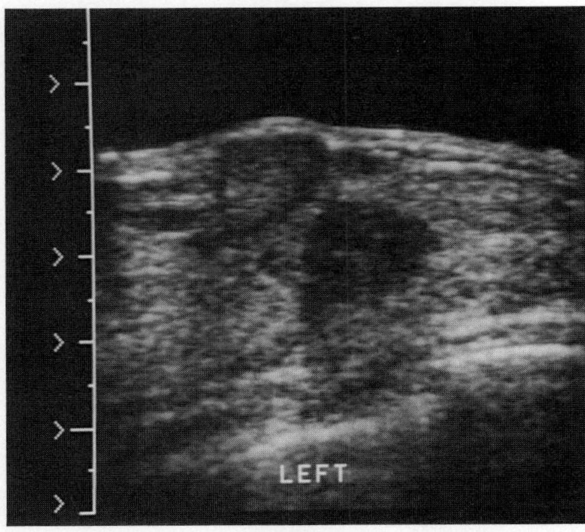

FIGURE 20-33. Infiltrating ductal carcinoma. Sonogram of a 50-year-old woman whose excisional biopsy revealed sclerosing adenosis. One year after biopsy, the patient presented with a palpable mass at the biopsy site that bulged the skin. The skin was also retracted. Mammography revealed a 1.7-cm lobulated mass with surrounding architectural distortion. Sonography verified the solid nature of the lesion and demonstrated deeper extension of the mass into the breast than was detected by mammography. The second (posterior) mass was more hypoechoic than the anterior, palpable mass. Mild acoustic shadowing was present. Biopsy and subsequent mastectomy confirmed the lesion was carcinoma.

Secondary findings

Adjacent tissue: Highly echogenic secondary to reactive fibrosis

Cooper's ligaments: Thickened, straightened, retracted

Skin: Thickened, retracted, flattened, bulging

Nipple: Flattened, inverted

Subcutaneous fat: Increased echogenicity; loss of normal fat/parenchymal border

Retromammary space: Interruption of fascial planes

The entire mass must be carefully inspected. Some tumors demonstrate attenuation shadowing, wall irregularities, and textural inhomogeneity in only a small portion of the mass. The degree of attenuation depends on the amount of fibrous tissue within and around the tumor.[13,44] Not all cancers cause acoustic shadowing.

Skin changes may be localized, diffuse, or distant from the primary site. Clinical correlation is important, since skin changes and acoustic shadowing can result from benign etiologies. Microcalcifications are not routinely detected by ultrasound but are occasionally seen with high-resolution scanners (Figs. 20-34, 20-35).

Occasionally, lymph node metastasis can be detected when sonographic interrogation is performed in the axillary and lateral subclavian regions. Rounded, hypoechoic masses measuring 5 mm or more, located near the pectoral muscles, and axillary and subclavian vessels are suspicious for metastatic involvement and can be confirmed with biopsy.[54]

Differential diagnosis. Some invasive ductal and multilobular carcinomas may be relatively well-marginated and may be difficult to differentiate from fibroadenoma unless reactive changes are seen (Fig. 20-36). Comedocarcinoma may present, not as a specific mass, but more as an area of architectural distortion and fibrotic change.[19,26] A necrotic ductal carcinoma may appear as a cystic mass.

Benign conditions that mimic scirrhous carcinoma include traumatic fat necrosis,[1] hyperplastic fibrosis,[19] radial scar, granular cell tumors,[58] hyalinized fibroadenoma,[64] and old hemorrhagic or inflammatory changes.

Well-Marginated Carcinoma. Medullary, colloid, papillary, certain duct carcinomas, and sarcomas represent a small percentage of malignancies that display relatively well-defined margins.[19] Although these lesions compress peripheral tissues as they grow, they usually elicit little or no reactive fibrosis. Attenuation effects, if present, are minimal. Some lesions demonstrate acoustic enhancement. Sonography cannot reliably differentiate these well-marginated cancers from benign solid lesions. Prognosis is usually better for these lesions than for other invasive malignancies, since metastatic involvement is less common.

Intracystic and solid papillary carcinomas tend

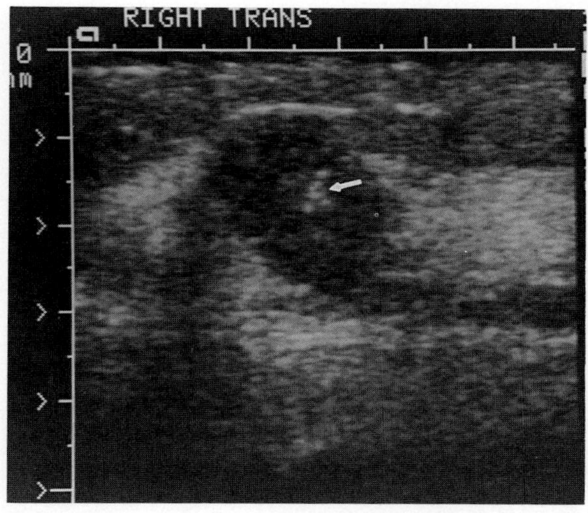

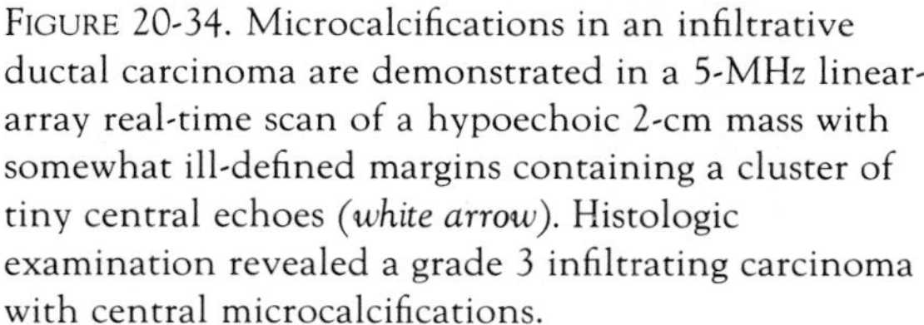

Figure 20-34. Microcalcifications in an infiltrative ductal carcinoma are demonstrated in a 5-MHz linear-array real-time scan of a hypoechoic 2-cm mass with somewhat ill-defined margins containing a cluster of tiny central echoes (*white arrow*). Histologic examination revealed a grade 3 infiltrating carcinoma with central microcalcifications.

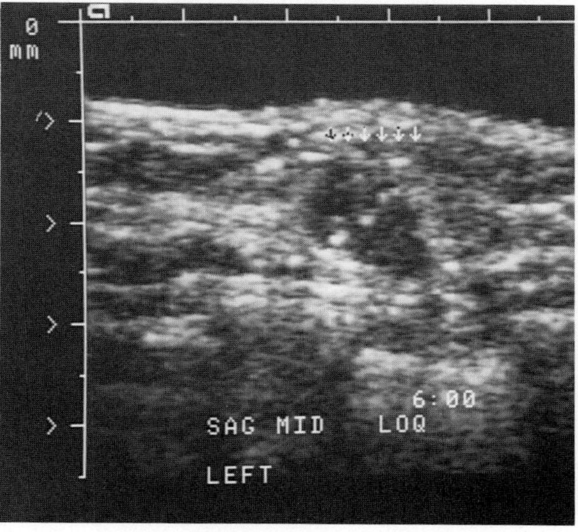

Figure 20-35. Microcalcifications. Real-time image displays a 1.5-cm solid mass with nonuniform internal echoes. Borders of the mass are mildly ill-defined. Bright central echoes suggest microcalcifications. Although no attenuation shadowing was present, the findings suggested malignancy. Two other lesions were found in the same breast quadrant. Histologic examination revealed poorly differentiated, multicentric carcinoma.

Figure 20-36. Well-marginated ductal carcinoma with degeneration (*arrow*). Real-time image of 39-year-old woman with a palpable mass. The differential diagnosis included fibroadenoma with cystic degeneration, cystosarcoma phylloides, and degenerating, well-marginated carcinoma. Biopsy revealed malignancy.

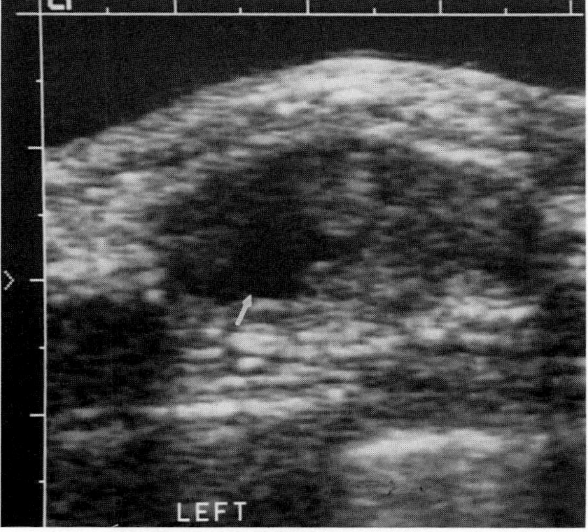

to occur in older women. Sonographically, they may not differ significantly from their benign counterparts, although intracystic carcinoma can become invasive when the mass spreads beyond the confines of the cyst. Any loss of wall definition, wall thickening, or extension of the tumor beyond the cyst wall suggests malignant change (see Fig. 20-16).

Medullary Carcinoma. Medullary carcinoma is a cellular tumor containing predominantly epithelial tissue. This uncommon lesion grows relatively fast. It tends to occur earlier than other breast cancers and to be less common after menopause.[29] Tumors can be multiple or bilateral.

Signs and symptoms. Palpable masses are discrete but softer than intraductal cancers and are usually centrally located. A larger mass may cause skin bulging and discoloration.

Mammographic features.[19] The wall definition of this circumscribed, highly dense lesion varies with the degree of infiltration into surrounding tissues. Typically it is not calcified. Some fibrous tissue strands may be present.

Sonographic features (Fig. 20-37).[6,10,13,21,26,44,49]

DIAGNOSTIC CRITERIA OF MEDULLARY CARCINOMA

Shape: Round or lobulated

Borders: Well-marginated, smooth or slightly irregular

Internal echoes: Uniform or nonuniform texture of low- to medium-level echoes

Attenuation: None or minimal

Distal echoes: Variable posterior enhancement

Associated findings: Variable lateral refractive shadowing, skin bulging

As the tumor enlarges, a wide band of increased echoes may be imaged anterior to the mass.[44] Central hemorrhage and necrosis is relatively common, causing a complex sonographic appearance.

Differential diagnosis. Other well-marginated cancers and benign solid tumors such as fibroadenoma, cystosarcoma, or necrotic tumors can have similar imaging patterns. Occasionally, medullary carcinoma may appear relatively anechoic and mimic a cyst. Increasing the gain setting demonstrates the solid nature of the mass.

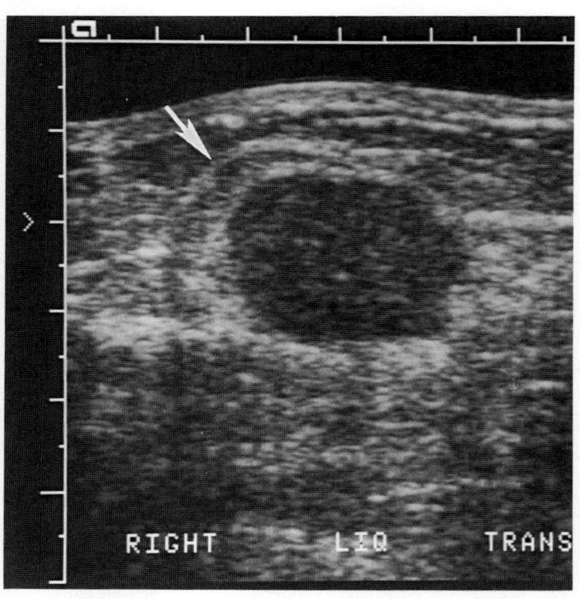

FIGURE 20-37. Medullary carcinoma with lymphoid stroma. Real-time sonogram of a 45-year-old woman who noticed a "growing" mass 3 weeks before seeking medical consultation. Mammography revealed a radiopaque lesion with slightly irregular margins. Sonography confirmed a solid, hypoechoic mass with slightly lobulated margins and evenly distributed low-level internal echoes. Anterior and lateral tissues peripheral to the mass appeared compressed *(arrow).*

Colloid Carcinoma. Colloid (mucinous) carcinoma is an uncommon, slow-growing lesion containing tumor cells dispersed in a gelatinous secretion.[29,44] This lesion presents in most women during their late fifties or sixties.[19] Although infrequent, tumors may be bilateral and multiple.

Signs and symptoms.[19] When palpable, the mass is sometimes soft and may feel like an area of thickening. Skin changes are not common.

Mammographic features. Colloid carcinoma can appear as a low-density, radiopaque, circumscribed tumor, depending on the tissue background.[64] Some trabecular distortion is noted on close inspection.

Sonographic features.[21,44]

DIAGNOSTIC CRITERIA OF COLLOID CARCINOMA
Shape: Round or oval
Borders: Well-marginated, smooth
Internal echoes: Low-level echoes, fine distribution
Distal echoes: Posterior enhancement possible
Associated findings: Occasional calcifications

Secondary changes are not prominent features with this cancer. Internal hemorrhage is not common as it is with medullary carcinoma.[19]

Differential diagnosis. Colloid carcinoma can resemble other well-marginated, solid, benign and malignant masses, mucocele-like tumors,[57] and some fluid lesions containing low-level echoes.

Multicentric and Inflammatory Carcinoma. Multicentric carcinoma refers to the spread of primary malignant nodules to various sites in the breast by way of the ducts.[19] Multiple histologic types may coexist in the same breast. Sonographically, multiple lesions or areas of architectural distortion may be seen (Fig. 20-38).

Diffuse or inflammatory carcinoma occurs when a highly invasive cancer invades the lymphatics of the skin.[19,21,26] Since spread is rapid, prognosis is poor. The skin becomes red, hot, and edematous. The breast is painful and hard. Sonographically, the texture of the breast is extremely disrupted, and a focal tumor may not be seen. The skin is thickened and lymph vessels may be dilated.

Evaluation of both breasts is necessary to compare architecture. Biopsy is necessary to differentiate inflammatory carcinoma from benign causes of infection.

Metastatic Carcinoma. The sonographic appearance of metastatic breast disease is variable. Metastasis of cancer to the breast from distant sites is uncommon. Malignant lymphoma, melanoma, and cancer of the lung, ovary, cervix, prostate, or bladder are the most common distant primary lesions.[29] Sonographically, the lesions are fairly discrete masses with relatively smooth walls and nonuniform, low-level, internal echoes. Sound attenuation is usually minimal, if present. Metastatic lesions generally are found in the subcutaneous tissues, unlike most primary malignancies (Fig. 20-39).[1]

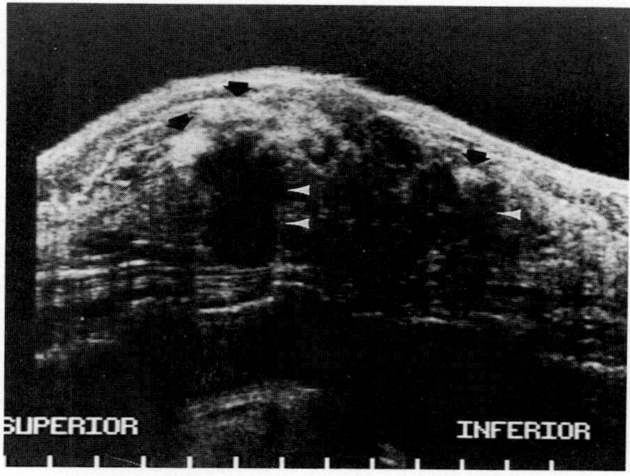

FIGURE 20-38. Multicentric carcinoma. Supine water-path scan demonstrates marked architectural distortion. Multiple areas of increased echogenicity *(black arrow heads)* are displayed with distal acoustic shadowing *(white arrow heads)*. Findings suggest desmoplasia with secondary sound absorption. The other breast was unremarkable. Surgery revealed four primary tumors in the left breast, proven at pathology to be invasive ductal carcinoma (scirrhous type). (Courtesy Margaret Washburn, MD, Sedro Woolley, WA.)

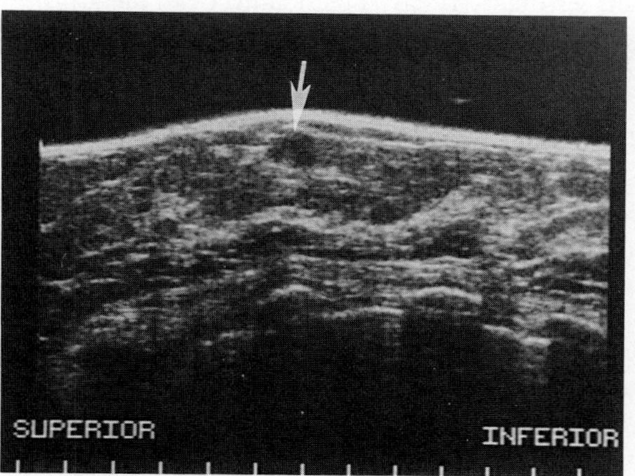

FIGURE 20-39. Lymphoma. Supine scan shows a subcutaneous, hypoechoic lesion. Lymph node was positive for lymphoma. (Courtesy Margaret Washburn, MD, Sedro Woolley, WA.)

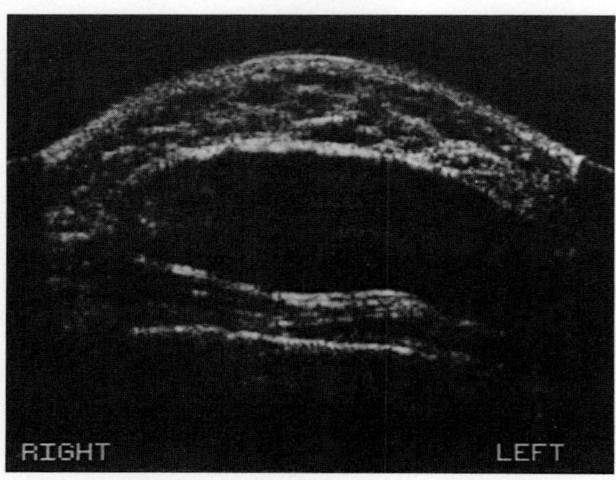

FIGURE 20-40. Saline bag prosthesis. Sagittal supine linear scan of a saline prosthesis positioned anterior to the pectoral muscles. (Courtesy Margaret Washburn, MD, Sedro Woolley, WA.)

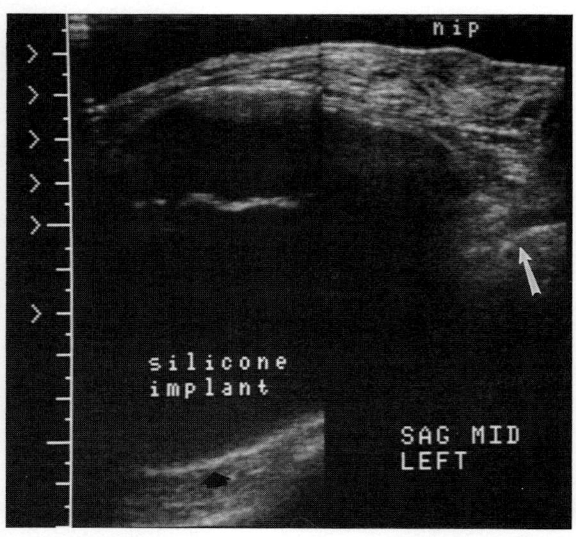

FIGURE 20-41. Silicone implant. Dual-mode real-time sonogram of the augmented breast made with a 5-MHz linear-array probe. The back wall *(black arrow)* of the implant appears to extend deeper into the chest than is possible. The true level of the chest wall is shown *(white arrow)*. This depth distortion occurs because the sound travels slower in silicone than in the breast tissue. A linear band of echoes within the implant is from a wrinkle in the bag. The breast tissue and nipple are seen overlying the implant.

Metastatic cancer from a primary source in the opposite breast produces diffuse architectural change without focal mass, not unlike inflammatory carcinoma. Spread is by way of the lymphatic system. Malignant calcifications and retraction of the skin and nipple are not common features in this setting.[19] Primary breast cancer can metastasize to distant organs. The most frequent sites are the nodes, liver, lung, bone, and brain.[29,50]

THE AUGMENTED BREAST

Sonography is particularly helpful in evaluating patients who have undergone augmentation mammoplasty. Mammography is often suboptimal and technically difficult in these patients. Sonography, however, allows evaluation of overlying breast tissues for masses and examines for changes in and around the prosthesis.

The most common implants are the saline implant, the silicone gel bag, and the silicone gel surrounded by a saline bag (double-bag) implant (Figs. 20-40, 20-41).[12,55] Implants are positioned behind the glandular tissue and in front of the pectoral muscle (submammary) or beneath the muscle (subpectoral). Injection of liquid silicone into the breast is no longer performed because of numerous problems and resultant fibrosis (Fig. 20-42).

Sonographically, most implants appear as large, oval, relatively echo-free structures behind the gland. Certain imaging artifacts may be seen when scanning implants. The speed of sound through silicone is slower than through soft tissue.[10,12,21] Therefore, on sonography the posterior wall of silicone implants appears to extend deeper into the chest wall than the surrounding tissue (see Fig. 20-41). This depth distortion is not seen with saline prostheses. Reverberation artifacts are commonly seen parallel to the scanning surface of the implant. Depending on the prosthesis, echoes from retention valves, closure pumps, and bag membranes may be demonstrated within the fluid background of the implant.

Complications associated with breast augmentation can be evaluated by sonography. These conditions include changes in the contour and place-

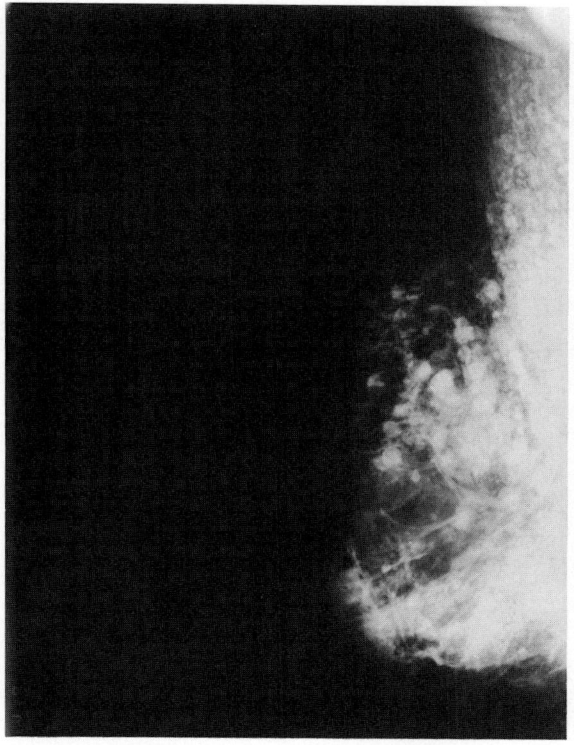
A

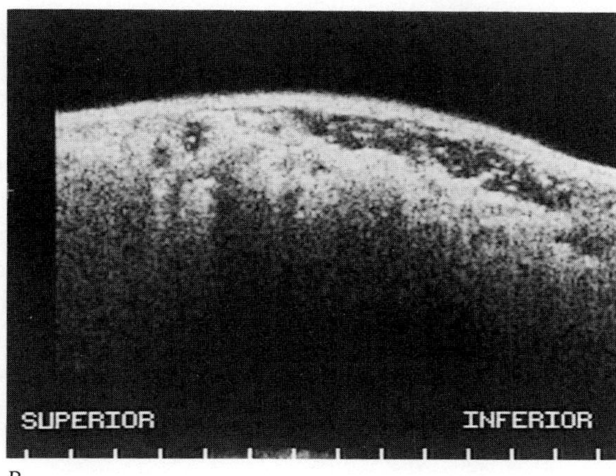

B

Figure 20-42. (*A*) Mammogram shows numerous droplets of silicone that were injected into the breast many years before. (*B*) Silicone injection. Sonogram of the same patient shows marked scattering of the sound beam by the silicone droplets. The breast is difficult to penetrate and only the subcutaneous fat is seen. (Courtesy Margaret Washburn, MD, Sedro Woolley, WA.)

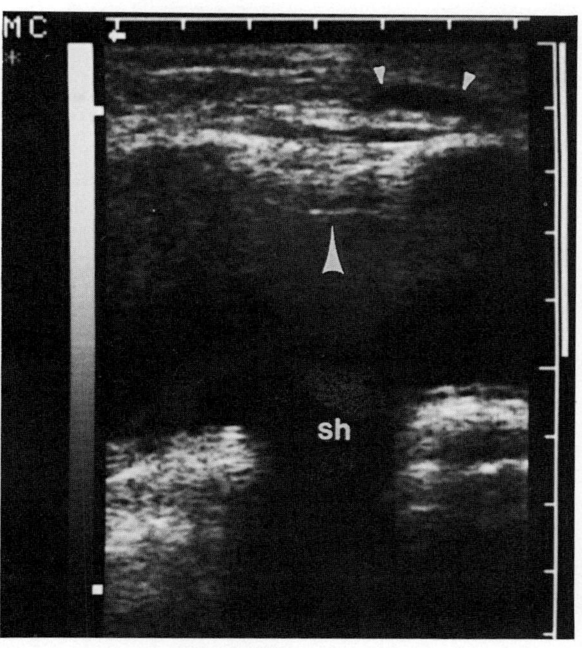

Figure 20-43. Sonographic demonstration of an expander valve (*large arrow head*) within a saline prosthesis. Acoustic shadowing is seen posterior to the valve. An oval, anechoic seroma (*small arrow head*) is noted anterior to the implant. (From Darnell EK, DeMars RV: Ultrasonographic localization of breast tissue expander valves. J Ultrasound Med 1987, 6:533.)

ment of the implant, capsular fibrosis, pericapsular leaks and abscess formation, granuloma formation, and cracks or wrinkles in the implant.[12,19,55] Sonography can be used to locate expander valves on saline implants for postsurgical inflation (Fig. 20-43).[15] Mass lesions detected within the overlying tissues are classified according to their imaging characteristics.

The Irradiated Breast

Alternatives to mastectomy, such as lumpectomy followed by radiation therapy, have become more common in recent years because of earlier diagnosis of breast cancer. The treated breast is often difficult to evaluate by physical examination and mammography, secondary to fibrosis and lack of compressibility.[8]

Sonography can detect changes in the irradiated breast that are not seen in the normal healthy breast. The amount of change depends on the extent of surgery and treatment and on the interval since irradiation. Initially, skin changes are most notable, showing varying degrees of thickening, which may be marked. With time, the thickening becomes milder and localized and the skin may return to normal.[25,55] Skin retraction may result from ligamentous contraction or from tumor recurrence. The subcutaneous fat layer may be altered, showing increased echogenicity. Secondary to post-irradiation fibrosis or surgical scarring, Cooper's ligaments may be thickened and the parenchyma may appear distorted, highly echogenic, and attenuative.[8,25,55] Residual effects may be minimal or result in scar formation in the tissues.

Most sonographic findings seen in the irradiated breast are similar to those seen in patients with secondary signs of malignancy. Since these changes are usually secondary to the effects of surgery and irradiation, tumor recurrence may be difficult to identify in the absence of a localized mass.

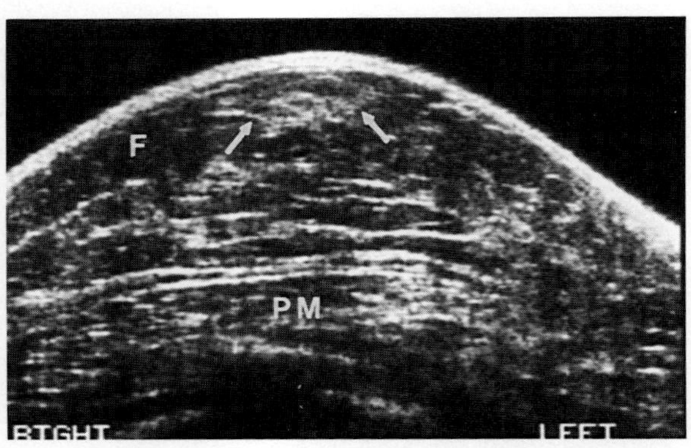

FIGURE 20-44. Gynecomastia. Transverse scan using an automated supine scanner on a 27-year-old male with breast enlargement. The majority of the breast displays hypoechoic fatty tissue (F). An area of increased echogenicity beneath the nipple *(arrows)* represents fibroglandular tissue, indicative of gynecomastia. The pectoralis muscle (PM) is seen behind the breast. (Courtesy Valerie P. Jackson, MD, Indianapolis, IN.)

THE MALE BREAST

The normal male breast is comprised mainly of fatty tissue and some rudimentary ducts surrounded by connective tissue.[18,26] The skin is thicker and the muscle larger than that usually seen in the female breast.

Males with breast enlargement, nipple discharge, tenderness, or a palpable mass are candidates for sonography. Mammography is often technically difficult in small male breasts, and magnification views are recommended for adequate evaluation.

Gynecomastia refers to male breast enlargement characterized by an abnormal proliferation of fibroglandular tissue and an increased volume of subcutaneous fat.[10,19] Hormones, antihypertensive and antidepressant medications, and other factors can lead to growth of the ducts and supporting connective tissues.[19,55] The breast is often painful. A palpable, firm mass of tissue may be felt beneath the nipple. This condition may be temporary and is more likely to present around puberty or after age 50 years.

Sonographic features diagnostic of gynecomastia include demonstration of (1) fibroglandular tissue, seen as a triangular area of increased echogenicity beneath the areola, and (2) ductal structures, seen as tubular lucencies converging toward the nipple.[26,34] Increased fat is noted in the breast. Clear demonstration of the hyperechoic glandular tissue, alone, is sufficient for diagnosis (Fig. 20-44).

Breast cancer is rare in men, accounting for about 1% of all malignancies.[9,26,34] Advanced disease can result in skin ulceration, chest wall invasion, and lymph node metastasis. Men with prostate cancer may develop metastatic lesions to the breast or gynecomastia from long-term estrogen therapy. In the male breast benign and malignant masses have the same imaging characteristics as in women.

Real-Time Fine-Needle Aspiration and Biopsy Techniques

High-resolution sonography provides an alternative to mammography for localization of certain breast masses during fine-needle aspiration and biopsy procedures. Real-time systems allow direct visualization of the needle tip as it approaches and enters a mass.

Indications for sonographic needle guidance are both diagnostic and therapeutic: (1) aspiration of a simple cyst; (2) aspiration biopsy of a solid or atypical cystic mass; (3) drainage of a hematoma or abscess; and (4) preoperative dye or wire localization of an nonpalpable mass. These procedures can be performed on an outpatient basis and are generally tolerated well by patients. Before the needle is introduced, the mass is scanned to determine its solid or cystic nature, its size, and its location in the breast. All previous mammograms and sonograms are reviewed.

Materials

What supplies are needed depends on the type of procedure to be performed. They may include the following: 20- to 25-gauge needle at least 40 mm long, syringe, connective tubing, local anesthetic (optional), sterile container, sterile set-up, slides, 95% alcohol or fixative spray, methylene- or Evan's blue dye, xylocaine, spring hook-wire, tape and sterile gauze.

Patient Preparation

The patient is fully informed of the procedure and its possible complications and signs a consent form. Complications are uncommon but include hematoma, infection, and possibly fainting. Premedication is not recommended. A relative or other person should accompany the patient to provide support after the procedure.

The patient is positioned so as to maximize access to the mass, usually supine or slightly oblique. For large-breasted patients, the C-C position may help stabilize the breast during needle puncture. This seated position allows the needle to be directed away from the chest wall.

The skin and transducer are sterilized with an antiseptic solution. If needed, a sterile sleeve is draped over the probe. Sterile gel or additional antiseptic solution is used as a coupling agent during scanning. Local anesthesia is not always necessary.

Guidance Techniques

Some real-time transducers have built-in or attachable biopsy guides. On some systems, electronic calipers mark the path and the distance to the mass.

When a biopsy guide is not used, the following techniques can be used for proper needle guidance. The methods described utilize a linear-array real-time probe.

Method 1. The transducer is positioned so that the greatest cross-section of the mass is lying under the center of the probe. The distance from the skin to the center of the mass is measured. The needle is placed adjacent to the center of the transducer's side and the needle is inserted obliquely into the breast along a path and to the depth necessary to intersect the mass. The needle tip is seen as it enters the mass (Fig. 20-45).[23]

Method 2. The transducer is positioned so that the mass is under the outer portion of the probe. The needle is inserted adjacent to the corresponding edge of the transducer. The needle tip and distal shaft are imaged passing obliquely toward and into the mass. Necessary adjustments in angulation are made under direct real-time visualization (Fig. 20-46).[23]

Another variation is to place the transducer centrally over the mass and advance the needle along a path parallel to the long axis of the transducer at the depth of the mass.[45]

Method 3. The transducer is positioned over the center of the mass. An acoustic marker, such as a thin straw or needle, is slid between skin and transducer and is moved until its acoustic shadow is overlying the center of the mass. The transducer is removed and the skin is marked. This procedure is done in two perpendicular planes. The distance from the skin to the mass is measured. The biopsy needle is inserted at the depth and angle indicated.[20,39] This technique can be modified for use with a dedicated supine scanner (see Figs. 20-30, 20-47).

Procedures

Cyst Aspiration.[2,39] The aspiration needle is attached to the syringe with connective tubing, which allows easier manipulation of the needle. The needle is guided into the dependent portion of the cyst, and the fluid is aspirated. Evacuation is assisted by applying gentle pressure over the cyst with the hand. After removing the syringe, pressure is applied over the puncture site to prevent formation of a hematoma. Sonography is used to verify complete or incomplete evacuation. A sample of the fluid is

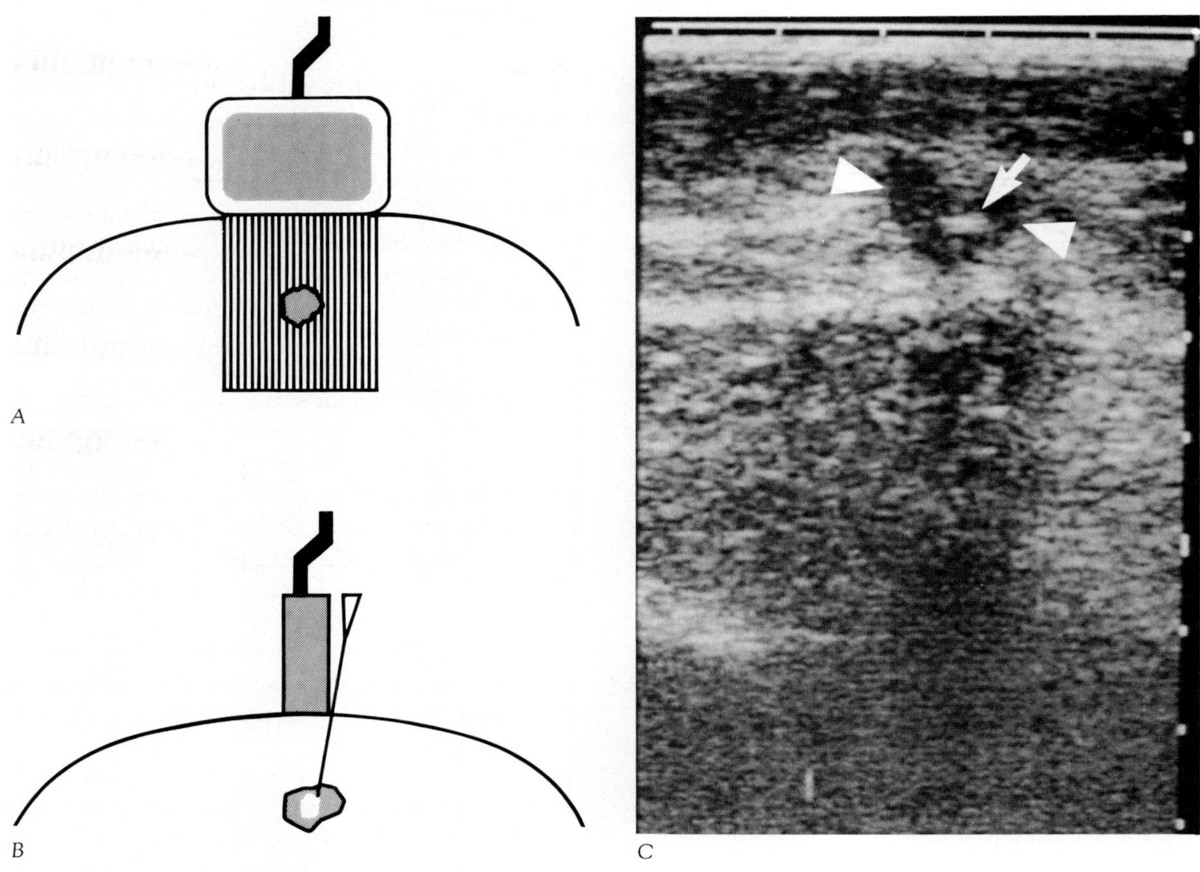

Figure 20-45. Method 1 for ultrasound-guided aspiration biopsy of the breast. (*A*) Frontal view of the linear-array probe in relation to the suspicious mass to be sampled by biopsy. (*B*) Side view shows the oblique needle tangential to the probe. The needle tip has reached the mass in the scan plane. (C) Sonogram shows the bright needle tip echo *(arrow)* within the hypoechoic nonpalpable carcinoma, 13 mm in maximal diameter *(arrowheads)*. (Reprinted with permission from Fornage B, Faroux M, Simatos A: Breast masses: US-guided fine-needle aspiration biopsy. Radiology 1987, 162:410.)

sent for cytologic evaluation. Cyst fluid is rarely clear, and evidence of old hemorrhage may warrant surgical excision.

If pneumocystography is desired, the needle is left in place and another syringe is filled with a volume of air equal to or greater than that of the fluid removed. The air is injected into the cyst cavity through the needle. The needle is removed when resistance is felt. A mammogram is taken to document the cyst wall cavity.

Aspiration Biopsy.[2,23,39] The biopsy needle is guided into the mass. Several forceful, back-and-forth, needle passes inside the mass are made while intermittent suction is applied with the syringe. The needle is withdrawn after releasing negative pressure in the syringe. Aspirated material is spread onto glass slides and a fixative is applied. The choice of fixative depends on the staining technique to be used. Failure of cytologic analysis to identify malignant cells may not obviate the need

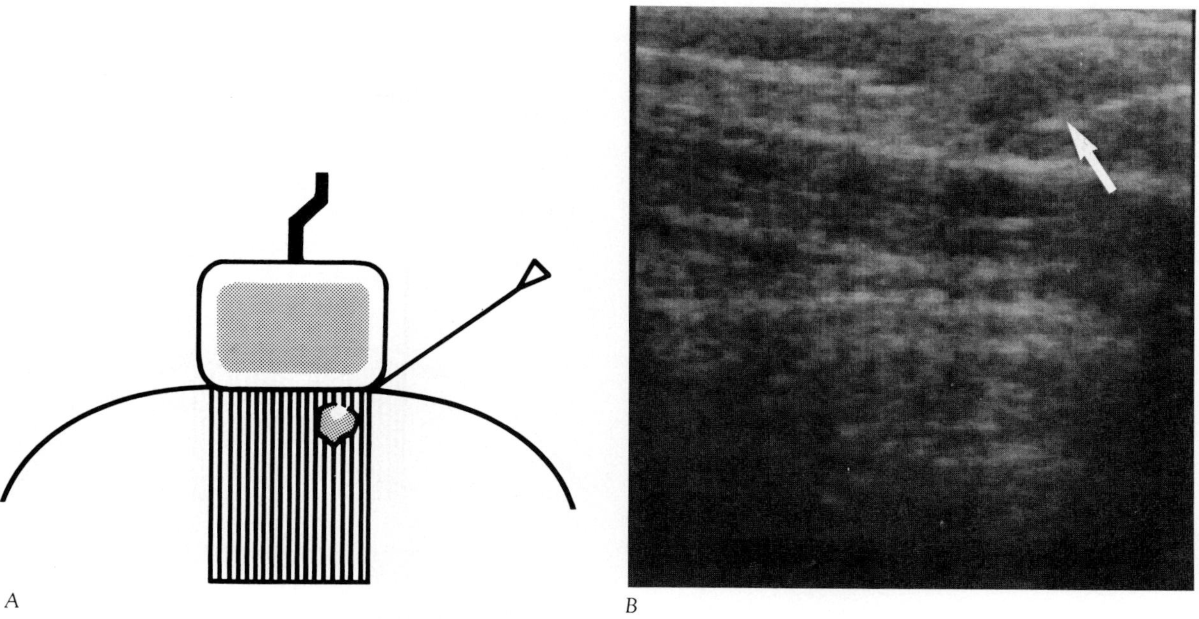

FIGURE 20-46. Method 2 for ultrasound-guided aspiration biopsy of the breast. (*A*) Frontal view shows the suspicious mass under the outer extremity of the probe. The needle is inserted into the scan plane at an oblique angle toward the mass. The tip and distal portion of the needle are clearly seen in the scan plane. (*B*) Sonogram obtained with a 7.5 MHz linear-array probe shows the obliquely oriented needle (*arrow*) within a smoothly marginated, homogeneous, hypoechoic, 12 × 16 mm fibroadenoma. (Reprinted with permission from Fornage B, Faroux M, Simatos A: Breast masses: US-guided fine-needle aspiration biopsy. Radiology 1987, 162:410.)

for excisional biopsy of a suspicious mass. Since the needle biopsy sample is small, malignant cells in a mass may not always be aspirated.

Preoperative Localization.[39] A spring hook-wire needle is inserted into the lesion under ultrasound guidance. The shortest path to the lesion is chosen. The guide is removed and a 0.5- to 1-ml mixture of blue dye and xylocaine is injected along the entire needle track. The syringe is removed and the hook-wire is inserted through the same needle. The needle is removed, keeping the wire in place. The end of the wire is taped to the skin, and sterile gauze is taped over the site. During subsequent excision the wire or dye acts as a surgical guide to the nonpalpable mass. A mixture of blue dye and xylocaine can be injected along a standard fine-needle track to the site of the mass without placement of a hook-wire, but surgery must be performed soon after localization (within ½ to 4 hours), before the dye diffuses in the parenchyma.[20]

Mammography is still the principal technique chosen to localize most nonpalpable solid breast masses and clustered microcalcifications. When mammography has limited efficacy, as in a dense breast, other imaging modalities, including sonography, can be utilized to detect and to localize solid breast masses.

Summary

On occasion, breast abnormalities detected by physical examination or mammography require further diagnostic evaluation by sonography. So-

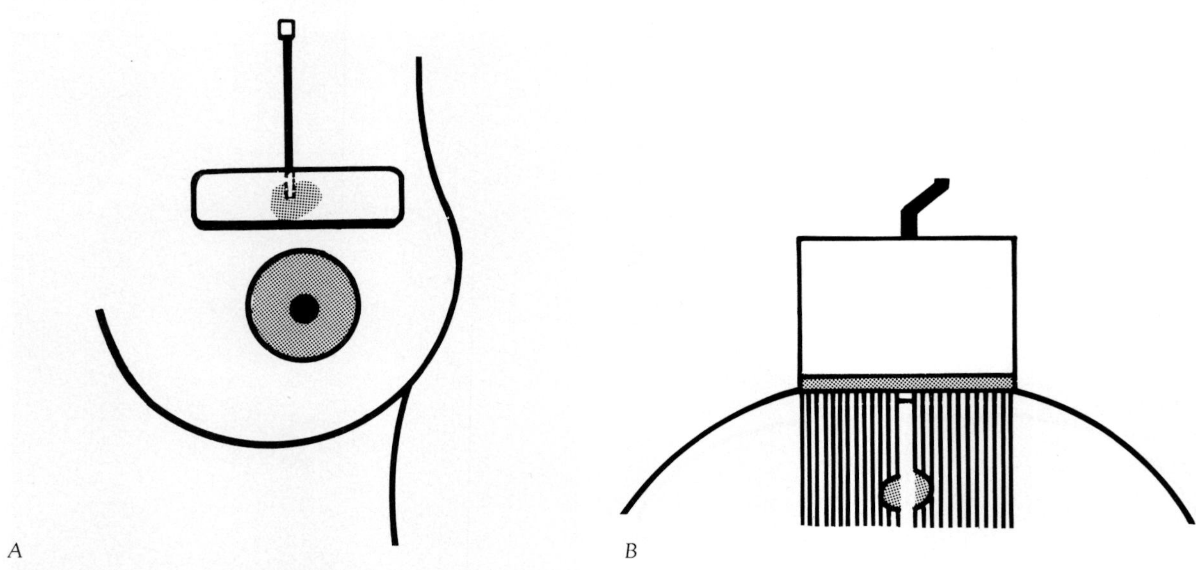

FIGURE 20-47. Method 3 for ultrasound localization of a breast mass. (*A*) The transducer is centered over the middle portion of the mass. A thin straw or needle is slid beneath the skin and transducer to a point where it overlies the center of the mass. (*B*) The straw or needle casts an acoustic shadow over the mass when it is in the correct location. The tip of the acoustic marker is shown on end in the drawing.

nography is advantageous in that it provides a painless, noninvasive, tomographic study of the breast without known biologic effects. The principal role of sonography is in differentiating cysts and solid breast masses, which distinction has a direct effect on patient management. When the two are used in conjunction, the strengths of sonography offset the weaknesses of mammography, providing greater diagnostic confidence.

Research into the utility of Doppler techniques in the evaluation of breast disease is encouraging, although sensitivity and specificity are still variable. Continuous-wave, pulsed-wave, and color flow Doppler studies are used to characterize blood flow within and around tumors.[47,60] Malignant tumors may show increased border vascularity associated with abnormal Doppler waveforms. Preliminary findings show that some cancers display spectral patterns with moderate to high velocities secondary to increased neovascularity and arteriovenous shunting. Not all cancers have detectable Doppler signals. Benign masses typically show no associated Doppler signal, although fibroadenomas, fibrocystic disease, and inflammatory processes may elicit a Doppler response. Doppler angiography combined with continued improvements in high-resolution sonography may someday play a greater role in distinguishing between benign and malignant breast disease.

References

1. Andersson I: Mammography in Clinical Practice. Medical Radiology and Photography 1986, 62(2).
2. Annonier C: Female Breast Examination. New York, Springer-Verlag, 1986.
3. Aquaflex Ultrasound Gel Pad Standoff. Orange, NJ, Parker Laboratories.
4. Ausonics Prone Breast Scanner Promotional Material. Milwaukee, WI, Ausonics Corporation.
5. Bassett L, Gold R, Kimme-Smith C: Breast Ultrasound. *In* Sarti DA (ed): Diagnostic Ultrasound Text and Cases, 2nd ed. Chicago, Year Book Medical Publishers, 1987.
6. Bassett L, Kimme-Smith C, Sutherland L, et al: Automated and hand-held breast US: Effect on patient management. Radiology 1987, 165:103–108.

7. Burgener FA, Kormano M: Localized lesions in mammography. *In* Verlag GT: Differential Diagnosis in Conventional Radiology. New York, Thieme-Stratton, 1985.
8. Calkins A, Jackson V, Morphis J, et al: The sonographic appearance of the irradiated breast. J Clin Ultrasound 1988, 16:406–415.
9. Case C (ed): The Breast Cancer Digest, 2nd ed. Bethesda, MD, National Cancer Institute, 1984.
10. Cole-Beuglet C: The breast. *In* Sabbagha R (ed): Diagnostic Ultrasound, 2nd ed. Philadelphia, JB Lippincott, 1988.
11. Cole-Beuglet C: The use of ultrasound in breast evaluation. *In* Sanders R, James E (eds): The Principles and Practice of Ultrasonography in Obstetrics and Gynecology, 3rd ed. Norwalk, CT, Appleton-Century-Crofts, 1985.
12. Cole-Beuglet C, Schwartz G, Kurtz A: Ultrasound mammography for the augmented breast. Radiology 1983, 146:737–742.
13. Cole-Beuglet C, Soriano R, Kurtz A, et al: Ultrasound analysis of 104 primary breast carcinomas classified according to histopathic type. Radiology 1983, 147:191–196.
14. Cole-Beuglet C, Soriano R, Kurtz A, et al: Ultrasound, x-ray mammography, and histopathology of cystosarcoma phylloides. Radiology 1983, 146:481–486.
15. Darnell EK, DeMars RV: Ultrasonographic localization of breast tissue expander valves. J Ultrasound Med 1987, 6:531–534.
16. Dempsey PJ: Breast sonography: Historical perspective, clinical application, and image interpretation. Ultrasound Quart 1988, 6:69–90.
17. Echo Acoustic Standoffs, Echo Ultrasound, Imaging Supply Center, Lewiston, PA.
18. Egan RL: Breast Imaging, 3rd ed. Baltimore, University Park Press, 1984.
19. Egan RL: Breast Imaging, Diagnosis and Morphology of Breast Disease. Philadelphia, WB Saunders, 1988.
20. Elyaderani M: Aspirations performed for miscellaneous conditions. *In* Letoureau J, Elyaderani M, et al: Percutaneous Biopsy Aspiration and Drainage. Chicago, Year Book Medical Publishers, 1987.
21. Ezo MG, Hagen-Ansert S: Breast. *In* Hagen-Ansert SL (ed): Textbook of Diagnostic Ultrasonography, 3rd ed. St. Louis, CV Mosby, 1989.
22. Fleischer A, Muhletaler C, Reynolds V, et al: Palpable breast masses, evaluation by high-frequency, hand-held real-time sonography and xeromammography. Radiology 1983, 148:813–817.
23. Fornage B, Faroux M, Simatos A: Breast masses: US-guided fine-needle aspiration biopsy. Radiology 1987, 162:409–414.
24. Gordon L: The utility of hand-held real-time scanners for breast sonography. J Diagn Med Sonogr 1986, 2:266–270.
25. Grant E, Richardson J, Olcay OS: Sonography of the breast: Findings following conservative surgery and irradiation for early carcinoma. Radiology 1983, 147:535–539.
26. Harper AP (ed): Ultrasound Mammography. Baltimore, University Park Press, 1985.
27. Harper P, Kelly-Fry E: Ultrasound visualization of the breast in symptomatic patients. Radiology 1980, 137:465–469.
28. Harper AP, Kelly-Fry E, Nor JS, et al: Ultrasound in the evaluation of solid breast masses. Radiology 1983, 146:731–736.
29. Harris JR, Hellman S, Henderson IC, et al (eds): Breast Diseases. Philadelphia, JB Lippincott, 1987.
30. Heywang S, Dunner P, Lipsit E, et al: Advantages and pitfalls of ultrasound in the diagnosis of breast cancer. J Clin Ultrasound 1985, 13:525–532.
31. Hilton S, Leopold G, Olson L, et al: Real-time breast sonography, application in 300 consecutive patients. AJR 1986, 147:479–486.
32. Homer MJ: Breast imaging pitfalls, controversies and some practical thoughts. Radiol Clin North Am 1985, 23:459–471.
33. Homer MJ: Benign diseases of the breast. *In* Putnam C, Ravin C (eds): Textbook of Diagnostic Imaging. Philadelphia, WB Saunders, 1988.
34. Jackson V, Gilmor R: Male breast carcinoma and gynecomastia. Radiology 1983, 149:533–536.
35. Jackson V, Kelly-Fry E, Rothschild P, et al: Automated breast sonography using a 7.5-MHz PVDF transducer. Radiology 1986, 159:679–684.
36. Kersschot EA, Hermans M, et al: Juvenile papillomatosis of the breast; Sonographic appearance. Radiology 1988, 169:631–633.
37. Kimme-Smith C, Bassett L, Gold R: High-frequency breast ultrasound, hand-held versus automated units. J Ultrasound Med 1988, 7:77–81.
38. Kitecko Standoff Pads, 3M Medical Surgical Division, St. Paul, Minnesota.
39. Kopans DB: Clinically occult breast lesions and interventional procedures in the breast. *In* Taveras JM (ed): Radiology: Diagnosis—Imaging—Intervention. Philadelphia, JB Lippincott, 1987.
40. Kopans DB: Introduction to breast imaging. *In* Taveras JM (ed): Radiology: Diagnosis-Imaging-Intervention. Philadelphia, JB Lippincott, 1987.
41. Kopans DB: Other breast modalities. *In* Taveras JM (ed): Radiology: Diagnosis-Imaging-Intervention. Philadelphia, JB Lippincott, 1987.
42. Kopans DB, Meyer J, Lindfors K: Whole-breast US

imaging, 4-year follow-up. Radiology 1985, 157:505–507.

43. Labsonics Supine Breast Scanner Operations Manual and Promotional Materials, Labsonics/Labeco, Inc., Mooresville, Indiana, and conversations with Amy Lex and Nancy Luther, Mooresville, Indiana.
44. McSweeney M, Murphy C: Whole breast sonography. Radiol Clin North Am 1985, 23:157–167.
45. Matalon T, Silver B: Ultrasound guidance of interventional procedures. Radiology 1990, 174:43–47.
46. Maturo VG, Zusmer N, Gilson A, et al: Ultrasound of the whole breast utilizing a dedicated automated breast scanner. Radiology 1980, 137:457–463.
47. Merritt C: Breast imaging techniques. *In* Putnam C, Ravin C (eds): Textbook of Diagnostic Imaging. Philadelphia, WB Saunders, 1988.
48. Merritt C: Doppler color flow imaging. J Clin Ultrasound 1987, 15:591–597.
49. Meyer J, Amin E, et al: Medullary carcinoma of the breast: Mammographic and ultrasound appearance. Radiology 1989, 170:79–82.
50. Moore KL: Clinically Oriented Anatomy, 2nd ed. Baltimore, Williams & Wilkins, 1985.
51. Nelsen M: Breast care. *In* Thompson DS (ed): Every Woman's Health, rev. ed. New York, Doubleday, 1982.
52. Netter FH: Anatomy and Pathology of the Mammary Gland. *In* Oppenheiner E (ed): The Ciba Collection of Medical Reproductions, vol. 2. Summit, NJ, CIBA Pharmaceutical, 1954.
53. Omoto R, Kobyayashi M: Breast. *In* Amoto R, Kobyayashi M: Atlas of Essential Ultrasound Imaging. Tokyo, Igaku-Shoin, 1981.
54. Pamilo M, Soiva M, Lavast E: Real-time ultrasound, axillary mammography, and clinical examination in the detection of axillary lymph node metastases in breast cancer patients. J Ultrasound Med 1989, 8:115.
55. Porrath S: A Multimodality Approach to Breast Imaging. Rockville, MD, Aspen 1986.
56. Reuter K, D'Orsi C, Reale F: Intracystic carcinoma of the breast: The role of ultrasonography. Radiology 1984, 153:233–234.
57. Rosen PP: Mucocele-like tumors of the breast. Am J Surg Pathol 1986, 10:464–469.
58. Scatarige J, Hsiu J, de la Torre R, et al: Acoustic shadowing in benign granular cell tumor (myoblastoma) of the breast. J Ultrasound Med 1987, 6:545–547.
59. Schneider JA: Invasive papillary breast carcinoma: Mammographic and sonographic appearance. Radiology 1989, 171:377–379.
60. Schoenberger SG, Sutherland CM, Robinson AE: Breast neoplasms: Duplex sonographic imaging as an adjunct in diagnosis. Radiology 1988, 168:665–668.
61. Sickles EA: Overview of the Breast Cancer Problem. *In* Putman C, Ravin C (eds): Textbook of Diagnostic Imaging. Philadelphia, WB Saunders, 1988.
62. Sickles E, Filly R, Callen P: Benign breast lesions: Ultrasound detection and diagnosis. Radiology 1984, 151:467–472.
63. Tabar L: Teaching Course in Mammography {Student Manual}. Conference held June 10–12, 1988, Seattle, WA.
64. Tabar L, Dean PB: Teaching Atlas of Mammography, 2nd ed. New York, Thieme-Stratton, 1983.
65. vanDam P, Van Goethem, Kersschot E, et al: Palpable solid breast masses: retrospective evaluation of 201 lesions. Radiology 1988, 16:435–439.
66. Walter JP: Physics of high-resolution ultrasound—practical aspects. *In* McGahan J (ed): Radiol Clin North Am 1985, 23:3–12.

CHAPTER 21

Scrotum

WAYNE C. LEONHARDT

The diagnosis of scrotal disease often begins with clinical palpation and transillumination. After the clinical examination, however, the cause of the patient's symptoms may still be an enigma. Before the advent of scrotal sonography in the mid-1970s, accurate diagnosis of most testicular masses required surgical exploration.[42] Today, with the exception of a few entities, diagnostic ultrasound is the imaging modality of choice in the evaluation of scrotal disease.

Ultrasound is particularly useful. Its accuracy rate approaches 100% for determining the location (whether a lesion is intratesticular or extratesticular) of a scrotal abnormality and for defining its characteristics, especially in determining whether a lesion is cystic or solid.[10,12,41,43] Testicular sonography is also useful in the repeat examination of benign lesions such as infections and varicoceles.[35,41] The diagnosis of testicular torsion is currently evaluated with Tc^{99m} radionuclide scan.[11] Recent studies using color Doppler sonography to assess testicular blood flow, show that color Doppler sonography can reliably display normal blood flow in the testis, and demonstrate the absence of blood flow in patients with testicular torsion.[8,35,36] The accuracy of color Doppler sonography in the evaluation of torsion and ischemia is as good as scintigraphy, ninety-seven percent.[8] Undescended testis can be evaluated with ultrasound; however, an undescended testis in the abdomen is better evaluated with magnetic resonance imaging (MRI) or computed tomography (CT).[13] Because ultrasound offers excellent diagnostic efficacy without risk or discomfort to the patient, scrotal sonography is widely accepted, especially in the evaluation of acute pain in the scrotum.

Sonographic Imaging Techniques

In general, the range of high-frequency transducers used to evaluate the scrotum are 5, 7.5, and 10 MHz. The highest-frequency real-time transducer (10 MHz) has the capability to resolve structures as small as 0.5 mm.[31] Conventional Doppler and color-flow Doppler duplex scanning are useful in many cases. The rate of blood flow in the vessels of the scrotum can be measured, which aids in distinguishing epididymitis from torsion. Vascular abnormalities such as varicocele can be characterized. The ability to detect flow can determine whether fluid collections are vascular or nonvascular. Color flow imaging has recently increased the diagnostic efficacy in the evaluation of the acute painful scrotum because of its ability to quantify perfusion in small vessels (between 1 and 2 mm) and to better define morphology.

REAL-TIME SCROTAL ULTRASOUND

High-resolution real-time ultrasound has improved the diagnostic utility of ultrasound evaluation of the scrotum.[10,29] Because real-time sonography can detect movement, the sonographer can correctly

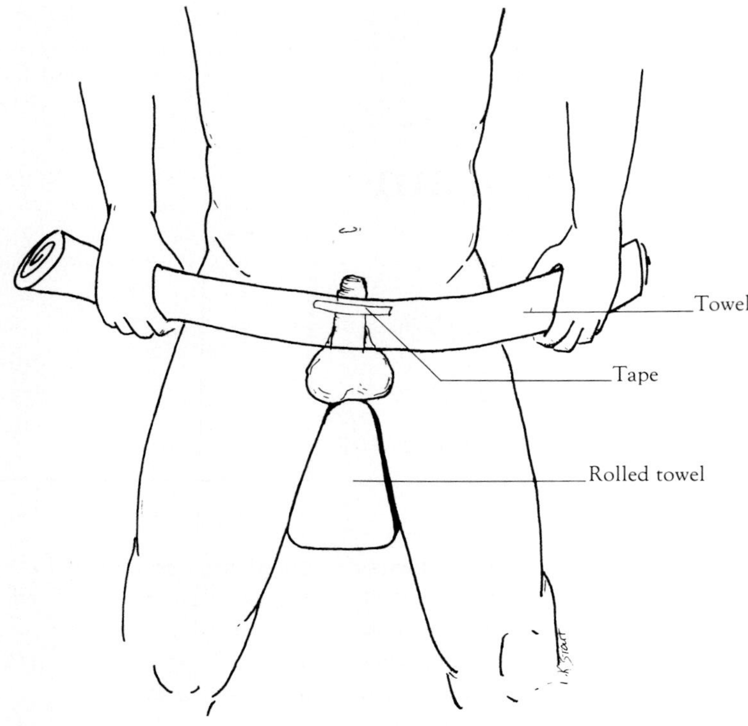

FIGURE 21-1. Patient positioning and preparation for scrotal ultrasound examination.

identify herniation of bowel by identifying the peristalsis of the herniated bowel. With high-resolution real-time sonography, it is easy to correlate a palpable mass with the real-time sonographic image.[10,28] Real-time sonography also decreases the time needed to image the entire scrotum. Color-flow Doppler instrumentation adds another dimension and allows the sonographer to determine the direction and velocity of blood flow and to evaluate small vessels in superficial structures.

Protocol. Before scanning the scrotum, the examiner takes a careful history and palpates the lesion to locate the area of interest.[26,28] The scrotum is then supported on a rolled towel placed between the thighs to isolate and immobilize it and its contents for scanning (Fig. 21-1).[26] The penis is lifted onto the anterior abdominal wall, immobilized with paper tape, and covered with a towel. Warm gel is applied to the scrotal skin as a couplant. The sonographer's gloved fingers are placed underneath the scrotum, and the thumb over the scrotum. This hand position stabilizes the scrotum and allows the fingers to be used as reference points for the lesion as the scan progresses.[28] (The fingers are identified as echogenic bands; Fig. 21-2.) Scanning planes include longitudinal, transverse, and oblique projections.[28] The sonographer must be careful to be consistent in producing each scanning plane, since small changes in angulation can make it difficult to recognize structures. A consistent scanning protocol precludes ambiguity and errors of omission.

The real-time scrotal sonographic evaluation begins with longitudinal oblique scans of the spermatic cord (with both quiet respiration and the Valsalva maneuver to check for varicocele), the epididymal head, and the testis (upper pole, middle portion, and lower pole, (Fig. 21-3).[28] The testis examination includes the body and tail of the epididymis. Longitudinal testicular measurement is made

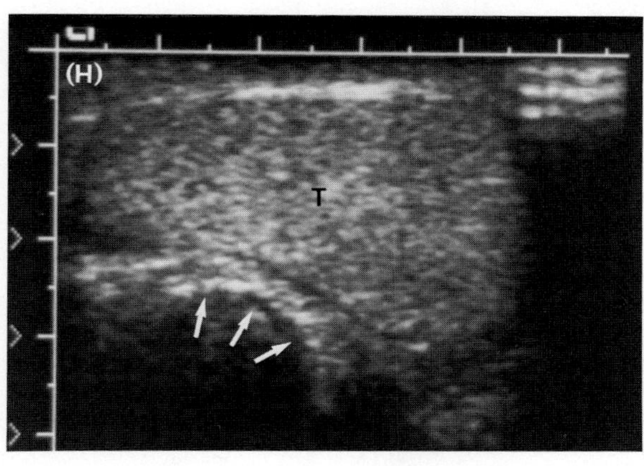

FIGURE 21-2. Longitudinal scan of normal testis (T) using gloved-hand technique. The echogenic, crescent-shaped area *(arrows)* represents the finger, which is used as a reference point for localizing lesions (H, toward patient's head).

at the middle portion of the testis.[4] In the transverse projection, scans are obtained of the cord (with both quiet respiration and the Valsalva maneuver); the epididymal head, body, and tail; and the testis (upper pole, middle portion, and lower pole; (Fig. 21-4).[4] Transverse testicular measurement is made at the middle portion of the testis. A transverse scan that demonstrates both testes together should be obtained to facilitate evaluation of testicular echogenicity and size (Fig. 21-5).[26] In patients with severe testicular pain, the contralateral testicle can be used as a window to scan the painful testicle, which minimizes the discomfort (Fig. 21-6).[25] A stand-off pad is useful for anterior lesions such as those in the tunica vaginalis.

Normal Anatomy and Sonographic Appearance

It is paramount in the study of any organ system to know the normal anatomy and the range of normal variation. It is not possible to correctly identify

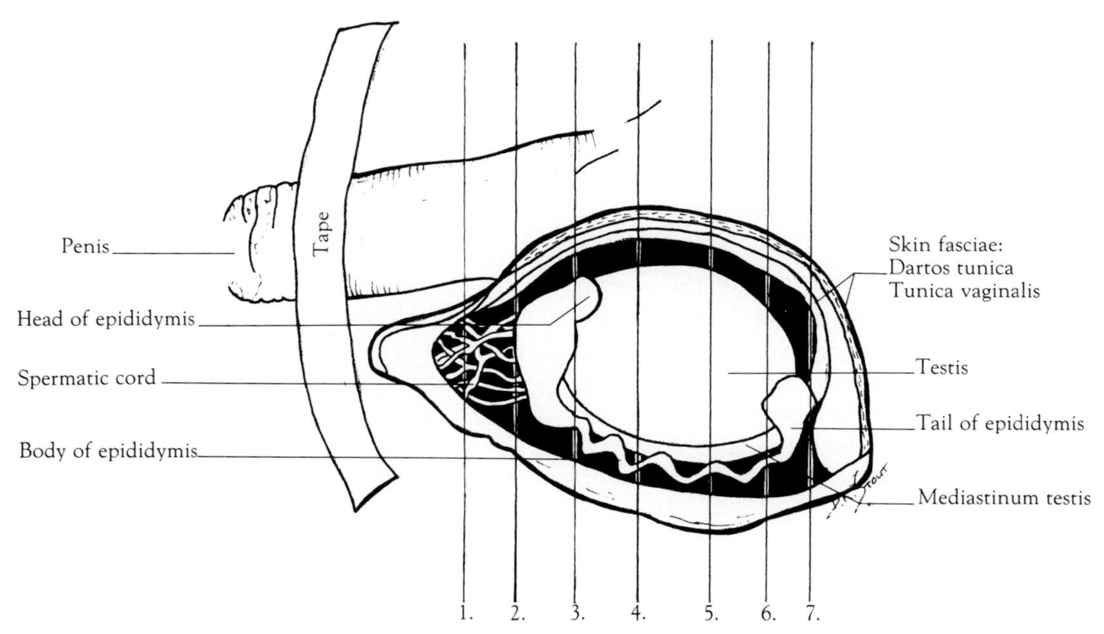

FIGURE 21-3. Schematic illustration of longitudinal scanning survey protocol for the testis. 1. Spermatic cord—rest; 2. Spermatic cord—Valsalva; 3. Head of epididymis; 4. Testis—superior; 5. Testis—mid; 6. Testis—inferior; 7. Tail of epididymis. Note that the body of the epididymis is seen in sections 4–6.

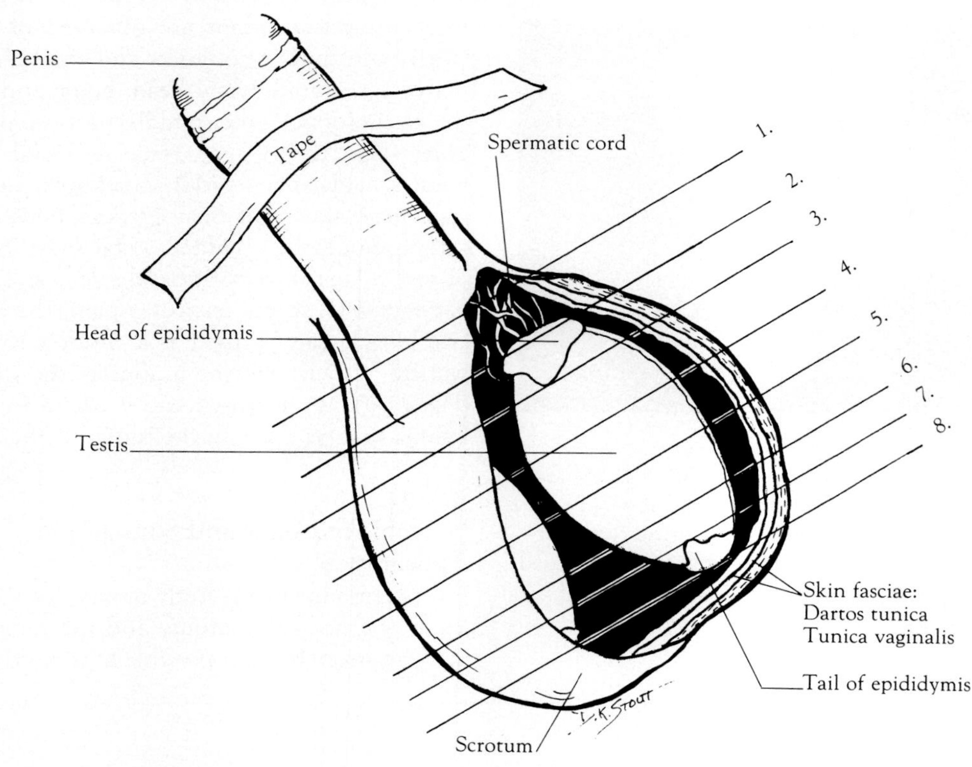

FIGURE 21-4. Schematic illustration of transverse scanning survey protocol for the testis. 1. Spermatic cord—rest; 2. Spermatic cord—Valsalva; 3. Head of epididymis; 4. Testis—superior; 5. Testis—mid; 6. Testis—inferior; 7. Tail of epididymis; 8. Bilateral testis. The body of the epididymis is seen in sections 4–6.

disease without having a clear idea of the normal baseline anatomy of the structure for each age group. Without this clear concept of the normal, pathologic processes may be missed or a normal variant may be mistaken for disease.

Three major structures are contained in the scrotum: the spermatic cord, the epididymis (head, body, and tail), and the testes (Fig. 21-7).[1] The scrotum is a musculocutaneous pouch composed of several layers of tissue: Dartos tunica, external spermatic fascia, middle spermatic fascia, cremaster muscle, internal spermatic fascia, and tunica vaginalis (Fig. 21-7).[21] The thickness of the scrotal wall varies from 2 to 8 mm; some variation in thickness may be attributed to the Dartos muscle (Fig. 21-8).[31] The scrotal pouch is divided into two compartments by the raphe, a fibrous band of tissue that runs ventral to the undersurface of the penis and dorsal along the middle of the perineum to the anus.[21]

SPERMATIC CORD

The spermatic cord is composed of arteries, veins, nerves, lymphatics, and the seminal duct.[22] It is located between the abdomen and the scrotum and is surrounded by three layers of fascia (Fig. 21-7).[21]

Blood flow to the testis is supplied by several arteries. The testicular arteries arise from the anterior aspect of the aorta just below the level of the renal arteries. They enter the spermatic cord at the internal inguinal ring with the other cord structures. At the posterior superior aspect of the testis the testicular artery divides into branches that pierce the tunica albuginea that run along the periphery of the

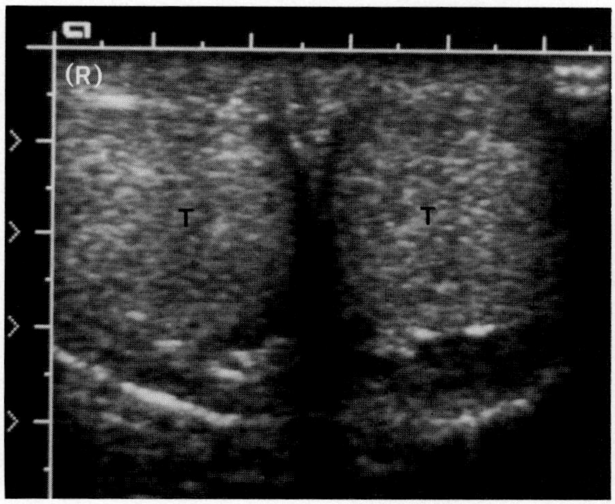

FIGURE 21-5. Transverse scan of normal bilateral testes (T) shows a homogeneous midline echogenicity (R, patient's right side).

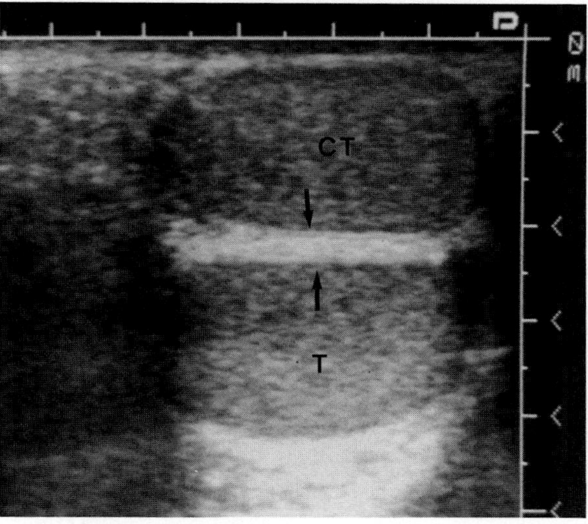

FIGURE 21-6. The normal testis (T) is seen on a longitudinal scan, and the contralateral testis (CT) is used as an acoustic window. The echogenic band (*arrows*) represents the scrotal septum.

testis in a layer known as the tunica vasculosa. These capsular arteries in the tunica vasculosa supply centripetal branches that enter the testicular parenchyma and run toward the mediastinum testis. At the mediastinum the centripetal arteries arborize into recurrent rami arteries that run in the opposite direction away from the mediastinum testis. The cremasteric and deferential arteries primarily supply the epididymis and peritesticular tissues; however, they also contribute a variable amount of blood to the testis via anastomoses with the testicular artery.[21,38] Venous drainage of the scrotum is via the pampiniform plexus, which empties into the cremasteric and internal spermatic veins (Fig. 21-7).[21] These veins drain into the inferior vena cava on the right and the left renal vein on the left.

Sperm travels in the seminal duct to the vas deferens, which then empties into the ejaculatory ducts.[21] The spermatic cords are bilateral and run between the scrotum and abdominal cavity in the inguinal canal.[21] Each spermatic cord lies above and parallel to the inguinal ligament and suspends the testis in the scrotum.[21] (The inguinal ligament lies just below the oblique fold seen on the anterior body surface between the abdomen and the leg.)

The sonographic appearance of the normal spermatic cords is of numerous linear structures, 1 to 2 mm in diameter.[22] The normal spermatic cord is less echogenic than the epididymis or the testis and the echo pattern is heterogeneous (Fig. 21-9).[44]

EPIDIDYMIS

The epididymides store small quantities of sperm prior to ejaculation, convey sperm from testis to seminal vesicles, and secrete a small portion of the seminal fluid.[1] They are bilateral and are divided anatomically into three parts: head, body, and tail. The head of the epididymis is called the globus major and is normally 7 to 8 mm in diameter,[28] the average overall dimensions being 7 × 11 × 6 mm.[31,44] The body (corpus) and the tail (cauda or globus minor) of the epididymis are normally 1 to 2 mm in diameter. With age, the organ shrinks. Small epididymides tend to be associated with small testes.[22] The head of each epididymis lies superior to the testis, the body posterior to it, and the tail posterior and inferior to the testis.[22,28]

The normal sonographic appearance of the epididymal head varies. On longitudinal scans it may have a triangular, crescent, or teardrop shape.[22,31]

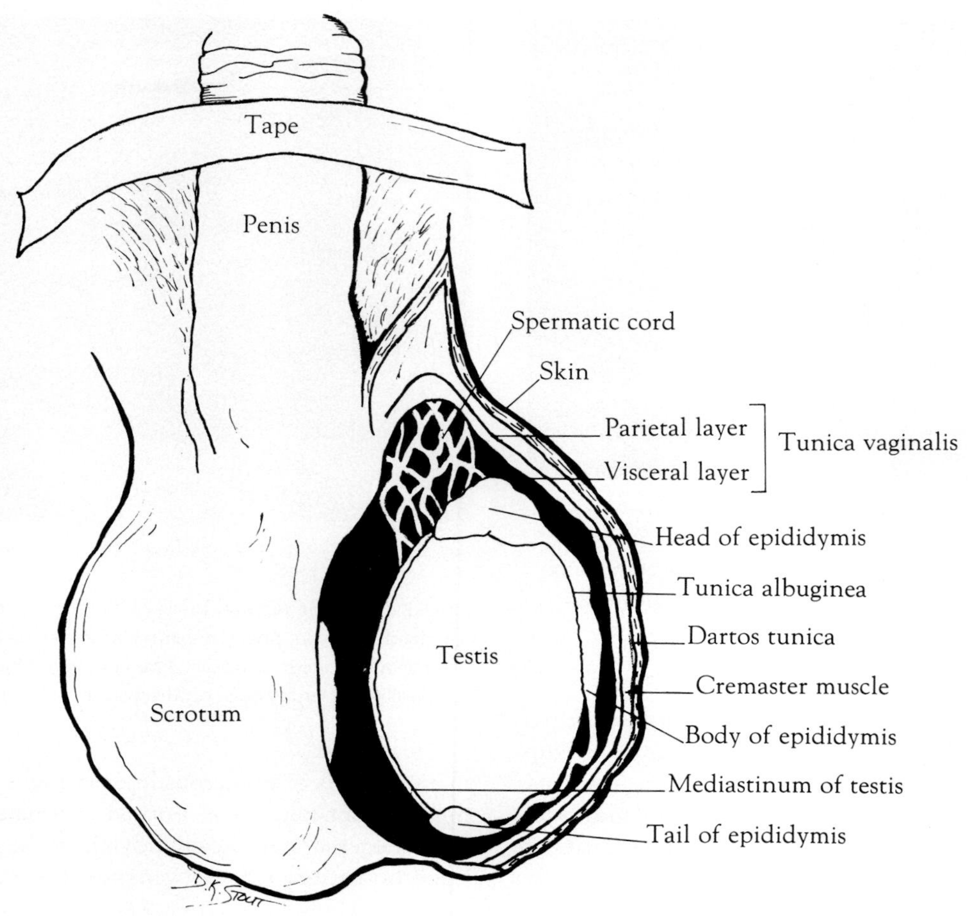

Figure 21-7. Schematic drawing of sagittal anatomic section of normal testis.

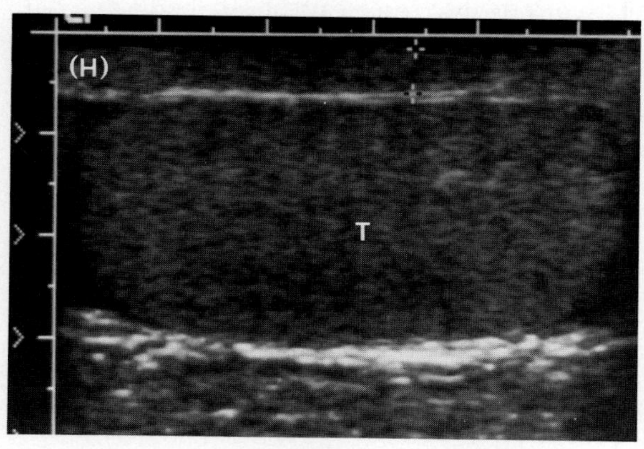

Figure 21-8. Longitudinal scan of normal testis (T). Cursors measure scrotal skin thickness (H, toward patient's head).

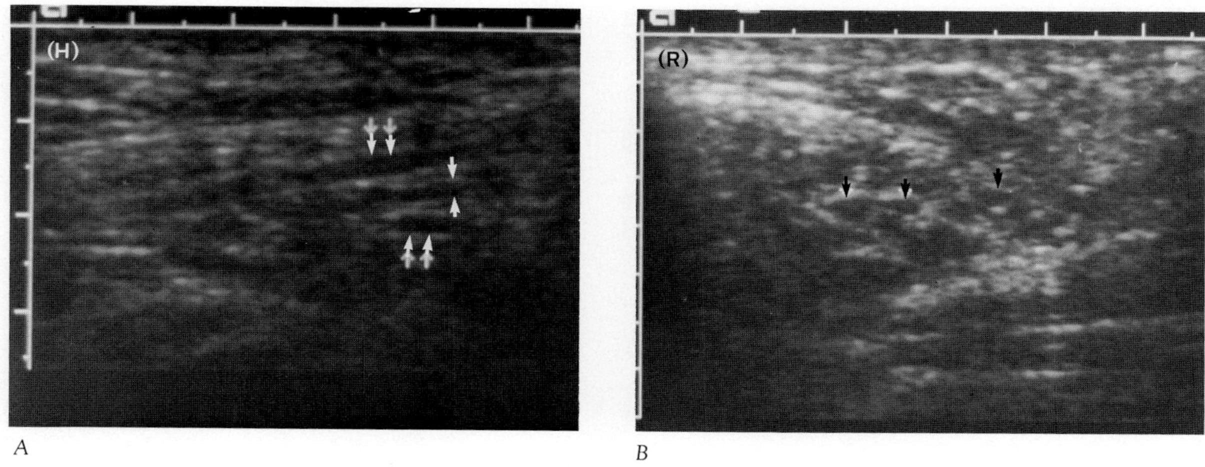

Figure 21-9. (*A*) The longitudinal sonogram of the normal spermatic cord shows the pampiniform plexus as numerous tubular hypoechoic structures *(arrows)* measuring 1 to 2 mm in diameter (H, toward patient's head). (*B*) In the transverse scan of the same normal spermatic cord, the pampiniform plexus is seen as ovoid hypoechoic structures (*arrows;* R, patient's right side).

The echogenicity of the normal epididymis is homogeneous, equal to or greater than that of the testis, but coarser (Fig. 21-10).[28,29]

A vasectomy is a common method of male contraception; therefore a significant proportion of men referred for sonography will have had a vasectomy. In a study conducted at the Royal Naval Hospital in the United Kingdom in 1988, Jarvis and Dubin scanned 31 men before and after a vasectomy. The sonographic appearance of the testis was unchanged after vasectomy. However, in 14 men (45%) there were persistent changes in the epididymis: all 14 had an enlarged epididymis, 11 patients had also developed cysts, and 5 had an inhomogeneous echo pattern. These sonographic changes were unrelated to symptoms. This study demonstrated three aspects of change in the epididymis seen after vasectomy: the epididymis increased in size, cysts were present, and the echogenicity of the epididymis was changed. The enlargement of the epididymis was consistent with congestion and dilatation of epididymal tubules seen pathologically.[27]

Testis

The testes' primary functions are the creation of sperm, which drains into the epididymides, and the secretion of hormones. Androgens, chiefly testosterone, are the main testicular hormones, and they determine male sex characteristics.[1]

The testes develop between the posterior abdominal wall and the peritoneum. The testes begin to pass through the inguinal ring during the seventh month of gestation and lie in the scrotum by the eighth month. During testicular descent, in the inguinal region, the caudal genital ligament is continous with a band of mesenchyme extending into the genital swellings. This mesenchyme band, including the caudal genital ligament, is known as the gubernaculum. The gubernaculum anchors the fetal testis to the inguinal region to prevent upward movement. The gubernaculum testis in the adult becomes much reduced and constitutes the scrotal ligament which extends from the inferior pole of the testis and the tail of the epididymis to the skin of the scrotal wall.[14,40]

As the testes descend, they become covered with

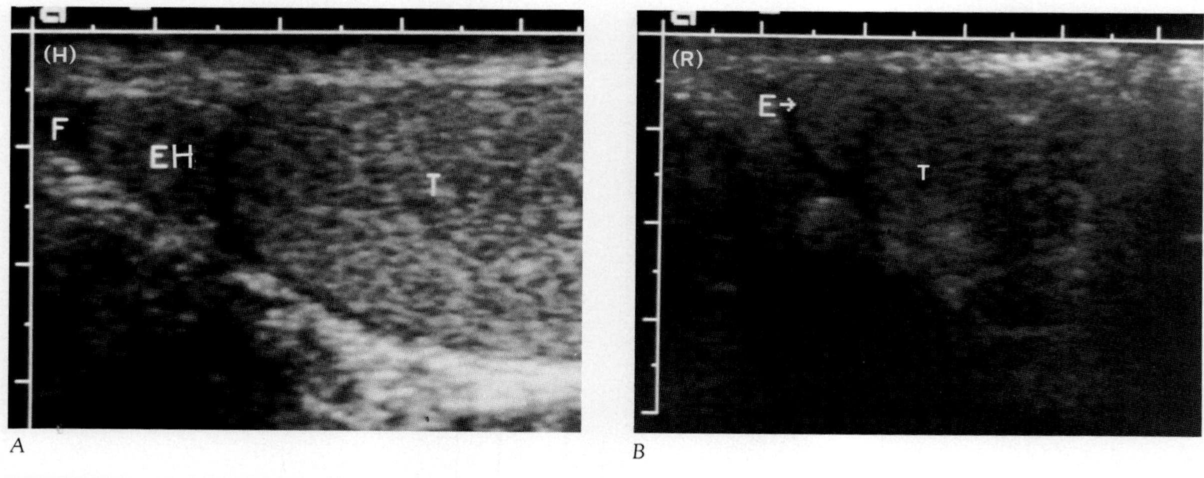

FIGURE 21-10. (*A*) Longitudinal sonogram of normal scrotal contents. The epididymal head (EH), superior to the testis'(T), is surrounded by a minimal amount of fluid (F; H, indicates toward patient's head). (*B*) Transverse scan of the same normal scrotum. The epididymal head (E) is superior and lateral to the testis (T; R, patient's right side).

a portion of peritoneum called the processus vaginalis. After birth, the processus vaginalis is referred to as the tunica vaginalis as it closes and forms a pouch within the scrotum which prevents abdominal contents from entering. The tunica vaginalis covers and surrounds the testis except on its posterior aspect in the region of the head of the epididymis (see Fig. 21-7).[10,41] Also, the tunica vaginalis contains a visceral layer, closely applied to the testis, and a parietal layer outside the visceral layer. A potential space exists between the visceral and parietal layer. In the normal scrotum, it is common to visualize small amounts (1 to 2 ml) of fluid surrounding the upper pole of the testis and the epididymal head (see Fig. 21-10).[28,31,41] If this space becomes abnormally enlarged, bowel can herniate into the potential space (scrotal hernia) and large amounts of serous fluid (hydrocele) or blood (hematocele) can accumulate in the space.[28]

The tunica albuginea is a fibrous capsule that covers the testes. A sagittal cross-section of the testis shows lobules (approximately 250) containing seminiferous tubules, which join straight seminiferous tubules, which drain into the rete testis, a series of anastomosing channels. The efferent ducts of the seminiferous tubules drain into the ductus epididymis.[28,41]

The mediastinum testis lies posterior and represents an invagination of tunica albuginea into the posterior testis and a coalescence of arteries, veins, and seminiferous tubules. In the longitudinal scanning plane, the sonographic appearance of the mediastinum testis is an echogenic line parallel to the epididymis, and it should not be mistaken for disease (Fig. 21-11). The appendix testis is a fibrous band superior to the testis, but usually it is seen only when a hydrocele is present (Fig. 21-12).[28]

The testes are bilateral and are normally located in the scrotum in adult males. The testicles of a fetus lie in the peritoneal cavity near the inguinal canal. Most boys' testes are descended at birth, but occasionally they descend later. The incidence of undescended testis in preterm infants is 30.3%, compared to 3.4% for term infants, and 0.8% 1 year after birth.[42] Because retraction of the cremaster muscle can give the appearance of undescended testis the best time to detect undescended testis is shortly after birth, when the cremasteric reflex is

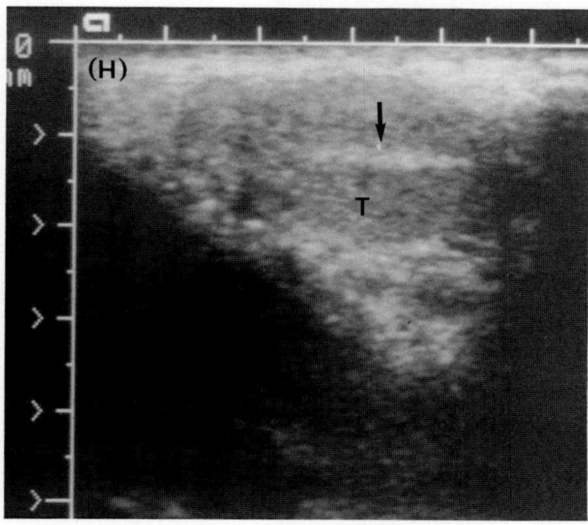

FIGURE 21-11. On this longitudinal sonogram, the mediastinum testis *(arrow)* is seen as an echogenic band running parallel to the testis (T; H, toward patient's head).

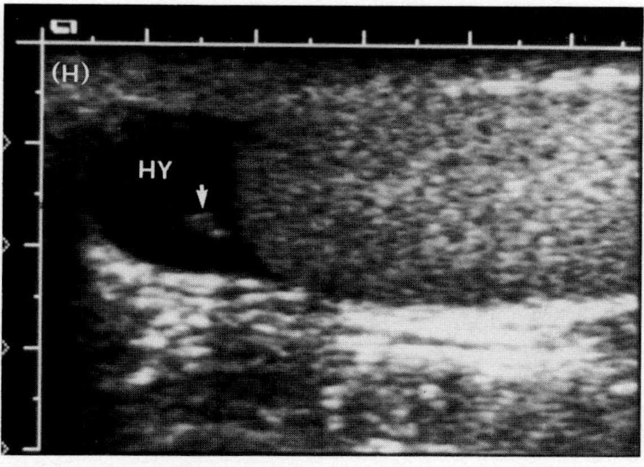

FIGURE 21-12. This longitudinal scan demonstrates a simple hydrocele (Hy). The appendix testis is clearly seen *(arrow)* as an echogenic protuberance superior to the testis (H, toward patient's head).

absent, the scrotum is relatively large, and there is minimal subcutaneous fat.[42]

The testicles attain maximum size around puberty. The normal size of adult testicles is 3 to 5 cm in length and 2 to 3 cm in both width and anteroposterior diameter (Figs. 21-13, 21-14).[21] The normal sonographic appearance of the testes is of ovoid structures of the size described above, which tend to shrink somewhat with age.[31] The testicles are of medium-level echogenicity and homogeneous texture (see Fig. 21-14).[12,31]

Sonography of Scrotal Disease

Common presenting symptoms for which ultrasound can assist in making a diagnosis include decreased size or absence of a testicle, acute painful scrotum, and scrotal or testicular mass. The common scrotal lesions are shown in Table 21-1.

DECREASE IN SIZE OF TESTIS

Decrease in the size of a testis may be a cause of infertility or a symptom of a pituitary tumor (the pituitary gland secretes a hormone that stimulates the testicles, and a tumor in the pituitary may stop the flow of testicle-stimulating hormones). Chronic testicular atrophy is usually painless, but acute testicular atrophy can be painful. Scrotal atrophy may be associated with infertility, renal transplantation, endocrine disease, senility, or schizophrenia.[19,21] Testicular atrophy can also be seen following testicular torsion or trauma.[22] The sonographic finding in testicular atrophy is of a small testicle that has a homogeneous echo texture and may be hypoechoic,[22] however, the epididymis is normal (Fig. 21-15).[28]

UNDESCENDED OR ABSENT TESTIS

Absence of a testicle may be an important finding, since an undescended testicle has 48 times the normal potential for development of cancer. An undescended testicle may also cause infertility, probably because the sperm are exposed to abnormally high temperatures.[28] When the undescended testis is located and brought into the scrotum by age 6, the chances of sterility are lessened.

Absence of a testicle may represent a congenital anomaly or an undescended testicle. Undescended testes are bilateral in 10% of cases. An undescended testicle is in the inguinal canal 80% of the time and in the peritoneal cavity 20% of the time.[28] Undescended testis occurs in 30.3% of premature infants,

(text continues on page 592)

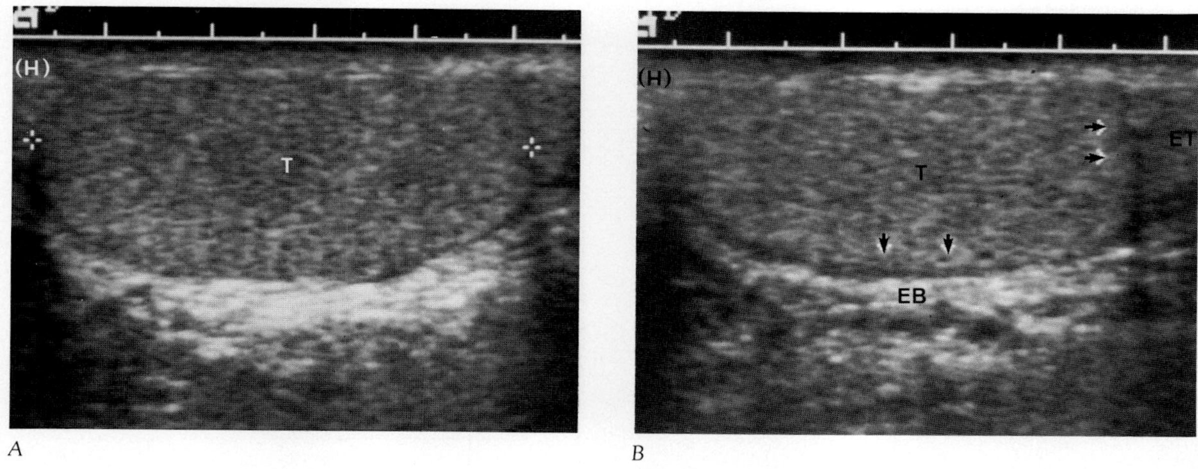

FIGURE 21-13. (*A*) Longitudinal sonogram of a normal testis (T) shows the homogeneous normal echogenicity of the testis. Cursors placed inferior and superior measure the length of the testis (H, toward patient's head). (*B*) This longitudinal sonogram of the same normal testis (T) shows the body (EB) and tail (ET) of the epididymis (H, toward patient's head).

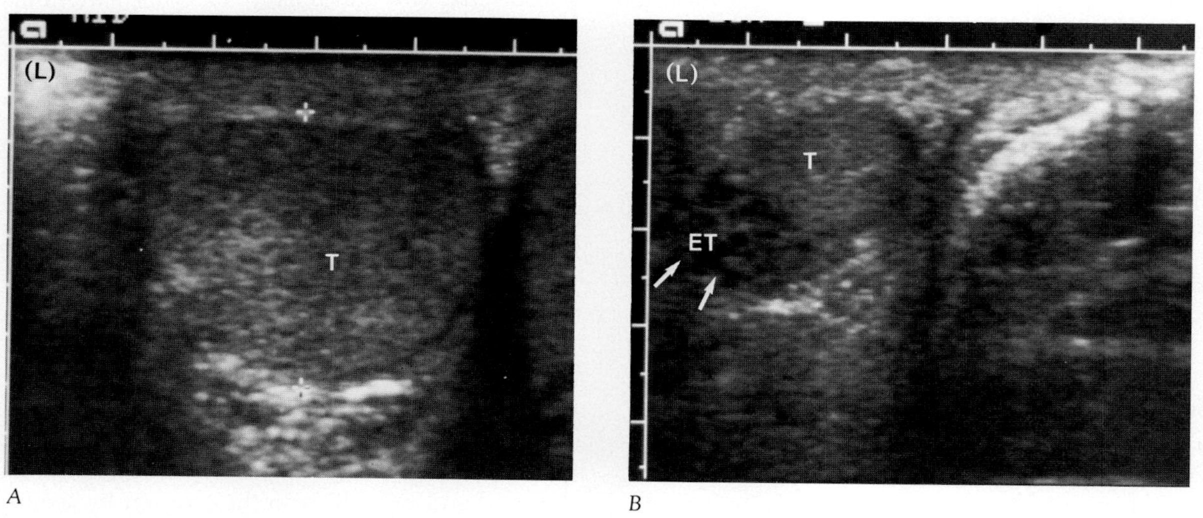

FIGURE 21-14. (*A*) On this transverse sonogram of a normal testis (T), cursors measure the width of the midportion of the testis. (Since the patient is supine, the width appears in the vertical dimension.) (L, lateral aspect of the testis.) (*B*) A lower transverse sonogram of the same testis (T) shows the tail of the epididymis (ET and *arrows;* L, lateral aspect of testis).

Table 21-1. Sonographic appearance of scrotal lesions

Lesion	Sonographic Appearance	Reference
Spermatic Cord		
Varicocele	Tubular, serpiginous, anechoic fluid collection in the region of the epididymis	21, 23, 24
Hematoma/seroma	Discrete, heterogeneous areas of increased and decreased echoes that extend the length of the cord	13
Sperm granuloma	Focal hypoechoic solid mass	23
Hydrocele	Anterior fluid collections along the cord	13
Hernia	Complex mass with echogenic and anechoic areas representing air- and fluid-filled segments of bowel; characteristic haustral appearance and peristalsis	19, 41
Benign neoplasms		
Lipoma	Solid, homogeneous mass with medium to low echo intensity, distinct from both testis and epididymis	13
Adenomatoid tumor	Solid mass, variable echogenicity, equal to or greater than that of testis	8, 21, 23, 42
Hemangioma, cholesteatoma, leiomyoma	Solid mass, variable echogenicity, hyperechoic to hypoechoic	8
Malignant neoplasms from the mesenchyme: fibrosarcoma, liposarcoma, rhabdomyosarcoma	Solid, heterogeneous echo texture with echogenic areas and focal anechoic areas of necrosis	13, 19
Epididymis		
Epididymitis	Enlargement of the epididymis with variable echogenicity, depending on the stage of the disease; normal testis; a reactive hydrocele is often seen, with scrotal skin thickening	1, 19
Acute	Epididymis enlarged with diffuse hypoechogenicity	5, 11, 21, 22, 23
Chronic	Epididymis enlarged, focal or diffuse hyperechogenicity; tunica thickened; shadowing from calcification may be seen	11, 22, 23, 42
Spermatocele	Cystic mass with well-defined walls and few internal echoes secondary to spermatozoa or debris in the region of the epididymis, most often in the globus major; unilocular or multilocular	19, 11
Epididymal cyst	Anechoic cystic mass with well-defined walls occurring anywhere along the epididymis	19, 22, 23, 25, 35
Tuberculosis	Epididymal enlargement with diffuse or focal areas of hypoechogenicity	19, 31
Sarcoidosis	Epididymal enlargement with solid, irregular, hypoechoic focal areas; foci of high-level echoes with shadowing caused by calcification may be seen	19
Sperm granuloma	Solid hypoechoic mass	19, 23
Abscess	Complex intrascrotal mass with focal or diffuse areas of inhomogeneity and increased echogenicity, usually in tail of the epididymis	19, 21
Adenomatoid tumor	Solid mass, well-circumscribed, with variable echogenicity, hyperechoic to hypoechoic	8, 21, 23, 24

(continued)

Table 21-1. Sonographic appearance of scrotal lesions *(continued)*

Lesion	Sonographic Appearance	Reference
Tunica Vaginalis		
Simple hydrocele	Echo-free fluid collection anterolateral to testis with strong sound transmission	8, 19, 21, 23
Chronic hydrocele	Sonolucent fluid collection anterolateral to testis with echogenic septations, calcification, and diffuse scrotal wall thickening	19, 21
Scrotal calculus in hydrocele (simple or chronic)	Highly echogenic spherical focus with associated acoustic shadowing moving freely in the hydrocele	19, 26
Acute hematocele	Anechoic fluid collection with distal acoustic enhancement	21, 36
Chronic hematocele	Thickened tunica vaginalis with dense fibrous tissue, appearing as a thick-walled fluid collection; indistinguishable from chronic hydrocele or abscess	21, 36
Pyocele	Thick hemiscrotal wall; echogenic fluid collection with septations and occasionally focal mural calcifications; similar to chronic hydroceles and hematoceles	23, 36
Hematoma	Appearance of hematoma varies with age; acutely, the scrotal wall is thickened; after 2–3 days, hypoechoic areas are seen (liquefaction); extratesticular hematoma can be solid or septate cystic mass	19, 22, 36
Abscess	Complex intrascrotal mass with focal hypoechoic or mixed areas	19, 21, 22
Tunica albuginea cyst	Defined anechoic area(s) with posterior enhancement	13, 19
Testicular Focal—Benign		
Hematoma	Appearance of hematoma varies with time: Early it is hyperechoic; after 2–3 days, hypoechoic areas (liquefaction)	19, 36
Rupture	Irregular tunica with focal hypoechoic areas early, which become hyperechoic with time	22, 31, 36
Abscess	Complex intrascrotal mass with focal hypoechoic or mixed areas	19, 21, 22
Focal orchitis	Focal hypoechoic mass	8, 16, 21
Liquefactive necrosis (seen in subacute torsion)	Focal echofree areas	5, 8
Focal ischemic infarction (following infection and torsion)	Initially hypoechoic; becomes hyperechoic with age	5, 8, 19, 22
Adenomatoid tumor	Uniform hyperechoic or isoechoic solid mass with well-defined margin	19, 42
Sarcoidosis	Solid, focal hyperechoic mass	19, 23
Sperm granuloma	Hypoechoic solid mass	19, 23
Benign gonadal stromal tumors (Leydig, Sertoli)	Focal, hyperechoic solid mass	8, 19

TABLE 21-1. *(continued)*

LESION	SONOGRAPHIC APPEARANCE	REFERENCE
Epidermoid cysts	Cystic mass with well-defined echogenic walls; may have calcifications appearing as echogenic foci	19
Dermoid cyst	May simulate simple cyst or may have echogenic areas along periphery; occasionally cyst itself is echogenic	19
Cystadenoma	Multiseptate cystic mass	19
Testicular Diffuse—Benign		
Orchitis	Enlarged, diffusely hypoechoic testis	11, 19
Infarcts (after trauma, infection, and torsion)	Small, diffusely hypoechoic testis	6, 8, 23
Granulomatous disease	Enlarged, irregular, hypoechoic testis; may have calcifications	19
Sarcoidosis	Echogenic irregular testis; may have calcifications	19
Acquired atrophy	Small, hypoechoic testis	19, 21
Testicular Focal—Malignant		
Seminoma	Uniformly hypoechoic mass; may have scattered hyperechoic areas; echogenic band representing pseudocapsule often surrounds mass	7, 8, 16, 37
Embryonal cell	Hypoechoic mass, less well-circumscribed than seminoma; texture is heterogeneous with areas of hemorrhagic necrosis or cystic change	8, 11, 16, 23
Choriocarcinoma	Complex mass with areas of increased echogenicity representing hemorrhage, necrosis, and calcification	8, 16, 23
Teratocarcinoma	Complex mass may have sonolucent and echogenic components reflecting heterogeneous composition	8, 11, 16, 23
Teratoma	Complex mass with multiple cystic areas representing bone, cartilage, smooth muscle and other tissues	11, 23, 31, 37
Lymphoma	Enlarged testis with focal areas of decreased echogenicity	8, 11, 31
Leukemia	Enlarged testis with focal areas of decreased echogenicity	16, 31
Metastases	Multiple hypoechoic (less often echogenic) masses; rarely, both are seen together	8, 23
Testicular Diffuse—Malignant		
Leukemia	Enlarged, hypoechoic testes	8, 16, 23
Lymphoma	Enlarged, hypoechoic testes	8, 16, 23
Diffuse embryonal cell	Enlarged, hypoechoic testis with irregular margins and focal echogenic areas due to hemorrhage or necrosis	8, 11, 16, 23, 31
Diffuse seminoma	Enlarged, hypoechoic testis with irregular or lumpy margins	31, 37

but in only 3.4% of normal term infants. Undescended testis is present in only 0.28% of adult men.[25]

The sonographic appearance of an absent testicle depends on the cause. In congenital absence, no testicle is seen. With undescended testicle, ultrasound may show a soft tissue mass in the inguinal canal or the peritoneal cavity with an oval or elongated shape. The undescended testicle may be mobile on palpation or under the transducer. It is usually smaller than the normal testicle but has normal echogenicity (Fig. 21-16).[22,25,28]

High-resolution ultrasound has an accuracy of 91% in locating undescended testis.[28] Because ultrasound is relatively inexpensive and delivers no ionizing radiation, it should be the initial imaging method for undescended testis, with adjunctive CT or MRI when sonography cannot definitively localize the testis.[28] In some cases, enlarged lymph nodes may mimic an undescended testis on ultrasound or the body habitus of the patient may make ultrasound technically inadequate.[13] CT produces excellent delineation of undescended testis, but it has the disadvantages of radiation and cost, and boys younger than 5 years must be sedated. MRI has an accuracy of 94% in locating undescended

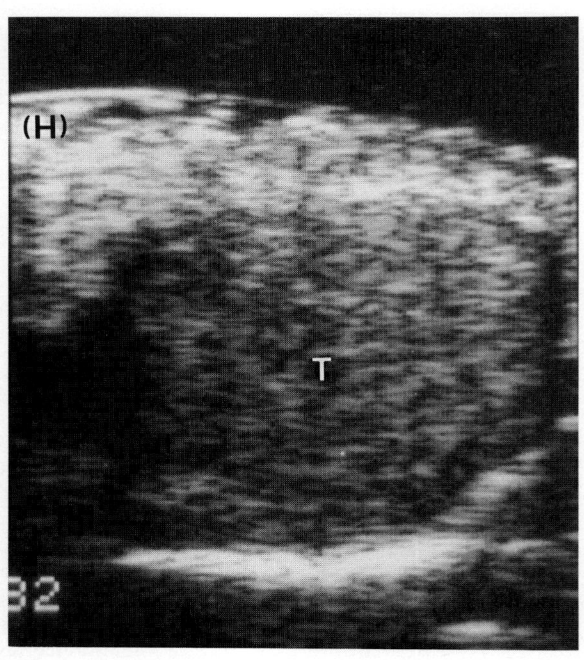

FIGURE 21-15. The longitudinal sonogram of this atrophic testis (T) shows a small, hypoechoic gland (H, toward patient's head).

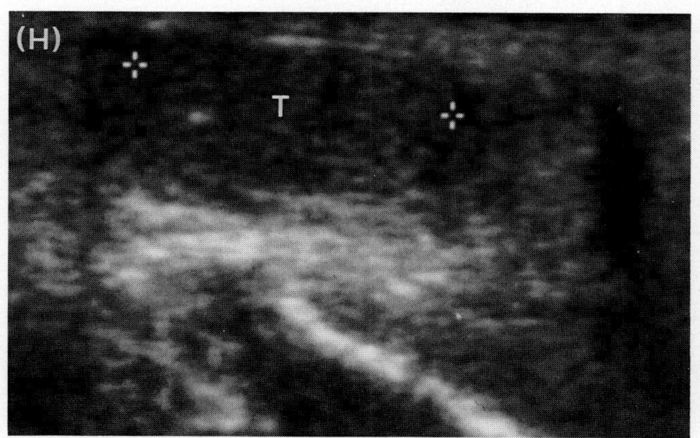

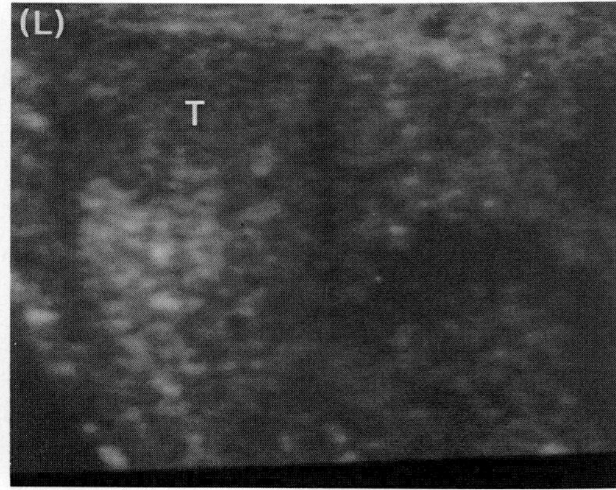

FIGURE 21-16. (*A*) Longitudinal sonogram shows a small, undescended testis (T) located in the inguinal canal. The echogenicity is homogeneous, with medium-level echoes (H, toward patient's head). (*B*) A small, undescended testis (T) in the inguinal canal in a transverse scan is ovoid (L, lateral aspect of testis).

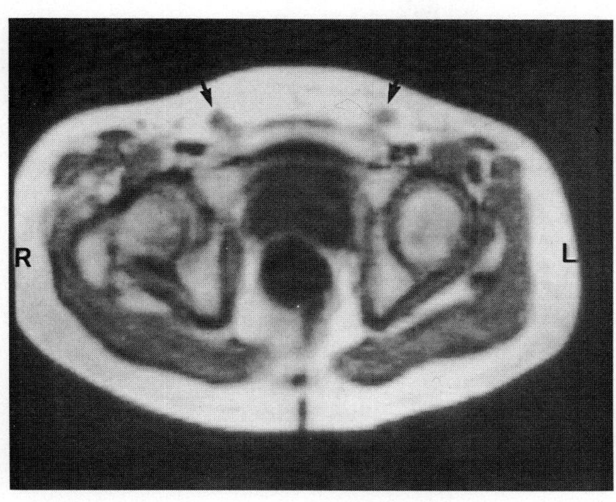

Figure 21-17. On this transaxial MR image, undescended testes *(arrows)* are seen in the inguinal canals bilaterally.

testis (Fig. 21-17).[13] Like ultrasound, MRI uses no ionizing radiation and can provide multiplanar imaging.[3] MRI is, however, more expensive than ultrasound and requires sedation for children younger than 5 years, to minimize motion during the long examination.

Acute Painful Scrotum

Acute painful scrotum is often a serious presenting symptom. Epididymitis is the most common cause of the acute painful scrotum. It is critical to differentiate patients with epididymitis from those with suspected torsion. Grey-scale sonography with color flow Doppler is the diagnostic tool of choice in assessing perfusion to the testis and distinguishing inflammatory from ischemic processes. With prompt diagnosis, conditions such as ischemic necrosis and abscess can be surgically corrected to preserve testicular viability and function.[35,37]

Causes of acute painful scrotum include torsion (spermatic cord torsion), rupture, epididymitis, epididymoorchitis, and abscess. Since arterial flow is occluded and only surgical restoration of blood flow can prevent loss of the testicle, testicular torsion is a surgical emergency. Abscess is also a surgical emergency, since drainage of an abscess can prevent loss of the testicle. Epididymitis is painful, but antibiotic treatment resolves the symptoms fairly rapidly. Left untreated, epididymitis may develop into an abscess.[22]

Testicular Torsion

Testicular torsion (twisting) represents 20% of the scrotal disease in postpubertal males.[28] It is due to a developmental weakness of the mesenteric attachment from the spermatic cord onto the testis and epididymis (Fig. 21-18). A short mesenteric attachment allows the testis to fall forward within the scrotum and rotate freely, like a swing on a rope.[42] Treatment to correct testicular torsion must occur within 6 hours, to avoid irreversible damage to the testis.[45]

Although testicular torsion may occur at any age, it is most common during adolescence, between age 12 and 18 years.[42] Because of the twisted cord, a rotated testis sits higher in the scrotum than the normal contralateral one.[6] There are two types

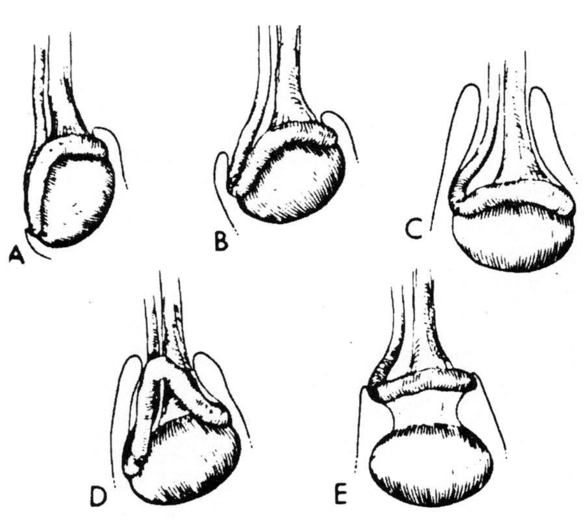

Figure 21-18. Attachment and suspension of the testis: (*A*) Normal attachment and suspension of the processus vaginalis. (*B–D*) Variations in the bell-and-clapper deformity of the mesenteric attachment of the epididymal pedicle to the testis. (*E*) Abnormal attachment of the pedicle between the epididymis and the testis. (From Allen TD: Disorders of the male external genitalia. *In* Kelalis PP, King LR (eds): Clinical Pediatric Urology. Philadelphia, WB Saunders, 1985.)

of testicular torsion. In the intravaginal type, the torsion is of the spermatic cord only. Extravaginal torsion involves twisting of the spermatic cord and the tunica vaginalis. Intravaginal testicular torsion can be seen in children or adults, but it is more common in children. Extravaginal testicular torsion usually occurs in newborns.[28]

Clinical signs of testicular torsion include sudden onset of severe pain, which usually begins when the patient is at rest or asleep. Nausea and vomiting accompany the pain in 50% of cases. Also in 50% of cases, the symptoms mimic epididymitis.[22,25,28] After 24 to 48 hours the pain usually disappears, generally indicating that the testicle is dead. In newborns, testicular torsion may present with only painless swelling and redness.[28]

The sonographic findings in testicular torsion vary as the time from the onset of the torsion increases. Bird divides testicular torsion into acute (24 hours' duration or less), subacute (24 hours to 10 days), and chronic (more than 10 days).[6]

The sonographic appearance of acute testicular torsion also has subphases. At 1 to 2 hours, Doppler ultrasound shows decreased arterial flow. A critical element that differentiates acute torsion from acute epididymitis is that in testicular torsion, flow in the cord is decreased or diminished, whereas, in acute epididymitis, blood flow in the cord is increased.[25] At 1 to 6 hours, ultrasound shows epididymal and testicular enlargement. The testis shows decreased echogenicity, which is accompanied by scrotal skin thickening and sometimes by hydrocele.[6,25] In a study by Middleton and associates in 1990 at the Mallinckrodt Institute of radiology in St. Louis, Missouri, using color Doppler, five of seven patients with surgically confirmed torsion with symptoms lasting less than six hours had no intratesticular flow and had normal testicular parenchyma.[37] The accuracy of color Doppler sonography in detecting absent intratesticular flow in acute torsion is 97% accurate and therefore is the preferred imaging modality for patients with suspected acute torsion.[8] At 24 hours to 10 days (subacute torsion), the testis and epididymis are enlarged. Sonography also shows a hypoechoic testis with localized anechoic areas, which represent liquefactive necrotic areas in the testis.[6] The epididymis has foci of increased and decreased echogenicity (Fig. 21-19).[6] With color Doppler sonography, patients with delayed torsion more than 24 hours (non-salvageable testis) will show peritesticular hyperemia and absent intratesticular flow.[8,37] After 10 days (chronic torsion), ultrasound shows a small hypoechoic testis with a large, uniformly echogenic epididymis (Fig. 21-20).[6]

TESTICULAR RUPTURE

Testicular rupture is rare.[46] It occurs when the capsule (the tunica albuginea, a fibrous band that surrounds the testis) is torn by trauma.[26,46] Testicular rupture is associated with athletic injuries and industrial and vehicular accidents.[46] Early diagnosis is critical. Within 72 hours, the salvageability rate is 90%; later it drops to 45%.[22,46] Surgical treatment is either repair of the tunica albuginea or orchiectomy.[46] Failure to repair the testis may result in the loss of spermatogenesis and hormonal function, chronic scrotal pain, and secondary anaerobic infection (scrotal gangrene).[46]

Sonographic findings in testicular rupture may include an irregular fibrous capsule (tunica albuginea), extrusion of the testicular contents into the scrotal sac, hematocele between the tunica vaginalis and parietalis,[46] and intratesticular hematoma or infarction (which appears on the sonogram as hypoechoic or hyperechoic focal abnormalities in the testicle; Fig. 21-21).[26,41] In general, acute scrotal hematoma manifests as increased scrotal wall thickness.[25] Owing to liquefaction of the hematoma, hypoechoic focal areas within the testis or scrotal wall can be seen after 3 days.[25] Disruption of testicular echogenicity, with focal hyperechoic and hypoechoic areas in the testicle, along with an ill-defined tunica albuginea, must be considered suggestive of testicular rupture.[46]

EPIDIDYMITIS AND EPIDIDYMOORCHITIS

Epididymitis (inflammation of the epididymis) represents 75% of all acute inflammatory processes in the scrotum.[22,35] The most common cause is bacterial infection, but a number are idiopathic.[45] Bacterial epididymitis arises through the spread of organisms from an infection of the lower urinary tract, especially prostatitis.[22,35] Less frequently, epididymitis can be seen following trauma.[45] Epididymitis can affect the head, body, or tail of the epididymis or the entire organ. The inflamed

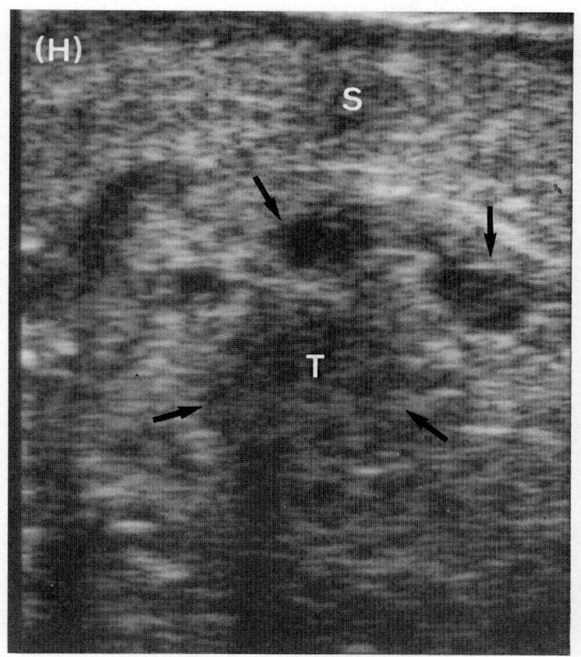

FIGURE 21-19. Early subacute testicular torsion. The longitudinal sonogram demonstrates a diffusely enlarged testis (T) with hypoechoic focal areas *(arrows)* representing hemorrhage and liquefactive necrosis. There is prominent scrotal skin thickening (S; H, toward patient's head).

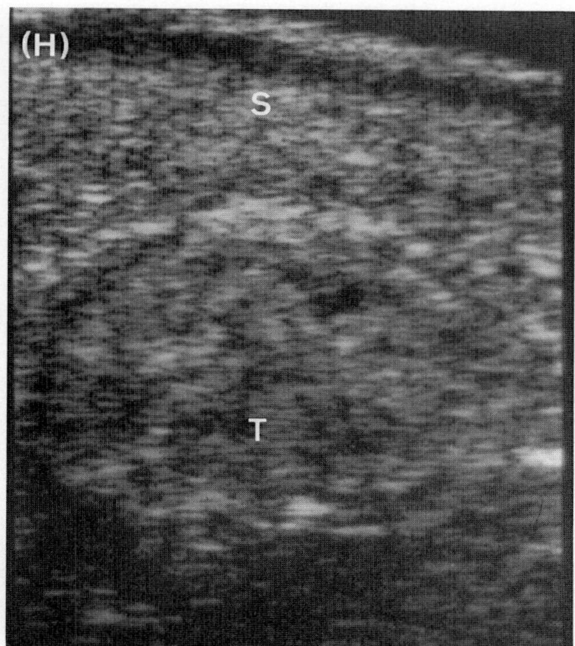

FIGURE 21-20. This longitudinal sonogram of a patient with chronic testicular torsion shows a small, hypoechoic testis (T) with minimal scrotal skin thickening (S; H, toward patient's head).

FIGURE 21-21. The longitudinal sonogram of a testicular rupture shows the site of fragmentation *(black arrows)*. Intratesticular hypoechoic areas *(small arrows)* represent subsequent hemorrhage. Normal testicular parenchyma is seen on either side of the hematoma (He). The tunica albuginea *(small, open arrows)* is ill-defined (H, toward patient's head). (Courtesy Richard H. Steinberg, Daytona Beach, FL.)

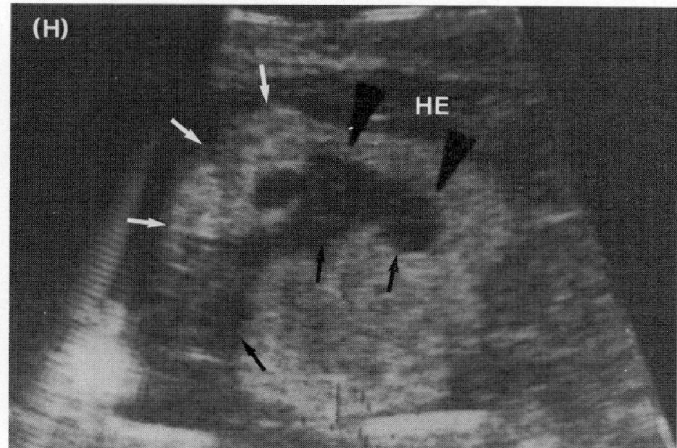

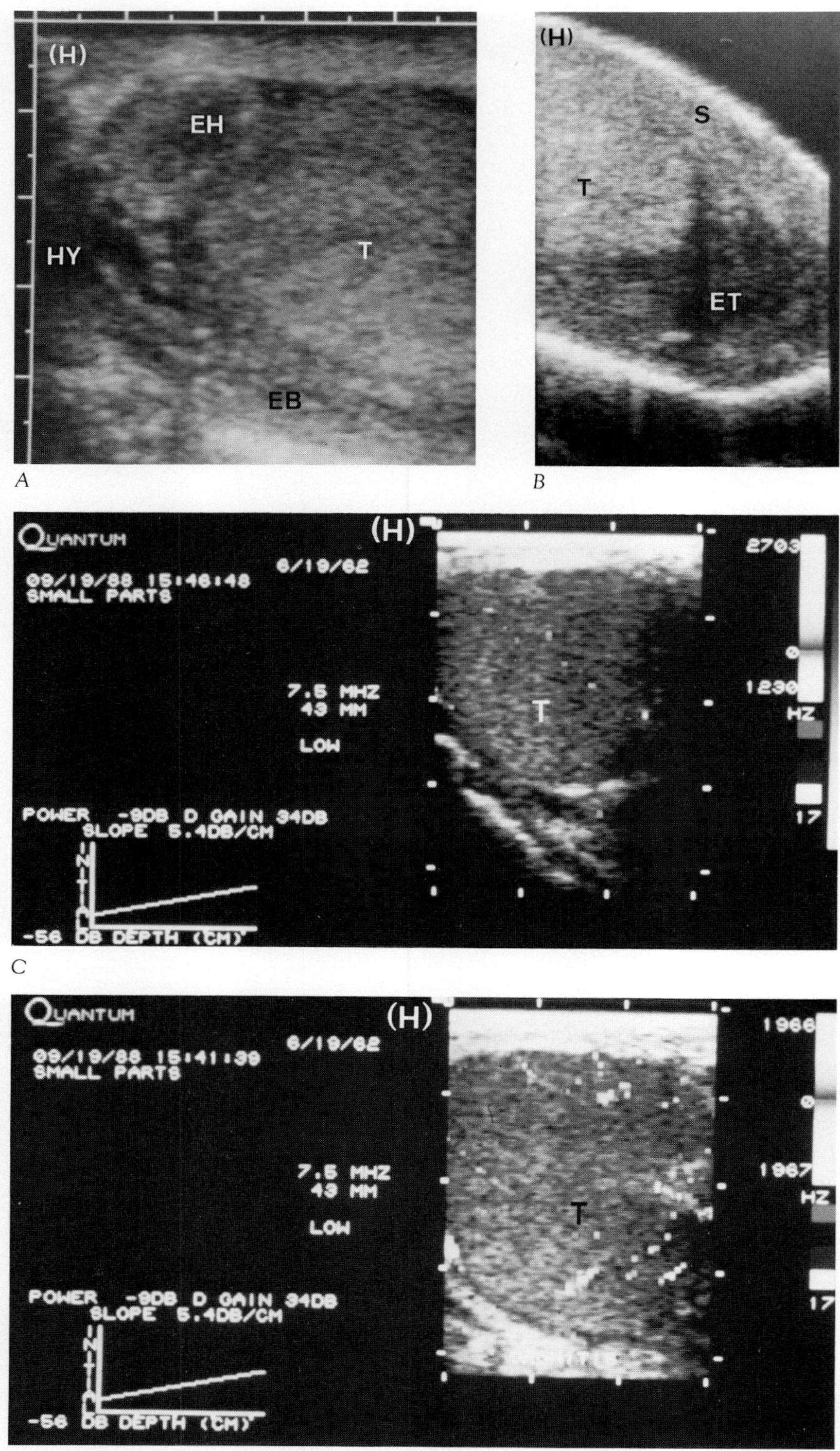
(H)
EH
HY
T
EB
A
(H)
S
T
ET
B
QUANTUM
(H)
09/19/88 15:46:48
SMALL PARTS
6/19/62
7.5 MHZ
43 MM
LOW
T
2703
0
1230
HZ
17
POWER -9DB D GAIN 34DB
SLOPE 5.4DB/CM
-56 DB DEPTH (CM)
C
QUANTUM
(H)
09/19/88 15:41:39
SMALL PARTS
6/19/62
7.5 MHZ
43 MM
LOW
T
1966
0
1967
HZ
17
POWER -9DB D GAIN 34DB
SLOPE 5.4DB/CM
-56 DB DEPTH (CM)
D

epididymis is tense and swollen. Epididymitis is usually unilateral but can be bilateral.[35] The epididymis is usually palpable as a hard cord posterior to the testis. If epididymitis is not treated, it may progress to involve the testis, producing epididymoorchitis (inflammation of both epididymis and testicle).[22]

Epididymoorchitis represents 15% of the acute inflammatory processes of the scrotum.[35] Untreated, acute epididymoorchitis may progress to abscess formation.[22] Epididymitis and epididymoorchitis are most common after puberty.[28] Clinical signs include fever, a swollen, tense, and tender epididymis, and hemiscrotum.

Sonographic findings of acute epididymitis, epididymoorchitis, and orchitis are enlargement and decreased echogenicity of the affected structure (Fig. 21-22).[22,25,28] With chronic epididymitis and epididymoorchitis, increased echogenicity may be seen, probably secondary to microabscesses.[22] The tunica albuginea becomes thickened, and shadowing from calcifications may be seen. Other sonographic findings include scrotal skin thickening and a reactive hydrocele (fluid between the parietalis and vaginalis fascia). In patients with epididymitis, epididymoorchitis, and isolated orchitis, color Doppler will show increased blood flow due to tissue hyperemia.[37] With focal orchitis, there are areas of decreased echogenicity and patchy hyperemia (increased flow) using color Doppler (Fig. 21-23).[23] In epididymitis, the testicle is usually sonographically normal[35]; however, if the inflammation is severe enough, testicular infarcts or diffuse testicular infarction may be seen.[5] Testicular infarcts appear sonographically as focal hypoechoic masses; with time, they show echogenic areas representing fibrosis. Diffuse testicular infarction shows a small, hypoechoic testis.[9]

In severe chronic epididymoorchitis, sonography of the testicle shows focal hypoechoic or mixed areas, which represent abscesses (Fig. 21-24).[26] If the abscess involves the entire scrotum, the epididymis and testis may be replaced by a complex mass and may be indistinguishable (Fig. 21-24C).[22] This appearance is often seen with chronic tuberculous epididymoorchitis, discussed later.[22] In chronic or recurrent epididymoorchitis, calcifications may be present, which appear on the sonogram as areas of increased echogenicity in the epididymis and tunica vaginalis (Fig. 21-24D).[22]

Scrotal or Testicular Mass

A scrotal or testicular mass can be an ominous sign. Both benign and malignant lesions can present as scrotal masses. Because the majority of intratesticular lesions are malignant, it is especially important to differentiate intratesticular from extratesticular lesions. In practice, intratesticular lesions are considered malignant until proven otherwise.[28] Having 90 to 95% accuracy in differentiating intratesticular from extratesticular masses, ultrasound is especially effective in the evaluation of scrotal masses.[28]

Benign Scrotal Masses

Benign scrotal masses include hydrocele, spermatocele, varicocele, scrotal hernia, abscess, hematoma, hematocele, pyocele, granulomatous disease, tunica albuginea cyst, epididymal cyst, intratesticular cyst, and sperm granuloma.

Figure 21-22. (*A*) The longitudinal scan shows a normal testis (T). The patient has epididymitis. The epididymal head (EH) and body (EB) are diffusely enlarged, with both increased and decreased echogenicity, representing inflammation, and a small, reactive hydrocele (Hy). There is minimal scrotal skin thickening (H, toward patient's head). (*B*) A longitudinal scan low in the testis (T) of a patient with epididymitis shows an enlarged, hypoechoic epididymal tail (ET) with scrotal skin thickening (S). (C) Color-flow Doppler study (angiodynography) in the longitudinal plane of a normal scrotum demonstrates normal vascular flow to the testis (T; H, toward patient's head). (*D*) On a longitudinal color-flow Doppler sonogram of a patient with orchitis, the testis (T) is diffusely enlarged, with increased vascular flow and minimal scrotal skin thickening (H, toward patient's head). (*C*, *D*, Courtesy of Kay Lambert, Quantum Medical Systems.)

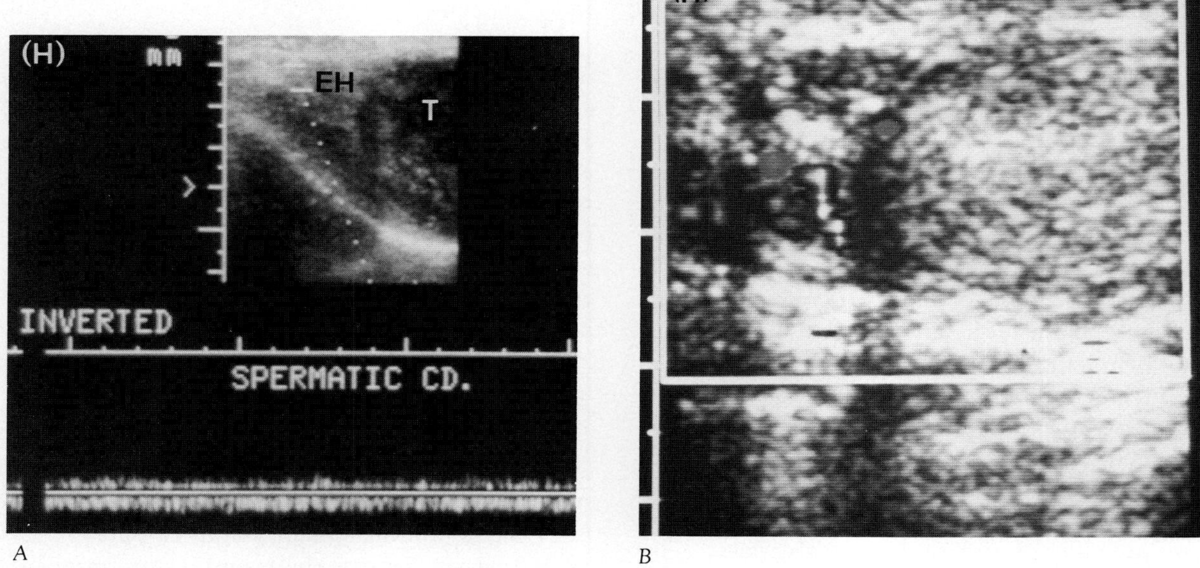

FIGURE 21-23. (*A*) This longitudinal scan using conventional pulsed-wave Doppler and spectral analysis samples the spermatic cord just proximal to the epididymal head (EH). In this patient with diffuse enlargement and complex echogenicity of the testis (T) and epididymis, the spectrum shows increased flow in the cord. This helps to differentiate inflammatory processes from testicular torsion, which would show no flow in the cord (H, toward patient's head). (*B*) Color-flow Doppler study in a patient with epididymitis. The epididymis is enlarged. Vascular flow in the epididymal head is increased, indicating that this is inflammation, not torsion (H, toward patient's head). (Courtesy Kathy Cislo, Acuson.)

FIGURE 21-24. (*A*) The longitudinal scan of epididymoorchitis with microabscess in the epididymal head and intratesticular abscess shows the epididymal head (EH) is enlarged, with areas of increased (microabscesses) and decreased echogenicity. A testicular abscess (TA) is just inferior to the epididymal head (H, toward patient's head). (*B*) The transverse scan of the same testis shows a large, complex mass representing intratesticular abscess (Ab) with a border of normal-looking medium-level echoes—the unaffected testis (T; R, patient's right side). (C) On this transverse scan of a trauma patient with epididymoorchitis, there is prominent scrotal skin thickening (S), enlargement of the head of the epididymis (EH) with focal areas of hypo- and hyperechogenicity representing early abscess formation *(arrows)*, and a reactive hydrocele (Hy; R, patient's right side; T, testicle). (*D*) On this longitudinal scan of a patient with recurrent epididymoorchitis there is scrotal skin thickening (S) and enlargement of the epididymal head (EH) with areas of increased and decreased echogenicity *(arrows)* suggesting early abscess formation. An echogenic band *(open arrows)* represents thickening of the visceral and parietal layers of the tunica vaginalis. Thickening of the tunica is characteristic of recurrent epididymoorchitis. Fluid (Hy) superior to the testis represents a reactive hydrocele, which is often associated with inflammatory processes.

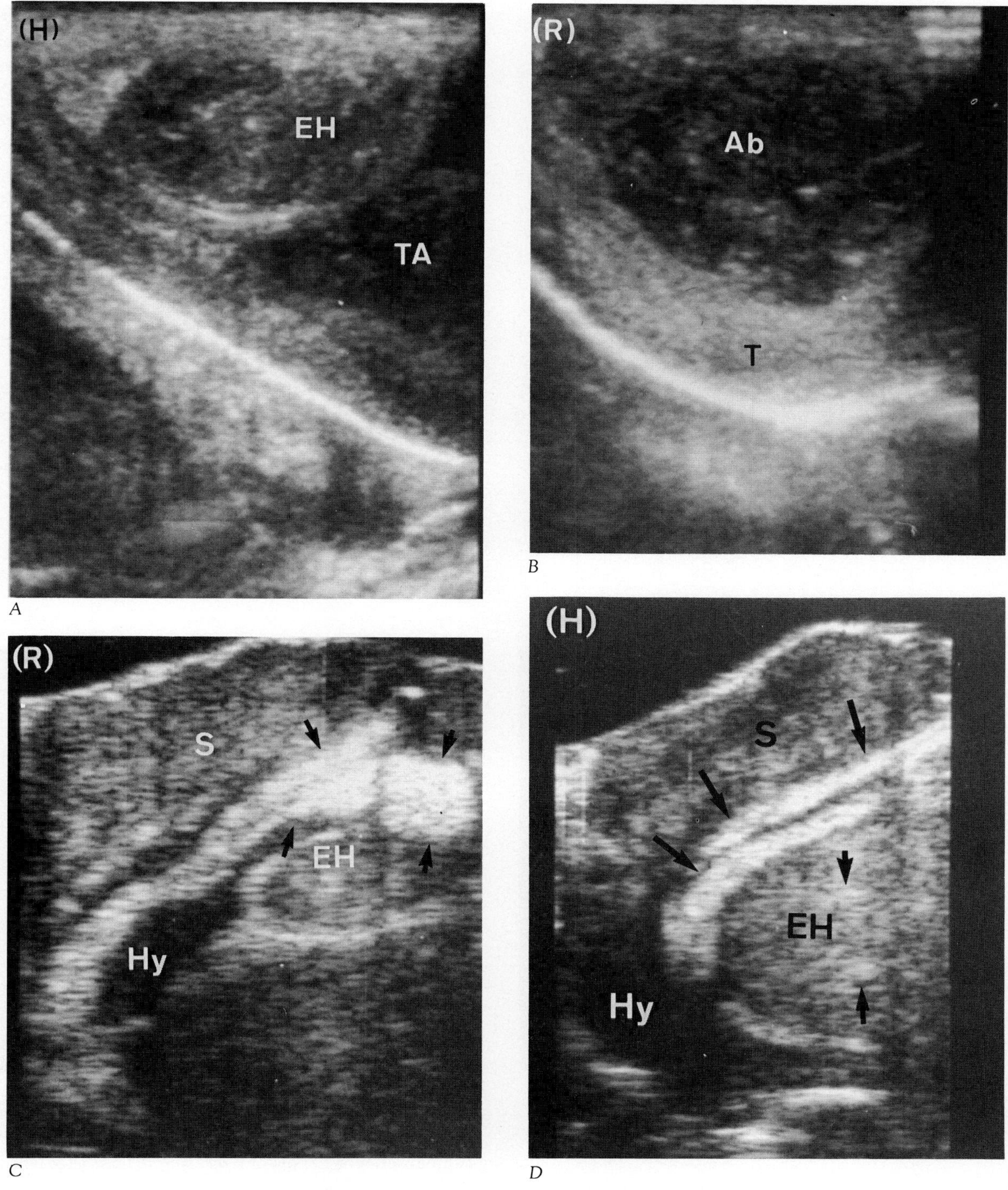
(H)
EH
TA
A
(R)
Ab
T
B
(R)
S
EH
Hy
C
(H)
S
EH
Hy
D

Hydrocele. A hydrocele is an abnormal accumulation of serous fluid in the potential space between the visceral and parietal layers of the tunica vaginalis, which surround the testis.[25,28] Hydroceles, the most common fluid collection of the scrotum,[35] occur in both children and adults. Hydrocele is most common in newborns (congenital hydrocele), since the processus vaginalis, which connects the scrotal sac with the peritoneum, is still open.[22] Hydroceles are often idiopathic. Fifty percent of patients with acquired hydrocele have a history of trauma.[28] Acquired hydrocele is often associated with infection (epididymis and epididymoorchitis), infarction, and torsion,[22,28] and is seen with 10% of malignant testicular neoplasms.[28]

The clinical sign of hydrocele is a scrotal mass, which may or may not be painful. Sonographic findings of a simple acute hydrocele are a fluid collection (anechoic area) anterolateral to the testis,[22,28] with strong sound transmission affording excellent visualization of the underlying testis (Fig. 21-25).[22,25] An acute hydrocele has a thin wall and always transilluminates (light is transmitted through it).[25] The hydrocele may have calcifications that produce acoustic shadows. These calcifications, known as scrotal pearls, may be seen after inflammation of the tunica vaginalis testis and are associated with acquired hydroceles (Fig. 21-26).[22,32] Scrotal calcifications are benign lesions and may be singular or multiple, filling the potential space between the layers of the tunica vaginalis testis.[32] Hydroceles can be unilateral or bilateral. In chronic hydrocele the sonographic finding may include diffuse scrotal wall thickening and echogenic septations resulting from old hemorrhage or infection (Fig. 21-27).[22] Chronic hydroceles cannot be transilluminated.[25]

Spermatocele. A spermatocele is a retention cyst of small tubules that contain sperm.[26,28] The most common location for spermatoceles is the head of the epididymis; less frequently they occur in the body and tail.[22,25] Spermatoceles may displace the testis anteriorly, distinguishing them from a hydrocele, in which fluid surrounds the testis.[25]

The clinical finding in spermatocele is a scrotal

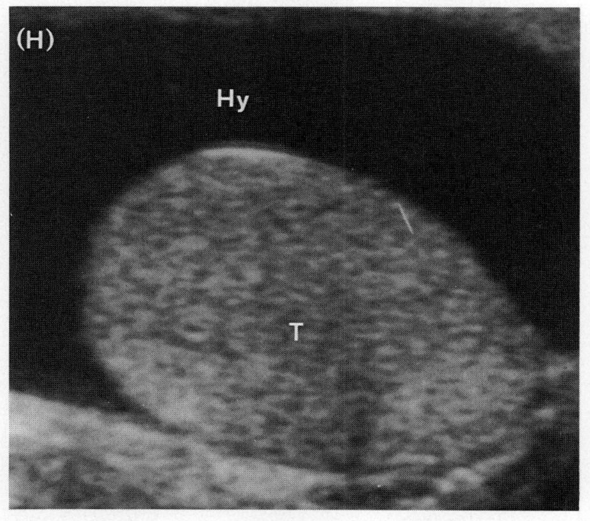

A

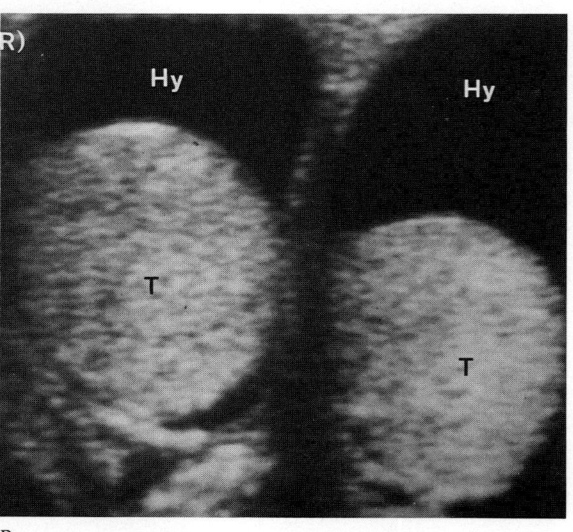

B

Figure 21-25. (*A*) This longitudinal sonogram shows a large, simple hydrocele (Hy) surrounding the normal testis (T; H, toward patient's head). (*B*) Bilateral hydroceles are seen in this patient. On the transverse sonogram, the testes (T) are normal, but are surrounded by a simple collection of fluid (Hy) characteristic of hydrocele. (R) indicates the patient's right side.

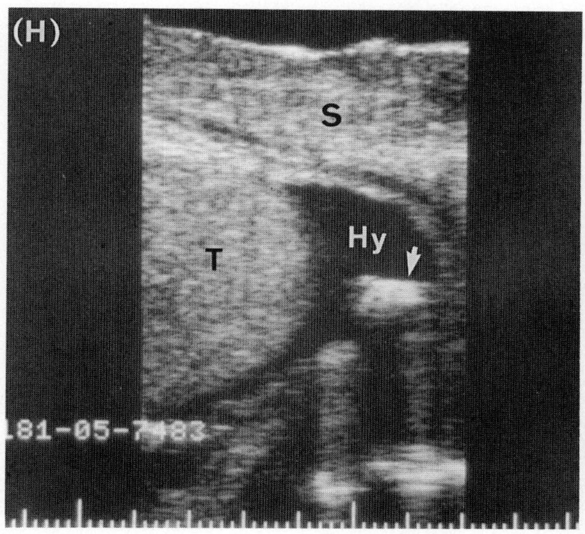

FIGURE 21-26. On this longitudinal scan low in the testis (T), scrotal skin thickening (S) is seen, accompanied by a hydrocele (Hy) and calcification (*arrow*), which represents the "scrotal pearl" seen with chronic hydrocele (H, direction toward patient's head).

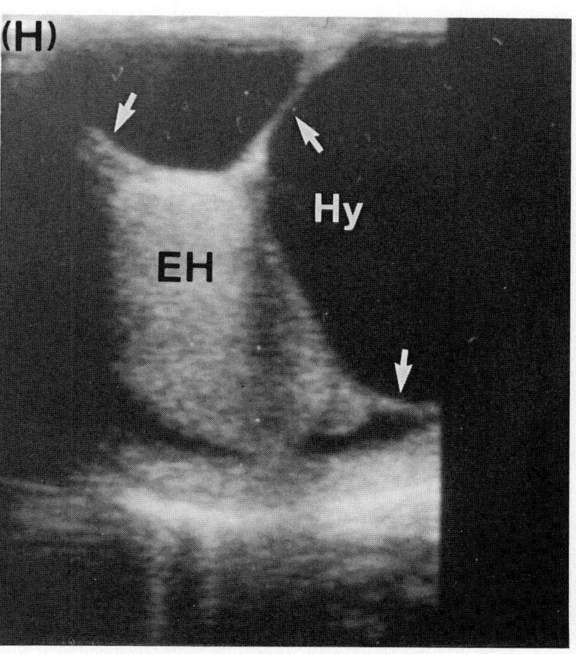

FIGURE 21-27. This longitudinal sonogram of the epididymal head (EH) shows a septate hydrocele (Hy) surrounding the epididymis. The hydrocele contains septate bands (*arrows*). Bands are usually seen in chronic hydrocele (H, direction toward patient's head).

mass, which is usually painless. Spermatoceles are treated surgically if they cause pain or are a cosmetic problem.

Sonographically, a spermatocele is a cystic mass that displaces the testicle anteriorly (Fig. 21-28).[25] The mass may have septations, which represent sediment composed of cellular debris, fat, or spermatozoa. Spermatoceles are sonographically indistinguishable from epididymal cysts, although needle aspiration can distinguish the two: spermatoceles yield creamy fluid and epididymal cysts, clear fluid.[22] Spermatoceles can be unilateral or bilateral, unilocular or multilocular.[25] They can vary in diameter from 0.2 to 9 cm.[45]

Varicocele. A varicocele is formed by dilatation of the veins of the pampiniform plexus greater than 2 mm.[44,49] There are two types of varicocele, primary and secondary. Primary varicoceles are idiopathic and occur between ages 15 and 25 years. They are thought to result from incompetent valves in the internal spermatic veins.[41] Secondary varicoceles may result from elevated pressure in the internal spermatic vein produced by tumor, hydronephrosis, or muscle strain.[25] Varicoceles occur in 8 to 15% of adult men,[44] and they are more common on the left side.[22,25,43] This may occur because the left spermatic vein drains into the left renal vein, whereas the right spermatic vein drains into the vena cava. Patients should be examined by ultrasound in both the supine and the upright positions. The veins of the pampiniform plexus normally have a diameter between 1 to 2 mm. They change little in size with the patient in the erect position, with abdominal compression, or with the Valsalva maneuver. The primary type of varicocele may disappear with the patient in the supine position, so upright scanning may be necessary for its detection. With a varicocele, the veins increase in size with abdominal compression, in the erect position, and with the Valsalva maneuver. Secondary varicoceles do not

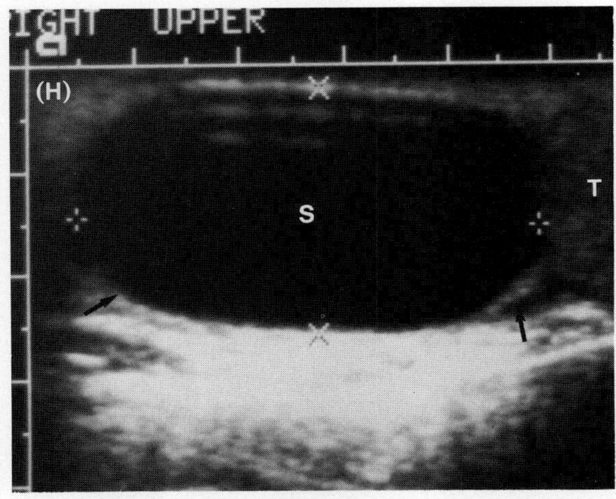

A

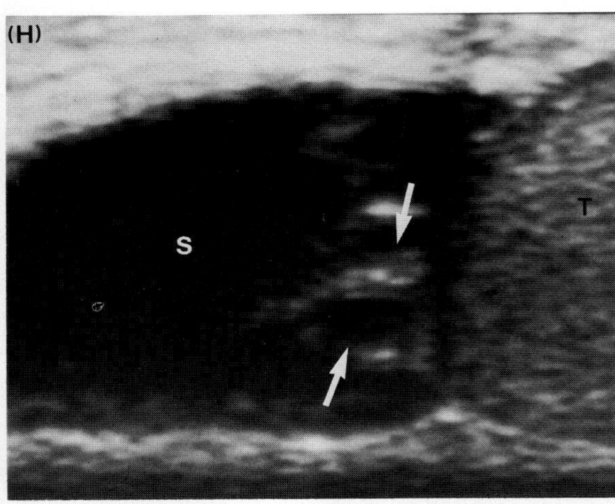

B

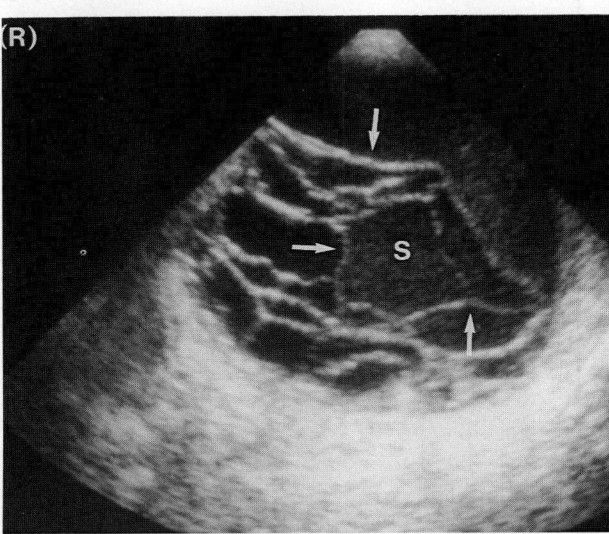

C

FIGURE 21-28. (*A*) Longitudinal scan at the level of the head of the epididymis shows a large fluid collection, the spermatocele (S), which is superior to the testis (T). An echogenic band *(arrows)* surrounds the epididymis (H, toward patient's head). (*B*) In this patient, a collection of fluid is seen craniad to the testis (T), which represents a spermatocele (S). Cystic areas are also seen within the epididymis *(arrows)*, which also represent smaller spermatocele (H, direction toward patient's head). (C) A transverse scan at the level of the head of the epididymis shows a fluid collection with multiple septations *(arrows)* representing a septate spermatocele (S; R, patient's right side). (Courtesy R. Brooke Jeffrey, MD, San Francisco, CA.)

disappear with the patient in the supine position. In this situation the abdomen and pelvis should be scanned carefully to exclude a mass compressing the spermatic vein on the involved side.[22]

Clinical signs of varicocele, in addition to the scrotal mass, may include infertility and an abnormally warm scrotum, which is due to increased blood flow.[44,48] The sonogram of a varicocele shows veins greater than 2 mm in the pampiniform plexus, which should change with the Valsalva maneuver (expiration against a closed glottis; Fig. 21-29).[44] The veins in the varicocele appear as tubular serpiginous anechoic structures in the region of the epididymis.[25,41,44] Doppler duplex sonography can detect venous flow in varicoceles, which can help to differentiate varicoceles from spermatoceles, which show no flow.[28] Color flow imaging of varicoceles will show prominent veins with increased flow with the Valsalva maneuver.[33]

Scrotal Hernia. Scrotal hernias are inguinal hernias that descend into the scrotum, receiving coverings

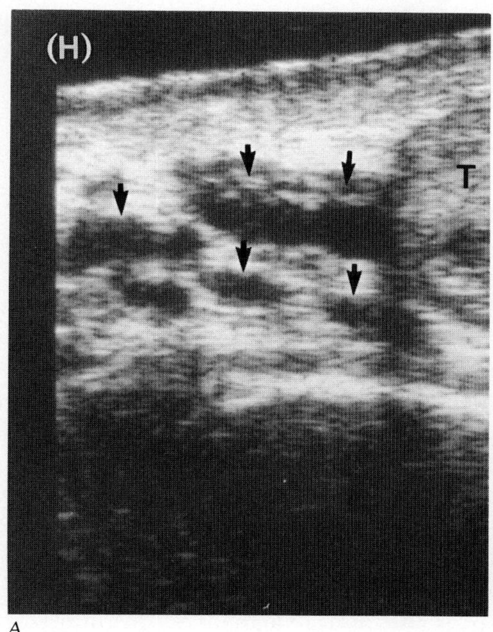

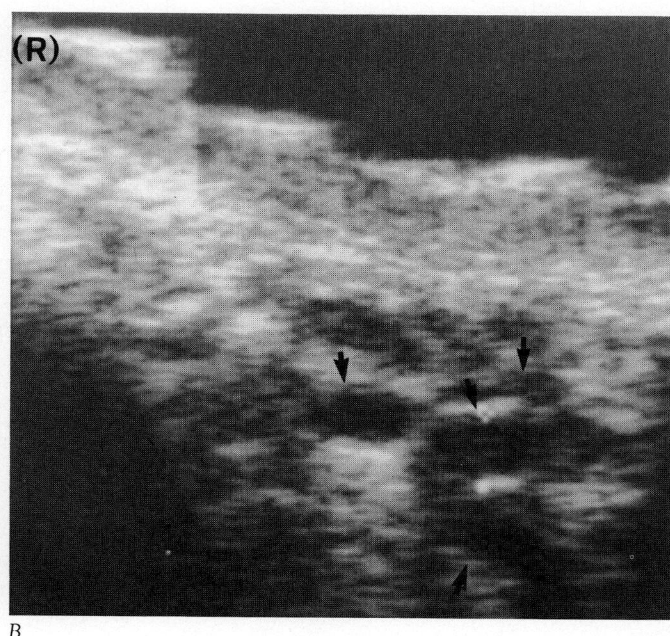

A B

FIGURE 21-29. (*A*) On this longitudinal scan, the varicocele *(arrows)* appears as dilated, anechoic, serpiginous vessels superior to the testis (T; H, towards patient's head). (*B*) In this patient, the transverse scan of a varicocele shows multiple ovoid, fluid-filled structures *(arrows)* in the region of the spermatic cord; (R, patient's right side).

from the superficial fascia and the integument.[20,51] There are two types of inguinal hernia: external (indirect) and internal (direct).[20,28] Indirect inguinal hernias are more common than the direct type.[20] In an indirect inguinal hernia, the intestine escapes from the abdominal cavity, passes via the external inguinal ring into the inguinal canal (which lies parallel to the inguinal ligament and is about 2.5 to 4 cm long), and then into the scrotum.[1,51] Direct inguinal hernias result from a weakness in the floor of the inguinal canal in Hesselbach's triangle, formed medially by the lateral border of the rectus sheath, laterally by the inferior epigastric artery, and inferiorly by the inguinal ligament.[51]

Inguinal hernias are usually associated with persistent patency of the processus vaginalis,[51] the canal that connects the peritoneal cavity to the tunica vaginalis. Normally it closes between the eighth month of fetal life and the first month after birth.[34,42] Scrotal hernias can occur at any age and may be associated with heavy lifting.

Clinical examination can diagnose most scrotal hernias.[22] The clinical sign of scrotal hernia is a persistent or intermittent scrotal mass; the patient may have abdominal pain, and there may be blood in the stool.[34]

The sonographic image in scrotal hernia shows an extratesticular scrotal mass with echogenic and anechoic areas representing air- and fluid-filled loops of bowel, which can be traced to the inguinal canal (Fig. 21-30).[22] The characteristic sonographic appearance of haustra can be seen. If omentum alone is present in the hernia, an echogenic mass is seen.[22,51] The presence of bowel in the scrotum is confirmed if real-time examination demonstrates

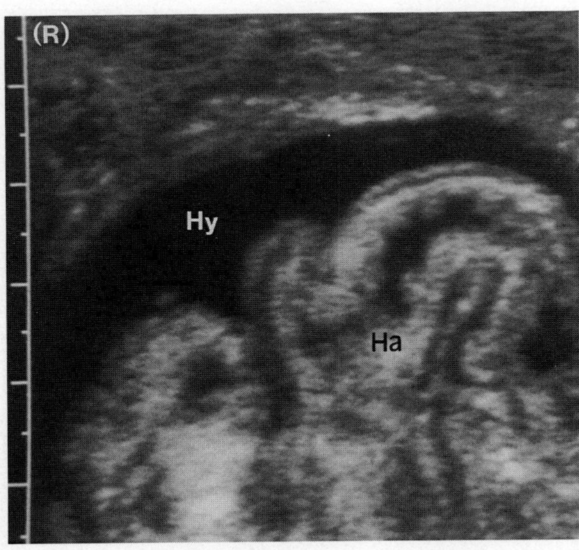

FIGURE 21-30. This transverse scan of a scrotal hernia demonstrates echogenic haustra (Ha) surrounded by a hydrocele (Hy). (Courtesy R. Brooke Jeffrey, MD, San Francisco, CA.)

peristalsis. Extratesticular masses such as multiloculated hydrocele and hematocele with fibrous septations may mimic fluid-filled segments of bowel.[51]

Incarcerated hernias are irreducible hernias the blood supply of which is obstructed. If not relieved within a few hours, the incarcerated bowel becomes gangrenous.[34] Clinically, they present as very painful masses in the groin accompanied by scrotal swelling, pressure, and inflammation. Pain may be referred to the abdomen.[34]

The sonographic appearance of incarcerated hernia is similar to that of reducible scrotal hernia, but real-time evaluation will not show peristalsis. Differential diagnosis of incarcerated scrotal hernia includes testicular torsion. If the diagnosis is in doubt, color flow Doppler is accurate in assessing normal or absent flow characteristic with spermatic cord torsion.[8]

Scrotal Abscess. Scrotal abscesses are commonly a consequence of untreated epididymoorchitis.[22] The clinical presentation is usually a painful and swollen scrotum. On ultrasound, a scrotal abscess appears as a complex intrascrotal mass (Fig. 21-31).[22,25] With epididymal involvement, the mass is usually in the tail of the epididymis.[22,25] Color Doppler imaging in patients with scrotal abscess will show hyperemia (increased flow) around the periphery of the abscess, with flow void centrally.[23]

Scrotal Hematoma. Scrotal hematomas can be either extratesticular or intratesticular. Both are usually associated with a history of trauma.[22] In extratesticular hematoma, blood collects beneath the tunica Dartos and tunica vaginalis.[25,26] In intratesticular hematoma, the blood is contained in the testis itself. In both conditions, the scrotum is swollen, painful, and sometimes discolored.[22]

The sonographic appearance of hematomas varies with their age. In acute extratesticular hematoma, the scrotal wall becomes thickened (Fig. 21-32A).[25,26,46] After 2 or 3 days, hypoechoic areas are seen, which represent liquefaction of the hematoma (Fig. 21-32B).[26,46] Late extratesticular hematomas may show a solid or septate cystic mass.[22]

Intratesticular hematomas are less common than extratesticular hematomas and may be associated with testicular rupture.[46] Sonography of an intratesticular hematoma shows focal areas of either increased or decreased echogenicity, depending on the age of the hematoma.[22] Initially the intratesticular hematoma appears as a focal hyperechoic area, which later becomes hypoechoic as it liquefies (Fig. 21-33).[22,46] Disease processes that can mimic intra-

FIGURE 21-32. (*A*) In this patient with acute blunt trauma to the scrotum, the transverse sonogram shows diffuse scrotal wall thickening (S). The testis (T) has a heterogeneous echo pattern, with increased and decreased echogenicity (*arrows*) representing an acute intratesticular hematoma (R, patient's right side). (*B*) A transverse scan of the same patient made 1 week later demonstrates a marked decrease in the echogenicity of the hematoma (H), which represents liquefaction. The testis (T) is compressed by the hematoma (R, patient's right side).

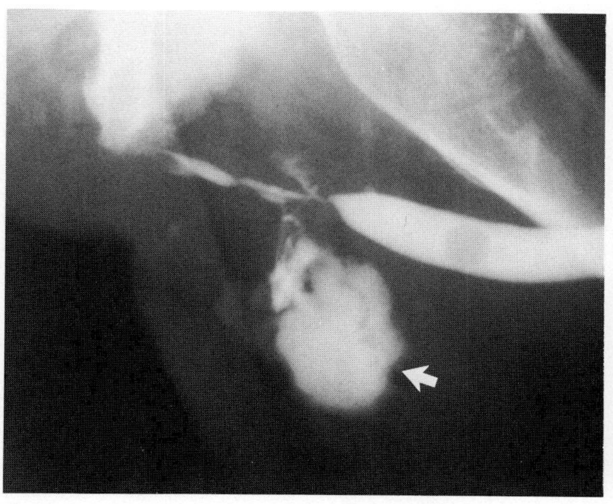

A

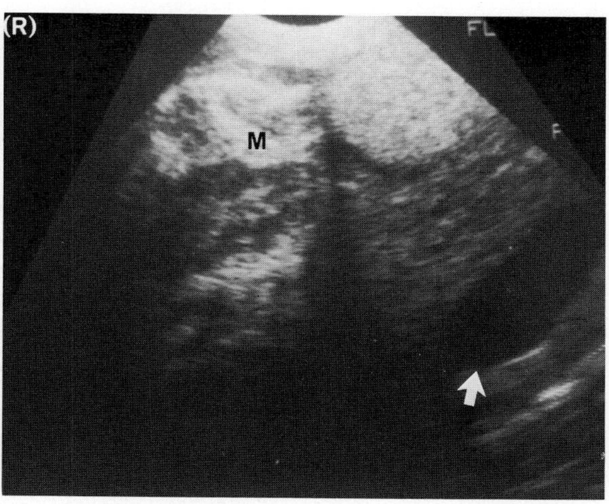

B

FIGURE 21-31. (*A*) On this retrograde urethrogram, there is filling of a scrotal abscess cavity *(arrow)*, which communicates via a fistulous tract with the proximal urethra. (Courtesy R. Brooke Jeffrey, MD, San Francisco, CA.) (*B*) By ultrasound, a transverse scan of the same patient with the scrotal abscess shows a complex mass (M), with increased and decreased anechoic regions *(arrow)* which represent the fistulous tract. (R) indicates the patient's right side. (Courtesy R. Brooke Jeffrey, MD, San Francisco, CA.)

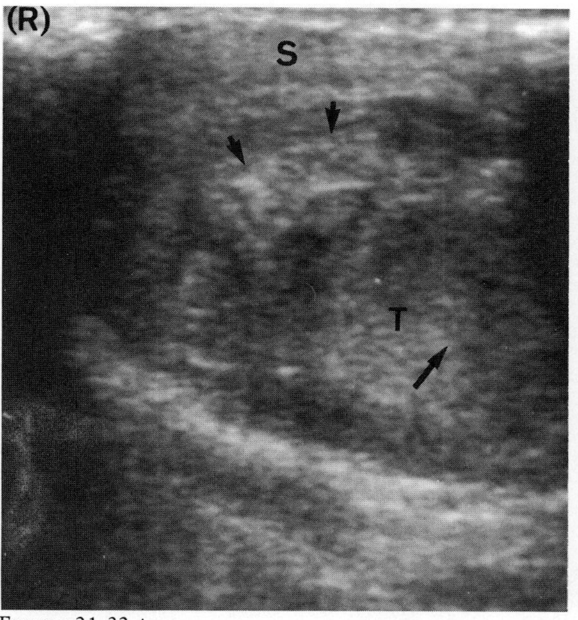

FIGURE 21-32 *A*

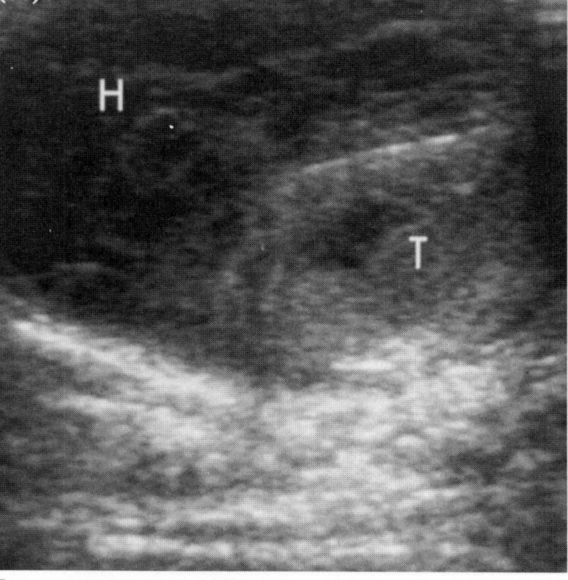

B

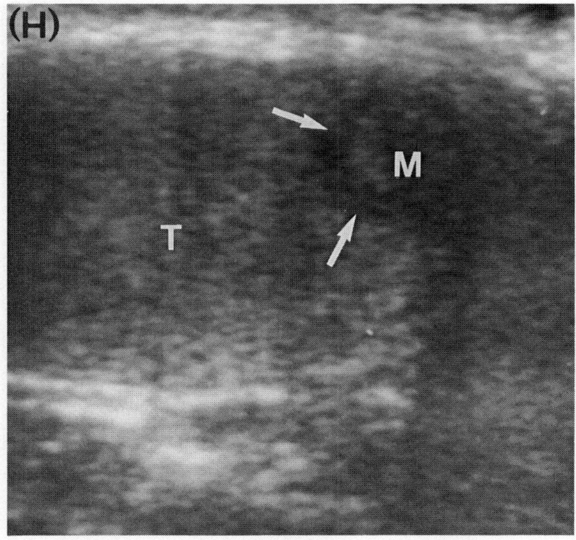

A

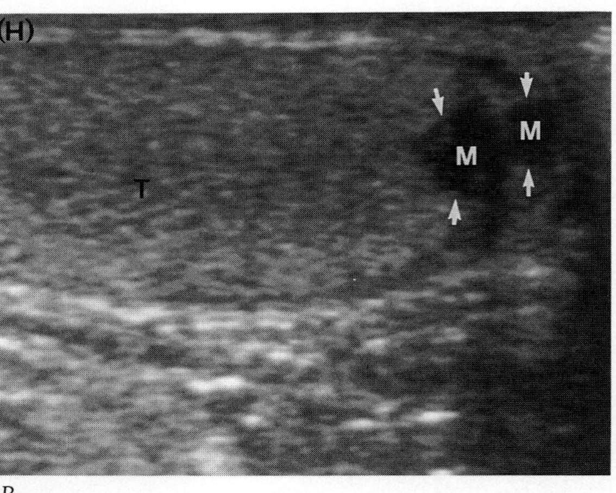

B

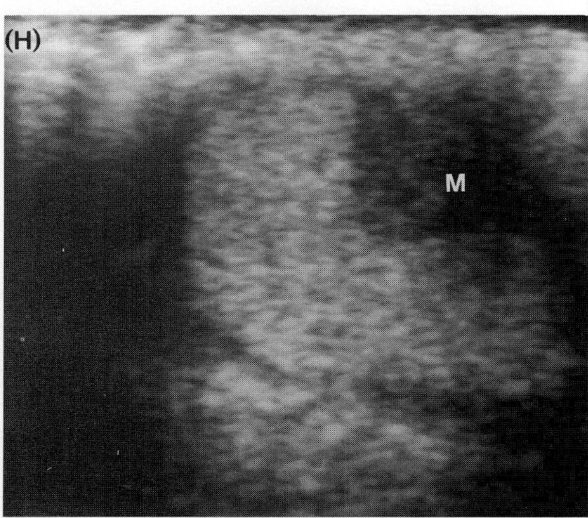

C

FIGURE 21-33. (*A*) The longitudinal scan demonstrates a focal echogenic mass (M, *arrows*), which represents the acute focal intratesticular hematoma in the anterior inferior aspect of the testis (T; H, toward patient's head). (*B*) One week later, a longitudinal sonogram of the testis (T) of the same patient shows that the hematoma (M) has become hypoechoic as it liquefies (H, toward patient's head). (*C*) In a different patient with a subacute focal intratesticular hematoma, the longitudinal sonogram shows the hematoma (M) as a well-defined hypoechoic mass in the anterior margin of the otherwise normal-looking testis. Without the history of trauma, this could be misinterpreted as a primary neoplasm of the testis (H, toward patient's head). (Courtesy R. Brooke Jeffrey, MD, San Francisco, CA.)

testicular hematoma include focal orchitis, testicular infarct, and testicular neoplasm.[43,46] With focal intra- and extratesticular hematomas, color Doppler will show normal perfusion to the testis and/or peritesticular tissues, with focal areas of absent vascularity.[30]

Hematocele. Hematoceles are usually a result of trauma to the scrotum and often accompany testicular rupture.[21,22,28] Hematoceles also can result from surgery, diabetes, neoplasia, or atherosclerotic disease.[28] A hematocele arises when hemorrhage occurs in the space between the tunica parietalis and tunica vaginalis.[25,26] They usually present as a painful scrotal mass surrounding the testicle.[24] The clinical signs may mimic epididymitis or torsion of the spermatic cord.

Sonographic findings of acute hematocele are thickening of the scrotal wall and fluid (hemorrhage) without echoes in the space between the parietalis and vaginalis fascia.[25,28,46] In the acute stage, hematoceles can mimic hydroceles, but unlike hydroceles they do not transilluminate.[26,46]

In chronic hematocele, sonography demon-

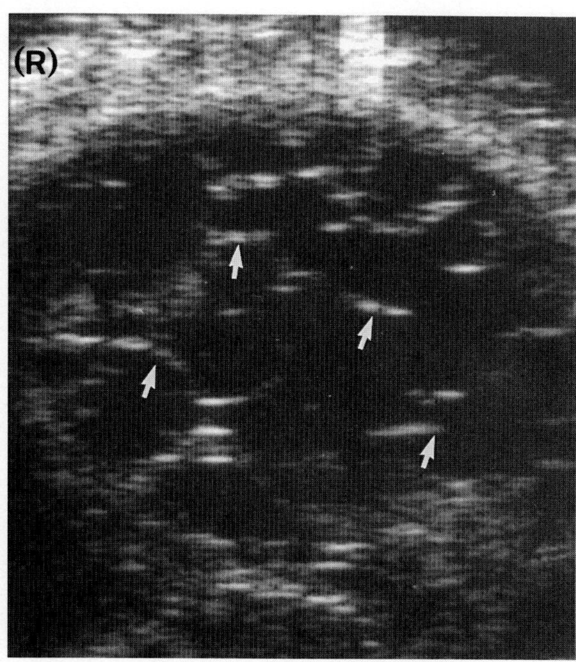

FIGURE 21-34. This transverse scan of a patient with a chronic hematocele following trauma shows a mass with multiple septations which represents a hematocele. The echogenic septa (*arrows*) probably represent clot formation (R, patient's right side).

strates a thick, fibrous scrotal wall, internal septation from clot formation, and occasionally focal mural calcifications within the tunica vaginalis (Fig. 21-34).[26,46] Chronic hematoceles may be difficult to distinguish from chronic hydroceles and pyoceles.[26,46]

Pyocele. The clinical signs of pyoceles may mimic those of infection and inflammation, with hemiscrotal swelling and pain.[46] After trauma or following rupture of a testicular abscess, pus fills the potential space between the tunica parietalis and vaginalis.[28] Sonographic findings in pyocele include a thick hemiscrotal wall, echogenic fluid collections with septations, and occasionally focal mural calcifications.[46]

Granulomatous Disease. Granulomatous disease of the testis and epididymis is usually secondary to the spread of tuberculosis from the kidneys, prostate, or seminal vesicles.[22] Granulomatous disease of the testis is usually unilateral but can be bilateral.[22] Initially, granulomatous disease involves the epididymis, but if left untreated it spreads to the testis in 60 to 80% of cases.[22] Tuberculous orchitis without epididymitis is rare.[18] Tuberculosis of the epididymis usually starts in the globus minor, probably because this structure has a richer blood supply than other parts of the epididymis.[18] The peak incidence of granulomatous disease in the scrotum occurs in men 20 to 45 years of age; however, recent studies indicate a notable increase in men older than 45.[18]

Clinical symptoms may include those of urinary tract infection (e.g., frequency, with or without pain) and a swollen scrotum that is painful and inflamed.[18]

On sonography, granulomatous orchitis may appear as a focal hypoechoic mass, although the testis may also be diffusely involved, becoming enlarged, irregular, and homogeneously hypoechoic (Fig. 21-35).[22] In chronic scrotal tuberculosis, the epididymis and testis may be inseparable on the sonogram, appearing as a complex mass, sometimes accompa-

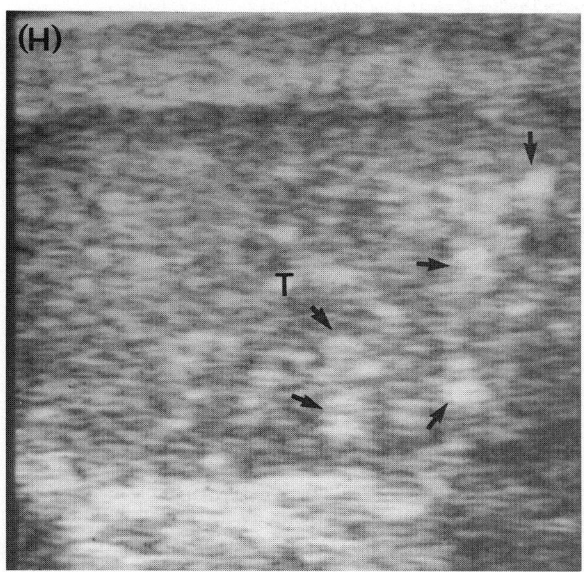

FIGURE 21-35. On a longitudinal scan of a patient with granulomatous orchitis, the testis (T) is hypoechoic, with multiple echogenic foci representing calcifications (*arrows*; H, toward patient's head).

nied by scrotal wall thickening and fistulous tracts.[22] Calcifications may be seen in the epididymis or testis (see Fig. 21-35).[22]

Focal lesions of granulomatous disease in the testis may mimic testicular neoplasia. Tubercular epididymitis and orchitis appear similar to these conditions caused by other infectious organisms or sarcoid.[18]

Sarcoidosis can involve the scrotum, usually the epididymis, less often the testis.[22] Scrotal sarcoid is found in 1% of patients with acute sarcoidosis. With scrotal swelling and enlargement of the testes and epididymis, scrotal sarcoid may be painful or painless.

The sonographic appearance of scrotal sarcoid is epididymal enlargement, an irregular hypoechoic mass in the testis, or a diffusely enlarged and irregular testis. Echogenic foci with high-level echoes representing calcifications may be present in the testis or epididymis.[22]

Tuberculosis and AIDS. Tuberculosis occurs in approximately 10% of patients with AIDS and involves at least one extrapulmonary site in nearly 50% of the cases. Tuberculous infection of the testicle in AIDS is rarely seen; however, the various viral, bacterial, fungal, and parasitic infections must be considered in the differential diagnosis of orchitis or epididymitis and testicular abscess. With the increasing incidence of AIDS and associated tuberculosis, it is important to consider tuberculosis orchitis, epididymitis, and abscess in the differential diagnosis of diffuse and focal testicular lesions. A case report in 1990 from University of Texas Medical School described tuberculosis abscess of the testicle in a patient with AIDS. A patient with acquired immune deficiency presented with right testicular swelling. Sonography demonstrated diffuse enlargement and inhomogeneity of the testis with central hypoechoic areas.[17]

Tunica Albuginea Cyst. Cysts arising in the tunica albuginea are rare.[40] Clinically, tunica albuginea cysts may present as a painless scrotal lump or may be associated with testicular pain and swelling.[40] The cause of these cysts is not known, although it is felt that trauma and subsequent hemorrhage into the albuginea could lead to cyst formation.[40] Tunica cysts are generally seen in men in the fifth and sixth decades.[40]

Sonographically, tunica albuginea cysts appear as well-circumscribed anechoic areas that have posterior wall acoustic enhancement (Fig. 21-36).[16] The cysts are small, may be single, multiple, or multilocular,[40] and are situated in the anterior and lateral aspects of the testis. Tunica albuginea cysts can invaginate into the testicular parenchyma and simulate an intratesticular cyst.[22]

Epididymal Cysts. Epididymal cysts are uncommon.[45] Like spermatoceles, they are felt to be secondary to cystic dilatation of the epididymal tubules.[45] Leung and colleagues reported epididymal cystic structures in 29% of their patients.[31] Rifkin and coworkers reported that of 27 cystic structures in the epididymis diagnosed by ultrasound with pathologic correlation, only six were epididymal cysts.[45] Epididymal cysts and spermatoceles are sonographically indistinguisable.[31,45] Epididymal cysts are clinically asymptomatic and are usually

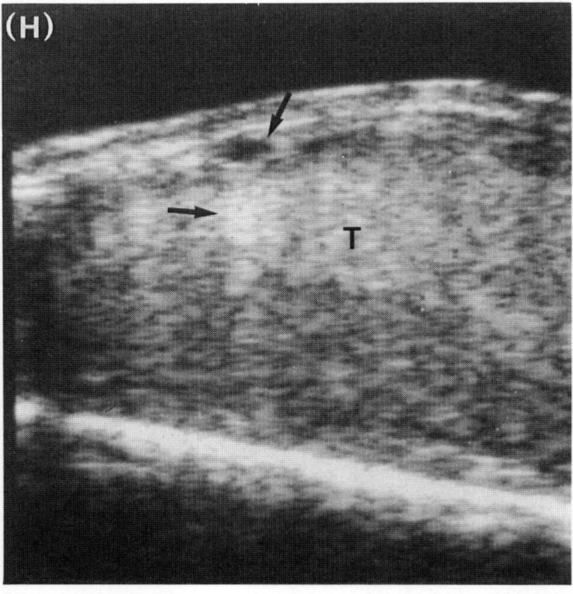

FIGURE 21-36. The longitudinal scan of the testis (T) shows a focal anechoic structure *(arrow)* located in the anterior surface of the tunica albuginea. The posterior enhancement *(arrow)* is typical of a cyst. The location is also indicative of a tunica albuginea cyst (H, toward patient's head).

discovered as an incidental finding during a sonographic examination or as a palpable mass on a physical examination.

On a sonogram an epididymal cyst is an anechoic structure with a sharp back wall and posterior enhancement (Fig. 21-37).[45] Epididymal cysts range in diameter from 0.2 to 9 cm.[45] The differential diagnosis of epididymal cyst includes spermatocele and varicocele.[45] Epididymal cysts can be seen throughout the epididymis, whereas spermatoceles almost always arise in the head.[45] Varicoceles may appear cystic in one scanning plane, and tubular on the orthogonal projection.[45]

Simple Testicular Cysts. Simple testicular cysts were once considered rare;[40] however, a recent study indicates they occur in 10% of the male population. Simple testicular cysts are asymptomatic and sonographically appear as well-circumscribed anechoic areas in the testis with smooth walls and posterior acoustic enhancement (Fig. 21-38).[16] Testicular cysts range in size from 2 mm to 2 cm.[16] Most (45%) occur in the upper pole of the testis, 27% in the middle, and 27% in the lower pole.[16]

Sperm Granuloma. Following trauma or infection, sperm may be extravasated into the surrounding tissues and produce necrosis, resulting in granuloma formation.[28] Such granulomas are often found in asymptomatic men.[22] They can be intratesticular or extratesticular.[9,28] Sperm granulomas are composed of fibrous connective tissue with well-defined necrotizing granulomas containing a few degenerated spermatozoa in their necrotic centers.[22] Sonographically, these lesions usually have the appearance of a solid hypoechoic mass.[22,28]

Neoplasms of the Scrotum

EXTRATESTICULAR NEOPLASMS

Primary solid neoplasms outside the testes are rare.[22] The majority arise from the spermatic cord and are benign.[22]

Benign Neoplasms. Adenomatoid tumors are the most common extratesticular tumors,[9] accounting for approximately 30% of extratesticular tumors in the scrotum.[40] The tumors are benign, slow growing, and are generally located in the epididymis (most often the globus minor),[23] and less often in the spermatic cord[40] and testis.[52] Adenomatoid tumors are usually asymptomatic, present as a small, solid mass in the scrotum, and are generally benign.[40]

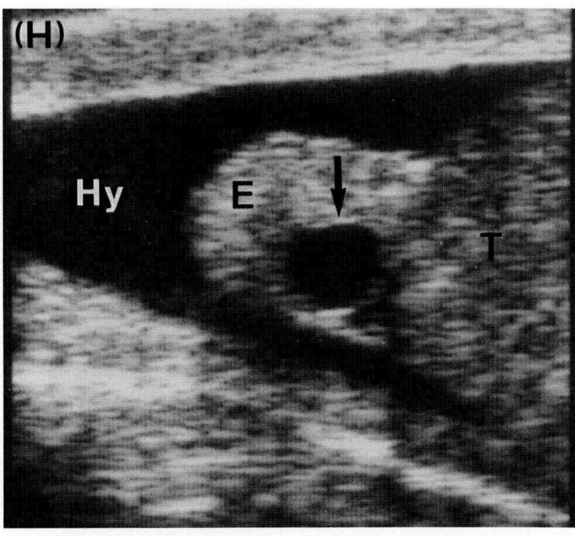

FIGURE 21-37. On this longitudinal scan, a small epididymal cyst *(arrow)* is seen in the head of the epididymis (E), outside the normal testis (T). The testis is surrounded by a hydrocele (Hy; H, toward patient's head).

Sonography of adenomatoid tumors shows well circumscribed solid masses with variable echogenicity (hyper to hypoechogenicity) (Fig. 21-39).[9,22,25,28,52] This appearance is indistinguishable from other benign tumors such as spermatic granulomas, leiomyomas, fibromas, and lipomas of the spermatic cord.[9]

Malignant Neoplasms. Primary malignant extratesticular neoplasms are uncommon.[28] Spermatic cord neoplasms represent the majority of malignant lesions.[41] Approximately 30% of spermatic cord neoplasms are malignant.[12,42] The most common malignancies are fibrosarcoma and liposarcoma in adults and rhabdomyosarcoma in children.[41]

Few malignant extratesticular neoplasms have been reported in the sonographic literature.[41] The cases of rhabdomyosarcoma and myxoliposarcoma

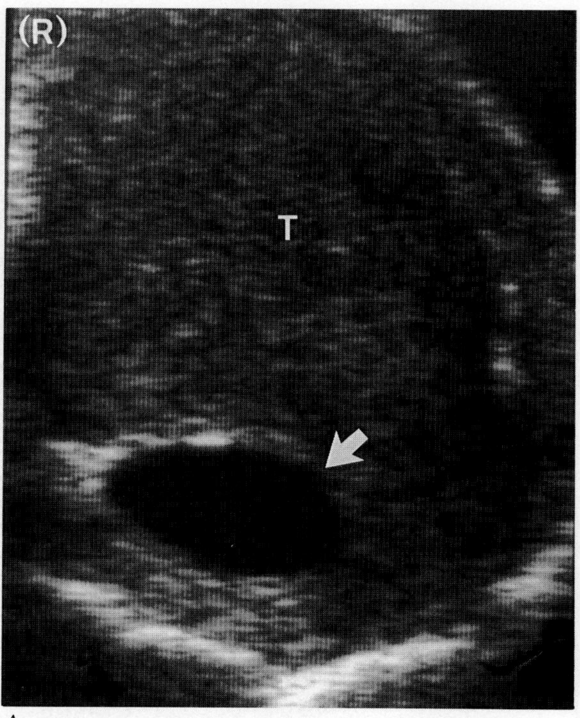

A

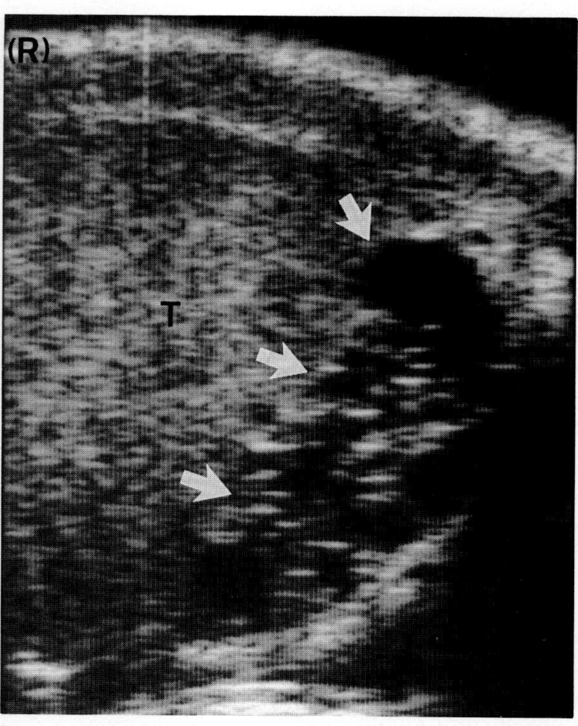

B

FIGURE 21-38. (*A*) On this transverse sonogram, a single intratesticular cyst *(arrow)* is seen in the inferior aspect of the testis (T; R, patient's right side). (*B*) A transverse scan of this testis (T) shows a cluster formation of tiny anechoic structures *(arrows)*, which represent intratesticular cysts (R, patient's right side).

sonographically illustrated have focal echogenic areas, anechoic areas representing necrosis, and occasional calcifications, with or without acoustic shadowing.[41]

INTRATESTICULAR NEOPLASMS

The majority (95%) of testicular neoplasms are malignant.[22] All intratesticular lesions should be considered potentially malignant until proven otherwise.[28]

Benign Neoplasms. Non–germ cell neoplasms of the testis are Leydig cell tumors, Sertoli cell tumors,[28] epidermoid cysts,[22,39] dermoid cysts, cystadenomas,[22] and adenomatoid tumors.[52] Leydig cell tumors (also called interstitial cell tumors) are the most common non–germ cell neoplasm of the testis.[22] Although considered in the benign group, 10% of Leydig cell tumors are malignant.[39] Leydig cell tumors comprise between 1% and 3% of all testicular neoplasms. They generally occur in men between the ages of 20 and 60 years.[39] Clinical features of Leydig cell tumors may include endocrine imbalance, impotence, decreased libido, and gynecomastia.

True Sertoli cell mesenchymal tumors account for fewer than 1% of all testicular tumors. The majority of Sertoli cell tumors are benign; 10% are malignant.[39] Sertoli cell tumors may be painless or painful. Gynecomastia can be a symptom.

The benign Leydig and Sertoli cell tumors are usually well-circumscribed, whereas the malignant forms of these neoplasms are larger and have less defined borders.[39] These neoplasms are seen sonographically as a solid mass in the testis.[22] The echogenicity of the mass varies, but it is usually hypoechoic relative to normal testicular parenchyma.[22] Very large neoplasms may develop cystic areas, occasionally giving the appearance of a multiseptate cystic mass.[22]

Epidermoid cysts represent 1% of testicular neoplasms; they generally develop between ages 20 and 40 years.[22,39] Epidermoid cysts are usually asymptomatic and are discovered incidentally.[22] The sonogram shows a cyst with well-defined echogenic walls, which may be thickened.[22] The cyst may contain calcifications, which appear as echogenic foci.[22]

Less common benign neoplasms are dermoid cysts, cystadenomas, and adenomatoid tumors. Dermoid cysts may simulate a true simple testicular cyst,[22] or echogenic areas may be present along the peripheral border of the cyst. Occasionally, the cyst is completely echogenic, owing to the presence of fat, sebum, and hair.[22] Sonographically, cystadenomas of the testis appear as multiseptate cystic masses.[22] Adenomatoid tumors are uncommon in the testis. The sonographic appearance is the same as for extratesticular adenomatoid tumors—a well circumscribed solid mass with variable echogenicity (hyper to hypoechogenicity).[22,52]

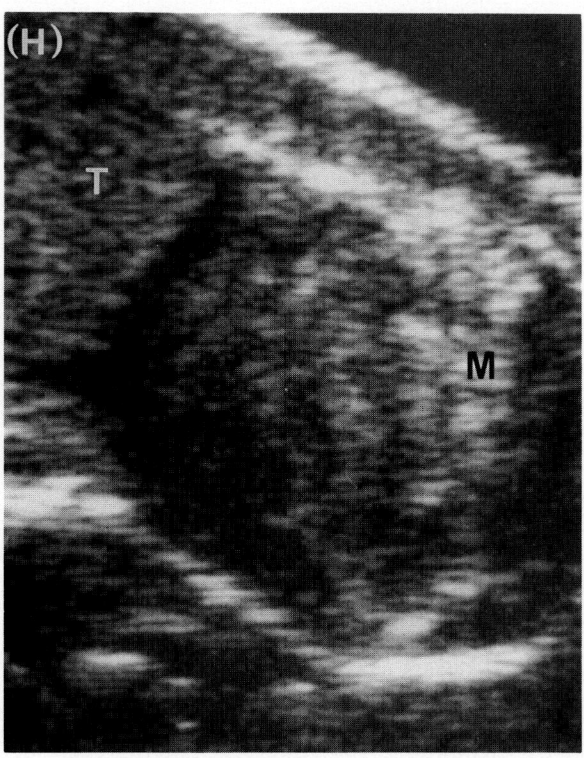

FIGURE 21-39. On longitudinal scan, an isoechoic mass (M) with hyperechoic areas represents an adenomatoid tumor of the epididymis in its tail, just inferior to the testis (T; H, toward patient's head). Adenomatoid tumors are the most common benign neoplasms in the scrotum. (Courtesy Gretchen A. W. Gooding, MD, San Francisco, CA.)

Malignant Neoplasms. Malignant testicular neoplasms most often present as a painless scrotal mass or hardness of the testis with unilateral enlargement.[28,39] Ten percent of testicular neoplasms present with acute pain and simulate an inflammatory process.[26,35,39]

Some 90% to 95% of scrotal neoplasms[28,39] are primary germ cell neoplasms: seminoma, embryonal cell carcinoma, choriocarcinoma, and teratoma.[28,39] Of scrotal neoplasms, 5% to 10% are of non–germ cell origin.[28,39] Forty percent of malignant neoplasms have a mixture of cell types.[28] The most common mixed neoplasm, teratocarcinoma, contains both teratoma and embryonal cells.[28]

Most testicular neoplasms are unilateral, but approximately 8% of patients with a history of one testicular neoplasm develop neoplasm in the contralateral testis.[28] Testicular neoplasms are most common between age 20 and 34 years.[39]

The sonographic appearance of malignant intratesticular masses is most often focal and hypoechoic.[19,26,28,47] Less often, neoplasms can appear as focal hyperechoic masses, diffuse infiltration of the testicular parenchyma, or mixed lesions containing focal anechoic areas with echogenic foci.[12,19,43,47] If the tumor is confined to the tunica albuginea, the testis usually retains its oval shape. Invasion of the testis and epididymis distorts the smooth contour of the testis, making it irregular and lumpy.[40,47] Ultrasound is sensitive for detecting malignant testicular masses, but it cannot distinguish the cell type of malignancies.[19,28,34,41,50] Color Doppler imaging of malignant testicular neoplasms larger than 1.5 cm in diameter has been reported exhibiting hypervascularity when compared with normal testicular parenchyma. Infiltrated or diffuse malignancies, such as leukemia and lymphoma, may appear similar to diffuse orchitis, making it difficult to differentiate between them. In the latter situation, clinical history is extremely important.[23]

Other pathologic processes that may mimic testicular neoplasms include abscess, hematoma, focal orchitis, testicular infarcts, and torsion.[43,46] Features that tend to distinguish neoplasms (benign or malignant) from inflammatory processes are the scrotal wall thickness, the character of the epididymis,[2,43,46] the margination of the lesions, and the surrounding testicular parenchyma.[7]

In general, with malignancy the thickness of the scrotal wall is normal. The appearance of the epididymis is normal, too, except in the rare cases when the neoplasm invades the epididymis.[43,46] Inflammatory processes usually show thickening of the scrotal wall and fluid.[43] In 5% to 10% of patients with a testicular neoplasm, there is concurrent epididymitis or epididymoorchitis[39]; reactive hydroceles accompany 10% of testicular neoplasms.[28] Neoplasms are generally well-marginated, whereas inflammatory processes have indistinct margins.[7] With neoplasms, the testicular parenchyma surrounding the lesion and the contralateral testis are usually normal. In inflammatory processes, the testicular parenchyma around the lesion differs from normal testis, and the contralateral testis is often abnormal as well.[7]

Seminoma. Like other testicular neoplasms, seminoma presents as a gradual enlargement, usually of one testicle.[41] In 10% to 15% of cases, the testicle is painful, conceivably owing to hemorrhage into the tumor.[41] Seminoma occurs mostly in men 35 to 39 years of age.[39] Seminoma accounts for 40% of primary testicular neoplasms,[28,39] and it is the testicular neoplasm that is most often detected by ultrasound.[28,41] Nonseminomatous elements can occur in seminoma.[9] On sonography a seminoma appears as a mass with a hypoechoic homogeneous pattern that may contain scattered hyperechoic areas (Fig. 21-40).[9,47] The epididymis is usually spared, at least in part.[41] Seminomas often have a pseudocapsule, which is demonstrated sonographically as an echogenic band surrounding the neoplasm.[7] Most of the testis can be replaced by seminomas,[9] and a reactive hydrocele may be associated (Fig. 21-40C).[28]

Embryonal cell carcinoma. Embryonal cell carcinoma occurs primarily in men between ages 25 and 35[39] and represents 25% of primary testicular neoplasms.[28,39] Often invading the tunica albuginea and distorting the testicular contour, embryonal cell carcinoma is the most aggressive of the primary scrotal malignancies.[9,28] Sonographic findings in embryonal cell carcinoma are a hypoechoic mass in the testicle that is less homogeneous in echo pattern than seminoma.[9,28] The mass may be focal or may be diffuse or have indistinct boundaries (Fig. 21-41).[9,28] The tunica albuginea may be invaded, the testicle may be distorted, and focal hyperechoic areas due to hemorrhage or necrosis may be found.[9,12,19,28]

Choriocarcinoma. Choriocarcinoma is a rare neoplasm that accounts for 3% or fewer of testicular neoplasms[28,39] and usually occurs in men between the ages of 20 and 30.[39] All patients with choriocarcinoma have elevated levels of human chorionic gonadotropin (hCG). This may be a useful way to follow these tumors; however, it is not useful in the differential diagnosis since 60% of all patients with testicular neoplasms have an elevated hCG value.[39] Choriocarcinoma may appear as a mixed neoplasm with embryonal cell carcinoma, teratoma, or seminoma. With metastatic choriocarcinoma there may be no evidence of choriocarcinoma in the primary lesion,[23] and often there is no palpable testicular mass.[28] Sonographically, the choriocarcinoma may be small and show a mixed echo pattern that reflects hemorrhage, necrosis, and calcification.[9,28]

Teratoma. Most common in men between ages 25 and 35 years, teratomas account for 5% to 10% of scrotal neoplasms.[28,39] Previously, they were considered benign, but it is now known that about a third of the teratomas that are left untreated metastasize within 5 years.[28] Teratomas contain multiple tissue elements—bone, soft tissue, skin, among others.[28] Sonographically, teratomas show a mixed pattern, areas of increased and decreased echogenicity reflecting the various tissue elements.[28]

Mixed neoplasms. Forty percent of testicular neoplasms are of the mixed type.[28] Teratocarcinoma is the most common mixed neoplasm and the second most common of all testicular neoplasm, seminoma being first.[28] Teratocarcinomas contain both teratoma and embryonal carcinoma cells.[28] These neoplasms are aggressive and contain cysts, hemorrhage, and areas of necrosis; sonographically they are complex masses with anechoic areas (Fig. 21-42).[9,12,19,28]

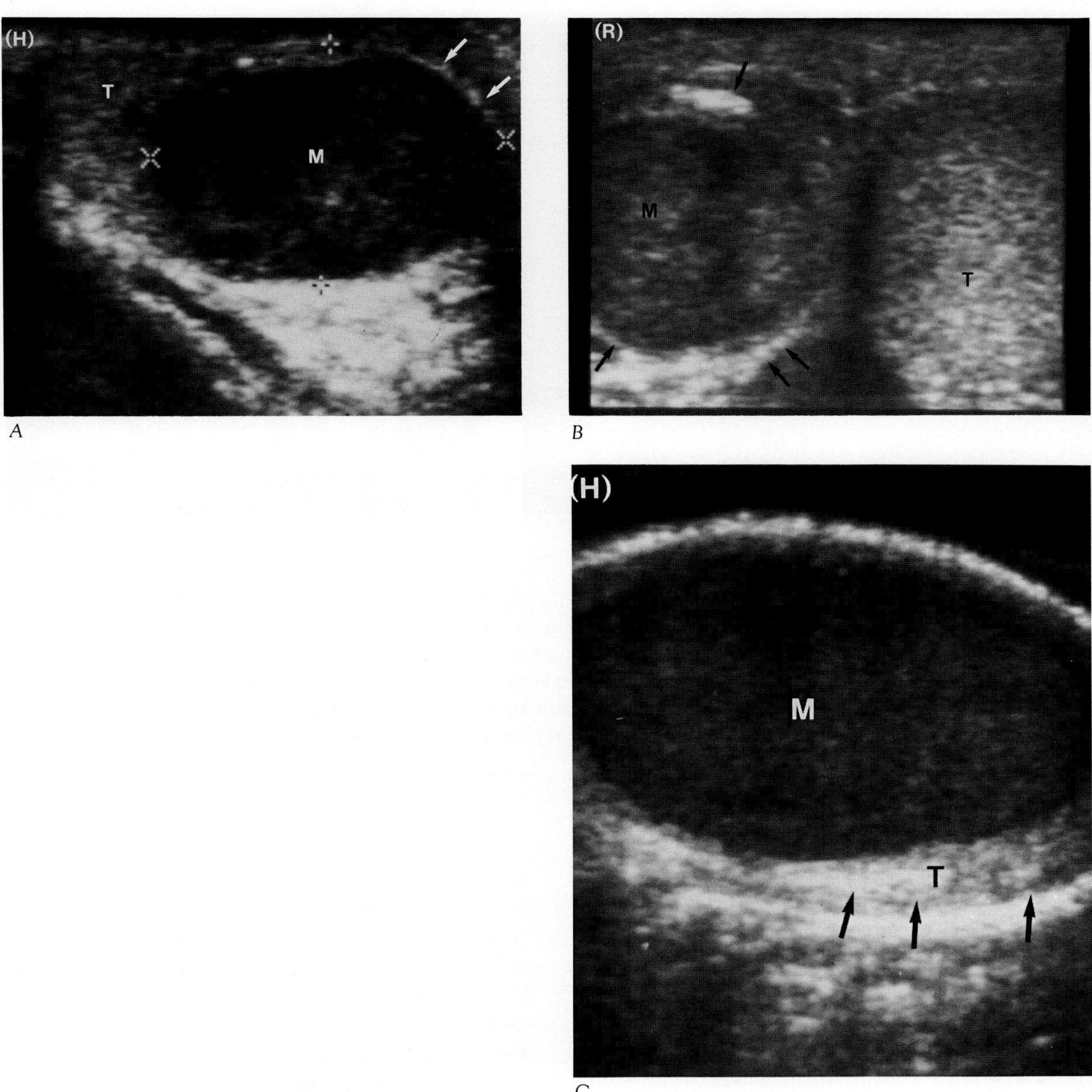

FIGURE 21-40. (*A*) This seminoma on longitudinal scan appears as a solitary hypoechoic solid mass (M), surrounded by an echogenic band *(arrows)*. This band represents a pseudocapsule. Normal testis (T) is seen at the periphery (H, toward patient's head). (*B*) In another patient, a transverse scan of both testes shows a solid, hypoechoic mass (M) with a pseudocapsule *(arrows)* in the right testis. The mass was shown to be a seminoma at operation. The normal contralateral testis (T) can be valuable for comparison, to detect subtle alterations in the testis. (C) In a different patient a seminoma appears as a large, hypoechoic mass (M) that virtually replaces the testis. Only a thin rim of testicular parenchyma (T, *arrows*) remains at the periphery of the gland (H, toward patient's head).

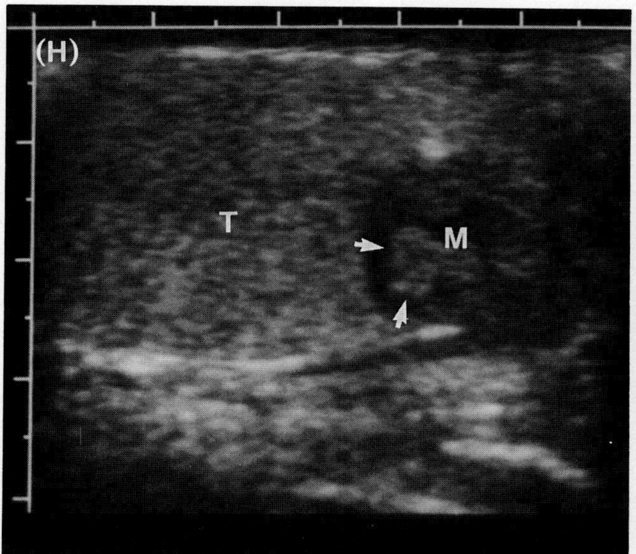

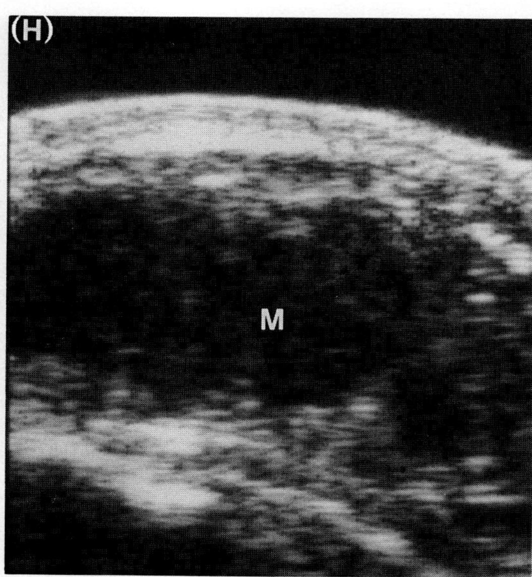

FIGURE 21-41. (*A*) On a longitudinal scan of a patient with a focal embryonal cell carcinoma, the neoplasm is shown as a mass (M) in the inferior aspect of the testis (T). The tumor is principally hypoechoic but has areas of increased echogenicity (*arrows;* H, toward the patient's head). (*B*) In a different patient with diffuse embryonal cell carcinoma, this tumor appears as a large, lumpy, heterogeneous mass (M) distorting the testicular architecture (H, toward patient's head).

Metastases to the testis. Metastasis to the testes is rare, and generally occurs late in life, between age 60 and 70 years.[39] The prostate and the kidney are the most common primary sites; less frequent are bowel, bladder, lungs (bronchogenic carcinoma), pancreas, thyroid, skin (melanoma), and nerve (neuroblastoma).[28] Metastases are more common than germ cell tumors in patients older than 50 and are often multiple and bilateral. The sonographic appearance is usually a solid, hypoechoic mass; less often it is hyperechoic. A patient with single tumor type concurrently may have lesions with both sonographic characteristics.

Lymphoma and leukemia. In lymphoma and leukemia, infiltration of the testis is uncommon; however, clinical recognition is important, as testicular involvement may be the first manifestation of extramedullary disease in the absence of bone marrow involvement.[41]

Lymphoma accounts for 5% of all testicular neoplasms; approximately 2.5% of patients with lymphoma have testicular lymphoma.[39] The incidence of secondary testicular lymphoma peaks in men around age 60, although primary lymphoma may affect children.[39] Approximately 25% of patients experience weight loss, weakness, and anorexia.[39] The sonographic appearance of testicular lymphomas is nonspecific (Fig. 21-43). One or both testes may be enlarged, and there are areas of decreased echogenicity, either diffuse or focal.[28,41] In male children with acute lymphocytic leukemia the testis is a prime site of relapse.[39] Testicular enlargement is bilateral in 50% of cases and is commonly associated with scrotal discoloration.[39]

Like lymphoma, the sonographic appearance of testicular leukemia is nonspecific, with areas of decreased echogenicity, either diffuse or focal (Fig. 21-44).[19,28]

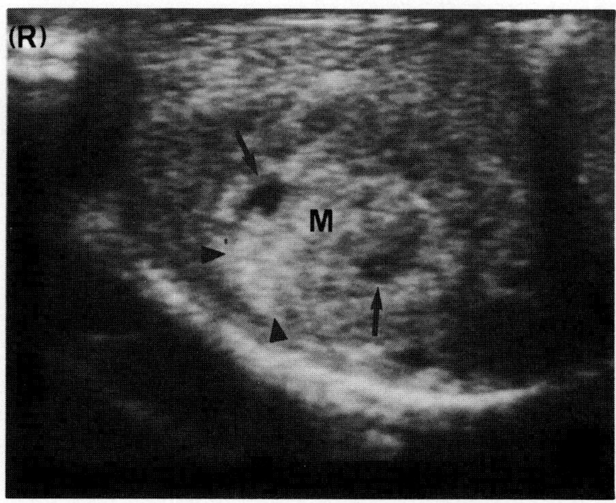

Figure 21-42. On a transverse scan of a patient with teratocarcinoma, the tumor appears as a large, complex mass (M) with areas of increased echogenicity (*arrowheads*) and cystic areas (*arrows*; R, patient's right side). (Courtesy R. Brooke Jeffrey, MD, San Francisco, CA.)

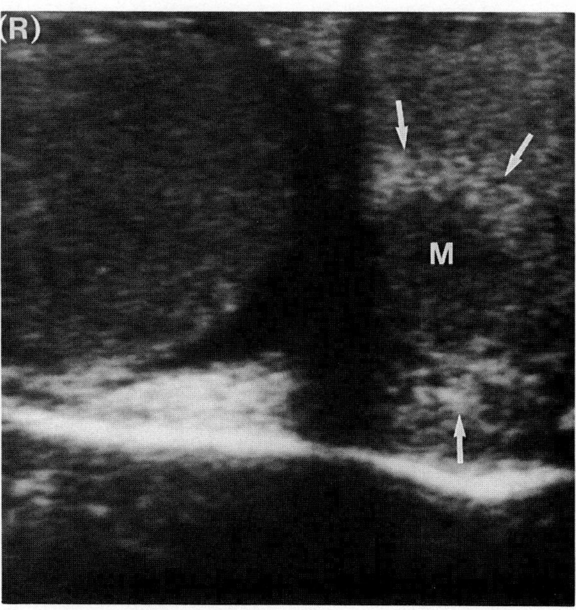

Figure 21-43. On transverse scan of a patient with non-Hodgkin's lymphoma both testes are enlarged. The parenchyma of the right testis is diffusely abnormal. The left testis shows a focal hypoechoic mass (M) and increased echogenicity (*arrows*) in the remainder of the left testis (R, patient's right side). (Courtesy R. Brooke Jeffrey, MD, San Francisco, CA.)

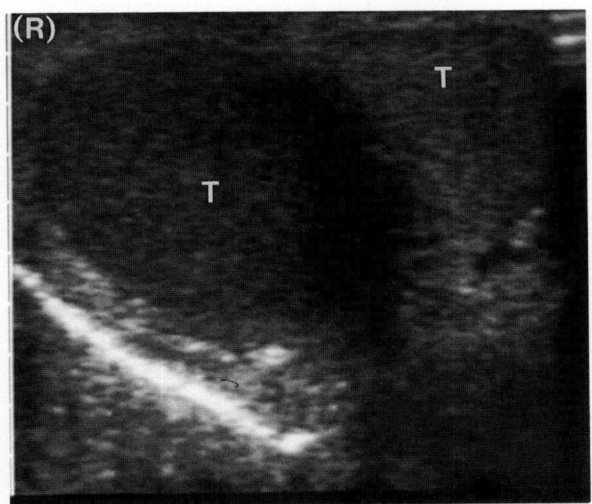

Figure 21-44. A bilateral transverse testicular scan of a 12-year-old boy with leukemic infiltration of the testis (T), demonstrates that the right testis is diffusely enlarged, with decreased echogenicity compared to the normal parenchyma of the left testis (R, patient's right side). (Courtesy Paul Nancarrow, MD, Oakland, CA.)

Diagnosis of Scrotal Lesions by Ultrasound

An approach to the diagnosis of scrotal lesions by ultrasound is shown in Figure 21-45. Scrotal wall thickness is a useful first indicator. If this parameter is normal, the assessment of testicular size is the next most useful observation. With scrotal wall thickening, it is important next to determine whether there is a history of trauma. The decision tree highlights many of the differential aspects mentioned in this chapter.

Conclusion

High-resolution real-time sonography is a reliable diagnostic imaging adjunct for localizing, detecting, and differentiating intratesticular from extratesticular lesions of the scrotum. Its sensitivity for disease, lack of ionizing radiation, easy repeatabil-

(*text continues on page 618*)

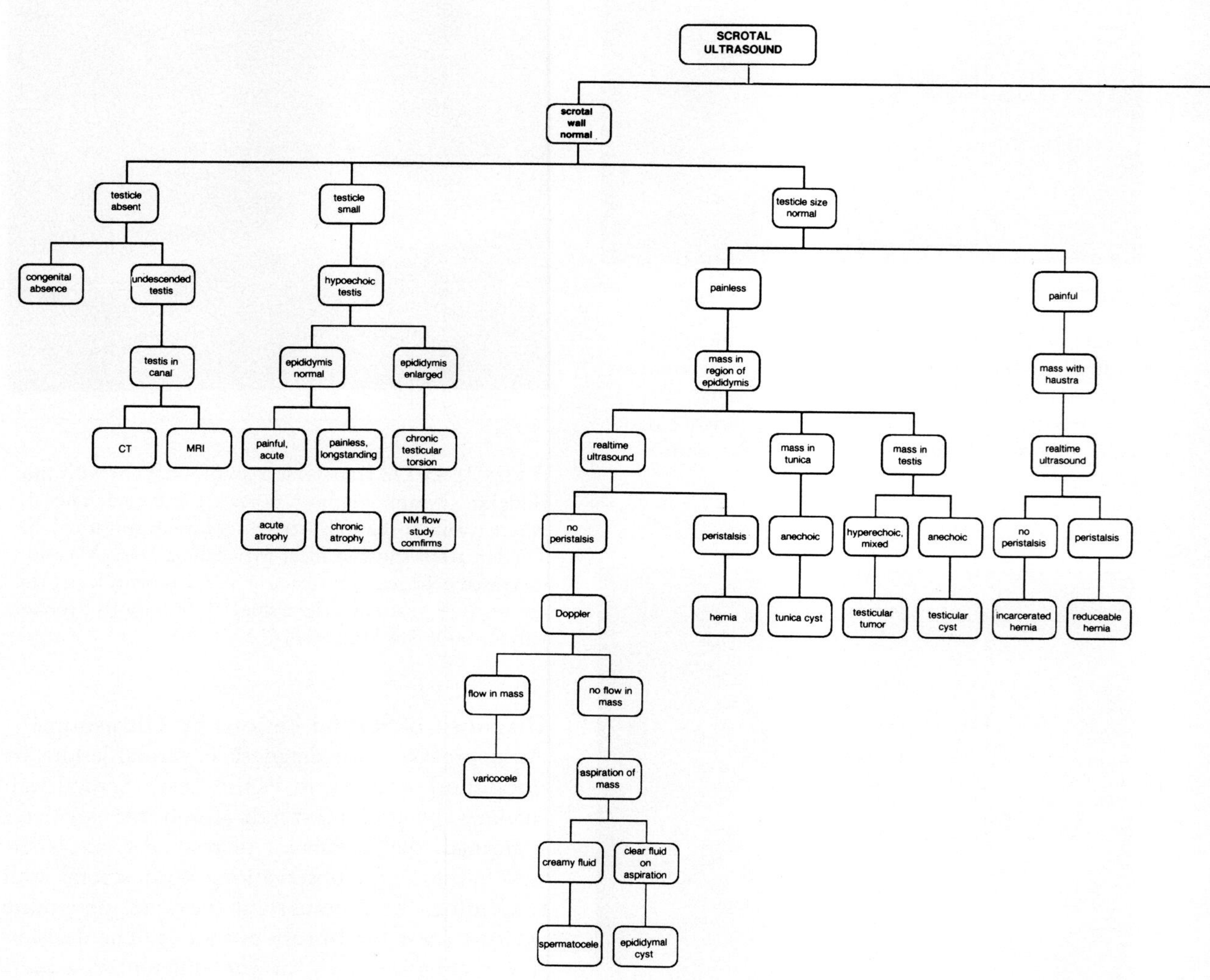

SCROTAL ULTRASOUND
scrotal wall normal
testicle absent
testicle small
testicle size normal
congenital absence
undescended testis
hypoechoic testis
painless
painful
testis in canal
epididymis normal
epididymis enlarged
mass in region of epididymis
mass with haustra
CT
MRI
painful, acute
painless, longstanding
chronic testicular torsion
realtime ultrasound
mass in tunica
mass in testis
realtime ultrasound
acute atrophy
chronic atrophy
NM flow study comfirms
no peristalsis
peristalsis
anechoic
hyperechoic, mixed
anechoic
no peristalsis
peristalsis
Doppler
hernia
tunica cyst
testicular tumor
testicular cyst
incarcerated hernia
reduceable hernia
flow in mass
no flow in mass
varicocele
aspiration of mass
creamy fluid
clear fluid on aspiration
spermatocele
epididymal cyst

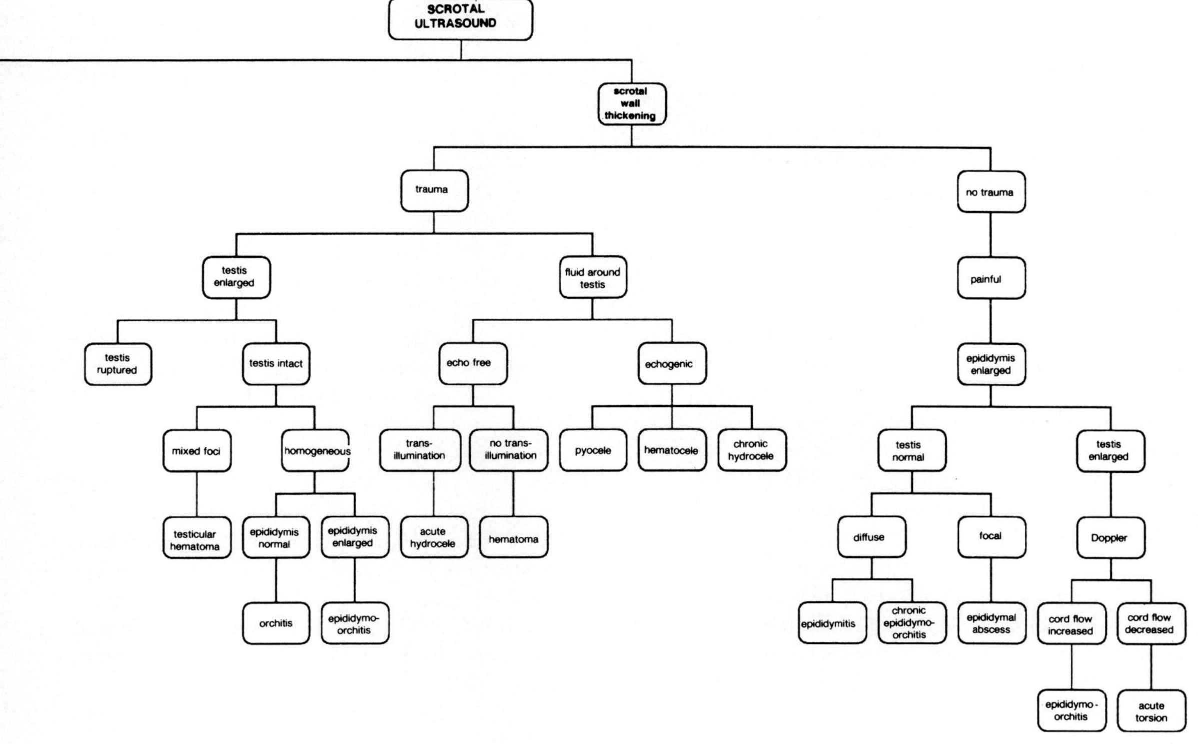

FIGURE 21-45. Approach to the differential diagnosis of scrotal lesions by sonography.

ity, and relatively low cost make sonography the imaging modality of choice for the evaluation of most scrotal pathology. Color-flow Doppler investigation has shown value in evaluating fluid collections (differentiating vascular from nonvascular) and vascular abnormalities such as varicocele and for differentiating epididymitis from testicular torsion.

Acknowledgments

The author wishes to thank Frida Q. Trevett, RDMS, for her assistance in conceptualizing and developing the scrotal scanning protocol and Marcus W. Hedgcock, MD, for assistance in preparing the manuscript.

References

1. Anthony CP, Kolthoff NJ: Textbook of Anatomy and Surgery. St. Louis, CV Mosby, 1981.
2. Arger PH, Mulher CB, Coleman BG, et al: Prospective analysis of the value of scrotal ultrasound. Radiology 1981, 141:763–766.
3. Baker LL, Hajek PC, Burkhard TK, et al: MR imaging of the scrotum: Pathologic condition. Radiology 1987, 163:93–98.
4. Bell BJ, Nowers C: SDMS suggested scanning techniques. J Diagn Med Sonogr 1986, 2:343–347.
5. Bird K, Rosenfield AT: Testicular infarction secondary to acute inflammatory disease: Demonstration by B-scan ultrasound. Radiology 1984, 152:785–788.
6. Bird K, Rosenfield AT, Taylor KJ: Ultrasonography in testicular torsion. Radiology 1983, 147:527–534.
7. Blei L, Sihelnik S, Bloom D, et al: Ultrasonographic analysis of chronic intratesticular pathology. J Ultrasound Med 1983, 2:17–23.
8. Burks DD, Markey BJ, Burkhard TK, et al: Suspected testicular torsion and ischemia: Evaluation with color Doppler sonography. Radiology 1990, 175:815–821.
9. Carroll BA: Ultrasonography of the scrotum. *In* Sarti DA (ed): Diagnostic Ultrasound: Text and Cases. Chicago, Year Book Medical Publishers, 1987
10. Carroll BA, Gross DM: High-frequency scrotal sonography. AJR 1983, 140:511–515.
11. Chen CD, Holder LE, Kaplan GN: Correlation of radionuclide imaging and diagnostic ultrasound in scrotal disease. J Nucl Med 1986, 27:1774–1781.
12. Fowler RC, Chennells PM, Ewing R: Scrotal ultrasonography: A clinical evaluation. Br J Radiol 1987, 60:649–654.
13. Fritzsche PJ, Hricak H, Kogan BA, et al: Undescended testis: Value of MR imaging. Radiology 1987, 164:169–173.
14. George FW, Wilson JD: Embryology of the genital tract. *In* Walsh P, Gittes RF, Perlmutter AD, et al (eds): Campbell's Urology, 5th ed. Philadelphia, WB Saunders, 1986.
15. Gooding GAW: Sonography of the spermatic cord. AJR 1988, 151:721–724.
16. Gooding GAW, Leonhardt WC, Stein R: Sonography of testicular cysts. Radiology 1987, 163:537–538.
17. Goodman P, Maklad NF, Verani RR, Gottlieb HE: Tuberculous abscess of the testicle in AIDS: Sonographic demonstration. Urol Radiol 1990, 12:53–55.
18. Gow JG: Genitourinary tuberculosis. *In* Walsh P, Gittes RF, Perlmutter AD, et al (eds): Campbell's Urology, 5th ed. Philadelphia, WB Saunders, 1986.
19. Grantham GJ, Charboneau WJ, James ME, et al: Testicular neoplasms: 29 tumors studied by high-resolution ultrasound. Radiology 1985, 55:775–780.
20. Gray H: The surgical anatomy of hernia. *In* Gray H (ed): Anatomy, Descriptive and Surgical. New York, Bounty Books, 1977.
21. Healey JE, Seybold WD: A Synopsis of Clinical Anatomy. Philadelphia, WB Saunders, 1969.
22. Hill MC, Sanders RC: Sonography of benign disease of the scrotum. *In* Sanders, RC, Hill MC (eds): Ultrasound Annual. New York, Raven Press, 1986.
23. Horstman WG, Middleton WD, Melson GL: Scrotal inflammatory disease: Color Doppler US findings. Radiology 1991, 179:55–59.
24. Howards SS: Surgery of the scrotum and its contents. *In* Walsh P, Gittes RF, Perlmutter AD, et al (eds): Campbell's Urology, 5th ed. Philadelphia, WB Saunders, 1986.
25. Hricak H, Frilly RA: Sonography of the scrotum. Invest Radiol 1983, 18:112–121.
26. Hricak H, Jeffrey RB: Sonography of the acute scrotal abnormalities. Radiol Clin North Am 1983, 21:595–603.
27. Jarvis LJ, Dubbins PA: Changes in the epididymis after vasectomy: Sonographic findings. AJR 1989, 152:531–534.
28. Krone KD, Carroll BA: Scrotal ultrasound. Radiol Clin North Am 1985, 23:121–139.
29. Leopold GR, Woo VL, Scheible FW, et al: High-resolution ultrasonography of scrotal pathology. Radiology 1979, 131:719–722.
30. Lerner RM, Mevorach RA, Hulbert WC, Rabinowitz R: Color Doppler in the evaluation of acute scrotal disease. Radiology 1990, 176:355–358.

31. Leung ML, Gooding GA, Williams RD: High-resolution sonography of scrotal contents in asymptomatic subjects. AJR 1984, 143:161–164.
32. Linkowski GD, Avellone A, Gooding GA: Scrotal calculi: Sonographic detection. Radiology 1985, 156:484.
33. McCann J: Researchers find novel applications for color Doppler. Diagnostic Imaging 1988, 10:11–13.
34. McVay CB: The hernias. *In* Davis L (ed): Christopher's Textbook of Surgery. Philadelphia, WB Saunders, 1968.
35. Martin B, Conte J: Ultrasonography of the acute scrotum. J Clin Ultrasound 1987, 15:34–44.
36. Middleton WD, Melson GL: Testicular ischemia: Color Doppler sonographic findings in five patients. AJR 1989, 152:1237–1239.
37. Middleton WD, Siegel BA, Melson GL, et al: Acute scrotal disorders: Prospective comparison of color Doppler ultrasound and testicular scintigraphy. Radiology 1990, 177:177–181.
38. Middleton WD, Thorne DA, Melson GL: Color Doppler of the normal testis. AJR 1989, 152:293–297.
39. Morse MJ, Whitmore WF: Neoplasms of the testis. *In* Walsh P, Gittes RF, Perlmutter AD, et al (eds): Campbell's Urology, 5th ed. Philadelphia, WB Saunders, 1986.
40. Murphy GP, Gaeta JF: Tumors of the testicular adnexal structures and seminal vesicles. *In* Walsh P, Gittes RF, Perlmutter AD, et al (eds): Campbell's Urology, 5th ed. Philadelphia, WB Saunders, 1986.
41. Philips GN, Abrams HJ, Kumari-Subaija S: Scrotal ultrasonography. *In* Sauders RC, Hill MC (eds): Ultrasound Annual 1983. New York, Raven Press, 1983.
42. Rajfer J: Congenital anomalies of the testis. *In* Walsh P, Gittes RF, Perlmutter AD, et al (eds): Campbell's Urology, 5th ed. Philadelphia, WB Saunders, 1986.
43. Rifkin MD: Scrotal ultrasound. Urol Radiol 1987, 9:119–126.
44. Rifkin MD, Foy PM, Kurtz AB, et al: The role of diagnostic ultrasonography in varicocele evaluation. J Ultrasound Med 1983, 2:271–275.
45. Rifkin MD, Kurtz AB, Goldberg BB: Epididymis examined by ultrasound. Radiology 1984, 151:187–190.
46. Schaffer RM: Ultrasonography of scrotal trauma. Urol Radiol 1985, 7:245–249.
47. Schwerk WB, Schwerk WN, Rodeck O: Testicular tumors: Prospective analysis of real-time US patterns and abdominal staging. Radiology 1987, 164:369–374.
48. Sherins RJ, Howard SS: Male infertility. *In* Walsh P, Gittes RF, Perlmutter AD, et al (eds): Campbell's Urology, 5th ed. Philadelphia, WB Saunders, 1986.
49. Sigmund G, Gall H, Bahren W: Stop-type and shunt-type varicoceles: Venographic findings. Radiology 1987, 163:103–110.
50. Smith EH, Raptopoulos V: Ultrasound. *In* Walsh P, Gittes RF, Perlmutter AD, et al (eds): Campbell's Urology, 5th ed. Philadelphia, WB Saunders, 1986.
51. Subramanyam BR, Balthazar EJ, Raghavendra BN, et al: Sonographic diagnosis of scrotal hernia. AJR 1982, 139:535–538.
52. Vick CW, Bird KI, Rosenfield AT, et al: Scrotal masses with a uniformly hyperechoic pattern. Radiology 1983, 148:209–211.

Index

Note: Italic numerals indicate figures.

ISBN 0-397-50954-5